McGraw-Hill Specialty Board Review

# Cardiology

*Edited by*

**Ragavendra R. Baliga, MD, MBA, FACP, FACC, FRCP (Edin)**
Editor-in-Chief, *Heart Failure Clinics of North America,*
Associate Editor, *American College of Cardiology Cardiosource Review Journal,*
Vice-Chief & Assistant Director, Division of Cardiovascular Medicine,
Professor of Internal Medicine, The Ohio State University,
Attending Cardiologist, Richard M. Ross Heart Hospital,
Columbus, Ohio

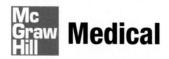

New York   Chicago   San Francisco   Lisbon   London   Madrid   Mexico City
Milan   New Delhi   San Juan   Seoul   Singapore   Sydney   Toronto

**McGraw-Hill Specialty Board Review: Cardiology**

1 2 3 4 5 6 7 8 9 0    CTP/CTP    14  13  12  11


Set ISBN 978-0-07161408-5;     MHID 0-07-161408-7
Book ISBN 978-0-07-161410-8;   MHID 0-07-161410-9
DVD ISBN 978-0-07-161411-5;    MHID 0-07-161411-7


This book was set in Goudy Oldstyle by Thomson Digital.
The editors were Jim Shanahan and Regina Y. Brown.
The production supervisor was Sherri Souffrance.
Project management was provided by Aakriti Kathuria, Thomson Digital.
The designer was Mary McKeon.
Cover: Specialist for cardiology, cardiograph, and cardiogram. Credit: © Friedrich Stark / Alamy.
China Translation & Printing, Ltd. was the printer and binder.


This book is printed on acid-free paper.

**Library of Congress Cataloging-in-Publication Data**
Cardiology / edited by Ragavendra R. Baliga.
    p. ; cm. — (McGraw-Hill specialty board review)
  Includes bibliographical references and index.
  ISBN-13: 978-0-07-161410-8 (pbk. : alk. paper)
  ISBN-10: 0-07-161410-9 (pbk. : alk. paper)
  1. Cardiology—Examinations, questions, etc.  I. Baliga, R. R. II. Series: McGraw-Hill specialty board
review.
  [DNLM: 1.  Cardiovascular Diseases--Examination Questions. 2.  Cardiology—methods—Examination
Questions.  WG 18.2]
  RC669.2.C373 2011
  616.1'20076—dc22
                                                          2010032799

McGraw-Hill books are available at special quantity discounts to use as premiums and sales
promotions, or for use in corporate training programs. To contact a representative please
e-mail us at bulksales@mcgraw-hill.com.

**Dedicated to**

*The memory of my paternal grandparents*
*Bantwal Vaikunta and Sharada Baliga*
*who had the courage to eat food with the 'untouchables' in 1920's when it was anathema*
*to do so and for having the courage to actively participate in India's freedom movement.*
*The memory of my maternal grandparents*
*Kochikar Sanjiv and Girija Pai*
*who actively participated in the underground movement during India's pursuit for freedom.*
*The memory of my father*
*Ram Krishna Baliga*
*who envisioned The Electronic City in Bangalore, India in*
*the 1970's making it a modern day global powerhouse.*
*My mother*
*Shanthi Baliga*
*who till this day continues to pursue her lifetime social mission that*
*includes emancipation of women and providing for indigent children.*
*My wife*
*Jayashree*
*for her solid support over the last two decades.*
*My siblings*
*Narendra and Lathika.*
*My children*
*Anoop and Neena.*

# Contents

# Section Editors

**Alex J. Auseon, DO, FACC**
Director, Cardiology Fellowship Program
Associate Professor of Clinical Internal Medicine
The Ohio State University Medical Center
*Section XI: Valvular Heart Disease*

**Quinn Capers, IV, MD, FACC, FSCAI,**
Associate Dean for Admissions
The Ohio State University College of Medicine
Director, Peripheral Vascular Interventions
Assistant Professor of Internal Medicine
The Ohio State University Medical Center
*Section XIII: Aorta and Vascular Disease*

**Curt Daniels, MD**
Director of the Adolescent and Adult Congenital
Heart Disease Program and the Pulmonary Hypertension
Program, Associate Professor of Clinical Cardiovascular Medicine
The Ohio State University
*Section XII: Congenital Heart Disease*

**Emile G. Daoud, MD, FACC**
Chief, Electrophysiology Section
Richard M. Ross Heart Hospital
Professor, Internal Medicine
The Ohio State University Medical Center
*Section X: Electrophysiology*

**Veronica Franco, MD, MSPH**
Director of the Exercise Physiology/Metabolic
Exercise Testing Program, Assistant Professor of Clinical
Medicine, The Ohio State University
*Section III: Pulmonary and Critical Care*

**Richard Gumina, MD**
Director of Interventional Cardiovascular Research and
Co-Director of the Ischemia and Metabolism
Thematic Research Davis Heart and Lung Institute, Assistant
Professor of Internal Medicine, The Ohio State University
*Section VII: Interventional Cardiology*

**Ayesha Hasan, MD, FACC**
Medical Director, Cardiac Transplant Program
Director, Heart Failure Devices Clinic
The Ohio State University
*Section IX: Heart Failure*

**Albert J. Kolibash, MD**
Medical Director of Medical Specialties at
Stoneridge in Dublin, Associate Professor of Medicine
The Ohio State University
*Section VI: Acute Coronary Syndrome*

**John Larry, MD**
Section Chief, OSU East Cardiovascular Medicine
Associate Professor of Medicine
Ohio State University Medical Center
*Section V: Coronary Artery Disease*

**Krishnan Marar, MD**
Director, Non-Invasive Laboratories
OSU University Hospital East
Assistant Professor of Medicine
Ohio State University Medical Center
*Section I: General Topics*

**Ernest L. Mazzaferri, Jr., MD, FACC**
Associate Medical Director
Richard M. Ross Heart Hospital
Assistant Professor, Interventional Cardiology
The Ohio State University
*Section VII: Interventional Cardiology*

**Laxmi S. Mehta, MD, FACC**
Director, Women's Cardiovascular Health Clinic
Assistant Professor, Clinical Internal Medicine
The Ohio State University
*Section VIII: Imaging*

**Vasudevan A. Raghavan, MBBS, MD, MRCP(UK)**
Director, Cardiometabolic and Lipid Clinic Services
Division of Endocrinology, Scott & White Hospitals
and Texas A&M Health Sciences Center
Temple, Texas
*Section IV: Preventive Cardiology*

**Raul Weiss, MD, FACC**
Director of the Electrophysiology Fellowship Program
Richard M. Ross Heart Hospital
Professor, Internal Medicine
The Ohio State University Medical Center
*Section X: Electrophysiology*

# Contributors

George S. Abela, MD, MSc, MBA, FACC
Professor and Chief Division of Cardiology
Michigan State University
East Lansing, Michigan

Elsayed Abo-Salem, MD, MSc
Echocardiography Laboratory
University of Southern California and Cardiology Division
Keck School of Medicine, Los Angeles, California
and Mansoura University
Dekahlia, Egypt

Theodore Abraham, MD
Director, Hypertrophic Cardiomyopathy Clinic
Associate Professor of Medicine, Johns Hopkins
University School of Medicine
Associate Director of the Echocardiography
Laboratory at Johns Hopkins Hospital
Baltimore, Maryland

Abinash Achrekar, MD
Assistant Professor of Medicine
University of New Mexico School of Medicine
Cardiology Division
Albuquerque, New Mexico

Jonathan Abrams, MD
Distinguished Professor of Medicine
University of New Mexico
Cardiology Division
Albuquerque, New Mexico

Kul Aggarwal, MD, MRCP(UK), FACC
Chief, Cardiology Section
Harry S. Truman Veterans Hospital
Professor of Clinical Medicine
University of Missouri
Columbia, Missouri

Aman M. Amanullah, MD, PhD, FACC, FAHA
Section Chief, Noninvasive Cardiology
Albert Einstein Medical Center
Clinical Professor of Medicine
Jefferson Medical College
Philadelphia, Pennsylvania

Amrut V. Ambardekar, MD
Division of Cardiology
University of Colorado
Denver Aurora, Colorado

Anish K. Amin, MD
Fellow in Cardiovascular Medicine
Division of Cardiovascular Medicine
Ohio State University
Columbus, Ohio

Asimul H. Ansari, MD
Clinical Instructor, Department of Internal
Medicine, Division of Cardiology
Northwestern Feinberg School of Medicine
Chicago, Illinois

Najamul H. Ansari, MD
Assistant Professor, Department of Internal
Medicine, Division of Cardiology
Rush Medical College; Attending Physician
Section of Adult Cardiology, John H. Stroger, Jr.
Hospital of Cook County
Chicago, Illinois

Raluca Arimie, MD
Attending Cardiologist
Ronald Reagan UCLA Medical CenterSanta
Monica-UCLA Medical Center
Los Angeles, California

**Julian M. Aroesty, MD**
Associate Clinical Professor of Medicine
Harvard Medical School, Director of Quality
Assurance and Improvement
Cardiovascular Institute
Boston, Massachusetts

**Ralph Augostini, MD, FACC**
Co-Director, Electrophysiology Fellowship Program
Assistant Professor of Clinical Medicine
Department of Cardiovascular Medicine
The Ohio State University
Columbus, Ohio

**Eric H. Awtry, MD, FACC**
Boston Medical Center
Assistant Professor of Medicine
Boston University School of Medicine
Director of Education, Division of Cardiology
Boston, Massachusetts

**Aaron Baggish, MD**
Associate Director for the Cardiovascular
Performance Program at the Massachusetts
General Hospital Heart Center
Massachusetts General Hospital
Harvard Medical School
Boston, Massachusetts

**Kara Barnett, MD**
Department of Anesthesiology and
Critical Care, University of Pennsylvania
School of Medicine
Philadelphia, Pennsylvania

**Craig T. Basson, MD, PhD**
Gladys and Roland Harriman Professor of Medicine
Director, Cardiovascular Research, Cardiology Division
Weill Medical College of Cornell University
New York, New York

**Melike Bayram, MD**
Fellow, Cardiovascular Medicine
Division of Cardiology Ohio State University
Medical Center
Columbus, Ohio

**Richard C. Becker, MD**
Professor of Medicine, Duke University
Medical Center, Director
Duke Cardiovascular Thrombosis Center
Duke Clinical Research Institute
Durham, North Carolina

**R. Michael Benitez, MD, FACC**
Professor of Medicine
Director, Cardiology Fellowship Program
Division of Cardiology, University
of Maryland School of Medicine
Baltimore, Maryland

**Daniel S. Berman, MD**
Chief, Cardiac Imaging, Cedars-Sinai Heart Institute
Professor of Imaging, Cedars-Sinai Medical Center
Professor of Medicine, David Geffen School
of Medicine at UCLA
Los Angeles, California

**Advay G. Bhatt, MD**
Fellow, Section of Cardiology
Boston University School of Medicine
Boston, Massachusetts

**John D. Bisognano, MD, PhD**
Director of Outpatient Cardiology
Professor of Medicine
University of Rochester Medical Center
Rochester, New York

**Sonia Blome, MD**
Department of Cardiology
University of Maryland Medical College
Baltimore, Maryland

**Lawrence M. Boxt, MD, FACC**
Professor of Clinical Radiology
Albert Einstein College of Medicine
Director of Cardiac MRI and CT
North Shore University Hospital
Manhasset, New York

**Kelley R. Branch, MD, MS**
Assistant Professor in Cardiology
University of Washington
Seattle, Washington

**Angela G. Brittsan, MD, PhD**
Cardiology Fellow, Division of Cardiovascular
Medicine, The Ohio State University
Medical Center
Columbus, Ohio

**Katharina M. Busl, MD**
Neurology Chief Resident
Brigham and Women's Hospital
Massachusetts General Hospital
Harvard Medical School
Boston, Massachusetts

**Peter J. Cawley, MD**
Acting Assistant Professor of Medicine
Division of Cardiology, University
of Washington School of Medicine
Seattle, Washington

**Amar R. Chadaga, MD**
Division of Internal Medicine
Evanston Northwestern Healthcare
Instructor of Medicine, Northwestern
Feinberg School of Medicine
Evanston, Illinois

**Konstantinos Charitakis, MD**
Cardiology Fellow, Greenberg Division of Cardiology
Department of Medicine, New York Presbyterian Hospital
Weill Medical College of Cornell University
New York, New York

**Melvin D. Cheitlin, MD, MACC**
Emeritus Professor of Medicine
University of California, San Francisco
Former Chief of Cardiology
San Francisco General Hospital
San Francisco, California

**Christopher V. Chien, MD**
Cedars Sinai Medical Center &
University of California
Los Angeles
Los Angeles, California

**Gary W. Chune, MD**
Assistant Professor of Internal Medicine
Division of Endocrinology, Scott & White Hospitals,
Texas A&M Health Sciences Center
Temple, Texas

**Michael Craig, MD**
Assistant Professor Division of Cardiology
Medical University of South Carolina
Charleston, South Carolina

**Eric S. Davidson, MD**
Boston Medical Center, Cardiology Section
Boston University School of Medicine
Boston, Massachusetts

**Hossein Dehghani, MD**
Cardiology Fellow, Tulane Heart
and Vascular Institute
New Orleans, Louisiana

**Anita Deswal, MD, MPH**
Associate Professor of Medicine
Section of Cardiology and Winters
Center for Heart Failure Research
Michael E. DeBakey VA Medical Center
and Baylor College of Medicine
Houston, Texas

**Marcelo F. Di Carli, MD, FACC**
Chief, Division of Nuclear Medicine-PET
Director, Noninvasive Cardiovascular Imaging Program
Department of Medicine and Radiology
Associate Professor of Radiology and Medicine
Harvard Medical School
Boston, Massachusetts

**Sharmila Dorbala, MD, FACC**
Director of Nuclear Cardiology
Brigham and Women's Hospital
Assistant Professor of Radiology
Harvard Medicial Schol
Boston, Massachusetts

**Amit A. Doshi, MD**
The Ohio State University
Division of Cardiology
Columbus, Ohio

**Robert T. Eberhardt, MD**
Director of Medical Vascular Services
Associate Professor of Medicine
Department of Medicine
Section of Cardiovascular Medicine
Boston University School of Medicine,
Boston Medical Center
Boston, Massachusetts

**William P. Fay, MD**
JW and Lois Winifred Stafford Distinguished
Chair in Diabetes and Cardiovascular Research
Professor of Internal Medicine
Medical Pharmacology and Physiology
Director, Division of Cardiology
University of Missouri
Columbia, Missouri

**Savitri E. Fedson, MD**
Medical Director, Cardiac Care Unit
Associate Vice Chair for Inpatient Operations
Associate Professor of Medicine
University of Chicago Medical Center
Chicago, Illinois

**Valerian Fernandes, MD, MRCP, FACC**
Director of the Cardiac Catheterization Laboratories
Ralph H. Johnson VA Medical Center
Associate Professor, Department of Medicine
Division of Cardiology, Medical
University of South Carolina
Charleston, South Carolina

**Peter J. Fitzgerald, MD, PhD**
Professor of Medicine and Engineering
Stanford University School of Medicine
Director, Center for Cardiovascular Technology
Division of Cardiovascular Medicine
Stanford University Medical Center
Stanford, California

**Lee A. Fleisher, MD**
Robert D. Dripps Professor and Chair
of Anesthesiology and Critical Care
Professor of Medicine
University of Pennsylvania School of Medicine
Philadelphia, Pennsylvania

**JoAnne M. Foody, MD, FACC, FAHA**
Editor-in-Chief, CardioSmarts.org
Director of the Cardiovascular Wellness Center
Staff Physician, Chief of the Division of
Preventive Medicine, Brigham and Women's Hospital
Associate Professor of Internal Medicine
Harvard Medical School
Boston, Massachusetts

**Ashish Gangasani, MD**
Attending Cardiologist
OhioHealth Medical Speciality Foundation
Columbus, Ohio

**Rajeev Garg, MBBS, FACP**
Division of Cardiology
University of Missouri
Columbia, Missouri

**Guido Germano, PhD, MBA**
Professor of Medicine, UCLA School of Medicine
Director, Artificial Intelligence Program
Cedars-Sinai Medical Center
Los Angeles, California

**Thomas D. Giles, MD, FACC, FAHA**
Professor of Medicine
Chief Medical Service and
Cardiology at the Veterans Administration
Medical Center in New Orleans
Director of Cardiovascular Research
Heart & Vascular Institute
Tulane University School of Medicine
Metairie Lousiana

**Shawn A. Gregory, MD, MMSc**
Assistant Director, Nuclear Cardiology
Consultant Cardiologist Cardiology Division
Massachusetts General Hospital and
Harvard Medical School
Boston, Massachusetts

**Rory Hachamovitch, MD, FACC**
Attending Cardiologist
Cleveland Clinic
Cleveland, Ohio

**David T. Hart MB, BS FACC**
Assistant Professor Cardiovascular Medicine
Ohio State University Medical Center
Ohio State University
Columbus, Ohio

**Rajiv S. Hede, FACC, FASE**
Chief of Cardiology
St. Ann's Hospital Mount Carmel Health System
Columbus, Ohio

**William B. Hillegass, MD, MPH, FACC, FSVMB**
Associate Professor, Interventional Cardiovascular
Section, University of Alabama at Birmingham
Birmingham, Alabama

**Brian D. Hoit, MD**
Director of Echocardiography
University Hospitals Health System
Professor of Medicine, Physiology and Biophysics
Case Western Reserve University
Cleveland, Ohio

**Yasuhiro Honda, MD, FACC, FAHA**
Co-Director, Cardiovascular Core Analysis
Laboratory, Center for Cardiovascular Technology
Division of Cardiovascular Medicine, Stanford University
Medical Center
Stanford, California

**Mahmoud Houmsse, MD, FACP, FACC**
Director, Heart Station
Assistant Professor of Clinical Medicine
Department of Cardiovascular Medicine
The Ohio State University
Columbus, Ohio

**John D. Hummel, MD**
Director of Clinical Electrophysiology Research
Professor of Clinical Medicine
The Ohio State University Medical Center
Columbus, Ohio

**Sanja Jelic, MD**
Herbert Irving Assistant Professor of Medicine
Division of Pulmonary, Allergy and
Critical Care Medicine
Columbia University College of Physicians
and Surgeons
New York, New York

**Rami Kahwash, MD**
Assistant Professor of Clinical Medicine
Department of Cardiovascular Medicine
The Ohio State University
Columbus, Ohio

**Steven J. Kalbfleisch, MD, FACC**
Medical Director of Cardiac Electrophysiology
Professor of Clinical Medicine
Cardiovascular Medicine
The Ohio State University Medical Center
Columbus, Ohio

**Jason N. Katz, MD**
Medical Director, Cardiac Intensive Care Unit
Assistant Professor of Medicine
Divisions of Cardiology and Pulmonary/
Critical Care Medicine, University
of North Carolina
Chapel Hill, North Carolina

**Stuart D. Katz, MD**
Helen L. and Martin S. Kimmel Professor of Advanced
Cardiac Therapeutics; Chair Cardiovascular Medicine
Director Heart Failure Program
New York University Lagone Medical Center
Leon H. Charney Division of Cardiology
New York City, New York

**Joseph D. Kay, MD, FACC**
Program Director, UC Denver
Adult Congenital Cardiology
Assistant Professsor of Medicine & Pediatrics
University of Colorado
at Denver School of Medicine Aurora
Denver, Colorado

**Amit Khera, MD, MSc**
Director, Preventive Cardiology
Assistant Professor
Department Inernal Medicine/Cardiology
UT Southwestern Medical Center
Dallas, Texas

**Luke Kim, MD**
Clinical Fellow in Cardiology
Greenberg Division of Cardiology
Department of Medicine, New York
Presbyterian Hospital, Weill Medical College
of Cornell University
New York, New York

**James N. Kirkpatrick, MD**
Associate Professor of Medicine
Cardiovascular Division, Non Invasive Imaging/
Echocardiography; Associate Fellow
Center for Bioethics, University of Pennsylvania
School of Medicine
Hospital of the University of Pennsylvania
Philadelphia, Pennsylvania

**Michelle M. Kittleson, MD, PhD**
Director of Post Graduate Medical Education
in Heart Failure and Transplantation at
Cedars-Sinai Heart Institute
Assistant Clinical Professor of Medicine/Cardiology
at the David Geffen School of Medicine at the
University of California, Los Angeles (UCLA)
Los Angeles, California

**Jon A. Kobashigawa, MD**
Associate Director of the Cedars-Sinai Heart Institute
Director of Advanced Heart Disease and Director of the
Heart Transplant Program at Cedars-Sinai
DSL/Thomas D. Gordon Chair in Heart Transplantation
Medicine, Clinical Professor of Medicine and Cardiology
at the David Geffen School of Medicine at the University
of California, Los Angeles (UCLA)
Los Angeles, California

**Bon-Kwon Koo, MD, PhD**
Postdoctoral Fellow, Center for Cardiovascular
Technology, Division of Cardiovascular Medicine
Stanford University Medical Center, Stanford
California; Assistant Professor, Division of Cardiology
Seoul National University Medical College
Seoul, South Korea

**Itzhak Kronzon, MD, FACC, FASE**
Director Non-Invasive Cardiology Laboratory
Professor of Medicine, New York University
School of Medicine
New York, New York

**Saravanan Kuppuswamy, MD**
Assistant Professor, Department of Internal Medicine
University of Missouri
Columbia, Missouri

**L. Veronica Lee, MD, FACC, FAHA**
Director, Cardiology Fellowship Program
Assistant Professor of Medicine
Section of Cardiology, Yale University
School of Medicine
New Haven, Connecticut

**Thierry H. Le Jemtel, MD**
Henderson Chair Professor of Medicine
Director, Heart Failure and Transplant Program
Tulane University Heart and Vascular Institute
New Orleans, Louisiana

**Michael J. Lim, MD, FACC, FSCAI**
Interim Director, Division of Cardiology
Director Cardiac Catheterization Laboratory
Associate Professor of Internal Medicine
St. Louis University
St. Louis, Missouri

**Zhenguo Liu, MD, PhD**
Associate Professor, Division of Cardiovascular Medicine
The Ohio State University Medical Center
Columbus, Ohio

**Charles Love, MD**
Professor of Medicine, Director of Arrhythmia
Device Services, Department of Cardiovascular Medicine
The Ohio State University
Columbus, Ohio

**Calum A. MacRae, MD, PhD**
Brigham and Women's Hospital
Formerly, Director of Cardiology Fellowship
Program, Massachusetts General Hospital
Harvard Medical School
Boston, Massachusetts

**Alan S. Maisel, MD, FACC**
Professor of Medicine
Director, Coronary Care Unit
University of California - San Diego
Division of Cardiology
San Diego, California

**Amgad N. Makaryus, MD, FACC**
Assistant Professor of Clinical Medicine
New York University School of Medicine
Division of Cardiology
North Shore University Hospital
Manhasset, New York

**Peter A. McCullough, MD, MPH, FACC, FACP**
Chief Academic and Scientific Officer
Medical Director, Preventive Cardiology
St. John Providence Health System
Providence Park Heart Institute
Novi, Michigan

**Mandeep R. Mehra, MD**
Dr. Herbert Berger Professor and Head of Cardiology
University of Maryland School of Medicine, Baltimore
Maryland and Editor in Chief, The Journal of Heart
and Lung Transplantation
Baltimore, Maryland

# Preface

Increasingly medical education and assessment is focusing on the clinicians ability to "*connect-the-dots*" across pieces of information (JAMA, 2009;302:1332–1333). Acquiring new information requires both verbatim memory and gist memory. Verbatim memory includes recollection of facts (for example. reversible causes of pericardial effusion) whereas gist memory involves interpretation (for example that the elevated TSH is due to hypothyroidism and may be the cause of a pericardial effusion and bradycardia). Experienced clinicians rely on such gist-based reasoning and their clinical reasoning is superior because they are able to recognize the gist of clinical symptoms. This book has been put together keeping this in mind.

They key goals of this book and the accompanying CD (containing over 600 questions) is to provide a comprehensive review of core cardiovascular medicine curriculum to enhance not only verbatim memory but also improve the ability to 'connect the dots' and thereby prepare the reader for certification and re-certification examinations in cardiology including the American Board of Internal Medicine (ABIM) boards in cardiovascular medicine, British Cardiovascular Society/European Cardiac Society Knowledge Based Assessment Exam, Royal College of Physicians and Surgeons of Canada (RCPSC) certification examination in cardiology, Fellow of Royal College of Australasian Physicians (FRACP) cardiology, Doctor of Medicine (DM) Cardiology and Diplomate of the National Board of Medicine (Cardiology).

This book should also be a valuable reference text for ABIM boards in Internal Medicine, Fellow of College of Physicians and Surgeons of Canada (FRCPSC) Internal Medicine certification exam, MD (General Medicine), MRCP (UK), MRCP (Ireland), FRACP internal medicine certification, Diplomate of the National Board of Medicine (General Medicine) and Postgraduate Diploma in Cardiology at various universities in the UK.

This book should be a valuable reference text for internists, family physicians, anesthesiologists, critical care physicians and nurses, cardiovascular nurse practitioners, nurses and physician assistants and all physician extenders with an interest in cardiovascular care.

The book is best used at the bedside soon after or before the clinician sees the index patient. This allows correlating facts in the book with bedside clinical findings. I encourage readers of this book to follow this '*Book-to-Bedside-to-Book*' approach to maximize their ability to 'connect the dots' and derive the best out of this book. I encourage readers to start using this book at least eighteen months before their board exams or ideally the month they start their cardiology fellowship program.

The unique quality of this book is that it includes contributors from several institutions allowing it to have a broad perspective. Contributors include faculty from Harvard Medical School (Massachusetts General Hospital, Beth Israel Deaconess Hospital, Brigham and Women's Hospital), Johns Hopkins, Baylor, Boston University, Cleveland Clinic, Columbia, Cornell, Duke, Northwestern, NYU, Stanford, SLU, Tulane, Vanderbilt, Yale, Medical University of South Carolina (MUSC), University of Alabama, University of California Los Angeles (UCLA), University of California San Diego (UCSD), University of Colorado, University of Maryland, University of Missouri, University of New Mexico (UNM), University of North Carolina (UNC), University of Pennsylvania (UPenn), University of Southern California, University of Texas Southwestern Medical Center, University of Washington, Seattle and The Ohio State University. The style of this book reflects this diversity of authors and follows an 'open source' format. The Section Editors role included soliciting articles and actively editing the articles to reflect the key goals of this book.

We hope that this book will help the reader to improve the ability to 'connect-the-dots' between theoretical aspects of cardiovascular medicine and the clinical management of the patient by the bedside with the ultimate goal of providing superior patient care.

Sincerely
Ragavendra R. Baliga, MD, MBA, FACP, FACC, FRCP (Edin)
Editor-in-Chief, *Heart Failure Clinics of North America*,
Associate Editor, *American College of Cardiology Cardiosource Review Journal*,
Vice-Chief & Assistant Director,
Division of Cardiovascular Medicine,
Professor of Internal Medicine,
The Ohio State University,
Attending Cardiologist, Richard M. Ross Heart Hospital,
Columbus, Ohio

# Acknowledgments

First and foremost I would like to thank each contributor and section editor for their patience and untiring efforts as this huge project, involving contributors from several organizations, matured to fruition.

This book was possible because several chiefs of cardiology encouraged their faculty to contribute to this book, including G. William Dec Jr, MD, Massachusetts General Hospital; Robert Bourge, MD, University of Alabama; James N. Weiss, MD, University of California, Los Angeles; Peter Buttrick, MD, University of Colorado; William P. Fay, MD, University of Missouri, Columbia, Missouri, Mandeep R. Mehra, MD, University of Maryland; Joseph Hill, MD, UT Southwestern Medical Center; and Douglas B. Sawyer, MD, Phd, Vanderbilt University and I also thank Talmadge E. King, Jr, MD, Chair of Internal Medicine at University of California, San Francisco, and Richard L. Page, MD, Chair of Internal Medicine, University of Wisconsin for their support for this book.

I would like to thank my leadership here at The Ohio State University including William T. Abraham, MD, Chief of Cardiology, Michael Grever, MD, Chair of Medicine, Thomas J. Ryan, MD, Director of Heart and Vascular Center, Catherine R. Lucey, MD, Dean of The Ohio State University Medical School, Vice-President for Medical Education, University of California San Francisco (UCSF) and President of American Board of Internal Medicine, James N. Allen, MD, Vice-Chair of Medicine, Joel G. Lucas, MD, Director of University Hospitals East, Charles A. Bush, MD, Director of Ross Heart Hospital Hagop S. Mekhjian, MD, Chief Medical Officer, Ohio State University Medical Center and Garrie J Haas, MD, Director of Heart Failure and Cardiac Transplant, The Ohio State University Medical Center for their support.

Others supporters include Kim A. Eagle, MD, Director of University of Michigan, Cardiovascular Center, James B. Young, MD, Executive Dean, Lerner School of Medicine at Cleveland Clinic, and Jagat Narula, MD, Philip J. and Harriet L. Goodhart Chair in Cardiology, Professor of Medicine and Associate Dean for Global Health, Mount Sinai School of Medicine.

I would like to thank the Editorial Team at McGraw Hill, James Shanahan, Editor-in-Chief, Christine Diedrich, Editor, Regina Y. Brown, Senior Developmental Editor, Barbara Holton, Editor for CD, Sherri Souffrance, Laura Libretti for their support and Ruth Weinberg, Commissioning Editor who persuaded me to take on this project. At Thomson Digital, Aakriti Kathuria and Sandeep Pannu, Anand Kumar, and Roni Mathew patiently copyediting this book.

Finally, I would like to thank Rebecca Abbott for her assistance.

# General Topics I

# General Topics 1

# The Cardiovascular History and Physical Exam

Jonathan Abrams and Abinash Achrekar

## ● PRACTICAL POINTS

- The pain of myocardial ischemia is usually described as pressure, burning or indigestion.

- Women have atypical symptoms compared to men.

- Atypical symptoms like dyspnea, diaphoresis, nausea, emesis, dizziness and fatigue are more often seen in diabetics, the elderly, and women.

- Location is typically substernal but radiation can occur to the shoulders, jaw, neck and interscapular and epigastric regions.

- Abnormal jugular venous pulse waves are seen in several cardiac conditions: prominent A waves in tricuspid stenosis, pulmonary stenosis, and pulmonary hypertension; rapid x and y descent in cardiac tamponade and constrictive pericarditis, respectively; and prominent V waves in tricuspid regurgitation.

- Abnormal carotid pulse patterns include pulsus parvus et tardus in aortic stenosis; pulsus bisferiens in combined aortic stenosis and regurgitation; pulsus paradoxus in cardiac tamponade, and bifid pulse in hypertrophic cardiomyopathy.

- A loud S1 is typical of mitral stenosis, though it may also be heard with a short P-R interval.

- A single S2 is heard in pulmonic and aortic stenosis.

- Paradoxic splitting of S2 is typical of left bundle branch block (LBBB) but can also be heard in aortic stenosis, hypertrophic cardiomyopathy, patent ductus, and systemic hypertension.

- Accentuation of P2 is indicative of pulmonary hypertension.

- Systolic ejection murmurs may be benign or pathologic. The latter are usually grade 3 or louder, associated with abnormal carotid upstroke, abnormal S2, or an ejection click.

- Pansystolic murmurs are usually due to ventricular septal defect and mitral or tricuspid regurgitation. The latter is augmented by inspiration.

- Diastolic murmurs are almost always pathologic and are usually due to mitral or tricuspid stenosis and aortic or pulmonary regurgitation.

- Continuous murmurs are usually due to patent ductus arteriosus, coronary or pulmonary arteriovenous fistulas, or peripheral pulmonary artery stenosis.

## INTRODUCTION

Taking a patient's cardiovascular history and performing a physical exam are the oldest and arguably most important initial diagnostic tools in the evaluation of heart disease. A careful and thorough history and physical exam will screen for common cardiovascular diseases, guide further noninvasive and invasive testing, and may obviate needless expensive exams by pointing supporting a noncardiac diagnosis or a low severity of cardiovascular disease. In addition to obtaining details of the presenting complaint, a good history should include a detailed past medical assessment. Such an assessment could suggest vascular disease as well as provide a survey of cardiac risk factors, a social history, including recreational drug and tobacco use, a family history of heart disease, including sudden death, stroke, and current medications. This chapter will focus on those common presenting complaints suggestive of cardiovascular disease, as well as physical diagnostic findings that suggest or confirm underlying cardiac abnormalities.

# CHEST PAIN

Chest pain remains the most common cardiac complaint in the outpatient clinic or emergency room setting. Chest discomfort encompasses a plethora of diagnoses ranging from innocuous to critical. Obtaining a good history is a diagnostic challenge for the clinician.

## Coronary Artery Disease (CAD)

### History

Myocardial ischemia or infarction most commonly presents as chest pain or discomfort. From patient history an examiner should be able to ascertain the character, location, radiation pattern, and associated symptoms of the chest discomfort. Emphasis should be placed on provocative and palliative features and frequency of the chest pain. The pain of myocardial ischemia typically is described as chest tightness, pressure, burning, indigestion, or heaviness. The classic description of "it feels like someone sitting on my chest," while commonly heard, need not be present. Women often may have less typical chest discomfort than men. Anginal discomfort is usually deep rather than superficial, located substernally and

supramammary. The pain may sometimes radiate to the arms, shoulders, interscapular region, epigastrum, jaw, and/or neck. The diagnostic value of particular characteristics of chest discomfort is given in (**Table 1-1**). Radiation of the discomfort is often manifest as numbness and tingling. Associated symptoms, or sometimes atypical symptoms (especially in diabetics, women, and the elderly), include dyspnea, diaphoresis, nausea, vomiting, lightheadedness, weakness, lethargy, and apprehension. These same associated symptoms may be anginal equivalents. Dyspnea caused by elevated left ventricular filling pressures or ischemic mitral regurgitation may be prominent. Silent or asymptomatic ischemia may occur in 25% or more of patients, most commonly in diabetics, women, the elderly, and those in the postoperative state.

Stable angina is often brought on by exertion, emotional stress, cold or hot weather, or after a large meal is consumed. Anginal discomfort is gradual in onset, lasts minutes rather than seconds, and is typically promptly relieved with rest and/or sublingual nitroglycerin. Reproducibility of chest pain at a given threshold level of activity is a hallmark of chronic stable angina. The Canadian Cardiovascular Society (CCS) classification of grading the functional severity of angina is practical and commonly accepted. (**Table 1-2**).

Unstable angina (ACS) is usually associated with increase in the frequency, intensity, and/or duration of ischemic chest discomfort. Chest pain may occur at rest or at a lower threshold of activity than previously noted. The discomfort of ACS is usually more severe (CCS class III or IV), lasts longer (>20 minutes), and is not as readily relieved by rest or sublingual nitroglycerin.

**Table 1-1 • Value of Specific Components of the Chest Pain History for the Diagnosis of Acute Myocardial Infarction (AMI)**

| Pain Descriptor | No. of Patients | Positive Likelihood Ratio (95% CI) |
|---|---|---|
| Increased likelihood of AMI | | |
| Radiation to right arm or shoulder | 770 | 4.7 (1.9–12) |
| Radiation to both arms or shoulders | 893 | 4.1 (2.5–6.5) |
| Associated with exertion | 893 | 2.4 (1.5–3.8) |
| Radiation to left arm | 278 | 2.3 (1.7–3.1) |
| Associated with diaphoresis | 8426 | 2.0 (1.9–2.2) |
| Associated with nausea or vomiting | 970 | 1.9 (1.7–2.3) |
| Worse than previous angina or similar to previous MI | 7734 | 1.8 (1.6–2.0) |
| Described as pressure | 11504 | 1.3 (1.2–1.5) |
| Decreased likelihood of AMI | | |
| Described as pleuritic | 8822 | 0.2 (0.1–0.3) |
| Described as positional | 8330 | 0.3 (0.2–0.5) |
| Described as sharp | 1088 | 0.3 (0.2–0.5) |
| Reproducible with palpation | 8822 | 0.3 (0.2–0.4) |
| Inframammary location | 903 | 0.8 (0.7–0.9) |
| Not associated with exertion | 893 | 0.8 (0.6–0.9) |

Modified from Swap CJ, Nagurney JT. Value and limitations of chest pain history in the evaluation of patients with suspected acute coronary syndromes. JAMA. 2005;294(20):2623–2629.

> **Table 1-2 • Canadian Cardiovascular Society (CCS) Classification of Angina Pectoris**
>
> - *Class I*: Ordinary physical activity, such as walking or climbing stairs, does not cause angina. Angina occurs with strenuous, rapid, or prolonged exertion at work or recreation.
> - *Class II*: Slight limitation of ordinary activity. Angina occurs on walking or climbing stairs rapidly, walking uphill, walking or climbing stairs after meals, or in cold, in wind, or under emotional stress, or only during the few hours after awakening. Angina occurs on walking more than 2 blocks on the level and climbing more than 1 flight of ordinary stairs at a normal pace and in normal condition.
> - *Class III*: Marked limitations of ordinary physical activity. Angina occurs on walking 1 to 2 blocks on the level and climbing 1 flight of stairs in normal conditions and at a normal pace.
> - *Class IV*: Inability to perform any physical activity without discomfort—anginal symptoms may be present at rest.

Acute myocardial infarction (AMI) usually presents with symptoms of severe chest pain, with similar but worse characteristics and associated symptoms similar to angina. Chest discomfort is more intense, longer lasting, and not relieved with rest or sublingual nitroglycerin. Infarction pain is often quite unexpected and may occur at rest, not infrequently during the morning hours. The discomfort of acute myocardial infarction is often gradual in onset, but quickly reaches a severe and unrelenting level, which can last up to several hours. The patient may not report "chest pain" but chest heaviness, pressure, discomfort, and/or arm and jaw discomfort may be the presenting complaints.

A detailed history of prior ischemic events and cardiac procedures is essential in the evaluation of a patient with symptoms suggestive of cardiac ischemia. Previous ischemic events include prior angina, myocardial infarction, cerebral vascular accident, or peripheral artery (PA) disease. The latter two are considered coronary artery disease equivalents; those with prior history of cerebral ischemia or peripheral artery disease have a very high likelihood of having significant coronary artery disease. Knowledge of previous coronary artery anatomy and function, if present, is very helpful in assessment of a patient with symptoms suggestive of ischemia.

A detailed history of a patient with suggestive symptoms of ischemia must include the possible presence of coronary artery disease risk factors, such as tobacco abuse, hypertension, dyslipidemia, diabetes mellitus, obesity, and a family history of premature coronary heart disease. The metabolic syndrome is a recent candidate for unsuspected CAD. The presence of one or more of these risk factors increases the likelihood of underlying coronary artery disease and also provides important targets for subsequent risk reduction.

## Physical Exam

It would be quite helpful if coronary artery disease (CAD) could be diagnosed on a standard physical examination, but this is not the case. Most individuals with CAD have a completely normal cardiovascular examination, even those who have had a myocardial infarction (MI). Abnormalities may be present in some patients who have had a MI, particularly if significant myocardial damage is present. Large or polyinfarcts often result in left ventricular enlargement, papillary muscle dysfunction, significant wall motion abnormalities, left ventricular hypertrophy, or mitral regurgitation, which may appear in physical findings upon cardiac exam.

*Blind Alleys*  An earlobe crease or arcus senilus have formerly achieved notoriety as being markers of coronary artery disease (CAD) and hyperlipidemia. Such observations, never proven to be reliable, do not deserve further discussion.

*Noncardiac Physical Exam Abnormalities*  As atherosclerosis is a multiorgan problem, evidence of arterial narrowing in noncardiac structures can suggest patients who are at increased risk for coexisting CV disease, such as carotid artery or peripheral artery disease (PAD). Atheromatous deposits outside the coronary bed signal patients at high risk for CAD. Carotid stenosis or abdominal aneurysm can be discovered upon exam, often with little effort. Findings of a decreased carotid pulse or peripheral artery arterial upstroke suggest coexisting CAD. Abdominal aneurysm should be sought in all older subjects, especially those with a history of coronary disease, PAD, or a known pre-existing aneurysm.

## Pericarditis—An Unusual Cause of Chest Pain

### History

Pericarditis can present rapidly or slowly, depending on the etiology. Infectious pericarditis, usually viral, manifests with severe symptoms, while uremic pericarditis presents quietly or even silently. The patient typically describes a variable intensity of sharp pleuritic precordial pain radiating to the back near the trapezius. The pain can radiate in almost any direction with a similar pattern to ischemic pain, however the quality of pericardial pain is very different. Such pain is usually improved by sitting up and leaning forward. Gastrointestinal symptoms of odynophagia, dysphagia, nausea, and vomiting are sometime associated with pericarditis.

### Physical Exam

*Pericardial Rub*  The classic pericardial friction rub is well known to physicians, but often missed. It typically is a "close to the ear" scratchy sound, frequently with murmur-like properties. The friction rub may be heard only in systole, but a rub in both systole and diastole provides more reassuring evidence that the sound in question is truly pericardial and not a heart murmur.

While pericardial rubs are often ephemeral and difficult to hear, a change in body position and respiration may alter the qualities of the rub. It is taught that diagnosis requires a 3-component rub, but this may be too rigorous a criterion. When a pericardial rub is suspected, the examiner should immediately have a colleague listen for the rub to confirm the diagnosis.

Whether or not a rub is truly present may be a matter of some debate. A rub associated with right ventricular enlargement, fluid retention, or edema may suggest pericardial effusion; in general, with increasing pericardial fluid, the rub softens or disappears, only to reappear after pericardiocentesis or a decrease in size of the effusion. Jugular vein distension is a likely partner to a rub.

## DYSPNEA, FATIGUE, AND EDEMA

Patients with symptoms of dyspnea, fatigue, and/or edema may be in congestive heart failure (see **Table 1-3**). The severity and rapidity of onset of symptoms (see **Table 1-4**) may suggest a specific cardiac diagnosis, such as left- and or right-sided heart failure. The history should focus on likely causative factors of heart failure (see **Table 1-5**). Left ventricular dysfunction from any cause results in neurohormonal compensatory mechanisms to support cardiac output at the expense of elevated left ventricular filling pressures. Elevated filling pressures consequently lead to increased interstitial pulmonary edema. Etiologies of left ventricular dysfunction include coronary ischemia, cardiomyopathies, valvular lesions, and right heart disease will be discussed below.

### Table 1-3 • Symptoms of Congestive Heart Failure

| Symptom | Description |
|---|---|
| Dyspnea | Discomfort with breathing |
| Peripheral edema | Fluid retention seen in lower extremities, sacrum, and abdomen; increased weight or abdominal girth |
| Orthopnea | Supine dyspnea |
| Paroxysmal nocturnal dyspnea | Dyspnea that occurs several hours after sleeping that awakens the patient |
| Nocturia | Multiple awakenings during the night to urinate |
| Fatigability | General or muscular weakness with activity |
| Anorexia | Loss of appetite |
| Chest discomfort | Angina |
| Presyncope/ syncope | Near or total loss of consciousness lasting seconds to a few minutes |
| Palpitations | Sensation of extra or rapid heart beats |

### Table 1-4 • New York Heart Association Functional Classification of Heart Failure

- *Class I*: Patients with no limitation of activities; they suffer no symptoms from ordinary activities.
- *Class II*: Patients with slight, mild limitation of activity; they are comfortable with rest or with mild exertion.
- *Class III*: Patients with marked limitation of activity; they are comfortable only at rest.
- *Class IV*: Patients who should be at complete rest, confined to bed or chair; any physical activity brings on discomfort and symptoms occur at rest.

## Mitral Regurgiutation

### History

The clinical symptoms of a patient with mitral regurgitation will be dependent on the speed of onset and degree of hemodynamic disturbance. Acute severe mitral regurgitation, such as from papillary muscle ischemia or rupture, may cause the patient to complain of profound dyspnea,

### Table 1-5 • The Evaluation of the Cause of Heart Failure: The History

History to include inquiry regarding:
  Hypertension
  Diabetes
  Dyslipidemia
  Valvular heart disease
  Coronary or peripheral vascular disease
  Myopathy
  Rheumatic fever
  Mediastinal irradiation
  History or symptoms of sleep-disordered breathing
  Exposure to cardiotoxic agents
  Current and past alcohol consumption
  Smoking
  Collagen vascular disease
  Exposure to sexually transmitted diseases
  Thyroid disorder
  Pheochromocytoma
  Obesity

Family history to include inquiry regarding:
  Predisposition to atherosclerotic disease
    (Hx of MIs, strokes, PAD)
  Sudden cardiac death
  Myopathy
  Conduction system disease (need for pacemaker)
  Tachyarrhythmias
  Cardiomyopathy (unexplained HF)
  Skeletal myopathies

*HF indicates heart failure; Hx, history; MI, myocardial infarction; and PAD, peripheral arterial disease.*
*ACC/AHA 2005 Guideline Update for the Diagnosis and Management of Chronic Heart Failure in the Adult: A Report of the American College of Cardiology/ American Heart Association Task Force on Practice Guidelines (Writing Committee to Update the 2001 Guidelines for the Evaluation and Management of Heart Failure) J Am Coll Cardiol. 2005;46:1–82.*

orthopnea, chest discomfort, and/or systemic signs of shock. Conversely, chronic mitral regurgitation from myxomatous or rheumatic disease has a more insidious presentation, with patients typically complaining of easy fatigability and progressive dyspnea over months to years.

### Physical Exam

*Precordial Exam* The range of precordial motion findings in mitral regurgitation is dependent on the severity of the regurgitation and the status of left ventricular size and function. Hemodynamically significant mitral regurgitation in the presence of relatively normal left ventricular function will result in a normal or increased prominence of the point of maximal (apical) impulse (PMI). Left ventricular systolic dysfunction typically results in increased size and strength of the PMI. With left ventricular dysfunction and moderate to severe mitral regurgitation, elevated pulmonary capillary or wedge pressure is typically present. Thus, resulting pulmonary hypertension can be mild to severe, possibly resulting in right ventricular dysfunction, typically with tricuspid regurgitation. A right ventricular lift is common in such patients, but often missed because of physician failure to search for the impulse, which typically denotes right ventricular hypertension or a large right ventricle. To allow detection of a right ventricular impulse, the patient should be supine and the lower sternum examined using firm pressure with the heel of the hand and breath held in expiration. The patient also should be examined in the left lateral decubitus position, palpating the apical impulse (which is typically more prominent in this position). A palpable S4 is common, along with an enlarged left ventricle, in acute mitral regurgitation. If the patient has depressed left ventricular function, the left ventricular apical impulse is likely to be quite prominent and displaced leftward.

*Auscultation* The murmur of mitral regurgitation or insufficiency is highly variable, depending on systemic blood pressure, the degree or left ventricular dilation (if any), left ventricular function, the timing of the murmur, and the regurgitation volume per beat. In mitral regurgitation blood returns to the left atrium with each left ventricular contraction. The "shape" or length of the systolic murmur may be holosystolic, systolic, or even early systolic with no murmur vibrations in late systole (**Figure 1-1** and **Figure 1-2**). Classic mitral regurgitation results in a holosystolic murmur. The classic murmur of mitral valve prolapse or papillary muscle dysfunction is a mid to late systolic murmur extending to the first heart sound; early systole is silent in such cases.

*Mitral Click* In mitral valve prolapse, one or more of a series of high frequency clicks may be heard (**Figure 1-3**). These appear "close together" and may sound like an unusual crackling from multiple clicks, or there may be a single loud click. These sounds signify mitral valve prolapse, or less

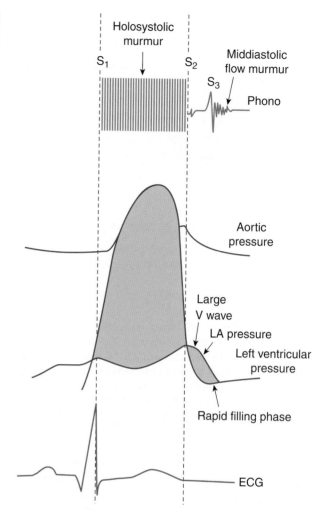

**Figure 1-1.** Pressure-sound correlations in mitral regurgitation. There is a large pressure gradient between the left ventricle and the left atrium that begins before the aortic valve opens and ends during isovolumic relaxation. This pressure difference results in a holosystolic murmur with sound vibrations beginning with S1 and extending to S2. The murmur classically is even or plateaulike in configuration, although many variants exist. An S3 frequently is present when there is a significant degree of mitral regurgitation; the S3 reflects the excessive blood volume traversing the mitral valve in early diastole. Such voluminous left ventricular filling may produce a short mid-diastolic flow murmur in patients with severe mitral regurgitation. (From: *Synopsis of Cardiac Physical Diagnosis.* 2nd ed. p. 187, Figure 13-2.)

likely, papillary muscle dysfunction; both typically manifest as a late systolic crescendo murmur only.

## Mitral Stenosis

### History

A careful history of a patient with mitral stenosis includes discovery of whether rheumatic disease or childhood in a rheumatic fever endemic area. Patients with multiple sclerosis (MS) typically complain of slow progressive symptoms of dyspnea and often heart failure. Dyspnea is the

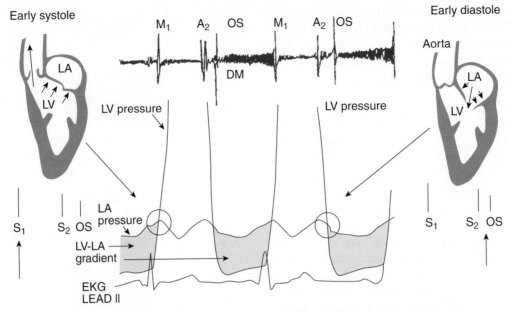

Early systole

Early diastole

**Figure 1-2.** Intracardiac pressure and sound relationships in mitral stenosis. Pressure crossover between the left atrium (LA) and left ventricle (LV) always precedes the cardiac sounds generated by mitral valve closure ($M_1$).and opening (opening snap), the persistence of a late diastolic gradient between the left atrium and left ventricle in combination with the thickened mitral valve apparatus results in an accentuated S1. Similarly, the maximal opening excursion of the rigid fibrotic valve generates an opening snap (OS), which immediately precedes early diastolic filling of the left ventricle and the resultant diastolic murmur (DM). (From: *Synopsis of Cardiac Physical Diagnosis.* 2nd ed. p. 223, Figure 14-2.)

most common symptom of mitral stenosis, followed by orthopnea. Atrial fibrillation may accompany signs of heart failure in the mitral stenotic patient. The stenotic mitral valve leads to left atrial hypertension and dilation resulting in atrial fibrillation.

## Physical Exam

Mitral stenosis, uncommon and often missed by physicians, has a Plethora of cardiac physical exam findings. Mitral stenosis is common in impoverished countries, such as India; it is often found in Native Americans and Hispanics as well.

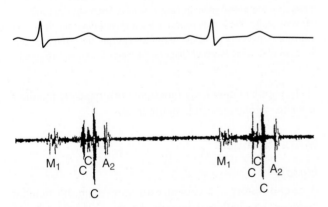

**Figure 1-3.** Multiple systolic clicks in a patient with mitral valve prolapsed. There are at least three dominant clicks, with the loudest in late systole. (From: Cheitin, Mel MD, Byrd, RC; *Curr Probl Cardiol.* 1984;8:1. p. 249, Figure: 15-2.)

The cardiac exam in mitral stenosis may change over time as valve inflammation and thickening increases, resulting in more severe obstruction to mitral inflow. The diastolic opening snap of mitral stenosis allows a "make my day" diagnosis if it has not been previously discovered.

*General Inspection* Patient appearance may be normal in the absence of severe mitral stenosis. Experts of cardiac physical diagnosis in years past have noted "mitral facies" in patients with severe mitral stenosis and high right heart pressures; mitral facies is a characteristic reddened facial skin, often accompanied by a shiny appearance. It would be most unusual to see patients with such advanced valvular disease in countries with accessible well-trained physicians.

*Jugular Venous Pulse* Normal in mild valve disease, but likely to be elevated in patients with moderate to severe mitral stenosis with pulmonary hypertension. The classic finding is a dominant V wave, which in severe cases is very obvious to most examiners. The holosystolic measure of tricuspid insufficiency is common in such patients. One can typically see the jugular venous pulsating from the foot of the bed in these patients. Inspiration will produce a more prominent jugular venous pulse with a taller V wave.

*Precordial Exam* In mild mitral stenosis usually no abnormality can be found. However, as peripheral artery (PA) pressure increases to significant levels, a right ventricular heave or lift is common, especially if the patient is examined in held expiration with firm pressure on the lower sternum, with the patient in the left lateral position.

*Cardiac Rhythm* Most—but not all—individuals with mitral stenosis ultimately develop atrial fibrillation. This arrhythmia, with beat to beat variation of the pulse, is common in such patients and is a hallmark of significant mitral stenosis, suggesting left atrial enlargement and tricuspid regurgitation due to pulmonary hypertension.

*Auscultation* The classic physical diagnostic exam in mitral stenosis is the opening snap (OS) in diastole, followed by a low pitched diastolic murmur or rumble (**Figure 1-2**). The OS is often missed by physicians, even when patient diagnosis is known. The OS is "close to the ear," variable in distance from S2, and initiates the mitral stenosis murmur. The P2-OS interval is a valuable clue to the severity of mitral stenosis. While not a perfect indicator, in general a short P2-OS interval is associated with a significantly diseased mitral valve structure and a small mitral valve area, whereas a long interval suggests mild disease. It takes skill and patience to learn how to use these general principles, but the reward of a proper physical finding and diagnosis of mitral stenosis is worth the effort.

The diastolic murmurs of mitral stenosis are usually hard to hear unless the heart rate is slow and the P2-OS clicks are readily audible. This murmur is typically low frequency (e.g., "rumble") and of variable audibility, especially in the presence of coexisting mitral regurgitation. The long systolic murmur of The long systolic is often audible and suggests both stenosis and regurgitation of the mitral valve.

Furthermore, in advanced disease, right-sided tricuspid regurgitation murmurs are often present, along with an OS, a mitral murmur, and a short P2-OS (typically heard), culminating in a virtual cardiac symphony!

## Aortic Sclerosis and Stenosis

### History

Aortic sclerosis in isolation is asymptomatic and usually found during evaluation for an unrelated complaint. In fact, patients with aortic stenosis only become symptomatic after valve area is reduced by at least 50%. The hallmark symptoms of severe aortic stenosis are angina, presyncope/syncope, and heart failure. The aortic outflow obstruction may be progressive over time; cardiac output is maintained by left ventricular hypertrophy. Patents should be carefully questioned about the onset of symptoms of dyspnea or exertion-related chest discomfort; reduction of activity from symptoms may be almost imperceptible to patients. In severe aortic stenosis about two-thirds of patients will complain of angina. Presyncope may occur in many patients with fixed cardiac output and systemic vasodilatation. Presyncope/syncope may also be a result of atrioventricular block, atrial, and/or ventricular arrhythmias. Patients should be questioned about dyspnea, orthopnea, and dizziness, which, unfortunately, are very late and poor prognostic features of aortic stenosis.

### Physical Exam

*Blood Pressure* Blood pressure is often elevated, as aortic stenosis is a coexisting condition most common in older hypertensive individuals. Hypertension itself may result in leaflet stiffening and produce a systolic stenosis murmur indistinguishable from aortic stenosis. Blood pressure, if elevated, is a potential contributor to progression of aortic stenosis.

*Pulse* A classic finding in aortic stenosis is in the carotid artery exam, demonstrating a decreased pulse volume and a vibratory sensation on direct palpation on top of the carotid artery. The classic "parvus and tardus" description of the aortic pulse in severe aortic sclerosis remains true, but it is recognized only with careful examination. One practical problem is that aortic stenosis is common in the elderly, as is hypertension. Thus, the carotid artery upstroke may be more brisk than expected in a younger subject, considerably decreasing the sensitivity of the carotid exam, and falsely masking aortic obstruction.

It is obligatory to include the carotid artery exam in all older patients, as a rough or prominent systolic murmur or bruit can suggest atherosclerosis, aortic sclerosis, or intrinsic sclerosis of aortic artery itself, i.e., significant aortic sclerosis.

*Jugular Venous Pulse* The venous pulsations are normal in aortic stenosis.

*Precordial Exam* In mild aortic stenosis or aortic sclerosis, there is no PMI perturbation as there is in moderate to severe aortic stenosis, where the left ventricular apical impulse may be prominent due to left ventricular hypertrophy (**Figure 1-4**). In subjects with depressed left ventricular systolic function, the PMI may be displaced to the left; the apical impulse may be increased in size and strength, all findings suspicious for left ventricular failure.

*Auscultation* The cardinal finding is a harsh systolic murmur at or above the right clavicle, which usually radiates to the head vessels. Surprisingly, this murmur can be very prominent at the cardiac apex; if present, the apical systolic murmur of aortic stenosis is less harsh and more musical than at the aortic area, and may often be confused with mitral regurgitation.

The severity of aortic stenosis may be predictable by auscultation. The length of the murmur increases with the severity

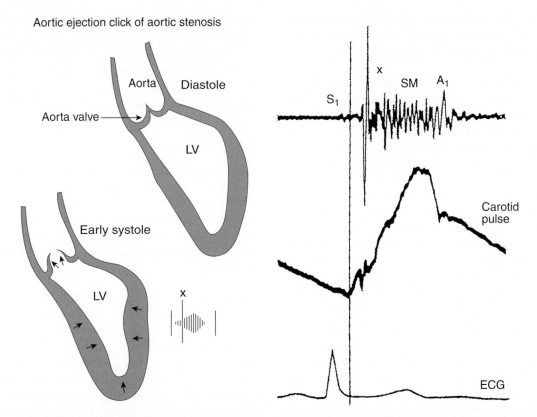

**Figure 1-4.** Ejection click associated with aortic stenosis due to a congenitally bicuspid valve. Note the high-frequency, high-amplitude sound that follows S1 and is coincident with the onset of the ejection into the aorta. The aortic ejection sound is formed by sudden cessation of the opening motion of the abnormal valve leaflets (doming). Note also the delayed carotid upstroke and long systolic murmur. (From: *Synopsis of Cardiac Physical Diagnosis*. 2nd ed. p. 135, Figure 10-3.)

of the aortic value obstruction. Thus, in severe aortic stenosis the murmur is quite long, extending to S2. Conversely a short aortic murmur is less likely to reflect severe obstruction to left ventricular outflow.

It is important to listen closely for a prominent systolic, often rough murmur at the right sternal border and superior chest in all patients, particularly the elderly. Such a murmur suggests either aortic valvular obstruction or possibly carotid artery atherosclerosis. Both murmurs can be quite harsh or grunting.

## Aortic Regurgitation

### History

Many patients with moderate or even severe aortic regurgitation have no complaints. The patient with chronic aortic regurgitation usually remains asymptomatic until the left ventricle dilates. After this occurs, the patient may complain of classic symptoms of congestive heart failure, such as exertional dyspnea. Patients should be asked about a pounding sensation or palpitations; this is a reflection of the wide pulse pressure that develops with significant aortic regurgitation. Patients are also questioned about symptoms of angina that may develop late in the disease process as a result of

left ventricular hypertrophy and decreased coronary perfusion pressure. Patients with acute aortic regurgitation may not exhibit the compensatory mechanisms of left ventricular hypertrophy and dilation and, therefore, present with severe congestive heart failure and masked physical findings.

### Physical Exam

*Auscultation* Aortic insufficiency or regurgitation is commonly seen on 2-D echocardiography as typically trace or mild; but these small jets of blood flow returning to the left ventricle are infrequently audible. Aortic regurgitation murmurs are usually high frequency and soft. Thus, when a high pitched diastolic murmur of aortic regurgitation is heard, the degree of reflux of blood in to the left ventricle is likely to be at least moderate. An aortic regurgitation murmur starts with S2 and is usually the only audible murmur. An accompanying early systolic murmur can also be present, reflecting increased left ventricular blood flow and in Left ventricular stroke volume. It is most important to listen for aortic regurgitation in a quiet room, using firm pressure of the stethoscope on the diaphragm, while the patient is leaning forward with breath held. Increasing degrees of aortic regurgitation correspond to a murmur that becomes lower in frequency, louder, and often accompanied by a systolic ejection murmur. An ejection click in early systole may be noted with careful auscultation.

## Right Heart Failure

### History

There are a plethora of diseases which lead to right heart dysfunction; however the advanced state of these processes result in similar symptoms and history. The interviewer should ask about easy fatigability, whether leg swelling is present, and how the patient's energy level has changed. Patients may report of pulsations in the neck from jugular venous distention, increased abdominal girth, anorexia, and lower extremity edema. Presyncope and syncope can occur as result of left ventricular compression by the right ventricle. These complaints are ubiquitous in right heart failure and do not point toward a precise etiology. A history of angina may suggest coronary disease, while complaints of exertional dyspnea but not orthopnea may suggest a primary pulmonary process.

### Physical Exam

Tricuspid regurgitation or insufficiency is a very common finding on 2-D echo and almost ubiquitous in hearts with valvular disease or abnormal left ventricular function. Pulmonary hypertension of any cause typically results in tricuspid regurgitation. Most physicians do not make the appropriate diagnosis when tricuspid regurgitation is present.

*Jugular Venous Pulse* The jugular venous pulse is highly likely to be elevated in subjects with tricuspid regurgitation, cardiovascular disease, severe mitral regurgitation, pulmonary hypertension, or right ventricular failure. A prominent V wave may be noted in the jugular venous pulse (JVP); and when tricuspid regurgitation is severe, the neck veins bulge conspicuously, reflecting high jugular venous and right atrial pressure. The normal, more dominant, A wave often is smaller than the V wave of tricuspid regurgitation.

*Precordial Exam* Pulmonary hypertension is the cause of a large jugular wave, often associated with a palpable right ventricular heave over or just leftwards of the sternum. This is most likely to be present in severe mitral regurgitation, mitral stenosis, or COPD.

*Auscultation* The murmur, if present, is best heard adjacent to left sternal border or directly over the midsternal area. Often silent, an audible tricuspid regurgitation murmur suggests a significant degree of reflux of blood from the right ventricle to the right atrium. The classic physical exam findings are of a holosystolic, medium-to-high pitched murmur, heard best over or adjacent to the sternum, which increases in loudness during inspiration (**Figure 1-5**). The degree of respiratory variation may be virtually inaudible or quite prominent. Tricuspid regurgitation generally reflects moderate to severe pulmonary hypertension. Isolated tricuspid regurgitation can be a result

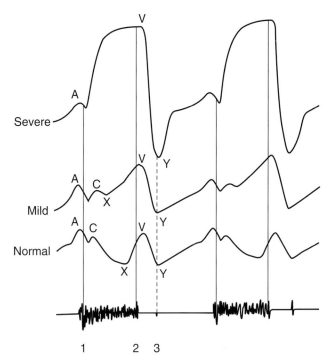

**Figure 1-5.** Jugular venous pulse in tricuspid regurgitation. Alterations of the venous contour in mild tricuspid regurgitation are depicted in the middle tracing. The V Wave is augmented and the Y descent is more prominent; the X descent is attenuated markedly. With severe tricuspid regurgitation (top tracing), there is a plateaulike systolic regurgitant C-V wave, which in part represents "ventricularization" of the right atrial and jugular venous pulses. Notice the right ventricular $S_3$ coinciding with the nadir of the Y descent. A normal venous pulse is depicted in the bottom. (From: *Synopsis of Cardiac Physical Diagnosis.* 2nd ed. p. 264, Figure: 16-2.)

of tricuspid valve endocarditis. In general, the louder the tricuspid regurgitation murmur, the greater the degree of reflux of blood from the right ventricle to the right atrium.

*Other Signs of Tricuspid Regurgitation* Severe tricuspid regurgitation is frequently noted in patients with pulmonary hypertension and right heart failure. Thus, an increased amount of blood is propelled backward from the right ventricle, resulting in mild to vigorous neck vein pulsations, as mentioned, but also a pulsatile liver. This is usually missed by the exam, but is quite common in biventricular failure and severe pulmonary hypertension. Ruptured chordae tendinae of the tricuspid valve can produce a hepatic V wave. In the proper technique for detecting this often ignored phenomenon the patient hold his or her breath while the examiner palpates the liver edge that extends distally with each cardiac pulsation. The hepatic pulsations are subtly noted at the hepatic inferior border and are usually missed. The distal fingers should be positioned with the fingers coming up from below to feel the hepatic impulse. This finding confirms severe elevation of right heart pressure and/or volume, and significant tricuspid regurgitation.

# Ethics in Cardiovascular Medicine

JAMES N. KIRKPATRICK AND SAVITRI E. FEDSON

## ● PRACTICAL POINTS

- Increasing relevance of ethics in the practice of cardiovascular medicine.

- Large number of elderly patients with chronic heart failure and end-of-life decision issues.

- Explosion of diagnostic and therapeutic modalities e.g., ICDs, LVADs, raises dilemmas regarding informed consent, costs (individual, social) and resource utilization.

- Increasing industry financing of research leading to conflicts of interest.

- Ethical issues related to preservation of patient confidentiality in an era of electronic medical records.

- Basic principles of bioethics include Autonomy, Beneficence, Nonmaleficence and Justice of which

- Autonomy is the most important in American medical ethics.

- The exercise of autonomy presupposes decision making capacity (particularly relevant in informed consent) which is determined by medical providers, unlike competency which is decided by the courts.

- Important to consider cultural and religious background when approaching end-of-life issues.

- Ethical considerations are particularly important in decisions regarding withdrawal of life sustaining therapies like pacemakers, ICDs and LVADs.

- Genetic testing should be done only after informed consent and availability of genetic counseling.

## INTRODUCTION

Ethics has always played an important part in medicine, but medical ethics as a discipline has received particular attention only in the last 50 years. Even more recently, ethics has been officially recognized as an important component of cardiovascular medicine. The 1989 and 1997 American College of Cardiology (ACC) Bethesda Conferences were devoted entirely to the application of ethical standards to the practice of cardiovascular medicine. In 2004, the ACC and the American Heart Association (AHA) sponsored a conference on Professionalism and Ethics. Nonetheless, studies have shown that cardiovascular journals publish few articles dealing with ethics topics, such as end-of-life issues, in comparison to other medical specialties.

Several features of modern cardiovascular medicine make ethics increasingly important. As the population ages and the prevalence of patients with chronic heart failure skyrockets, cardiologists will encounter increasing numbers of patients facing end-of-life decisions. The explosion of diagnostic and therapeutic technologies raises ethical dilemmas concerning informed consent, cost (both public and private), resource utilization and financial conflicts of interest. Frequent media reports about the unethical behavior of some cardiovascular specialists emphasize the importance of medical professionalism. Ethics and monitoring of clinical research will become increasingly important as cardiovascular research continues to move out of academia and into private practice (and research itself continues to be heavily financed by industry). The challenge of preservation of patient confidentiality cannot be underestimated with the profusion of electronic medical records and genetics-driven "personalized medicine." And, as with every important aspect of modern medicine that garners attention from the educational establishment, questions concerning ethics will be more and more likely to appear on cardiovascular certification examinations.

## PRINCIPLES OF MEDICAL ETHICS

The field of medical ethics encompasses a wide range of perspectives; most address the essential distinction between what "can" be done in medicine and what "should" be done. Two of the more recognized general approaches to ethical reasoning include *principlism* and *casuistry*. Advocates of principlism look to time-honored, immutable principles to help them decide what to do in a given situation. Various sets of principles have been proposed, but the most well known include autonomy, beneficence, nonmaleficence, and justice (see **Table 2-1**). Of the four, autonomy is generally regarded as the most important principle in American medical ethics, although beneficence and nonmaleficence can be found in the writings of Hippocrates, and justice in the earliest known religious writings. Casuistry involves drawing parallels between a present case and similar cases of the past. By referring to the outcomes of prior cases and the reasoning used in those cases, casuistic analysis derives guidance for decision about one should do, using precedents. In the practice of clinical ethics, both approaches are often employed.

A well-known formula for resolving ethical dilemmas, specifically in the clinical setting, is the "four box model."(see **Table 2-2**) The four box model uniquely recognizes the importance of the medical facts of the case in ethical analysis. These "medical indications" include diagnosis, prognosis, treatment options, and recommendations based on medical knowledge and judgment. Patient preference is very similar to autonomy, but the ability of patients to make autonomous choices is based on what they know about the medical indications (hence, it is the second box, not the first). Below the line, "quality of life" refers to an external observer's assessment of the patient's quality of life, not how the patient

| Table 2-1 • Principles of Bioethics | |
|---|---|
| Autonomy | Respecting the right of patients to decide what is done to them |
| Beneficence | Acting to do what is best for the patients |
| Nonmaleficence | Avoiding what is harmful for the patient |
| Justice | Ensuring equal and fair distribution of medical resources |

| Table 2-2 • The Four Box Model | |
|---|---|
| Medical indications | Patient preferences |
| Quality of life | Contextual features |

assesses her or his own quality of life. "Contextual features" include considerations of cost, research or educational interests, and issues related to the patient's familial, social, religious, cultural or ethnic group. The two top boxes are considered more important than the bottom boxes, because there is more controversy about how much of a role quality of life and, especially issues of cost, should play in making decisions. However, in the absence of clear medical indications or patient preferences, the bottom two boxes may become the essential factors by which an ethical dilemma is resolved.

## DECISION-MAKING CAPACITY, INFORMED CONSENT, AND SURROGATES

The exercise of autonomy presupposes **decision-making capacity (DMC)**. DMC must be distinguished from **competency**, which can only be determined by the law courts. Medical providers cannot declare a patient incompetent, but must determine whether a patient has the DMC to be able to make his or her own medical decisions. Patients may have transiently impaired DMC (as in cardiac arrest) or be permanently impaired (end-stage dementia). Although no universally accepted definition for DMC exists, most definitions include ability to understand relevant information and appreciate the consequences of decisions or lack of decision (see **Table 2-3**). Patients may have adequate decision-making capacity for making certain decisions but not for others, based on their relative ability to understand relevant information. Decisions should not be influenced by medical conditions such as delirium, organic brain conditions, or other medical conditions affecting brain function. Even with regard to patients with intact DMC, both

| Table 2-3 • Elements of Decision-Making Capacity |
|---|
| Patients must be able to: |
| • Express a choice |
| • Understand information relevant to decisions about treatment |
| • Appreciate the significance of the situation and the information disclosed |
| • Reason about information in a way that allows one to make comparisons and weigh options |
| *Grisso T, Appelbaum PS. Comparison of standards for assessing patients' capacities to make treatment decisions. Am J Psych. 1995;152(7):1033–1037.* |

| Table 2-4 • Emancipated Minors |
| --- |
| Married |
| Joined military |
| Obtained court order |
| Had a child (in some states) |

intentional and unintentional coercion, recognized or un-recognized by the patient, may influence decisions.

Children (people under age 18 years) are presumed to lack DMC, but those in the legal category of **emancipated minor** can make their own medical decisions (see **Table 2-4**).

Determination of DMC (and freedom from coercion) must be made on a case-by-case basis, sometimes with the assistance of psychiatrists, lawyers, and ethicists. Some ethicists believe there is an appropriate double standard in clinical practice: A higher level of DMC is required of a patient to be able to refuse medically indicated therapies, while it is often assumed that a patient has appropriate DMC when in agreement with his or her doctor. However, disagreement with doctors is not a sign of lack of DMC.

## INFORMED CONSENT

DMC is particularly relevant in **informed consent**. (**Table 2-5**) In brief, "informed consent = proper information + voluntary decision." Proper information is sometimes hard to define, but generally uses the "reasonable person standard" (defined by what a reasonable person in the same situation would want to know in order to make a decision). As such, informed consent does not include an exhaustive list of all possible outcomes but does require a discussion of the more probable outcomes. Informed consent is not necessary for standard procedures involving minimal risk (e.g., although it is possible that placing an IV might cause a catastrophic infection resulting in limb loss, the risk is extremely low). Importantly, informed consent does *not* consist of cajoling a patient into signing a form ("getting consent") but, rather, of an ongoing dialogue and exchange of information that allows the patient to make an educated decision. The informed consent form provides a means to record this

| Table 2-5 • Elements of Informed Consent |
| --- |
| • Description of the procedure or intervention |
| • Description of any reasonable foreseeable risks or discomforts |
| • Description of any benefits to the patient |
| • Disclosure of appropriate alternative procedures or courses of treatment |
| • Documentation of the process of informed consent |

process in the medical record; it is *not* a waiver of rights or a document that absolves clinicians from legal action. Even though minors cannot provide informed consent, clinicians should seek **assent**, or agreement, from them.

## SURROGATES

Patient who lack DMC require a surrogate decision-maker to provide informed consent. In general, surrogates should make **substituted judgments**, essentially, the decisions that *the patient* would have made if he or she had DMC. The surrogate is not to make decisions based on his or her own values and wishes. Emphasizing this fact not only may prevent surrogates from making inappropriate decisions but may also relieve them from some of the emotional stress of making life and death decisions for another person. A patient may have mentioned what he or she would want done in a certain situation or may have expressed values or beliefs which can guide the surrogate's decisions. In the absence of a court-appointed guardian or person appointed in a durable power of attorney for healthcare document (DPAHC), many states authorize a hierarchy of family members and friends to be surrogates, generally following next of kin order. Such an order reflects presumed familiarity with the patients' values, beliefs, and wishes. A surrogate in the hierarchy may defer to those below him or her. Problems can arise, as in the case of estranged family members (e.g., separated but not divorced spouses), close friends who are more familiar with a patient's values than are family members, and disagreement with an even split between surrogates at the same level (e.g., four adult children, two on each side). Furthermore, studies have repeatedly demonstrated a relatively high rate of values discordance between patients and their potential surrogates.

If no one knows what the patient would have wanted, if there is suspicion that surrogates are not properly conveying the patient's wishes, or if a suitable surrogate cannot be found, substituted judgment gives way to **best interests**. Preservation of life and alleviation of suffering are presumed to be in a patient's best interests. If a clinician believes that a surrogate is not acting in the patient's best interests or in cases when a surrogate is necessary but not available, a judge can assign a **court-appointed guardian** who generally uses a best interests standard to make medical decisions. A best interests standard must be employed for patients who never had DMC (e.g., children and adults with severe mental retardation from childhood). Although parents or guardians usually make medical decisions for children, some states allow minors to receive medical care for sexually transmitted diseases, pregnancy and mental illness without parental consent. Such statutes presume that parental notification for these conditions may dissuade some minors from seeking medical care (which is in their best interest). In the provision of emergency care, patients without DMC or surrogates are treated under **implied consent**—the assumption that a reasonable person would chose to undergo medical interventions to reduce the chance of serious morbidity or mortality.

## CULTURAL AND RELIGIOUS ISSUES

End-of-life care must take into account different cultural and religious beliefs. Autonomy is not as important as an ethical principle in some non-Western cultures, and physicians should allow patients to defer to family members to make decisions and even receive diagnoses and prognoses. Many Jehovah's Witnesses (JW) will not accept blood products or derivatives (such as clotting factors) on religious grounds. Many Christian Scientists avoid modern medicine and instead rely on faith healing. The legal system recognizes the rights of competent adults to follow such cultural and religious beliefs, even if death ensues. The issue is more complicated with regard to children— pitting parental autonomy against the government's interest in protecting children. The courts have reasoned that children have not yet made an adult decision to refuse care on religious grounds and therefore should be given necessary life-sustaining care, even over the objections of the parents. Exceptions have been made for mature minors with sincere religious beliefs. It can be helpful to involve religious leaders in discussions with patients. On the other hand, some patients may not hold strongly to specific beliefs. It is advisable, at some point, to discuss patients' specific beliefs without other members of the culture or religion present, in order to prevent possible coercion.

## ADVANCE DIRECTIVES

In 1990, the U.S. Congress passed the **Patient Self Determination Act (PSDA)**. This act required health care practitioners to provide adult patients with information about their rights to:

- Participate in one's health care decisions
- To accept or refuse medical or surgical treatment
- To prepare an advanced directive

Advance directive documents include **living wills (LW)** and **durable powers of attorney for healthcare (DPAHC)**. Simply stated, a LW outlines what a patient would want done, and a DPAHC specifies a person who should make medical decisions in an end-of-life situation in which the patients lacks DMC. Individual states have specific regulations concerning these documents. Patients must have had DMC when they made the decisions in the documents, and the advance directives become operational when patients lose DMC (and are faced with an end-of-life situation).

Advance directives are valid across state lines and do not require a lawyer to draft. Some states require that they be notarized, but most simply require one or two witnesses.

Official guidelines now recommend advance directives for patients with end-stage heart failure. Some centers require advance directives before the implantation of ventricular assist devices. In practice, few cardiology patients have advance directives, even patients with established, life-threatening cardiovascular problems.

Another form of advance directive is a **do not resuscitate (DNR)** order. It differs from an LW in that it is written by a physician and does not state the wishes of the patient; the wishes expressed in an LW or by a DPAHC may be applied through a DNR order. Unfortunately, patient wishes concerning resuscitation are frequently not followed. The SUPPORT investigation studied whether a nurse educator could facilitate communication and improve adherence to the resuscitation preferences of end-stage patients, but it showed no benefit. There was also no difference in cost and other utilization outcomes. Complicating the issue: A significant proportion of patients changed their minds during the study period. End-stage cardiomyopathy patients were more likely than other patients to do so.

Advance directives (ADs) are a part of **advance care planning (ACP)**, which involves preparations for end-of-life care and death, including financial preparations, plans about extended care facilities and hospice, funeral preparations, and special communications to family members and friends.

It is increasingly evident that there is a growing population of patients with heart failure who would benefit from ACP. Many, if not most, of these patients or their surrogates will face hard choices about aggressive medical support, heart transplantation and/or device implantation. Some will suffer complications from these interventions, potentially leaving them with severely reduced quality of life. Improved longevity from recent advances in cardiac care will ensure that many cardiac patients survive long enough to contract cancer and other diseases. Others will progress to end-stage heart failure symptoms, which are hard to treat.

Cardiologists are not as diligent about discussing end-of-life issues with patients as are other specialists. Sensitive discussion with the patient, surrogates and other physicians is vital in end-of-life care. Studies suggest that specialists believe it is the role of primary care physicians to discuss end-of-life issues, but primary care physicians believe the same about specialists. For patients with serious cardiovascular problems, it seems logical for a cardiovascular specialist at least to be involved in, if not lead, such discussions. For instance, cardiologists can provide the best input about medical futility in settings such as un-revascularizable coronary artery disease and heart failure with vasodilatory shock.

## Withdrawing and Withholding of Life-sustaining Therapies

We chose to avoid the standard term "withdrawal of *care*" because of the greater recognition in recent years that patients for whom life-sustaining interventions are no longer appropriate still require aggressive palliation of symptoms and intensive psychological, social, and religious interventions. There is general ethical consensus that no meaningful difference exists between withdrawing and withholding life-sustaining interventions. The right to withdraw life-sustaining therapies is well established as an application of autonomy by multiple legal cases. Withdrawal of therapies such as hemodialysis and mechanical ventilation is well established. Although more controversial, there are legal precedents to support the decision specifically to withdraw hydration and nutrition. Brain death or a persistent/permanent vegetative state is not a necessary criterion for withdrawing or withholding life-sustaining therapy. Medical and surgical interventions can be specifically evaluated in light of the patient's overall goals of care. The ability of surrogate decision-makers is limited in some states unless the desires of the patient are clearly apparent, such as in a living will. When appropriate, these decisions can be made with the input of legal counsel or an ethics consultant.

Withdrawing life support has unique considerations within cardiology, specifically in reference to deactivation of specialized implantable devices. This issue is complicated by the specific effects of each device and the likely results of deactivation. Depending on a patient's underlying condition, deactivation of a pacemaker may not prevent death but rather make the patient suffer from light-headedness, fatigue, or dyspnea. Maintaining pacemaker function, therefore, is generally consistent with the goals of palliative care. Implantable cardioverter defibrillators (ICD), however, can impede the natural dying process through the delivery of shocks for malignant arrhythmias. The backup pacing function of ICDs should not be deactivated. Deactivation of ICDs is similar to withholding external defibrillation. Death from ventricular fibrillation is generally a quick and painless process, though often unexpected. Depending on patient goals, this type of death may be preferable to lingering with stage IV congestive heart failure. Others may want to stay alive as long as possible (e.g., until a grandchild is married). In palliative care, active defibrillators can cause suffering, as electrolyte and other metabolic disturbances can lead to arrhythmias that ICDs will detect and try to treat. There have

been multiple media reports of patients in hospice writhing from repeated ICD shocks, to the horror of onlooking family members.

CRT devices may extend life as well as relieve symptoms, so they generally should not be deactivated in the palliative care setting (unless they are causing diaphragmatic stimulation).

With ventricular assist devices (VADs) the decision to withdraw support is more ethically challenging. Although some operations can be palliative to relieve symptoms, performing an operation to remove a VAD in order to discontinue life-sustaining treatment may induce suffering. Turning off a VAD is usually a terminal event because it can cause stasis and backpressure in the VAD circuit, impeding residual heart function. In essence, rather than "letting nature take its course," discontinuing VADs actually hastens death. VAD discontinuation, therefore, requires detailed discussion with patients or surrogates and probably should be anticipated in AD discussions before destination VADs are inserted. In general, the complexities involved in withdrawal of implanted cardiac devices argue for multidisciplinary input from primary care physicians, general and specialized cardiovascular clinicians, and palliative care specialists.

## Physician-assisted Suicide and Euthanasia

There may be concern that the withdrawal of pacing, defibrillation, or VADs constitute physician-assisted suicide (PAS), euthanasia or murder. The key distinction in this matter is that the death of the patient is a natural consequence of their underlying disease process. The devices are, in a sense, an "unnatural" way of prolonging life.

In PAS, a physician enables a patient to end his or her own life (as in providing a prescription for a lethal combination of medications). In voluntary euthanasia, a physician directly ends the patient's life at the patient's request (in involuntary euthanasia, there is no request by the patient). The ethical justification for both involves extension of the principle of autonomy to cover decisions about time and manner of death. Euthanasia is legal in the Netherlands. In 1997, the U.S. Supreme Court established that there is no constitutional right to physician-assisted suicide, but it did not specifically prohibit the practice. It outlined a clear distinction between allowing a patient to die and intentionally hastening death by an intervention, stating that patients have a right to withdrawal of medical interventions. Oregon legalized PAS in the same year, and the Supreme Court upheld the Oregon law in 2005. The issue remains hotly debated on moral, legal, and medical grounds. The ACC/AHA did not advocate or support PAS in its 29th Bethesda Conference document.

## Cost Considerations at the End-of-life

It is increasingly recognized that part of a physician's responsibility is to involve cost consciousness in end-of-life decisions. There should be a reasonable expectation of good outcome and/or knowledge gain from any diagnostic test or therapy. In the care of terminally and critically ill patients, the ACC/AHA has outlined a goal of "ensuring that patients do not receive care that is both expensive and unwanted." Patients should also not receive care that is expensive and futile. However, care must also be taken to insure patients receive medically indicated care, including palliation. Decisions against interventions should not be made covertly, but, rather, they should involve full discussion with the patient or surrogate.

## Futility

A physician does not have an obligation to provide a specific treatment if it is not in agreement with his or her medical judgment. Some patients or surrogates may insist on interventions that have no or little chance of providing any benefit. Examples include request for an angiogram for non-cardiac chest pain after a normal thallium stress test or for a VAD in refractory shock if there is irreversible multisystem organ failure. Some hospitals have instituted policies that permit "unilateral" withholding of therapies in futile cases, in which a DNR order is placed despite objections by the patient or surrogate. Such policies often require ethics or legal consultation, and some require that transfer of care to another institution be offered.

There are important caveats to determining futility. Prognosis plays an important role, yet is extremely difficult. Studies suggest that family members tend to be overly optimistic, but physicians are overly pessimistic, compared with actual outcomes. Furthermore, the definition of futility is inherently subjective. Should an intervention be considered futile if the chance of a favorable outcome is 1%? 5%? 10%? 20%? How should a favorable outcome be defined?

There are many underlying reasons for potential conflict between patients/surrogates and physicians over futility. Physicians should acknowledge concerns and feelings and provide education in a sensitive manner. Fears of abandonment should be addressed. Emphasizing "aggressive" palliative care is almost always appropriate. Sometimes a **time-limited trial** to see if patients improve before a certain date can give families or patients the necessary time to come to grips with a medically futile situation.

## Palliation and Hospice

Aggressive palliative care and appropriate and informed discussions of hospice referral may prevent some of the problems that spawn requests for PAS and conflicts over futile care.

| Table 2-6 • Medicare/Medicaid Hospice Benefit Eligibility Requirements |
| --- |
| 6 months or less prognosis certified by 2 physicians |
| Patient agreement not to pursue life-sustaining or curative therapies |
| Enroll in Medicare-certified hospice |

There are important issues related to cardiovascular patients and hospice. Despite accurate prognostication models in acute decompensated heart failure, it remains challenging for a physician to predict whether end-stage patients will live beyond 6 months (**Table 2-6**). Differentiating between life-sustaining and palliative therapies can also be difficult (e.g., oral heart failure medications, CRT devices, and destination left ventricular assist devices (LVADs) prolong life <u>and</u> improve symptoms). Inotropes are sometimes very important parts of palliative regimens in heart failure. But they are expensive and may only be covered by larger hospices, since the Medicare hospice benefit consists of a per diem, capitated payment. There should be clear directives concerning devices (e.g., deactivate shock therapy in ICDs while maintaining backup pacemaker function). While end-stage heart failure patients predominantly suffer from dyspnea, a significant percentage report severe pain, severe weakness, anxiety, and depression. An important concept in palliative care is the **principle of double effect**. It is not physician-assisted suicide or euthanasia to administer a medical intervention that relieves suffering, but which also has the unintended consequence of hastening death. The second effect (death) is not the primary goal of the intervention. As in the decision to deactivate implanted devices, optimal palliative care of cardiovascular patients often requires multidisciplinary input from primary care physicians, general and specialized cardiovascular clinicians, and palliative care specialists.

# ORGAN TRANSPLANTATION

Ethics of organ transplantation center on definitions of death and altruism. Medical, philosophical and ethical discussions of the definition of death date back thousands of years. Not until recent legislation codified definitions, such as in the Uniform Death Act, has organ transplantation begun to flourish without fear of legal prosecution for murder. Controversies surrounding definition of death, altruism, and true voluntary consent to donation persist. The issues in transplantation can be divided into deceased donor, living donor, and recipient categories.

## Deceased Donor

Before the invention of mechanical ventilation and other means of life support, irreversible loss of cardiorespiratory function

| Table 2-7 • Criteria for Brain Death |
| --- |
| Presence of coma, with known cause |
| Absence of confounders—including drugs, hypothermia, electrolyte, endocrine disorders |
| No brainstem reflexes |
| No motor responses |
| Apnea |
| *From American Academy of Neurology.* |

was considered the main criterion that death had occurred. But, since the widespread use of life support, and in postcardio-pulmonary resuscitation patients, **brain death criteria (Table 2-7)** have played a more significant role in this regard. There is general consensus that irreversible loss of brainstem function constitutes death, even if external means are able to support vital organs. Irreversible loss of higher cortical function with an intact brain stem constitutes **persistent vegetative state (Table 2-8)** and does not meet most definitions of death.

Most donations come from brain dead individuals, but there has been a return to cardiopulmonary definitions of death in the practice of **donation after cardiac death (DCD)**. Although rare, hearts can be procured in this way. In DCD, life support measures are withdrawn from patients who do not meet brain death criteria, allowing them to die a cardiac death. The patient is taken to the operating room and support is withdrawn. After 2–5 minutes of asystole (depending on the local protocol), the patient is pronounced dead, and the organs are harvested. If the patient does not die within 30–60 minutes (depending on the organ), the procurement is aborted. Heparin is often administered to prevent thrombotic damage to organs, and large-bore catheters are sometimes inserted to infuse organ-preserving solutions after death. These measures generate questions about potential harm to donors (risks of heparin and discomfort of catheters). Protocols prohibit transplant teams from participating in the removal of life support or declaration of death. **Table 2-9** gives an overview of potential donor physiologic function.

Prior authorization to donate organs is becoming an increasingly contentious issue. Many states allow driver's license

| Table 2-8 • Criteria for Vegetative State |
| --- |
| No evidence of awareness of self/environment |
| Inability to interact with others/environment |
| No sustained, reproducible, or purposeful responses to stimuli |
| Preservation of sleep/wake cycle |
| Preserved brainstem and midbrain autonomic functioning |
| Variable response of cranial and spinal reflexes |
| *Guidelines of the U.S. Multi-Society Task Force on Persistent Vegetative State, 1994.* |

holders to state that they wish to be organ donors, but many also allow families to override this decision. Several European countries and a number of states have passed laws related to universal implied consent to donation. Although specifics vary, the general idea is that everyone who dies is assumed to be an organ donor unless otherwise specified. Some legislation authorizes physicians to override advance directives to keep patients alive and organs functional until harvested.

## Living Donor

The living donor highlights a set of ethical concerns that center on coercion and secondary gain. Coercion can exist between blood relatives, loved ones, or even business relations. Transplant centers have developed donor advocacy groups and established that the health care providers for recipient should be different from those of the donor to minimize coercion from the medical establishment. In China, publicity about the sale and use of organs from executed prisoners brought worldwide attention to the wider and more grievous possibilities of coercion.

Transplant tourism and paid organ donation have complicated the concept of altruism, historically the main motivation of transplantation. Many transplant advocates and ethicists see paid donation as a "win-win" situation for donor and recipient and highlight its great potential to increase the number of organs for transplant while lifting donors out of poverty. A recent study of living donors in the developing world, however, uncovered a significant incidence of coercion and found that few donors actually derived any substantial financial benefit. The World Health Organization states that the donation of organs, tissues, and cells should ideally remain an unpaid practice.

## Recipient

Selection of organ recipient is based largely on medical criteria. However, considerations such as patient compliance, habits such as smoking or alcohol use, use of illicit substances, social support, and finances are considered in the determination of candidacy for organ transplantation. It may be argued that prospective recipients have an ethical duty to care for the organ as a scarce resource, since it might otherwise go to someone else. Along similar lines, transplant programs have an ethical duty to ensure that organs do not go to patients who will not comply with medical regimens. Using social criteria, however, always runs the risk of social bias. The committees deciding who would receive hemodialysis when it was first available tended to discriminate in favor of patients from same socio-economic strata of the committee members. More blatantly, recent well-publicized cases involve physicians helping celebrities and wealthy persons to "jump the line" to receive organs ahead of more medically deserving candidates.

| Table 2-9 • Physiologic Function in Potential Donor States | | | | |
|---|---|---|---|---|
| | "Alive" Patients | Vegetative State | Brain Death | Cardiac Death |
| Heart beating | Yes | Yes | Yes | No |
| Spontaneous breathing | Yes | Yes | Usually assisted | No |
| Vital organ function intact | Yes | Yes | Yes | No |
| Consciousness | Yes | No | No | No |

## PROFESSIONALISM

Principles for behavior for medical professionals are based on the idea that medicine is set apart from other professions in several ways: There exists an inherent power differential between physicians and patients, which physicians are obligated not to exploit for personal gain; physicians are endowed with a significant amount of trust by society; there is a **social contract** between physicians and society, by which physicians are given a degree of autonomy by which they govern themselves; and physicians receive generally high salaries and a certain measure of prestige in exchange for acting in accordance with professional standards. The text box lists one set of professional standards (**Table 2-10**). Other sets of standards explicitly describe a physician's commitment to put the needs of the patient above his or her own.

**Fraud** is inconsistent with professional behavior and can take many forms, including lying to patients to avoid a lawsuit (e.g., intentionally failing to disclose medical errors), billing for work not performed (e.g., coding for a higher level office visit than justified by the history and physical examination performed), falsely claiming to have supervised a trainee, or misrepresenting a diagnosis in order to justify performing a procedure.

**Patient confidentiality** springs directly from autonomy but also involves nonmaleficence, as disclosure of sensitive health information can have consequences for a patient's employment, insurance status, or social relationships. Patient confidentiality has received special attention since the passage of the Health Insurance Portability and Accountability Act of 1996 (HIPAA). The HIPAA privacy rule safeguards "individually identifiable health information," which includes medical information that might be used to identify patients, along with common identifiers such as name, social security number, birth date, and address. When any information is disclosed, it should be the "minimum necessary" to meet the purposes of the disclosure. Information may be used and disclosed with a patient's authorization, or in a limited number of circumstances (**Table 2-11**). The most common permitted uses of information fall into HIPPA's "Treatment, Payment, and Health Care Operations" category: Treating a patient, determining payment, insurance underwriting, and performing quality improvement are specifically permitted.

## CONFLICTS OF INTEREST

A **conflict of interest (COI)** involves a clash between any two or more competing interests; it does not have to involve financial conflicts. The concern over COI relates to compromise of important and valuable interests, such as the good of the patient, medical objectivity or academic

| Table 2-10 • Charter on Medical Professionalism |
|---|
| Physicians should have a commitment to: |
| • professional competence |
| • honesty with patients |
| • patient confidentiality |
| • maintaining appropriate relations with patients |
| • improving quality of care |
| • improving access to care |
| • a just distribution of finite resources |
| • scientific knowledge |
| • maintaining trust by managing conflicts of interest |
| • professional responsibilities |
| *Charter on Medical Professionalism, Medical Professionalism Project. ABIM Foundation, the ACP–ASIM Foundation, and the European Federation of Internal Medicine. Medical professionalism in the new millennium: a physician charter. Ann Int Med. 2002;136(3):243–246.* |

| Table 2-11 • HIPAA-permitted Categories of Disclosure |
|---|
| 1. To the individual patient |
| 2. Treatment, payment, and health care operations |
| 3. To give the patient the opportunity to agree or object to what is written in the medical records |
| 4. Incident to an otherwise permitted use and disclosure |
| 5. Public interest and benefit activities (legal requirements, authorized public health uses/organizations, situations of abuse and neglect, health oversight activities, judicial or administrative proceedings, law enforcement, funeral directors/coroners, cadaveric organ donation, serious threat to health and safety, essential government functions, workers compensation) |
| 6. Limited data set for the purposes of research, public health or health care operations |
| *Code of Federal Regulation 45 164.502(a)(1).* |

# 3

# Biomarkers in Cardiovascular Disease

KABIR J. SINGH, PAM RAJENDRAN TAUB, AND ALAN S. MAISEL

## ● PRACTICAL POINTS

- Troponin is a sensitive but not specific marker of myocardial injury.

- Elevated troponin with a characteristic rise and fall in the appropriate setting is the current gold standard for the diagnosis of acute myocardial infarction.

- Serial measurements of troponin are essential since in only a minority of patients will the initial value be abnormal.

- In patients with ACS, elevated troponins constitute a marker of 30-day mortality and infarction and identify those who would benefit from an early invasive strategy.

- CK-MB is most useful in the diagnosis of re infarction.

- Myoglobin is the earliest detectable biomarker of myocardial injury and has a high negative predictive value.

- A multimarker strategy may be superior in the early diagnosis, detection of recurrence, and prognosis after myocardial injury.

- BNP and NT proBNP (NP) are increased in volume and pressure overload states and are superior to clinical judgment in the initial evaluation of patients with dyspnea.

- Elevated BNP is not pathognomonic of heart failure. Age, gender, BMI, and renal function can all affect NP levels.

- Low level elevation of CRP is associated with presence of atherosclerotic disease and is an indicator of elevated risk of MI, stroke and death in patients with stable angina, ACS, post CABG, and post PCI.

## INTRODUCTION

Biomarkers—a variety of enzymes, hormones and other biomolecules that can be measured and evaluated as indicators of disease presence and activity—have emerged as essential tools in clinical decision-making, particularly in cardiovascular diseases. They can provide valuable diagnostic and prognostic information above and beyond existing modalities, such as physical exam, radiographic data, and routine laboratory studies. In some cases, they have even proven superior to the clinical judgments formed in their absence. Some biomarkers are intimately involved in the disease process itself, and thereby can provide insight into pathogenesis, offer new treatment targets, and guide the use of potent medications.

For each biomarker, multiple unique factors affect their serum or plasma concentration, and multiple biologic processes, both normal and pathologic, may lead to their elevation. As such, proper interpretation of a biomarker level requires a comprehensive understanding of the many complex factors that govern their levels.

# BIOMARKERS OF MYOCARDIAL NECROSIS

The biomarkers of myocardial necrosis include troponin I and T, creatinine kinase (CK) and its myocardium-specific isoenzyme creatine kinase-muscle and brain (CK-MB), and myoglobin. Elevated concentrations of these biomarkers have become the cornerstone of diagnosis in acute coronary syndrome (ACS), offering powerful prognostic information and guiding treatment in many critical scenarios. Each of these markers has unique physiology, metabolism, strengths, and limitations. In light of their differences, concurrent measurement of these biomarkers and a multimarker strategy is currently optimal in the management of patients with ACS.

## Troponin I and T

### Physiology

The troponins (Tn) along with tropomyosin form the thin filament component of the contractile apparatus of striated muscle. Three troponin subtypes, TnT, TnI, and TnC, each serve a unique function in facilitating the interaction between actin and myosin, including $Ca^{2+}$ binding (TnC), inhibition (TnI), and tropomysin binding (TnT). Cardiac-specific isoforms of TnT and TnI are released in myocardial necrosis, rendering these proteins both highly sensitive and specific tools in the detection of cardiac injury. Elevated levels of these biomarkers are now considered the gold standard in diagnosis of myocardial infarction.

Troponin elevations above upper reference ranges are typically detectable 4-6 hours after injury, though with modern high-sensitivity assays, elevations can be detected as early as 2-3 hours after the onset of symptoms (**Figure 3-1**). Levels peak within 24 hours, though this time course may be shorter with successful reperfusion. Troponin is cleared by the kidney and levels remain elevated for 10-14 days after myocardial injury, allowing for diagnosis even in cases of delayed presentation (**Figure 3-2**).

| | Timing after onset of chest pain | | | Strengths | Weaknesses |
|---|---|---|---|---|---|
| | Initial elevation | Peak | Duration | | |
| Troponin I & T | 6 hours | 24 hours | 10–14 days | 1. High sensitivity and specificity<br>2. Gold standard for diagnosis of MI<br>3. Most important prognosticator<br>4. Guides adjunctive treatment | 1. Delay in elevation<br>2. Long half decreases utility of serial monitoring once diagnosis of MI is made<br>3. May be chronically elevated in cerain cinditions i.e CKD, and heart failure |
| CK/CKMB | 4–6 hours | 18–24 hours | 36–48 hours | 1. Useful in the diagnosis of reinfarction and reperfusion | 1. Detectable around the same time as troponin, but inferior in terms of sensitivity & specificity<br>2. May be elevated in muscle injury |
| Myoglobin | 1 hour | 6 hours | 24 hours | 1. High negative predictive value.<br>2. Useful in the diagnosis of reinfarcation and reperfusion | 1. Non-specific marker.<br>2. Undulating pattern of release makes trends difficult to interpret |

**Figure 3-1.** Kinetics, strengths and weakness of the biomarkers of myocardial necrosis.

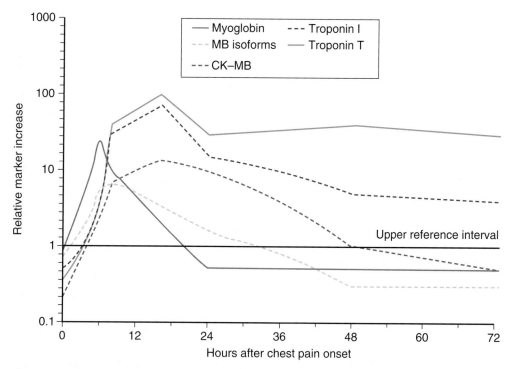

**Figure 3-2.** Time course after symptom onset for various biochemical markers of myocardial necrosis. *Abbreviation:* CK-MB, creatine kinase-MB isoenzyme. (From Newby LK. Markers of cardiac ischemia, injury, and inflammation. *Prog Cardiovasc Dis.* 2004 Mar-Apr;46(5):404–416.)

## Diagnosis of Acute Myocardial Infarction (MI)

In 2000, a consensus group between the European Society of Cardiology (ESC) and American College of Cardiology (ACC) provided recommendations that redefined the diagnosis of myocardial infarction, making an elevated troponin the cornerstone of diagnosis. A rise and fall in troponin above the diagnostic cutpoint in the setting of clinical symptoms (chest pain, shortness of breath, etc.), pathologic electrocardiograph (ECG) changes, or imaging evidence of ischemia fulfill ESC/ACC criteria for acute MI. In order to optimize sensitivity, the 99th percentile of an asymptomatic reference control population is typically used as the diagnostic cutoff for an elevated troponin, and recommended serial measurements beginning at presentation followed by measurements at 6 to 9 hours, and again at 12 to 24 hours if earlier markers are negative and clinical suspicion remains high. Based on these recommendations, serial markers 6 hours apart after onset of chest pain have become a typical protocol in many emergency rooms and coronary care units. This strategy is validated by data from the Global Use of Strategies to Open occluded coronary arteries (GUSTO) IIa study, in which serial assays provided incremental diagnostic and prognostic information. In that study, only 45% of patients with an elevated troponin on serial examination had a troponin elevation on initial presentation. Further, patients with negative troponin on serial testing had a 0% 30-day mortality. Using newer assays with higher sensitivity

and lower cutoff values, recent evidence suggests that up to 80% of patients with acute MI will have a positive troponin within 2-3 hours from the onset of symptoms. However, these assays remain in the research stage and have not yet been incorporated into the recommended diagnostic protocol. In patients with chronically elevated troponin, such as those with end-stage renal disease (ESRD) or structural heart disease, the presence of a rising pattern over time may be necessary for diagnosis.

## Risk Stratification in Acute MI

Elevated troponin levels risk-stratify patient presenting with ACS. Multiple studies have demonstrated that patients presenting with an ACS and found to have an elevated troponin are at greater risk of short-term cardiac events and death (**Figure 3-3**), and that this risk is proportional to the degree of troponin elevation at presentation (**Figure 3-4**). In one meta-analysis, surveying 21 studies with a total of 18,982 patients with ACS, an elevated troponin was associated with an increased risk of 30-day mortality or MI (odds ratio 2.86, 95% confidence interval [CI] 2.35-3.47). This association was even more robust in patients presenting with ST-elevation MI (odds ratio 4.93, 95% CI 3.77- 6.45). Initially, the value of troponin in risk stratification of patients with renal dysfunction was in doubt based on troponin's renal clearance. However, in a subset analysis of the GUSTO-IV trial, troponin elevation remained predictive of short-term

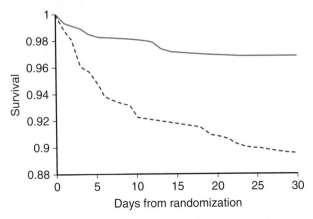

**Figure 3-3.** Kaplan–Meier estimates of survival during first 30 days for baseline cTnT-positive (dashed line) and -negative (solid line) patients. Troponin-positive patients have a worse prognosis. (From Newby LK, et. Al. Value of serial troponin T measures for early and late risk stratification in patients with acute coronary syndromes. *Circulation.* 1998;98:1853–1859.)

MI and death, regardless of creatinine clearance, thereby validating its use in patients with renal failure.

### Management of Acute MI

Elevated troponin helps identify those patients who will benefit from use of particular therapeutics and thereby guides management in ACS. The Fragmin during Instability in Coronary Artery Disease (FRISC) trial and a substudy of the Thrombolysis in Myocardial Infarction (TIMI) 11b study demonstrated that among patients with non-ST-elevation ACS, use of a low molecular-weight heparin (LMWH) therapy in those with elevated troponin resulted in significantly lower rates of short-term MI and mortality. Patients without troponin elevations did not benefit

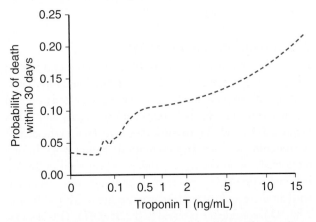

**Figure 3-4.** Mortality within 30 Days According to the Baseline Troponin T Level in patients presenting with symptoms and ECG changes of acute ischemia. The degree of troponin elevation at baseline correlates with prognosis. (From Ohman EM, et al. Cardiac troponin T levels for risk stratification in acute myocardial ischemia. *N Engl J Med.* 1996;335:1333–1342. Copyright © [year of publication] Massachusetts Medical Society. All rights reserved.)

from LMWH. Studies of glycoprotein IIb/IIIa inhibitors have had similar results (**Figure 3-5**). The Chimeric 7E3 Antiplatelet Therapy in Unstable Angina Refractory to Standard Treatment (CAPTURE), Platelet-Receptor Inhibition for Ischemic Syndrome Management (PRISM), and Delaying and Preventing Ischemic Evens in Patients with Acute Coronary Syndromes Using the Platelet GP IIb/IIIa Inhibitor Lamifban (PARAGON B) studies demonstrated that among patients with an ACS, only those with elevated troponins benefit from use of LMWH with reduced short-term rates of recurrent MI or death.

Troponin-elevation may be used to guide the decision to pursue an early-invasive catheterization strategy in ACS patients. In the Treat Angina with Aggrastat and Determine Cost of Therapy with an Invasive or Conservative Strategy (TACTICS)–TIMI 18 trial, patients with ACS and an elevated baseline troponin T > 0.1 ng/mL were found to be at increased risk for recurrent ischemia and mortality at 30 days and 6 months post-event as compared to those without a troponin elevation. Among patients with a troponin elevation, those randomized to receive an early invasive strategy had a reduced event rate. In fact, patients who had a troponin elevation and underwent early intervention faced near-equivalent risk for recurrent MI and death as those who did not have an initial elevation troponin. No treatment benefit was observed in patients without a troponin elevation at presentation. The Fragmin and Fast Revascularization During Instability in Coronary Artery Disease (FRISC II) study had similar findings, demonstrating decreased incidence of recurrent ischemia and death at 1 year in troponin T-positive patients who underwent an early-invasive strategy, while those with a negative troponin did not benefit from this therapy (**Figure 3-5**).

### Differential Diagnosis of Elevated Troponin

Proper interpretation of an elevated troponin requires recognition that it is a biomarker of myocardial injury, which has many etiologies aside from ischemia. Therefore, an elevated level must always be interpreted in the clinical context with respect to this principle (**Table 3-1**).

## Creatinine Kinase and CK-MB

Creatinine kinase (CK) facilitates the transport of high-energy phosphates across the mitochondrial membrane in multiple cell types including striated muscle. Different isoenzymes of CK have been identified and are distinguished by their constituent protein subunits. Though CK is present in both skeletal and cardiac muscle, the CK-MB isoform is found in highest concentrations in myocardium and thereby has improved specificity for myocardial necrosis. However, CK-MB still constitutes 1-3% of CK in skeletal muscle. Further, in response to skeletal muscle damage or chronic inflammation, there can be re-expression of proteins synthesized during

## A. Cardiac Troponin I (cTnI)

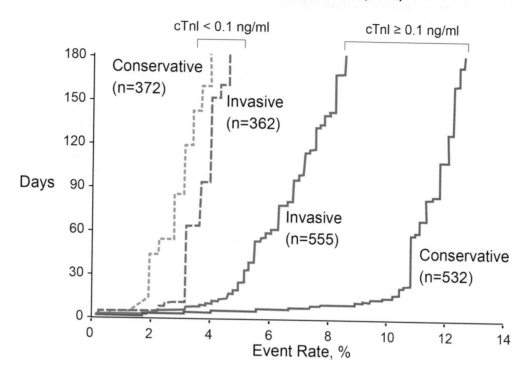

## B. Cardiac Troponin I (cTnT)

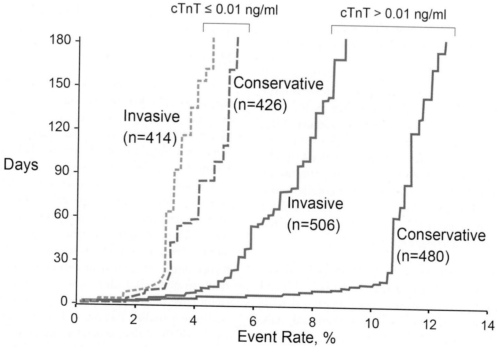

**Figure 3-5.** Probability of Death or MI in ACS Patients Through 6 Months of Follow-up, Stratified by Treatment Strategy. Only patients with an elevated troponin benefited from an early-invasive treatment strategy.

## Table 3-1 • Nonthrombotic Causes of an Elevated Troponin Level

**Nonthrombotic myocardial ischemia**
 Coronary vasospasm
 Intracranial hemorrhage or stroke
 Ingestion of sympathomimetic agents

**Direct myocardial damage**
 Cardiac contusion
 Direct current cardioversion
 Cardiac infiltrative disorders
 Chemotherapy
 Myocarditis
 Pericarditis
 Cardiac transplanation

**Demand ischemia**
 Sepsis/systemic inflammatory response syndrome
 Hypotension
 Hypovolemia
 Supraventricular tachycardia/atrial fibrillation
 Left ventricular hypertrophy

**Myocardial strain**
 Congestive heart failure
 Pulmonary embolism
 Pulmonary hypertension or obstructive disease
 Strenuous exercise

**Chronic kidney disease**

*Adapted from Jeremias A, Gibson CM. Narrative review: alternative causes for elevated cardiac troponin levels when acute coronary syndromes are excluded. Ann Intern Med. 2005, May 3; 142(9):786–791.*

ontogeny including the MB isoform, thereby limiting its specificity particularly when cardiac and skeletal injury coexist.

CK and CK-MB begins to rise as early as 4-6 hours after myocardial injury, though levels may not be elevated until as long as 12 hours. These levels peak within 18-24 hours, and return to baseline within 36-48 hours (**Figure 3-2**). Prior to the routine use of troponin, CK-MB was the biomarker of choice in the diagnosis of acute MI. A rise in CK to twice the maximum of normal range with a concurrent increase in CK-MB fulfills typical diagnostic criteria. Some have suggested utilizing a ratio of CK-MB to CK to improve specificity, but this approach has not been well evaluated and is not part of formal diagnostic criteria.

Still, it is notable that patients with an elevated CK-MB but a normal CK have been shown to be more at risk for MI and mortality. In a meta-analysis of the 25,960 patients with non-ST elevation MI examined in four large-scale clinical trials, patients with an elevated CK-MB were at increased risk. In that analysis an elevated CK-MB was defined as above the upper limit of normal as determined by each participating sites clinical laboratory. Patients with a CK within normal range but elevated CK-MB, carried an increased relative risk of 55% for 180-day death or recurrent MI.

CK and CK-MB find additional utility in the detection of successful reperfusion after thrombolysis and in the diagnosis of reinfarction. After successful reperfusion, the rate of CK release from myocardium transiently increases, likely a result of improved blood flow to damaged myocardium and "washout" of released CK and CK-MB. This phenomenon leads to higher and earlier peak values. A time to peak CK of less than 4 hours indicates successful reperfusion with achievement of TIMI 2- or 3-grade flow. Another model using the ratio of CK-MB one hour after thrombolysis and baseline CK-MB demonstrated that a ratio greater than 3.3 was predictive of TIMI 2 or 3 flow, with sensitivity and specificity of 70% and 63%, respectively. Other models utilize the slope of CK-MB rise with additional clinical variables to improve predictive capability. Importantly though, models using CK or CK-MB have not been shown to be predictive of TIMI-3 flow alone, which is the only level of reperfusion associated with improved survival after thrombolysis.

In regards to reinfarction, the short half-life of CK and CK-MB and their relatively quick release into serum allow these markers to be useful in diagnosis. Similarly, a decline in CK or CK-MB even in the face of continually rising troponin still suggests completion of an infarct. The 2004 ACC/AHA task force made specific recommendations for diagnosis of reinfarction after acute ST-elevation MI using CK-MB. Within the first 18 hours post-infarct, symptoms of ischemia along with a recurrent elevation in CK-MB to above three times the upper limit of normal range or 50% greater than the previous value meets criteria.

## Myoglobin

Myoglobin is a ubiquitous heme protein that is present in cardiac muscle. It is released rapidly from damaged tissue, and with existing assays it can potentially be the earliest detectable biomarker of cardiac injury. Concentrations in serum may begin to rise as soon as 1 hour after myocardial injury. They peak within 6 hours, and return to baseline within about 24 hours. However, as myoglobin is present in high concentration in multiple other tissues and abundantly in skeletal muscle, elevations are not specific to cardiac injury and limit its utility. Further, owing to its rapid release and metabolism (half-life in serum of 8-10 minutes), serial myoglobin levels may demonstrate an undulating pattern that can prove difficult to interpret. Assessments of sensitivity have ranged widely, varying between 60 and 100% in different studies. Its principal utility is found in its negative predictive value, which has been found to be as high as 97.4%. Myoglobin also provides prognostic data independent of that provided by other biomarkers. In an analysis of data collected in TIMI 11B and TACTICS-TIMI 18, myoglobin elevations >100 mg/L, independent of other markers of cardiac damage or ST-changes, have been found to be prognostic in patients with ACS, predicting the presence of an occluded culprit artery, visible thrombus, and absence of TIMI-3 flow. Further, myoglobin elevations are associated with increased mortality 6 months post-event.

## Multimarker Strategy in ACS

Given the complex interaction between the timing of patient presentation to the emergency department for evaluation of ischemic symptoms and the varying timing of release, metabolism, sensitivity, and specificity of the biomarkers of myocardial necrosis, a multimarker strategy combining early-appearing markers with high negative predictive value with more specific but late-appearing markers provides a better evaluation tool than any individual biomarker alone. This approach was validated in the Chest Pain Evaluation by CK-MB, Myoglobin and Troponin I (CHECKMATE) study, in which 1005 patients with chest pain were evaluated with a panel of markers including myoglobin, CK-MB, and troponin. This multimarker strategy detected more marker-positive patients and did so earlier in the evaluation process. Similarly, another study found that the sensitivity and negative predictive value for point-of-care combination of myoglobin and troponin I was 96.9% and 99.6%, respectively, within 90 minutes of presentation. This was superior to the results provided by either marker individually. Further, once the diagnosis of MI is made with a positive troponin, CK-MB and myoglobin with their shorter half-lives become the superior markers for monitoring the evolution and termination of an infarct, as well as monitoring for recurrent ischemia. Thus, the information provided by individual markers is synergistic and complementary in the evaluation of patients with ischemic symptoms and in subsequent monitoring for resolution of MI and reinfarction.

# BIOMARKERS OF CARDIOVASCULAR STRESS

Biomarkers of cardiovascular stress are released in volume or pressure overload states. They have become valuable tools in the diagnosis, monitoring, and treatment of patients with congestive heart failure. Further, they provide powerful prognostic data not only in acute and chronic heart failure, but in a variety of cardiovascular conditions.

## Natriuretic Peptides: BNP & NT-proBNP

### Physiology

Several natriuretic peptides (NPs) have been identified, all with similar chemical structure and physiologic function. However, currently only B-type natriuretic peptide (BNP) and NT-proBNP are routinely used clinically. BNP is synthesized and secreted primarily from the ventricular myocardium in response to wall stress from volume expansion or pressure overload. NPs serve to counteract the physiologic abnormalities of heart failure by causing vasodilation, natriuresis, and diuresis, thereby exerting protective effect in volume or pressure overload states. The clearance of BNP is thought to be primarily via binding to a membrane-bound natriuretic receptor, with some contribution of active renal secretion and passive excretion as well. NT-proBNP, on the other hand, is thought to be cleared principally by the kidneys (**Figure 3-6**).

### Diagnosis of Acute Dyspnea

The clinical utility of BNP and NT-proBNP is best established in the diagnosis of acute dyspnea. In the Breathing Not Properly Multinational Study, 1587 patients presenting to the emergency department (ED) with acute dyspnea were

| | BNP | NT-proBNP |
|---|---|---|
| **Half-life (minutes)** | 22 | 60–120 |
| **Clearance**<br>**Primary mechanism**<br>**Hemodialysis** | Neutral endopeptidase<br>No | Renal<br>No |
| **Cut point for diagnosing heart failure in acute dyspnea** | 100 pg/mL | 300 pg/mL to "rule out" 900 pg/mL to "rule in" or age-adjusted cutpoints (see text) |
| **Recommended fluctuation for diagnosing acute on chronic HF** | 50–70% increase from baseline | 25% increase from baseline |
| **Correlation with GFR** | Moderate | Strong |
| **Clinical range (pg/mL)** | 0–5000 | 0–35000 |

**Figure 3-6.** Comparison of BNP and NT-proBNP. (Adapted from Daniels LB, Maisel AS. Natriuretic peptides. *J Am Coll Cardiol.* 2007 Dec 18;50(25):2357–2368.)

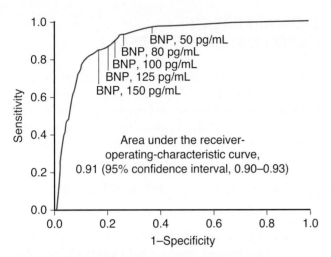

**Figure 3-7.** Receiver-operating characteristic curve for various cutoff levels of B-type natriuretic peptide (BNP) in differentiating between dyspnea due to congestive heart failure and dyspnea due to other causes. (From Maisel AS, et al. Rapid measurement of B-type natriuretic peptide in the emergency diagnosis of heart failure. *N Engl J Med.* 2002;347:161–167. Copyright © [year of publication] Massachusetts Medical Society. All rights reserved.)

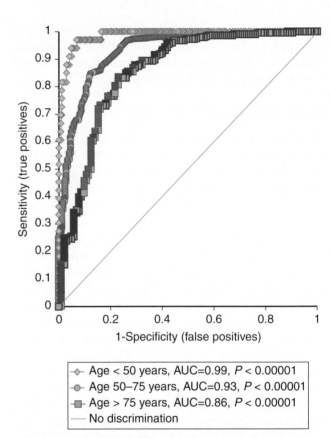

**Figure 3-8.** ROC curves for NT-proBNP-based diagnosis of acute HF across three age groups. NT-proBNP had high AUC in each age group. (From Maisel AS, et al. Rapid measurement of B-type natriuretic peptide in the emergency diagnosis of heart failure. *N Engl J Med.* 2002;347:161–167. Copyright © [year of publication] Massachusetts Medical Society. All rights reserved.)

evaluated by an ED physician and bedside BNP assay. BNP on arrival was shown to be superior to clinical judgment in the diagnosis of acute heart failure, with an area under the receiver-operator curve (AUC) of 0.91 (**Figure 3-7**). A BNP of 100 pg/mL was 90% sensitive and 76% specific in diagnosing dyspnea due to acute heart failure. Studies of the physiologic variability of BNP levels in stable heart failure patients suggest that an increase in BNP by about 50-70% from baseline or "dry" BNP accompanied with symptoms is most useful in the in the diagnosis of HF exacerbation in known chronic HF.

The strongest evidence for utility of NT-proBNP is provided by the ProBNP Investigation of Dyspnea in the Emergency Department (PRIDE) and International Collaborative of NT-proBNP (ICON) studies. In the PRIDE study, NT-proBNP levels measured on arrival in 599 patients presenting with acute dyspnea was found to be superior to clinical judgment, with an AUC of 0.94. Rather than a single cutpoint as identified for utilization of BNP, the PRIDE investigators found a dual cutpoint strategy optimal in the interpretation of NT-proBNP levels. A cutpoint of 300 ng/L had a 99% negative predictive value in excluding a diagnosis of acute HF. A cutpoint of 900 ng/L for NT-proBNP was found to be comparable to the BNP cutpoint of 100 pg/mL with a positive predictive value of 79%. The ICON study examined 1256 patients and was designed to evaluate the need for age-dependent cutoffs for optimal utilization of NT-proBNP. That analysis verified the findings of PRIDE, and demonstrated value of an age-adjusted cutpoint strategy. Using cutpoints of 450 ng/L, 900 ng/L, and 1800 ng/L for ages less than 50, 50 to 75, and greater than 75,

respectively, improved the positive predictive value to 88% (**Figure 3-8**). In patients with prior history of HF, an increase of greater than 25% over baseline "dry" NT-proBNP is recommended for diagnosis of acute exacerbation.

### Prognosis in Heart Failure

Several studies have shown that NP levels predict outcomes in both acute and chronic heart failure. A systematic review of studies assessing BNP for prognosis in patients with heart failure or asymptomatic patients found that each 100 pg/mL increase in BNP was associated with a 35% in the relative risk of death. In the prospective Rapid ED Heart Failure Outpatient Trial (REDHOT), patients presenting to the ED with acute shortness of breath and found to have a BNP > 200 mg/mL had a higher rate of CHF-related events and mortality (9% vs. 29% p = 0.006). In chronic heart failure, BNP also provides powerful prognostic information. In data collected in the Valsartan Heart Failure Trial (Val-HeFT), in which 4300 patients were followed for 3 years following a measurement of baseline BNP, patients with an initial BNP greater than the median value of 97 pg/mL were at higher risk (RR 2.1, 95% CI 1.79-2.42) for morality and first morbid event. Further, BNP showed a significant, quartile-depending increase in mortality and first morbid event.

## Monitoring Therapy in Heart Failure

As the natriuretic peptides have been shown to correlate with clinical status including heart failure stage and offer prognostic information in heart failure patients, some have hypothesized that they may be useful in guiding treatment. Evidence in support of this approach comes in a study in which 72 patients admitted for exacerbation of HF were monitored with daily BNP assessments and followed for events. Patients found to have a fall in BNP levels were less likely to have a subsequent readmission or cardiac death within the 30-day follow-up period. Further, BNP levels at discharge have been shown to predict recurrent events. In that particular study, a BNP < 430 pg/mL had a strong negative predictive value for recurrent hospitalization. Another study demonstrated that predischarge BNP was the most powerful predictor of readmission for CHF and mortality at 6 months, with a discharge BNP 350 pg/mL suggesting good prognosis. In light of these findings, some have suggested that in the treatment of acute heart failure exacerbation BNP assessment at admission, shortly thereafter to ensure response to treatment, and just prior to discharge can guide treatment and optimize follow-up planning. The optimal utilization of NPs in the management of acute and chronic heart failure remains under investigation.

## Other Applications of NPs

Evolving data indicate that NP levels carry substantial prognostic information in a variety of acute and chronic cardiovascular disease aside from heart failure. Elevations in both BNP and NT-proBNP predict increased risk of cardiovascular events in patients across the spectrum of coronary artery disease, including stable angina and ACS. NPs have been shown to predict sudden cardiac death and predict response to cardiac resynchronization therapy in CHF patients. In aortic stenosis, NP levels rise with the severity of disease, predict symptom onset, and may predict surgical outcomes. How the additional information provided by NPs in these clinical scenarios will guide clinical decision-making remains an evolving area of research.

## Differential Diagnosis of Elevated NPs

In the interpretation of elevated natriuretic peptide levels, it is essential one keep in mind these levels are not pathognomonic for heart failure. BNP is secreted in response to multiple conditions that result in increased ventricular wall stress. Common acute causes, particularly pertinent to the differential diagnosis of breathlessness, include chronic but stable heart failure, valvular heart disease including aortic stenosis and regurgitation, acute coronary syndromes, pulmonary diseases including chronic obstructive disease, primary and secondary pulmonary hypertension, pulmonary

| Table 3-2 • Differential Diagnosis of Elevations in Natriuretic Peptides |
|---|
| Acute and chronic heart failure |
| Acute coronary syndromes |
| Valvular disease<br>    Aortic stenosis<br>    Mitral stenosis |
| Atrial fibrillation |
| Myocardial diseases<br>    Hypertrophic cardiomyopathy<br>    Infiltrative cardiomyopathies<br>    Apical ballooning syndrome<br>    Inflammatory disease, including myocarditis and<br>        chemotherapy |
| High-output sates:<br>    Sepsis<br>    Burns<br>    Hyperthyroidism<br>    Cirrhosis |
| Pulmonary heart disease/right heart dysfunction<br>    Pulmonary embolism<br>    Pulmonary hypertension<br>    Obstructive sleep apnea |
| Primary pulmonary disease<br>    COPD<br>    Asthma<br>    ARDS |
| Congenital heart disease |
| Stroke |

embolism, and atrial fibrillation. Several analyses from the Breathing Not Properly study have suggested that patients with these diagnoses do not have as marked elevations in their BNP levels (less than 500 pg/mL) as those with acute HF. Still, appreciation of the broad differential of an elevated NP level is critical to proper interpretation (**Table 3-2**).

## Other Factors Affecting NP levels

Factors aside from these pathologic conditions also affect baseline NP levels, though there effects are often more subtle (**Table 3-3**). Advanced age is associated with higher levels of BNP and NT-proBNP. The cause of this is unclear but may be related to evolving diastolic dysfunction or reduced metabolism and clearance. Female gender is also associated

| Table 3-3 • Factors Influencing Baseline NP Levels |
|---|
| **Factors increasing baseline NPs** |
| Advancing age<br>Female gender<br>Chronic kidney disease |
| **Factors decreasing baseline NP** |
| Obesity |

with higher NP levels, possibly as a consequence of higher levels of estrogen.

Renal dysfunction is an important and frequent confounder in the patients with elevated NPs, though the underlying mechanisms of this interaction are unclear. Patients with chronic kidney disease often have higher atrial and systemic blood pressure, and consequent increases in ventricular mass, all of which could contribute to higher NP levels as an appropriate compensatory mechanism. However, these patients may also have decreased renal filtration and decreased clearance by NP-receptors and end peptidases within renal tissue. Several studies have demonstrated that BNP levels increase with estimated glomerular filtration rate below 60 mL/min/1.7 m$^2$. Data from these trials suggest that higher cutpoints are not unreasonable for patients with renal function below this threshold. An exact cutpoint has not been well defined for BNP. Data from the PRIDE study indicate that the optimal cutpoint for NT-proBNP in renal dysfunction is 1200 ng/L. However, when using the age-stratified cutpoints, one need not make further adjustment aside from that for the unusually young patients with poor renal function.

Obesity, on the other hand, has been associated with decreased BNP and NTpro-BNP levels, likely due to increased clearance by NP receptors on adipocytes. Still, BNP likely has equivalent diagnostic value in this group of patients, albeit with lower cutpoints. A subgroup analysis of data from the Breathing Not Properly study demonstrated that, with lower cutpoint values determined by BMI, BNP retained both sensitivity and specificity in diagnosis of acute HF. Similarly, an analysis of data obtained in the ICON study showed that NT-proBNP concentration is lower in patients with higher BMI, but it retains its diagnostic and prognostic capacity across all BMI categories.

## BIOMARKERS OF INFLAMMATION

Atherosclerosis is now well recognized as a disease of inflammation. Biomarkers assessing inflammation may be markers of disease process and, in some cases, have been implicated in pathogenesis. As the information provided by these markers becomes better understood, the markers may offer new therapeutic targets for patients with cardiovascular disease.

### C-Reactive Protein (CRP)

CRP is an acute phase protein produced largely by hepatocytes in response to inflammatory cytokines. It is a nonspecific marker of inflammation that is synthesized most abundantly in acute infectious or inflammatory processes.

Despite this lack of specificity, multiple studies have demonstrated that low-level elevations of CRP are associated with the presence of atherosclerotic disease and predict cardiovascular events. Further, CRP may be an independent predictor, making it a potential tool to identify patients without traditional risk factors that remain at-risk for cardiovascular disease.

CRP has demonstrated predictive value in a broad spectrum of cardiovascular disease. Data from the Prevention of Events with Angiotensin-Converting Enzyme Inhibition (PEACE) trial showed prospectively that, in patients with stable coronary artery disease, those with CRP > 1.0 mg/L were at increased risk of MI, stroke, and cardiovascular disease, independent of more established risk factors. Elevated CRP has been demonstrated to be prognostic in patients with non-ST-elevation ACS and ST-elevation MI, predicting short-term mortality and recurrent ischemic events. Smaller studies have demonstrated predictive capability in many other clinical scenarios, including heart failure and patient's post-coronary artery bypass grafting or post-percutaneous intervention. Perhaps most importantly, in patients without prior cardiovascular disease, CRP is associated with increased risk.

Elevations in CRP are associated with many recognized cardiovascular disease risk factors, including hypertension, smoking, age, diabetes, and HDL levels, an observation that raises doubt that CRP can provide additional information over existing tools. Multiple studies have examined this issue and provide conflicting results.

Several existing therapies for cardiovascular disease such as aspirin and statins also have anti-inflammatory effect and reduce CRP. Further, there is evidence that the anti-inflammatory effects contribute to the benefit of these medications. In the Pravastatin or Atorvastatin Evaluation and Infection Therapy (PROVE-IT) study, independent of cholesterol reduction on statin therapy, those with lower CRP levels had better outcomes than those with higher levels (**Figure 3-9**). Furthermore, in the Cholesterol and Recurrent Events (CARE) trial, patients with a higher baseline CRP prior to initiation of statin therapy experienced greater reduction in recurrent events. Studies that will prospectively evaluate the efficacy of targeting treatment towards reducing CRP in patients with normal LDL levels are ongoing.

Based on these and other data, the Center for Disease Control (CDC) and American Heart Association (AHA) issued guidelines regarding the use of serum CRP in determining cardiovascular risk in 2003. CRP should be measured twice, two weeks apart, with the values averaged. Low, intermediate, and high risk values were defined as <1 mg/L, 1-3 mg/L, and >3 mg/L, respectively. A level greater than

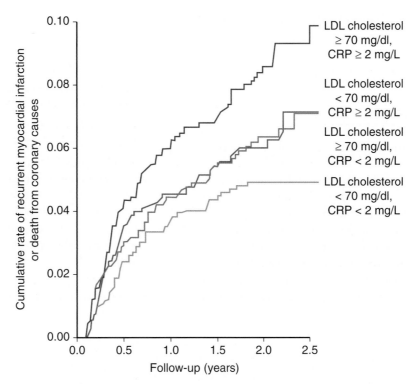

**Figure 3-9.** Cumulative incidence of recurrent myocardial infarction or death from coronary causes, According to the achieved levels of both LDL cholesterol and CRP. (From Ridker PM, et al. C-reactive protein levels and outcomes after statin therapy. *N Engl J Med.* 2005;52:20–28. Copyright © [year of publication] Massachusetts Medical Society. All rights reserved.)

10 mg/L should be repeated and the patient should be evaluated for an acute infectious or inflammatory process. In patients with intermediate risk for cardiovascular disease by Framingham risk score (10-20% at 10 years), an elevated CRP may, at the discretion of the treating physician, be treated as an additional risk factor when determining therapeutic targets for primary prevention such as blood pressure and LDL goals.

## SELECTED EMERGING BIOMARKERS

### Biomarkers of Oxidative Stress

Oxidative stress is thought to be a potential link between cardiovascular risk factors and inflammation in the development of cardiovascular disease. Powerful oxidants are routinely produced by endogenous enzymes such as MPO, and these agents play important roles in inflammatory processes and defense against infection. However, excessive oxidative stress results in modification of various fatty acids, lipoproteins, and amino acids into proinflammatory and atherogenic particles. Further, oxidative stress may directly damage cellular proteins and cause myocyte apoptosis. MPO is a heme enzyme present in the granules of inflammatory cells, and is released in response to infectious and inflammatory stimuli. MPO has been detected within

atherosclerotic lesions, and MPO mass has been shown to have independent predictive value in predicting the presence of angiographically defined coronary artery disease and cardiovascular events.

### Biomarkers of Ischemia

Biomarkers that reliably detect myocardial ischemia in the absence of necrosis would be extremely useful, particularly in the identification of patients with unstable angina and in differentiating patients with chest pain due to causes aside from cardiac ischemia. Further, if ischemia could be detected prior to myocardial necrosis, it may be possible to intervene earlier and prevent myocardial damage. Several such markers of ischemia are under investigation and include unbound free fatty acids (FFAu), heart-type fatty acid-binding protein, and ischemia-modified albumin (IMA). Ischemia is also associated with the release of free fatty acids (FFA) from muscle tissue. The majority of these fatty acids are bound to albumin, however, a fraction of unbound free fatty acids (FFAu) may be measured. In post-percutaneous coronary angioplasty (PCTA) patients, post-PCTA concentrations of FFAu were found to be several fold higher than baseline level, and the highest FFAu concentrations were observed in patients who exhibited periprocedural ST-elevations. Further, FFAu elevations are associated with additional risk of ventricular dysrhythmia and death in patients with acute

MI. Although far from definitive, current evidence suggests that, amongst patients presenting with symptoms of ischemia, FFAu levels may provide early evidence of ischemia prior to myocardial necrosis.

## CONCLUSION

Biomarkers have proven themselves invaluable tools in modern cardiovascular medicine. However, they are currently best validated in the diagnosis and management of myocardial necrosis, pressure overload, and remodeling—cardiovascular disease in its endgame. As recently identified biomarkers are better understood and new biomarkers are discovered, it will very likely be possible to detect cardiovascular disease in earlier, preclinical stages. As this incredible potential of biomarkers is realized, physicians will be increasingly better equipped to prevent the progression and consequent morbidity and mortality of cardiovascular diseases.

## Suggested Readings

1. Newby LK. Markers of cardiac ischemia, injury, and inflammation. *Prog Cardio Dis.* 2004;46:404–416.

2. Daniels LB, Maisel AS. Natriuretic peptides. *J Amer Coll Cardiol.* 2007;50:2357–2368.

3. Januzzi JL, Chen-Tournaoux AA, Moe G. Amino-terminal pro-B-type natriuretic peptide testing for the diagnosis or exclusion of heart failure in patients with acute symptoms. *Amer J of Cardiol.* 2008;101[suppl]:29A–38A.

4. de Ferranti SD, Rifai N. C-reactive protein: a nontraditional serum marker of cardiovascular risk. *Cardiovasc Pathol.* 2007;16:14–21.

5. Morrow DA, de Lemos JA. Benchmarks for the assessment of cardiovascular biomarkers. *Circulation.* 2007;115:949–952.

# 4

# Heart Disease in the Elderly

MICHAEL W. RICH

## ● PRACTICAL POINTS

- Cardiovascular reserve is decreased with aging due to increased vascular stiffness, impaired LV diastolic function, decreased beta-receptor responsiveness, endothelial dysfunction, and other factors.

- Systolic hypertension is the strongest risk factor for cardiovascular events in patients over the age of 65 years.

- Atypical presentation of ACS is common, resulting in delayed diagnosis and worse prognosis.

- Physical signs of aortic stenosis may be masked in the elderly.

- Percutaneous aortic valve replacement is an exciting new development particularly suitable for the older patient.

- HF is the leading cause of hospitalization in the elderly.

- Atypical presentation of HF is common and hence the diagnosis is more challenging.

- BNP less specific due to elevated levels with age.

- Treatment is more challenging because of increased incidence of concomitant renal and hepatic dysfunction and polypharmacy resulting in adverse drug reactions.

- Prevalence of atrial fibrillation is approximately 10% in octogenarians. The elderly have significantly increased risk of stroke as well as bleeding with anticoagulation though the benefits of warfarin generally outweigh the risks.

## EPIDEMIOLOGY

The prevalence of cardiovascular disease increases progressively with age (**Figure 4-1**), as a result of which persons 65 years of age or older account for more than 60% of hospitalizations for cardiovascular disease, including over 60% of admissions for acute myocardial infarction (MI) and over 75% of admissions for decompensated heart failure. In addition, over 50% of percutaneous and surgical coronary revascularization procedures, 55% of defibrillator implantations, 80% of arterial endarterectomies, and 85% of permanent pacemaker insertions occur in this age group. Importantly, with increasing age women comprise a progressively greater proportion of patients hospitalized with cardiovascular disorders as well as patients undergoing cardiovascular procedures.

## EFFECTS OF AGING ON THE CARDIOVASCULAR SYSTEM

The principal effects of aging on the cardiovascular system are summarized in **Table 4-1**.[1] The net effect of these changes is a marked reduction in cardiovascular reserve. As a result, increasing age is associated with an inexorable decline in maximum exercise capacity in healthy individuals (**Figure 4-2**). Older patients are also less able to maintain cardiac performance in response to a wide range of stressors, including ischemia, brady- and tachyarrhythmias, infections (e.g., pneumonia, sepsis), anemia, and metabolic disorders (e.g., thyroid disease). In turn, the impaired capacity to respond to stress accounts for the exponential increase in the incidence of heart failure with advancing age, as well as the markedly worse prognosis associated with acute and chronic cardiovascular disorders in older patients.

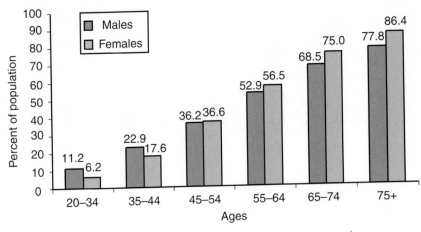

**Figure 4-1.** Prevalence of cardiovascular disease in the U.S. by age and sex. (*Source*: CDC/NCHS and NHLBI. These data include coronary heart disease, heart failure, stroke and hypertension.)

## EFFECTS OF AGING ON OTHER ORGAN SYSTEMS

Age-related alterations in other organ systems also impact the clinical presentation, response to therapy, and prognosis of cardiovascular diseases in elderly patients (**Table 4-2**). Impaired renal function predisposes older patients to electrolyte disturbances and intravascular volume overload, as well as to increased toxicity from renally excreted medications. Similarly, age-related changes in hepatic and gastrointestinal function further increase the risk of adverse drug effects, especially in patients receiving multiple medications. The ability of the central nervous system to maintain cerebral perfusion over a range of arterial blood pressures also declines with age, predisposing older patients to lightheadedness, falls, syncope, and impaired cognition in response to medications, alterations in position, and changes in cardiac output.

## CARDIOVASCULAR RISK FACTORS

As in younger patients, hypertension, dyslipidemia, diabetes mellitus, smoking, and possibly physical inactivity remain the most important modifiable risk factors for the development of cardiovascular disease in the elderly, and current guidelines advocate a generally similar approach to managing these risk factors irrespective of age. However, the combination of age-related cardiovascular changes in conjunction with a tendency to have more risk factors and a longer duration of exposure to these factors results in a greater number of incident cardiovascular events in older compared to younger individuals; i.e., the number of events "attributable" to prevalent risk factors is higher in the elderly.

### Hypertension

Systolic blood pressure tends to increase gradually with age, while diastolic blood pressure peaks in late middle-age

| Table 4-1 • Principal Effects of Aging on the Cardiovascular System |
|---|
| **Rest** |
| Increased arterial stiffness |
| Decreased myocardial relaxation and compliance |
| Impaired responsiveness to beta-adrenergic stimulation |
| Decreased sinus node function |
| Impaired endothelium-dependent vasodilation |
| Decreased baroreceptor responsiveness |
| **Exercise** |
| Progressive decline in maximum heart rate |
| Progressive decline in maximum cardiac output |
| Decreased peak coronary blood flow |
| Decreased peripheral vasodilation |
| **Net effect:** marked reduction in cardiovascular reserve |

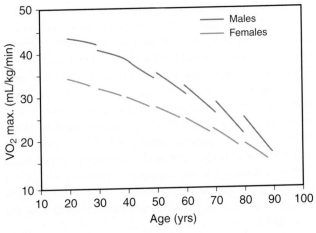

**Figure 4-2.** Age and VO$_2$max in healthy men and women. (*Source*: Circulation 2000;102(Suppl II):II-602.)

| Table 4-2 • Age-related Changes in Other Organ Systems |
|---|
| **Kidneys** |
| Decreased glomerular filtration rate |
| Diminished concentrating and diluting capacity |
| Impaired electrolyte homeostasis |
| **Lungs** |
| Decreased vital capacity |
| Increased ventilation-perfusion mismatching |
| **Central Nervous System** |
| Decreased autoregulatory capacity |
| Altered reflex responsiveness |
| Impaired thirst mechanism |
| **Musculoskeletal System** |
| Osteopenia |
| Sarcopenia |
| **Hematologic System** |
| Altered balance between thrombosis and fibrinolysis |
| **Gastrointestinal System** |
| Altered absorption and elimination of drugs |
| Altered hepatic drug metabolism |

pressure is also the most potent risk factor for cardiac disease and stroke in older individuals. Pulse pressure, a marker for age-related arterial stiffness, increases with age and has been shown to be an independent predictor of cardiovascular disease in some but not all studies.

Several prospective randomized clinical trials have shown that treatment of both systolic and diastolic hypertension is associated with a reduction in cardiovascular events in older patients, including octogenarians (**Table 4-3**).[2] In the recently published Hypertension in the Very Elderly Trial (HYVET), octogenarians with stage II systolic hypertension (systolic blood pressure ≥160 mm Hg) who were randomized to diuretic-based therapy with indapemide experienced a 30% reduction in stroke, 21% decline in total mortality, and 64% lower incidence of heart failure compared with patients randomized to placebo.

In the absence of a compelling indication for a specific antihypertensive drug class, the choice of a first-line agent for treatment of hypertension in the elderly remains controversial. In the ALLHAT trial, the diuretic chlorthalidone was at least as effective as the calcium antagonist amlodipine, the angiotensin-converting enzyme lisinopril, and the alpha-blocker doxazosin in reducing the risk of cardiovascular events. In addition, almost all large randomized trials that included patients over 80 years of age used a diuretic

and declines modestly thereafter (**Figure 4-3**). As a result, isolated systolic hypertension is the dominant form of hypertension in the elderly, accounting for over 90% of hypertension in patients over 70 years of age. Systolic blood

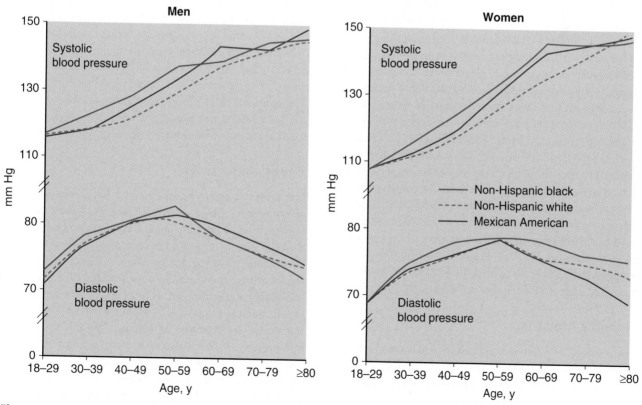

**Figure 4-3.** Age and blood pressure in the U.S. (*Source*: National Health and Nutrition Examination Survey.)

| Table 4-3 • Selected Trials of Antihypertensive Treatment in the Elderly | | | Risk Reduction | | | |
|---|---|---|---|---|---|---|
| Trial | N | Age, yrs | CVA | CAD | HF | All CVD |
| STOP-HTN | 1627 | 70-84 | 47% | 13% | 51% | 40% |
| SHEP | 4736 | ≥60 | 33% | 27% | 55% | 32% |
| Syst-Eur | 4695 | ≥60 | 42% | 26% | 36% | 31% |
| STONE | 1632 | 60-79 | 57% | 6% | 68% | 60% |
| Syst-China | 2394 | ≥60 | 38% | 33% | 38% | 37% |
| HYVET | 3845 | ≥80 | 30% | 28% | 64% | 34% |

HYVET: Hypertension in the Very Elderly Trial; SHEP: Systolic Hypertension in the Elderly Program; STONE: Shanghai Trial of Nifedipine in the Elderly; STOP-HTN: Swedish Trial in Old Patients with Hypertension; Syst-China: Systolic Hypertension in China Trial; Syst-Eur: Systolic Hypertension in Europe Trial.

as initial therapy. Therefore, until additional data become available, initiation of treatment with a diuretic is appropriate in most patients.

## Dyslipidemia

Average total serum cholesterol and low-density lipoprotein (LDL) cholesterol levels increase in men until approximately age 70 and then level off. In women, total serum cholesterol and LDL-cholesterol levels rise sharply after menopause and average 15–20 mg/dL higher than in men after age 60. High-density lipoprotein (HDL) cholesterol levels average about 10 mg/dL higher in women than in men throughout adult life. Although the strength of association of cholesterol levels with cardiovascular disease declines with age, in part due to the confounding effects of comorbid conditions and nutritional factors, low HDL-cholesterol levels and high total cholesterol to HDL-cholesterol ratios remain independent predictors of coronary events in older persons, including those over 80 years of age. In addition, observational studies and clinical trials indicate that statin therapy is associated with a reduction in cardiovascular events in moderate to high risk patients up to age 85.[3] In the PROSPER trial, for example, which randomized 5804 patients 70-82 years of age to pravastatin or placebo, those receiving pravastatin experienced a 15% reduction in the primary outcome of coronary death, nonfatal myocardial infarction, or nonfatal or fatal stroke during a mean follow-up period of 3.2 years. Conversely, limited data are available on statin therapy in lower risk patients and in patients over 85 years of age. Treatment of these subgroups must therefore be individualized based on an overall assessment of potential benefits and risks.

## Diabetes Mellitus

The prevalence of diabetes mellitus increases with age, and approximately half of all patients with diabetes in the U.S. are 65 years of age or older. As in younger individuals, the impact of diabetes on cardiovascular risk is greater in older women than in older men. Although very limited data are available on the effect of diabetes control on clinical outcomes in elderly patients, current guidelines recommend that functional, cognitively intact individuals with good life expectancy be managed in similar fashion to younger adults. In particular, hypertension and dyslipidemia should be treated in accordance with existing guidelines, as therapy for these conditions has been shown to reduce the risk of cardiovascular complications in older diabetics.

## Smoking

The prevalence of smoking declines with age, in part due to premature deaths attributable to smoking and in part due to successful smoking cessation. In 2006, 12.6% of men and 8.3% of women over 65 years of age in the U.S. were active smokers, declining to less than 5% among persons over age 85. In most studies, smoking is a strong risk factor for fatal and nonfatal cardiovascular events in older individuals, and several large observational studies indicate that smoking cessation is associated with substantial reductions in risk. Therefore, all older people who smoke should be strongly advised to quit, and appropriate resources should be provided to patients who express a desire to stop smoking.

## Physical Inactivity

Low levels of daily physical activity have been associated with increased risk for cardiovascular and all-cause mortality in patients of all ages, including the elderly, and initiation of a regular exercise program has been associated with a reduction in risk across the age spectrum. Additional benefits of regular aerobic exercise include improved functional capacity and quality of life, improved control of other risk factors (i.e., hypertension, diabetes, dyslipidemia, and obesity), and favorable effects on depressive symptoms. Strength and balance training have also been associated with a reduced risk for falls and fractures in older patients. In the absence of contraindications, older patients with or without cardiovascular disease should be encouraged to engage in a regular exercise program that includes both aerobic and strengthening activities.

## Other Risk Factors

Obesity is associated with increased cardiovascular risk in young and middle-aged people, but the importance of obesity as a risk factor in the elderly, especially persons over 80 years of age, is less clear. Among older patients with coronary artery disease, heart failure, or renal insufficiency, being overweight or mildly obese (body mass index [BMI] 25-35 kg/m²) has been associated with a more favorable prognosis than a BMI of 20–25 kg/m², and individuals with a BMI < 20 kg/m² have the highest mortality. There is also no evidence that weight reduction improves outcomes in older patients. Thus, although modest weight reduction may be desirable in elderly patients with moderate or severe obesity (BMI ≥ 35 kg/m²), significant weight loss in patients with lower BMIs should be undertaken cautiously or not at all.

Several biomarkers, including C-reactive protein, fibrinogen, and D-dimer, have been associated with increased cardiovascular risk in older adults, but the clinical utility of these markers in guiding management is unproven. Coronary artery calcium content assessed by computer tomography increases with age but the correlation of calcium scores with the severity of coronary artery stenoses declines with age. Nonetheless, higher calcium scores are associated with increased risk for incident coronary events in older adults. At present, routine quantitation of coronary artery calcium to screen for coronary artery disease (CAD) is not recommended.

# CORONARY ARTERY DISEASE

## Epidemiology

The incidence and prevalence of CAD increase with age, and autopsy studies indicate that up to 70% of persons 70 years of age or older have 50% or greater narrowing of one or more coronary arteries. The prevalence of clinical CAD also increases with age in both men and women (**Figure 4-4**), and

persons age 65 or older account for approximately two-thirds of hospitalizations for acute myocardial infarction (MI) and 80% of MI deaths in the U.S. Moreover, over 40% of MIs and up to 60% of MI deaths occur in the 6% of the population age 75 or older. In addition, the proportion of MIs occurring in women increases from 26% in the 45-64 year age group, to 35% in persons 65-74 years of age, and 55% in those 75 years or older.

## Acute Coronary Syndromes

Older patients with acute coronary syndromes (ACS) are less likely than younger patients to present with typical ischemic chest pain and more likely to present with altered mental status, confusion, dizziness, or syncope. Time from symptom onset to presentation also tends to be longer in older patients, and the initial electrocardiogram (ECG) is more likely to be nondiagnostic of ACS due to pre-existing conduction abnormalities, paced rhythm, left ventricular hypertrophy, prior MI, and higher prevalence of non-ST-elevation ACS. As a result of these factors, the diagnosis of acute MI in older adults is often delayed, resulting in a shorter "window of opportunity" for interventions aimed at reducing infarct size, thereby contributing to the worse prognosis of older patients with ACS.

### Therapy

In general, treatment of ACS in older and younger patients is similar.[4,5] Because mortality rates from acute MI increase exponentially with age, the potential benefits of pharmacological and mechanical interventions increase with age. Conversely, older patients are at increased risk for complications from both medications and invasive procedures. Therefore, treatment of older patients must be individualized based on a careful assessment of the benefits and risks.

Aspirin should be administered to all patients with suspected ACS, regardless of age. Hemodynamically stable patients should receive an oral beta-blocker, but these agents should

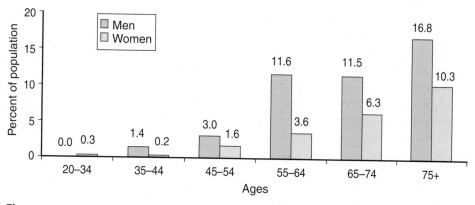

**Figure 4-4.** Prevalence of coronary artery disease in the U.S. by age and sex. (*Source*: CDC/NCHS and NHLBI.)

be given cautiously (if at all) in patients with systolic blood pressure <120 mm Hg, heart rate ≥110/minute, or Killip class III or IV heart failure, as these findings have been associated with increased risk for cardiogenic shock and death, especially in patients 70 years of age or older. An angiotensin-converting enzyme (ACE) inhibitor or angiotensin receptor blocker (ARB) should be initiated in hemodynamically stable patients with adequate renal function (est. creatinine clearance ≥30 cc/min), especially those with left ventricular (LV) systolic dysfunction. Early administration of high-dose statin therapy is also reasonable, although data are limited in patients over 75-80 years of age.

The role of adjunctive antithrombotic therapy in patients with ACS continues to evolve. The COMMIT study, which included 11,934 patients ≥70 years of age with suspected MI, showed that compared to aspirin alone, the addition of clopidogrel 75 mg to aspirin 162 mg was associated with a statistically significant 9% reduction in death, reinfarction, or stroke during a mean follow-up of 15 days; results were similar in younger and older patients. Unfractionated heparin or low molecular weight heparin (LMWH) is indicated in most patients with ACS, but older patients are at increased risk for bleeding, and dosage adjustment of LMWH is essential in patients with an estimated creatinine clearance of less than 30 cc/min. Bivalirudin and fondaparinux may be associated with improved outcomes relative to heparin, but data in the very elderly are limited, and dosage adjustment based on estimated creatinine clearance is required for both of these agents. Glycoprotein IIb/IIIa inhibitors are indicated in selected patients with ACS, particularly those undergoing percutaneous coronary intervention (PCI), but the risk of bleeding complications in older patients is increased, and limited efficacy data are available in patients over 75-80 years of age; eptifibatide and tirofiban also require dosage adjustment for renal impairment.

Reperfusion therapy is recommended for patients with ST-elevation MI (including MI associated with new left bundle branch block), and PCI is preferable to fibrinolytic therapy provided that the procedure can be performed within 90-120 minutes of the patient's arrival at the hospital. Compared to fibrinolytic therapy, PCI has been associated with improved outcomes in patients up to 85 years of age, but data are limited in patients over age 85. The value of PCI in patients over age 75 with cardiogenic shock remains controversial. The risk of intracranial hemorrhage among patients treated with a fibrinolytic agent increases significantly after age 75, and is also greater with the more potent, fibrin-specific agents (e.g., alteplase, reteplase) than with streptokinase.

Early PCI has been associated with improved outcomes in high-risk patients with non-ST-elevation MI, including the elderly, especially those with ongoing ischemia, extensive ECG changes, decreased LV systolic function, or hemodynamic instability. In elderly patients who are hemodynamically stable without evidence for extensive or ongoing ischemia, an initial strategy of optimal medical therapy is appropriate.

## Chronic CAD

Older patients with CAD are less likely than younger patients to present with typical angina pectoris, but more likely to complain of exertional fatigue or shortness of breath. Since the incidence and prevalence of CAD increase with age in both men and women, it is important to maintain a high index of suspicion in older patients who report new or worsening exercise intolerance.

Management of chronic CAD is similar in older and younger patients, including appropriate management of prevalent risk factors in accordance with guideline recommendations. Aspirin 75-162.5 mg daily is indicated in the absence of aspirin intolerance, and statin therapy is recommended for all patients with CAD, including the elderly and those with untreated low density lipoprotein cholesterol (LDL-C) levels within the desirable range. Although altered hepatic metabolism and the use of multiple medications may place older patients at risk for statin-related side effects, studies have not consistently shown an increased risk for statin toxicity in older individuals.

All patients with prior MI or symptomatic LV systolic dysfunction should be treated with a beta-blocker, and beta-blockers are also first line therapy for ischemia in patients with chronic CAD. Calcium channel blockers and long-acting nitrates can be used alone or in combination with other anti-ischemic agents. In addition, ranolazine has recently gained approval as a first line agent for treatment of angina pectoris in patients with chronic CAD.

In patients with inadequate symptom control despite combination anti-anginal therapy, revascularization with PCI or coronary artery bypass grafting (CABG) is appropriate, and both procedures have been associated with a reduction in symptoms and improved quality of life in older patients. However, procedural complication rates, including death, increase with age, especially after age 80. Compared to CABG, PCI is associated with fewer major complications, shorter length of hospital stay, lower cost, and more rapid recovery, but with somewhat lower efficacy with respect to symptom control and with a higher likelihood of repeat revascularization procedures. Long-term survival is similar after PCI or CABG. Importantly, up to 50% of older patients undergoing CABG experience some degree of cognitive dysfunction post-operatively, which may result in increased length of stay and delayed recovery. In most cases, cognitive function returns to baseline within 3 to 6 months, but a small proportion shows persistent cognitive impairment.

# VALVULAR HEART DISEASE

## Aortic Stenosis

The prevalence of aortic stenosis (AS) increases with age, approaching 15% in octogenarians. As in younger patients, the symptoms of AS in older adults include exertional shortness of breath progressing to overt heart failure, angina pectoris, light-headedness, and syncope. However, symptom onset is often delayed due to sedentary lifestyle. Physical findings associated with severe calcific AS include a loud, harsh, late-peaking systolic ejection murmur radiating to the carotids, diminished A2 component of the second heart sound, an S4 gallop, and an LV heave. In contrast to younger patients, the carotid upstrokes are often brisk in elderly patients with severe AS as a result of increased arterial stiffness.

At the present time, aortic valve replacement remains the treatment of choice in elderly patients with severe AS.[6] Operative mortality in octogenarians is less than 5% in experienced centers, and long-term outcomes are excellent. Bioprosthetic valves have excellent durability in this age group and obviate the need for long-term anticoagulation.

Percutaneous balloon aortic valvuloplasty is associated with relatively high complication rates and poor long-term outcomes and is therefore not a suitable alternative to valve replacement. Recently, percutaneous approaches to aortic valve replacement have been developed and preliminary reports have been favorable. Ongoing studies will help clarify the role of percutaneous valve replacement in elderly patients with severe AS.

## Aortic Regurgitation

The prevalence of chronic aortic regurgitation (AR) increases with age, and up to 30% of older adults have at least mild AR by echocardiography. In most cases, chronic AR is mild or moderate in severity, and only rarely is it severe enough to require surgical intervention.

The incidence of acute AR also increases with age, and the most common causes include type A aortic dissection, infective endocarditis, malfunction of a prosthetic aortic valve, and chest trauma. Management of acute AR is similar in older and younger patients,[6] but operative mortality is generally higher in the elderly, especially those with multiple co-existing medical illnesses.

## Mitral Stenosis

Rheumatic mitral stenosis (MS) is relatively uncommon in older adults in the U.S., but occasionally patients in their 70s or 80s will present with symptoms attributable to rheumatic MS. More commonly, MS in older adults is caused by non-rheumatic calcification of the mitral valve annulus leading to a narrowed orifice and decreased excursion of the valve leaflets. Whether rheumatic or non-rheumatic, MS in older adults tends to progress very gradually, and conservative management is appropriate in most patients in the absence of debilitating symptoms.[6] Patients with MS who develop atrial fibrillation are at high risk for thromboembolism; therefore, anticoagulation with warfarin to maintain the international normalized ratio (INR) in the range of 2.0-3.0 is indicated in almost all cases.

Patients with severe symptomatic rheumatic MS should be considered for interventional therapy. Percutaneous balloon mitral valvuloplasty is safe and effective, but the majority of older patients are not suitable candidates for this procedure due to extensive calcification and commissural fusion or concomitant moderate or severe mitral regurgitation. Therefore, most patients will require mitral valve replacement with a bioprosthesis. In experienced centers, mitral valve replacement is associated with a 5-10% perioperative mortality in older patients, but mortality may exceed 15% in low volume centers. In patients with severe calcific non-rheumatic MS, operative mortality rates and long-term outcomes following surgery tend to be less favorable than in those undergoing valve replacement for rheumatic disease.

## Mitral Regurgitation

Mitral regurgitation (MR) of at least mild severity is present in up to one-third of older adults, but only a small proportion require surgical intervention. Management of acute and chronic MR is generally similar in older and younger adults, except that medical therapy may be preferable to surgery in older patients with severe chronic MR and mild symptoms due to shorter life expectancy and higher perioperative mortality.[6] If surgery is indicated, mitral valve repair is preferable to valve replacement in patients of all ages because it is associated with preservation of ventricular integrity, improved functional outcomes, and lack of requirement for long-term anticoagulation. When valve replacement is necessary, bioprosthetic valves are preferable to mechanical valves for most patients over 65 years of age. As noted above, mortality rates from mitral valve surgery in older adults range from about 5% to more than 15% depending on the experience of the surgeon and the hospital's surgical volume.

## Infective Endocarditis

The incidence of infective endocarditis (IE) increases with age due to the increased prevalence of valvular abnormalities in conjunction with the increased risk for bacteremia related to poor dentition, urinary tract and pulmonary infections, and invasive procedures. The organisms associated

### Table 4-4 • Summary of Revised Recommendations for Endocarditis Prophylaxis

**Cardiac conditions warranting endocarditis prophylaxis**

Prosthetic cardiac valve or prosthetic material used for cardiac valve repair

Cardiac transplantation associated with valvulopathy

Previous documented infective endocarditis

Selected forms of congenital heart disease:

- Unrepaired cyanotic congenital heart disease
- Repaired congenital heart defect with prosthetic material or device for 6 months after the procedure
- Repaired congenital heart disease with residual defects at the site of prosthetic material

**Procedures for which endocarditis prophylaxis is recommended***

- All dental procedures that involve manipulation of gingival tissue or the periapical region of teeth or perforation of the oral mucosa
- Respiratory tract procedures
- Procedures involving infected skin, skin structures, or musculoskeletal tissue

*i.e., in patients with the cardiac conditions listed above
Source: Wilson W, Taubert KA, Gewitz M, et al. Prevention of infective endocarditis: guidelines from the American Heart Association. Circulation. 2007;116(15):1736–1754.

with IE are similar in older and younger patients, but up to 10% of older patients with IE are culture-negative, most commonly due to prior treatment with antibiotics. The clinical manifestations of IE are similar in older and younger patients, except that peripheral manifestations, such as petechiae and embolic phenomena, tend to occur less frequently in the elderly. Management of IE, including indications for surgical intervention, is unaffected by age, but the prognosis is worse in older patients. Guidelines for IE prophylaxis have recently been revised (**Table 4-4**), and prophylaxis is no longer recommended for gastrointestinal or genitourinary tract procedures, including endoscopy, cystoscopy, and biopsies, or for routine dental work, even in patients with valvular heart disease.

## HEART FAILURE

### Epidemiology

In the U.S., the prevalence of heart failure (HF) increases exponentially with age, roughly doubling with each decade after age 45, and reaching about 10% among octogenarians (**Figure 4-5**). HF is the leading cause of hospitalization in the Medicare age group and it is also the most costly medical illness among older adults. The median age of HF patients in the U.S. is 75 years, and two-thirds of HF deaths occur in patients 75 years of age or older. The incidence of HF is higher in men than in women at all ages, but women comprise slightly more than half of all HF patients due to their longer life expectancy. In older women, HF is most often attributable to hypertension, whereas in older men, CAD and hypertension contribute equally to the development of HF. Among HF patients 65 years of age or older, approximately 50% have preserved LV systolic function, including about two-thirds of women and up to 40% of men.

### Clinical Features

Compared to younger patients, older HF patients are less likely to present with exertional dyspnea and lower extremity edema but more likely to exhibit atypical symptoms such as decreased mental acuity, confusion, lethargy, anorexia, or altered bowel function. In addition, due to the higher prevalence of preserved LV systolic function, older HF patients are less likely to manifest an S3 gallop or signs of right heart failure, including increased jugular venous pressure, hepatomegaly, and pitting edema. B-type

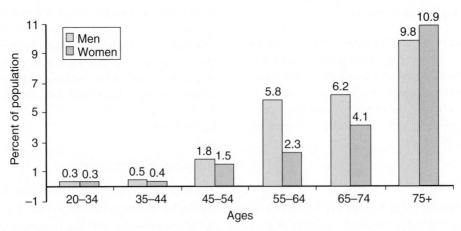

**Figure 4-5.** Prevalence of heart failure in the U.S. by age and sex. (*Source*: CDC/NCHS and NHLBI.)

natriuretic peptide (BNP) levels increase with age, especially in women, resulting in reduced specificity and positive predictive value of elevated BNP levels for diagnosing HF in older adults.

## Management

Despite the fact that HF is predominantly a disorder of the elderly, most clinical trials have excluded patients over 75 to 80 years of age as well as patients with multiple comorbid conditions, as are typically present in older HF patients. In addition, older patients are at increased risk for significant medication side effects due to polypharmacy and diminished renal and hepatic function. As a result, management of HF in older adults must be individualized, and older patients with advanced HF in the context of multiple coexisting illnesses or significant socioeconomic issues may benefit from participation in a structured HF management program, as such programs have been associated with a reduction in HF hospitalizations and improved quality of life.[7]

### Pharmacotherapy of Systolic HF

Despite the paucity of data from clinical trials, drug therapy of systolic HF is generally similar in older and younger patients.[7] In the absence of contraindications or limiting side effects, an angiotensin converting enzyme (ACE) inhibitor or angiotensin receptor blocker (ARB) in combination with a beta-blocker is indicated in most cases. In patients with severe renal dysfunction (est. creatinine clearance <30 cc/min), hydralazine/isosorbide dinitrate provides a reasonable alternative to an ACE inhibitor or ARB. The addition of spironolactone should be considered in patients with severe LV systolic dysfunction (ejection fraction <30%), persistent New York Heart Association class III-IV symptoms, and adequate renal function (est. creatinine clearance >30-45 cc/min), but close monitoring is required in older patients due to an increased risk for worsening renal function and hyperkalemia. Judicious use of diuretics to maintain euvolemia is appropriate, but over-diuresis should be avoided and renal function and serum electrolytes should be assessed periodically. Digoxin has no effect on mortality in HF patients but reduces HF hospitalizations and should be considered as adjunctive therapy in patients who fail to respond adequately to the above measures. Based on recently published data, the optimal serum digoxin concentration appears to be in the range 0.5-0.9 ng/mL, and levels above this range should be avoided.

### Pharmacotherapy of Diastolic HF

To date, no interventions have been shown to reduce mortality in HF patients with preserved LV systolic function, and management of this condition remains empiric. Hypertension, CAD, atrial fibrillation, and other comorbid conditions should be treated in accordance with current guidelines.[7] Recent studies suggest that the ARB candesartan,

the ACE inhibitor perindopril, and the beta-blocker nebivolol may be associated with fewer hospitalizations and/or improved quality of life in older patients with HF and preserved LV systolic function. Conversely, in the recently completed I-PRESERVE trial, the ARB irbesartan failed to improve clinical outcomes in patients with diastolic HF.

### Device Therapy

The implantable cardioverter-defibrillator (ICD) has been shown to reduce mortality from sudden cardiac death in patients with an LV ejection fraction ≤35% and New York Heart Association class II or III HF symptoms.[8] Although few older patients were enrolled in the ICD trials, observational studies indicate that the benefits of ICDs are similar in older and younger patients, and in the U.S. 40-45% of ICD implantations are in patients 70 years of age or older. ICDs have not been shown to improve outcomes in patients with class I or IV HF symptoms, and there is no survival benefit within the first 12-18 months after ICD implantation. In addition, older HF patients are at relatively higher risk than younger patients to die from other illnesses, thereby reducing the potential benefit of an ICD. Furthermore, ICD shocks are associated with diminished quality of life, and up to 20% of shocks are inappropriate, i.e., occurring in the absence of a life-threatening tachyarrhythmia. In light of these factors, elderly patients with reduced life expectancy (<18 months) should not receive an ICD, and ICD implantation in older patients who fulfill criteria for a device should be undertaken only after thorough discussion of the potential benefits and risks.

Cardiac resynchronization therapy (CRT) improves symptoms, exercise tolerance, quality of life, and survival in selected patients with advanced HF and evidence for LV dyssynchrony.[8] Although few older patients have been enrolled in CRT trials, observational studies suggest that older patients, including octogenarians, derive significant benefit from CRT. Therefore, CRT is a reasonable option in appropriately selected elderly patients who remain markedly symptomatic despite optimal medical therapy.

## Prognosis and End-of-life Care

The median survival of older patients with HF is 2-3 years, with similar survival rates in patients with systolic or diastolic HF. Factors adversely affecting prognosis include older age (esp. ≥85 years), male gender, more severe symptoms (e.g., higher New York Heart Association class), lower systolic blood pressure, prevalent CAD, diabetes (esp. in women), peripheral arterial or cerebrovascular disease, cognitive dysfunction, renal insufficiency, anemia, hyponatremia, low BMI (esp. <20 kg/m$^2$), and persistently elevated BNP levels.

The prognosis of HF is worse than for most forms of cancer. Therefore, it is appropriate to discuss end-of-life care early in the course of treatment and to readdress preferences as clinical circumstances evolve. Patients should be advised to develop an advance directive, designate an individual to serve as power of attorney, and explicitly indicate what interventions they would or would not wish to undergo in the event that death seemed imminent. In patients with ICDs, there should also be a discussion about disabling the device near the end of life in order to avoid repetitive painful shocks. In patients with a life expectancy of less than 6 months, transition to palliative care and hospice should be offered.

## CARDIAC ARRHYTHMIAS

### Epidemiology

The incidence and prevalence of both supraventricular and ventricular tachyarrhythmias increase progressively with age. In the Baltimore Longitudinal Study on Aging, over 90% of men and women 65 years of age or older demonstrated supraventricular ectopy and over 75% demonstrated ventricular ectopy on a 24-hour ambulatory electrocardiogram (ECG). In addition, almost 50% of men and women exhibited short runs of supraventricular tachycardia, but less than 0.5% had 5 or more beats of ventricular tachycardia. With the exception of atrial fibrillation, in the absence of structural heart disease the presence of supraventricular and ventricular arrhythmias on ambulatory ECG does not predict cardiac events or mortality.

Age-related changes involving the sinoatrial and atrioventricular (AV) nodes result in an increase in bradyarrhythmias with age. Although resting heart rate is unaffected by age in healthy individuals, the prevalence of sinus node dysfunction ("sick sinus syndrome") and AV-nodal block increase progressively with age. In addition, the prevalence of infranodal conduction system disorders, including bundle branch block and left anterior fascicular block, increases with age. Consequently, over 75% of permanent pacemakers are implanted in patients 65 years of age or older, and approximately half are in patients age 75 or older.

### Atrial Fibrillation

The incidence and prevalence of atrial fibrillation (AF) increase exponentially with age, and the prevalence of AF in octogenarians is approximately 10% (**Figure 4-6**). As a result, over 50% of patients with AF are 75 years of age or older. The proportion of strokes attributable to AF also increases with age, from <2% in patients less than 60 years, to over 20% in octogenarians. In addition, women with AF are at increased risk for stroke relative to men, especially after age 75.

In patients with asymptomatic or minimally symptomatic paroxysmal or persistent AF, multiple clinical trials have demonstrated that a strategy directed at rate control with AV-nodal blocking agents (i.e., beta-blockers, diltiazem, verapamil, digoxin) in conjunction with anticoagulation to maintain the INR in the range of 2.0-3.0 is associated with fewer hospitalizations and favorable trends in stroke and mortality rates relative to a strategy aimed at maintaining sinus rhythm with antiarrhythmic drugs.[9] Conversely, patients who experience significant shortness of breath, fatigue, or exercise intolerance attributable to AF may benefit from restoration and preservation of sinus rhythm, either with antiarrhythmic drugs or, in select cases, with catheter ablation of AF or the surgical Maze procedure. For patients who remain in sinus rhythm for a minimum of 6-12 months following catheter ablation or surgery for AF, it may be safe to discontinue anticoagulation, but older patients treated with medications alone to maintain sinus rhythm should continue to receive warfarin to achieve a therapeutic INR.

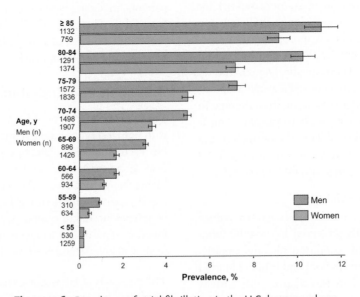

**Figure 4-6.** Prevalence of atrial fibrillation in the U.S. by age and sex.

Although age over 75 is a strong independent risk factor for stroke in patients with AF, patients in this age group are also at increased risk for bleeding complications with long-term anticoagulation. In most cases, the benefits of warfarin, i.e., 60-70% reduction in the risk of stroke and other embolic events, outweigh the risk of major bleeding, including intracranial hemorrhage.[9] Among patients at high risk for major bleeding with warfarin, aspirin 75-325 mg/day is a reasonable alternative, but aspirin is much less effective than warfarin and only reduces stroke risk by 20-25%.

## Bradyarrhythmias

In the absence of symptoms, most sinus bradyarrhythmias and AV-nodal conduction disorders do not require pacemaker implantation.[8] However, patients with severe bradycardia (heart rate <40 bpm) or asystolic pauses of 3 seconds or longer while awake, as well as patients with significant symptoms clearly associated with bradycardia (e.g., marked light-headedness, syncope, angina, or exercise intolerance) that can not be attributed to medications, hypothyroidism, or other causes, should be considered for pacemaker therapy.[8] Pacing is also indicated in patients with high degree infranodal block, whether or not symptoms are present.

In patients with sinus rhythm and preserved AV conduction (i.e., normal PR interval and narrow QRS) who require permanent pacing, atrial pacing is the preferred mode. Conversely, patients with sinus rhythm and impaired AV conduction are often best served by dual chamber pacing (i.e., atrial and ventricular), whereas patients with AF should receive a ventricular pacemaker. Compared to single-chamber ventricular pacemakers, dual chamber devices do not decrease the risk of stroke or improve survival, but reductions in the incidence of AF and hospitalization for HF have been demonstrated.

## Tachy-brady Syndrome

Tachy-brady syndrome is a common variant of "sick sinus syndrome" in which patients manifest both supraventricular tachyarrhythmias and bradyarrhythmias, either or both of which may be symptomatic. Treatment of the tachyarrhythmias with medications often exacerbates symptoms related to bradycardia, as a result of which pacemaker implantation may be required.

## Peripheral Arterial Disease

The prevalence of peripheral arterial disease (PAD), including disorders of the abdominal aorta and its branches, increases with age and is higher in men than in women. In one study, the prevalence of PAD increased from 5.6% in persons 38-59 years of age, to 15.9% in persons 60-69 years of age, and to 33.8% among those 70-82 years of age.

Current guidelines recommend a formal history and physical examination to screen for PAD in patients 50-69 years of age with risk factors for atherosclerosis, and in all patients 70 years of age or older.[10] In addition, men 60 years of age or older with a family history of abdominal aortic aneurysm (AAA) and men 65-75 years of age who have ever smoked should undergo an abdominal ultrasound to screen for AAA.[10]

Patients with symptoms or signs suggestive of PAD should undergo assessment of the ankle-brachial index (ABI), the ratio of the systolic blood pressure obtained below the knee to that obtained over the ipsilateral brachial artery. A normal ABI is 0.9-1.3, and an ABI < 0.9 has over 90% sensitivity and specificity for diagnosing lower extremity PAD. However, older patients with stiff arteries may have artifactually high systolic blood pressure readings resulting in a falsely normal or even elevated ABI. An ABI < 0.40 is usually associated with severe PAD and impaired perfusion of the distal limb.

PAD is a coronary risk-equivalent, and most deaths in patients with PAD are related to concomitant CAD. Management of PAD therefore includes aggressive treatment of cardiovascular risk factors, including aspirin 75-325 mg/day and a statin to maintain the LDL-cholesterol level below 100 mg/dL.[10] Walking for at least 30-45 minutes at least 3 times a week for a minimum of 3-6 months has been associated with significant improvement in patients with symptomatic PAD. Cilostazol, a type III phosphodiesterase inhibitor, has been shown to improve maximum walking distance by 40-60% in patients with significant claudication; however, cilostazol is not recommended for patients with HF.

Revascularization is indicated for patients with severe symptoms that have not responded to conservative therapy and for patients with critical limb ischemia, defined as rest pain, ulceration, or gangrene.[10] The choice of revascularization procedure, i.e., percutaneous transluminal angioplasty with or without stenting versus surgery, is dependent on lesion location and severity, likelihood of success, risk of major complications, and the experience and technical expertise of the interventionalist and surgeon. Indications for AAA repair include development of symptoms, aneurysmal dilatation ≥1 cm in 1 year, and aneurysms ≥5.5 cm in diameter. Patients with asymptomatic AAAs 4.0-5.4 cm in diameter should undergo serial evaluations at 6-12 month intervals. For patients who require AAA repair, surgery is the preferred treatment for both suprarenal and infrarenal lesions, but endovascular repair is a reasonable option for patients with infrarenal AAA who are at high risk for complications from an open procedure. Additional indications for endovascular repair await the results of ongoing studies.

# References

1. Lakatta EG. Age-associated cardiovascular changes in health: impact on cardiovascular disease in older persons. *Heart Failure Rev.* 2002;7(1):29–49.

2. Chobanian AV, Bakris GL, Black HR, et al. The Seventh Report of the Joint National Committee on Prevention, Detection, Evaluation, and Treatment of High Blood Pressure: the JNC 7 report. JAMA. 2003;289(19):2560–2572.

3. National Cholesterol Education Program (NCEP) Expert Panel on Detection, Evaluation, and Treatment of High Blood Cholesterol in Adults (Adult Treatment Panel III). Third Report of the National Cholesterol Education Program (NCEP) Expert Panel on Detection, Evaluation, and Treatment of High Blood Cholesterol in Adults (Adult Treatment Panel III) final report. *Circulation.* 2002;106(25):3143–3421.

4. Alexander KP, Newby LK, Cannon CP, et al. Acute coronary care in the elderly, part I: Non-ST-segment-elevation acute coronary syndromes: a scientific statement for healthcare professionals from the American Heart Association Council on Clinical Cardiology: in collaboration with the Society of Geriatric Cardiology. *Circulation.* 2007;115(19):2549–2569.

5. Alexander KP, Newby LK, Armstrong PW, et al. Acute coronary care in the elderly, part II: ST-segment-elevation myocardial infarction: a scientific statement for healthcare professionals from the American Heart Association Council on Clinical Cardiology: in collaboration with the Society of Geriatric Cardiology. *Circulation.* 2007;115(19):2570–2589.

6. Bonow RO, Carabello BA, Chatterjee K, et al. ACC/AHA 2006 guidelines for the management of patients with valvular heart disease: a report of the American College of Cardiology/American Heart Association Task Force on Practice Guidelines. *J Am Coll Cardiol.* 2006;48(3):e1–e148.

7. Hunt SA, Abraham WT, Chin MH, et al. ACC/AHA 2005 Guideline Update for the Diagnosis and Management of Chronic Heart Failure in the Adult: a report of the American College of Cardiology/American Heart Association Task Force on Practice Guidelines. *Circulation.* 2005;112(12):e154–e235.

8. Epstein AE, DiMarco JP, Ellenbogen KA, et al. ACC/AHA/HRS 2008 Guidelines for Device-Based Therapy of Cardiac Rhythm Abnormalities: a report of the American College of Cardiology/American Heart Association Task Force on Practice Guidelines. *Circulation.* 2008;117(21):e350–e408.

9. Fuster V, Ryden LE, Cannom DS, et al. ACC/AHA/ESC 2006 Guidelines for the Management of Patients with Atrial Fibrillation: a report of the American College of Cardiology/American Heart Association Task Force on Practice Guidelines and the European Society of Cardiology Committee for Practice Guidelines. *Circulation.* 2006;114(7):e257–e354.

10. Hirsch AT, Haskal ZJ, Hertzer NR, et al. ACC/AHA 2005 Practice Guidelines for the management of patients with peripheral arterial disease (lower extremity, renal, mesenteric, and abdominal aortic): a collaborative report from the American Association for Vascular Surgery/Society for Vascular Surgery, Society for Cardiovascular Angiography and Interventions, Society for Vascular Medicine and Biology, Society of Interventional Radiology, and the ACC/AHA Task Force on Practice Guidelines. *Circulation.* 2006;113(11):e463–e654.

# 5

# Performance Measures in General Cardiology

L. Veronica Lee and JoAnne M. Foody

## INTRODUCTION

Performance measures are designed to accurately gauge and improve the current standard of health care delivery based on current updated guidelines. Such measures provide a means to quantify how well an individual provider, group of providers, hospital, or hospital system is delivering what is considered to be current optimal care. Several organizations have developed performance measures, including National Committee for Quality Assurance (NCQA), Health Plan Employer Data and Information Set (HEDIS), Joint Commission on Accreditation of Healthcare Organizations (JCAHO) through its initiative ORYX, the Centers for Medicare & Medicaid Services (formerly HCFA) through the Peer Review Organization 6th Scope of Work. The American Medical Association's (AMA's) Division of Clinical Quality Improvement has created a Physician Consortium for Performance to identify, define, and develop performance measures targeting the practicing physician, and to create tools for quality improvement. This chapter

will focus on the physician level performance measures developed jointly by the American Heart Association and American College of Cardiology (ACC/AHA Task Force on Performance Measures), as well as those proposed jointly by the AMA/PCPI/ACC/AHA and that are National Quality forum(NQF)-endorsed. Current available national performance guidelines for both inpatients and outpatients include stable angina, acute myocardial infarction, atrial fibrillation, heart failure, and cardiac rehabilitation.

## PERFORMANCE MEASURES: METHODOLOGY AND SPECIAL CONSIDERATIONS

Performance measures are distinct from guidelines in that they are a limited set of criteria that one must be able to measure, and they are items that may be reported. They promote both health quality improvement and cost-effective care. Only the clearest, most important and accepted evidence-based guidelines are included, and these must be flexible to allow the exercise of a physician's professional judgment in individual clinical scenarios. The measures must allow for variations in access to care and resources and assess patient satisfaction, access, and outcome. In addition the difficulty of added data collection needs to be balanced with the potential gain of additional measures.

The ACC/AHA Task Force has summarized the methodology used for creating and selecting performance measures that quantify the quality of care given to cardiovascular patients as defined by adherence to specific well-founded guidelines. This will lead to improvement in quality through a better measured understanding of current deficiencies.

| Table 5-1 • Summary of Performance Measure Development | |
| --- | --- |
| **Task Description** | **Measurement Sets** |
| **Phase I: Constructing** | |
| Task 1: Defining the target population and observational period | Develop a clear, concise, and implementable definition of the sample (e.g., adults >29 yrs of age, discharged alive with a principal diagnosis of heart failure (ICD-9: 398.91, 402.01, 402.11, 402.91, 428.0, 428.1, 428.9), with a length of stay of ≥1 day, excluding patients with an AMI in the previous month continuously enrolled for 6 months after discharge. |
| Task 2: Identifying dimensions of care | Explicitly define each aspect of care that should be quantified to ensure a valid assessment of the most meaningful aspects of care. Potential dimensions include diagnosis, risk stratification and patient education, treatment, self-management, and reassessment of patient's health status. |
| Task 3: Synthesizing and reviewing the literature | Review published literature (including guidelines and other performance measurement systems) with a team of clinicians and researchers with expertise in meta-analysis. |
| Task 4: Defining and operationalizing potential measures | For each measure, determine which data sources are available and define the data elements needed to construct it (including period of care). |
| Task 5: Selecting measures for inclusion in the performance measures set | Present information based on tasks 1–3 to writing group and other relevant individuals, and put in place a formal mechanism to decide upon the measures that will be selected for inclusion. |
| **Phase II: Determining Measure Feasibility** | |
| Definition of sample | Calculate sensitivity and specificity of selection criteria whenever possible. Document sources of case attrition (e.g., medical record never sent, not continually enrolled, died during period of care). Develop an algorithm to assign patients to providers (e.g., primary care provider, specialist) and validate the accuracy of the algorithm. |
| Feasibility of measures | Report validity, reliability, and completeness of collected data. If chart abstraction is used, then interabstractor reliability needs to be measured; if patient survey is used, then item and unit nonresponse must be measured. Data lags in identifying and surveying patients need to be assessed. |
| **Phase III: Measuring Performance** | |
| Determining reporting unit | Determine at what level information will be reported (e.g., physician-level data will typically require longer accrual period, even if only for internal monitoring). |
| Determining number and range of measures | Cost constraints may dictate how many measures can be measured. For quality improvement, how many measures will be evaluated and/or whether a combined measure is necessary will need to be determined. |
| Evaluating performance | *Caution*: To determine whether a provider has "improved" care over time or whether a provider is sufficiently different from others, a sample size calculation that incorporates the relevant statistical features of the "test" (within- and between-provider variability, size of test, significance of test) should be undertaken. |

*ICD, International Classification of Diseases; AMI, acute myocardial infarction*

Performance measures are not designed to be used as a quality instrument for either rewarding or punishing lack of adherence, since such a use may impact open reporting of adherence to these measures. Three phases are outlined in the development and implementation of performance measures:

I. Initial definition of the performance measure set
II. Evaluation of reliability and feasibility of data collection
III. Actual measurement of performance of the provider, hospital, or hospital system.

The details of these phases are outlined in **Table 5-1**.

## CRITERIA FOR PERFORMANCE MEASURES

In addition to its defining methodology, the ACC/AHA Task Force also has developed criteria for those attributes which a satisfactory performance measure should have. These are summarized in **Table 5-2**. Essentially, the criteria require performance measures to be evidence-based, interpretable, actionable, well-constructed, and feasible.

The basis for any performance measure is found in national guidelines. In cardiology, the guideline process is robust and

| Table 5-2 • ACC/AHA Attributes for Satisfactory Performance Measures |
| --- |
| **ACC/AHA Attributes for Satisfactory Performance Measures** |
| **Useful in improving patient outcomes** <br> 1. Evidence-based <br> 2. Interpretable <br> 3. Actionable |
| **Measure design** <br> 1. Denominator precisely defined <br> 2. Numerator precisely defined <br> 3. Validity <br>    a. Face validity <br>    b. Content validity <br>    c. Construct validity <br> 4. Reliability |
| **Measure implementation** <br> 1. Feasibility <br>    a. Reasonable effort <br>    b. Reasonable cost <br>    c. Reasonable time period for collection |
| **Overall assessment** |

exacting. All the performance measures discussed below are based on guidelines previously developed for treatment of a specific disease. These guidelines are ranked based on anticipated benefit as compared to risk (Class I, IIa, IIb, III), as well as anticipated certainty of treatment effect (Level-A, B, and C); they are summarized in **Figure 5-1**. The majority of performance measures support the performance of Class I indications and the avoidance of Class III indications. **Table 5-3** outlines the current status of available and developing performance measure sets for cardiology.

# PERFORMANCE MEASURES BY DISEASE STATE

## Chronic Stable Coronary Artery Disease

The leading cause of death, that which accounts for almost 20% of mortality in the United States, is chronic stable coronary artery disease (CAD). The incidence of CAD as measured by short-stay hospital discharges has increased by 18% in the past 20 years. Recurrent CAD is significant and the cost is over $130 billion a year. Although there is much information regarding how to treat and prevent CAD, there are still high rates of patient receipt of suboptimal care. For example, using Medicare database information, only half of patients at hospital discharge for an acute myocardial infarction have been counseled to stop smoking, only 79% are prescribed beta-blocker, and only 74% are prescribed an angiotensin-converting enzyme inhibitor. Performance

measures for chronic stable CAD are based on recommendations from the American College of Cardiology, American Heart Association, American College of Physicians— American Society of Internal Medicine, American College of Endocrinology, American Diabetes Association, and the National Heart, Lung and Blood Institute. The following performance measures are designed for an office-based practice and the physician who longitudinally manages a patient with chronic stable CAD. **Table 5-4** is a summary of the established performance measures for chronic stable coronary artery disease.

## Acute Myocardial Infarction

Coronary artery disease is the number one killer of men and women in the United States, accounting for 652,091 deaths in 2005. Of patients with an acute myocardial infarction (AMI) many will not make a full recovery, and about 30% of women and 20% of men will die during the first year of the first MI. Although there has been decline in mortality through better utilization of the current guidelines, ongoing improvements in performance are anticipated to translate into even greater reductions in mortality and morbidity. AMI is defined by the ICD-9 codes used in **Table 5-5**.

The guidelines given in **Table 5-6** were reviewed to develop the performance measures: 1999 ACC/AHA Guidelines for the Management of Patients with Acute Myocardial Infarction (AMI guideline), the ACC/AHA 2002 Guideline Update for Management of Patients with Unstable Angina and Non–ST-Segment Elevation Myocardial Infarction (UA/NSTEMI guideline), and the 2004 ACC/AHA Guidelines for the Management of Patients with ST-Elevation Myocardial Infarction (STEMI guideline), as well as sets previously developed by CMS and JCAHO. Measures made involving the initial hospitalization are typically made over the length of the hospitalization unless otherwise noted. Typically only guidelines with Class I evidence are used; however it was decided to incorporate the ARB guideline into the performance measure for ACE-I, although it is Class IIa because of the anticipated value of including this alternate therapy in the overall performance assessment. Measures involving the time it takes to reperfusion (primary PCI or fibrinolysis) are expressed as a median as opposed to mean in order to avoid the skewing of data by measures at the extremes. Previously, time to PCI first balloon inflation was ≤120 minutes; this has been changed to reflect the updated guidelines to ≤90 minutes. The reperfusion measure that combines primary PCI and fibrinolysis is expected to clarify performance issues relating to optimal identification and treatment of all patients that are eligible for reperfusion. Use of clopidogrel and ACE-I in patients with LVEF >40% have not been incorporated as yet. Data-to-decision

| | Class I | Class II | Class IIb | Class III |
|---|---|---|---|---|
| | *Benefit >>>Risk* | *Benefit >>>Risk*<br>*Additional studies with focused objectives needed* | *Benefit ≥ Risk*<br>*Additional studies with broad objectives needed; additional registry data would be helpful* | *Risk ≥ Benefit*<br>*No additional studies needed* |
| | **Procedure/treatment SHOULD be performed/ administered** | **IT IS REASONABLE to perform procedure/ administer treatment** | **Procedure/treatment MAY BE CONSIDERED** | **Procedure/treatment should NOT be performed/ administered SINCE IT IS NOT HELPFUL AND MAY BE HARMFUL** |
| **Level A**<br><br>*Multiple (3–5) population risk strata evaluated*<br>*General consistency of direction and magnitude of effect* | • Recommendation that procedure or treatment is useful/effective<br>• Sufficient evidence from multiple randomized trials or meta-analyses | • Recommendation in favor of treatment or procedure being useful/effective<br>• Some conflicting evidence from multiple randomized trials or meta-analyses | • Recommendation's usefulness/efficacy less well established<br>• Greater conflicting evidence from multiple randomized trials or meta-analyses | • Recommendation that procedure or treatment not useful/effective and may be harmful<br>• Sufficient evidence from multiple randomized trials or meta-analyses |
| **Level B**<br><br>*Limited (2–3) population risk strata evaluated* | • Recommendation that procedure or treatment is useful/effective<br>• Limited evidence from single randomized trial or nonrandomized studies | • Recommendation in favor of treatment or procedure being useful/effective<br>• Some conflicting evidence from single randomized trial or nonrandomized studies | • Recommendation's usefulness/efficacy less well established<br>• Greater conflicting evidence from single randomized trial or non-randomized studies | • Recommendation that procedure treatment not useful/effective and may be harmful<br>• Limited evidence from single randomized trial nonrandomized studies |
| **Level C**<br><br>*Very limited (1–2) population risk strata evaluated* | • Recommendation that procedure or treatment is useful/effective<br>• Only expert opinion case studies, or standard-of-care | • Recommendation in favor of treatment or procedure being useful/effective<br>• Only diverging expert opinion, case studies, or standard-of-care | • Recommendation's usefulness/efficacy less well established<br>• Only diverging expert opinion, case studies, or standard-of-care | • Recommendation that procedure or treatment not useful/effective and may be harmful<br>• Only expert opinion, case studies, or standard-of-care |
| **Suggested phrases for writing recommendations** | Should<br>Is recommended<br>Is indicated<br>Is useful/effective/beneficial | Is reasonable<br>Can be useful/effective/beneficial<br>Is probably recommended or indicated | May/might be considered<br>May/might be reasonable<br>Usefulness/effectiveness is unknown/unclear/uncertain or not well established | Is not recommended<br>Is not indicated<br>Should not<br>Is not useful/effective/beneficial<br>May be harmful |

**Figure 5-1.** Estimate of certainty (precision) of treatment effect.

## Table 5-3 • ACC/AHA Performance Measure Sets

| Topic | Publication Date | Partnering Organizations |
|---|---|---|
| Chronic heart failure | 2005 | ACC/AHA—Inpatient measures<br>ACC/AHA/PCPI—Outpatient measures |
| Chronic stable coronary artery disease | 2005 | ACC/AHA/PCPI |
| Hypertension | 2005 | ACC/AHA/PCPI |
| ST-elevation and non-ST-elevation Myocardial infarction | 2006* | ACC/AHA |
| Atrial fibrillation | 2008 | ACC/AHA/PCPI |
| Primary prevention of cardiovascular disease | Pending | ACC/AHA |
| Peripheral arterial disease | Pending | ACC/AHA/ACR/SCAI/SIR/SVM/SVN/SVS |

*At time of publication, undergoing update
PCPI, American Medical Association—Physician Consortium for Performance Improvement; ACR, American College of Radiology; SCAI, Society for Cardiac Angiography and Interventions; SIR, Society for Interventional Radiology; SVM, Society for Vascular Medicine; SVN, Society for Vascular Nursing; SVS, Society for Vascular Surgery

## Table 5-4 • Performance Measure Summary for Chronic Stable Coronary Artery Disease CAD

**Performance Measures Based on Known Risk Factors for CAD**

| | |
|---|---|
| **Hypertension** | Class I, Level-A |
| Blood pressure readings recommended every visit with target blood pressure of:<br><br>  <130/85 mm Hg (CAD and DM, renal or HF)<br><br>  <140/90 mm Hg (CAD and no DM, renal or HF) | % patients with blood pressure taken at last office visit |
| **Lipid profile** | Class I, Level-C |
| Lipid profile performed and include total cholesterol, high-density (HDL-C), low-density lipoprotein cholesterol (LDL-C), and triglycerides | % patients with >1 lipid profile |
| **Smoking cessation** | Class I, Level-C |
| Smoking history and intervention including counseling and therapy with goal of cessation implemented | % patients asked >1 time about smoking at office visit<br><br>% patients who smoke and had an intervention to stop smoking |
| **Symptom and activity assessment** | Class I, Level-C |
| Periodic review of activity level & anginal symptoms | % patients with determination of anginal symptoms & activity level at >1 office visit |
| **Diabetes screening** | Class I, Level-A |
| All high risk CAD patients screened for diabetes | % patients screened for diabetes |

**Performance Measures Based on Medical Therapy for CAD to Reduce Risk**

| | |
|---|---|
| **Antiplatelet** | Class I, Level-A |
| Antiplatelet therapy with aspirin is recommended for CAD patients without contraindications<br><br>If contraindication specific to aspirin substitution with other antiplatelet medications suggested | % patients prescribed antiplatelet therapy<br><br>% patients prescribed antiplatelet therapy, without documented medical reason for not prescribing |
| **Elevated LDL-C** | Class I, Level-A |
| LDL-C treatment target is <100 mg/dL in patients with chronic stable CAD<br><br>If baseline LDL-C ≥130 mg/dL, cholesterol-lowering drug should be prescribed<br><br>All stable CAD patients have lifestyle modification and nonlipid risk factors addressed | % patients prescribed lipid-lowering therapy<br><br>% patients prescribed lipid-lowering therapy, without contraindications (e.g., documented medical or patient reason for not treating is to achieve lower lipid level targets) |
| **Beta-blocker** | Class I , Level-A |
| Recommended that patients with prior MI receive beta-blocker therapy in absence of contraindications | % patients with prior MI prescribed beta-blocker therapy<br><br>% patients with prior MI prescribed beta-blocker therapy, without documented medical or patient reason for not taking |
| **ACE-I or ARB** | A)  Class I, Level-A<br>B)  Class IIa, Level-B |
| A)  All CAD patients with either left ventricular systolic dysfunction (LVSD) and/or diabetes should be prescribed ACE-I (angiotensin converting enzyme inhibitor).<br><br>B)  CAD patients or other vascular disease receive ACE-I treatment.<br><br>If patient intolerant or unable to take ACE-I then angiotensin receptor blocker (ARB) in STEMI patients with either clinical or radiological signs CHF or measured LVEF <40% | % patients with LVSD and/or diabetes prescribed ACE-I or ARB therapy<br><br>% patients with LVSD and/or diabetes prescribed ACE-I or ARB therapy, without medical contraindications or patient reasons for not taking either medication |

| Table 5-5 • Relevant ICD-9-CM Diagnosis Codes for STEMI/NSTEMI | |
|---|---|
| **ICD-9-CM** | **Description** |
| 410.01 | Anterolateral wall, acute myocardial infarction—initial episode |
| 410.11 | Other anterior wall, acute myocardial infarction—initial episode |
| 410.21 | Inferolateral wall, acute myocardial infarction—initial episode |
| 410.31 | Inferoposterior wall, acute myocardial infarction—initial episode |
| 410.41 | Other inferior wall, acute myocardial infarction—initial episode |
| 410.51 | Other lateral wall, acute myocardial infarction—initial episode |
| 410.61 | True posterior wall, acute myocardial infarction—initial episode |
| 410.71 | Subendocardial, acute myocardial infarction—initial episode |
| 410.81 | Other specified sites, acute myocardial infarction—initial episode |
| 410.91 | Unspecified site, acute myocardial infarction—initial episode |

time and decision-to-delivery time as yet have no specific ACC/AHA guidelines, and therefore have no specific performance measures.

**Table 5-6** summarizes the performance measure set for acute myocardial infarction-ST elevation myocardial infarction (AMI-STEMI) and non-ST elevation myocardial infarction (NSTEMI).

## Atrial Fibrillation

Atrial fibrillation (AF) is defined as an arrhythmia that is the result of uncoordinated atrial activity causing a supraventricular tachyarrhythmia that later leads to further deterioration of mechanical function of the atria. The diagnosis of atrial fibrillation is made by ECG criteria of evidence of disorganized atrial activity with the loss of P waves and the presence of fibrillatory waves that vary in amplitude, timing, and duration, as well as an irregular ventricular response. For the performance measures, atrial flutter is included with atrial fibrillation in terms of thromboembolic risk. Only people 18 years of age or older with atrial fibrillation or atrial flutter of nonvalvular cause are included in the guidelines.

Over 2.2 million Americans have been diagnosed with AF, and approximately 9% of people in their eighties have it. There has been a marked increase in incidence over the past two decades as the population ages. Atrial fibrillation

is associated with a high risk of morbidity (heart failure and stroke) and mortality. Its deleterious effects are more pronounced in women. The high and increasing incidence, morbidity, and mortality of AF make it an excellent choice upon which to develop performance measures, per the guidelines for performance measures discussed above.

Atrial fibrillation can be isolated, recurrent ($\geq 2$ episodes), persistent or paroxysmal (self-terminates without cardioversion or pharmacologic treatment), longstanding ($>1$ year) or permanent (episodes last for $>30$ seconds at a time). The set of performance measures given here was developed for AF that lasts for $>30$ seconds an episode and is not the result of a reversible cause (such as hyperthyroidism, pneumonia, pulmonary embolism, other acute pulmonary disease, acute myocardial infarction, myocarditis, pericarditis, cardiac surgery, or other acute illness). For the purposes of the performance measures patients are $\geq 18$ years of age.

The performance measurement set established for atrial fibrillation and atrial flutter, are summarized in **Table 5-7**.

**Table 5-7** shows three key areas:

1. Assessment of thromboembolic risk factors for non-valvular atrial fibrillation.
2. Chronic anticoagulation therapy with warfarin for patients with $>1$ moderate risk factors or any high risk factors. Risk factors for systemic embolism or ischemic stroke were determined from 5 primary prevention randomized trials with untreated control groups. Moderate risk factors are: a history of hypertension (relative risk RR = 1.6), heart failure of reduced LVF ($<35\%$) (RR = 1.4), age $>75$ (RR = 1.4; risk increases by decade, but so does risk of bleeding related to anticoagulation), and diabetes mellitus (RR = 1.7). A history of CVA or TIA (relative risk, RR = 2.5) or systemic embolism is considered at high risk for recurrence. (**Table 5-8** summarizes these performance measures.)
3. Monthly international normalized ratio (INR) measurement quality of anticoagulation such as time maintained within goal INR is not included.

**Table 5-9** summarizes the recommendations for antithrombotic therapy for nonvalvular AF patients based on the guidelines published by the 2006 ACC/AHA/ESC. Weaker or less validated risk factors such as female gender, age 65-74, coronary artery disease (RR = 1.5), and thyrotoxicosis are not considered in the performance measures. A moderate risk translates into a stroke rate of 3-5% a year, high risk is $>5\%$. Performance measures were not established for cardioversion at this time. Performance measures are to be reported for a period of one year.

## Table 5-6 • Summary of AMI-STEMI and NSTEMI

| | |
|---|---|
| **Aspirin on arrival** | Class I, Level-A 162 mg STEMI<br>Class I, Level-C 325 mg STEMI<br>Class I, Level-A USA/NSTEMI |
| Aspirin ≤24 h before or after hospital arrival for AMI-STEMI and NSTEMI patients without aspirin contraindications | % of AMI-STEMI or NSTEMI patients treated with aspirin ≤24h before or after hospitalization. The following patients are excluded: transfers to or form another hospital or emergency room during assessment period, patients left, discharged or expired ≤24 h, contraindication to aspirin therapy (allergy, active bleeding ≤24 h, warfarin use on arrival), or other medical reason documented |
| **Aspirin at discharge** | Class I, Level-A |
| Patients at discharge for AMI-STEMI and NSTEMI prescribed aspirin without aspirin contraindications | % of AMI-STEMI or NSTEMI patients prescribed aspirin at hospital discharge with the following exclusions: transfers to or form another hospital or emergency room during assessment period, patients left, discharged to hospice or expired ≤24 hours, contraindication to aspirin therapy (allergy, active bleeding ≤24 h, warfarin use on arrival, or other medical reason documented) |
| **Beta-blocker on arrival** | Class I, Level-A STEMI<br>Class I, Level-B USA/NSTEMI |
| Beta-blocker ≤24 hours before or after hospital arrival for AMI-STEMI and NSTEMI patients without beta-blocker contraindications | % of AMI-STEMI or NSTEMI patients prescribed beta-blocker ≤24 h of hospitalization for AMI with the following exclusions: transfers to or form another hospital or emergency room ≤ first 24 h, patients left, discharged or expired ≤24 h, contraindication to beta-blocker therapy: allergy, heart rate ≤60 bpm second or third degree heart block on ECG (without pacemaker), shock or CHF ≤24 h or other documented medical reasons |
| **Beta-blocker on discharge** | Class I, Level-A (except low risk post-STEMI)<br>Class IIa, Level-A (low risk post-STEMI) |
| Patients at discharge for AMI-STEMI & NSTEMI prescribed beta-blocker without contraindications for beta-blocker | % of AMI-STEMI or NSTEMI patients prescribed beta-blocker at hospital discharge with the following exclusions: transfers to or from another hospital, patients left, discharged to hospice or expired, contraindication to beta-blocker therapy: allergy, heart rate ≤60 bpm second or third degree heart block on ECG (without pacemaker), or other documented medical reasons |
| **LDL-C assessment** | Class I, Level-C (STEMI only) |
| Patients with AMI-STEMI & NSTEMI recommended to have LDL-C assessment during hospitalization or documented as planned after discharge | % of AMI-STEMI or NSTEMI patients with LDL-C measured during hospitalization or planned post-discharge with following exclusions: transfers to or form another hospital, patients left, discharged to hospice or expired, use of lipid-lowering medication on admission or documented medical reason |
| **Lipid-lowering therapy at discharge** | Class I, Level-A (LDL-C in STEMI >100 mg/dL and USA/NSTEMI >130 mg/dL)<br>Class I, Level-B (LDL-C USA/NSTEMI >100 mg/dL) |
| Patients at discharge for AMI-STEMI & NSTEMI prescribed lipid-lowering therapy for elevated LDL-C ≥100 mg/dL without contraindications to therapy | % of AMI-STEMI or NSTEMI patients prescribed lipid-lowering therapy at hospital discharge with the following exclusions: transfers to or form another hospital, patients left, discharged to hospice or expired, or documented medical reason |
| **ACE-I or ARB for LVSD at discharge** | Class I, Level-A (ACE-I)<br>Class I, Level-C (ARB if not tolerant ACE-I)*:<br>  STEMI ≤24 h if anterior wall, HF or LVEF <40% (without SBP <100 or <30 mm Hg of baseline)<br>Class I, Level A (ACE-I)<br>Class I, Level-B (ARB if not tolerant ACE-I)*:<br>  During recovery from STEMI<br>Class IIA, Level-B:<br>  STEMI substitution of ARB for ACE-I (not intolerant) if signs of HF or LVEF <40%*<br>Class I, Level-A:<br>  UA/NSTEMI long-term medical therapy with ACE-I if HF, LVEF <40%, hypertension or DM<br>  *valsartan or candesartan |
| AMI-STEMI & NSTEMI patients with LVSD should receive ACE-I or ARB at discharge who do not have contraindications | % AMI-STEMI & NSTEMI patients prescribed either ACE-I or ARB at hospital discharge with following exclusions: transfers to or from another hospital, patients left, discharged to hospice or expired, or documented medical reason for not using both ACE-I or ARB (allergy to both, moderate or severe aortic stenosis) |

*(continued)*

| Table 5-6 • (continued) | |
|---|---|
| Time to fibrinolytic therapy | Class I, Level-B:<br>  Initiation of fibrinolytic ≤30 min or PCI ≤90 min<br>Class I, Level-A:<br>  STEMI with rapid evaluation and reperfusion<br>Class I, Level-A:<br>  Acute coronary syndrome with STEMI patients should have assessment for immediate reperfusion therapy<br>Class I, Level-A:<br>  STEMI and new or presumed new LBBB should receive fibrinolytic therapy <12 h of presentation |
| Time measured from arrival of the AMI-STEMI and LBBB patients to administration of fibrinolytic therapy with goal of ≤30 min | AMI-STEMI and new or presumed new LBBB patients with time from presentation at hospital to administration of fibrinolytic therapy <30 min with following exclusions: patients transferred from another hospital or emergency room, or documented medical reason or patient preference. Time period of evaluation is <6 h |
| Time to PCI | Class I, Level-C:<br>  Interpreted 12-lead ECG ≤10 min) of arrival of patient with symptoms of possible STEMI or acute coronary syndrome<br>Class I, Level-A:<br>  STEMI with rapid evaluation and reperfusion<br>Class I, Level-A:<br>  Acute coronary syndrome with STEMI patients should be assessed for immediate reperfusion therapy<br>Class I, Level-B STEMI:<br>  If PCI chosen time from presentation to balloon inflation ≤90 min<br>Class I, Level-A ACS and STEMI:<br>  If PCI, time from presentation to balloon inflation ≤90 min and <12 h of symptom onset by skilled personnel (>75 PCI/year) and experienced lab (>200 PCI/yr, 36 primary PCI for STEMI) and cardiac surgery capability |
| Time measured from arrival of the AMI-STEMI and LBBB patients to administration of PCI therapy with a goal of ≤90 min | % of AMI-STEMI and LBBB patients with PCI ≤90 min of presentation with the following exclusions: patients transferred from other hospital or emergency room, prior administration of fibrinolytic for presenting episode, nonprimary PCI, or other medical or patient reason documented |
| Reperfusion therapy | Class I, Level-A |
| Patients with ST-segment elevation on the electrocardiogram (ECG) with AMI-STEMI should receive prompt fibrinolytics therapy or primary PCI | % of AMI-STEMI patients with reperfusion using fibrinolytic therapy or primary PCI with the following exclusions: medical or patient reason for not using reperfusion therapy |
| Smoking cessation | Class I, Level-C STEMI:<br>  Should receive counseling and medical therapy for smoking cessation during hospitalization, discharge, and cardiac rehabilitation<br>Class I, Level-B STEMI:<br>  Patients with a history of smoking cigarettes should be counseled to stop smoking and avoid secondhand smoke, as well as pharmacological therapy and smoking cessation programs<br>Class I, level B evidence UA/NSTEMI:<br>  All should receive information on smoking cessation<br>Class I, Level-A evidence UA/NSTEMI:<br>  All should be referred to smoking cessation program |
| All AMI-STEMI & NSTEMI patients who smoke cigarettes should receive smoking cessation counseling | % of AMI-STEMI & NSTEMI patients who smoke cigarettes who get smoking cessation counseling during hospitalization with the following exclusions: patient transferred to or form another hospital, patient left, discharged to hospice or expired |

# 6

# Biostatistics for the Clinical Cardiologist

LAURA F. WHITE AND LISA M. SULLIVAN

---

### ● PRACTICAL POINTS

- The basic approach to collection of data is sampling, i.e., obtaining data from a subset of the study population.

- The larger the sample the more accurately it estimates the population values.

- Of the various study designs, the randomized clinical trial is the gold standard.

- Data variables are classified as discrete, e.g., gender, presence or absence of a disease state, etc.; or continuous e.g., body weight, cholesterol level, etc.

- Data can be summarized in various ways, e.g., mean and standard deviation for continuous data, odds ratio or risk ratio for dichotomous data, and hazard ratio for time-to-event outcomes.

- Confidence interval estimates help to quantify uncertainty.

- Hypothesis testing involves stating the null and alternative hypotheses, setting the Type 1 error rate, calculating the appropriate test statistic and determining $p$-value.

- Bias and confounding can lead to erroneous conclusions. Appropriate randomization and blinding of subjects and researchers is important. Regression analysis is a method of decreasing confounding.

- An important medical application of statistical and probability theory is the assessment of the performance of diagnostic medical tests.

---

Research attempts to study and learn more about the unknown. Statistical analysis is a powerful tool, assisting the researcher in making statements about that which is unknown using available data; it also provides a way to describe how confident the researcher can be about these statements, using the concepts of probability. For instance, one might wish to study the efficacy of a new drug proposed to reduce systolic blood pressure (SBP). It is not known prior to the study how effective this drug might be, so the researcher designs a study to test whether the new drug is more effective than a placebo or another drug that is currently in use (i.e., an active control). She might wish to assess whether a new biomarker is useful in predicting whether a patient is likely to develop cardiovascular disease. In what follows, we outline key issues and general approaches to conducting

statistical analyses. Many other issues and details are left uncovered. Interested readers should see D'Agostino et al. (2005) and Pagano and Gavreau (2000) for more in-depth discussion.

## UNIT OF ANALYSIS

To begin a research study, it is important one identify the *unit of analysis*. The unit of analysis is the entity on which data are measured. In many instances, data are measured on people. It is important to understand whether there are relationships among the units (people) under study, because most statistical procedures assume that each data element or observation is measured in an independent unit (i.e., in unrelated persons). It is important to know whether data come from families where there are important genetic and environmental similarities between family members that must be considered. As an example, there are familial relationships in the Framingham Heart Study (mother-father-child and among siblings). If a father has a myocardial infarction (MI), his child may have an elevated risk of experiencing an MI as compared to the risk in an unrelated individual. Analysis of genetic predictors of future disease explicitly account for familial relationships in statistical models (see Lange, 1999; Ott, 1997 for more information).

Another situation that creates lack of independence is one in which multiple observations are obtained on the same person in a study. For example, in the Framingham Heart Study clinical examinations are performed on each member of the original cohort approximately every 2 years and on each member of the offspring cohort approximately every 4 years (Dawber et al. 1951). Measurements within the same individual tend to be correlated (e.g., systolic blood pressure measured at one point in time is related to SBP measured 2 or 4 years earlier in the same individual). In the analysis of such data we need to account for these dependencies. Independent data arise from subjects or objects that are chosen at random and have no apparent relationships with one another. A key question that one can ask in determining if the data are independent is whether knowledge about one data point in the study influences knowledge about another data point.

## GENERAL APPROACH: SAMPLING

Once we have identified what we are going to study, we must determine how to obtain data. In order to study and better understand the unknown, statistical analysis focuses on working with samples. For example, we might be interested in estimating the average systolic blood pressure (SBP) for all females between the ages of 45 and 65 in the United States. The population is the collection of all units, and thus, females between the ages of 45 and 65 make up the population. It would be too expensive, time-consuming, and likely not possible to collect the SBP for all of the women in the population. **Figure 6-1** illustrates the approach. We take a random sample (a subset of females between the ages of 45 and 65) of 30 women from the population and measure their individual SBPs. From the average of these SBPs we can estimate the population level SBP. While this value is not likely to exactly estimate the true SBP in the population, it is our best estimate. The number of units (in this case, women) we select to obtain this estimate depends on several factors. These include the variability of the outcome (estimating outcomes that are more variable requires more individuals to ensure that estimates are sufficiently precise) and how precise the estimate needs to be (specifically, how close does the estimate need to be to the true population

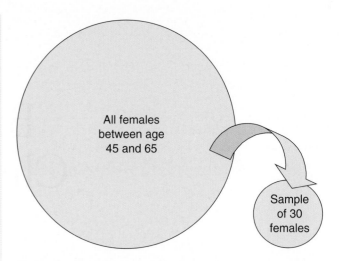

**Figure 6-1.** Sampling from the population.

value for it to be useful). In general, the more data collected, the less variable the estimates, and so the estimates obtained from the sample more precisely estimate the true population values. Sample size determination for studies is discussed in detail in Lenth (2001). In what follows we provide an overview of methods for obtaining samples (study designs), techniques for estimation, and general approaches to testing hypotheses.

## STUDY DESIGNS

To initiate data collection we must carefully select a method for obtaining data that will minimize bias, confounding (see Multivariable Methods Section) and other systematic errors in our data. We now discuss some of the more common study designs and refer the interested reader to Rothman and Greenland (2008) for more detailed discussion. Study designs can be grouped into two major categories: observational studies and experimental studies. There are limitations and strengths with each study design.

### Case Series

Case series involve a summary of the common features of a small sample of cases with the intent of isolating their unique and similar features. Among the main uses of these studies are identifying new diseases and generating hypotheses for further study. Case series are typically simple to implement, inexpensive, but also unplanned and lacking controls for comparison.

### Case-control

Case-control studies identify participants for a sample based on their outcome status (e.g., patients with brain aneurysm versus those without). Specifically, one set of individuals that are diseased (cases) is selected, while another set of individuals who are not diseased but are otherwise similar to the diseased participants (controls) is selected. Information is then collected on all the participants with regard to potential exposures retrospectively.

This design is particularly useful in studying rare outcomes because it allows one to identify an adequately large number of cases for study. Case-control studies are also relatively inexpensive to carry out and do not tend to require a long time to perform. From these studies we can identify potential exposures that are correlated with the outcome of interest.

There are several issues with case-control studies, including the tendency for bias to be introduced. Misclassification, selection, and recall bias are all potential problems in these studies (see Confounding and Bias Section). Additionally, it is often not possible to infer temporal relationships between exposures and outcomes because the data on exposure and outcomes are collected at the same time. It is also not possible to estimate incidence of the outcome in these studies.

## Cohort

Cohort studies are performed by identifying a group of individuals for the study sample who meet specific inclusion criteria and following them for a period of time to identify associations between risk factors and disease. For instance, we might wish to study a group of individuals who are at high risk of MI, or we might wish to follow a group that would be representative of the general population. Examples of large cohort studies of representative populations include the Framingham Heart Study, the Nurses' Health Study, and the Black Women's Health Study (Dawber et al., 1951; Belanger et al., 1978; Rosenberg et al., 1995). Once the cohort is identified, information is collected on participants periodically and the data can be analyzed. These studies are useful in that they do not put participants at risk by exposing them to new drugs or interventions; rather, they allow for assessment of temporal relationships between exposures and outcomes and they estimate incidence of disease.

Cohort studies must be designed to be large enough so that researchers can be confident they will observe an adequate number of outcome events or diseased individuals for a study. For this reason these studies are not ideal for rare outcomes. Loss to follow-up is a challenge as it can be difficult to keep participants enrolled over time since people move, die, or lose interest in participation. Additionally, these studies are subject to confounding, because it is challenging to understand and control for all the factors that contribute to disease acquisition. We can observe associations in these studies, but these are always subject to unmeasured confounding. For an interesting commentary on some of the weaknesses of these studies, see Taubes (2007).

## Randomized Clinical Trials (RCT)

Randomized clinical trials are the gold standard from a statistical point of view in experimental designs. Here the researcher controls the exposure status of the individuals by randomly assigning participants to either a particular intervention or the control group, which receives the standard of care or a placebo. In theory, if there is an effect of the intervention, it is due to that intervention because all other factors that can lead to disease development are randomly distributed between the comparison groups. Randomized trials can investigate one intervention or several interventions against a control group. When ethically possible and feasible, a placebo can be used for the control group. When this is not possible then the standard of care should be used for the control group (an active control).

Bias can be reduced in these studies by *blinding*. Ideally, *double blinding* should be used, wherein both the subject and the researcher measuring the outcome are blinded as to which group the participant is assigned. Blinding is not always feasible; for example, when one of the interventions is a surgical intervention and the other is not. Because we are able to control confounding and reduce bias, the analysis of randomized trials allows us to be more certain that differences in the outcomes between intervention groups can be attributable to the differences in the intervention.

The major disadvantages of these studies are that they are expensive and can be time-consuming. However, when they are appropriately performed, randomized trials are the means for establishing the efficacy of new treatments and interventions. For more information see Chow and Liu (2004).

## CLASSIFICATION OF VARIABLES

Statistical procedures differ depending on how the data are measured, specifically how variables are classified. There are typically three categories of data: discrete, continuous, and time-to-event data. *Discrete data* are data that assume only a finite number of values, for instance, gender (male or female), presence of hypertension (yes or no), and level of agreement with a statement (strongly agree, agree, neutral, disagree, strongly disagree). By contrast, *continuous data* can take on any value within a range of values. For instance, body weight, cholesterol level, and systolic blood pressure are examples of continuous variables. Time-to-event data are data that reflect the time between some prespecified starting point and the occurrence of a specific outcome. For instance, we might study the time until a patient has an MI or the time until patients with hypertension on treatment return to nonhypertensive status. In studies that measure time-to-event data, we are not likely to observe the event in every patient. There is usually a specified observation period, for example 10 years. The fact that some patients go the entire study time without the event is informative. *Time-to-event data* include the time the patient was in the study as well as an indicator of whether he or she experienced the outcome of interest (having an MI or recovery) or not. If participants do not have the event during the observation period, this is termed *censoring* (see Hosmer and Lemeshow, 1999, for more details).

# SUMMARIZING DATA

The first step in any statistical analysis is to appropriately summarize the data collected sample. We describe appropriate measures for summarizing single variables and then for comparing groups. These measures depend on the type of data collected.

## Continuous Data

Continuous variables are summarized using a measure of central tendency and of variability. The mean and standard deviation of the data are appropriate when there are no outliers; when outliers exist, the median and the interquartile range (Q1 to Q3) are most appropriate.

For example, consider an RCT designed to test the effectiveness of a new treatment to reduce systolic blood pressure. **Table 6-1** provides a description of patients in terms of characteristics measured at the start of the study (i.e., baseline).

When comparing groups with respect to a continuous variable, we typically compare the means between groups. Let $\mu_1$ and $\mu_2$ be the true, unknown population means of the two groups that we wish to compare. We estimate the difference in the true means $\mu_1 - \mu_2$ by examining the difference in the observed sample means. For example, we might want to estimate the difference in mean systolic blood pressures between those receiving an intervention and those in a control group. To best do this, we estimate the mean SBP for both groups from our sample data and take the difference.

## Dichotomous Outcomes

Appropriate summaries of dichotomous data include the *number of the units* with a specified response, the *proportion* of units with this response, and the *odds* of the response.

Let $x$ denote the number of individuals in a sample who develop MI over 5 years and n denote the total number of individuals in the sample (with and without MI at the start of the study). The proportion who develop MI is $p = x/n$. The odds of MI for this sample is defined as the ratio of the number of persons who develop MI to the number who do not, odds = $x/(n - x)$. Equivalently, the odds $= p/(1 - p)$.

There are several ways to express differences in outcomes between two groups (for instance, the proportions of diabetics versus nondiabetics who develop MI). Here, the goal is to compare the proportions between groups. First, let $p_1$ and $p_2$ be the respective proportions of diabetics and nondiabetics in the population who develop MI. There are several commonly used *measures of effect* for dichotomous outcomes:

- risk difference: $p_1 - p_2$
- relative risk: $p_1/p_2$
- odds ratio: $[p_1/(1 - p_1)]/[p_2/(1 - p_2)]$.

We estimate these using the observed sample data, specifically observed proportions in the two comparison groups. Of the ratio measures (relative risk and odds ratio), relative risk is more intuitive. However, in case-control studies, it is not possible to estimate a relative risk. Rather, the odds ratio can be estimated and used to summarize the association between the exposure or risk factor and the outcome. When the proportion of outcome events is low in the total sample, the odds ratio is close in value to the relative risk.

## Time-to-Event Outcomes

A common way to summarize time-to-event data is through the hazard rate. The *hazard rate* is the rate of a particular outcome (for instance, dying) conditional on time. For instance, if we have a study with 100 individuals and 15 of them die in the first month, then the hazard rate for the first month is 15/100. If another 5 pass away in the second month, then the hazard rate for that month is 5/85.

| Table 6-1 • Baseline Characteristics of RCT for High Blood Pressure Treatment* | | |
|---|---|---|
| **Baseline Characteristics** | **Treatment** (*n* = 100) | **Control** (*n* = 100) |
| Age, years | 54.2 (4.6) | 52.9 (4.7) |
| % male | 47% | 43% |
| Total serum cholesterol | 209.3 (202–275) | 212.4 (200–282) |
| Systolic blood pressure, mm Hg | 125.3 (15.9) | 127.3 (16.1) |
| % hypertensive | 24% | 22% |

*Mean and standard deviation (SD) or median and interquartile range (Q1 to Q3) are shown for continuous variables (age, total serum cholesterol, and systolic blood pressure); percent is shown for dichotomous outcomes (gender and hypertensivity). Because total serum cholesterol can be skewed due to extremely high values, both median and Q1 to Q3 are presented.

To compare two groups with respect to the time-to-event, we use the *hazard ratio*, which is the ratio of the hazard rates for each group. For instance we might wish to compare the rate of recovering from hypertension for those on a placebo or active control versus those on a new drug. Once the study is complete, we can calculate the hazard rate for each treatment group and then calculate the ratio of these rates.

## GENERAL APPROACH TO ESTIMATION

We have just described measures that can be used to summarize data. Summary measures from a sample are estimates of unknown population parameters. These estimates are called *point estimates*, and are the best single-valued estimates of the unknown population values. For instance, in the General Sampling Section we described a sample of 30 females between 45 and 65 years was used to obtain an estimate of the SBP for *all* women between 45 and 65 years old. This is our best estimate of the true SBP in the population. It is clear that this estimate is likely not equal to the true value of the SBP in the population, so it is important that we quantify the *precision* of the estimate.

The precision of an estimate is based on its variability and the sample size. Many analysts produce *confidence interval* estimates as a means of quantifying uncertainty. The confidence interval takes the form of a point estimate ± margin of error; the margin of error is the product of the *confidence level* and the *standard error* (or the *variability* of the point estimate). To generate a confidence interval, we select a confidence level. Usually confidence levels of 90%, 95%, or 99% are used. The confidence level can be interpreted in the following manner. If we were to assemble 100 different samples and create a separate confidence interval for each (i.e., 100 confidence intervals) the confidence level would describe the percentage of the intervals that would contain or cover the true value of the population mean. The confidence interval is then a range of values that are likely to include the true unknown SBP in the population at the confidence level stated. For more details see Sullivan (2006).

## GENERAL APPROACH TO HYPOTHESIS TESTING

Hypothesis testing is a systematic procedure to discover the truth of a statement about a population using sample data. Consider again our example in which we want to test whether a new drug is effective in reducing systolic blood pressure when compared to a placebo.

- *State the null and alternative hypotheses.* The *null hypothesis* is a statement of no effect or status quo. It implies that any observed effect might be due to chance alone (sampling variability). The alternative hypothesis is typically a statement of effect or what we would like to prove. In our example, the null hypothesis reflects no difference in mean systolic blood pressures in subjects taking the new drug versus placebo; the alternative hypothesis states there is an effect of lower systolic blood pressure in patients taking the new drug.
- *Set the Type I error rate (or alpha level, or level of significance).* The *Type I error rate* indicates the probability of rejecting the null hypothesis when it is really true. This is usually set at 0.05.
- *Calculate an appropriate test statistic.* The *test statistic* is a single-number summary of the data that is measured in the sample. For instance, in our randomized clinical trial example the test statistic would quantify the difference in the mean systolic blood pressures in patients taking the new drug versus placebo. The test statistic also incorporates an estimate of the variability of this difference.
- *Determine the p-value.* The *p-value* indicates the chance of observing the data (or test statistic) by chance alone if the null hypothesis is true. If the p-value is less than the Type I error rate, then we reject the null hypothesis in favor of the alternative. In our example, the p-value is computed by comparing the observed test statistic to the distribution of all possible test statistics, assuming that the null hypothesis is true. In our example, the observed test statistic essentially reflects the observed difference in the mean SBPs between groups.

As an alternative example, we might wish to test in an observational study whether the proportion of diabetics who develop MI is different from the proportion of nondiabetics who develop MI. In this case we would use as our test statistic the risk difference, relative risk, or odds ratio to summarize the effect. If we use relative risk or odds ratio, our null hypothesis would indicate that these measures have a value of one (no effect) in the population. The alternative hypothesis would be that the relative risk or odds ratio is different from one. If we use the risk difference then the null hypothesis would be that the risk difference is zero and the alternative would state that it is not. The steps of hypothesis testing outlined above would again be followed to test this hypothesis.

When a test of hypothesis is significant (e.g., $p < 0.05$), we can be comfortable that the data support the alternative hypothesis because we control the probability that this conclusion is in error (by selecting a small Type I error rate). However, if we fail to reach significance, it may be that, in fact, there is no effect, or it may be that we have committed a Type II error. A *Type II error* is a failure to reject the null hypothesis when it is false. When a test fails to reject the null hypothesis this conclusion may be in error. Unfortunately, we cannot simply set a Type II error rate at the outset as it depends on the Type I error rate, the sample size, and the effect. The best safeguard is to plan the study carefully to ensure that the sample size is large enough to minimize the Type II error rate or to maximize the *power* of the test, which is the probability that the test will reject a null hypothesis when in fact it is false. The power of a test is equal to 1 – Type II error rate.

We have discussed the general approach to estimation and hypothesis testing for comparing two groups. The procedures can be extended to make comparisons among more than two groups. In general the procedures to compare two groups assume that the groups being compared are independent (i.e., the participants in one group are different from participants in the other, as discussed in the randomized clinical trial example. There are situations where this is not true. For example, a *crossover study* is one in which participants are measured under both the experimental treatment and then the control. Thus, the two comparison groups are correlated since they are composed of the same individuals, and this needs to be reconciled in the analysis.

## CONFOUNDING AND BIAS

*Bias* is a systematic error in a study that leads to uncertainty about the estimates generated from the study. Bias can be introduced into a study through the following: the way information is collected on subjects; the methods used to select subjects for inclusion in a study; the attitudes and preconceived ideas and beliefs of researchers; failure to adjust for confounders in the analysis. There are many types of bias, some examples are:

- *Recall bias.* Often in studies, subjects are asked to recall information about their past. The bias here is introduced when different groups that are being compared recall information differently. For instance it might be that those who are diseased are more likely to accurately recall exposures to potentially harmful sources than those who are healthy.
- *Interviewer bias.* This bias occurs when subjects are interviewed and the interviewer and/or the questions are not completely objective and guide the participant to favor particular responses.
- *Selection bias.* This arises when those who agree to participate in a study are somehow different than the population that they are presumed to represent. For instance, it may be that only those who are less sick

decide to participate and the reason that they are not as sick is because the exposure that is being studied does not have as severe of an impact on them as those who decide not to participate in the study.
- *Misclassification bias.* Here subjects are incorrectly classified as cases or controls or their exposure status may be incorrectly classified. This type of bias can either dampen the observed effect (if it is done equally systematically) or can exaggerate the effect (if one group is misclassified more often than another).

Bias can be reduced in studies by using appropriate randomization techniques, blinding subjects and researchers to the interventions being studied, and collecting adequate amounts of data so that confounding variables can be controlled for in the analysis (see *Sica, 2006*, for more information). The latter approach is described in the Multivariable Methods Section.

In RCTs, assuming that the randomization is effective in creating comparison groups that are similar in all ways except for the intervention, we can be confident that an observed effect is attributable to the intervention and not to another factor. However, in other designs we may wish to quantify the association between a specific risk factor or exposure and an outcome; and participants with and without the risk factor may be different. For example, suppose we wish to assess the association between total serum cholesterol and coronary heart disease (CHD). We may find that individuals with higher total serum cholesterol are far more likely to suffer CHD. However, this crude or unadjusted analysis may be misleading. We must consider whether there might be other characteristics or risk factors that explain or account for this association. In **Figure 6-2** we can see that cholesterol is correlated with age as an older person is more likely to have higher cholesterol. Additionally, age is correlated with CHD. So, if we were to only consider the relationship between cholesterol and CHD, it might be somewhat exaggerated since the impact of age is absorbed in cholesterol. These kinds of complex relationships among variables are called *confounding*.

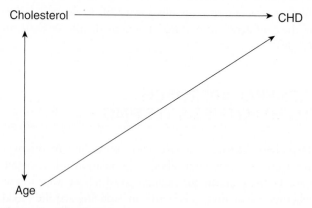

**Figure 6-2.** Confounding.

In the Framingham Heart Study, for example, participants indicated, among other things, their age, and whether they had diabetes. Their SBP was also measured. The average SBP for diabetics was 148.3 mm Hg and for nondiabetics it was 132.5 mm Hg. However the average age was 55.4 years for diabetics and 49.8 for nondiabetics. When we account for the age differences, the average SBP is 142.8 mm Hg for diabetics and 136.2 mm Hg for nondiabetics (See the Multivariable Methods Section for more details). Accounting for the age difference, sometimes called "adjusting for age," leads to a significant change in the estimated means for each group, indicating that age is a confounder of the relationship between diabetes and SBP. This is likely because diabetics tend to be older and older individuals tend to have higher SBP.

## MULTIVARIABLE METHODS

Multivariable statistical methods can be used to adjust for confounding. Specifically, *multivariable methods* allow us to consider the impact or relationship between many variables simultaneously. Typically this is done through a *regression model*. These models have one variable that we wish to predict or study in greater depth, for example systolic blood pressure, incidence of disease, or time until death. This variable is call the *outcome* or *dependent variable*. We are interested in determining its relation to *predictors* of interest, for instance the treatment regime, a biomarker, or some behavioral attribute, such as smoking. These predictors of interest are called the *independent variables*. In some applications we are interested in the association between each independent variable and the outcome, adjusting for other variables, and in other applications, we are specifically interested in one predictor but recognize that to assess its association with the outcome, we need to adjust for potential confounders. Regression analysis follows a general framework, outlined below.

Specific regression models are used depending on the type of outcome variable considered (see **Table 6-2** below).

### Linear Regression

Linear regression is used when the outcome variable is continuous. For instance, suppose we want to determine the

| Table 6-2 • Common Regression Models by Type of Outcome | |
|---|---|
| **Type of Outcome Variable** | **Regression Model Used** |
| Continuous | Linear |
| Dichotomous | Logistic |
| Time-to-event | Cox proportional hazards |

effect of smoking on systolic blood pressure. We would use a linear regression model and could control for important confounders, such as age and gender. In this framework, we would construct the following model:

$$SBP = \beta_0 + \beta_1 \, smoking + \beta_2 \, age + \beta_3 \, gender + error$$

Linear regression methods would use the data we collect from our study sample to generate estimates of the regression coefficients $\beta_0$, $\beta_1$, $\beta_2$, $\beta_3$. The regression coefficients reflect the change in the outcome ($SBP$) relative to a one unit change in the predictor, controlling for other variables in the model (or assuming that the other variables are held constant). A positive regression coefficient indicates that the predictor is directly associated with the outcome, whereas a negative regression coefficient indicates that the predictor is inversely associated with the outcome. For instance, if the estimate of $\beta_2$ is positive, then a one-unit increase in age is associated with a $\beta_2$-unit increase in SBP, holding smoking status and gender constant. If the estimate of $\beta_1$ is positive, then, on average, smokers' SBP is $\beta_1$ units higher than nonsmokers' SBP, holding age and gender constant.

### Logistic Regression

Logistic regression is used when the outcome variable is dichotomous. Logistic regression models are slightly more complicated in that they model the natural logarithm of the odds of the outcome. Suppose that we are interested in determining variables that are associated with the incidence of MI; a logistic regression model is appropriate. If we use the same predictor variables as above for SBP, our model looks like the following:

$$\log(odds \, of \, \mathrm{MI}) = \log\left(\frac{p_{\mathrm{MI}}}{1 - p_{\mathrm{MI}}}\right) = \beta_0 + \beta_1 \, smoking + \beta_2 \, age + \beta_3 \, gender + error$$

where $p_{\mathrm{MI}}$ is the probability of developing myocardial infarction. Again we use the data we collect from our study sample to generate estimates of the regression coefficients, $\beta_0$, $\beta_1$, $\beta_2$, $\beta_3$. The regression coefficients in logistic regression reflect the change in the log odds of the outcome relative to a one unit change in the predictor, controlling for other variables in the model (or assuming that the other variables are held constant). To promote interpretability, we generally exponentiate the estimates of the $\beta_i$ which produce odds ratios. For instance, $\exp(\beta_1)$ expresses the odds of having an MI for smokers as compared to nonsmokers. Similarly, $\exp(\beta_2)$ expresses the odds of having an MI taking into consideration a one-year increase in age. Again, a positive coefficient indicates an increase in the odds of the outcome relative to a one-unit change in the predictor.

## Cox Proportional Hazards Regression

Finally, *Cox proportional hazards regression models* are used for time-to-event data. These models consider the natural logarithm of the hazard function $h(t)$ of the outcome on the left hand side of the regression equation. For instance, consider a 10-year clinical trial involving patients with a history of MI in which the subjects are randomized to a new intervention or control treatment, and the outcome of interest is time-to-death. In addition to treatment regime, we might control for age, gender, and smoking status. Our model would look like:

$$\log(h(t)) = h_0(t) + \beta_1 \, smoking + \beta_2 \, age + \beta_3 \, gender + \beta_4 \, treatment + error$$

In this model, $h(t)$ is the hazard at time $t$ in the study, and $h_0(t)$ is the baseline hazard and is interpreted as the hazard of dying when all of the predictor variables are zero. In this model, treatment is an indicator of receiving the new intervention, and $\exp(\beta_4)$ is the hazard ratio comparing the hazard of dying for those receiving the new intervention versus those in the control group, controlling for age, gender and smoking status.

Regression models are powerful statistical tools, but they must be used with care. There are several assumptions required for the appropriate use of each model. The assumptions must be tested and analyzed prior to estimating models and most importantly in interpreting the model results (see Vittinghoff, 2005, for more details).

## DIAGNOSTIC TESTS

Lastly, we discuss an important medical application of statistical and probability theory to assess the performance of diagnostic tests, which are essential tools in clinical practice. For example, creatine kinase (CK) is routinely measured in emergency patients as a marker for MI, injury, and several other conditions where muscle is damaged. The clinical cutoff for a high level of CK has been previously set at 200 U/L. However not all patients with an elevated level of CK will have muscle damage, and not all patients with muscle damage will have an elevated level of CK. This is a limitation of all diagnostic tests.

There is no test that will perfectly determine every time whether a patient has a given illness or condition. It is important to understand how well the tests perform, and there are several measures that we discuss to understand performance. Cutoffs used to determine whether someone is sick or not are chosen so as to optimize *sensitivity* and *specificity*. Sensitivity is defined as the probability that a test comes back positive for disease given that the individual is

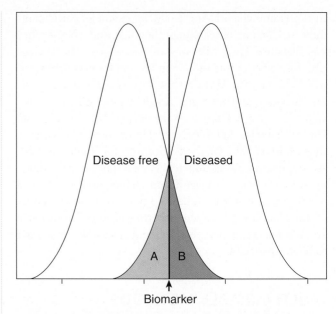

**Figure 6-3.** Illustration of the trade-off between sensitivity and specificity. The distributions of a particular biomarker are shown for those with disease and those without. The arrow indicates the cutoff to be used by the diagnostic test. Those with values of the biomarker higher than the cutoff are considered positive for disease, while those with values less are considered negative for disease. By choosing a cutoff for the test as indicated, region A indicates the false negatives and region B the false positives.

truly sick. Specificity is the probability that the test comes back negative given that the individual is not sick. There is inevitably a trade-off between sensitivity and specificity of a test. **Figure 6-3** illustrates this challenge and the inevitable misclassification that will arise. As the figure shows, there are individuals who are not correctly classified as diseased or nondiseased. Ideally, we want a test that has high sensitivity *and* high specificity. This is not always possible. The acceptability of a test depends on the implications of errors, specifically false positives and false negatives, which are quantified by 1-specificity and 1-sensitivity, respectively.

Patients are generally more interested in the positive and negative predictive values of a test. The *positive predictive value* is the probability that a patient who tests positive actually has the disease. This value depends upon the prevalence of the disease, or proportion of diseased individuals in the population, and can be calculated as:

$$PPV = \frac{Number\ of\ True\ Positives}{Number\ of\ True\ Positives + Number\ of\ False\ Positives}$$

$$= \frac{(sensitivity)(prevalence)}{(sensitivity)(prevalence) + (1 - specificity)(1 - prevalence)}$$

Similarly the *negative predictive value* defines the probability that a patient with a negative test is actually disease free. It is calculated as:

$$NPV = \frac{Number\ of\ True\ Negatives}{Number\ of\ True\ Negatives + Number\ of\ False\ Negatives}$$

$$= \frac{(specificity)(1 - prevalence)}{(specificity)(1 - prevalence) + (1 - sensitivity)(prevalence)}$$

For further information on diagnostic testing see Altman (1994) and Altman and Bland (1994).

## CONCLUSION

Statistical analysis is critical in medical research. Attention to study design, classification of variables, and details of specific techniques is important. It is extremely important that researchers recognize the limitations of statistical analysis, and most importantly, addressing of bias and confounding at the design and analysis stages. While certainly not comprehensive, this chapter has discussed some of the key issues in designing studies, summarizing data that is obtained from the study, and performing analyses in the sample data in order to better understand the population.

### References

1. Altman, DG. Statistics Notes: Diagnostic tests 2: predictive values, *BMJ.* 1994;309:102.

2. Altman DG, Bland JM. Statistics Notes: Diagnostic tests 1: sensitivity and specificity. *BMJ.* 1994;308:1552.

3. Belanger CF, Hennekens CH, Rosner B, Speizer FE. The Nurses' Health Study. *Am J Nurs.* 1978;78:1039–1040.

4. Chow SC, Liu JP. *Design and Analysis of Clinical Trials: Concepts and Methodologies.* New York: John Wiley and Sons; 2004.

5. D'Agostino R, Sullivan L, Beiser A. *Introductory Applied Biostatistics.* Florence, KY: Brooks Cole; 2005.

6. Dawber TR, Meadors GF, Moore FE Jr. Epidemiological approaches to heart disease: the Framingham Study. *Am J Public Health.* 1951;41 (3):279–286.

7. Hosmer DW, Lemeshow S. *Applied Survival Analysis: Regression Modeling of Time to Event Data.* NewYork: John Wiley and Sons; 1999.

8. Lange K. *Mathematical and Statistical Methods for Genetic Analysis.* Springer-Verlag, New York; 1997.

9. Lenth RV. Some practical guidelines for effective sample size determination. *Am Statistic.* 2001;55, 187–193.

10. Ott J. *Analysis of Human Genetic Linkage.* 3rd ed. Johns Hopkins University Press, Baltimore; 1999.

11. Pagano M, Gauvreau K. *Principles of Biostatistics.* Pacific Grove, CA: Duxbury Press; 2000.

12. Rosenberg L, Adams-Campbell L, Palmer JR. The Black Women's Health Study: a follow-up study for causes and preventions of illness. *J Am Med Wom Assoc.* 1995;50:56–58.

13. Rothman KJ, Greenland S, Lash TL. *Mod Epidemiol.* 3rd ed. Lippincott Williams & Wilkins; 2008.

14. Sica GT. Bias in research studies. *Radiology.* 2006;238: 780–789.

15. Sullivan LM. Statistical primer for cardiovascular research: estimation from samples. *Circulation.* 2006;114:445–449.

16. Taubes, Gary. "Do We Really Know What Makes Us Healthy?" *New York Times Magazine,* 16 Sept 2007.

17. Vittinghoff E, Glidden D, McCulloch CE, Shiboski SC. *Regression Methods in Biostatistics: Linear, Logistic, Survival, and Repeated Measures Models.* New York: Springer; 2005.

# $\cdot 7$

# Molecular Biology of Cardiovascular Disease

CALUM A. MACRAE

## ● PRACTICAL POINTS

- The ability to interpret genomic information will be an important part of clinical care in the near future.

- A careful family history is critical for the diagnosis and management of inherited disease even if genetic testing is available.

- The presence of a Mendelian disease in a first-degree relative dramatically changes the prior probability of the same disease in the patient.

- Genotyping, like any other testing, must be interpreted in the context of the relevant clinical information.

- Family history remains the most robust risk predictor for inherited cardiomyopathies or arrhythmias associated with sudden death.

- Clinical assessment of the entire patient is a key factor in the diagnosis of inherited cardiac disease as diagnostic features may be present outside the cardiovascular system.

- Genetic association studies have identified only a small fraction of the known inherited risk for most cardiovascular conditions.

- Genetic testing for the prediction of drug responses is already in clinical use, and will become more prevalent.

- Federal online genetic testing resources offer the most up-to-date information on the availability and utility of genetic testing.

- Care must be taken in the delivery of genetic information to the patient as there are many unanticipated consequences, and genetic counseling is often required over a prolonged period of time.

## MOLECULAR BASIS OF CARDIOVASCULAR DISEASE

There is a growing body of knowledge regarding the specific molecular determinants of clearly familial (Mendelian or "monogenic") cardiovascular conditions, such as familial hypercholesterolemia, hypertrophic cardiomyopathy, and the long QT syndrome. For such rare, Mendelian, diseases mutations in a single gene may lead to profound clinical manifestations in individual families. However, more common "complex" cardiovascular diseases, such as coronary heart disease, are the leading cause of death and disability in men and women. For these complex diseases, the overall contribution of genetic factors to disease onset and severity may be modest relative to the contribution from environmental determinants.

The National Institutes of Health-sponsored Human Genome Project completed the sequencing of the human genome in 2001. This achievement has dramatically enhanced the capacity to examine associations between common, "complex" diseases and genetic variation across the entire genome. The discovery of specific genotype–cardiovascular disease associations may have uses in the development of new and improved drug therapies as well as novel strategies for diagnosis, screening, and prevention. The resulting exponential growth

71

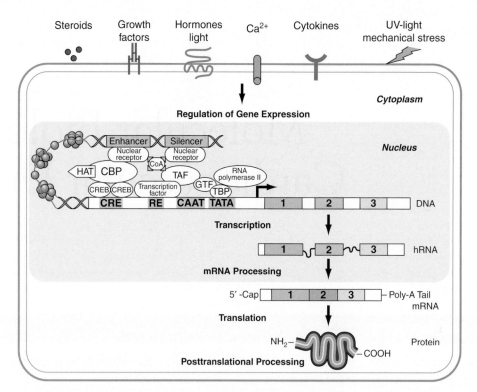

**Figure 7-1.** Flow of genetic information. Multiple extracellular signals activate intracellular signal cascades that result in altered regulation of gene expression through the interaction of transcription factors with regulatory regions of genes. RNA polymerase transcribes DNA into RNA that is processed to mRNA by excision of intronic sequences. The mRNA is translated into a polypeptide chain to form the mature protein after undergoing posttranslational processing. HAT, histone acetyl transferase; CBP, CRED-binding protein; CREB, cyclic AMP response element–binding protein; CRE, cyclinc AMP responsive element; CoA, Co activator; TAF, TBP-associated factors; GTF, general transcription factors, TBP, TATA-binding protein; TATA, TATA box; RE, response element; NH$_2$, aminoterminus; COOH, carboxyterminus.

of genetic information is generating new opportunities for advances in diagnosis and treatment. Understanding basic genetic terminology and the current and future applications of genetics and genomics is critical for physicians diagnosing and treating cardiovascular disease.

## CHROMOSOMES GENES AND DNA

The human genome is encoded in two sets (male and female) of 23 chromosomes; each chromosome consists of a polymer of deoxyribonucleic acid (DNA) (**Figure 7-1**). Four bases make up the DNA: adenine (A), thymine (T), cytosine (C), and guanine (G) (**Figure 7-2**). Chromosomes 1 through 22 are numbered from largest to smallest. Each somatic cell contains these 22 pairs of autosomes, one copy from the father and the other copy from the mother. In addition to the autosomes each cell contains two sex chromosomes. Females have two X chromosomes (XX), and males only one (XY).

A gene consists of coding DNA sequences (exons), intervening noncoding sequences (introns), and regulatory sequences (**Figure 7-3**). The introns and exons form a continuous DNA sequence from which transcription generates a messenger RNA molecule. Posttranscriptional modification, including RNA splicing, results in removal of the intron regions and production of an mRNA template for protein synthesis. In the exons, each triplet of DNA bases forms a codon, the genetic code for one of the 20 amino acids found in all proteins. Based on the published analysis of the human genome, there appear to be 20,000-30,000 protein-encoding genes in the human genome. The size of genes is highly variable, and less than 1.5% of the total DNA in the human chromosomes is sequence that encodes proteins. Recent work has identified large numbers of genes that encode RNAs of diverse function that do not form proteins. These include short microRNAs, which regulate the stability and translation of multiple other RNAs, as well as long noncoding RNAs of unknown function. It has also become evident that large parts of the genome between known genes are also actively transcribed. Together these data suggest that the so-called "junk DNA," which occupies much of the genome, is far from inert.

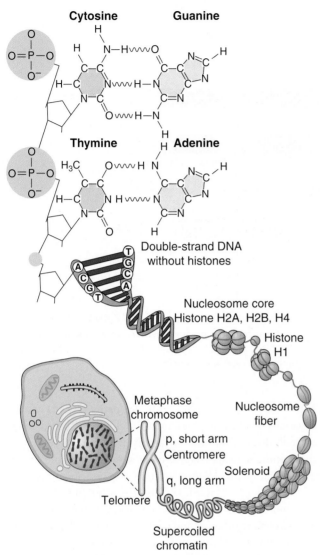

**Figure 7-2.** Structure of chromatin and chromosomes. Chromatin is composed of double-strand DNA that is wrapped around histone and nonhistone proteins forming nucleosomes. The nucleosomes are further organized into solenoid structures. Chromosomes assume their characteristic structure, with short (p) and long (q) arms at the metaphase stage of the cell cycle.

Any given segment of DNA that is inherited is called a *locus*. Differences in the DNA sequence at any given gene locus are called *alleles*. The genetic information at a given gene locus is defined as the *genotype*. If there are two alleles at a locus, then there are three possible genotypes, with the locus either the same (*homozygous*) for one or the other allele or different (*heterozygous*) for the two alleles.

An alteration in the primary nucleotide sequence of DNA that results in an abnormal phenotype is called a *mutation*. Mutations at the level of the chromosome structure may include deletions, duplications, or inversions of segments of DNA. Mutations at the level of the gene may include insertions, deletions, or point mutations, which may result in an amino acid alteration. DNA variation may have no functional consequence and then is known as *polymorphism*. A polymorphism is a region of the genome that varies between individual members of the population. A polymorphism caused by the change of a single nucleotide is a *single nucleotide polymorphism (SNP)*. Millions of SNP variants have been identified to date and made publicly available through the Human Genome Project (**Figure 7-4**). The initial efforts to develop comprehensive catalogs of SNPs have revealed some of the fine structure of the human genome. It is now known that chromosomes are inherited as unique combinations of ancient building blocks of the order of only a few kilobases of DNA. These regions of low recombination, where only a few different alleles might encompass all the variation that has ever existed, are interspersed with local regions of high recombination. This block structure allows much of a population's common variation to be captured by the typing of a relatively small proportion of the polymorphic sites and has accelerated the advent of comprehensive genome mapping on a single "chip" or microarray. The intensive study of the basis for the noncontinuous nature of the genome is revealing other insights into human biology and disease. It is expected that SNP discovery will lead to the discovery of common DNA variations that lead to alterations in the amount or function of the expressed protein and then to downstream cardiovascular disease.

Perhaps the most important and influential consequence of the completion of the Human Genome Project is the potential to study biologic processes in a global and unbiased manner. For the first time, it is possible to study not just one gene, but all genes, and to relate variation in these genes directly to phenotype. In addition, the availability of complete sequence allows the expression levels of all the genes to be studied in parallel. Finally, it is feasible to understand in many ways how a genome functions, as a whole, using comparisons with the genomes of other organisms. This ability to define orthologous segments of DNA (both within coding sequences and beyond) in animal models also makes possible faithful recapitulation of the mechanisms of human genetic diseases. Although far from complete, the success of global strategies in the analysis of human sequence (genomics) has heralded similar comprehensive approaches in whole tissues and organisms to the study of proteins (the proteome), metabolic pathways (metabolome), and noncoding RNA structure and function (the RNAome).

## GENETICS AND CARDIOVASCULAR DISEASE

Genetic techniques have been applied to cardiovascular disease (CVD) and have been successful in dissecting the Mendelian disorders of lipids, cardiomyopathies, and arrhythmias. The comprehensive study of genes, expression, and SNPs does not

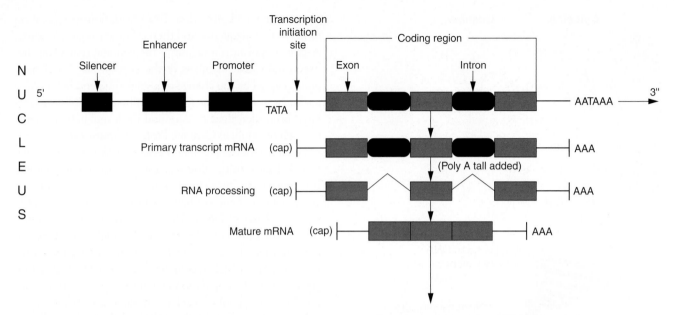

**Figure 7-3.** Transcription. Transcription occurs in the nucleus, producing mRNA that is processed into mature mRNA and transported to the cytoplasm. In the cytoplasm, translation occurs, with the mRNA coding for specific amino acids that are linked together to form a polypeptide and ultimately to form a mature protein. (Source: Mares A Jr, Towbin J, Bies RG, Roberts R. Molecular biology for the cardiologist. *Curr Probl Cardiol.* 1992;17:9–72. Reproduced with permission from the publisher and authors.)

offer major theoretical advantages over conventional genetic markers but will affect classic human genetics in several ways. First, the ready availability of genomic data will ease the application of proven genetic strategies, allowing the relatively rapid identification and study of genes that were previously difficult or impossible to clone. The tools that the genomics revolution has spawned have already made mapping and mutation detection much faster and cheaper. Second, there is the potential that, if common alleles do cause common diseases, genomics will dramatically affect the mapping and cloning of common disease. Paradoxically, as noted above, the greatest legacy of genomics may be its role as a foundation for other "omics," ultimately influencing phenotyping more than genotyping.

## MONOGENIC DISEASE

Substantial progress has been made in defining the molecular basis for a number of monogenic cardiovascular diseases, including familial hypercholesterolemia, hypertrophic cardiomyopathy, and long QT syndromes.

Familial hypercholesterolemia is an archetypal monogenic disorder characterized by elevated LDL cholesterol and premature coronary artery disease in heterozygotes. Homozygous individuals exhibit a more extreme phenotype, with coronary disease appearing in the first two decades of life. The discovery of mutations in the LDL receptor in this disorder has been central to our understanding of cholesterol transport and metabolism, but it has also greatly informed the diagnosis and therapy of more common forms of coronary artery disease.

Patients with hypertrophic cardiomyopathy (HCM) exhibit a variety of clinical phenotypes, including a broad range of wall thickening and variability in progression to life-threatening sequelae, such as congestive heart failure or sudden cardiac death. There is substantial genetic heterogeneity in the etiology of HCM, because the syndrome may result from mutations in any one of several genes that encode cardiac sarcomere proteins, including beta-myosin heavy chain, cardiac troponin T, troponin I, alpha-tropomyosin, and myosin-binding protein C. There is also substantial intragenic or allelic heterogeneity, meaning that several of the sarcomere protein genes have been found to contain multiple disease-causing mutations. Diagnosis of this condition is still largely clinical, although genetic tests have the potential to improve diagnostic reliability. While there are data suggesting that particular families may have distinct prognoses, to date there is no available evidence to recommend significant preventive or therapeutic interventions based on genotype.

Long QT syndrome is a rare, familial disease that is manifested by syncope and sudden cardiac death, often mediated through polymorphic ventricular tachycardia or ventricular fibrillation. The syndrome is characterized by a prolonged, heart-rate-adjusted QT (QTc) interval. QTc prolongation beyond 0.50 second provides evidence for long QT syndrome, but QTc intervals associated with this condition may be less marked. There is substantial genetic heterogeneity in the long QT syndrome. Five genes for sodium and potassium ion channels have been implicated in Romano–Ward syndrome, the autosomal dominant form of long QT syndrome: KVLQT1, HERG, SCN5A, KCNE1, and KCNE2. In addition, several

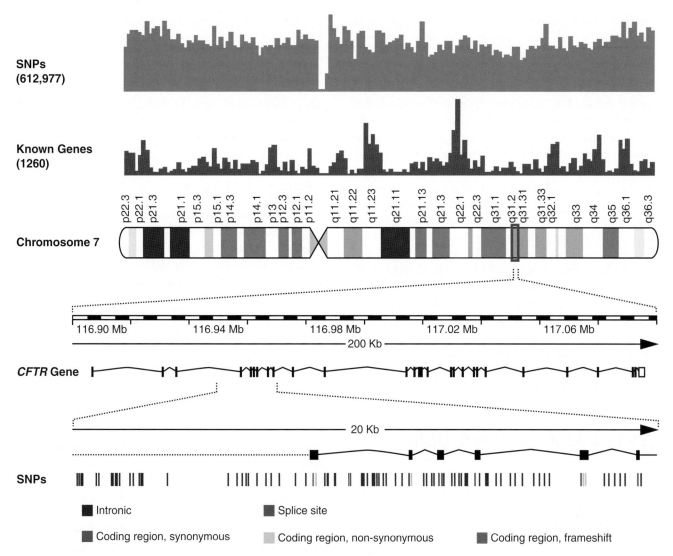

**Figure 7-4.** Chromosome 7 is shown with the density of single nucleotide polymorphisms (SNPs) and genes above. A 200-kb region in 7q31.2 containing the *CFTR* gene is shown below. The *CFTR* gene contains 27 exons. More than 1420 mutations in this gene have been found in patients with cystic fibrosis. A 20-kb region encompassing exons 4–9 is shown in further amplified in order to illustrate the SNPs in this region.

isolated cases of LQT have been associated with mutations in a number of other channel trafficking or scaffolding proteins. Mutations in KVLQT1 and KCNE1, when present in the homozygous state, are also associated with the Jervell and Lange–Nielsen syndrome, an autosomal recessive form of long QT syndrome associated with deafness. Mutations in the SCN5A gene may cause the long QT syndrome, Brugada syndrome, or conduction disease. A variety of different types of mutations are found, including missense mutations (most common), frameshift mutations, deletions, nonsense, and splice-site mutations. However, family members of patients with symptomatic long QT syndrome may have no QTc prolongation, despite carrying the causative mutation. Molecular diagnosis may enhance diagnostic accuracy for long QT syndrome. However, the appropriate use of genetic tests remains under investigation. There is not yet consensus on therapeutic

recommendations for persons who are genotype-positive and phenotype-negative (or borderline). At present, there are insufficient data regarding use of these tests for screening.

Recent human molecular genetic studies are beginning to shed light on other cardiac syndromes with large heritable components, such as dilated cardiomyopathy, atrial fibrillation, arrhythmogenic right ventricular cardiomyopathy or dysplasia, aortic dissection, and congenital heart disease.

## COMMON CARDIOVASCULAR DISEASES

In contrast to inherited diseases caused by specific rare mutations, common polymorphisms in a variety of genes may be associated with more subtle increases in susceptibility to complex cardiovascular diseases, such as coronary heart disease. Although there is generally no evidence for clearly dominant or recessive transmission of most common cardiovascular traits through families, there is compelling evidence for familial aggregation of, and risk factors for, cardiac and vascular disease. For "qualitative' traits, such as myocardial infarction or stroke, evidence for familiality has been demonstrated by calculation of simple sibling recurrence risk ratios or more sophisticated modeling of potential inheritance patterns. For "quantitative" traits such as low-density lipoprotein (LDL) cholesterol or systolic blood pressure, correlations among siblings or first-degree relatives can be calculated to estimate heritability, the proportion of variability in the quantitative trait that is attributable to shared genetic factors. Using these methods, a moderate (30-50%) degree of heritability has been demonstrated for several risk factors, including LDL cholesterol, systolic blood pressure, glucose levels, and body mass index, as well as quantitative subclinical vascular disease measures, such as carotid intima media thickness or coronary artery calcification. Common cardiovascular syndromes that appear to have a heritable component include hypertension, left ventricular hypertrophy, myocardial infarction, atrial fibrillation, and sudden cardiac death.

## GENETIC ASSOCIATION STUDIES

Not all phenotypes segregate in large families and so other genetic techniques have been developed that do not use transmission probability, but rely on simple association of genotypes with phenotypes within a population. These studies are qualitatively different from linkage analyses and have proliferated as the technologies for dense genotyping have become widely available. The most commonly used association study design is the case-control study. A potential problem is confounding bias from population stratification, which results in spurious association of a polymorphism with disease, simply because the disease and the unlinked sequence variant are found in the same population subgroup. This can be partly addressed by replicating the findings in large study cohorts drawn from genetically distinct populations. Another potentially important problem in multiple testing is the prior probability that any observed effect results from the specific polymorphism(s) studied is usually extremely low, resulting in a high false positive rate (through Bayesian inference). Confirmation associations in independent case-control studies provide increased support for the hypothesized genotype and phenotype association. As a result of these limitations, and the generally small effect sizes observed, case-control association studies are generally regarded as hypothesis generating.

Because segregation information is absent from these studies, it also is impossible to infer causality from the relationship between specific variants and a particular phenotype. If the genotype–phenotype association in question is not spurious, it may result from a functional variation within the candidate gene, but more commonly the association results from functional variation within a nearby or linked gene, in so-called "linkage dysequilibrium" with the tested polymorphism. These issues would partly be dealt with by using extended haplotypes of markers in large populations. Parallel evidence for a functional role of the putative variant is essential. These studies, which may use cell culture or model organisms, are possible much earlier because of the ready availability of detailed sequences for cognate genes in other genomes.

Association study designs may be used to analyze qualitative or quantitative traits. Large-scale screening studies of "complex" disease traits, such as myocardial infarction or congestive heart failure, have yielded interesting hypotheses regarding gene variants that may confer disease risk. However, very few genetic variants are strongly and consistently associated with a common CVD outcome in multiple studies. Among the possible explanations, most common genetic variants may confer relatively small effects on a population scale (thus, larger sample sizes may be needed) and important unmeasured environmental modifiers may play a substantial role, but be substantially different in different populations. Further, clinically apparent disease traits, while heritable, may be heterogeneous. By contrast, quantitative preclinical disease phenotypes, such as decreased levels of high density lipoprotein cholesterol, increased levels of hemostatic factors, or subclinical vascular disease, may represent more tractable measures for dissecting the role of specific genetic variants. Ideal quantitative phenotypes are heritable and strongly related to prospective risk for CVD. Some candidate gene variants have been consistently noted to explain a significant proportion of the interindividual variability of these "upstream" phenotypes, despite less consistent associations of the same variants with disease phenotypes. For example, although the angiotensin-converting enzyme (ACE) deletion/insertion polymorphism is clearly associated with levels of serum ACE, there are only modest associations of this polymorphism with blood pressure and inconsistent associations in dozens of studies with CVD outcomes such as coronary heart disease and congestive heart failure.

## GENETIC TESTING (FIGURES 7-5 AND 7-6)

Genetic testing for common cardiovascular disease may be informative for identifying patients at increased risk of disease who would benefit most from prevention strategies such as drug treatment or reduction of risk factors, rather than for prediction or diagnosis of disease. For common diseases, there has been little evidence to date that a given genetic variant is diagnostic of disease or highly predictive of disease onset. Variants associated with disease normally contribute only

# 8

# Pre-Op Evaluation of Noncardiac Surgery

ADVAY G. BHATT AND ERIC H. AWTRY

## ● PRACTICAL POINTS

- On an annual basis, there are greater than 1 million perioperative cardiovascular complications, including myocardial infarction, congestive heart failure, and arrhythmia; these cost greater than $20 billion in healthcare expenditures.

- Perioperative cardiovascular events generally occur either intra-operatively or within the first 72 hours post-operatively, and are associated with increased mortality: 10-15% and 1.6% mortality associated with preoperative myocardial infarction and heart failure, respectively.

- High risk clinical predictors that should delay elective surgery include unstable coronary syndromes, decompensated heart failure, symptomatic valvular disease, and significant arrhythmias.

- Intermediate risk clinical predictors include the presence of ischemic heart disease, congestive heart failure, cerebrovascular disease, diabetes mellitus, chronic kidney disease, and high risk surgery. These factors are known as the Revised Cardiac Risk Index.

- Individuals undergoing major vascular surgery are at two- to threefold higher risk for perioperative events than those undergoing major nonvascular surgery.

- Impaired functional capacity, i.e., the patient has less than 4 METS, is associated with a twofold increase in postoperative cardiac complications.

- Preoperative echocardiography is recommended for individuals with dyspnea of unclear etiology and a history congestive heart failure with a recent change in clinical status.

- Noninvasive stress testing should be considered for individuals with symptoms of ischemia in whom testing is indicated, even in the absence of surgery and in patients with greater than 3 clinical risk predictors who are undergoing vascular surgery. It should also be considered in patients with 1-2 clinical risk predictors undergoing vascular surgery or with poor functional capacity, undergoing intermediate risk surgery.

- Elective preoperative revascularization does not improve outcomes and is only recommended in the setting of acute coronary syndromes, significant left main stenosis, and high risk 2-vessel disease.

- Perioperative beta-blockade is recommended for individuals undergoing vascular surgery who have evidence of ischemia on noninvasive stress testing and for those previously treated with beta-blockers for ischemic heart disease, hypertension, and arrhythmia.

## INTRODUCTION

Assessment of perioperative cardiovascular risk is an increasingly important aspect of consultative cardiology, as the number of surgical procedures performed steadily rises and improved surgical techniques and anesthetics allow for surgery in higher risk populations. As of 2000, estimates of annual numbers of procedures performed include:

- Nearly 40 million surgical procedures
- Greater than 10 million major noncardiac procedures

- 4 million major noncardiac procedures in individuals over the age of 65
- 2-3 million procedures in individuals with risk factors for coronary artery disease (CAD)
- 1 million procedures in individuals with known CAD.

The annual economic and social cost associated with perioperative cardiovascular morbidity and mortality includes:

- Greater than $20 billion in healthcare expenditures
- Greater than 1 million perioperative cardiovascular complications.

The preoperative evaluation provides an opportunity for the treating physician to intensify/maximize treatment of a patient's known cardiac condition and to identify and institute therapy for previously unrecognized cardiovascular disease. Important questions to be asked/answered during the preoperative cardiac assessment include:

- What is the patient's overall risk of adverse cardiac events?
- For what specific adverse event is the patient at risk (e.g., ischemia, CHF, etc.)?
- Does the patient require further testing to clarify risk?
- Is the patient's risk so high that canceling/postponing surgery is warranted?
- What can be done to decrease the patient's perioperative risk (e.g., medications, monitoring procedures, invasive procedures, etc.)?

## ADVERSE CARDIAC EVENTS

### Myocardial Infarction (MI)

The incidence of perioperative MI is highly variable and depends in part on the prevalence of CAD in the population being studied. The event rate for a healthy individual is below 1%, whereas the event rate for an individual with risk factors for CAD or with documented CAD ranges from 3 to 19%. In a recent study of one series of patients over the age of 40 undergoing a variety of elective noncardiac surgeries, the event rate for postoperative ischemia was as follows:

- 4.1% in patients with known CAD
- 0.8% in patients with peripheral vascular disease but no evidence of CAD
- 0% in patients with risk factors but no clinical evidence of atherosclerosis.

The majority of postoperative MIs are clinically silent, owing in part to the use of analgesics and sedation. Hence, postoperative ischemia is often identified by ST depressions or new Q waves on ECG monitoring or by measurement of cardiac biomarkers such as creatinine kinase (CK) and/or troponin. Postoperative infarcts predominately occur 24 to 72 hours following surgery, as the hemodynamic effects of anesthesia wane. Pathophysiology is thought to reflect both supply/demand mismatch and plaque instability. Overall, the mortality of postoperative MI is approximately 10 to 15%, with survivors having reduced long-term survival.

### Congestive Heart Failure (CHF)

The incidence of CHF following noncardiac surgery ranges from 5 to 20% during the first 24 to 72 hours following surgery. Perioperative event rates are substantially higher in patients with CHF than it is in individuals with CAD alone. Also:

- Approximately 17% of individuals with perioperative CHF require readmission.
- Approximately 1.6% of individuals with perioperative CHF die within 30 days of surgery.

Risk factors for the development of postoperative heart failure include:

- S3 gallop and elevated jugular venous pressure (JVP)
- Prior pulmonary vascular congestion
- Stenotic valvular disease
- Uncontrolled systemic or pulmonary hypertension (HTN)
- Depressed LV systolic function (LVEF <40%).

The precipitants of postoperative CHF include increased venous return, owing to perioperative hydration and volume resuscitation, cessation of positive pressure ventilation and vasodilatory anesthetics, reabsorption of third-space fluid, and myocardial ischemia.

### Cardiac Arrest and Death

Overall perioperative mortality varies depending on the population studied and the nature of the surgery, and ranges from 0.6 to 6.3%. However, high risk individuals who undergo the highest risk surgeries (i.e., abdominal aorta aneurism (AAA) repair) have substantially greater mortality. Ventricular fibrillation (VF) and cardiac arrest may complicate up to 0.5% of surgical procedures, most frequently relate to perioperative myocardial ischemia, and are associated with a mortality of 50-90%.

## PHYSIOLOGICAL BASIS FOR ADVERSE EVENTS

There are several physiologic changes that occur in the surgical setting and contribute to the development of perioperative adverse cardiac events. These are outlined in **Table 8-1.**

| Table 8-1 • Physiologic Alterations That Contribute to Postoperative Adverse Events | |
|---|---|
| **Contributing Factors to Perioperative Events** | **Physiologic Basis/Effect** |
| Postoperative procoagulable state | Platelet activation<br>Increased fibrinogen<br>Reduced intrinsic fibrinolytic activity |
| Supply and/or demand mismatch | Tachycardia<br>Hypertension<br>Hypoxemia<br>Fluid shifts<br>Blood loss |
| Elevated catecholamines | Vasospasm<br>Tachycardia<br>Hypertension |
| Activation of the renin-angiotensin System | Hypertension<br>Water and sodium retention |
| Anesthetic effects | Vasodilation<br>Negatively inotropic |
| Withdrawal of positive pressure Ventilation | Increased venous return<br>Increased afterload |

## PATIENT-SPECIFIC FACTORS THAT IMPACT PERIOPERATIVE RISK

Specific aspects of a patient's history and physical examination may provide significant insight into perioperative risk. This risk stratification was initially performed by qualitative assessment of an individual's medical and functional status using the American Society of Anesthesiology (ASA) physical status classification system. However, this model failed to adequately integrate patient specific and surgery specific factors to predict the risk of perioperative events. This led to the development of multiple multivariable risk models to quantify perioperative risk:

- Original Cardiac Risk Index (Goldman criteria)
- Modified Cardiac Risk Index (Detsky criteria)
- Revised Cardiac Risk Index (RCRI).

Of the 3 models, the RCRI appears to have the greatest accuracy for predicting perioperative adverse cardiac events.

### High Risk Clinical Predictors

High risk clinical predictors reflect active cardiac conditions that warrant delay or cancellation of surgery to allow further cardiovascular evaluation and preoperative treatment of the condition. These predictors fall into the following categories:

- Unstable coronary syndromes
  - CCS (Canadian Cardiac Society) class III or IV angina

- Unstable angina
- MI within previous 30 days
- Decompensated CHF
  - New-onset or worsening CHF
  - NYHA (New York Heart Association) class IV CHF
- Significant arrhythmias
  - Symptomatic bradycardia
  - Mobitz II atrioventricular ventricular (AV) block
  - High-grade AV block
  - Third-degree AV block
  - Uncontrolled SVT with ventricular rates >100 bpm
  - Newly diagnosed ventricular tachycardia
- Valvular heart disease
  - Symptomatic aortic stenosis
  - Asymptomatic aortic stenosis with an AV are $\leq 1.0$ cm$^2$ or a mean transaortic gradient >40 mm Hg
  - Symptomatic mitral stenosis

### Intermediate Risk Clinical Predictors

Individuals without the active cardiac conditions defined above may still be at increased risk for adverse events and require careful evaluation prior to intermediate or high risk surgical procedures. Current guidelines stratify risk in these patients based upon the presence of a subset of the following six criteria (the RCRI):

1. Ischemic heart disease
   - History of MI
   - History of positive stress test
   - Current complaint of chest pain considered to be secondary to myocardial ischemia
   - Use of nitrate therapy
   - ECG with pathological Q waves
2. Congestive heart failure
   - History of congestive heart failure
   - Pulmonary edema
   - Paroxysmal nocturnal dyspnea
   - Bilateral rales or S3 gallop
   - Chest radiograph showing pulmonary vascular redistribution
3. Cerebrovascular disease
   - History of TIA or stroke
4. Insulin-dependent diabetes mellitus
5. High risk surgical procedures
   - Intraperitoneal
   - Intrathoracic
   - Suprainguinal vascular
6. Chronic kidney disease (CKD) with a baseline creatinine >2.0 mg/dL.

An individual receives one point for each applicable category. Based on the total point score, the risk of major perioperative cardiac events (MI, pulmonary edema, VF, primary cardiac arrest, and complete heart block) can be estimated (**Table 8-2**).

| Table 8-2 • Estimation of Perioperative Cardiac Event Rate Based on the RCRI Point System ||||
| Risk Factors | Point Score | Class | Adverse Event Rate |
| --- | --- | --- | --- |
| Ischemic heart disease | 0 | I | 0.4% |
| CHF | 1 | II | 0.9% |
| TIA/CVA | 2 | III | 6.6% |
| Diabetes | ≥3 | IV | 11% |
| Creatinine >2.0 | | | |
| High risk surgery | | | |

## Minor Clinical Predictors

The presence of other risk factors may raise the possibility of underlying cardiac disease; however, they do not improve upon the predictive accuracy of the RCRI and are not incorporated into the preoperative risk assessment models. These minor predictors include:

- Advanced age (>70 years)
- Abnormal electrocardiogram (ECG)
  - Left ventricular hypertrophy (LVH)
  - Resting ST-T abnormalities
  - Left bundle branch block (LBBB)
  - Rhythms other than sinus (including atrial fibrillation)
- Uncontrolled HTN:
  - >180/110 mm Hg
- Depressed LV ejection fraction

## Impact of Functional Capacity

Cardiopulmonary impairment of functional capacity is one of the best clinical predictors of both perioperative and long-term events. Impaired functional capacity is associated with an overall twofold increase in adverse events and a fivefold increase in ischemia, postoperatively. A patient's functional capacity can be estimated based on his or her ability to perform a variety of common activities, as outlined in the Duke Activity Status Index (see **Table 8-3**):

- Ability to achieve >4 METS is associated with a positive predictive value (PPV) of 10% and negative predictive value (NPV) of 95% for perioperative events.
- Inability to climb 2 flights of stairs or walk 4 blocks is associated with a twofold increase in postoperative cardiac complications. One case series estimated that the inability to climb 2 flights of stairs indicates a PPV of 82% for postoperative cardiopulmonary events.

# SURGERY SPECIFIC FACTORS THAT IMPACT PERIOPERATIVE RISK

## Timing of Surgery

The incidence of perioperative cardiovascular complications is two- to fivefold higher in individuals undergoing emergent or urgent surgery, in part because time is not available for preoperative cardiovascular evaluation and treatment. Patients undergoing elective surgeries, on the other hand, should be fully evaluated and medically optimized preoperatively, and show a lower incidence of perioperative complications. Delay of surgery is often appropriate for patients with active cardiac conditions and for high risk individuals meeting criteria for preoperative noninvasive stress testing.

Special consideration regarding timing of surgery needs to be given following percutaneous coronary interventions (PCI) with bare-metal or drug-eluting stents (see section on revascularization below), and in patients after MI. Earlier guidelines recommended that elective surgery be delayed for

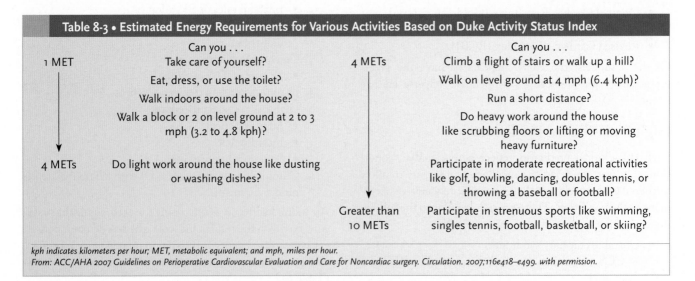

**Table 8-3 • Estimated Energy Requirements for Various Activities Based on Duke Activity Status Index**

|  | Can you . . . |  | Can you . . . |
| --- | --- | --- | --- |
| 1 MET | Take care of yourself? | 4 METs | Climb a flight of stairs or walk up a hill? |
|  | Eat, dress, or use the toilet? |  | Walk on level ground at 4 mph (6.4 kph)? |
|  | Walk indoors around the house? |  | Run a short distance? |
|  | Walk a block or 2 on level ground at 2 to 3 mph (3.2 to 4.8 kph)? |  | Do heavy work around the house like scrubbing floors or lifting or moving heavy furniture? |
| 4 METs | Do light work around the house like dusting or washing dishes? |  | Participate in moderate recreational activities like golf, bowling, dancing, doubles tennis, or throwing a baseball or football? |
|  |  | Greater than 10 METs | Participate in strenuous sports like swimming, singles tennis, football, basketball, or skiing? |

kph indicates kilometers per hour; MET, metabolic equivalent; and mph, miles per hour.
From: ACC/AHA 2007 Guidelines on Perioperative Cardiovascular Evaluation and Care for Noncardiac surgery. Circulation. 2007;116e418–e499. with permission.

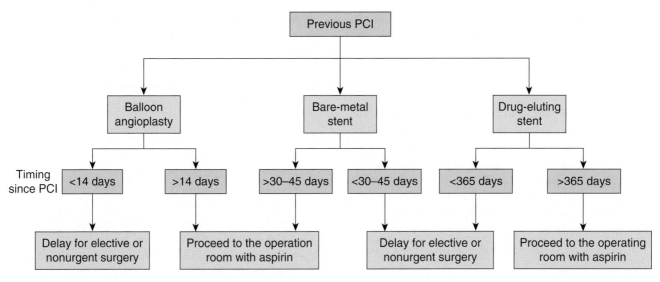

**Figure 8-3.** Proposed approach to the management of patients with previous PCI who require noncardiac surgery. Based on expert opinion. (From: ACC/AHA 2007 Guidelines on Perioperative Cardiovascular Evaluation and Care for Noncardiac surgery. *Circulation.* 2007;116e418–e499. with permission.)

4 to 6 weeks following placement of a bare-metal stent, and at least 1 year following implantation of a drug-eluting stent. However, the increased risk of postoperative bleeding in patients on antiplatelet agents (clopidogrel increases bleeding risk ~50%) raises substantial concern and frequently necessitates the cessation of one or both antiplatelet agents. The timing of elective surgery in relation to PCI should be carefully planned to minimize the risks of stent thrombosis and limit bleeding complications (see **Figure 8-3**).

Individuals who are status post-recent PCI and require elective noncardiac surgery should be managed by the following consensus guidelines:

- After balloon angioplasty: delay surgery for 2 to 4 weeks, then proceed on aspirin therapy.
- After bare-metal stent placement: delay surgery for 4 to 6 weeks of dual antiplatelet therapy, then proceed on aspirin therapy.
- After drug-eluting stent placement: delay surgery for 1 year of dual antiplatelet therapy, then proceed on aspirin therapy.

## The Role of Perioperative Medical Therapy

Beta-blockers: The physiological basis for the perioperative use of beta-blockade includes:

- Reduction in myocardial oxygen consumption
- Blunting of the adverse effects of elevated cate-cholamines
- Reduction of postoperative tachyarrhythmias
- Plaque stabilization due to anti-inflammatory effects.

Data regarding the use of perioperative beta-blocker therapy conflict; however, the weight of evidence suggests that beta-blocker use is associated with a reduction in postoperative MI

and mortality. Current guidelines recommend that perioperative beta-blocker therapy be used for the following patients:

- Individuals previously on beta-blockers for CAD, HTN, or arrhythmia.
- Individuals undergoing vascular surgery who have evidence of ischemia on preoperative testing.

Furthermore, perioperative beta-blocker therapy should be considered for:

- Individuals undergoing vascular surgery who have more than 1 RCRI risk factor.
- Individuals undergoing intermediate risk procedures who have more than 1 RCRI risk factor.

The utility of perioperative beta-blockade in individuals with zero or 1 RCRI risk factor is unproven, even for high risk vascular surgery, and there are insufficient comparative trials to support the use of one beta-blocker over another. Beta-blockade should be started as far in advance of surgery as possible and up-titrated to a goal heart rate of 60 to 65 bpm. However, care must be taken to avoid hypotension and profound bradycardia, as recent data suggest these may increase the risk of perioperative stroke. Additionally, withdrawal of beta-blockers prior to or immediately after surgery is associated with increased postoperative adverse events and should be avoided. The ideal duration of beta-blocker therapy following surgery is uncertain, but at least 1 to 4 weeks seems reasonable.

Alpha-2 agonists: Alpha-2 agonists, such as clonidine, blunt the central release of catecholamines and are associated with a reduction in postoperative MI and mortality. In addition, clonidine results in minimal hemodynamic effects and is available in both oral and transdermal formulations. This agent may be useful in patients who would otherwise benefit from perioperative beta-blocker therapy but are beta-blocker intolerant.

Statin: The physiological basis for the use of statins during the perioperative period may include plaque stabilization, decreased oxidative stress, and decreased vascular inflammation. Small studies suggest there may be a threefold reduction in the number of perioperative events in statin-treated patients. In general, statin therapy is indicated whenever long-term lipid therapy is appropriate. Current guidelines suggest that statin use should not be discontinued prior to surgery and initiation of statin therapy may be beneficial for the following patients:

- Individuals undergoing vascular surgery, irrespective of risk factors.
- Individuals undergoing intermediate risk procedures with 1 or more RCRI risk factors.

Calcium channel blocker (CCB): CCBs are considered safe in the perioperative period but have not been proven to reduce postoperative events. Use of CCBs may reduce the risk of postoperative tachyarrhythmias.

## Congestive Heart Failure

Routine assessment of LVEF prior to noncardiac surgery is recommended only in the setting of new or worsening CHF (see "Assessment of LV Function" above) and should prompt further investigation into the underlying etiology of congestive heart failure. Evaluation of new-onset CHF in the postoperative period should focus on potential ischemia. The medical therapy of perioperative CHF is similar to that in the nonoperative setting and includes careful volume management and afterload reduction through the judicious use of diuretics, vasodilators, and beta-blockers. Prophylactic hemodynamic monitoring with a pulmonary artery (PA) catheter does not appear to improve perioperative outcomes in patients with a history of CHF, although individuals with NYHA class III and IV CHF have not been thoroughly studied. Individuals with hypertrophic cardiomyopathy with obstructive physiology are at particular risk of perioperative hemodynamic instability, owing to their intolerance of volume shifts, vasodilation, and tachycardia.

## Valvular Heart Disease

### General Principles

Patients with severe aortic or mitral stenosis are prone to CHF and hemodynamic instability perioperatively; cancellation of noncardiac surgery and evaluation for valvular surgery should be considered in patients with symptomatic stenotic valve lesions. Valvular insufficiency is generally well-tolerated perioperative, owing to the vasodilatory effects of anesthetics.

### Antibiotic Prophylaxis for Valvular Disease

A recent update to the AHA guideline for the prevention of infective endocarditis narrowed the indications for antibiotic prophylaxis to patients undergoing high risk procedures (from the infectious standpoint) who have the following cardiac conditions:

- Prior infective endocarditis
- Prosthetic cardiac valves
- Unrepaired cyanotic congenital heart defects, including palliative shunts and conduits
- Congenital heart defects (ASD, VSD, PDA) that are repaired with prosthetic material or via implanted device, whether surgically or percutaneously, during the first 6 months after the procedure
- Repaired congenital defects with residual shunting at the site of repair
- Cardiac transplant.

### Anticoagulation of Mechanical Valves

In managing perioperative anticoagulation in patients with prosthetic valves, the physician needs to weigh the risk of valve thrombosis against the risk of bleeding. Procedures associated with a low risk of bleeding (i.e., skin procedures, most dental procedures, and ophthalmologic procedures) do not warrant discontinuation of anticoagulation. However, procedures associated with a high risk of bleeding may warrant cessation of warfarin and often require use of bridging anticoagulation with either unfractionated heparin (UFH) or low molecular weight heparin (LMWH).

Individuals with the following history are at the highest risk of thrombotic complications when anticoagulation is withheld perioperatively:

- Mechanical valve in the mitral or tricuspid position
- Bjork–Shiley or Starr–Edwards mechanical valve
- Recent prosthetic valve thrombosis or embolism
- Concomitant atrial fibrillation, history of prior thromboembolus, hypercoagulable state, and LVEF <30%.

The 2006 ACC/AHA Guidelines for the Management of Patients with Valvular Heart Disease recommend the following approaches for these patients:

- Individuals with a bileaflet aortic valve and no high risk factors are low risk, and bridging anticoagulation is unnecessary. Stop anticoagulation 48 to 72 hours prior to surgery and resume warfarin within 24 hours after the procedure.
- Individuals with any high risk features (as mentioned above) require bridging anticoagulation. Stop anticoagulation 3 to 5 days prior to surgery and initiate bridging anticoagulation when the INR falls below 2.0. Stop UFH 4 to 6 hours or LMWH 12 hours prior to the surgery. Resume bridging anticoagulation and warfarin as soon as possible postoperatively, and continue bridging for 24 hours after attaining a therapeutic INR.

## *Role of Prophylactic Valvuloplasty for Aortic or Mitral Stenosis*

Prophylactic valvuloplasty as a bridge to major noncardiac surgery may be considered for the following patients:

- Individuals with hemodynamically unstable aortic stenosis who are high risk for valve replacement or when delay of noncardiac surgery is unacceptable.
- Individuals with NYHA class II to IV CHF from moderate to severe mitral stenosis and favorable valve morphology.

## Arrhythmias

The combination of hypoxia, pain, bleeding, fever, infection, electrolyte derangements, medications, and underlying structural heart disease contribute to the development of postoperative bradyarrhythmias and tachyarrhythmias.

### *Bradyarrhythmias*

All individuals with class I indications for implantation of a permanent pacemaker should undergo the procedure prior to elective surgery. If emergent noncardiac surgery is required, a temporary transvenous pacemaker should be used perioperatively as a bridge to permanent pacemaker implantation.

### *Supraventricular Tachycardia (SVT)*

SVT, in particular atrial fibrillation, is the most common perioperative rhythm disturbance and complicates greater than 15% of thoracic surgical procedures. Atrial fibrillation often resolves spontaneously within 36 to 48 hours of the noncardiac surgery.

- Postoperative SVT is associated with a twofold increased risk of pulmonary edema.
- Preoperative use of calcium channel blockers or beta-blockers can reduce the incidence of atrial fibrillation by 50 to 60%.
- Limited data suggest that statin therapy is associated with a lower rate of postoperative atrial fibrillation.

### *Ventricular Tachycardia (VT)*

Nonsustained VT is not predictive of increased perioperative risk and is most often the result of electrolyte abnormalities. Sustained ventricular tachycardia in the perioperative setting is usually caused by ischemia and warrants a formal cardiac evaluation.

## PERIOPERATIVE DEVICE MANAGEMENT

Electrocautery and radiofrequency scalpels used in the surgical arena induce electromechanical interference (EMI) that may result in inhibition of pacemaker function or inappropriate therapies for VT/VF owing to device oversensing. Newer devices with bipolar leads are less prone to EMI because of a narrower sensing field width. Physicians managing pacemakers and ICDs perioperatively need to consider indication for the device and the device settings. General recommendations for the management of these devices include:

- Monitoring ECG.
- Turning off rate responsiveness in individuals who are not pacemaker-dependent in order to avoid incorrectly tracking EMI and pacing at the upper rate limit of the pacemaker.
- Reprogramming to asynchronous pacing modes (VOO or DOO) for pacemaker dependent individuals.
- Inactivating ICD therapies (magnets do not always turn off the pacing function of an ICD).
- Reprogramming back to the original settings as soon as possible postoperatively.
- Using bipolar/ultrasonic cautery, as it may lower the risk of EMI with compared to unipolar cautery.

## POSTOPERATIVE MONITORING

### Telemetry and ECG

Intraoperative and postoperative telemetry with ST-segment monitoring is indicated in patients at risk for, or known to have, atherosclerosis. ST segment changes frequently occur when patients are awakening from deep anesthesia, and prolonged ST-segment depression during the postoperative period is predictive of postoperative ischemia and death. An ECG should be obtained immediately after surgery and daily for 48 hours in patients with known or suspected CAD and in low risk patients only if they show evidence of cardiac dysfunction perioperatively.

### Cardiac Biomarkers

Cardiac troponin is a highly sensitive marker of myocardial injury; however, the clinical significance of a mildly elevated postoperative troponin without other evidence of MI is not clear.

- Nonetheless, cardiac enzymes should be assessed in patients who are clinically suspected of having a perioperative cardiac event.

### Pulmonary Artery (PA) Catheters

The use of perioperative hemodynamic monitoring with a PA catheter does not clearly improve clinical outcomes; however, it may be useful in high risk patients with severe coronary disease, cardiomyopathy, or valvular disease, providing expertise with its interpretation is available.

### Other Factors

Significant blood loss and the need for blood transfusions are associated with increased postoperative events. The goal should be to maintain a hematocrit greater than 30 in patients with known CAD.

# MANAGEMENT OF POSTOPERATIVE MI

The majority of postoperative MIs relate to supply/demand mismatch, are clinically silent, and do not have associated ECG changes to suggest plaque instability. If ST changes are present and plaque instability is suspected, then unfractionated heparin should be administered, providing the bleeding risk is acceptable. Glycoprotein IIb/IIIa inhibitors and fibrinolytics are generally contraindicated in the postoperative setting. Intensive medical therapy and stabilization is appropriate for the majority of postoperative non-ST-segment elevation MIs (NSTEMIs). However, individuals who are refractory to medical therapy or have an ST-segment elevation MI (STEMI) should be considered for coronary angiography and PCI, with acceptance of the bleeding potential in all but the highest risk patients.

## Suggested Readings

1. Brilakis ES, Banerjee S, Berger PB. Perioperative management of patients with coronary stents. *J Am Coll Cardiol.* 2007;49(22):2145–2150.

2. Fleisher LA, Beckman JA, Brown KA, et al. ACC/AHA 2007 Guidelines on Perioperative Cardiovascular Evaluation and Care for Noncardiac Surgery. A Report of the American College of Cardiology/American Heart Association Task Force on Practice Guidelines (Writing Committee to Revise the 2002 Guidelines on Perioperative Cardiovascular Evaluation for Noncardiac Surgery). *Circulation.* 2007;116:e418–e499.

3. Lee TH, Marcantonio ER, Mangione CM, et al. Derivation and prospective validation of a simple index for prediction of cardiac risk of major noncardiac surgery. *Circulation.* 1999;100:1043–1049.

4. McFalls EO, Ward HB, Moritz TE, et al. Coronary-artery revascularization before elective major vascular surgery. *N Engl J Med.* 2004;351:2795–2804.

5. Poldermans D, Hoeks SE, Feringa HH. Pre-operative risk assessment and risk reduction before surgery. *J Am Coll Cardiol.* 2008;51(20):1913–1924.

# 9

# Acute Brain Injury and Heart Disease

Katharina M. Busl and Martin A. Samuels

---

## • PRACTICAL POINTS

- Common ECG changes in the setting of brain injury include large, inverted T waves. These ECG changes do not reflect ischemic heart disease, but are a sign of autonomic dysregulation.

- Neurogenic cardiac disease, including sudden cardiac death, may occur in a structurally complete, normal heart and does not require preexisting heart disease; however, patients with preexisting cardiovascular disease may be more sensitive to neurogenic stress.

- Stress cardiomyopathy typically involves the left ventricular apex and midventricle, as these contain the greatest catecholamine terminal density.

- The most common clinically significant complication of neurogenic cardiomyopathy is left heart failure.

- Neurogenic cardiomyopathy can mimic a myocardial infarction and must be considered a differential diagnosis.

- Peak troponin release in subarachnoid hemorrhage is predictive of risk for left ventricular dysfunction, hemodynamic instability, and pulmonary edema.

- Seizures can mimic heart disease; arrhythmia may be the most prominent finding, and syncope may occur in cases of ictal bradycardia.

---

## INNERVATION OF THE HEART

The brain controls circulation primarily via the sympathetic and parasympathetic nervous systems. Afferent impulses are received from peripheral receptors, and parasympathetic and sympathetic efferent outflows are adjusted to enable the circulation to adapt appropriately.

### Cardiac Afferents

Baroreceptors (mechanoreceptors) are located in the carotid sinus and the aortic arch, and in heart and lungs. Their function is to maintain the blood pressure (BP) within normal range. They are activated by wall expansion in response to elevated blood pressure. Decreased blood pressure leads to decreased firing of these nerves. The baroreflex sensitivity increases during sleep and during rest (i.e., → BP falls),

and decreases during exercise, with chronic hypertension and with age (i.e., → BP rises).

Chemoreceptors serve to maintain oxygen delivery. They are located in the carotid arteries and the aortic bodies. Hypoxia leads to reflex bradycardia (vagally mediated) and vasoconstriction (sympathetically mediated). Both sympathetic and parasympathetic receptors are present in all four chambers of the myocardium.

Most afferent pathways from baroreceptors and from some of the mechanoreceptors terminate in the nucleus tractus solitarius (NTS), a nucleus in the lower brain stem, which receives a variety of primary visceral afferent signals. Neurons of the NTS relay information to the reticular formation (vasomotor center) and the vagal nuclei, from where the sympathetic and parasympathetic outflows pass to the blood vessels and the heart. Neural pathways from the NTS also regulate hormonal secretion (vasopressin) from the hypothalamus. Control from higher centers, such as the response to emotional stress, is exerted mainly via the hypothalamus by input to the NTS and the vasomotor center.

The insulae and thalamus have a sensory viscerotropic representation that includes the termination of cardiopulmonary afferents.

## Cardiac Efferents

### Sympathetic Efferents

The main sympathetic outflow originates in the paraventricular nucleus of the hypothalamus and in the rostral ventrolateral medulla (reticular formation). There are connections with the NTS and the dorsal motor nucleus of the vagal nerve providing sympathetic influence on parasympathetic output. Most sympathetic outflow travels to the intermediolateral cell column of the spinal cord, exits the upper thoracic (T1-5) spinal cord via the anterior root and white rami communicantes, travels in the sympathetic chain, and reaches the stellate and superior cervical ganglia, from which the sympathetic postganglionic fibers travel to the heart. Sympathetic innervation of the heart is asymmetrical. The efferents from the left stellate ganglion terminate at SA and AV nodes, and the efferents from the right stellate ganglion reach atria, septum, and ventricles. The main transmitter is norepinephrine. The sympathetic activity is largely reflex, based on afferent information processed by the brainstem's cardiovascular control centers.

### Parasympathetic Efferents

Parasympathetic outflow mostly originates in the vagal nuclei (dorsal motor nucleus and nucleus ambiguous in the brain stem) and reaches the intracardiac ganglia via the superior, middle, and inferior cardiac rami of the ipsilateral vagus nerve. Parasympathetic efferents from both sides reach the SA (right vagus > left) and AV (left vagus > right) nodes, cardiac vessels, and cardiac cells in all four chambers. Though the predominant effect of vagal activity is negatively chronotropic (i.e., slowing of the heart rate), there is also a negative inotropic effect (i.e., reduction of the contractile force) of vagal activity. Preganglionic neurons are stimulated by nicotine and are insensitive to atropine. Preganglionic parasympathetic and postganglionic sympathetic fibers combine within the cardiac plexus at the heart base (see **Table 9-1**).

The vagal input on the SA node can override maximal sympathetic (adrenergic) tone. While the parasympathetic action has a short latency of 200 msecs and reaches its maximal effect after 400 msecs, sympathetic action has a latency of 1-3 seconds and lasts longer.

### Table 9-1 • Sympathetic and Parasympathetic Effects in the Heart

|  | Sympathetic | Parasympathetic |
|---|---|---|
| SA node | acceleration, ↓ refractory period | deceleration |
| Atrial myocardium | positive inotropic | negative inotropic |
| AV node | acceleration | deceleration |
| His-Purkinje bundle | ↑ pacemaker activity, ↓ refractory period | little (↓pacemaker activity) or none |
| Ventricular myocardium | ↓ refractory period | slight negative inotropic effect |

The balance between sympathetic and parasympathetic cardiac modulation is regulated by two main influences: medullary reflexes triggered by activation of mechano- and chemoreceptors, and descending influences from the cerebral cortex, amygdala, hypothalamus, and periaqueductal gray matter, which mediate integrated responses to stressors.

## THE BRAIN–HEART CONNECTION

### Mechanisms of the Production of Neurogenic Heart Disease

There are several mechanisms for neurogenic cardiac damage: catecholamine effects, stress with or without steroid effect, nervous system stimulation, and reperfusion.

The most important mechanism for neurogenic cardiac damage seems to be direct catecholamine-induced damage. Catecholamine infusion into the heart causes a characteristic pathological picture in the cardiac muscle: contraction band necrosis (also known as myofibrillar degeneration, or coagulative myocytolysis). Cells die in a hypercontracted state (contraction bands). Calcification occurs rapidly (even immediately). The damage is predominantly subendocardial. Contraction band necrosis is the major lesion seen in the setting of acute neurological or psychiatric catastrophes. The likelihood and extent of myocardial necrosis is correlated with the severity of clinical neurological state (see **Figure 9-1**).

This form of cardiac damage is distinct from the damage in ischemic myocardial infarction (coagulation necrosis), which is characterized by cell death in a relaxed state, and late, if any, calcification.

Other mechanisms of neurogenic heart disease are stress (with or without the influence of steroids), nervous system stimulation (stimulation of hypothalamus, limbic cortex,

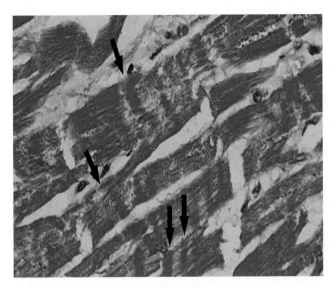

**Figure 9-1.** Myocardial muscle (H&E stain), with contraction band necrosis (arrows). Histopathology of contraction band necrosis: myocyte injury characterized by hypercontracted sarcomers, dense eosinophilic transverse bands, interstitial mononuclear inflammatory response.

mesencephalic reticular formation, stellate ganglion can lead to cardiac lesions), or after cardiac reperfusion following a period of ischemia (seen in patients who die after the use of the left ventricular assist pump, after coronary thrombolysis and angioplasty, or after extracorporal circulation). Cardiac necrosis is greatest near the nerve terminals in the left ventricular apical endocardium, simply because this is the location of greatest catecholamine terminal density.

At the cardiac cellular level, the norepinephrine released into myocardium from sympathetic nerve terminals acts to open a receptor-operated calcium channel. This leads to a rapid influx of calcium with corresponding changes in the electrocardiogram ("cerebral T waves"—see **Figure 9-2**). If the process continues, free radicals are activated, both from calcium entry and the catecholamine metabolites (e.g., adrenochrome), leading to peroxidation of the lipid of the cardiac cell membrane. Cardiac cells will leak enzyme (e.g., troponin, creatine kinase) and may die. If severe enough, there may be a rapid decrement in cardiac function, greatest in the left ventricular apex, producing the characteristic appearance of left ventricular apical ballooning (also known as the "tako-tsubo-like cardiomyopathy;" see neurogenic cardiomyopathy). This cascade is potentially reversible, provided a serious cardiac arrhythmia does not intervene, in which case the process may lead to sudden cardiac death.

## ECG Abnormalities in Neurocardiac Disease

A wide variety of ECG changes can be seen in neurological disease. The two most common ones are arrhythmias and repolarization changes. Typical ECG changes in cerebrovascular disease are long QT intervals, large, usually inverted T waves, and sometimes U waves. Less common are wide, deep Q waves, varying degrees of heart block, widening of the QRS complex, and asystole.

The changes are often best seen in anterolateral or inferolateral leads. The ECG pattern of neurocardiac disease is reminiscent of subendocardial ischemia, probably because intracardiac catecholamines are released into the endocardium and migrate toward the epicardium, dissipating as they go (**Figure 9-3**).

ECG changes seen in the context of neurological disease do not represent ischemic heart disease but are rather a

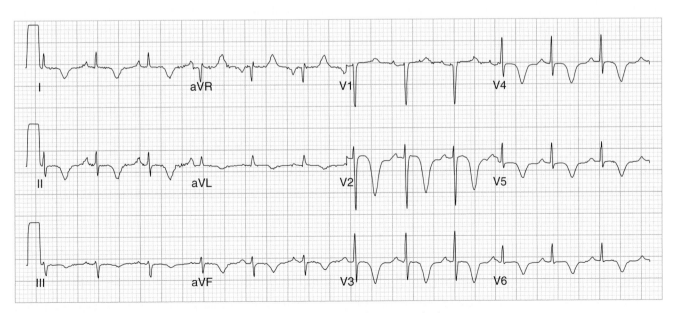

**Figure 9-2.** ECG of a 65-year-old patient with a left hemispheric stroke showing cerebral T waves.

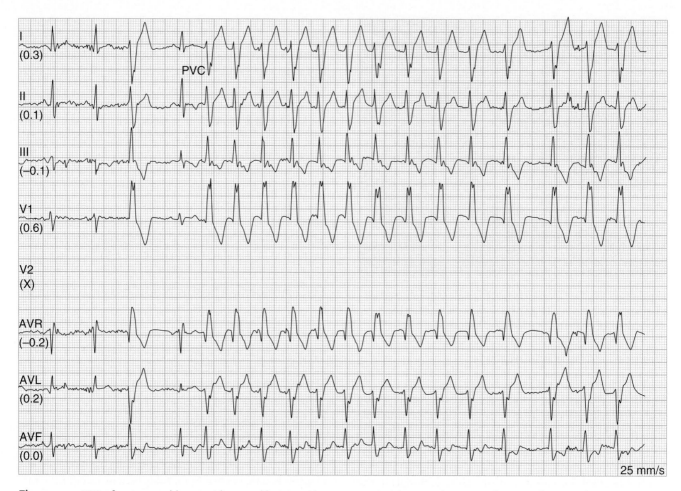

**Figure 9-3.** ECG of a 40-year-old man with normal heart and intense emotional stress, during recollection of events, showing sinus tachycardia and cerebral T waves.

manifestation of autonomic dysregulation, possibly caused by a lesion that affects the cortical or subcortical representations of the autonomic nervous system's cardiac outflow. A major ionic shift (calcium entry into cell) is probably the cause of ECG changes in the context of a neurological catastrophe. The risk of arrhythmias is high due to high catecholamine levels, and the mostly subendocardial location of the intracardiac lesions, thereby affecting the conducting system.

The ECG may be grossly abnormal, but microscopic changes might be minimal—due to reversibility of cardiac membrane abnormalities. ECG changes in neurological disease improve with any process that has the effect of disconnecting the brain from the heart (e.g., brain death, cardiac transplantation, severe autonomic neuropathy).

## Sudden Death

Sudden cardiac death may occur by neurogenic causes in a patient with a completely normal heart. It usually is the result of arrhythmia, but may also occur because of reduced cardiac output with secondarily reduced coronary blood flow. It is often associated with mental or physical stress. Sympathetic stimulation (as occurs under severe stress) lowers the threshold for ventricular fibrillation. An identifiable emotional trigger can be found in one-fifth of patients with life-threatening arrhythmias undergoing resuscitation.

Arrhythmias may also be the major immediate mechanism of sudden death in many neurological circumstances (subarachnoid hemorrhage, stroke, epilepsy). Cerebral hemispheric dominance (left: parasympathetic, right: sympathetic) also may contribute to the dominant mechanism of sudden death in a given person. Asymmetrical activation at the level of the midbrain is associated with an asymmetrical neural input to the heart, thus enhancing the repolarization inhomogeneities that predispose to arrhythmia.

Patients with preexisting cardiovascular disease may be more sensitive to stress-induced neurogenic arrhythmia. Certain neurological (epilepsy, subarachnoid hemorrhage, stroke) and psychiatric conditions (e.g., panic attacks) are associated with an enhanced risk of arrhythmia and sudden death.

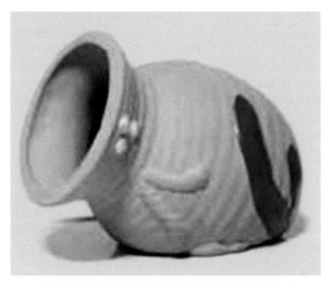

**Figure 9-4.** Tako-Tsubo (Japanese octopus trapping pot).

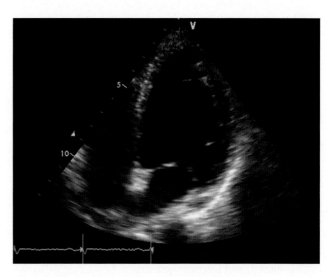

**Figure 9-6.** Repeat transthoracic echocardiogram two weeks later showing resolution of the apical ballooning.

The principles and mechanisms of neurogenic heart disease are applicable to the cardiac changes encountered in cerebrovascular disease (ischemic stroke, hemorrhagic stroke, subarachnoid hemorrhage), epilepsy, head trauma, psychological stress, increased intracranial pressure, encephalitis, and others, and also in the iatrogenic setting of electroconvulsive therapy. ECG changes and sudden death can occur in all of these circumstances.

## NEUROGENIC CARDIOMYOPATHY

Neurogenic cardiomyopathy is also known as *left ventricular apical ballooning syndrome*, or *tako-tsubo-like cardiomyopathy*. It is defined as acute transient left ventricular

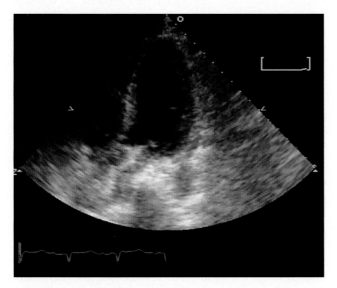

**Figure 9-5.** Transthoracic echocardiogram showing left ventricular apical ballooning.

dysfunction (LVD), with left ventricular apical ballooning. (See **Figures 9-4** and **9-5**). During systole, the shape of the left ventricle resembles a tako-tsubo (Japanese octopus trapping pot, similar to a flask with a short, narrow neck and wide, rounded body (see **Figure 9-6**)).

The most likely mechanism is a catecholamine excess: Catecholamines released directly into the heart by sympathetic nerve terminals lead to myocardial stunning (negative inotropic effect on myocyte contraction), microvascular dysfunction, and hyperdynamic contractility with midventricular outflow obstruction. Catecholamine levels are found to be many fold higher than what is seen in a normal resting person and significantly higher than in cases of acute myocardial infarction or cardiac failure. Common precipitants are severe, sudden emotional stress (e.g., news of an unexpected death, earthquakes), or physical stress (noncardiac medical events such as sepsis, subarachnoid hemorrhage). The pattern of dysfunction is most consistent with a neural rather than vascular distribution, and contraction band lesions may be found on endocardial biopsy.

Neurogenic cardiomyopathy may occur at any age, but proportionally few patients are younger than 50 years of age. There is a strong female predominance (>80%, mostly postmenopausal women). The precise incidence is unknown, but the diagnosis is becoming more common, probably because of increased recognition of the disease. A small number (perhaps about 2%) of patients with ST segment elevation, sudden onset heart failure, or acute coronary syndrome are ultimately found to have a stress cardiomyopathy.

The typical presentation includes chest pain (in about 70%) and dyspnea. It often mimics the acute coronary syndrome.

In a few patients, cardiogenic shock, ventricular fibrillation, and sudden cardiac death may ensue.

A potentially reversible regional wall motion abnormality beyond a single coronary artery distribution is found by echocardiography. Typically, the left ventricular apex and midventricle are affected, with relative sparing of the basal segment. However, neurogenic cardiomyopathy can involve any part of the myocardium. Right ventricle involvement, left and right ventricular apical akinesia and basal hyperkinesias, and left ventricular outflow obstruction due to hypercontractile basal myocardium can be observed, as can "inverted patterns" with basal ventricular suppression with apical sparing, or mid-ventricular ballooning. The most frequently affected right ventricular segments are apico-lateral, antero-lateral, and inferior segments.

Significant coronary artery disease is usually absent. However, stress cardiomyopathy and coronary artery disease are not mutually exclusive. The typical appearance is evident on ventriculography, echocardiography or cardiac MRI.

ECG changes are common in the acute stage: ST elevation (in 70-80%, commonly involving precordial leads), T wave abnormalities (~60%), Q waves, and QRS changes. T wave inversion can persist for several months.

Biomarkers for cardiac injury are also frequently abnormal. Troponin is elevated in 86%, creatine kinase myocardial band (CK-MB) in 74%. Pleural effusions are more common and more severe with right ventricular (RV) involvement (pleural effusions predictive of RV dysfunction). Reduced left ventricular ejection fraction (LVEF) is typically more obvious in patients with RV involvement.

Investigators at the Mayo Clinic have suggested the following criteria (all of which needed to be fulfilled) for diagnosis of tako-tsubo-like cardiomyopathy in 2004 (see **Table 9-2**).

---

**Table 9-2 • Proposed Mayo Criteria for the Clinical Diagnosis of the Transient Left Ventricular Apical Ballooning Syndrome**

1. Transient akinesis or dyskinesis of the left ventricular apical and mid-ventricular segments with regional wall motion abnormalities extending beyond a single epicardial vascular distribution
2. Absence of obstructive coronary artery disease and angiographic evidence of acute plaque rupture
3. New electrocardiographic abnormalities (either ST segment elevation or T wave inversion)
4. Absence of: recent significant head trauma, ICH, pheochromocytoma, obstructive epicardial coronary artery disease, myocarditis, hypertrophic cardiomyopathy

*From: Bybee KA, et al. Ann Intern Med. 2004;141:858–865, with permission.*

---

Treatment is supportive. There are no randomized controlled trials for treatment, but most experts use heart failure drugs including nitrates, diuretics, beta-blockers, ACE inhibitors, and aspirin. Controversy exists regarding vasopressors, because excessive levels of catecholamines are the basis for disease. Inotropic agents are counterintuitive due to worsening of epinephrine effects. Beta-blockers might be appropriate. Aortic balloon pump counterpulsation might be the best treatment for hemodynamic support.

The prognosis for patients who have suffered a neuropathic cardiomyopathy is overall excellent. Spontaneous improvement and return to normal function very often occur within days, and typically there is near complete resolution within a month. The most common complication is left heart failure with or without pulmonary edema. Rare complications include apical thrombus and left ventricular rupture. The in-hospital mortality is estimated as low as <1%.

## SUBARACHNOID HEMORRHAGE-INDUCED CARDIAC DYSFUNCTION

Subarachnoid hemorrhage (SAH) commonly causes cardiac dysfunction, probably because of a state of sympathetic nervous system hyperactivity. The mechanism likely is catecholamine-induced cardiac dysfunction. Patients with SAH have an increase in norepinephrine within 48 hours of the ictus, which persists during the first week, gradually normalizing by several months. Multivessel coronary artery spasm and microvascular dysfunction are other possible mechanisms, but convincing data to support these are lacking (coronary angiograms usually reveal normal coronary arteries even in the face of ongoing electrographic abnormalities).

Cardiac injury may be evident immediately or develop within hours after aneurysmal rupture. There is a fairly stereotyped sequence of hemodynamic changes after SAH. Initially, there is a dramatic rise in systemic blood pressure, and an extreme sinus tachycardia with various arrhythmias. This is followed by a rise in left ventricular pressure parallel to the systemic pressure, with an up to twofold increase in coronary blood flow.

Cardiac arrhythmias are frequent. Sinus tachycardia is the most common, but other supraventricular or ventricular arrhythmias can occur (e.g., supraventricular or ventricular tachycardia, bradycardia, asystole, atrial fibrillation, A-V block, premature ventricular beats, couplets). Stress cardiomyopathy with congestive heart failure and pulmonary edema can ensue (see "Neurogenic cardiomyopathy" above).

Sudden death occurs in up to 12% of patients with SAH. Pulmonary edema, partly cardiac, partly neurogenic, is found in the majority of those on autopsy. ECG abnormalities can be very transient and occur in 25-75% of patients with SAH, or even more on serial ECG monitoring. The most common are rate changes and ST segment abnormalities, T wave abnormalities (typically symmetrical T wave inversions), and QTc prolongation.

Cardiac biomarkers are often abnormal. Troponin I is elevated in 20-40%, highest on the day of ictus. Severe SAH (high Hunt–Hess score) is highly predictive of troponin I release. Troponin I is highly sensitive for detecting LV dysfunction in SAH. The peak troponin I levels are predictive of increased risk for hypotension, pulmonary edema, LV systolic dysfunction, and the need for vasopressors. The peak troponin I levels are also associated with increased risk of death or severe disability. CK-MB is elevated less often and is much less sensitive than troponin I for LV dysfunction.

The echocardiogram reveals regional wall motion abnormalities in 8% of patients with SAH. The wall motion abnormality often extends beyond the territory of a single coronary vessel, suggesting a stress cardiomyopathy. In some patients, there is a severely reduced ejection fraction with large regions of akinesis (accompanied by only modest troponin elevation, a pattern that is not reminiscent of myocardial infarction).

In summary:

- SAH-induced CHF can be mistaken as acute MI, which could delay the correct diagnosis,
- depressed cardiac index and presence of pulmonary complications are independent predictors of symptomatic cerebral vasospasm,
- in SAH patients, there is improvement in the ejection fraction within days to weeks,
- it is possible that prevention of the cardiac complications of SAH can be accomplished using early alpha-beta-blockade, but further investigation is necessary,
- at the moment, supportive therapy is all that is available.

## CARDIAC MANIFESTATIONS IN EPILEPSY

The propagation of cortical seizure activity to the insula may give rise to a number of autonomic manifestations through the numerous connections of the insula. Firing of hypothalamic cells in bursts has been observed to coincide with arrhythmias, and bursts of activity within cardiac autonomic nerves have been found synchronized with ictal and interictal spikes.

The lateralization of cardiac control is not entirely clear. Generally, bradycardia is caused by left—and tachycardia by right—insular stimulation, but bradycardia associated with right-sided stimulation has been reported. Changes in heart rate or rhythm occur in 90% of patients during seizures. Heart rate changes often precede seizure onset. In most cases, the heart returns to baseline within minutes. Cardiac parameters also are affected by motor activity during a seizure.

Ictal tachycardia is the most frequent cardiovascular change (64-100%). The ictal heart rate can exceed 190 bpm, but hemodynamic compromise is rarely seen. Ictal tachycardia is more often seen in temporal seizures, and when mesial temporal lesions are present. Ictal bradycardia is rare, with a prevalence rate of <6%. Bradycardia is seen primarily in temporal lobe seizures, mostly with complex partial seizures, and more often in medically refractory focal epilepsy. To detect ictal bradycardia, continuous cardiac loop monitoring may be necessary. Most patients with ictal bradycardia need both pharmaceutical seizure treatment and cardiac pacing. Antiepileptic drugs (AED) alone may not be sufficient due to the failure rate of pharmaceutical treatment (up to 37% of patients). Also, AEDs may affect AV conduction and increase the cardiac risk. The occurrence of ictal tachycardia and bradycardia can be quite variable from one seizure to another, even in a given patient with the same type of seizures. Other ECG abnormalities seen in epilepsy are: QT prolongation, R on T phenomenon, bundle branch block, ectopy, and asystole.

Heart disease mimicking seizures or presenting as seizures is a vexing clinical problem. Syncope is defined as the self-limited loss of consciousness of relative rapid onset and spontaneous prompt recovery. The underlying mechanism is transient global cerebral hypoperfusion. Sudden cessation of blood flow for 6-8 seconds or a 20% drop in cerebral oxygen delivery is the mechanism leading to transient anoxia-induced dysfunction or neurons in the reticular formation, giving rise to reticulospinal pathways that provide excitatory and inhibitory influences to the spinal motor neurons. Syncope can mimic a seizure, with myoclonus, tonic spasms, versive eye movements, or righting movements. It can be difficult for one to make the distinction between seizure and syncope. A carefully taken history and direct observation (if possible) will often help. Motor activity in syncope is typically brief. True post-ictal confusion makes a seizure more likely, but very short-lived confusion may occur after syncope. Aura speaks for seizure, but syncope can occur with visceral and experiential sensations. EEG findings in syncope are diffuse slowing, then attenuation, then back to normal.

Seizures can present *as* syncope in cases of ictal bradycardia (see **Table 9-3**).

Long QT syndromes usually present with ventricular tachyarrhythmia or sudden death. About 10% may present with

| Table 9-3 • Distinguishing Features: Seizure Versus Syncope | | |
|---|---|---|
| | **Seizure** | **Syncope** |
| Aura | yes | no |
| Motor activity | longer | brief (seconds) |
| Post-ictal confusion | longer | very short |
| EEG | ictal pattern → post-ictal slowing | diffuse slowing → attenuation → normal |

episodes, suggesting generalized seizures. Sudden unexpected death in epilepsy (SUDEP) has come to be recognized as a major cause of death among epileptics. The mortality rate from sudden death in people with epilepsy is 24 times higher than age-matched controls. SUDEP accounts for up to 17% of deaths in epilepsy. The precise cause of SUDEP is unknown and it is likely that there are several mechanisms, including ictal arrhythmias (mostly bradycardia), cardiac myocyte injury due to catecholamine excess, neurogenic pulmonary edema, and ictal respiratory suppression/central apnea.

Risk factors for SUDEP are high seizure frequency, generalized tonic clonic seizures, young age, subtherapeutic AED levels, long duration of epilepsy, and more than two AEDs.

### Electroconvulsive Therapy—Cardiac Aspects

Electroconvulsive therapy (ECT) involves seizure induction by electrical currents in anesthetized patients, for treatment of psychiatric diseases (mostly depression). About 1 million people worldwide receive ECT every year, usually as a course of 6-12 treatments administered 2 or 3 times a week. Initially, the ECT stimulus induces a parasympathetic response followed by sympathetic activity. During the seizure, there is an up to 15-fold rise in circulating epinephrine, and a 3-fold rise in circulating norepinephrine. Cardiac output increases by up to 80% and myocardial oxygen consumption by 30-140%. Numerous potentially serious cardiac side effects can occur in this setting.

The rate of complications during ECT is difficult to establish as it depends on a variety of factors, including pre-ECT assessment and patient condition, anesthesia, and definition of "complication." The estimated frequency of deaths from ECT is 2-4 out of 100,000—comparable to the rate with barbiturate anesthesia alone. The general anesthesia-related mortality is about 1/13,000. The estimated cardiac complication rates are 0.5% during the first treatment and 0.9% at some point during treatment. Very few of these complications result in permanent injury or disability. Patients with preexisting cardiovascular disease are at significantly higher risk to experience minor complications (57% versus 23% in one series).

Common cardiac side effects of ECT are transient hypertension (13%), transient cardiac arrhythmias (3.5%), ECG changes consistent with ischemia, and decreased heart rate variability (due to relative decrease of vagal activity during ECT). Most deaths in ECT are due to cardiac complications. Increased sympathetic activity associated with increased risk for sustained ventricular arrhythmias and sudden death may be the culprit.

## COGNITION AND HEART SURGERY

There are three categories of central nervous system complications of cardiac surgery: acute encephalopathy, overt stroke, and the chronic syndrome of cognitive decline (often associated with depression).

The predominant mechanism for intraoperative brain injury is cerebral embolism. Manipulation of the heart and great vessels and clamping of the aorta are likely enough stimuli to release embolic showers which can travel to and lodge in the brain. Generally, microembolism can lead to inattention, confusion, delirium in the acute setting (acute encephalopathy occurs if embolic burden is high: ≈10%); chronic effects are chronic depression, apathy, inattention, and dementia. Macroembolism causes focal cerebral damage (i.e., overt stroke). Most embolic strokes occur postoperatively when the perfusing blood pressure is adequate.

Borderzone ischemia from hypotension or loss of cardiac output is relatively rare. Borderzone is the area at the boundary between the territories of two major intracranial vessels. These infarcts are often hemorrhagic. They are cone-shaped with the base on the pial surface and typically very symmetric; however, they may be unilateral in cases of carotid stenosis, thereby making one hemisphere more vulnerable. Circulatory arrest leads to generalized damage in the neocortex and cerebellum, and more variable damage in the central gray matter, motor nuclei in brainstem, and hypothalamus. The anterior horn cells are least vulnerable. The risk for borderzone hypotensive damage is increased in chronically hypertensive patients where the cerebral autoregulation curve (normally 50-150 mm Hg MAP) is shifted to the right, and makes them more vulnerable to falls in cerebral blood flow even when the absolute blood pressure is only modestly hypotensive.

Major neurologic defects after cardiopulmonary bypass are found in 6% of patients. Acute encephalopathy occurs in less than 10%. Stroke incidence is about 5% (as low as 3% for the best surgeons), with 2-3% being major; strokes are more likely to develop when pump time is maintained for longer periods. Patients with neurological complications after cardiac surgery have an up to 10-fold greater mortality compared with neurologically intact patients.

| Table 10-3 • Evolutionary ECG Changes in Acute Pericarditis | |
|---|---|
| Stage 1 | ST segments elevate, typically within a few hours of the onset of chest pain and persist for hours or days. Depression of the PR segment occurs in this stage and differentiates acute pericarditis from early repolarization variants. |
| Stage 2 | ST segments return to baseline; at this point, the T waves may appear normal or exhibit a loss of amplitude. |
| Stage 3 | T waves invert; may persist indefinitely, particularly with tuberculous, uremic, or neoplastic pericarditis. |
| Stage 4 (variable) | ECG normalizes. |

the ST segment elevations caused by acute pericarditis from those caused by acute MI or normal early repolarization. The ST-T wave changes in acute pericarditis are diffuse and have characteristic evolutionary changes (**Table 10-3**). In a typical case of acute pericarditis, the approximate time frame for these ECG changes is two weeks. However, only about half of patients with acute pericarditis display all four ECG stages, and variations are very common.

As in this case of uncomplicated acute pericarditis, the chest radiograph is generally normal. However, the cardiac silhouette may be enlarged because of a moderate or large pericardial effusion. In addition, the chest radiograph may provide evidence of tuberculosis, fungal disease, pneumonia, or neoplasm.

Accumulation of transudate, exudate, or blood in the pericardial sac is a frequent complication of pericardial disease and should be sought in all patients with acute pericarditis. Some pearls to remember about the echocardiogram in pericarditis and pericardial effusions:

- Echocardiographic identification of pericardial effusion confirms the clinical diagnosis of acute pericarditis, but a patient with purely fibrinous acute pericarditis may have a normal echocardiogram.
- Echocardiography estimates the volume of pericardial fluid, identifies cardiac tamponade, suggests the basis of pericarditis, and documents associated acute myocarditis with congestive heart failure.
- While echocardiography is the procedure of choice for the diagnosis of pericardial effusion, computed tomography (CT) and magnetic resonance imaging (CMRI) may be useful to identify loculated or atypically loculated pericardial effusions and to characterize the nature of the effusion.
- Epicardial fat may mimic an effusion, but it is slightly echogenic and tends to move in concert with the

heart; these two characteristics help distinguish it from an effusion, which is generally echolucent and motionless.
- Chronic effusive pericarditis may be associated with large, asymptomatic effusions. Transudative effusions occur in heart failure and other states associated with chronic salt and water retention. Exudative effusions occur in a large number of the infectious and inflammatory types of pericarditis.
- Frank hemorrhagic effusions suggest recent intrapericardial bleeding, but sanguineous and serosanguineous effusions occur in many infectious and inflammatory disorders.
- Chylous pericarditis implies injury or obstruction to the thoracic duct, and cholesterol pericarditis is either idiopathic or associated with hypothyroidism, rheumatoid arthritis, or tuberculosis.
- The etiology of a pericardial effusion is difficult to determine on historical or clinical grounds. Specific diagnoses are possible using visual, cytologic, and immunologic analysis of the pericardial effusion and pericardioscopic-guided biopsy.

Nonspecific blood markers of inflammation usually increase in cases of acute pericarditis, and serum cardiac isoenzymes may increase with extensive epicarditis. Many patients presenting with acute, idiopathic pericarditis have increased serum troponin I levels, often within the range considered diagnostic for acute myocardial infarction.

Hospitalization is warranted for high risk patients that present with an initial episode of acute pericarditis in order to determine an etiology and to observe for the development of cardiac tamponade. Features indicative of high risk pericarditis include fever >38°C, subacute onset, an immunosuppressed state, trauma, oral anticoagulant therapy, myopericarditis, a moderate or large pericardial effusion, cardiac tamponade, and treatment failure. Some treatment pearls:

- Acute pericarditis usually responds to high doses of oral nonsteroidal anti-inflammatory agents (NSAIDs), such as ASA or ibuprofen. Indomethacin reduces coronary blood flow and should be avoided.
- Colchicine may be used as monotherapy or as a supplement to NSAIDs.
- Chest pain is usually alleviated in 1-2 days and the friction rub and ST segment elevation resolve shortly thereafter. Most mild cases of idiopathic and viral pericarditis are adequately treated with 1-4 days of treatment, but the duration of therapy is variable, and patients should be treated until an effusion, if present, has resolved.
- Narcotics may be required for severe pain.
- Corticosteroids should be avoided unless there is a specific indication (such as connective tissue disease or uremic pericarditis).

- Painful recurrences of pericarditis may respond to NSAIDs but commonly require high-dose corticosteroids. Using the lowest possible dose, alternate-day therapy, combinations with nonsteroidal drugs, or colchicine minimizes the risks of long term steroids.

## CARDIAC TAMPONADE

A 57-year-old female with metastatic breast cancer presented to the emergency room with complaints of increasing shortness of breath and fatigue, chest discomfort, and dizziness. The arterial blood pressure was 100/70 with a 20 mm Hg paradox. The respiratory rate was 30/min and the heart rate was 110/min. The jugular venous pulse was elevated, decreased with inspiration, and the Y descent was absent. The heart sounds were muffled. There was mild ankle edema. An enlarged cardiac silhouette was noted on chest radiogram. ECG revealed low voltage and electrical alternans. A large pericardial effusion with right atrial and ventricular collapse, respiratory variation of ventricular dimensions and transvalvular and venous flows, and vena caval plethora were seen on echocardiogram. The patient was admitted to the intensive care unit where an echo-guided pericardiocentesis yielded 1000 cc of bloody fluid and provided symptomatic relief.

Cardiac tamponade is characterized by the accumulation of pericardial fluid under pressure and may be acute or subacute, low pressure, or regional. It is a hemodynamic condition in which there is equalization of cardiac chamber and pericardial pressures, arterial hypotension, and an exaggerated decrease in systolic blood pressure with inspiration (pulsus paradoxus). Central venous pressures increase in tamponade to maintain filling pressures and prevent cardiac chamber collapse in the setting of increasing pericardial pressures. This results in a transmural pressure (diastolic pressure minus pericardial pressure) equal to zero or negative with a subsequent loss of preload (and consequently decreased cardiac output and arterial hypotension) despite elevated intracardiac pressures. Some pearls regarding etiology and pathophysiology of cardiac tamponade to consider:

- Pericardial effusion from any cause may eventuate in tamponade, but most commonly complicate neoplastic, idiopathic, tuberculous, and purulent pericarditis; anticoagulant therapy is an important risk factor.
- Tamponade can be a complication of a diagnostic procedure (cardiac catheterization, pacemaker/implantable defibrillator placement), myocardial infarction (cardiac rupture), and ascending aortic dissection. Thoracic trauma may also lead to tamponade.

- Acute bleeding (e.g., due to trauma) into a relatively stiff pericardium can rapidly lead to tamponade. As intrapericardial volume increases, there is an initial small increase in intrapericardial pressure followed by an almost vertical ascent. Tamponade in these instances occurs with relatively small pericardial effusions.
- In comparison, chronic accumulation of a pericardial effusion (e.g., neoplastic) allows the pericardial compliance to increase gradually. As a result, intrapericardial pressure increases more slowly until a critical point is reached when an almost vertical ascent is again seen. In this setting, tamponade may not occur until 2 L or more have accumulated.

Some diagnostic pearls:

- Electrical alternans on the ECG is characterized by beat-to-beat alterations in the QRS complex; although relatively specific, it is not very sensitive for tamponade.
- Low QRS voltage in patients with a pericardial effusion may actually be a specific manifestation of tamponade, not of the effusion per se.
- Echocardiographic findings suggesting hemodynamic compromise (right atrial and ventricular collapse) are the result of transiently reversed right atrial and right ventricular diastolic transmural pressures, respectively (**Figure 10-1**). Cardiac chamber collapse typically occurs before hemodynamic embarrassment.
- Reciprocal changes in left and right ventricular volumes that occur with respiration play a central role in the pathogenesis of pulsus paradoxus.
- The respiratory variation of mitral and tricuspid flow velocities is greatly increased and out of phase, reflecting the increased ventricular interdependence.
- Any chamber collapse has a sensitivity and specificity of ~90 and 65%.

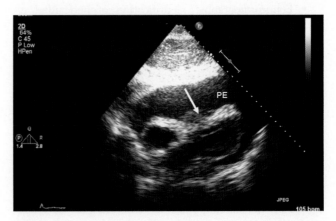

**Figure 10-1.** Two-dimensional echocardiogram in cardiac tamponade. There is a large effusion (PE) with marked compression of the right ventricle (arrow).

- The sensitivity is lower and specificity higher (75 and 91%) for abnormal right-sided venous flows (systolic predominance and expiratory diastolic reversal), but the latter cannot be evaluated in more than one-third of patients.
- The specificity is highest (98%) for right atrial and right ventricular collapse plus abnormal venous flow.

Other imaging techniques, such as computed tomography (CT) and cardiovascular magnetic resonance (CMR), are not necessary if 2-D and Doppler echocardiography are available and technically adequate. However, pericardial effusion may be detected, quantified, and characterized by CT and CMR.

Cardiac catheterization shows elevation (10-30 mm Hg) and equalization (within 4-5 mm Hg) of right atrial, pulmonary capillary wedge pressure and pulmonary artery diastolic pressures. Pericardial pressures are elevated and equal to right atrial pressure. Right atrial tracings and pulmonary capillary wedge tracings demonstrate a blunted or absent Y descent. Cardiac output is decreased and systemic vascular resistance is increased. Cardiac tamponade is defined as mild when pericardial pressure is <10 mm Hg and severe when pericardial pressure is >20 mm Hg.

Management of cardiac tamponade requires urgent pericardiocentesis to restore hemodynamic stability. Removal of small amounts of fluid produces considerable improvement in the clinical picture owing to a steep pericardial pressure-volume relationship. Pericardiocentesis may be done under echo guidance, fluoroscopic guidance, or surgically, depending on a center's resources and areas of expertise, as well as on the etiology, overall prognosis, and/or the need for diagnostic tissue sampling. Pericardial drainage should continue until drainage volume is <25 mL/day.

Medical management of tamponade (while awaiting definitive pericardial drainage) includes fluids to maintain preload and dobutamine to increase cardiac output. Recurrent effusions may be treated with pericardial window or sclerotherapy.

## CONSTRICTIVE PERICARDITIS

A 62-year-old male with a history of idiopathic pericarditis 10 years previously presented with several months of increasing fatigue, dyspnea, weight gain, abdominal discomfort, nausea, increased abdominal girth, and swollen legs. The blood pressure was normal without a pulsus paradox. The heart rate was irregularly irregular at a rate of ~90/min. There was temporal wasting and markedly elevated jugular venous pressure with prominent X and Y descents that did not decrease with inspiration. The intensity of S1 was variable and a third heart sound was heard. There was shifting dullness in the abdomen and 2+ lower extremity edema. The ECG revealed atrial fibrillation, low QRS voltage, nonspecific T wave changes, and P mitrale. Chest radiogram revealed a slightly enlarged cardiac silhouette and a ring of pericardial calcification. An echocardiogram revealed increased pericardial thickness, abrupt inspiratory posterior motion of the ventricular septum in early diastole, enlarged atria, an abnormal contour between the posterior left ventricular and left atrial posterior walls, plethora of the inferior vena cava and hepatic veins with expiratory diastolic reversals, but minimal respiratory variation of transmitral diastolic velocities. The annular tissue velocity was increased. The BNP was 138 ρg/mL. Cardiac catheterization confirmed the suspicion of pericardial constriction by demonstrating discordance of LV and RV pressure with respiration, an inspiratory decrease in the pulmonary capillary wedge-LV diastolic gradient, elevated and equal atrial pressures, Kussmaul's sign (the lack of an inspiratory decline in jugular pressure), and a "dip and plateau" of ventricular diastolic pressure. The patient was referred for pericardiectomy.

Constrictive pericarditis is the result of scarring and consequent loss of elasticity of the pericardial sac. Pericardial constriction is typically chronic, but may be subacute, transient, or occult. The pathological changes are chronic inflammation, sometimes with calcification. Grossly, the pericardium is considerably thicker than normal in approximately 80% of cases. Some pearls related to the pathophysiology of constrictive pericarditis to ponder:

- In constrictive pericarditis the upper limit of cardiac volume is constrained by the inelastic pericardium. Unlike tamponade, compression does not occur until the cardiac volume approximates the reserve volume of the pericardium, which occurs in mid through late diastole. Since there is no compression in systole and early diastole, the normal bimodal pattern of venous return is maintained.
- Venous return to the right heart does not increase during inspiration because the respiratory variation in intrathoracic pressure is not transmitted to the heart chambers. As a result of this dissociation of intrathoracic and intracardiac pressures, there is an inspiratory decrease in pulmonary venous, but not left ventricular pressure, and consequently a reduction in left ventricular volume.
- Another important pathophysiologic feature of constrictive pericarditis is greatly enhanced ventricular interaction or interdependence, in which the hemodynamics of the left and right heart chambers are directly influenced by each other to a much greater degree than normal. As a result of the inspiratory decrease in LV filling, the right heart volume expands via a leftward shift of the interventricular septum.

Constrictive pericarditis can occur after virtually any pericardial disease process. A few pearls regarding the etiology of constrictive pericarditis:

- Most data come from a few large series of patients with constrictive pericarditis diagnosed at pericardiectomy. The frequency of the various causes in these reports is influenced by referral bias.
- Most commonly, constrictive pericarditis results from idiopathic or viral pericarditis, cardiac surgery, radiation therapy, connective tissue disorder, or infectious pericarditis. Miscellaneous causes (malignancy, trauma, drug-induced, asbestosis, sarcoidosis, uremic pericarditis) account for a small percent.
- Tuberculosis once accounted for the majority of cases but is now only a rare cause of constrictive pericarditis in developed countries. However, this disorder may be increasing among immigrants from underdeveloped countries and patients with HIV infection.

Patients with pericardial constriction may present with two types of complaints: those related to fluid overload, ranging from peripheral edema to anasarca; and those related to diminished cardiac output response to exertion, such as fatigability and dyspnea on exertion. Pericardial constriction should be considered in any patient with an unexplained elevation in jugular venous pressure, particularly if there is a history of a predisposing condition. The case presented typifies the clinical features of constrictive pericarditis that occurred years after idiopathic pericarditis. Clinical pearls to remember:

- The X and Y descents are more prominent than the peaks of the jugular venous pulse, and the inspiratory decline in venous pressure is confined to the depth of the Y descent.
- Occult constriction has been described in patients who are volume-depleted; in this setting, the increase in venous pressure may not become apparent without rapid volume expansion.
- Common findings with more severe constriction include peripheral edema, ascites, pulsatile hepatomegaly, and pleural effusion. These findings may lead to the misdiagnosis of chronic liver disease. In patients with cirrhosis, the jugular pressure is normal or only slightly elevated, unless there is tense ascites.
- Pulsus paradoxus is not common in the absence of pericardial fluid or pulmonary disease.
- Kussmaul's sign may be present but does not distinguish constriction from severe tricuspid valve disease or right-sided heart failure.
- A pericardial knock (a third heart sound) may be audible and sometimes palpable.
- Profound cachexia occurs with late-stage disease; because of the associated ascites and hepatic dysfunction, the patient's appearance simulates that of severe malnutrition.

- The presence of a ring of calcification around the heart, best seen on a lateral chest radiograph, strongly suggests pericardial constriction in patients with symptoms of right heart failure, but pericardial calcification can occur in the absence of constriction.
- Plasma BNP is only slightly elevated in constrictive pericarditis; in contrast, in restrictive cardiomyopathy (which constriction resembles clinically), the BNP is markedly elevated.

Echocardiography is an essential adjunctive procedure in patients with pericardial constriction. One or more of the following findings may be seen:

- Increased pericardial thickness. Unlike transthoracic imaging, measurement of pericardial thickness by transesophageal echocardiography correlates strongly with that obtained by computed tomography.
- While no sign or combination of signs on M-mode is diagnostic of constrictive pericarditis, a normal study virtually rules out the diagnosis. One useful sign is the abrupt posterior motion of the ventricular septum in early diastole with inspiration (septal shudder or bounce), which results from underfilling of the left ventricle during inspiration.
- 2D-echocardiography reveals dilation and absent or diminished collapse of the inferior vena cava and hepatic veins (plethora), biatrial enlargement, a sharp halt in ventricular diastolic filling, and an abnormal contour between the posterior left ventricular and left atrial posterior walls (**Figure 10-2**). The left ventricular ejection fraction is typically normal.
- Doppler echocardiography is critically important for diagnosis and usually shows a high early diastolic velocity of right and left ventricular inflow (restrictive

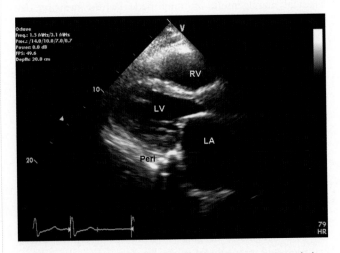

**Figure 10-2.** Two-dimensional echocardiogram in pericardial constriction. Note the thickened pericardium (peri), dilated left atrium (LA), and abnormal left ventricular (LV)-left atrial contour.

filling pattern); mitral inflow velocity falls at least 25 percent and tricuspid velocity greatly increases in the first beat after inspiration. Increased respiratory variation of mitral inflow may be missing in patients with markedly elevated left atrial pressure, as in our case, but can sometimes be brought out in such patients by preload reduction. Hepatic vein flow reversal increases with expiration, reflecting the ventricular interaction and the dissociation of intracardiac and intrathoracic pressures.

- Tissue Doppler shows a prominent mitral diastolic annular E' (in contrast to the low E' in restrictive cardiomyopathy, which shares clinical and hemodynamic features).

CT scanning of the heart is extremely useful in the diagnosis of constrictive pericarditis; findings include increased pericardial thickness (>4 mm) and calcification. CMR is claimed by some to be the diagnostic procedure of choice for the detection of constrictive pericarditis.

Cardiac catheterization is used to confirm the clinical suspicion of pericardial disease, uncover occult constriction, diagnose effusive-constrictive disease, and identify associated coronary, myocardial, and valvular disease. Some hemodynamic pearls:

- Discordance between peak right ventricular (RV) and left ventricular (LV) systolic pressures during inspiration is a sign of increased ventricular interdependence. During peak inspiration an increase in RV pressure occurs when LV pressure is lowest.
- Equalization of LV and RV diastolic plateau pressure tracings with a "dip and plateau" or "square root" appearance reflects rapid early diastolic filling of the ventricles, followed by lack of additional filling due to compression in mid and late diastole.
- Right atrial pressure is increased with prominent X and Y descents. In contrast, the Y descent of diastolic filling is absent in tamponade.
- A greater inspiratory fall in pulmonary capillary wedge pressure compared to left ventricular diastolic pressure is seen, reflecting dissociation of intrathoracic and intracardiac pressures.
- Effusive-constrictive pericarditis, an uncommon entity, occurs when pericardial fluid accumulates between the thickened layers of pericardium. The hemodynamic picture is consistent with tamponade prior to pericardiocentesis and constrictive pericarditis afterwards.

Pericardiectomy is the definitive treatment for constrictive pericarditis, but is unwarranted either in very early constriction or in severe, advanced disease (functional class IV), when the risk of surgery is excessive (30-40% mortality) and the benefits are diminished. Involvement of the visceral pericardium also increases the surgical risk. A few treatment pearls:

- Symptomatic relief and normalization of cardiac pressures may take several months after pericardiectomy; they occur sooner when the operation is carried out before the disease is too chronic and when the pericardiectomy is almost complete.
- Complete or extensive pericardial resection is desirable, as recurrences may be seen more frequently in patients who have undergone partial versus complete resection of the pericardium.
- Constriction may be transient with a course lasting weeks to a few months in patients recovering from acute effusive pericarditis. Therefore, it is reasonable that patients with subacute constrictive pericarditis who are hemodynamically stable be given a trial of conservative management for 2-3 months until it is clear that the constrictive process is permanent before pericardiectomy is recommended.

## Suggested Readings

1. Hoit BD. Diseases of the pericardium. In: Fuster V, O'Rourke RA, Walsh RA, Poole-Wilson PA, eds. *Hurst's The Heart*, 12th ed. New York: McGraw-Hill; 2008:1951–1974.

2. Hoit BD. Pericarditis. In: Antman E, ed. *Treatment of Pericardial Disease, in Cardiovascular Therapeutics*. 3rd ed. Philadelphia PA: W.B. Saunders; 2007:787–797.

3. Little, WC, Freeman, GL. Pericardial disease. *Circulation*. 2006;113:1622.

4. Maisch B, Seferovic PM, Ristic AD, et al. Guidelines on the Diagnosis and Management of Pericardial Diseases Executive Summary: The Task Force on the Diagnosis and Management of Pericardial Diseases of the European Society of Cardiology. *Eur Heart J.* 2004;25:587–610.

5. Shabetai R. *The Pericardium*. Norwell, MA: Kluver Academic Publishers; 2003.

# 11

# Cardiovascular Trauma as Seen by the Cardiologist

Melvin D. Cheitlin

## ● PRACTICAL POINTS

- Cardiac trauma is considered to be either penetrating or nonpenetrating injuries. Despite their mechanistic differences, both types of trauma can result in similar cardiovascular injuries.

- The degree of tissue damage caused by a penetrating missile depends on the missile's mass, shape, composition, and tumbling characteristics, as well as its velocity. The higher the velocity, the more extensive the tissue damage.

- It is not always possible by noting the point of entry of a missile to predict the path it takes and the structures it can injure since, especially with low velocity, the missile's path can be deflected by bone or even tissue planes.

- In deceleration or sternal compression accidents the most frequent site of aortic rupture is the proximal descending aorta. The second most common point of rupture is the ascending aorta, but due to the intrapericardial position of the ascending aorta, cardiac tamponade occurs rapidly and the patient usually dies at the scene of the accident.

- In penetrating injury to the chest or abdomen, when the patient develops hemodynamic instability and there is no evidence of significant hemorrhage, primary consideration should be given to the presence of cardiac tamponade. In injury where there is obvious significant loss of blood, cardiac tamponade can be present even in the absence of an elevated central venous pressure.

- With penetrating chest injury, fistulous connections between contiguous structures can occur. Examples are: aortic to right atrial or to right ventricular outflow tract fistulas; coronary cameral fistulas to right atrium or right ventricle; and coronary arteriovenous fistulas.

- With nonpenetrating injury, rupture of the mitral, tricuspid, or aortic valve can occur. In these cases of massive valvular regurgitation, the expected murmurs can be atypical or even absent, the patient in severe heart failure, and the cardiac silhouette on chest X-ray not enlarged.

- Myocardial contusion or blunt cardiac injury (BCI) can manifest as supraventricular and ventricular arrhythmias, ECG changes including nonspecific T wave changes, ST-segment elevated myocardial infarction (STEMI), and varying degrees of conduction defects.

- The preferred cardiac enzymes in evaluation of a patient for myocardial contusion are the myocardial-specific enzymes, troponin I and T. Creatine kinase, and even CK-MB, can be elevated due to skeletal muscle injury and, therefore, is nonspecific for myocardial necrosis.

- Retained foreign bodies in the cardiovascular system can migrate far from their point of entry.

# INTRODUCTION

Until the beginning of the twentieth century, trauma to the heart was believed to be almost invariably fatal. The famous German-Austrian surgeon Theodor Billroth, in 1888, is reported to have said that "the surgeon who attempts heart surgery loses the respect of his colleagues."[1] Although it was probably not what he meant when he belittled the procedure of pericardiocentesis by surgeons, it was the belief of surgeons at that time. As late as 1896 in Stephen Paget's classic textbook, *Surgery of the Chest*, he declared the heart to be off-limits to surgeons. Dr. Daniel Hale Williams, a black surgeon from Chicago, who reported it in the literature in 1897, performed the first successful surgery involving a stab wound to the heart in 1893. He repaired the pericardial tear but since the right ventricular puncture was not bleeding, didn't suture the heart wound.[2] In 1897 Dr. Ludwig Rehn, a surgeon from Frankfort Germany reported the first successful suture of a human heart wound in a 22-year-old man, who was stabbed in the heart.[3]

Rapid advances in surgery for cardiac trauma depended on the development of anesthesia, ventilatory support, blood preservation and banking, antibiotics, and cardiopulmonary bypass techniques. As is often the case with advances in trauma surgery, advances in cardiac trauma surgery were accelerated by experiences obtained in the twentieth century wars. It wasn't until World War II that it was possible to salvage with some regularity patients with abdominal or thoracic wounds.[4] In the Korean War rapid advances in techniques for repairing arterial injuries led to a marked decrease in the rate of limb amputations. Also, with rapid helicopter evacuations from the battlefield to treatment hospitals, mortality of those injured in battle was markedly decreased. In Vietnam, the mortality of an injured soldier found alive was <1%. Most wartime innovations have been applied to trauma management in civilian life. With knife and gunshot wounds, automobile accidents, and other traumatic incidents occurring daily, cardiovascular trauma will continue to be a problem.

Because trauma patients are first seen in the ER, the workup and management of the acutely injured patient is the province of the emergency physicians and surgical teams. A cardiologist is involved after initial resuscitation and stabilization, if cardiovascular trauma is suspected, usually by history, physical examination, or laboratory finding such as a chest X-ray.

# CLASSIFICATION AND PHYSICAL CAUSES OF TRAUMATIC INJURY

Cardiovascular trauma is usually divided into the categories "penetrating" and "nonpenetrating" injury.[5] However, it is important to realize that both can cause almost all

traumatic injuries. The features of each of these types are given here:

Penetrating injuries:

- low velocity objects; i.e., knife wounds, shrapnel, spent bullets;
- high velocity objects; i.e., gunshot wounds, shrapnel.

Nonpenetrating injuries:

- deceleration and acceleration; i.e., falls from a height, automobile accidents;
- direct compression or crush; i.e., heavy objects falling on the chest, steering wheel injuries;
- blast and concussion; i.e., explosions, IEDs (improvised explosive devices);
- lower body compression; i.e., heavy objects falling on the abdomen, cave-ins in a hole being dug;
- electrical; i.e., shocks from high power lines, lightning strikes;
- environmental; i.e., heat and cold.

Injury to tissues is the result of direct trauma of the object such as a knife or bullet and the energy released into the tissue by physical force contacting the body. In missile penetration damage done depends on the mass of the object, the shape and tumbling characteristics, fragmentation, and the velocity of the missile.[6] A low velocity missile causes little damage aside from the track of the missile in the body and the structures directly injured. Examples of low velocity trauma are those caused by knives and low velocity bullets and shrapnel. On entering the body, these weapons rapidly lose velocity, release little energy and frequently come to rest in the body forming intracardiac foreign bodies. Since they move slowly, these penetrating objects can be deflected off bones and even tissue planes, causing a path change in the body. For this reason it is not always possible for one to predict the path the missile by noting the point of entry. Therefore, the structures injured or where the missile finally came to rest are also not obvious. Low velocity missiles can enter cardiac chambers, arteries, or veins and migrate or embolize to some other point in the body distant from either the point of entry or from its known path. A high velocity missile releases a great deal of energy along its path through the body according to the equation:[7]

$$KE = \frac{m\,(V_1 - V_2)}{2\,g}$$

where KE = kinetic energy
  $m$ = mass of missile
  $V_1$ = entrance velocity
  $V_2$ = exit velocity
  $g$ = gravity constant

This results in a cylinder of energy release in the form of heat and gaseous expansion, causing tissue necrosis at variable, sometimes great, distances from the missile path. Also important in determining the degree of damage is the size and shape of the missile itself and how it tumbles as it moves when it enters the body and the tissue it passes through. With elastic tissue such as lung, the temporary cavity produces little damage away from the missile path. With liver or brain there can be substantial damage in the area of the temporary cavity. That explains the massive damage done by the so-called "dumdum" bullet that expands on impact.

In nonpenetrating injury due to compression—crush or concussion—the injury is produced when the heart strikes the sternum or spine. Here, two physical forces are involved: direct compression and transfer of energy to the body. In deceleration injuries, such as what occurs in car crashes, in which the body suddenly decelerates, the organs, including the heart and great vessels, continue to move at the velocity of the vehicle before the crash, striking the sternum or spine with force. Since the aorta and great vessels are variably restrained by intercostal vessels and the great arteries of the arch, differential movement at points of attachment at the time of the collision can cause aortic, arterial, and venous laceration.[8]

The mechanism by which the aorta is ruptured in vehicular accidents and steering wheel injury is still unclear. The most frequent sites of rupture are the root of the aorta as it arises from the heart and the proximal descending aorta at the ligamentus arteriosus, where differential movement would be greatest. Originally it was believed that this shearing stress was the cause of the rupture. However, experimental injury involving dogs and primates subject to sudden sternal compression simulating steering wheel injuries using high-speed cardioangiography have shown with massive chest compression there is marked posterior, caudal, and rightward displacement of the heart. There is also cranial displacement of the aortic arch with stretching of the thoracic aorta, resulting in shearing stress and rupture at the same sites as mentioned above.[9]

Another important feature involved in the effects of cardiac trauma is the timing of the impact during the cardiac cycle. There is a vulnerable period just before the peak of the T wave, at which time energy delivered to the heart can precipitate ventricular arrhythmias. Also in animal experiments, myocardial contusion and laceration are more likely to occur when the injury is delivered in diastole than in systole.[10] In diastole the heart is at its greatest mass and the wall's firmness and elasticity are least. In systole, the ventricular mass is at its smallest and the heart is firm and resilient and capable of moving away from the force, thereby limiting the distortion of the wall by the force.[10] Finally, compressive injuries to the lower extremities and abdomen as occurs when a heavy weight falls on the lower part of the body, can cause cardiovascular injury by suddenly compressing arteries and veins, causing a marked simultaneous increase in venous blood return to the heart and systemic vascular resistance. Together, these forces can result in atrial, ventricular, and valvular rupture.

## Penetrating Cardiac Injury

The severity of damage in penetrating injury depends on the track of the missile and its velocity and tumbling characteristics. Availability of a history describing the weapon responsible and the details of the attack is helpful. Estimating the track of the penetrating object is difficult, considering that a low velocity, penetrating missile can be deflected in the body, significantly altering the pathway and injuring organs not in the track presumed from the entrance wound. Therefore, cardiac injury can occur from penetrating injury in either the upper abdomen or the lateral chest wall.

The first consideration in the hemodynamically unstable patient must be cardiac tamponade. Therefore, before they can be diagnosed, patients with penetrating injury with a low blood pressure must have massive bleeding and cardiac tamponade ruled out. The most helpful differentiating feature is most often the central venous pressure, which can be estimated from examination of the cervical neck veins. In the presence of a low blood pressure, absence of venous waves is most often due to low blood volume and elevated venous pressure due to cardiac tamponade. One circumstance violates this rule: if there is major loss of blood and hypovolemia, cardiac tamponade can occur without an elevation in cervical venous pressure. In this case a paradoxical pulse is usually present. Confirmation of either tamponade or hemorrhage causing low blood pressure is obtained with a transthoracic echocardiogram (TTE).

### Complications of Penetrating Injury

Hemorrhage with subsequent hypovolemia is the most common result of a penetrating missile. High velocity bullets cause massive injury around the track of the missile, which must be extensively debrided. Laceration of the great vessels and the pericardium and heart occur, resulting in cardiac tamponade. If the laceration of the pericardium is relatively small and the chamber penetrated bleeds into the pericardial space relatively slowly, tamponade may occur gradually and late after the injury. If the bleeding into the pericardium is rapid, tamponade occurs very rapidly. If the pericardial laceration is large, the blood gathers in the pleural space. Even with rapid bleeding from a cardiac chamber laceration, blood cannot stay in the tight pericardial space and tamponade doesn't occur.

With laceration of either ventricle, if the laceration is completely through the ventricular wall, blood is ejected out of the chamber into the pericardial space. If the laceration does not create an extensive hole in the epicardium, blood can accumulate on the surface of the heart, trapped by the relatively intact epicardium and pericardium. This is the basis for the formation of a ventricular false aneurysm or pseudoaneurysm, with communication of the ventricular chamber with an aneurysmal sac composed of pericardium and thrombus. Diagnosis is made usually from observation of the deformity of the ventricular silhouette on the chest X-ray, although small false aneurysms can be discovered by TTE, MRI, or CAT scans. Since these false aneurysms can rupture at any time, even long after injury, usually they are repaired when discovered. If the damage to the ventricular myocardium is extensive, ventricular function is compromised and heart failure occurs.

Penetrating injuries can lacerate two adjacent structures and result in arteriovenous fistulae, aorto-cameral fistulae, and fistulae between adjacent chambers (interventricular, interatrial fistulae). If the shunt is large enough, murmurs can be heard. Depending on which chambers are connected and the size of the shunt, the murmur can be systolic, diastolic, continuous, or absent. If the shunt is small, there is little danger of late complications, although endocarditis has been reported. If the shunt is large enough, the chambers can become dilated and heart failure can ensue. If this occurs, repair is indicated. Repair usually means surgical repair. In the case of interventricular septal defects and aortocameral fistulae, it is possible to close some of these by interventional catheter techniques.[11-13]

Penetrating injury to any of the valves or papillary muscles can result in aortic, mitral, or tricuspid or pulmonary valve regurgitation. The clinical consequences of such injury depend on the severity of the regurgitation and the response of the ventricles to the volume overload. The treatment of such injury is similar to the treatment of a like amount of valvular regurgitation from any other cause.[14-17]

## Myocardial Contusion— Blunt Cardiac Injury (BCI)

The cardiac injury most often suspected in trauma is that of myocardial contusion. Since almost any pathologic cardiac damage is possible from nonpenetrating trauma including pericardial injury and laceration, myocardial rupture, development of aorto-cameral fistulae, coronary artery rupture or thrombosis, and valvular disruption, a better term—blunt cardiac injury (BCI)—has been introduced.[18] Nonpenetrating cardiac injury occurs most often as a result of motor vehicle accidents. However, falls, compressive injury due to heavy objects falling on the chest, and compression due to collapse of the walls onto a person who has been digging a hole have all been responsible for BCI. Blunt cardiac Injury can cause arrhythmias, conduction defects, and even sudden death without any detectable myocardial pathological injury, so-called *commotio cordis*.[19-21] This occurs in situations, frequently sporting events, where there is an impact imparting low energy to

the ventricle at a vulnerable window just before the T wave peak, causing ventricular tachycardia or fibrillation.[20]

If the heart is examined after BCI, myocardial necrosis, edema, and hemolytic infiltrate can be seen. The degree of injury depends on the mechanism of the BCI and the magnitude of the force.[19,22] In the classic study from the Armed Forces Institute of Pathology (AFIP) in 1958, Parmley and colleagues reported the spectrum of injury at autopsy of people who died with cardiovascular trauma in 546 nonpenetrating cardiac trauma cases.[23] Since they were all fatal, not necessarily from the cardiac injury, this series is not representative of all BCIs, only the most serious. They reported 64% with at least one cardiac chamber rupture, 20% with two or more chambers ruptured, 23% with myocardial contusion, 6% with pericardial laceration, 4% with papillary muscle rupture, 2% with valvular rupture, and 1% with coronary artery laceration.[23]

## The Clinical Picture of BCI and Penetrating Injury

Blunt cardiac injury is the result of compressive, concussive, or crushing forces to the chest. The most common mechanism responsible for BCI is the motor vehicle accident, but in the large city environment the type of trauma seen is very near what is seen in a war zone: gunshot and knife wounds, missile fragment wounds, and massive injury from falls or collisions.

# IMMEDIATE ASSESSMENT AND THERAPY[24]

The first priority must be rapid evaluation of the patient's injuries, evidence of hemorrhage, vital signs and hemodynamic stability.

*Rapid assessment of adequacy of airway, respiration, blood pressure, heart rate and cardiac output:*

- Establish airway and respiration: may need oral airway, tracheostomy, or assisted respiration. Rule out tension pneumothorax.
- If blood pressure and pulse are absent, start cardiopulmonary resuscitation. Although the prognosis for survival is poor, studies show that the results are similar to the results of cardiopulmonary resuscitation in medical out-of-hospital cardiac arrests.[25,26] In one study[25] more trauma than medical arrest patients lived to be admitted to the hospital (29.9% versus 23.5%), but there was no difference between the two groups at hospital discharge (2.2% versus 2.8%), although other studies[26] have reported survival rates of 9.7%.
- Insert at least 2 large bore needles or catheters for fluids. If blood pressure low, infuse 2 liters of fluids rapidly. May start with saline or Ringers solution, substitute with colloids (blood) as soon as possible.

- Assess central venous pressure (CVP): neck veins or central venous catheter. If CVP is elevated and injury capable of causing tamponade, make presumptive diagnosis and act on it.
- The patient who has an injury that could have caused tamponade and is pulseless, in shock, or without blood pressure should be assumed to be in cardiac tamponade and a thoracotomy should be performed in the emergency department, as a last resort toward saving patient's life.[24,27]
- If life-threatening arrhythmia is present: Start CPR. If asystole, infuse isoproterenol or place a temporary pacemaker. If ventricular tachycardia or fibrillation, cardiovert or defibrillate. If complete A-V block is present an external pacemaker is applied until more definitive treatment can be instituted.

*Once respiratory and circulatory support is adequate:*

- Take a brief history of the trauma. Obtain a description of the time and details of the trauma; if auto accident, was it a front-end or rear-end collision? Was patient wearing a seatbelt? If violent crime, what weapon was used? Gunshot? Type of knife?
- Get a past medical history; is the patient hypertensive, diabetic; does he have heart or lung disease and type?
- What medications is the patient taking? Any illicit drugs and type?

*Do a rapid physical examination:*

- Vital signs—BP, heart rate and rhythm, respiration rate, and signs of distress.
- Note presence of sites of contusions, hematomas, lacerations, missile entry, and exit wounds.
- Assess head and neck for cervical and cranial trauma. Palpate for depressed skull fractures, note blood or cerebrospinal fluid from nose and ear canals.
- Examine for face and extremity pallor or cyanosis as a clue to pulmonary or peripheral arterial or venous injury.
- Note cervical venous pressure.
- Examine lungs for dullness or resonance on percussion, absent breath sounds or rales.
- Cardiac examination: note position of PMI abnormal lifts, quality of heart sounds, presence of friction rubs, murmurs and gallops. Examine pulses and note pulsus alternans or paradoxus.
- Note abdominal and extremity injury
- Do a rapid neurological examination: state of consciousness, cranial nerve abnormalities, movements of eyes and limbs, quality of reflexes

After assessing the status of the airway and pulse and attending immediately to any life-threatening abnormalities, obtain a brief history addressing the circumstances of the trauma, whether external bleeding was seen and how extensive it was, and whether the patient has symptoms:

Pain, where, how severe, and what aggravates it, shortness of breath, light-headedness of syncope, and a brief assessment of other significant injuries. A past medical history and medications taken by the patient should be obtained. With myocardial rupture and tamponade, the patient may be dead at the scene or hemodynamically unstable or in shock. In the patient suspected of BCI, the commonest presentation is that of chest pain. In patients over the age of 40, especially in patients with coronary risk factors, acute myocardial infarction precipitated by the massive sympathetic and catecholamine stress that occurs with an accident must be considered and ruled out.[28,29] BCI can cause an increase in creatine kinase (CK) and the myocardial selective CK (CK-MB). Healey and colleagues found that a CK-MB level of >200 mg/dL had a 100% positive predictive value for cardiac complications.[30] However, CK-MB is found in a number of other tissues such as skeletal muscle, lung, liver, small intestine,[31] so most other investigators have found that CK-MB is not predictive of complications and is not a warranted study.[32,33] The preferred cardiac enzyme studies are the myocardium specific troponins I and T.[34,35] In a prospective study of 333 blunt thoracic injuries, Velmahos and colleagues identified 13% with significant BCI. BCI was diagnosed when there was hypotension in the absence of bleeding or neurogenic cause, cardiac arrhythmias, posttraumatic ECG abnormalities, or a cardiac index <2.5L/min/m². Combining a normal ECG and troponin I at 8 hours revealed a negative predictive accuracy of 100%, eliminating patients with clinically significant BCI.[35]

Drugs taken by the patient can modify the physical findings. As an example, beta-blockers and some calcium channel blockers can blunt the expected sinus tachycardia and even precipitate a drop in BP. Illegal drugs such as methamphetamines and cocaine can be responsible for sinus tachycardia or other arrhythmias, severe hypertension, and myocardial ischemia and even infarction.

## LABORATORY STUDIES

When cardiovascular trauma is suspected, an ECG and chest X-ray are essential.[32] The ECG is the quintessential laboratory technique to diagnose arrhythmias and support suspicion of myocardial contusion. Foil and colleagues retrospectively reviewed 524 suspected BCI patients and found that 85% who had complications, mostly arrhythmias, had an abnormal ECG, sinus tachycardia excepted, on admission.[36] Maenza and colleagues did a meta-analysis of 43 studies involving 4681 patients suspected of having BCI and found that an abnormal ECG predicted the risk of developing a cardiovascular complication, again mostly arrhythmias.[37] Biffl and colleagues reviewed 359 patients at high risk for BCI and found that an abnormal ECG, excluding sinus tachycardia, was the most significant independent predictor of cardiac complications, defined as arrhythmia requiring therapy, cardiogenic shock, traumatic valvular regurgitation, or pericardial tamponade.[33] There are no typical ECG abnormalities that are predictive of BCI. The most common findings are sinus tachycardia, otherwise not explained, followed by premature atrial and ventricular extrasystoles. Other findings less common and in decreasing frequency are T wave changes, atrial fibrillation/flutter, ST elevation or depression, conduction defects, ventricular arrhythmias, and new Q waves.[30,39] Fildes and colleagues prospectively evaluated 100 patients admitted to rule out BCI.[40] The patients were monitored for at least 24 hours. They found that if the patient was <55 years of age, lacked a history of heart disease, was hemodynamically stable, and did not need surgery or observation for other injuries, then no cardiac complications developed. They concluded that in the absence of one of these criteria, patients with a normal admission ECG could be safely sent home. With 1 or more of the criteria present, they recommend 24-hour observation. An ECG might also help identify preexisting cardiovascular disease by revealing left ventricular hypertrophy or an old myocardial infarction. The chest X-ray can show a hemopneumothorax, an enlarged cardiac silhouette, multiple rib or clavicular fractures often accompanying cardiac trauma. Most helpful is the finding of a widened mediastinum or obscuration of the aortic knob consistent with traumatic rupture of the aorta.[38]

Echocardiography has revolutionized rapid diagnosis in the ER, and increasingly so since the practice was established of having the echocardiographic equipment in the emergency room,, with ER personnel trained to do a rapid sonographic assessment for peritoneal and pericardial fluid and left ventricular function—the bedside Focused Assessment with Sonography for Trauma (FAST) examination.[41,42] Four windows are evaluated: subcostal, right and left upper quadrant, and suprapubic areas and can be evaluated in 1 to 2 minutes.[43] In a study by Mandavia et al.[41] the FAST examination was 97% accurate for myocardial injury and Rozycki et al. 247 penetrating chest injury patients demonstrated 100% sensitivity and specificity for hemopericardium with the use of FAST.[44]

Not all studies support the routine use of sonography in diagnosing myocardial contusion. In a meta-analysis of 18 studies in patients with suspected myocardial contusion, Christensen and Sutton[45] found no support for the use of routine echocardiography as a screening test in diagnosing clinically significant myocardial contusion. Karalis et al.[47] in a prospective series of 105 patients suspected of having myocardial contusion found that cardiac complications as a result of BCI were so infrequent that routine echocardiography

was of little value. They concluded that BCI is common after blunt chest trauma, rarely requires treatment, has a favorable prognosis, and that echocardiography should be reserved for patients who develop cardiac complications. Finally, Nagy et al., in an analysis of a prospective study of 315 patients, concluded that the echocardiogram added little to the diagnosis for patients with a normal ECG and blood pressure on admission.[47] The Eastern Association for the Surgery of Trauma recommends that echocardiography be reserved for those patients with hemodynamic instability or who suffer evident cardiac complications.[32] Transesophageal echocardiography (TEE) should be reserved for patients whose transthoracic echocardiogram (TTE) is technically inadequate or where aortic disruption is suspected.

In many institutions, multidetector row computed tomography (MDCT) is available 24 hours per day, 7 days a week, and is the fastest way to rule out aortic rupture. It is also very good way of assessing the presence of pericardial fluid, myocardial function, and valvular regurgitation. The presence of air, bone, blood, and metal fragments along the wound track allows visualization of the course of the bullet or knife.[48] MRI with gadolinium with delayed enhancement has been suggested as a way of differentiating myocardial contusion with viable but stunned myocardium from nonviable myocardium from an acute myocardial infarction.[29,49] Totally necrotic contused myocardium may react similarly to necrotic myocardium from an acute myocardial infarction, so the MRI may not be able to differentiate these two conditions. Although transesophageal echocardiography is an excellent way to assess these same problems, the truth is that it is not as rapidly available at all times as rapid computed tomography in many hospitals. Although computed tomography is most used in the diagnosis of aortic injury and disruption, it has also been used to differentiate between myocardial contusion and acute myocardial infarction precipitated by or causing the traumatic incident. Magnetic resonance imaging is also an excellent technique to image the heart and great vessels, but is used rarely in the immediate workup of the suspected BCI patient. Although radioisotopic imaging can identify nonviable and viable myocardium in areas of myocardial contusion, because it identifies relatively large transmural defects and can miss smaller areas of injury and because it images the thinner right ventricle poorly, it has relatively little role to play in the diagnosis of BCI.[37,50]

The introduction of myocardial specific enzymes such as troponins I and T has made the diagnosis of myocardial necrosis possible, whereas with creatine phosphokinase (CK), myocardial contusion could not be distinguished from skeletal muscle or other tissue trauma.[31] Obviously, serial hemoglobin and hematocrit levels and other chemistries such as serum electrolytes, liver, renal, and pancreatic function tests, as appropriate to the clinical picture, should be done.

49. Kim RJ, Fieno DS, Parrish TB, et al. Relationship of MRI delayed contrast enhancement to irreversible injury, infarct age, and contractile function. *Circulation.* 1999;100: 1992–2002.

50. Potkin RT, Werner JA, Trobaugh GB, et al. Evaluation of noninvasive tests of cardiac damage in suspected cardiac contusion. *Circulation.* 1982;66:627–631.

51. Pichakron KO, Perlstein J. Blunt traumatic pericardial rupture presenting with cardiac herniation. *Curr Surg.* 2006;63: 275–280.

52. Wall MJ Jr, Mattox KL, Wolf DA. The cardiac pendulum: blunt rupture of the pericardium with strangulation of the heart. *J Trauma.* 2005;59:136–141.

53. Rubin S, Falcoz PE, Poncet A, et al. Traumatic aorto-right atrial fistula and tricuspid valve rupture. Post-operative cardiac and respiratory support with extracorporeal membrane oxygenation. *Interact Cardiovasc Thorac Surg.* 2006;5:735–737.

54. Setoyama T, Furukawa Y, Abe M, et al. Acute pleuropericarditis after coronary stenting: a case report. *Circ J.* 2006;70: 358–361.

54. Egoh Y, Okoshi T, Anbe J, et al. Surgical treatment of traumatic rupture of the normal aortic valve. *Eur J Cardiothorac Surg.* 1997;11:1180–1182.

55. Thors A, Guarneri R, Costantini EN, et al. Atrial septal rupture, flail tricuspid valve, and complete heart block due to nonpenetrating chest trauma. *Ann Thorac Surg.* 2007;83: 2207–2210.

56. Sousa RC, Garcia-Fernandéz MA, et al. Value of transesophageal echocardiography in the assessment of blunt chest trauma: correlation with electrocardiogram, heart enzymes, and transthoracic echocardiogram *Rev Port Cardiol.* 1994;13:833–843, 807–808.

57. Dubrow TJ, Mihalka J, Eisenhauer DM, et al. Myocardial contusion in the stable patient: what level of care is appropriate? *Surgery.* 1989;106:267–273.

58. Symbas PN. Great vessels injury. *Am Heart J.* 1977;93: 518–22.

59. Dabbagh A, Mar'ashi AS, Malek B. Traumatic arteriovenous fistula due to an old gunshot injury: a victim from the Afghanistan War. *Mil Med.* 2007;172:1129–1131.

60. McGwin G Jr, Reiff DA, Moran SG, et al. Incidence and characteristics of motor vehicle collision-related blunt thoracic aortic injury according to age. *J Trauma.* 2002;52: 859–865

61. Merrill WH, Lee RB, Hammon JW Jr, et al. Surgical treatment of acute traumatic tear of the thoracic aorta. *Ann Surg.* 1988;207:699–706.

62. Fabian TC, Richardson JD, Croce MA. Prospective study of blunt aortic injury: Multicenter Trial of the American Association for the Surgery of Trauma. *J Trauma.* 1997;42:374–380.

63. Schmoker, J D, Lee C H, Taylor R G. et al. A novel model of blunt thoracic aortic injury: a mechanism confirmed? *J Trauma.* 2008;64: 923–931.

64. Roisinblit JM, Allende NG, Neira JA, et al. Local thrombus as an isolated sign of traumatic aortic injury. *Echocardiogr.* 2002;19:63–65.

65. Atik FA, Navia JL, Svensson LG, et al. Surgical treatment of pseudoaneurysm of the thoracic aorta. *J Thorac Cardiovasc Surg.* 2006;132:379–385.

66. Gundry SR, Burney RE, Mackenzie JR, et al. Assessment of mediastinal widening associated with traumatic rupture of the aorta. *J Trauma.* 1983;23:293–299.

67. Kirsh MM, Behrendt DM, Orringer MB, et al. The treatment of acute traumatic rupture of the aorta: a 10-year experience. *Ann Surg.* 1976;184:308–316.

68. Symbas PN, Tyras DH, Ware RE, et al. Traumatic rupture of the aorta. *Ann Surg.* 1973;178:6–12.

69. Dake MD, Miller DC, Semba CP, et al. Transluminal placement of endovascular stent-grafts for the treatment of descending thoracic aortic aneurysms. *N Engl J Med.* 1994;331: 1729–1734.

70. Demetriades D, Velmahos GC, Scalea TM, et al. American Association for the Surgery of Trauma Thoracic Aortic Injury Study Group. Operative repair or endovascular stent graft in blunt traumatic thoracic aortic injuries: results of an American Association for the Surgery of Trauma Multicenter Study. *J Trauma.* 2008;64:561–570.

71. Jahromi AS, Kazemi K, Safar HA, et al. Traumatic rupture of the thoracic aorta: cohort study and systematic review. *J Vasc Surg.* 2001;34:1029–1034.

72. von Oppell UO, Dunne TT, De Groot MK, et al. Traumatic aortic rupture: twenty-year metaanalysis of mortality and risk of paraplegia. *Ann Thorac Surg.* 1994;58:585–593.

73. Canaud L, Alric P, Branchereau P, et al. Lessons learned from midterm follow-up of endovascular repair for traumatic rupture of the aortic isthmus. *J Vasc Surg.* 2008;47:733–738.

74. Whitson BA, Nath DS, Knudtson JR, et al. Is distal aortic perfusion in traumatic thoracic aortic injuries necessary to avoid paraplegic postoperative outcomes? *J Trauma.* 2008;64: 115–120.

75. Fleming AW, Green DC. Traumatic aneurysms of the thoracic aorta. Report of 43 patients. *Ann Thorac Surg.* 1974;18: 91–101.

76. Midgley F, Behrendt DM. Surgical repair of chronic post-traumatic aneurysm of the aortic arch. *J Thorac Cardiovasc Surg.* 1974;67:229–232.

77. Symbas PN, Symbas PJ. Missiles in the cardiovascular system. *Chest Surg Clin N Am.* 1997;7:343–356.

78. Symbas PN, Picone AL, Hatcher CR, et al. Cardiac missiles. A review of the literature and personal experience. *Ann Surg.* 1990;211:639–647.

79. McLaughlin JS, Herman R, Scherlis L, et al. Sterile pericarditis from foreign body. Acute tamponade one month following gunshot wound. *Ann Thor Surg.* 1967;3:52–56.

80. Bland EF, Beebe GW. Missiles in the heart. A twenty-year follow-up report of World War II cases. *N Engl J Med.* 1966;274:1039–1046.

81. Al Halees Z, Abdoun F, Canver CC, et al. A right ventricle to aorta fistula caused by a fractured sternal wire. *Asian Cardiovasc Thorac Ann.* 2007;15:453–454.

82. Luedde M, Krumsdorf U, Zehelein J, et al. Treatment of iatrogenic femoral pseudoaneurysm by ultrasound-guided compression therapy and thrombin injection. *Angiol.* 2007; 58:435–439.

83. Bolad I, O'Meallie L. Spontaneous closure of an iatrogenic circumflex coronary artery-to-coronary vein fistula. *J Invasive Cardiol.* 2007;19:E125–127.

84. Lipiec P, Peruga JZ, Krzemińska-Pakula M, et al. Right coronary artery-to-right ventricle fistula complicating percutaneous transluminal angioplasty: case report and review of the literature. *J Am Soc Echocardiogr.* 2004;17:280–283.

85. Tisi PV, Callam MJ. Surgery versus non-surgical treatment for femoral pseudoaneurysms. Cochrane Database *Syst Rev.* 2006;1:1–22.

86. Reidy JF, Deverall PB, Sowton E. Successful late non-surgical removal of intracardiac catheter fragment. *Br Heart J.* 1982;48:407–409.

87. Leiter E, Gribetz D, Cohen S. Arteriovenous fistula after percutaneous needle biopsy—surgical repair with preservation of renal function. *N Engl J Med.* 1972;287:971–972.

88. Enghoff E, Cullhed I. Experiences with transseptal left heart catheterization. A review of 454 studies. *Am Heart J.* 1971;81:398–408.

89. Preis O, Digumarthy SR, Wright CD, et al. Atrioesophageal fistula after catheter pulmonary venous ablation for atrial fibrillation: imaging features. *J Thorac Imaging.* 2007;22:283–285.

# Twelve-Lead Electrocardiography

Sonia Blome, Keyur B. Shah, and R. Michael Benitez

## ● PRACTICAL POINTS

- Consider 2:1 sinoatrial exit block for sinus bradycardia with a rate <40 bpm.

- When a pause occurs of less than twice the usual RR interval, look for deformation of the T wave preceding the pause. If the T wave is of different morphology from the usual T wave, suspect a nonconducted APC.

- Distinguish a rhythm originating from a low atrial focus from an AV junctional rhythm by the PR interval! Although a low atrial focus may activate the atrium in a retrograde manner (resulting in inverted P waves in II, III, aVF), the PR interval will be greater than 0.11 second, differentiating it from an AV junctional rhythm.

- Be careful to distinguish multifocal atrial tachycardia from NSR with multifocal APCs. The key with MAT is the absence of any single dominant P wave morphology.

- Consider atrial flutter with 2:1 block if the rate of the SVT is 150 bpm.

- Consider Wolff–Parkinson–White syndrome if the atrial rate is >200 bpm with a QRS complex duration greater than 0.12 second, or in the presence of a "concertina effect"—constant variance of QRS duration.

- Identify the underlying sinus mechanism, if possible.

- Consider "digitalis toxicity" when a junctional rhythm is present, especially if atrial fibrillation is evident or a history of congestive heart failure is provided.

- If you see an electrocardiogram with frequent VPCs and fusion beats, measure the intervals between ectopic beats to ensure you have not missed ventricular parasystole.

- In addition to coding for VT, be sure to code for "AV dissociation," the underlying sinus rhythm, and the abnormal QRS axis, if they are present.

- If a P wave is associated with a QRS complex, even for only 1 beat, the patient is not in complete heart block. Look for complete heart block in patients with a ventricular pacemaker.

- Consider WPW with atrial fibrillation when there is a wide complex tachycardia with an irregular rhythm, especially if the QRS duration is variable.

- Remember to code for the associated findings of ventricular hypertrophy, including conduction delays, atrial abnormalities, and ST-segment abnormalities.

- Ventricular hypertrophy and myocardial infarction (Q waves) can still be interpreted in the presence of RBBB—look carefully for these!

- The two major causes of a right axis deviation are LPFB and RVH—the precordial leads can yield important clues to RVH (R>S lead V1, S>R lead V6)!

- In the presence of bundle branch blocks, do not forget to still code axis deviations, AV delay, and atrial abnormalities when present!

- ST-segment depression with T wave inversion in the early precordial leads may accompany RVH and should be coded separately as "secondary to hypertrophy."

- ST depression should be coded as "suggesting myocardial ischemia," ST elevation as "suggesting myocardial injury," and pathologic Q waves as "infarction." ST elevation/injury should always be considered the primary event, and if Q waves are present, infarction should also be coded.

(continued)

- The clinical history plays an integral role in the diagnosis for a clinical disorder.

- Do not forget to code for the individual abnormal intervals and repolarization abnormalities observed with digitalis.

- Digitalis toxicity is the most common cause of paroxysmal atrial tachycardia. PAT with atrioventricular block is pathognomonic of digitalis toxicity.

- Do not forget to code for the abnormal intervals, repolarization abnormalities, and rhythm disturbances observed with antiarrhythmic medications.

- Hypocalcemia is a common finding in end-stage renal disease patients. Note that *only* hypocalcemia and hypothermia result in QT prolongation with a normal T wave duration.

- Distinguish dextrocardia from lead reversal by identifying a decrease in R wave amplitude from V1-V6.

- Clues that distinguish pericarditis from abnormal repolarization include PR-segment deviation, reciprocal changes in aVR, decreased T wave amplitude, and a history of pleuritic chest pain.

Electrocardiographic interpretation is a skill that all cardiologists are expected to master. The integration of this information into clinical decision-making is as important as history and physical examination in the care of patients with complex heart disease. Because of its importance, the American Board of Internal Medicine (ABIM) incorporates a specific section on the board examination for ECG interpretation, which must be passed—regardless of performance on the remainder of the exam—for certification. Successful completion of this section requires both a working knowledge of the rules governing ECG diagnoses and familiarity with the ABIM coding algorithms. On most of the ECGs presented on the examination, there will be one to three major findings for coding, and points are given for correct identification of these. Overdiagnosis (checking off more major findings than are present) or misdiagnosis may result in either failure to accrue points or actual subtraction of points. Because of this system, guessing about a diagnosis is more likely to lead to point subtraction and should be avoided.

In order to correctly identify the most abnormalities and maximize scoring, it is essential the physician follow a plan, as outlined here:

- Devise a routine method of analyzing each tracing, starting with rate, rhythm, intervals, and axis.
- Follow with examination of the P waves for regularity, and morphology and axis as they relate to atrial enlargement and origin of activation respectively.
- Inspect the QRS morphology for infarction and hypertrophy.
- Evaluate the ST segment for acute injury, pericarditis, and— along with the T/U waves—electrolyte disorders.
- Lastly, look for important clues that are often given in the brief clinical vignettes supplied. For example, one should look carefully for signs of hyperkalemia if the clinical presentation is that of a noncompliant dialysis patient.

## GENERAL FEATURES

It is not uncommon for a normal ECG to be included on the examination, since it is as important to recognize what is "normal" as what is "abnormal." There are, however, several normal variants that should be recognized and coded accordingly:

- Juvenile T waves are small, asymmetric T wave inversions present in leads V1-V3. It is important to differentiate this from ischemia, where the T waves may be deeper (often ≥3 mm) and are symmetric. Most often, the clinical vignette is that of a young, healthy woman without chest pain.
- An rSr′ in V1 may be a normal variant, and it is important *not* to code this as an incomplete or complete RBBB if the QRS duration is <0.10 second, the r′ is the smallest of the peaks, and the entire complex is <7 mm in height.

The most common "borderline" ECG presented is that of early repolarization. The diagnosis is suggested by the presence of J point elevation, with a concave upwards ST segment, and perhaps a notch on the downstroke of the R wave in otherwise healthy, young individuals. This feature is most commonly appreciated in the precordial leads, and it should be differentiated from what is seen in pericarditis (widespread ST change, and perhaps PR depression) and acute injury (straight ST segment or concave downwards).

The most common examples of incorrect lead placement are right arm–left arm reversal (**Figure 12-1**) and misplacement of a precordial lead. Arm lead reversal should be suspected when the P wave, QRS complex, and T wave are upright in lead aVR, and inverted in lead I. It is important one distinguish this from dextrocardia, which demonstrates

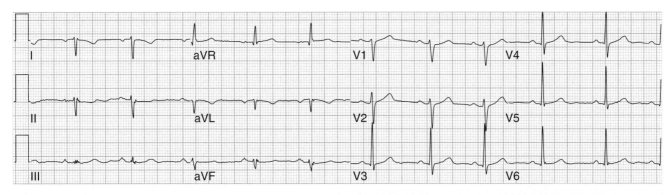

**Figure 12-1.** This ECG demonstrates arm lead reversal. Note the inverted P waves in lead I and inverted P waves in lead aVR.

the same limb lead findings, but in which R wave progression in the precordial leads is distinctly abnormal. In limb-lead reversal, the precordial leads are not affected and remain normal.

Precordial lead misplacement should be suspected when there is a sudden decrement in the R wave height present for only one lead with recovery in the next lead.

Far and away the most common artifact presented is that of the undulating baseline sometimes seen on the ECG of patients with Parkinson's disease. This is easily mistaken for atrial flutter. Differentiation can be made by recognizing the presence of P waves, most often in the early precordial leads, preceding each QRS, and by the tremor rate (500/min) which is much faster than usual atrial flutter (300/min).

## P WAVE ABNORMALITIES

Atrial activation is represented by the P wave. Right atrial activation precedes left atrial activation in normal depolarization resulting in a biphasic P wave in V1 and often a notched P wave in the limb leads.

## Right Atrial Abnormality or Enlargement (Figure 12-2)

Right atrial abnormality or enlargement is characterized by:

- P wave amplitude >than 2.5 mm in leads II, III, or aVF with normal P wave duration
- positive amplitude >than 1.5 mm in V1 or V2
- P wave frontal axis 70 or greater (rightward axis).

**CODING POINTER: Code for right atrial enlargement/ abnormality if *any* of the criteria above are present.**

## Left Atrial Abnormality or Enlargement

Left atrial abnormality or enlargement is characterized by:

- notched P wave with duration >0.12 second in leads II, III, or aVF
- downward terminal deflection of P wave in V1 with negative amplitude of 1 mm and duration of 0.04 second.

## ATRIAL RHYTHMS

This section reviews sinus rhythms as well as rhythms originating from ectopic pacemakers within the atria.

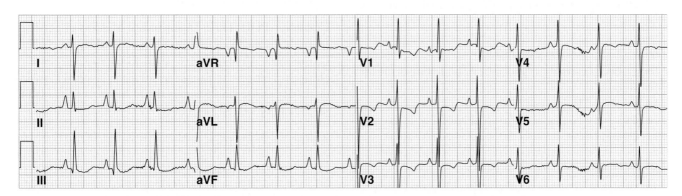

**Figure 12-2.** An ECG from a 65-year-old with emphysema has characteristics of a pulmonary disease pattern. Right atrial enlargement, right ventricular hypertrophy, and right axis deviation are present.

## Sinus Rhythm, Sinus Bradycardia, and Sinus Tachycardia

All sinus rhythms require a normal P wave axis (15 to 75°) and originate with depolarization of the sinus node. Sinus rhythm has a rate of 60-100 bpm. Sinus bradycardia has a rate <60 bpm. Sinus tachycardia has a rate >100 bpm and can demonstrate an *increase* in P wave amplitude and *decrease* in PR interval with increasing rates. Usually sinus tachycardia does not exceed 160 bpm in adults.

**CODING POINTER: Consider 2:1 sinoatrial exit block for sinus bradycardia with a rate <40 bpm.**

## Sinus Arrhythmia

While the impulse arises normally in the SA node, this arrhythmia is characterized by alternating periods of slower and more rapid heart rates:

- Normal P wave morphology and normal axis
- The PP interval varies by >0.16 second or 10%.

## Sinus Pause or Arrest

A sinus pause is defined as a pause >2.0 second without a P wave. The differential for this includes:

- Sinus arrhythmia: note a phasic gradual PP interval change
- Sinoatrial exit block: the pause is an exact multiple of the PP interval (2×, 3×)
- Nonconducted atrial premature complexes: evident by a P wave deforming the preceding t wave
- Sinus arrest.

## Sino-atrial Exit Block

When a sino-atrial block is present, the sinus node discharges, but there is no atrial depolarization because of the exit block. It is not possible to detect 1° and 3° sino-atrial exit block on an electrocardiogram. Distinguishing between 2° sino-atrial block type I and II requires an evaluation of the response of the perinodal tissues, or P waves.

Type I (Mobitz I) is characterized by:

- grouped beating with progressive shortening of the PP interval
- constant PR interval
- PP pause duration less than twice the normal PP interval.

Type II (Mobitz II) is characterized by:

- Constant PP interval followed by a dropped P wave
- Pause is a near multiple of the normal PP interval
- Interval pause may be slightly less than 2X normal PP interval, but usually within 0.1 second.

## Atrial Premature Complexes—Conducted

An atrial premature complex arises from an ectopic focus anywhere in either atrium and usually initiates a ventricular complex with a normal QRS configuration. It is characterized by:

- Premature P wave in relation to the normal sinus rhythm
- P wave differs in configuration from sinus P wave
- PR interval can be normal or can be increased or decreased
- QRS complex is similar in appearance to the QRS complex present during the sinus rhythm
- The post extrasystolic pause is generally noncompensatory. However, if sino-atrial entrance block is present and the SA node is not reset, the result can be an interpolated beat or fully compensatory pause.
- An APC can have aberrant intraventricular conduction, suggested by a P wave that occurs very early with a RBBB pattern. LBBB and variable QRS morphology can be seen but are not as common as a RBBB pattern.

## Atrial Premature Complexes—Nonconducted

Atrial premature complexes of the nonconducted type are characterized by:

- premature P wave that are abnormal in morphology but not followed by a QRS complex
- P waves often hidden in the T wave.

**CODING POINTER: When a pause occurs of less than twice the usual RR interval, look for deformation of the T wave preceding the pause. If the T wave is of different morphology from the usual T wave, suspect a nonconducted APC.**

## Ectopic Atrial Rhythms

Ectopic atrial rhythms are characterized by:

- P wave morphology or axis different from that in sinus rhythm
- rate <100 bpm
- PR interval >0.11 second.

**CODING POINTER: Distinguish a rhythm originating from a low atrial focus from an AV junctional rhythm by the PR interval! Although a low atrial focus may activate the atrium in a retrograde manner (resulting in inverted P waves in II, III, aVF), the PR interval will be greater than 0.11 second, differentiating it from an AV junctional rhythm.**

## Atrial Tachycardia

In contrast to atrial flutter or atrial fibrillation, atrial tachycardias arise from a single focus within the right or left atrium and are characterized by the following:

- A P wave with abnormal morphology, different than sinus P waves

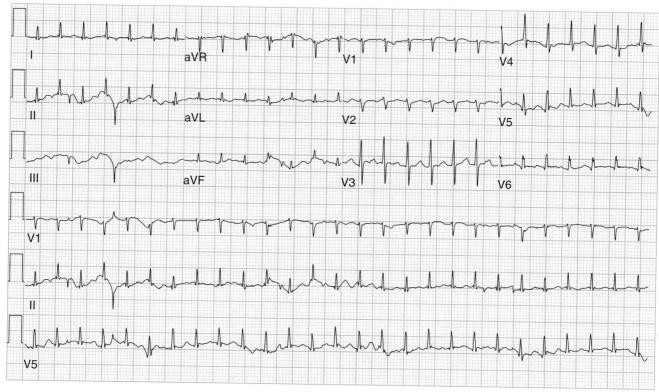

**Figure 12-3.** Supraventricular tachycardia.

- Each P wave is followed by a QRS complex that usually resembles the QRS morphology present during sinus
- 3 or more beats in succession
- An atrial rate that ranges from 100 to 180 bpm
- A regular rhythm with a constant RR interval (exception would be the warm-up period in automatic type AT)
- Atrial parasystole is characterized by recurring short runs of atrial tachycardia interrupted by, but not reset by, normal sinus rhythm.

## Atrial Tachycardia, Multifocal

Chaotic atrial tachycardia occurs when there are 3 or more different types of P waves activating the ventricles. It requires the following:

- at least 3 morphologically distinct P wave patterns with variable configuration and direction
- absence of 1 dominant atrial pacemaker
- variable length of PR, RR, and RP intervals
- an atrial rate >100 bpm
- an isoelectric baseline between P waves.

**CODING POINTER: Be careful to distinguish multifocal atrial tachycardia from NSR with multifocal APCs. The key with MAT is the absence of any single dominant P wave morphology.**

## Supraventricular Tachycardia (Figure 12-3)

The most common regular supraventricular tachycardia, atrioventricular nodal re-entract tachycardia occurs due to reentry within the compact AV node. It is characterized by:

- Regular rhythm
- Cannot easily identify P wave
- Narrow QRS complex (occasionally can be wide with aberrancy)
- Sudden onset and termination
- Possible retrograde P waves in the terminal portion of the QRS in V1.

**CODING POINTER: Consider atrial flutter with 2:1 block if the rate of the SVT is 150 bpm.**

## Atrial Flutter (Figure 12-4)

Atrial flutter is characterized by a regular atrial rate with a variable degree of AV block that rises from a single ectopic atrial focus:

- Rapid regular P waves with sawtooth pattern (F waves) seen best in the inferior leads and V1
- Atrial rate of 240-340 bpm
- AV conduction usually manifests with varying degrees of block (2:1, 4:1, or more), but complete block can also occur with or without an AV junctional tachycardia
- QRS complex can be normal morphology or aberrant

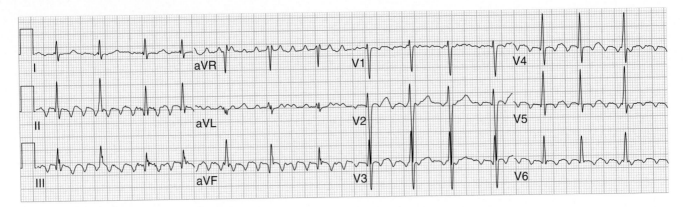

**Figure 12-4.** Atrial flutter with variable block.

- Rate and regularity of QRS complexes are variable and reflect varying AV block.

## Atrial Fibrillation (Figure 12-5)

Atrial fibrillation is commonly seen in patients with coronary artery disease, hyperthyroidism, and rheumatic mitral valve disease. It can also be found in normal patients. It is characterized by:

- Absence of P wave
- Atrial impulses appear as small, irregular waves with varying amplitudes, duration and morphology causing random oscillation of the baseline (fibrillatory or f waves)
- Irregularly irregular ventricular rhythm
- Rate is 100-180 bpm in the absence of drugs
- Differential includes multifocal atrial tachycardia, paroxysmal atrial tachycardia with block or atrial flutter.

CODING POINTER: Consider Wolff–Parkinson–White syndrome if the atrial rate is >200 bpm with a QRS complex duration greater than 0.12 second, or in the presence of a "concertina effect"—constant variance of QRS duration.

## AV JUNCTIONAL RHYTHMS

Impulses arising from the AV junction attempt to travel retrograde through the atrium and anterograde through the ventricle.

### AV Junctional Premature Complexes

An AV junctional premature complex is an ectopic beat arising from the AV node *before* the next expected sinus beat. It is characterized by:

- P wave location (if present):
  - Immediately prior to (<0.12 second)
  - Coincides with the QRS complex with beats arising high in the node
  - Follows the QRS complex if the beat arises lower in the AV junction
- P wave morphology (if present):
  - Inverted in the lateral lead (I, aVL)
  - Upright in the inferior lead (II, III, aVF)
- Usually associated with a noncompensatory pause
- QRS complex may exhibit aberration, depending on timing of beat.

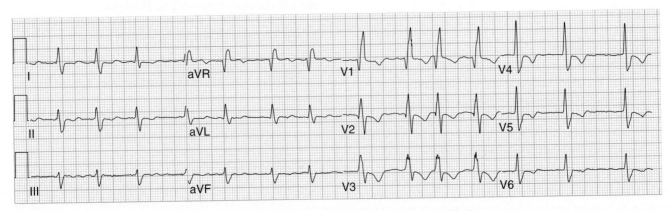

**Figure 12-5.** Atrial fibrillation. The P waves are absent. There is also a right bundle branch block.

## AV Junctional Escape Complexes

In contrast to premature junctional complexes, AV junctional escape complexes are produced due to the inherent automaticity of AV node. The AV node will function as a pacemaker when the sinus node fails to conduct a timely impulse to the AV node. The features of these complexes are:

- decreased sinus impulse formation or high-grade AV block
- normal QRS complex
- may or may not be associated with retrograde P wave conduction (depending on integrity of AV conduction)
- P wave location: the P wave may occur immediately prior to (<0.12 second) or coincide with the QRS complex with beats arising high in the node. The P-wave may follow the QRS complex if the beat arises lower in the AV junction.
- results in irregular rhythm.

## AV Junctional Rhythm

An AV junctional rhythm is simply a series of uninterrupted AV junctional escape complexes. The AV junction effectively takes over as the dominant pacemaker. This rhythm is observed with increased vagal tone, sinus node dysfunction, or heart block. it is characterized by:

- Normal QRS complexes, unless preexisting conduction disease present
- Rate of 40-60 bpm, constant RR interval
- P wave morphology: inverted in the lateral lead (I, aVL) and upright in the inferior lead (II, III, aVF)
- P wave location: the P wave may occur immediately prior to (<0.12 second) or coincide with the QRS complex with beats arising high in the node. The P-wave may follow the QRS complex if the beat arises lower in the AV junction.
- Isorhythmic dissociation may be present.

**CODING POINTER: Identify the underlying sinus mechanism, if possible.**

## AV Junctional Tachycardia (Nonparoxysmal)

Nonparoxysmal AV junctional tachycardia is a narrow complex tachycardia due to increased automaticity in the bundle of His. The arrhythmia is of gradual onset and slows, without terminating, with increased vagal tone. The ventricular rates range from 100 to 140 bpm. They are seen most often with inferior infarctions, myocarditis, open heart surgery, and especially *digitalis toxicity*.

This is a distinct entity from *paroxysmal* junctional tachycardias, which have a reentrant mechanism and present with higher ventricular rates (140-220 bpm),

**CODING POINTER: Consider "digitalis toxicity" when a junctional rhythm is present, especially if atrial fibrillation is evident or a history of congestive heart failure is provided.**

# VENTRICULAR RHYTHMS

## Ventricular Premature Complexes (Figures 12-6, 12-15, and 12-21)

Ventricular premature complexes (VPC) (**Figure 12-6**), premature ventricular contractions (PVC) (**Figure 12-15** and **12-21**), and extrasystoles all describe premature QRS complexes originating in the ventricle. VPC's are characterized by:

- Premature relative to RR interval
- Wide, slurred QRS complex, ≥0.12 second (unless ectopic focus near intraventricular septum)
- QRS vector markedly different from normal sinus beat
- Marked ST-segment and T-wave deviation in the direction opposite of the major deflection of the QRS complex
- Retrograde conduction possible, however, P wave often buried in ST segment or T wave
- Compensatory pause usually present (retrograde conduction may reset the sinus node or the VPC may be interpolated between two normally conducted QRS complexes).

## Ventricular Parasystole

Ventricular parasystole describes an ectopic ventricular pacemaker with an entrance block. The focus generates impulses at a fixed interval and depolarizes the ventricle whenever it is not refractory. It functions independently of the supraventricular pacemaker. On a surface electrocardiogram, it presents as VPCs occurring at a fixed interval or multiples of that fixed interval.

- VPC occurring at a fixed interval or multiples of the shortest fixed interval
- No relationship (grouped beating) with underlying sinus rhythm
- Fusion beats often present.

**CODING POINTER: If you see an electrocardiogram with frequent VPCs and fusion beats, measure the intervals between ectopic beats to ensure you have not missed ventricular parasystole.**

## Ventricular Tachycardia (Figure 12-7)

Ventricular tachycardia (VT) is defined as 3 or more consecutive premature ventricular complexes. *Monomorphic* VT

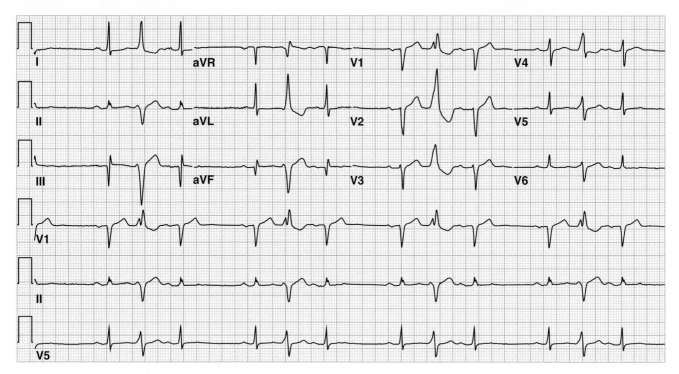

**Figure 12-6.** Interpolated ventricular premature complexes.

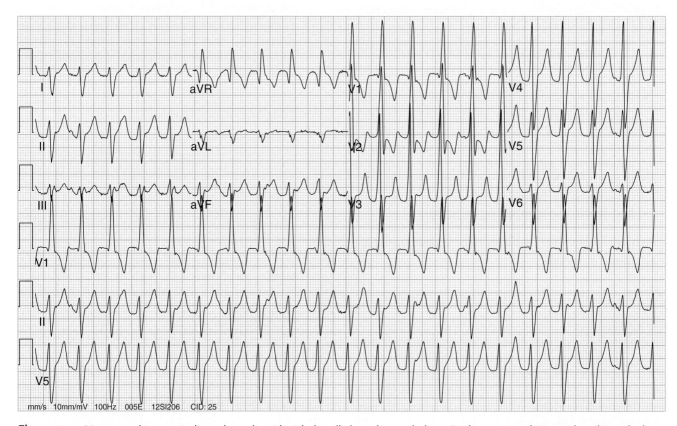

**Figure 12-7.** Monomorphic ventricular tachycardia with right bundle branch morphology. AV dissociation distinguishes this arrhythmia from a supraventricular tachycardia with aberrancy.

is a regular tachycardia with a constant QRS morphology. *Polymorphic* VT is an irregular tachycardia with QRS complexes of varying morphology.

It is challenging to distinguish monomophic VT from a supraventricular tachycardia with aberrant conduction or an antidromic A-V reciprocating tachycardia. The following characteristics favor the diagnosis of VT:

- wide complex, regular QRS complexes with secondary ST segment and T wave abnormalities (similar morphology to VPCs)
- aV dissociation commonly present 50% of the time (highly specific finding)
- capture beats and fusion beats
- concordance of QRS deflection in precordial leads
- northwest QRS axis
- initiated by VPC, abrupt onset
- morphology characteristics (**Table 12-1**).

**CODING POINTER: In addition to coding for VT, be sure to code for "AV dissociation," the underlying sinus rhythm, and the abnormal QRS axis, if they are present.**

## Accelerated Idioventricular Rhythm (Figure 12-8)

Accelerated idioventricular rhythm is a ventricular arrhythmia with a rate greater than the intrinsic ventricular escape rate and slower than ventricular tachycardia. It is often seen

| Table 12-1 • Morphology of QRS Complex Favoring Diagnosis of Ventricular Tachycardia | |
|---|---|
| **RBBB Pattern** | **LBBB Pattern** |
| QRS ≥ 0.14 sec<br>Left axis deviation | QRS ≥ 0.16 sec<br>Right axis deviation |
| V1<br>Monophasic R or<br>  qR complex<br>or<br>Rsr' pattern *only*<br>  if first R wave is<br>  dominant | V1 or V2<br>Broad (≥0.4 sec) R wave<br>or<br>Onset of QRC complex to nadir<br>  of S wave ≥ 0.6 sec<br>or<br>Slurred/notched downstroke of S wave |
| V6<br>rS complex<br>  (R wave < S wave) | V6<br>q or qS complex |

after *successful reperfusion* and *digitalis toxicity*. ECG characteristics are:

- 60-110 bpm
- AV dissociation
- fusion beats and capture beats usually present.

**CODING POINTER: An underlying sinus rhythm and AV dissociation may be present with this arrhythmia.**

## Ventricular Escape Complexes or Rhythm

A ventricular escape beat is a protective mechanism in response to a failure of upstream impulse generation and

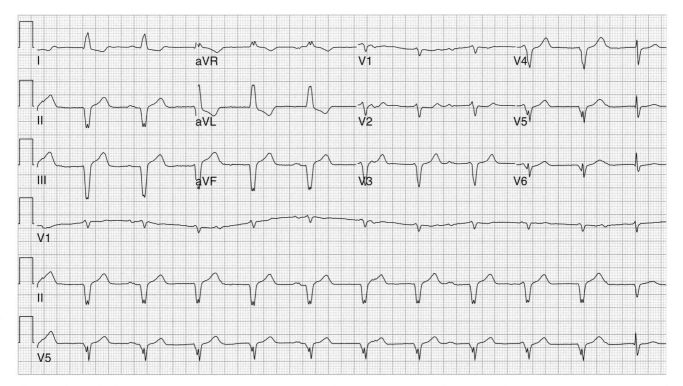

**Figure 12-8.** Accelerated idioventricular rhythm. (Note the very slow sinus rate – AV dissociation is also present.)

conduction. If a sinus beat or junctional escape beat fail to depolarize the ventricle, a focus originating in the ventricle generates an impulse. The features of a ventricular escape beat are:

- Wide, regular QRS complexes of similar morphology to VPC's
- Rate of 30 – 40 bpm
- Seen with sinus node disease or high-grade AV block, *after abrupt termination of atrial arrhythmia.*

**CODING POINTER: Identify the underlying conduction disease.**

## Ventricular Fibrillation

This is an easily recognized terminal rhythm. It presents in ECG as:

- chaotic, with no discernable wave forms
- irregular deflections.

# AV CONDUCTION

## AV Block, 1°

First degree AV block usually represents slowed impulse progagation from the sinus node through the AV node. It is characterized by:

- PR interval ≥0.20 second (1 large box)

- Every P wave is associated with a QRS complex at a fixed interval.

## AV Block, 2°-Mobitz Type I (Figure 12-9)

Mobitz type I block is characterized by progressive prolongation of the PR interval until a P wave is blocked from conducting a QRS complex. The block occurs at the level of the AV node and is benign in asymptomatic patients. ECG characteristics are:

- Grouped beating
- Progressive PR interval prolongation (*compare PR intervals immediately before and after blocked QRS complex*)
- Progressive RR interval shortening, fixed PP interval
- RR interval encompassing the nonconducted beat is less than 2 × PP interval.

## AV Block, 2°-Mobitz Type II

Mobitz type II block typically occurs within the bundle of His and has a high predeliction to progress to complete heart block. The PR interval in this arrhythmia is constant with intermittantly dropped QRS complexes. It is seen as:

- Fixed PR interval
- Intermittant nonconducted P wave
- RR interval encompassing the nonconducted beat is 2 × PP interval.

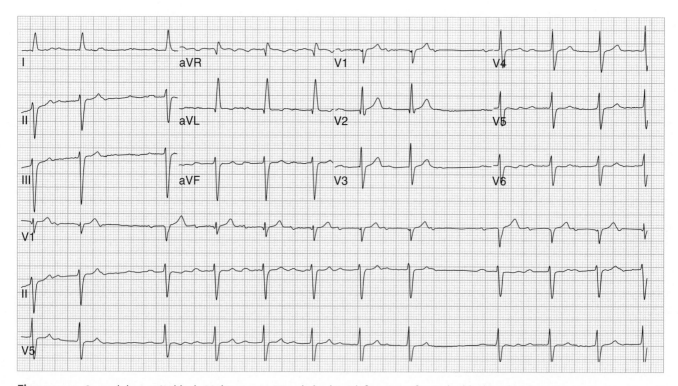

**Figure 12-9.** Second degree AV block, Mobitz type 1 (Wenchebach). A left anterior fascicular block is also present.

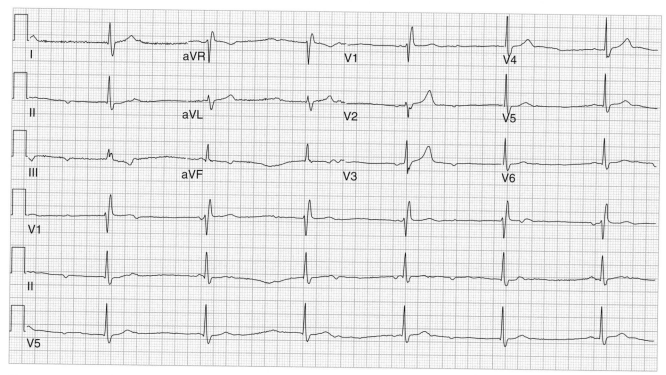

**Figure 12-10.** Complete heart block.

## AV Block, 2:1

When an atrial rhythm exhibits 2:1 conduction, it is not possible to distinguish between Mobitz Type I and Type II block:

- Regular atrial rhythm, conducting 1 QRS complex for 2 P waves.

## AV Block, 3° (Complete Heart Block Figure 12-10)

Complete heart block occurs when the atrial impulse consistently fails to reach the ventricle. ECG is characterized by:

- atrial and ventricular impulses conducting independently of each other
- constant PP and RR intervals
- variable PR intervals
- atrial rate greater than ventricular rate
- AV dissociation.

**CODING POINTER: If a P wave is associated with a QRS complex, even for only 1 beat, the patient is not in complete heart block. Look for complete heart block in patients with a ventricular pacemaker.**

## Wolf–Parkinson–White *Pattern*

Wolf–Parkinson–White (WPW) syndrome occurs when there is an accessory communication between atria to the ventricles, bypassing the AV node. The WPW pattern refers to the ECG findings associated with the accessory pathway. Anterograde conduction through the accessory pathway creates an early slurring in the QRS complex (delta wave) due to preexcitation of the ventricular myocardium. The delta wave can be a positive or negative deflection, giving clues to the location of the pathway. ECG includes:

- Short PR interval
- Delta wave from preexcitation of the QRS complex
- QRS complex can be narrow or widened
- Secondary ST-T wave changes, especially with higher degrees of preexcitation.

**CODING POINTER: Consider WPW with atrial fibrillation when there is a wide complex tachycardia with an irregular rhythm, especially if the QRS duration is variable.**

## AV Dissociation

AV dissociation is characterized by a failure of communication between the atria and the ventricles. Features include:

- No association between atrial and ventricular depolarizations
- Ventricular rate greater than atrial rate, as occurs in ventricular tachycardia, or
- Complete heart block

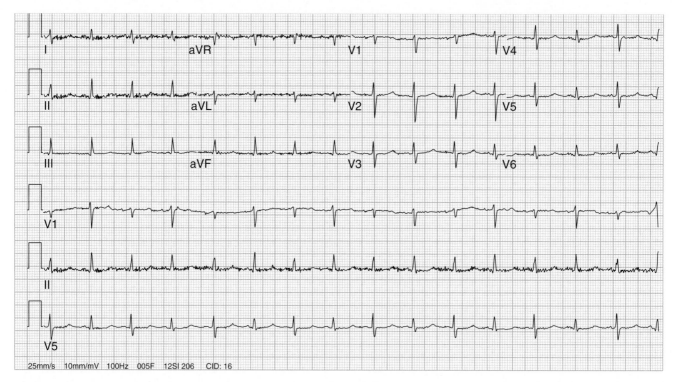

**Figure 12-11.** Pericardial effusion. The voltage is decreased and electrical alternans is present.

## ABNORMALITIES OF QRS VOLTAGE OR AXIS

Abnormalities such a low QRS voltage or deviation from normal axis can be clues to underlying clinical disorders.

### Low Voltage Present in Limb Leads Only

This coding may be used when voltage is normal in the precordial leads but low in the limb leads. It can be an important clue to the possibility of underlying chronic lung disease, the presence of a pericardial effusion, or myxedema. It is characterized by:

- QRS amplitude (R + S) less than 5 mm in all limb leads; normal amplitude in precordial leads.

### Low Voltage Present in Limb and Precordial Leads

- QRS amplitude (R + S) < 5 mm in all limb leads, and
- QRS amplitude (R + S) in each precordial lead is <10 mm.

### Left Axis Deviation (>−30°)

- Axis measured −30° to −105°
- Caution in diagnosing LAD in presence of inferior infarct.

### Right Axis Deviation (>+100° Figure 12-2)

- Axis measured 101° to −106°
- Causes include: right ventricle hypertrophy, vertical heart, chronic lung disease, pulmonary embolus, or left posterior fascicular block.

### Electrical Alternans (Figure 12-11)

- Height of P wave, QRS complex or T wave alternates with each beat
- Indication of organic heart disease and strongly suggestive of pericardial effusion.

## VENTRICULAR HYPERTROPHY

### Left Ventricular Hypertrophy (LVH)

The voltage criteria for diagnosing left ventricular hypertrophy (LVH) are listed in **Table 12-2**. While the criteria have limited sensitivity for clinical application, if any are present on the ECG, LVH must be diagnosed. Below are listed some of the key ECG features associated with LVH. In general, the limb lead criteria have higher specificities and the precordial lead criteria have higher sensitivities:

- Left axis deviation
- Left atrial enlargement
- Intraventricular conduction delay

| Table 12-2 • Criteria for Left Ventricular Hypertrophy | |
|---|---|
| Sokolow and Lyon criteria | S wave in V1 + R wave V5 or V6 <br> >35 mm (>30 y) <br> >40 mm (20-30 y) <br> >60 mm (<20 y) |
| Cornell criteria | R wave in aVL + S wave in V3 <br> >20 mm males <br> >24 mm females |
| Framingham criteria | R wave in aVL >11mm <br> R wave in V4-V6 >25mm <br> S wave V1-3 >25 mm <br> S wave in V1 or V2 + R wave <br> V5 or V6 >35 mm <br> R wave in I + S wave in III >25 mm |
| Other | R wave in aVF >20 mm <br> S wave in aVR >14 mm |

- Small R waves in early precordial leads
- Prominent R waves in lateral leads, with V6 >V5
- Intrinsicoid deflection in V5 or V6 greater than 0.05 second
- May be associated with ST segment and T wave changes in the direction opposite of the major deflection of the QRS complex (strain pattern).

## Right Ventricular Hypertrophy (RVH)

Prominent R waves in the early anterior precordial lead and prominent S waves in the lateral precordial lead suggest increased myocardial mass of the antero-medially situated right ventricle. Additionally, associated findings help distinguish RVH from other causes of right axis deviation (LPFB) or prominent R waves in V1 (posterior wall MI):

- R wave in V1 ≥7 mm
- R/S ratio in V1 >1
- R/S ratio in V5 or V6 ≤1
- If rsR' pattern present, R' >10 mm
- qR complex in V1
- R wave in V1 + S wave in V5/V6 ≥10.5.

Associated findings help distinguish RVH from other causes of right axis deviation (LPFB) or prominent R waves in V1 (posterior wall MI):

- right axis deviation
- right atrial enlargement
- incomplete RBBB (or an rSr' in lead V1)
- persistent precordial S waves
- "strain" in right ventricular leads.

## Combined Ventricular Hypertrophy

The diagnoses if biventricular hypertrophy is often difficult, as vectors from both hypertrophied ventricles cancel each other out. Usually, diagnostic criteria for LVH are met with additional ECG features that suggest RVH:

- LVH + RVH criteria met
- LVH criteria met +
  - right axis deviation *or*
  - right atrial enlargement *or*
  - aVR: R wave > S wave *and* V5: S wave > R wave *and* T wave inversion in V1 *or*
- LVH or RVH criteria met +
  - V3 or V4: large amplitude R wave and S wave that are of equal amplitude

**CODING POINTER: Remember to code for the associated findings of ventricular hypertrophy, including conduction delays, atrial abnormalities, and ST-segment abnormalities.**

# INTRAVENTRICULAR CONDUCTION

Right and left bundle branch blocks can be chronic or intermittent and usually reflect an intrinsic defect with conduction in the right or left bundle system.

## Right Bundle Branch Block (RBBB), Complete (Figure 12-12)

A common ECG finding, RBBB is not always indicative of underlying cardiac pathology. It requires all of the following:

- QRS prolongation ≥0.12 second
- Presence of R' in the right precordial leads with amplitude greater than initial R
- Wide S wave in I, V5, and V6
- Delayed intrinsicoid deflection in right precordial leads >0.05 second
- Demonstration of ST-T secondary changes in V1-V3
- QRS axis in the first .08 second should be normal unless a left anterior fascicular block (LAFB) is present as well

**CODING POINTER: Ventricular hypertrophy and myocardial infarction (Q waves) can still be interpreted in the presence of RBBB—look carefully for these!**

## Right Bundle Branch Block, Incomplete

- Presence of RBBB morphology (rSR') but with narrow QRS complex (0.09 to 0.11 second)

## Left Anterior Fascicular Block (LAFB) (Figures 12-9 and 12-13)

When a left anterior fascicular block is present, conduction spreads through the left posterior fascicle, resulting in

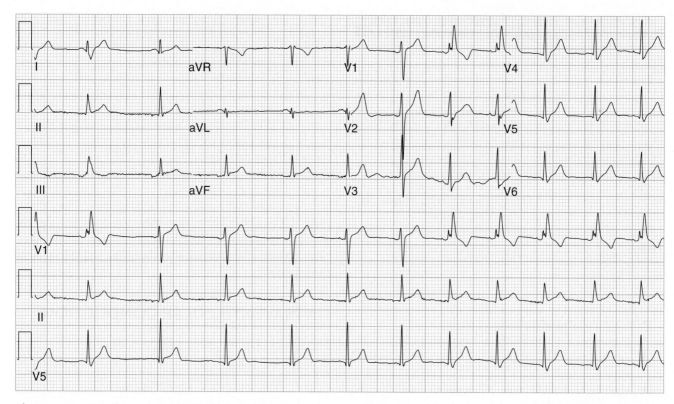

**Figure 12-12.** Rate-dependent right bundle branch block.

a QRS axis that is inferior and rightward. It requires all of the following:

- Mean QRS axis is displaced between −45° and −90°
- Normal or slightly longer QRS duration (0.08 to 0.10 second)
- qR complex in leads I and aVL
- rs in lead III
- No other factors responsible for LAD, including left ventricular hypertrophy, inferior infarct, emphysema (chronic lung disease)

## Left Posterior Fascicular Block (LPFB)

To diagnose LPFB, one must exclude other causes of right axis deviation such as right ventricular hypertrophy, lateral wall myocardial infarction, vertical heart, or emphysema (chronic lung disease). Diagnosis requires all of the following:

- normal or slightly longer QRS duration (0.08 to 0.10 second)
- deep S wave in lead I and Q wave in lead III ($S_1Q_3$ pattern)
- mean frontal plane QRS axis +110° or greater.

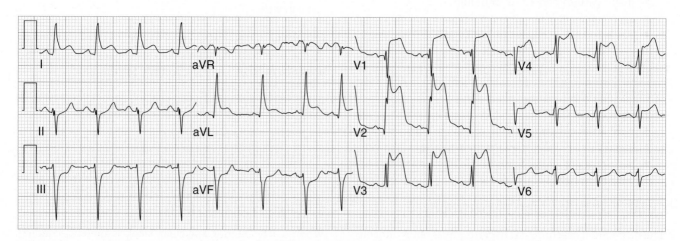

**Figure 12-13.** Anterolateral myocardial infarction (LAFB is also present).

CODING POINTER: The two major causes of a right axis deviation are LPFB and RVH—the precordial leads can yield important clues to RVH (R > S lead V1, S > R lead V6)!

## Left Bundle Branch Block (LBBB), Complete

In contrast to RBBB, left bundle branch block is seen commonly in patients with underlying coronary artery disease. It is characterized by *all* of the following:

- QRS duration ≥0.12 second
- slurred or notched broad R wave in leads I, V5, and V6
- delayed intrinsicoid deflection in left precordial leads and lead I >0.05 second.

CODING POINTER: In the presence of bundle branch blocks, do not forget to still code axis deviations when present, AV delay, and atrial abnormalities when present!

Complete LBBB may complicate acute myocardial injury or infarction. This should be considered in the presence of complete LBBB or an artificial pacemaker when the following ST changes are present:

- ≥1 mm ST elevation concordant with QRS complex
- ≥1 mm ST depression in leads V1 to V3
- ≥5 mm ST elevation discordant with the QRS complex.

## Left Bundle Branch Block, Incomplete

A delay or slowing through the conduction system can create a QRS morphology similar to LBBB. However, the QRS is usually <0.12 second in duration and septal activation is still normal.

## Intraventricular Conduction Disturbance, Nonspecific Type

When an intraventricular conduction defect (IVCD) is seen that cannot be placed in any of the above categories, then the disturbance is called *indeterminate* or *nonspecific* type. Such a defect is characterized by:

- QRS > 0.11 second, but morphology of the QRS complex does not fulfill criteria for LBBB or RBBB
- Can be used when QRS duration is not prolonged, but there is abnormal notching of the QRS complex.

CODING POINTER: Consider antiarrhythmic drug toxicity, hyperkalemia, or hypothermia.

## Functional (Rate-related) Aberrancy

This condition presents with the following traits:

- QRS complex is wider during a tachycardia (usually >0.12 second) compared to the QRS duration during a slower sinus rhythm
- Aberrated QRS complexes may have the appearance of RBBB, LBBB, or IVCD
- Expression is rate-related.

# Q WAVE MYOCARDIAL INFARCTION (FIGURES 12-13, 12-14, and 12-15)

A "transmural" myocardial infarction is defined by presence of Q waves with duration ≥0.04 second present in at least 2 contiguous leads. Associated ST and T changes can help define the timing of infarction (**Table 12-3**) and the leads involved can help determine infarct location (**Table 12-4**). ST elevations after myocardial infarction can persist for 48 hours to 4 weeks. Aneurysm should be considered if ST elevations remain present after 1 month. While Q wave criteria apply for all infarcts in RBBB, it is difficult to diagnose any infarct in presence of

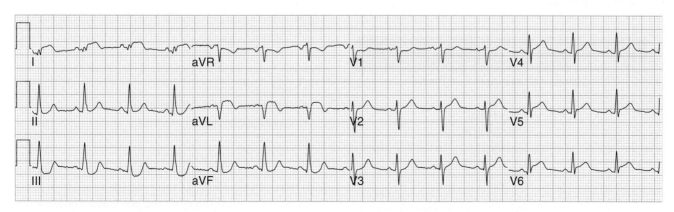

**Figure 12-14.** Lateral myocardial infarction.

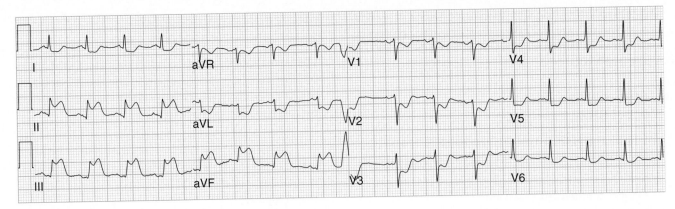

**Figure 12-15.** Inferior wall myocardial infarction (PVC also present).

LBBB. Lead aVF may have a Q wave present intermittently as a result of respiratory effects and low voltage inferiorly.

## REPOLARIZATION ABNORMALITIES

The T wave should normally be upright in all leads except lead aVR. When T waves are flattened or low (<0.5 mm), or mildly inverted (<3 mm), one should code for "nonspecific ST-T wave abnormality." Similarly, the ST segment should be horizontal, and at baseline, mild (<1 mm) elevation or depression should be coded as nonspecific.

Abnormally tall (≥10 mm precordial, ≥6 mm limb leads), symmetric T waves with mild prolongation of the QT interval ("hyperacute T waves") or symmetric and deep (≥3 mm) T wave inversion should be coded as "suggesting myocardial ischemia." The clinical scenario provided should help in differentiating hyperacute T waves of ischemia from those of hyperkalemia. Additionally, the latter may be associated with PR prolongation and/or QRS widening.

Flat or down-sloping ST depression should be coded as "suggesting myocardial ischemia." ST-segment depression associated with LVH should be coded when LVH is present and the ST segment is convex upwards with T wave inversion in lateral precordial leads.

| Table 12-3 • Electrocardiographic determinants of infarct age | | | |
|---|---|---|---|
| | **Q Waves** | **ST Segment** | **T Wave** |
| Acute MI | + | ST elevation +/−reciprocal ST depression | |
| Recent MI | + | Isoelectric ST | Ischemic T waves |
| Old MI | + | Isoelectric ST or normal ST | Nonspecific T wave abnormalities or normal t wave |

**CODING POINTER:** Convex upwards ST-segment depression with T wave inversion in the early precordial leads may accompany RVH and should be coded separately as "secondary to hypertrophy."

"Myocardial injury" should be selected when the ST segment is elevated ≥1 mm in a convex upwards pattern, with or without reciprocal ST depression in the opposing leads.

**CODING POINTER:** ST depression should be coded as "suggesting myocardial ischemia," ST elevation as "suggesting myocardial injury," and pathologic Q waves as "infarction." ST elevation/injury should always be considered the primary event, and if Q waves are present, infarction should also be coded.

"Prominent U waves" should be scored when the U waves, best seen in the early precordial leads, are >one-fourth the height of the associated T wave, or ≥1.5 mm.

## CLINICAL DISORDERS

**CODING POINTER:** The clinical history plays an integral role in the diagnosis for a clinical disorder.

### Digitalis Effect

Digitalis has a distinctive effect on the electrocardiogram. The ST segment appears "scooped out," downsloping, or sagging. The QT interval shortens and U waves become prominent. A summary of the features of digitalis effect:

- sagging ST segment
- prolongation of the PR interval
- shortening of the QT interval
- U waves
- T wave flattening or inversion.

**CODING POINTER:** Do not forget to code for the individual abnormal intervals and wave abnormalities observed with digitalis.

| Table 12-4 • Electrocardiographic determinants of infarct location | | |
|---|---|---|
| | **Age Probably Acute or Recent** | **Age Probably Old or Indeterminate** |
| **Anterolateral** | • Abnormal Q waves in leads V4-V6 with amplitude >15% total QRS complex<br>• ST elevation in V4-V6 | • Abnormal Q waves in leads V4-V6 with amplitude >15% total QRS complex<br>• No ST elevation |
| **Anterior or anteroseptal** | **Anterior:**<br>• rS in V1 followed by QS or QR in leads V2-V4<br>• ST elevation<br><br>**Anteroseptal**<br>• Q or QS deflection in V1-V3 and occ V4 with Q wave amplitude >25% of the QRS<br>• Q in V1 helps distinguish anteroseptal from anterior infarct<br>• ST elevation | **Anterior:**<br>• rS in V1 followed by QS or QR in leads V2-V4<br>• No ST elevation<br><br>**Anteroseptal**<br>• Q or QS deflection in V1-V3 and occ V4 with Q wave amplitude >25% of the QRS<br>• Q in V1 helps distinguish anteroseptal from anterior infarct<br>• No ST elevation |
| **Lateral** | • Q wave in lead I >10% of the amplitude of the QRS<br>• Q wave in lead aVL >50% of the amplitude of the QRS<br>• ST elevation | • Q wave in lead I >10% of the amplitude of the QRS<br>• Q wave in lead aVL >50% of the amplitude of the QRS<br>• No ST elevation |
| **Inferior** | • Q waves in leads II, III, aVF<br>• Q wave in aVF >25% amplitude of the R wave<br>• ST elevation | • Q waves in leads II, III, aVF<br>• Q wave in aVF >25% amplitude of the R wave<br>• No ST elevation |
| **Posterior** | • Initial R wave in leads V1 and V2 ≥0.04 sec with R ≥ S<br>• with ST depression<br>• Upright T wave in anterior precordial leads | • No ST changes |

## Digitalis Toxicity (Figure 12-16)

Digitalis has a narrow therapeutic window. Consider this diagnosis if the clinical history or ECG suggests digitalis use and the patient is presenting with symptoms of *headache, nausea, vomiting, malaise, fatigue, or altered color perception* and/or one of the following arrhythmias:

- atrial fibrillation with complete heart block (regular escape)
- paroxysmal atrial tachycardia
- junctional tachycardia
- complete heart block
- bidirectional ventricular tachycardia.

**CODING POINTER: Digitalis toxicity is the most common cause of paroxysmal atrial tachycardia, and the presence of PAT with heart block is pathognomonic.**

## Antiarrhythmic Drug Effect

Antiarrhythmic medications modulate myocyte ion channels leading to expected ECG changes. Present in the antiarrhythmic drug effect are:

- QT interval prolongation (mild)
- prominent U waves
- nonspecific ST segment and T wave abnormalities
- slowing of atrial flutter rate.

## Antiarrhythmic Drug Toxicity

Toxic levels of antiarrhythmic medication can lead to severe sinus node dysfunction or torsades de pointes. This is characterized by:

- sinus node dysfunction
  - sinus arrest
  - sinus bradycardia
  - SA exit block
- AV conduction bock
- QRS widening
- severe QT interval prolongation
- torsades de pointes

**CODING POINTER: Do not forget to code for the abnormal intervals, wave abnormalities, and rhythm disturbances observed with antiarrhythmic medications.**

## Hyperkalemia (Figure 12-17)

- hyperkalemia presents as: Mild
  - tall, narrow based T waves
  - QT interval shortening
  - left anterior or posterior fascicular block
- moderate
  - PR interval prolongation

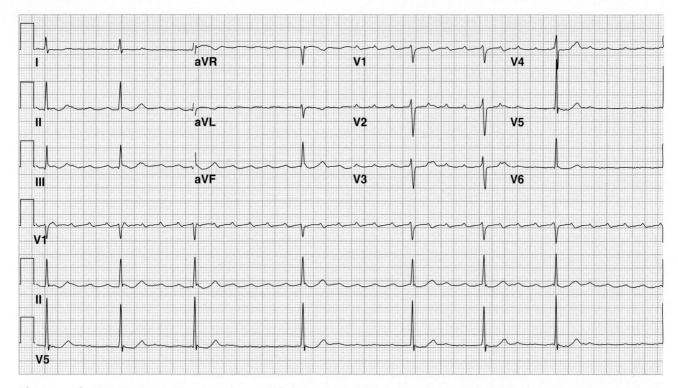

**Figure 12-16.** Digitalis toxicity. This patient has atrial flutter with significant bradycardia. Note the scooped out ST segments.

- ◦ flattening of the P wave
- ◦ QRS interval widening
- • severe
  - ◦ sinus node dysfunction
    - − sinus arrest
    - − sinoventricular conduction
  - ◦ significant widening of QRS complex (sine wave pattern)
  - ◦ ST-segment elevation
  - ◦ associated with ventricular arrhythmias, idioventricular rhythms, and asystole.

**CODING POINTER: If QT interval prolongation is also present, consider also the diagnosis of hypocalcemia (common in patients with end-stage renal disease).**

## Hypokalemia (Figure 12-18)

Hypokalemia presents as:

- • prominent U waves
- • ST-segment depression
- • T wave flattening

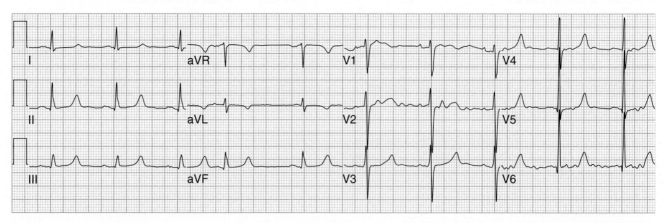

**Figure 12-17.** An electrocardiogram from a patient who missed dialysis and developed hypocalcemia (prolonged, flat QT interval) and hyperkalemia (peaked T waves).

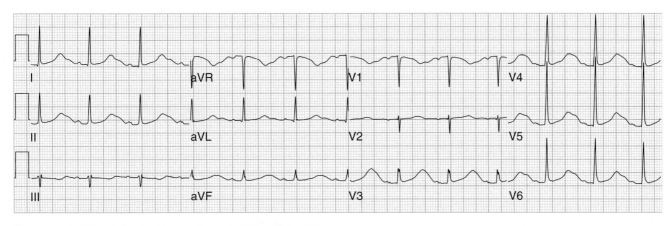

**Figure 12-18.** Hypokalemia. Note prolonged QT interval and U waves.

- increased P wave amplitude and duration
- QT interval prolongation
- associated with paroxysmal atrial tachycardia, AV block, and ventricular arrhythmias.

## Hypercalcemia

Increased extracellular calcium shortens ventricular action potential (phase 2), decreasing the QT interval. Thus, characteristics of hypocalcemia are:

- QT interval shortening (short ST segment)
- T wave flattening, notching or inversion in severe cases.

## Hypocalcemia (Figure 12-17)

Decreased extracellular calcium lengthens the ventricular action potential (phase 2), increasing the QT interval:

- QT interval prolongation (long ST segment), with normal T wave duration.

CODING POINTER: Hypocalcemia is a common finding in end-stage renal disease patients. Note that *only* hypocalcemia and hypothermia result in QT prolongation with a normal T wave duration.

## Atrial Septal Defect, Secundum (ASD–secundum)

Consider a diagnosis of atrial septal defect, secundum, if the patient is a young child presenting with a murmur and the following findings:

- incomplete RBBB
- right axis deviation
- associated findings
  - right ventricular hypertrophy
  - right atrial enlargement
  - 1° AV block.

## Atrial Septal Defect, Primum (ASD–primum)

Consider a diagnosis of atrial septal defect, primum, if the patient is a young child presenting with a murmur and the following findings:

- incomplete RBBB
- left axis deviation
- associated findings:
  - 1° AV block
  - biventricular hypertrophy.

## Dextrocardia, Mirror Image

This is seen in the following:

- left lateral leads (I, aVL) inverted waveforms
- right axis deviation
- decreasing R wave amplitude across precordium.

CODING POINTER: Distinguish dextrocardia from lead reversal by identifying a decrease in R wave amplitude from V1-V6.

## Chronic Lung Disease (Figure 12-2)

Consider a chronic lung disease diagnosis if the following constellation of ECG findings is present:

- right ventricular hypertrophy
- right atrial abnormality
- RBBB (complete or incomplete)
- right axis deviation
- PR-segment depression
- low voltage
- pseudoinfarction pattern in early precordial leads (mimics anterior wall myocardial infarction)
- poor R wave progression over the precordium
- rhythm disturbance

- ◦ sinus tachycardia
- ◦ multifocal atrial tachycardia
- ◦ junctional rhythm
- AV nodal and intraventricular conduction disease.

## Acute Cor Pulmonale Including Pulmonary Embolism

The changes on an electrocardiogram from an acute pulmonary embolism are related to the acute right ventricular dilation, right-sided strain, and rotation of the heart. The changes are often transient. ECG characteristics are:

- S1-Q3-T3 pattern
- RBBB (complete or incomplete)
- ST-segment depression and T wave inversion in early precordial leads
- right atrial dilation
- right axis deviation
- arrhythmia
  - ◦ sinus tachycardia
  - ◦ atrial fibrillation
  - ◦ atrial flutter.

## Pericardial Effusion

The features of pericardial effusion are:

- low voltage QRS complexes
- electrical alternans of QRS complexes
- often associated with ECG findings of pericarditis.

## Acute Pericarditis (Figure 12-19)

The ST segment and T wave changes observed in acute pericarditis represent epicardial injury that can be diffuse or localized. While evolution of the electrocardiogram can be observed in patients with pericarditis, the most likely presentation on the board examination will be stage 1.

- Stage 1
  - ◦ diffuse concave-down ST-segment elevation (ST-segment depression in aVR)
  - ◦ diffuse PR-segment depression (PR-segment elevation in aVR)
- Stage 2
  - ◦ ST segments return to baseline
  - ◦ T wave flattening
- Stage 3
  - ◦ T wave inversion (*after* ST segments return baseline)
- Stage 4
  - ◦ ECG returns to baseline
- Associated findings
  - ◦ sinus tachycardia
  - ◦ low voltage
  - ◦ electrical alternans of QRS complexes.

**CODING POINTER: Clues that distinguish pericarditis from abnormal repolarization include PR-segment deviation, reciprocal changes in aVR, decreased T wave amplitude, and a history of pleuritic chest pain.**

## Hypertrophic Cardiomyopathy

The diagnosis of hypertrophic cardiomyopathy should be considered in patients meeting criteria for ventricular hypertrophy. This is especially the case in patients of younger age presenting with a history of syncope, sudden cardiac death, or dyspnea on exertion.

In the apical variant, there are deep symmetrical T wave inversions in the lateral leads and:

- increased QRS amplitude
- left ventricular hypertrophy
- right ventricular hypertrophy
- left axis deviation

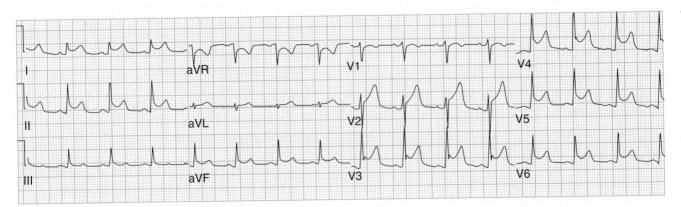

**Figure 12-19.** Acute pericarditis.

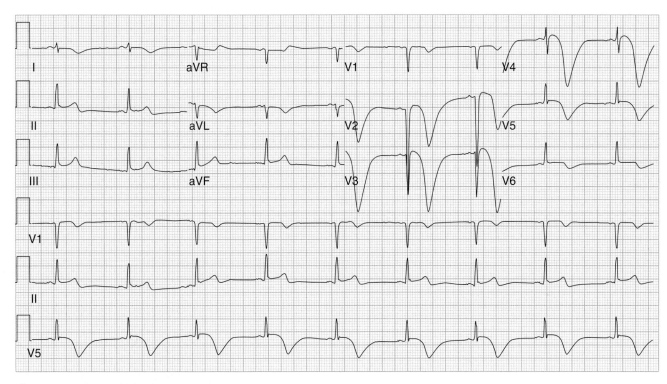

**Figure 12-20.** Central nervous system injury.

- markedly abnormal ST segment and T wave changes
- left or right atrial abnormalities.

## Central Nervous System Disorder (Figure 12-20)

This diagnosis should be considered if there are:

- deep inverted or large upright symmetrical T waves
- prolonged QT interval
- U waves
- ST-segment deviations (elevation or depression)
- Q waves
- broad range of rhythm disturbances.

## Myxedema

This disorder is marked by ECG characteristics of:

- low voltage
- PR interval prolongation
- sinus bradycardia
- T wave flattening
- electrical alternans (pericardial effusion).

## Hypothermia

A diagnosis of hypothermia should be considered for the following traits:

- sinus bradycardia
- osborne or J wave

- prolongation of PR, QRS and QT interval
- artifact (shivering/muscle tremor)
- rhythm disturbances
  - atrial fibrillation (often with slow ventricular response)
  - junction rhythm
  - ventricular tachycardia or fibrillation.

## Sick Sinus Syndrome

This diagnosis refers to any of the following disorders involving the sinus node:

- marked sinus bradycardia
- sinus arrest
- sinoatrial exit block
- tachy-brady syndrome
- prolonged sinus node recovery time after a premature atrial complex or cessation of an atrial tachycardia
- junctional escape rhythm.

## PACEMAKER FUNCTION

Once it is evident that a pacemaker is present, the clinician can identify the chambers that are sensed, paced, and the pacing intervals. With this information, pacemaker type and whether it is functioning correctly can be determined.

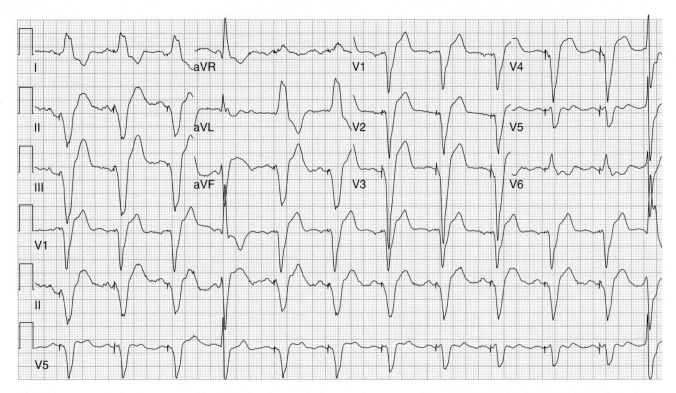

**Figure 12-21.** Dual chamber pacemaker, with normal sinus rhythm, atrial sensing and coupled ventricular pacing. A PVC is also present.

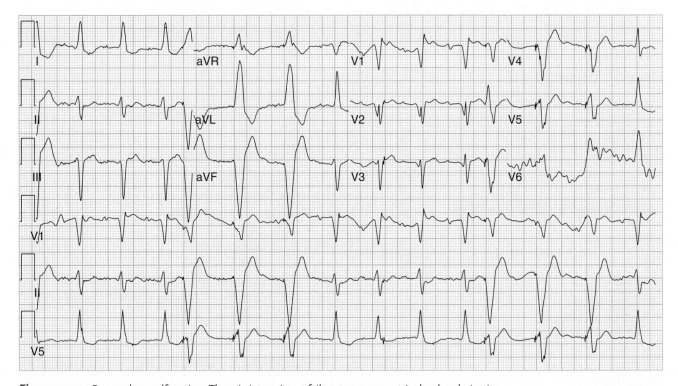

**Figure 12-22.** Pacemaker malfunction. There is intermittent failure to sense ventricular depolarization.

## Atrial or Coronary Sinus Pacing

With simple atrial pacing, a spike is followed by a P wave, which then conducts through the remainder of the heart. If the sensing function is activated, the pacemaker generates an impulse when it does not sense atrial depolarization after a programmed amount of time, the A-A interval (measured as the distance between two uninterrupted paced beats). On the ECG, a spike is followed by a P wave and QRS complex identical to the patient's native QRS complexes.

## Ventricular Demand Pacemaker (VVI), Normally Functioning

A ventricular demand pacemaker describes a pacemaker that senses and paces in the right ventricle. On the electrocardiogram, a pacer spike appears if an intrinsic ventricular depolarization is not sensed after a preprogrammed time interval, the V-V interval (measured as the distance between two uninterrupted paced beats). Thus, if the intrinsic rhythm should fall below a certain rate, the pacemaker is activated. On ECG, there is a spike that appears before a wide QRS complex with morphology similar to a VPC.

## Dual-chamber Pacemaker (DDD), Normally Functioning (Figure 12-21)

If the patient has a normally functioning dual chamber pacemaker, one will be able to identify either (1) a pacer spike preceding atrial and ventricular depolarization (atrial pacing, ventricular pacing) or (2) a pacer spike occurring at a fixed interval after the patient's native P waves (atrial sensing, ventricular pacing).

The programmed time interval from *atrial depolarization* to *ventricular pacing* is the A-V interval. The programmed time interval from *ventricular depolarization* to *atrial pacing* is the V-A interval.

## Pacemaker Malfunction, not Constantly Capturing (Atrium or Ventricle)

In this instance, pacemaker spikes are not followed by myocardial depolarization.

## Pacemaker Malfunction, not Constantly Sensing (Atrium or Ventricle)

Determining if a pacemaker is sensing inappropriately is simple once the programmed pacing intervals are identified. Sensing malfunction occurs if (1) the pacemaker attempts generate an impulse before the programmed time interval and the device has failed to sense the intrinsic rhythm (undersensing, **Figure 12-22**) *or* (2) the pacemaker fails to generate an impulse at the programmed interval because it has inappropriately sensed a native beat that never actually existed (oversensing). The ECG characteristics for these diagnoses are as follows:

- Atrial pacemaker sensing failure
  - Atrial pacemaker impulse occurs after a native P wave at an interval <A-A interval (*undersensing*)
  - No atrial pacemaker generated impulse at the A-A interval (*oversensing*)
- Ventricular demand pacemaker sensing failure
  - Ventricular pacemaker impulse occurs after a native QRS complex, at an interval <V-V interval (undersensing)
  - No ventricular pacemaker generated impulse at the V-V interval (oversensing)
- Dual chamber pacemaker sensing failure
  - Atrial component
    - No QRS complex associated with native P waves, atrial pacemaker impulse may be generated despite native P wave (undersensing)
    - Isolated paced ventricular complexes not associated with atrial depolarization (oversensing)
  - Ventricular component
    - Atrial pacemaker impulse generated <V-A interval (undersensing)
    - No atrial pacemaker generated impulse at the V-A interval (oversensing)

## ACKNOWLEDGEMENT

We are indebted to Dr. Robert W. Peters for his friendly guidance and seemingly endless supply of electrocardiograms.

# 13

# The Athlete's Heart

MALISSA J. WOODS, KIBAR YARED, AND AARON BAGGISH

## ● PRACTICAL POINTS

- Normal cardiac adaptations in athletes include atrial and ventricular enlargement.

- The presence of either symptomatic bradycardia or high degree AV block should prompt a thorough cardiac evaluation.

- There is a higher prevalence of lone atrial fibrillation in athletes compared to sedentary individuals. This appears to be related to heightened sympathetic and parasympathetic tone as well as presence of biatrial dilatation.

- Athletes frequently exhibit ECG changes including incomplete right bundle branch block, atrial enlargement, first degree AV block, and early repolarization.

- ECG changes, including high degree AV block, marked LVH with T wave inversion, should not be considered normal variants and thus require follow-up.

- The current ACC/AHA preparticipation evaluation in athletes includes a screening history and physical but not an ECG.

- Athletes with symptoms of chest pain, syncope, shortness of breath with exertion, or symptomatic tachycardia should undergo a thorough cardiac evaluation.

## HYPERTROPHIC CARDIOMYOPATHY

Hypertrophic cardiomyopathy (HCM) is a well-recognized cause of sudden cardiac death among athletic individuals. The prevalence of HCM in the general public is roughly 1/500 individuals. This condition is the most common cardiovascular cause of exercise-related sudden death among athletes in the United States and has the propensity to affect individuals at all levels of competition.

HCM is characterized by significant hypertrophy of the left ventricular (LV) free walls and the interventricular septum with normal to reduced LV cavity size. LV hypertrophy attributable to HCM can involve the entire LV in producing a symmetrically enlarged chamber. Alternatively, variants with hypertrophy confined to discrete regions are commonly encountered (**Figure 13-1**). The most common of these variants is one characterized by isolated interventricular septal hypertrophy with consequent obstruction of the LV outflow tract. This form of HCM is termed hypertrophic obstructive cardiomyopathy (HOCM). HOCM is commonly accompanied by mitral valve abnormalities including redundancy of subvalvular structures (chords and papillary muscles) leading to functional mitral valve abnormalities including regurgitation, prolapse, and systolic anterior motion.

It has been recently shown that HCM/HOCM is caused by mutations in genes that code for the production of myocardial proteins. Sporadic and heritable mutations in sarcomere proteins, including troponin, myosin, and actin, have been demonstrated to be causal. Histologic inspection of myocardium from afflicted individuals reveals characteristic myofibrillar disarray and patchy fibrocellular replacement (**Figure 13-2**).

Individuals with underlying HCM/HOCM often present with sudden cardiac death in the absence of antecedent symptoms. Such a catastrophe is thought to result from malignant ventricular tachyarrhythmia. Although precise mechanistic understanding of arrhythmias in the context of HCM/HOCM is elusive, most experts believe that they arise from reentry pathways that are facilitated by underlying myofibrillar disarray. Some individuals, most frequently those with the HOCM variant, do present with symptoms prior to sudden death. These symptoms are most frequently a consequence of dynamic, exercise-induced, LV outflow

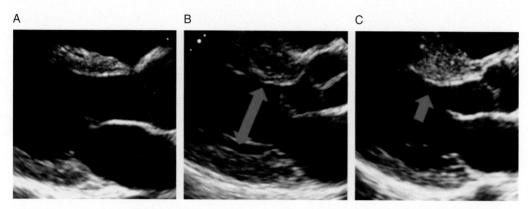

**Figure 13-1.** Transthoracic echocardiographic images demonstrating normal left ventricular architecture (A), hypertrophic cardiomyopathy (B) with symmetric enlargement of both the interventricular septum and the posterior left ventricular free wall (double red arrow), and hypertrophic obstructive cardiomyopathy (C) with asymmetric enlargement of involving only the interventricular septum (single red arrow).

tract obstruction and include syncope, chest pain, palpitations, and disproportionate dyspnea.

The diagnosis of HCM/HOCM requires a high index of suspicion. All individuals who participate in organized athletics should undergo a preparticipation medical history and physical examination as suggested by most recent ACC/AHA guidelines. A family history of unexplained syncope, "cardiac enlargement," or premature/exertional death should serve as suggestive of this diagnosis. Physical examination revealing a harsh cardiac systolic ejection murmur that increases in intensity with the Valsalva maneuver is suggestive of LV outflow tract obstruction. Individuals with any abnormality during preparticipation screening should be referred for further disease specific diagnosis.

Roughly 80% of individuals with HCM/HOCM have ECG abnormalities, including interventricular conduction delay,

voltage criteria for left ventricular hypertrophy, ST-segment depression, T wave inversion, and anterior/inferior Q waves producing a "pseudo-infarct" pattern. While such findings are typical of HCM, they are encountered commonly among trained athletes with no underlying structural heart disease. As such, the ECG can, at best, be considered suggestive of HCM/HOCM. The presence of any of the above findings is justification for transthoracic echocardiography (TTE).

TTE is the preferred test for confirming or excluding the diagnosis of HCM. Echocardiographic findings in HCM include increased wall thickness, normal or reduced LV cavity dimensions, altered indices of diastolic filling, and mitral valve abnormalities, including systolic anterior motion and regurgitation. The magnitude of wall thickness increase varies considerably among individuals with HCM. Severity classification schemes based on wall thickness have been proposed, and this metric has been shown to provide important prognostic information. Mild phenotypic expression of HCM can lead to wall thickness that exceeds sedentary population-based limits of normal (<12 mm) by only several millimeters. Similar-appearing hypertrophy can also as a component of adaptive remodeling in athletes without HCM.

Several studies have provided important data defining the magnitude of LV wall thickness increase that typically occurs in athletes without HCM. Current evidence suggests that a small but significant percentage of athletes (~2%) have LV wall thicknesses greater than or equal to 13 mm and that all of these individuals have concomitant LV cavity dilation, a combination not typically found among individuals with HCM. Although there may be a relatively low incidence of abnormally increased LV wall thickness measurements among athletes, a small but significant number of individuals do have wall thickness values in the 13-15-mm range. This finding may be particularly common among elite athletes, such

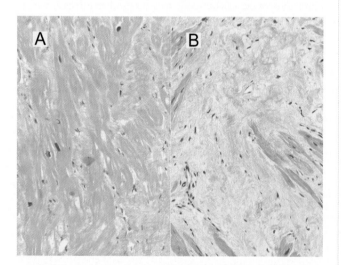

**Figure 13-2.** Post-mortem histopathologic specimen of LV ventricular myocardium from an athlete with hypertrophic cardiomyopathy showing (A) myofibrillar disarray and (B) patchy fibrosis.

as American National Football League players. Such athletes are often termed "gray zone" individuals, a term used to reflect the uncertainty of the cause of their LV hypertrophy.

Evaluation of the gray zone athlete can present a clinical challenge. The first step in the work-up of an athletic individual with LV enlargement is to define the magnitude of abnormality and to consider it in the context of other cardiac structural and functional imaging data. LV wall thickness greater equal to 16 mm is very rare among healthy athletes and this finding must be considered as highly suggestive of HCM. For individuals with mild LV wall thickness increase, adaptive remodeling can be differentiated from structural heart disease by concomitant consideration of LV cavity dimensions. Either isolated LV wall thickness increase or isolated LV dilation should prompt further assessment for potential pathology.

Several recently developed echocardiographic imaging techniques provide information that complements basic structural measurements in the assessment of individuals with suspected HCM/HOCM. One such technique is tissue Doppler imaging, which provides a direct measure of tissue velocities, and thus tissue function, during the systolic and diastolic phases of the cardiac cycle. Several studies have shown that diastolic tissue velocities are reduced among individuals with HCM/HOCM but normal or elevated among athletic individuals even in the context of LV enlargement and low-normal LV ejection fraction. Echocardiographic strain and strain rate imaging also provide valuable information about tissue function. Strain measurements define changes in muscle fiber length as they contract and relax during the cardiac cycle, while strain rate measures these length changes as a function of time. Individuals with HCM have lower LV systolic strain values than normal controls, while individuals with athletic remodeling have strain values that are normal or higher than those found in sedentary healthy controls. Both tissue Doppler and strain imaging can be performed during routine echocardiographic examination and should performed in all athletes with LV hypertrophy of indeterminate cause.

Occasionally, TTE does not provide sufficient information for definitive diagnosis and risk assessment of HCM/HOCM. Complementary options in the assessment of individuals with suspect HCM/HOCM included exercise stress testing, Holter-monitoring, prescribed deconditioning, and magnetic resonance imaging. MRI has emerged as a valuable option in such cases. Although the cost and time commitment of MRI do not compare favorably with TTE, it may serve as a valuable step in the assessment of athletes with suboptimal echocardiographic acoustic windows or in those whose with ECGs that show cause for concern or otherwise indeterminate echocardiograms. Ongoing work promises to define the optimal role of MRI in this context.

Management of the athlete diagnosed with HCM/HOCM presents a challenge. Athletes who present following a clinically relevant event attributable to HCM/HOCM should be prohibited from further athletic activity once diagnosis and causality have been established as HCM/HOCM-related sudden death appears to occur most frequently during periods of exercise. Some forms of sport that require only low level exertion may be appropriate for individuals with HCM/HOCM, and consensus committee guidelines have been developed to assist with decision-making regarding further athletic participation. In addition, family members of afflicted individuals should be screened for asymptomatic disease. The decision to prohibit athletic participation among individuals found to have HCM/HOCM during preparticipation screening can be difficult. Until more is learned about prognosis in this patient population, a cautious approach centered on sport avoidance is recommended.

Beyond avoidance of athletic participation, clinical management of athletes with HCM/HOCM must focus on the relief of symptoms and prevention of malignant arrhythmias. The use of medications with negative inotropic and antiarrhythmic action such as nondihydropyridine calcium channel blockers and beta-blockers may reduce HCM/HOCM symptoms. These medications have, however, not been shown to affect the likelihood of arrhythmia or sudden death. Athletes with HOCM and medication refractory symptoms such as heart failure or recurrent syncope may be considered for surgical or percutaneous septal reduction therapy. It must be emphasized that these therapies should be reserved for management of medication refractory symptoms and do not reduce risk adequately to permit return to athletic activity.

Prevention of malignant arrhythmias among athletes with HCM/HOCM may be accomplished with the use of automatic implantable cardiac defibrillators. Defibrillator implantation is clearly indicated for individuals with HCM/HOCM who present following survival of cardiac arrest or in those with documented ventricular arrhythmias. Such secondary prevention has been shown to reduce the likelihood of future catastrophe. While defibrillator placement leads to a reduction in arrhythmic complications, it does not reduce risk adequately to make return to athletics a completely safe option. Further work is needed to examine the long-term prognosis of individuals afflicted with HCM/HOCM that receive defibrillator implants.

The decision to place a defibrillator in individuals who have not experienced an arrhythmic episode is controversial. Risk factors including absolute LV wall thickness, family history of HCM/HOCM-related complications, unexplained syncope, and exercise-induced hypotension are commonly used to risk-stratify patients in this situation. At the present time there are insufficient data to provide recommendations regarding primary prevention

becoming increasingly important in confirming the diagnosis in probands and family members; however, it still does not play a role in the risk stratification of a person with ARVD/C. Pharmacologic treatment remains useful, but radiofrequency ablation and implantable cardioverter-defibrillator therapy are increasingly important therapeutic approaches in these patients.

ARVD/C has been shown to contribute a significant percentage of sudden cardiac death in athletes. A high level of clinical suspicion should be maintained once one is faced with an athlete who complains of unexplained palpitations, presyncope, syncope, or aborted sudden death, especially if accompanied by a positive family history or an abnormal ECG or imaging study. However, uncertainties remain about the specific etiology of the disease, the genetic basis, the clinical course of patients, and the appropriate diagnosis and therapy. Large clinical trials of ARVD/C patients such as the European ARVD Registry and the Multidisciplinary Study of Right Ventricular Dysplasia will hopefully improve our knowledge of ARVD/C.

## PART III SUGGESTED READING

1. Corrado D, Basso C, Thiene G. Arrhythmogenic right ventricular cardiomyopathy: diagnosis, prognosis, and treatment. *Heart*. 2000;83(5):588–595.
2. Frances RJ. Arrhythmogenic right ventricular dysplasia/cardiomyopathy. A review and update. *Int J Cardiol*. 2006;110(3):279–287.
3. Hedrich O, Estes NA, Link. MS. Sudden cardiac death in athletes. *Curr Cardiol Rep*. 2006;8(5):316–322.
4. Maron BJ. Sudden death in young athletes. *N Engl J Med*. 2003;349(11):1064–1075.
5. McKenna WJ, Thiene G, Nava A, et al. Diagnosis of arrhythmogenic right ventricular dysplasia/cardiomyopathy. Task Force of the Working Group Myocardial and Pericardial Disease of the European Society of Cardiology and of the Scientific Council on Cardiomyopathies of the International Society and Federation of Cardiology. *Br Heart J*. 1994;71(3):215–218.
6. Yoerger DM, Marcus F, Sherrill D, et al Echocardiographic findings in patients meeting task force criteria for arrhythmogenic right ventricular dysplasia: new insights from the multidisciplinary study of right ventricular dysplasia. *J Am Coll Cardiol*. 2005;45(6):860–865.

## PART IV ARRHYTHMIAS IN ATHLETES

Case presentation: VP is a 21-year-old elite swimmer who presented with the complaint of new onset palpitations noted at rest and immediately following exercise. He reported that he experienced dizziness and lightheadedness with the symptoms but denied chest pain, shortness of breath, or syncope. His physical exam was unremarkable and his resting electrocardiogram revealed a heart rate of 40 bpm but was otherwise normal. An event monitor was placed and revealed evidence of a narrow complex supraventricular arrhythmia at a rate of 180 bpm, consistent with atrioventricular (AV) node reentrant tachycardia. Due to his high level of athletic activity and resting bradycardia the decision was made not to medically manage his arrhythmia but to refer him for electrophysiologic (EPS) evaluation and possible ablation. EPS indeed revealed an inducible AV nodal reentrant which was successfully treated with radiofrequency ablation. He remains asymptomatic.

The notoriety associated with the death of a prominent athlete attracts a great deal of media attention and leads to the assumption by many that the arrhythmic death in athletes is common. While the risk of sudden cardiac death is rare, electrocardiographic abnormalities or the presence of cardiac arrhythmias may herald the presence of underlying heart disease, which could place an athlete at risk of sudden cardiac death. In this section we will review common physiologic electrocardiographic features of athletes, common arrhythmias in athletes, and less common arrhythmias which, when present, should lead to further cardiovascular diagnostic investigation.

The incidence of supraventricular and ventricular tachyarrhythmias as well as bradyarrhythmias is increased in athletes and cardiac arrhythmias remains one of the major reasons for disqualification from athletic participation. Differentiation of the physiologic from pathologic substrates is imperative in the athlete who presents with an arrhythmia. Thankfully, few athletes die every year due to underlying cardiac arrhythmias; however, those responsible for the healthcare of athletes need to understand the types of arrhythmias and ECG abnormalities that may be present both in healthy athletes and in those with cardiovascular disease.

### Bradyarrhythmias

Sinus bradyarrhythmias are frequently encountered in athletes and are rarely a cause for concern. The cardiovascular adaptations of athletic training include atrial and ventricular enlargement and resting bradycardia. While some athletes may exhibit first and second degree heart block, the presence of symptomatic bradycardia or high degree heart block should lead to a thorough cardiovascular evaluation (Thompson 2007).

### Ventricular Arrhythmias

The clinical presentation of ventricular tachyarrhythmias in athletes can vary from rare palpitations and isolated PVCs to sudden death in athletes with arrhythmic right ventricular cardiomyopathy (ARVC), hypertrophic, or other cardiomyopathy. It is estimated that fewer than 10% of athletes who present with symptomatic ventricular tachyarrhythmias have structurally normal hearts, thus, the presence of a ventricular arrhythmia in an athlete should prompt a thorough clinical investigation. There does not appear to be any association between training-associated left ventricular hypertrophy and the degree of left ventricular arrhythmias, in fact there was a great frequency and complexity of ventricular arrhythmias in those with lower left ventricular mass (Biffi et al. 2008).

The types of arrhythmias that may be present in structurally normal hearts include right ventricular monomorphic extrasytoles, right ventricular outflow tract (RVOT) and left ventricular outflow tract (LVOT) tachycardia, idiopathic left ventricular tachycardia, idiopathic propanolol sensitive (automatic) ventricular tachycardia, catecholaminergic polymorphic ventricular tachycardia, Brugada syndrome, and long QT syndrome.

It is important to identify ARVC when present due to the increased risk of sudden cardiac death it presents. RVOT ventricular tachycardia (VT), in contrast, carries a benign prognosis and is characterized by a LBBB pattern and inferior axis. RVOT VT can present as either nonsustained repetitive monomorphic VT or paroxysmal exercise-induced sustained ventricular tachycardia. When present, the resting extrasystoles decrease or disappear during exercise while sustained VT can be induced by physical activity. Treatment of the RVOT tachycardia includes IV adenosine in the acute setting, beta-blockers, and calcium channel blockers, while the highest degree of treatment success is associated with radiofrequency ablation. The presence of chronic sustained or nonsustained ventricular tachycardia can result in biventricular systolic dysfunction which improves following successful ablation of the arrhythmia (Bauce et al. 2008).

ARVC is associated with both structural and functional abnormalities of the right ventricle due to fibrofatty replacement of the myocardium, and affected individuals are predisposed to developing reentrant ventricular tachyarrhythmias. Diagnostic criteria for ARVC have been developed and include clinical, electrocardiographic, and structural features. While echocardiographic imaging with intravenous echo contrast is helpful in identifying focal right ventricular wall motion abnormalities, chamber dilatation and sacculations, magnetic resonance imaging remains the gold standard for diagnosing ARVC.

Electrocardiographic features of ARVC include T wave inversion in the right precordial leads and epsilon waves in V1-V2. The resting electrocardiogram in RVOT ventricular tachycardia is usually normal. While morphologic features of VT associated with ARVC may resemble those of RVOT, the tachycardia associated with ARVC usually exhibits a QRS duration >120 ms and an axis <30 degrees.

## Atrial Fibrillation in Athletes

Several studies have demonstrated a higher prevalence of athletic activity in individuals with lone atrial fibrillation. One study demonstrated up to a three-fold increase in the incidence of atrial fibrillation in athletes compared with sedentary controls. The potential mechanisms responsible for the predisposition to atrial fibrillation include both the heightened sympathetic and parasympathetic tone as well as biatrial dilatation, which are present in many well-trained athletes. The presence of both increased sympathetic and vagal tone results in a reduction in a reduction in the RR interval, increased heart rate variability, and reduced effective atrial refractory period, all of which lead to the increased incidence of atrial fibrillation (Lampert 2008).

The presence of atrial fibrillation in athletic individuals results in reduced quality of life and impaired athletic performance. The success of pulmonary vein isolation in the treatment of atrial fibrillation in athletes with resultant improvement in exercise capacity has recently been reported (Pellicia et al. 2008). This method of treatment is favored in many athletes who prefer to avoid cardiovascular medications and their associated side effects.

## Electrocardiography in Athletes

Electrocardiographic (ECG) screening has been recommended as part of preathletic participation screening by many international, national, and regional organizations. The implementation of ECG screening in Italy has resulted in decreased mortality in a population of competitive athletes. In Italy, ECG screening of 32,652 athletes revealed that the ECG was normal in 88%. Of the abnormalities encountered, the most common abnormalities encountered included first degree AV block, incomplete RBBB, and early repolarization. Less frequently encountered abnormalities included evidence of left ventricular hypertrophy, RBBB, LAF, LBBB, increased QTc, and pre-excitation. Such abnormalities in the absence of clinical or echocardiographic evidence of structural heart disease are generally considered to be innocent consequences of athletic training. While the prevalence of QTc prolongation in elite athletes is 0.4%, a QTc <0.50 msec in the absence of symptoms or familial disease is unlikely to represent long QT syndrome.

Pellicia and colleagues examined the clinical significance of deep precordial T wave inversion in 12,550 athletes without other evidence of cardiovascular disease. The athletes were followed for a mean of 9+/–3 years, and during that time 5 athletes (6%) developed evidence of a cardiomyopathy, including one with sudden cardiac death and ARVD, three with hypertrophic cardiomyopathy, and one with a dilated cardiomyopathy (Furlanello et al. 2008). The authors concluded that this individuals with deep T wave inversion warranted long term clinical follow-up.

The evaluation of cardiac arrhythmias in the athlete who presents a structurally normal heart and normal resting electrocardiogram should also include a detailed history of medication use, including use of possible performance-enhancing drugs. Many illicit drugs taken by athletes to enhance performance are associated with cardiac arrhythmias. Potentially arrhythmogenic illicit drugs include anabolic steroids (atrial and ventricular arrhythmias), beta agonists (particularly in individuals with underlying cardiomyopathies), stimulants (atrial and ventricular arrhythmias, QTc prolongation), cannabinoids (atrial fibrillation), glucocorticoids (arrhythmias secondary to metabolic perturbations), alcohol (atrial and ventricular arrhythmias), and beta-blockers (bradycardia and heart block) (White et al. 2008).

## Suggested Readings

1. Biffi A, Maron BJ, Di Giacinto B, et al. Relation between training-induced left ventricular hypertrophy and risk for ventricular tachyarrhythmias in elite athletes. *Am J Cardiol.* 2008;101(12):1792-1795. Epub 2008 Apr 15.

2. Bauce B, Frigo G, Benini G, et al. Differences and similarities between arrhythmic right ventricular cardiomyopathy and athlete's heart adaptations. *Br J Sports Med.*, 2008; 2010 Feb; 44(2): 148–154

3. Lampert R. Atrial fibrillation in athletes: toward more effective therapy and better understanding. *J Cardiovasc Electrophysiol.* 2008;19 463–465.

4. Pellicia A, DiiPaolo F, Quatterini F, et al. Outcomes in athletes with marked ECG repolarization abnormalities. *NEJM.* 2008;358:152–161.

5. Furlanello F, Lupo P, Pittalis M, et al. Radiofrequency catheter ablation of atrial fibrillation in athletes referred for disabling symptoms preventing usual training schedule and sport competition. *J Cardiovasc Electrophysiol.* 2008;19:457–462.

6. Whyte G, Stephens N, Senior R, et al. Differentiation of RVOT- VT vs. in ARVC in an Elite Athlete. Med Science Sports Exercise 2008 Aug; 40 (8):1357.

# Pulmonary and Critical Care

# 14

# Perioperative Management of Patients with Cardiovascular Disease

KARA BARNETT AND LEE A. FLEISHER

- ECG is not indicated in low risk patients undergoing low risk surgery.

- Emergency surgeries should not be delayed for cardiac evaluation.

- Low risk patients with stable or no heart disease can undergo low risk surgery without further testing or intervention

- For those with a left bundle branch block, a pharmacological stress test is preferred over an exercise stress test.

- Perioperative beta-blockade should be used in patients previously on beta-blockers (Class I) and considered for those with a positive stress test undergoing major vascular surgery (Class IIa). Statins and clonidine should be continued perioperatively, and aspirin should be continued, unless the risks outweigh the benefits.

## INTRODUCTION

With the growing elderly population, in the number of patients with heart disease undergoing surgery will increase. The purpose of the cardiologist's preoperative consultation is to thoroughly evaluate and address any questions suggested by the patient, surgeon, or anesthesiologist. In many cases the patient will be well known to the cardiologist, and

therefore the goal of the evaluation may simply be communication of known information. In other patients, the cardiologist may be asked specific questions by members of the perioperative team in order to modify care. A cardiologist should not "clear" a patient for surgery, but rather should communicate the information from the consultation with the anesthesiologists and surgeons.

## PREOPERATIVE MANAGEMENT

### Assessment

As part of the evaluation, the consultant should be able to communicate the extent and stability of the patient's cardiovascular disease, assess the implication of the cardiovascular disease on perioperative risk, and perhaps suggest changes in medical management of the patient, including the need for further testing. In some cases, this evaluation may lead to delay or cancellation of surgery. Further testing should only be performed if the results may affect the patient's perioperative management.

An overall assessment of risk can be performed utilizing the American Society of Anesthesiologists (ASA) Physical Status Index (**Table 14-1**). The ASA index, or score, is a simple way to communicate the severity of disease, but it does not directly address disease-specific risk. The specific identification of perioperative cardiac risk has been an area of active study for three decades, and much of the work has focused on the development of clinical risk indices. The most recent Index was developed in a study of 4315 patients aged 50 years or older undergoing elective major noncardiac procedures in a tertiary-care teaching hospital.

| Table 14-1 • ASA Physical Status Index |
| --- |
| ASA-I: Healthy patient without systemic disease (e.g., 21-year-old patient undergoing breast augmentation.) |
| ASA-II: Mild systemic disease without functional limitations (e.g., 45-year-old patient with mild hypertension and well-controlled diabetes mellitus undergoing a breast augmentation.) |
| ASA-III: Moderate to severe systemic disease that has some functional limitations (e.g., Morbidly obese 45-year-old patient with hypertensive kidney disease and diabetes mellitus undergoing an exploratory laparotomy.) |
| ASA-IV: Severe systemic disease that is incapacitating and a constant threat to life (e.g., Morbidly obese 45-year-old patient with necrotizing fasciitis and decreased mental status undergoing an exploratory laparotomy.) |
| ASA-V: Moribund patient who is not expected to survive >24 hours without surgery (e.g., 45-year-old patient with a ruptured aortic aneurysm in severe shock.) |
| ASA-VI: Brain-dead patient undergoing organ harvest |
| *Add the letter "E" to the classification for a surgery that is an emergency (e.g., The patient with the ruptured aortic aneurysm going into surgery is a ASA-VE)* |

Six independent predictors of complications were identified, and included in a Revised Cardiac Risk Index (RCRI): (1) high risk type of surgery, (2) history of ischemic heart disease, (3) history of congestive heart failure, (4) history of cerebrovascular disease, (5) preoperative treatment with insulin, and (6) preoperative serum creatinine >2.0 mg/dL Cardiac complication rates were noted to increase with an increasing number of risk factors. The RCRI has become the standard tool in the literature in assessing the prior probability of perioperative cardiac risk in a given individual and has been used to direct the decision to perform cardiovascular testing and implement perioperative management protocols in the most recent American College of Cardiology/American Heart Association (ACC/AHA) Guidelines on Perioperative Cardiovascular Evaluation. The Revised Cardiac Risk Index will be discussed throughout the rest of the chapter.

## Approach to the Patient

The preoperative evaluation/consultation begins with a thorough history and physical examination. Frequently, patients are evaluated because of the presence of overt coronary artery disease. It is critical the examiner ensure that the patient's underlying disease is stable. The perioperative period is associated with a hypercoagulable state, and therefore the presence of unstable coronary artery disease is associated with a very high rate of perioperative cardiac morbidity and mortality. In one study the presence of unstable angina was associated with a 28% risk of perioperative myocardial infarction (MI) and death. For patients with stable coronary

artery disease (CAD), it is important one assess the amount of myocardium in jeopardy, ischemic threshold, and ventricular function. This information may already have been gathered from previous evaluations or by history or physical examination, but further diagnostic testing to obtain more objective data may be warranted if the results might change perioperative management. It is also important the cardiologist assess the patient's current medication regimen.

Traditionally, coronary risk assessment for noncardiac surgery in patients with a prior myocardial infarction was based upon the time interval between the MI and surgery. The AHA/ACC Task Force on Perioperative Evaluation of the Cardiac Patient undergoing Noncardiac Surgery currently suggests that the highest risk cohort, those with active cardiac conditions, are patients who are within 6 weeks of their MI, a time period during which plaque and myocardial stabilization occur. Other active cardiac conditions that warrant further evaluation before noncardiac surgery include those found in **Table 14-2.**

In virtually all studies to date, the presence of symptomatic heart failure (HF) preoperatively has been associated with an increased incidence of perioperative cardiac morbidity. Stabilizing symptoms of pulmonary congestion is a prudent move prior to elective surgery. It is important to determine the etiology of the left heart failure since the type of perioperative monitoring and treatments would be different for such conditions as ischemic or nonischemic cardiomyopathy, systolic or nonsystolic HF, or mitral or aortic valvular insufficiency and/or stenosis. Diastolic filling abnormalities are particularly common in older patients and may point to an increased risk of these patients developing symptomatic heart failure or atrial fibrillation in the perioperative period.

In patients undergoing elective noncardiac surgery, the presence of aortic stenosis places the patient at the same level of increased risk. The presence of any of the classic triad of angina, syncope, and heart failure in a patient with aortic stenosis should alert the clinician to the need for further evaluation and potential interventions, usually valve replacement. However, many patients with severe or critical aortic stenosis may be asymptomatic, and preoperative patients with aortic systolic murmurs warrant a careful history and physical examination and often further evaluation. Mitral valve disease tends to cause less risk of perioperative complications than aortic stenosis. However, occult mitral stenosis from rheumatic heart disease is still encountered on occasion and can lead to severe left heart failure in the presence of tachycardia and/or volume loading.

In the perioperative patient with a functioning prosthetic heart valve, the major issues are antibiotic prophylaxis and

**Table 14-2 • Active Cardiac Conditions for which the Patient Should Undergo Evaluation and Treatment Before Noncardiac Surgery**[**]

| Condition | Examples |
| --- | --- |
| Unstable coronary syndromes | Unstable or severe angina* (CCS class III or IV)[†] <br> Recent MI[‡] |
| Decompensated HF (NYHA functional class IV; worsening or new-onset HF) | |
| Significant arrhythmias | High-grade atrioventricular block <br> Mobitz II atrioventricular block <br> Third-degree atrioventricular heart block <br> Symptomatic ventricular arrhythmias <br> Supraventricular arrhythmias (including atrial fibrillation) with uncontrolled ventricular rate (HR greater than 100 bpm at rest) <br> Symptomatic bradycardia <br> Newly recognized ventricular tachycardia |
| Severe valvular disease | Severe aortic stenosis (mean pressure gradient greater than 40 mm Hg, aortic valve area less than 1.0 cm², or symptomatic) <br> Symptomatic mitral stenosis (progressive dyspnea on exertion, exertional presyncope, or HF) |

CCS, Canadian Cardiovascular Society; HF, heart failure; HR, heart rate; MI, myocardial infarction; NYHA, New York Heart Association.
*According to Campeau.[10]

[†] May include "stable" angina in patients who are unusually sedentary.

[‡] The American College of Cardiology National Database Library defines recent MI as more than 7 days but less than or equal to 1 month (within 30 days).
**From the ACC/AHA 2007 guidelines.

anticoagulation. For most surgical procedures, oral anticoagulation should be stopped three days before surgery with the goal of an international normalized ratio <1.5. Patients may receive heparin perioperatively with discontinuation 4 to 6 hours prior to surgery. Current recommendations regarding both perioperative anticoagulation and endocarditis prophylaxis should be reviewed in the appropriate AHA/ACC and American College of Chest Physician Guidelines.

Although hypertension is a risk factor for CAD, it has only been shown to be a risk factor for developing perioperative myocardial ischemia and not perioperative cardiac morbidity or mortality. Based upon one randomized trial, one may conclude that there is no benefit in delaying surgery in hypertensive patients without overt CAD with blood pressure greater than 180/110 (stage 3 hypertension). If necessary, antihypertensives can be administered intravenously in the perioperative period to acutely lower blood pressure. Patients with signs of unstable hypertension such as angina or headache should have surgery delayed and the blood pressure treated first.

Patients with congenital heart disease should be evaluated for Eisenmenger syndrome and pulmonary hypertension. These patients may not tolerate hypoxia during surgery. Prophylaxis for endocarditis is also an important part of their management. A full review of this topic is beyond the scope of this chapter; it can be found elsewhere.

Asymptomatic ventricular arrhythmias have not been associated with an increase in cardiac complications. Patients with ventricular arrhythmias should only be treated if the arrhythmia causes hemodynamic compromise. Cardioversion should be performed for those with unstable arrhythmias; otherwise, rate control with medication is sufficient. Beta-blockade should be considered for rate control of arrhythmias.

## Decision to Perform Preoperative Diagnostic Testing

In the decision of whether to perform additional diagnostic testing, the consultant needs to evaluate the patient's functional status/exercise tolerance and identify clinical predictors and risks of surgery (**Figure 14-1**). The figure presents in algorithmic form a framework for determining which patients are candidates for cardiac testing. Given the availability of this evidence, the ACC/AHA Writing Committee chose to include the level of the recommendations and strength of evidence for many of the pathways:

- Step 1: The consultant should determine the urgency of noncardiac surgery. In many instances, patient- or surgery-specific factors dictate an obvious strategy (e.g., emergent surgery) that may not allow for further cardiac assessment or treatment.
- Step 2: Does the patient have one of the active cardiac conditions? In patients being considered for elective noncardiac surgery, the presence of unstable

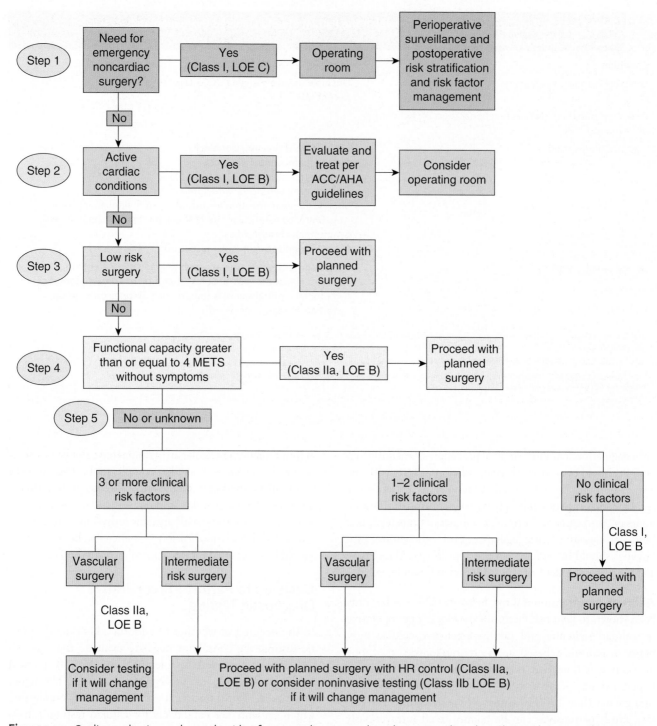

**Figure 14-1.** Cardiac evaluation and care algorithm for noncardiac surgery based on active clinical conditions, known cardiovascular disease, or cardiac risk factors for patients 50 years of age or older. (Reproduced with permission from Fleisher LA et al. *Circulation.* 2007;116:e418–499.)

coronary disease, decompensated heart failure, or severe arrhythmia or valvular heart disease usually leads to cancellation or delay of surgery until the cardiac problem has been clarified and treated appropriately. Examples of unstable coronary syndromes include previous MI with evidence of important ischemic risk by clinical symptoms or noninvasive study, unstable or severe angina, and new or poorly controlled ischemia-mediated heart failure. Depending on the results of the test or interventions and the risk of delaying surgery, it may be appropriate to proceed to the planned surgery with maximal medical therapy.

- Step 3: Is the patient undergoing low risk surgery? In these patients, interventions based on cardiovascular testing in stable patients would rarely result in a change in management, and it would be appropriate to proceed with the planned surgical procedure.
- Step 4: Does the patient have moderate functional capacity without symptoms? In highly functional asymptomatic patients, management will rarely be changed on the basis of results of any further cardiovascular testing and it is therefore appropriate to proceed with the planned surgery. If the patient has poor functional capacity, is symptomatic, or has unknown functional capacity, then the presence of clinical risk factors will determine the need for further evaluation. If the patient has no clinical risk factors, then it is appropriate to proceed with the planned surgery, and no further change in management is indicated.
- Step 5: If the patient has one or two clinical risk factors, then it is reasonable either to proceed with the planned surgery, with heart rate control, or to consider testing, if the outcome of testing could change management. In patients with three or more clinical risk factors or if the patient is undergoing vascular surgery, recent studies suggest that testing should only be considered if its outcome could change management. In nonvascular surgery in which the perioperative morbidity related to the procedures ranges from 1 to 5% (intermediate risk surgery), there are insufficient data to determine the best strategy (proceeding with the planned surgery with tight heart rate control with beta-blockade or further cardiovascular testing if it could change management).

## Tests

An ECG should be performed within 30 days if the patient has stable cardiovascular disease. It is not indicated in low-risk patients undergoing low-risk surgery. However, many anesthesia departments continue to have indications for a preoperative ECG based upon patient age or some other criteria, and a local discussion to determine best practice should be performed.

There are no Class I recommendations for performing a static assessment of ventricular function. It is reasonable to order this for patients with dyspnea of unknown origin or current or prior heart failure with worsening symptoms or other change in clinical status if an assessment has not been performed within 12 months.

Exercise stress testing is rarely a diagnostic benefit for patients with good exercise tolerance. For those who cannot exercise, a pharmacologic stress test is necessary. Stress nuclear perfusion imaging has a high sensitivity for detecting patients at risk for perioperative cardiac events, with the risk being proportional to the amount of myocardium at risk. It has a low positive predictive value, so it is best used in those with high clinical risk for cardiac events. For those with a left bundle branch block, a pharmacological stress test is preferred over an exercise stress test. The optimal test is best left to the discretion of the cardiologist based upon local expertise, although several meta-analyses have suggested that dobutamine stress echocardiography has the best sensitivity and specificity for predicting perioperative cardiovascular complications.

## Permanent Pacemakers and Cardioverter Defibrillators

Electromagnetic interference (EMI) from the widely used unipolar electrocautery during surgery can interfere with permanent pacemakers (PPMs) and automatic implantable cardioverter defibrillators (AICDs). Electrocautery uses radiofrequency current with cut and coagulation. The amount of interference depends on the amount of current near the PPM or AICD. The grounding pad or indifferent plate is usually placed on the thigh away from unit so that the current does not pass through the PPM or AICD.

The ASA 2005 advisory recommends that if EMI will be used during surgery, the PPM should be reprogrammed to an asynchronous mode (VOO or DOO) with the rate-responsive function disabled. The original program should be resumed after surgery. The AICD should have the antitachyarrhythmia function suspended. A magnet may be useful during surgery to disable the unit; however, not all units behave in the same manner with magnet placement, and an electrophysiologist or the manufacturer of the device should be contacted for information. EMI will be decreased significantly with a bipolar unit or harmonic scalpel; thus, the ASA recommends using these devices instead of the unipolar electrocautery if possible. If a unipolar unit must be used, then short, intermittent, and irregular bursts should be employed as far as is possible from the unit and leads. Temporary pacing and defibrillation equipment should also be available. If a patient is pacer-dependent, then the device and battery status should be evaluated within 3 to 6 months before the surgical procedure. The unit may also need a postoperative evaluation to ensure its integrity.

## Medications

There is increasing evidence that patients should continue to take their cardiovascular medications in the perioperative period. Specifically, beta-blockers and statins should be continued throughout the perioperative period. Medications should be taken on the day of surgery, with small sips of water with anticoagulation and aspirin per the surgeon's request. Diuretics, ACEIs, and ARBs may be held on the day of surgery, since the interaction of these agents and anesthetics can lead to profound hypotension.

There has been a great deal of controversy regarding the risks and benefits of administering beta-blockers in the perioperative period for patients not already taking these agents. Multiple studies have demonstrated improved outcome in patients that are given perioperative beta-blockers, especially if heart rate is controlled. However, newer studies have demonstrated that beta-blockers may not be beneficial if heart rate is not well-controlled or in lower risk patients. Recently, the POISE trial was published, in which 8351 high risk beta-blocker-naive patients were randomized to high dose metoprolol CR versus placebo. There was a significant reduction of the primary outcome of cardiovascular events, associated with a 30% reduction in MI rate, but with a significantly increased rate of 30-day all-cause mortality and stroke. The current ACC/AHA Guidelines on perioperative beta-blockade advocate that perioperative beta-blockade is a Class I indication and should be used in patients who had previously been on beta-blockers. In the 2009 update, beta blocked titrated to heart rate and blood pressure are probably recommand in those with a positive stress test undergoing major vascular surgery, although acute administration without titration may be associated with harm. (Class IIa) The use of these agents in those without active CAD or undergoing less invasive procedures is currently being reviewed in light of the POISE results.

The cholesterol lower statins also have antiinflammatory and plaque-stabilizing properties. Therapy should be continued in the perioperative period because of the statins' protective effect on cardiac complications. Durazzo and colleagues published a randomized trial of 200 vascular surgery patients in which statins were started an average of 30 days prior to vascular surgery. A significant reduction in cardiovascular complications was demonstrated using this protocol. Le Manach and colleagues demonstrated that statin withdrawal greater than 4 days was associated with a 2.9 odds ratio of increased risk of cardiac morbidity in vascular surgery. It is reasonable to prescribe statins for those undergoing vascular surgery or those with at least one clinical risk factor and undergoing intermediate risk. Poldermans and colleagues demonstrated reduced perioperative cardiac morbidity with administration of 30 days of preoperative fluvastatin compared to placebo in intermediate risk patients.

Central alpha-2-agonists, such as clonidine, may be useful in those who cannot tolerate beta-blockers. These drugs are associated with better hemodynamic stability, suppress sympathetic stimulation, and also have a sedating effect. There is a reduced mortality in intermediate and vascular surgery and for those with at least one clinical risk factor with clonidine use.

There is not enough evidence to support the use of calcium channel blockers. They do not decrease myocardial ischemia; however, verapamil is associated with a decreased incidence of supraventricular tachycardia.

There is anecdotal evidence that aspirin discontinuation is associated with an increased incidence of perioperative cardiac complications. This has been shown in patients with drug-eluting stents, but may also be true in other patients with high risk coronary lesions. The perioperative of aspirin withdrawal between 7 and 14 days may be associated with hypercoagulability.

## Coronary Revascularization

McFalls and colleagues reported the results of a multicenter randomized trail in the Veterans Administration Health System in which patients with documented coronary artery disease on coronary angiography, excluding those with left main disease or severely depressed ejection fraction (<20%), were randomized to coronary artery bypass grafting (CABG) (59%) or percutaneous coronary interventions (PCI) (41%) versus routine medical therapy. At 2.7 years after randomization, mortality in the revascularization group was not significantly different (22%) percent compared to the no-revascularization group (23%). Within 30 days after the vascular operation a postoperative myocardial infarction, defined by elevated troponin levels, occurred in 12% of the revascularization group and 14% of the no-revascularization group (p = 0.37). The authors suggested that coronary revascularization is not indicated in patients with stable coronary artery disease. However, in a follow-up analysis Ward and colleagues reported improved outcome in the subset that underwent CABG compared to PCI. Additionally, patients with left main disease have a long-term survival benefit from coronary revascularization. Poldermans and colleagues randomized 770 patients having major vascular surgery and considered as having intermediate cardiac risk, defined as the presence of one or two cardiac risk factors, to either undergo further risk stratification with stress imaging or proceed right to surgery. All patients received preoperative bisoprolol with a targeted heart rate (HR) of 60-65 initiated before and continued after surgery. The 30-day incidence of cardiac death and nonfatal MI was similar in both groups (1.8% in the no-testing group versus 2.3% in the tested group). The conclusion of the authors was that further risk stratification in this group of patients considered at intermediate risk based on clinical history alone was unnecessary as long as perioperative beta-blockers were used, and testing only delayed necessary vascular surgery.

The current evidence does not support the use of percutaneous transluminal coronary angioplasty (PTCA) beyond established indications for nonoperative patients, since the incidence of perioperative complications does not appear to be reduced in those patients in whom PTCA was performed less than 90 days prior to surgery. Based upon the prevailing evidence, the indications for CABG and PTCA are identical to those in the nonoperative setting, and simply performing coronary revascularization to "get the patient through surgery" is not indicated. Coronary stent placement may be a unique issue, and several studies suggest that a minimum of 30 days is required before the rate of perioperative complications is low. Several reports suggest that drug-eluting stents may represent an additional risk over a prolonged period (up to 12 months), particularly if antiplatelet agents are discontinued. The new guidelines suggest continuing aspirin therapy in all patients with a coronary stent and discontinuing clopidogrel for as short a time interval as possible for patients with bare-metal stents <30 days or drug-eluting stents <1 year.

# INTRAOPERATIVE MANAGEMENT

## Monitors

Intraoperative monitors are selected to fit the patient disease and surgery. Standard monitors include ECG rhythm (commonly II and V5), noninvasive blood pressure, pulse oximetry, and temperature.

Pulmonary artery catheters (PACs) in major surgery are a point of contention. Per the ASA 2003 practice guidelines, the anesthesiologist should take into account the patient, surgery, and practice setting. PAC placement should not be performed routinely, but is useful in those with an increased risk of hemodynamic disturbances and significant disease, such as cardiac, pulmonary, renal, older age, septic, and trauma. Surgeries with hemodynamic changes, damage to heart, lung, vasculature, kidney, liver, and brain are also important in the consideration of PAC use. One should take into account the level of training of those using the equipment and interpreting the information, and type of equipment available. Adverse effects of PAC placement includes malposition and damaging vessels, bleeding, embolism, pneumothorax, pulmonary infarction, arrhythmias, pulmonary artery hemorrhage, and endocardial damage. Because of the potential complications, using less invasive monitoring is best when possible.

Transesophageal echocardiography (TEE) is of minimal value over standard monitors for routine monitoring for myocardial ischemia. It may be useful in emergencies since it detects wall motion abnormalities before ECG changes are evident and can be very helpful in directing perioperative management. Some anesthesiologists avoid PAC placement and utilize TEE if diagnostic dilemmas develop.

## Blood Pressure and Heart Rate Management

Hypertensive patients tend to have exaggerated intraoperative blood pressure fluctuations and lability. Low blood pressure should be avoided because of the shift of the autoregulation curve of cerebral perfusion in hypertensive patients. **Table 14-3** lists the optimal management of blood pressure, heart rate, and contractility for those with several difference kinds of heart lesions.

## Anesthesia Technique

The type of anesthesia technique should be tailored to the type of surgery and patient and should be left to the discretion of the anesthesiologist. Advantages and disadvantages are listed in **Table 14-4**. General anesthesia is drug-induced amnesia, analgesia, unconsciousness, paralysis, and autonomic system control. The patient is unarousable, even to painful stimuli, and often needs ventilation either with a mask, laryngeal mask airway, or endotracheal tube. Intravenous and/or inhalational agents are used as a balanced anesthetic technique. Most general anesthetic drugs are cardiac depressants.

Inhalational agents in addition to nitrous oxide are used most commonly and include desflurane, isoflurane, and sevoflurane. They depress cardiac output in a concentration-dependent manner by decreasing systemic vascular resistance, preload, afterload, and contractility. There is no increase in myocardial ischemia or infarction with inhalational versus noninhalational techniques. Inhalational agents may possess a protective effect on the myocardium similar to ischemic preconditioning. Propofol, which is a common induction agent and maintenance infusion drug, can decrease heart rate, preload, afterload, and contractility. Opioids can decrease heart rate, preload, and afterload; this is especially the case with opioids that cause histamine release such as morphine.

### Table 14-3 • Optimal Management of Patients with Valve Lesions and Hypertrophic Obstructive Cardiomyopathy (HOCM)

| Lesion | Preload | Afterload | Rate | Rhythm | Contractility | PVR |
|---|---|---|---|---|---|---|
| Mitral stenosis | Normal to high | Normal to high | Low | Sinus rhythm | Normal | Decreased |
| Aortic stenosis | Normal to high | Normal to high | Normal to low | Sinus rhythm | Normal | No difference |
| Mitral regurgitation | Low | Low | High | Sinus rhythm | High | No difference |
| Aortic regurgitation | Low | Low | High | Sinus rhythm | High | No difference |
| HOCM | High | High | Low | Sinus rhythm | Low | No difference |

*PVR, pulmonary vascular resistance*

**Table 14-4 • Advantages and Disadvantages of the Different Anesthetic Techniques in Relation to Cardiovascular Disease**

| Type of Anesthetic Technique | Advantages | Disadvantages |
|---|---|---|
| General anesthesia | • Needed for most major surgeries (e.g., vascular, cardiac)<br>• Amnesia, analgesia, unconsciousness, paralysis, control of autonomic nervous system<br>• Airway protection | • Many drugs cause cardiac depression<br>• Positive pressure ventilation can decrease preload |
| Regional anesthesia: epidural | • May provide better post-operative pain control with epidural catheter (except for labor and delivery, usually use in conjunction with general anesthesia | • Decrease in sympathetic activation may lower blood pressure and slow heart rate<br>• May be patchy and one-sided, causing the need for general anesthesia<br>• Toxicity may cause dysrhythmias, cardiac collapse and seizures |
| Regional anesthesia: spinal | • Quicker onset than epidural anesthesia, will know if it is working right away | • Faster onset and decrease in sympathetic activation may lower blood pressure and slow heart rate quickly<br>• Toxicity may cause dysrhythmias, cardiac collapse and seizures<br>• One-time dose that may wear off before procedure is completed<br>• May get a "total spinal," causing the diaphragm paralysis and loss of the cardiac accelerator fibers |
| Monitored anesthesia care | • Decrease in medication and avoid use of ventilator and positive pressure ventilation | • Limited to minimally invasive and less painful procedures<br>• May not give adequate anesthesia and have sympathetic stimulation<br>• Overdosing anesthesia can cause an emergent need for general anesthetic and airway because loss of airway control |

Regional anesthesia includes peripheral nerve blocks and spinal or regional anesthesia. There are minimal hemodynamic effects with nerve blocks and they may be supplemented with sedation or general anesthesia. Spinal or epidural anesthesia causes a sympathetic blockade with vasodilation, in turn causing a drop in blood pressure and inhibition of the cardiac acceleration fibers slowing the patient's heart rate. Treatment includes pressor support with ephedrine or phenylephrine and intravascular fluid support. High levels above a T4 dermatomal level have the greatest effect on sympathetic stimulation of the heart. Contraindications to epidural and spinal anesthesia include patient refusal, coagulopathy, allergy to the agents used, systemic or local infection, and neurological abnormalities. If there is inadequate nerve blockade, the anesthesiologist may have to convert to a general anesthetic. Epidural catheters are also useful for postoperative pain relief in some abdominal, orthopedic, and thoracic surgeries.

Monitored anesthesia care (MAC) is sedation with local anesthesia. The patient is arousable and spontaneously ventilating. Tachycardia will occur with inadequate local anesthesia. There is also a high incidence of respiratory complications because of sedation without airway protection. Conversion to a general anesthetic is a possibility if the patient is unable to tolerate the procedure under MAC or the patient has received too much medication and is experiencing airway obstruction.

## Other Considerations During Surgery

Normothernia can reduce perioperative morbidity. Preoperative antibiotics are routine before almost all surgeries. Aggressive glucose control may reduce postoperative wound infections and other morbidities, although this remains controversial.

In the absence of randomized trials, current nonrandomized evidence suggests that hemoglobin should be maintained at greater than 9 mg/dL in those with active cardiovascular disease. Fluid overload should be avoided especially in those with a low ejection fraction.

Several randomized trials in patients undergoing noncardiac surgery have not demonstrated that intraoperative prophylactic use of nitroglycerin is associated with a reduced incidence of perioperative myocardial infarction. The decrease in preload associated with nitroglycerin may lead to hypotension, and therefore use of this agent is not recommended prophylactically.

## POSTOPERATIVE MANAGEMENT

Surgery is a stress, but postoperative ECG and cardiac bio markers are unnecessary in low risk patients with low risk surgery. Postoperative troponin levels should be measured in those with ECG changes or chest pain typical of acute coronary syndromes. The levels are not necessarily useful in those with clinically stable disease who have had vascular or intermediate risk surgery.

Postoperative myocardial infarctions are multifactorial in origin. They may be caused by plaque disruption and coronary thrombosis in a critical fixed stenotic area or noncritical stenotic area, as seen with tachycardia and the hypercoagulable postoperative state. The nidus may be associated with an area of noncritical stenosis and may not be detected before surgery. Noncritical stenotic areas do not have collateral coronary flow and a prolonged increase in myocardial oxygen demand may result in ischemia or infarction.

Postoperative arrhythmias may be due to infection, hypotension, metabolic derangements or hypoxia. Premature ventricular contractions are not worrisome if the patient is hemodynamically stable. Magnesium or potassium repletion may be useful.

Pain control is important in avoiding the tachycardia and sympathetic surge after surgery. Pain management should be tailored to the patient and procedure when one is choosing between a patient-controlled analgesia pump versus an epidural catheter.

Blood pressure-lowering agents, especially beta-blockers and clonidine, should be continued postoperatively.

The benefit versus risk of anticoagulation after surgery must be taken into account when a patient develops a postoperative MI. Anticoagulation may be more beneficial for medical management with heart rate and blood pressure control. Left ventricular evaluation, angiography, and the assessment of long term risk should take place during the same hospital stay.

## CONCLUSIONS

- Emergency surgeries should not be delayed for cardiac evaluation.
- Preoperative testing should only be ordered with a purpose and if the results might affect the management of the patient.

- Low risk patients with stable or no heart disease can undergo low risk surgery without further testing or intervention.
- Patients with unstable heart disease should undergo cardiac evaluation and possibly treatment before surgery.
- Aortic stenosis is the highest risk of all valvular lesions.
- Statins, beta-blockers, and clonidine should be continued perioperatively, and aspirin should be continued, unless the risks outweigh the benefits.
- Postoperative pain management is important in order to avoid high sympathetic stimulation.

## Suggested Readings

1. Fleisher LA, Beckman JA, Brown KA, et al. ACC/AHA 2007 guidelines on perioperative cardiovascular evaluation and care for noncardiac surgery: a report of the American College of Cardiology/American Heart Association Task Force on Practice Guidelines (Writing Committee to Revise the 2002 Guidelines on Perioperative Cardiovascular Evaluation for Noncardiac Surgery): developed in collaboration with the American Society of Echocardiography, American Society of Nuclear Cardiology, Heart Rhythm Society, Society of Cardiovascular Anesthesiologists, Society for Cardiovascular Angiography and Interventions, Society for Vascular Medicine and Biology, and Society for Vascular Surgery. *Circulation*, 2007;116:e418–499.

2. Geerts WH, Bergqvist D, Pineo GF, et al. Prevention of venous thromboembolism: American College of Chest Physicians Evidence-Based Clinical Practice Guidelines (8th ed.). *Chest.* 2008;133:381S–453S.

3. Lee TH, Marcantonio ER, Mangione CM, et al. Derivation and prospective validation of a simple index for prediction of cardiac risk of major noncardiac surgery. *Circulation*, 1999;100:1043–1049.

4. Nishimura RA, Carabello BA, Faxon DP, et al. ACC/AHA 2008 guideline update on valvular heart disease: focused update on infective endocarditis: a report of the American College of Cardiology/American Heart Association Task Force on Practice Guidelines: endorsed by the Society of Cardiovascular Anesthesiologists, Society for Cardiovascular Angiography and Interventions, and Society of Thoracic Surgeons. *Circulation.* 2008;118:887–896.

5. Poldermans D, Bax JJ, Boersma E, De Hert S, Eeckhout E, Fowkes G, Gorenek B, Hennerici MG, Lung B, Kelm M, Kjeldsen KP, Kristensen SD, Lopez-Sendon J, Pelosi P, Philippe F, Pierard L, Ponikowski P, Schmid JP, Sellevold OF, Sicari R, Van den Berghe G, Vermassen F, Hoeks SE, Vanhorebeek I. Guidelines for preoperative cardiac risk assessment and perioperative cardiac management in non-cardiac surgery: the Task Force for Preoperative Cardiac Risk Assessment and perioperative cardiac Management in Non-cardiac Surgery of the European Society of Cardiology (ESC) and endorsed by the European Society of Anaesthesiology (ESA). *European heart journal.* 2009;30:2769–2812.

# 15

# Pulmonary Arterial Hypertension

VERONICA FRANCO

## ● PRACTICAL POINTS

- The only method to diagnose pulmonary arterial hypertension is right heart catheterization (mean PAP ≥25 mm Hg and wedge pressure ≤15 mm Hg).

- High right atrial pressure and low cardiac index are associated with worse prognosis.

- Walking <300 minutes during the 6-minute walk test is associated with worse prognosis.

- Epoprostenol is the only medication that has been shown to improve survival in clinical trials.

- Calcium channel blockers are beneficial only in those patients that are responders in a vasodilator study.

## DEFINITION

*Pulmonary arterial hypertension* (PAH) is defined as a mean pulmonary artery pressure (mPAP) >25 mm Hg, in the setting of normal pulmonary capillary wedge pressure (PW ≤ 15 mm Hg) (**Figure 15-1** and **15-2**). The *pulmonary vascular resistance* (PVR) is not require for the diagnosis but is monitor during follow-up and is obtained by the following equation:

$$PVR = \frac{\text{pulmonary artery pressure} - \text{pulmonary venous pressure}}{\text{cardiac output}}.$$

The criterion of pulmonary hypertension (PH) when detected by Doppler echocardiography is a right ventricular systolic pressure (RVSP) >40 mm Hg or a resting tricuspid regurgitant velocity of 2.8-3.4 m/s. However, the echocardiographic criterion is not precisely defined, as careful

### Cardiac catheterization to assess severity and prognosis of PAH

- To measure wedge pressure or LVEDP:
  - Scrutinize wedge tracings!
  - Wedge saturation; end expiration
- To exclude or evaluate CHD
- To establish severity and prognosis
- To test vasodilator therapy

### Catheterization is required for every patient with suspected pulmonary HTN.

LVEDP = left ventricular end diastolic pressure.

**Figure 15-1.** Cardiac catheterization to assess diagnosis and severity of PAH.

Doppler examination by experienced sonographers yields quantifiable tricuspid regurgitant signals in only 74% of cases, and the estimation of PH is dependent on an estimated value from jugular venous distention. Further, an RVSP > 40 mm Hg per echocardiogram is present in 6% of otherwise normal individuals older than 50 years and 5% of people with body mass index (BMI) >30 kg/m². Therefore, *right heart catheterization is required to confirm a diagnosis of pulmonary arterial hypertension*.

### Diagnosis PAH

- Mean pulmonary artery   ≥25 mm Hg (rest)
    ≥30 mm Hg (exercise).
- **Wedge pressure, LVEDP, LAP ≤15 mm Hg**

**Figure 15-2.** Diagnosis of PAH.

# CLASSIFICATION

## Pulmonary Arterial Hypertension

The nomenclature and classification of PH was revised in 2009 by the World Health Organization (**Table 15-1**). Idiopathic PAH is now used, instead of primary PH. The classification is easy to remember if one thinks of PH as a "disease of triggers." In either idiopathic or familial PAH, the trigger is a mutation or polymorphism. In PAH associated with connective tissue disease, congenital disease, HIV, anorexigens, or portal hypertension, the trigger is permissive phenotype. This also helps one differentiate PAH from non-PAH etiologies (**Figure 15-3**).

| Table 15-1 • WHO Classification of Pulmonary Hypertension |
|---|
| **Pulmonary arterial hypertension** |
| Idiopathic<br>Heritable<br>Drug- and toxin-induced<br>Associated with:<br>    Collagen vascular disease<br>    Congenital systemic-to-pulmonary shunts<br>    HIV infection<br>    Schistosomiasis<br>    Chronic hemolytic anemia<br>Persistent pulmonary hypertension of the newborn<br>Pulmonary veno-occlusive disease and pulmonary capillary<br>    hemangiomatosis |
| **Pulmonary hypertension with left heart disease** |
| Heart Failure (systolic or diastolic)<br>Valvular heart disease |
| **Pulmonary hypertension associated with lung disease and/or hypoxemia** |
| Chronic obstructive pulmonary disease<br>Interstitial lung disease<br>Sleep-disordered breathing<br>Alveolar hypoventilation disorder<br>Chronic exposure to high altitude<br>Developmental abnormalities |
| **Pulmonary hypertension due to chronic thromboembolic disease** |
| **Pulmonary hypertension with unclear multifactorial mechanisms** |
| Hematologic disorders: myeloproliferative disorders,<br>    splenectomy<br>Systemic disorders: sarcoidosis, pulmonary Langerhans<br>    cell histiocytosis: lymphangioleiomyomatosis,<br>    neurofibromatosis, vasculitis<br>Metabolic disorders: glycogen storage disease, Gaucher<br>    disease, thyroid disorders<br>Others: tumoral obstruction, fibrosing mediastinitis,<br>    chronic renal failure on dialysis |

### Non-PAH pulmonary hypertension

- Pulmonary hypertension (PH) with left heart disease – **WHO Class 2** *Trigger: High LA Pressure*

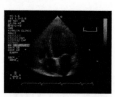

- PH with lung disease/hypoxemia – **WHO Class 3** *Trigger: Hypoxemia and Parenchyma Distortion*

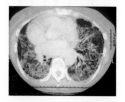

- PH due to chronic thrombotic and/or embolic disease – **WHO Class 4** *Trigger: Obstruction*

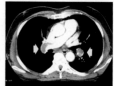

**Figure 15-3.** Non-PAH pulmonary hypertension.

### Idiopathic

Idiopathic PAH has an undetermined cause. It is a rare disease, with a prevalence <0.2%. It is more common in women, predominantly of child-bearing age. The mean age at onset is 35 years old. The natural course of this disease is of inevitable progression toward death. Studies have shown that among patients that do not undergo lung transplantation or treatment with specific PAH medications, survival is 68-77% at 1 year, and 22-38% at 5 years. One of the most important determinants of survival is functional capacity and the most common cause of death is right ventricular failure.

### Familial (Genetic)

Families with PAH exhibit a pattern of autosomal dominant inheritance. The mutation has been found on the chromosome 2q31-32, which codes for bone morphogenetic protein receptor 2 (BMPR2), a member of the TGF-β family.

Expression of this mutation is quite variable and incomplete. Siblings or children of familial PAH patients have a risk of 50% of inheriting the gene; with an overall penetrance of only 20%, therefore, their risk of actually acquiring the disease is 10%.

Females are more commonly affected and the disease has a tendency to develop at earlier ages in subsequent generations (genetic anticipation). The natural history of familial PAH is identical to that of idiopathic PAH, including response to treatment. Mutations of the BMPR2 gene have been reported in PAH associated with fenfluramine derivates, suggesting that some individuals have the genetic substrate but the disease does not develop until they are exposed to triggers such as diet pills.

### Associated with Collagen Vascular Disease

PAH has been associated with all of the connective tissue diseases, and if it develops, it is the most common cause of death in individuals so afflicted. It is most common and severe in patients with limited scleroderma (CREST) and presents in up to 60% of the population. Systemic scleroderma patients have a 16-33% risk of developing PAH, usually not isolated but in association with the antinuclear antibody anti-U3-RNP. PAH is less frequently observed in patients with systemic lupus erythamatosus (4-14%), rheumatoid arthritis (up to 21% but mild), or polymyositis. Anticardiolipin antibodies are associated with PAH in up to 68% of patients with lupus. Importantly, 40% of patients with idiopathic PAH and no other signs of connective tissue disease have positive antinuclear antibodies. Treatment for PAH associated with connective tissue disease is that of idiopathic PAH, although their prognosis is not as good.

### Associated with Congenital Heart Disease

The severity of the intracardiac defect is the major determinant of development of pulmonary arterial hypertension. Eisenmenger syndrome refers to left-to-right shunts that lead to PAH and as a consequence reverse the shunt from right-to-left. Patients with ventricular septal defects develop PAH more frequently than those with atrial septal defects. The likelihood of developing PAH is correlated with the severity and site of the defect. Rarely, PAH develops after the defect is corrected, although some have proposed that atrial septal defect is a trigger for PAH, which could develop even after the defect has been closed.

### Other Associations

Appetite suppressants and stimulants, like amphetamines, have been linked to pulmonary arterial hypertension. Dexfenfluramine increases the risk of developing PAH by 20 times if taken for more than 3 months. Twenty percent of patients with portal hypertension due to liver disease develop PAH, usually discovered when they undergo liver transplant evaluation. The mortality after liver transplantation increases if mPAP > 35 mm Hg and in some centers is considered a contraindication for transplantation. A minority of patients with HIV develops PAH (0.5%), and screening for HIV infection is done routinely for new patients with elevated pulmonary pressures. Schistosomiasis and hemolytic anemias are now considered associated causes of PAH.

### Pulmonary Venous Hypertension (Associated with Left Heart Disease)

Left heart disease, including congestive heart failure, valvular abnormalities, pericardial disease, and left atrium disorders, raise pulmonary venous pressures leading to an elevated pulmonary artery pressure. Initially, left heart disease produces elevated filling pressures but the transpulmonary gradient remains normal. However, chronically

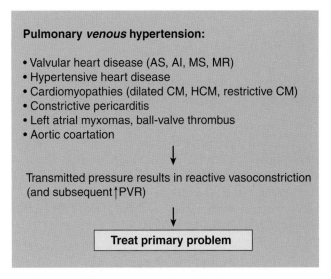

**Figure 15-4.** Pulmonary venous hypertension.

elevated wedge pressure leads to arterial remodeling and results in a high transpulmonary gradient due to high PVR. In the current cardiovascular clinical practice, this is the most common form of PH and must be excluded with cardiac imaging and hemodynamic measurements in patients with suspected PAH (**Figure 15-4**). Specific PAH medications are not indicated in this patient population, and if used they produce further increase of the wedge pressure and could precipitate episodes of pulmonary edema.

## Pulmonary Hypertension Associated with Hypoxemia

Pulmonary diseases must be excluded as well in the evaluation of patients with PH (**Figure 15-5**). Chronic hypoxia produces mild to moderate elevations of pulmonary pressures, and usually mPAP is <35 mm Hg. Pulmonary function

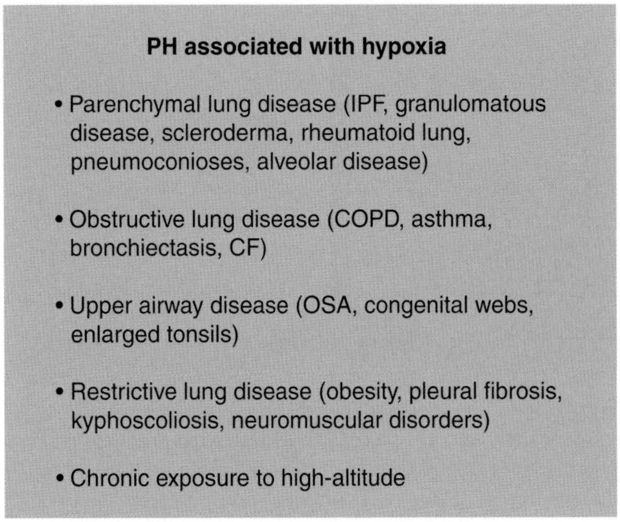

**PH associated with hypoxia**

- Parenchymal lung disease (IPF, granulomatous disease, scleroderma, rheumatoid lung, pneumoconioses, alveolar disease)

- Obstructive lung disease (COPD, asthma, bronchiectasis, CF)

- Upper airway disease (OSA, congenital webs, enlarged tonsils)

- Restrictive lung disease (obesity, pleural fibrosis, kyphoscoliosis, neuromuscular disorders)

- Chronic exposure to high-altitude

**Figure 15-5.** Pulmonary hypertension associated with hypoxia.

tests and exclusion of interstitial lung disease and sleep disorders are part of the diagnostic evaluation in patients with suspected pulmonary arterial hypertension.

## Pulmonary Hypertension Associated with Chronic Thromboembolic Disease

Up to 4% of survivors of acute pulmonary embolism will develop PH within 2 years. Importantly, patients with chronic thromboembolic PH (CTEPH) usually do not recall an acute event. A ventilatory perfusion scan should be part of every evaluation in patients with PH, even in the absence of history of pulmonary embolism, as proximal CTEPH could be cure with surgical intervention.

## PATHOPHYSIOLOGY OF PAH

This disease is believed to be a result of "two hits": an underlying susceptibility for PAH (i.e., BMPR2 mutation) and an associated risk factor (i.e., HIV, cirrhosis, anorexic drugs). Pulmonary vasoconstriction is the earliest component of the process, promoted by overexpression of vasoconstrictors, such as endothelin (ET)-1 and reduced production of vasodilators, such as nitric oxide (NO) and prostacyclin (**Figure 15-6**). There is endothelial dysfunction and over time, vasoconstriction leads to vascular remodeling and loss of vasodilator responsiveness (**Figure 15-7**).

The plexiform lesion is a focal proliferation typical of idiopathic pulmonary arterial hypertension. It may be found also in other disorders associated with PAH, as HIV and portopulmonary hypertension. Thickening of medial and adventitial layers and proliferation of endothelial cells within the intima characterize the plexiform lesion. This

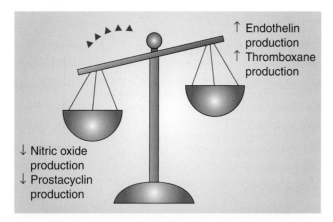

**Figure 15-6.** Pathophysiology of PAH. Dysfunctional pulmonary artery endothelial cells have decreased production of prostacyclin and endogenous nitric oxide, with an increased production of endothelin-1— a condition promoting vasoconstriction and proliferation of smooth-muscle cells. (Adapted from Gaine S. *J Am Med Assoc.* 2000;284:3160–3168.)

results in obliteration of the pulmonary arteriole and is also associated with in situ thrombosis of the narrowed vascular channels. The plexiform lesions of idiopathic PAH have been reported to be monoclonal in origin and express vascular endothelial growth factor (VEGF), and they are thought to represent a neoplastic-like disordered angiogenesis.

## ASSESSMENT OF THE PATIENT WITH SUSPECTED PH

### Prevention

#### Genetic Screening
Screening for mutations in BMPR2 screening is available, though such screening must be accompanied by full counseling. Screening is recommended in patients without other identifiable PAH-associated diseases (e.g. idiopathic and heritable PAH).

#### Echocardiogram for High Risk Populations
Echocardiogram (ECG) screening is recommended for those with known genetic defect, first degree relatives in familial PAH, connective tissue disease, liver transplant candidates and known intracardiac shunts. Patients that abuse amphetamine derivates are at a higher risk and should be encouraged to avoid known toxins. Echocardiographic screening is not recommended in these cases.

### Treat Underlying Cause

Identification and treatment of contributing factors can have an important effect on symptoms; these factors include supplemental oxygen for hypoxemia, continuous positive airway pressure therapy for sleep apnea, anticoagulation and possible thromboendarterectomy for pulmonary embolism. Importantly, the adequate recognition of type of PH will prevent potentially lethal complications. Indeed, the use of epoprostenol therapy in patients with prominent pulmonary vein involvement, such as pulmonary veno-occlusive disease, pulmonary capillary hemangiomatosis, or left-side heart disease, can be harmful as severe pulmonary edema and death may occur, presumably because of increased pulmonary perfusion in the presence of downstream vascular obstruction.

### Detection

Exertional dyspnea is present in 99% of patients at the time of initial diagnosis. Angina is reported in 40% of patients and syncope may develop in 30% of them. Signs of PH include: loud P2, right ventricular (RV) lift, tricuspid regurgitation (systolic) murmur, pulmonary regurgitation (diastolic) murmur, and RV S4. Signs that are suggestive of RV failure are JVD with V waves, RV S3, hepatomegaly or pulsatile liver, edema, and ascites. The typical chest x-ray

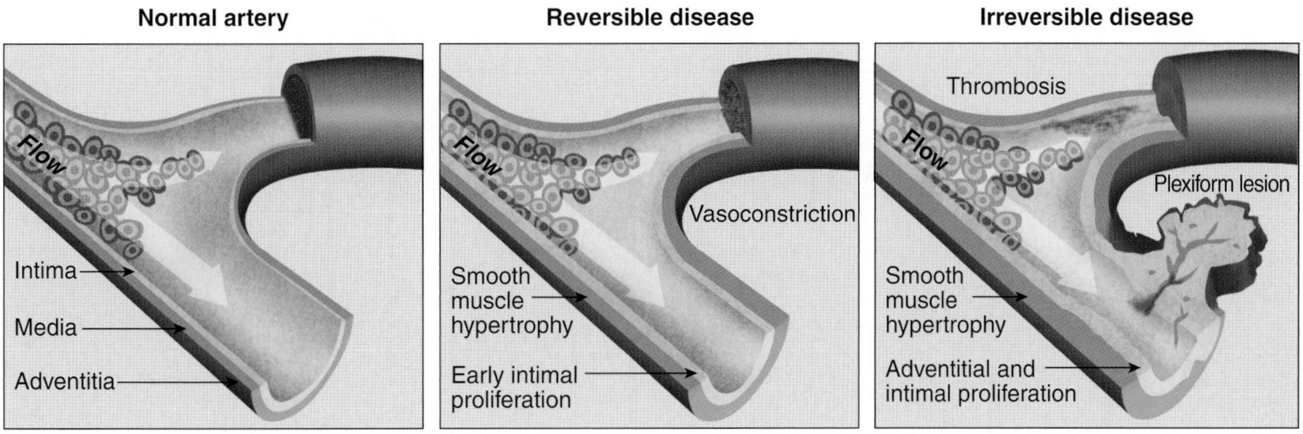

**Normal artery**          **Reversible disease**          **Irreversible disease**

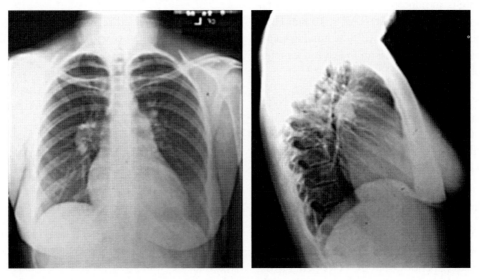

**Figure 15-7.** Stages in the development of pulmonary arterial hypertension.

shows peripheral pruning, dilated hilar pulmonary arteries and RV enlargement, particularly noted in the lateral x-ray, where it occupies the retrosternal area (**Figure 15-8**). The typical ECG has signs of RV enlargement and strain, right axis deviation , and P pulmonale (**Figure 15-9**).

## Diagnosis

Initial evaluation should be oriented to confirm the diagnosis, identify the underlying cause and/or associated disease, determine the prognosis, and identify the most appropriate therapy (**Figure 15-10**). Echocardiogram is a good and initial screening test, as it can estimate systolic pulmonary arterial pressure. Importantly, systolic pressure is extrapolated from RVSP only in the absence of pulmonary stenosis. The right atrial pressure (RAP) can either be a standardized value (10 mm Hg), or it can be estimated from characteristics of the inferior vena cava ultrasound or from degree of JVD:

$$RVSP = 4 \, [TR \text{ velocity}]^2 + RAP.$$

Pulmonary arterial pressure estimated by ECG is an observation but does not represent a diagnosis of pulmonary arterial hypertension. A right heart catheterization is mandatory to confirm the diagnosis of PAH (see **Figure 15-1**). Important hemodynamic measurements that should be obtained are pulmonary wedge pressure, cardiac output, and pulmonary vascular resistance. Cardiac output usually is calculated by Fick method (using pulmonary artery saturation) because significant TR may alter the result using thermodilution method. Intracardiac shunting should be ruled out by measuring SVC, IVC, PA and occasionally pulmonary vein saturations.

A vasodilatory study is performed routinely after confirmation of PAH, typically with inhaled nitric oxide or intravenous epoprostenol. A decrease in mPAP ≥ 10 mm Hg to mPAP ≤ 40 mm Hg, with a preserved cardiac output, is determined

**Figure 15-8.** Chest x-ray in PAH. Evidence of RV enlargement (retrosternal area), prominent hilar pulmonary arteries and peripheral pruning.

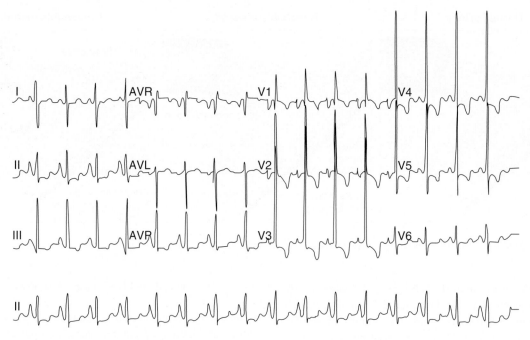

**Figure 15-9.** ECG in pulmonary arterial hypertension. Evidence of RV hypertrophy and strain, P pulmonale, and right axis deviation.

as a "responder" and only those patients who present with this may benefit from the use of calcium channel blocker treatment. The abrupt development of pulmonary edema or rise in wedge pressure during vasodilatory testing suggests pulmonary venopathy or microvasculopathy and is a contraindication to specific PAH vasodilator therapy.

## PROGNOSTIC FACTORS IN PAH

### Hemodynamic Measurements

Right atrial pressure is an important prognosticator as it reflects decompensated RV failure. An RAP < 10 mm Hg is associated with better survival; an RAP > 20 mm Hg points to median survival of 1 month and is an indication for referral to lung transplantation.

A cardiac index $\geq 4$ L/m$^2$/min is associated with a better outcome, while a cardiac index <2 L/m$^2$/min with a median survival of 17 months. Mean PAP is also important, and those with mPAP $\geq$ 85 mm Hg have a median survival of 12 months (**Figure 15-11**).

### Six-Minute Walk Test

The Six-Minute Walk Test (6MWT), in which the patient walks as far as possible in 6 minutes, is a simple, safe, and highly reproducible tool performed in the outpatient setting for the assessment of exercise capacity. Patients who walk <332 meters have significantly lower survival rate than those who walk farther, and is an independent predictor of mortality in PAH patients. Oxygen desaturation >10% during the 6MWT increases mortality risk by a factor of 3 over a median in a follow-up of 26 months.

Observations from cardiopulmonary exercise testing indicate that the mechanisms of exercise limitations in PAH include V/Q mismatching, lactic acidosis at a low work rate, arterial hypoxemia, and inability to adequately increase stroke volume and cardiac output.

### Functional Capacity

There is a linear correlation between functional capacity and 6MWT. Patients with WHO class I-II have a median survival of 59 months, WHO class III of 32 months, and WHO class IV is associated with very poor prognosis and median survival of only 6 months. The WHO classification uses similar parameters as the NYHA functional classification for heart failure patients.

## TREATMENT OF PAH

### General Measures

The guidelines recommend low-graded aerobic exercise to avoid exertional syncope. Avoidance of exposure to high altitudes is warranted because such exposure may produce hypoxic pulmonary vasoconstriction; the use of oxygen on commercial aircraft is recommended. Other medications that

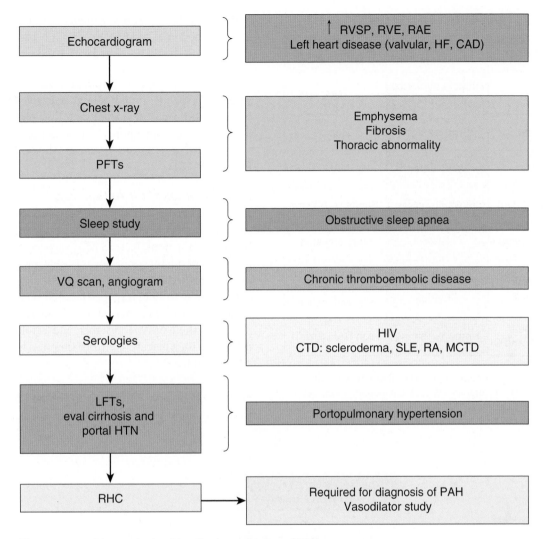

**Figure 15-10.** Diagnostic algorithm for the evaluation of PAH.

produce vasoconstriction, like sinus or cold therapies, should be avoided. Patients are advised to follow a low salt diet to prevent RV failure, and to lose weight if needed. Immunizations against influenza and pneumocco are recommended.

The hemodynamic fluctuations of pregnancy, labor, and delivery are potentially life-threatening in PAH, resulting in 30-50% mortality rate. Most experts recommend that pregnancy should be avoided or terminated early in women with severe pulmonary arterial hypertension. The ideal type of contraceptive is controversial. Finally, the risk of elective surgery should be carefully examined, as patients with PAH are prone to vasovagal events, hemodynamic fluctuations and ventilatory compromise, which could increase mortality.

## Pharmacological Treatment

### Conventional Therapy

Oxygen supplementation is suggested in patients with hypoxemia to maintain $O_2$ saturation $\geq 90\%$, to prevent pulmonary

vasoconstriction. Diuretics are indicated for the treatment of RV failure and volume overload, with close monitoring of electrolytes and renal function. Digoxin has not been studied extensively in patients with RV dysfunction, but it is generally recommended in RV failure or low cardiac output.

Idiopathic PAH is a prothrombotic state, and oral anticoagulation has proven to improved survival. The target international normalized ratio (INR) varies from center to center, but generally it is 1.5-2.5. Anticoagulation is controversial in associated conditions, like portopulmonary hypertension and congenital or collagen vascular disease, as the risk of bleeding may be higher (**Figure 15-12**).

### Calcium Channel Blockers

Only 6% of patients with PAH respond to calcium channel blockers (CCBs). Patients with a positive vasodilator study are considered responders to CCBs. This test is performed with inhaled nitric oxide, IV epoprostenol or IV adenosine. Positive studies are those where the final mPAP is at least

**PAH determinants of risk**

| Lower risk | Determinants of risk | Higher risk |
|---|---|---|
| No | Clinical evidence of RV failure | Yes |
| Gradual | Progression | Rapid |
| II, III | WHO class | IV |
| Longer (>400 m) | 6MW distance | Shorter (<300 m) |
| Minimally elevated | BNP | Very elevated |
| Minimal RV dysfunction | Echocardiographic findings | Pericardial effusion, significant RV dysfunction |
| Normal/near normal RAP and CI | Hemodynamics | High RAP, low CI |

**Figure 15-11.** Risk assessment in PAH. (Reproduced with permission from McLaughlin VV, et al. *Circulation*. 2006;114: 1417–1431.)

= < 40 mm Hg and there is a difference of at least 10 mm Hg between the initial and final mPAP. Only patients that meet this criterion should be treated with CCBs.

Long-acting nifedipine, diltiazem, or amlodipine are suggested. Verapamil should be avoided, given its potential negative inotropic effects. Close follow-up is crucial, and if a patient has not improved to functional capacity I-II with CCBs, alternative therapies should be used (see **Figure 15-12**).

### Endothelin Receptor Antagonists

There are two endothelin (ET) receptor antagonists approved for treatment of PAH: *bosentan* and *ambrisentan*. Bosentan is a nonselective ET receptor antagonist with potent vasodilator and antimitogen properties, taken twice a day. Ambrisentan is a selective type A receptor antagonist, with similar properties, that is taken once a day (**Figure 15-13**). Patients taking ET receptor antagonists improved their 6MWT distance and cardiac index, over those who took placebo controls; they also had lower PVR, mPAP, and RAP.

Side effects include volume retention and hepatotoxicity (more common with bosentan than with ambrisentan).

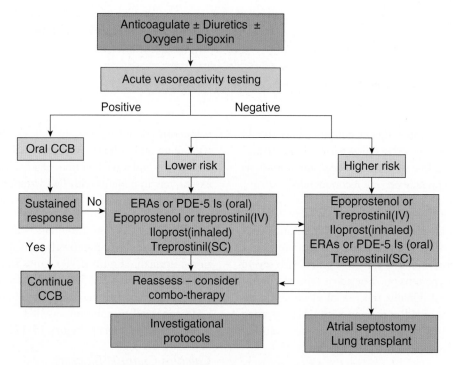

**Figure 15-12.** Algorithm for the medical treatment of PAH. Patients at highest risk, based on clinical assessment, should be considered for intravenous therapy as first-line therapy. Patients at lower risk are candidates for oral therapy. Patients should be followed up closely, and response to therapy should be assessed within several months. If treatment goals are not met, consider addition of a second agent. (Reproduced with permission from McLaughlin VV, et al. *Circulation*. 2006;114:1417–1431.)

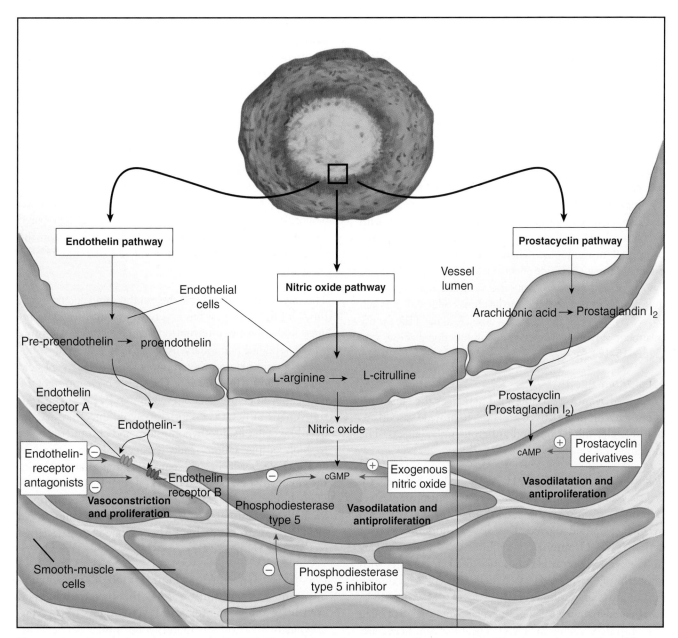

**Figure 15-13.** Targets for current therapies in PAH. Three major pathways involved in abnormal proliferation and contraction of the smooth-muscle cells of the pulmonary artery in patients with pulmonary arterial hypertension are shown. These pathways correspond to important therapeutic targets in this condition: endothelin-receptor antagonists, phosphodiesterase type 5 inhibitors, and prostacyclin derivatives. (Reproduced with permission from Humbert M et al. Treatment of pulmonary arterial hypertension. *N Engl J Med.* 2004;351:1425–1436. Copyright © 2004 Massachusetts Medical Society. All rights reserved.)

Bosentan exhibits a dose-dependent reversible risk of elevated transaminases. Liver function tests are required at least monthly in patients receiving bosentan and ambrisentan. A monthly pregnancy test is recommended for those at risk. The drugs may also be associated with mild anemia and have potential teratogenic effects. Importantly, these medications decrease the efficacy of hormonal contraceptives, and for this reason such contraceptives should not be used without a nonbarrier or permanent surgical method.

Long-term benefits of bosentan were demonstrated in a retrospective analysis and suggest a survival benefit with this medication. Overall survival estimates were 87%; incidences of event-free status (survival without transplantation, prostanoid initiation, or hospitalizations for right heart failure) were 61 and 44% at 1 and 2 years, respectively. In addition, estimates of survival in the patients with idiopathic PAH treated initially with bosentan were not inferior to a matched historical cohort of patients treated with intravenous epoprostenol.

The ACCP and European Guidelines recommend ET receptor antagonist therapy in low risk, functional class II-IV patients with idiopathic PAH or PAH related to collagen vascular disease without significant interstitial lung disease (see **Figure 15-12**).

### Phosphodiesterase Inhibitors

Phosphodiesterase (PDE)-5 inhibitors selectively inhibit the degradation of cGMP and augment the vascular response to endogenous or inhaled nitric oxide (NO) in PH (see **Figure 15-13**). Sildenafil, a highly specific PDE-5 inhibitor, improves exercise capacity, functional capacity, 6MWT and hemodynamics in patients, functional class I-IV, with idiopathic PAH or PAH secondary to collagen or repaired congenital heart disease. There is no mortality data with Sildenafil therapy. Its side effects include headache, flushing, dyspepsia, and epistaxis. Importantly, there is a significant drug interaction with HIV medications. Sildenafil was approved by the FDA in 2005, at a dose of 20 mg TID, for the treatment of patients with PAH of all functional classes (see **Figure 15-12**).

### Prostanoid Agonists

Prostanoid agonist use is intended to replace the deficiency of prostacyclin in patients with PAH, to provide vasodilatation, platelet inhibition, and antiproliferative effects. The mechanism is via the cyclic AMP pathway.

*Iloprost* Patients with PAH have reduced levels of prostacyclin, a potent vasodilator and antiproliferative. Iloprost is a prostacyclin analog that can be delivered by an aerosolized device. Due to its short duration of action of 20-25 minutes, it requires 6-9 inhalations/day to achieve long-term benefits. It is used in patients with idiopathic PAH or PAH associated with collagen disease and improves functional class ≥1 level, 6MWT ≥ 10%, and hemodynamic variables. Survival benefit has not been demonstrated. Common side effects are cough, headache, flushing, and jaw pain. The main limitation with this medication is the frequency of inhalations. Iloprost is recommended for functional class III-IV PAH patients (see **Figure 15-12**).

*Trepostinil* Treprostinil is a prostacyclin analog with a half-life of 4 hours, available for continuous subcutaneous or intravenous use. Like epoprostenol, it improves symptoms and, modestly, hemodynamics, but a definite survival benefit has not been compellingly demonstrated. Intravenous use is preferred, particularly as this drug is stable at room temperature, unlike epoprostenol.

Adverse effects include headache, diarrhea, flushing, jaw pain, and foot pain, as with epoprostenol. Because of the longer half-life of this drug, interruptions of trepostinil due to dislodgment of the catheter or pump malfunction tend to be less serious than with epoprotenol. Subcutaneous use's main limitation is pain and erythema at the site of infusion, reported as high as 85%; therefore, it is not used frequently in current practice. Intravenous trepostinil is recommended for high risk patients, particularly those with functional class IV or syncope (see **Figure 15-12**).

*Epoprostenol* Intravenous epoprostenol was the first medication that showed improvement in survival, functional capacity, 6MWT, and hemodynamics in patients with idiopathic pulmonary arterial hypertension. Importantly, long-term benefit and improved survival has been demonstrated with intravenous epoprostenol compared to historical controls and predicted survival based on the NIH equation, with 85-88% survival at 1 year and 55-56% survival at 5 years.

The important limitation is the cumbersome epoprostenol infusion. Epoprostenol has a very short half-life, <6 minutes, and infusion interruptions can be life-threatening, due to rebound pulmonary hypertension. The drug is unstable at acid pH and room temperature, is best kept cold prior and during the infusion. The sterile preparation of the medication, operation of the pump, and care of the central venous catheter is essential to avoid infections. Acute overdose could lead to hypotension, and chronic overdose to high output failure. Side effects are dose-dependant and include headache, jaw pain, flushing, diarrhea, rash, thrombocytopenia, musculoskeletal pain, and catheter-related infections or thrombosis. Epoprostenol is approved for high risk patients, particularly those with functional class III-IV, with idiopathic PAH or related to scleroderma (see **Figure 15-12**).

Due to the complexity of administration of epoprostenol, intravenous treprostinil is now the preferred method used in severely symptomatic PAH patients. Acute improvement in PVR was found to be similar between intravenous treprostinil and epoprostenol, and successful transition from epoprostenol to treprostinil has been demonstrated.

## Surgical Treatment

Atrial septostomy is used as a palliative measure or as a bridge to lung transplantation in selected patients with refractory RV failure or syncope/near syncope despite appropriate medical therapy. Mortality up to 13% has been reported secondary to this procedure, and it should be performed only at institutions with significant experience.

Referral for lung transplantation is generally reserved for those failing the best available therapy, but factoring into account the time needed to complete a transplant evaluation and time spent on the list of those awaiting suitable organs is important, as death while awaiting transplantation is high in patients with poor functional capacity. Survival in patients with PAH who undergo lung transplantation is 70% at 1 year, 40% at 5 years, and 25% at 10 years. Most centers prefer double lung transplantation. Combined heart/lung transplant is preferred in patients with complex congenital disease.

## Treatment Algorithm

Current treatment algorithms for PAH recommend oral medications as a first line treatment for PAH patients with low risk features, i.e., functional class II and III, whereas intravenous prostacyclins should be reserved for patients with high risk features, functional class IV, 6MWT < 300 m, high RAP, low cardiac output, and significant RV dysfunction (see **Figure 15-12**). Constant surveillance and reassessment of risk are very important during evaluation of response to therapy or need for combination treatment. If goals of therapy have not been met after 43-44 months of therapy, combination therapy should be considered (**Figure 15-14**). Combination therapy is necessary in almost 50% of patients to achieve these goals.

**Goals of therapy**
- **Improve symptoms**
  - 6-minute walk (>380 m)
  - functional class (I or II)
  - CPET ($VO_2$ max >10.4)
  - quality of life
- **Improve hemodynamics**
- **Improve survival**

**FIGURE 15-14.** Goals of therapy in PAH.

## Suggested Readings

1. Badesch D, Abman SH, Ahearn GS, et al. Medical treatment for pulmonary arterial hypertension. ACCP evidence-based clinical practice guidelines. *Chest.* 2004;126:35S-62S.

2. McLaughlin VV, McGoon MD. Pulmonary arterial hypertension. *Circulation.* 2006;114:1417–1431.

3. Advances in pulmonary hypertension. Available from: http://www.phaonlineuniv.org/Journal/Vol8No2Summer09. Accessed 6/10/10.

4. Simonneau G, Robbins IM, Beghetti M. Updated Clinical Classification of Pulmonary Hypertension. *J Am Coll Cardiol.* 2009;54:43–54.

# 16

# Sleep Apnea and Heart Disease

Sanja Jelic and Thierry H. Le Jemtel

## ● PRACTICAL POINTS

- Sleep apnea is an independent risk factor for cardio-vascular diseases.

- Sleep apnea is highly prevalent in cardiac patients but frequently remains unrecognized and untreated.

- Patients with obstructive sleep apnea are 2.2 times more likely to develop heart failure.

- Prompt recognition and treatment of sleep apnea lowers morbidity and may improve the life expectancy of patients with cardiovascular diseases.

- Routine implementation of CPAP as a standard of care for patients with heart failure and central sleep apnea cannot be recommended at present.

## INTRODUCTION

Sleep apnea, commonly referred to as sleep disordered breathing (SDB) may be due to repetitive collapse of the upper airway during sleep resulting in transient cessation of breathing as occurs in obstructive sleep apnea (OSA) or to alternation of diminished ventilatory drive and compensatory hyperventilation despite patent airway as occurs in central sleep apnea (CSA). Both OSA and CSA are associated with increased cardiovascular morbidity and possibly mortality (**Table 16-1**). The association between OSA and cardiovascular diseases will be reviewed first. The implications

and treatment of CSA in patients with chronic heart failure (CHF) will then be discussed.

## OBSTRUCTIVE SLEEP APNEA AND CARDIOVASCULAR DISEASES

Obstructive sleep apnea is a highly prevalent disorder that exerts a huge financial burden on society and negatively affects overall morbidity and possibly mortality. OSA is characterized by repetitive episodes of cessation of breathing called apnea and hypopnea, followed by arousals from

| Table 16-1 • Two Forms of Sleep Apnea | | |
|---|---|---|
| | **Obstructive Sleep Apnea (OSA)** | **Central Sleep Apnea (CSA)** |
| **Mechanism** | Collapse of upper airway during sleep | Oscillations in ventilatory drive |
| **Clinical Implications** | Risk factor for cardiovascular diseases | Consequence of heart failure or stroke |
| **Treatment** | CPAP* (rarely surgery) | Rx** of underlying disease and possibly CPAP |

CPAP* = continuous positive airway pressure
Rx** = treatment

sleep. Although increased incidence of OSA parallels the increasing prevalence of obesity in Western society, OSA remains largely unrecognized and untreated. Prevalence of previously unrecognized OSA exceeds 60% in subjects with BMI >30. A likely explanation for the low rate of OSA recognition is that only a minority of OSA patients experience daytime symptoms such as excessive sleepiness. While 5% or less of adults in Western countries report daytime sleepiness and experience episodes of apnea and hypopnea during sleep, up to 28% adults suffer from OSA as defined by more than 5 episodes of apnea and/or hypopnea per hour of sleep. Untreated OSA is associated with adverse health outcomes regardless of the presence of daytime sleepiness and, consequently, the true prevalence of OSA can only be determined by polysomnography documenting the presence of abnormal breathing during sleep. Utilization of health-care resources and economic cost are 50% greater among untreated OSA patients compared with age-matched subjects. When effective, treatment of OSA considerably lowers the cost of caring for patients with OSA. A major reason for the negative impact of OSA on morbidity and possibly mortality is the high prevalence of cardiovascular diseases in patients with OSA. OSA is clearly an independent risk factor for developing hypertension, myocardial ischemia, and stroke.

### Definition of Obstructive Apnea and Hypopnea

Obstructive apnea is defined by cessation of upper airway flow for at least 10 seconds despite continued respiratory effort. Obstructive hypopnea is defined by discrete airflow reduction for at least 10 seconds that results in decreased oxyhemoglobin saturation ≥4% despite the presence of thoracoabdominal ventilatory efforts. Electroencephalography (EEG) arousal is defined by an abrupt and discrete change in EEG frequency, with or without increased electromyography (EMG) activity. Apnea plus hypopnea index (AHI) is defined as the number of obstructive apnea plus hypopnea episodes per hour of sleep.

### Determining the Severity of Obstructive Sleep Apnea

The severity of OSA is assessed by the AHI as follows:
- normal = AHI <5 per hour of sleep,
- mild OSA = AHI 5-14 per hour of sleep,
- moderate OSA = AHI 15-29 per hour of sleep,
- severe OSA = AHI ≥30 per hour of sleep.

### Importance of Diagnosing and Treating OSA in Patients with Cardiovascular Conditions

Obesity is a frequent comorbid condition in patients with OSA who, after adjustment for obesity, remain at increased risk for developing hypertension, heart failure, stroke, and dying from a cardiovascular condition. Adherence with continuous positive airway pressure (CPAP) therapy has a beneficial effect on blood pressure control, cardiovascular morbidity, insulin resistance, and circulating levels of inflammatory cytokines in the absence of any weight change. Furthermore, adherence with CPAP therapy appears to improve survival in patients with chronic heart failure and coexistent OSA. Thus, diagnosis and treatment of underlying OSA significantly improves morbidity in patients with cardiovascular diseases. It may also enhance life expectancy.

## OBSTRUCTIVE SLEEP APNEA AND SYSTEMIC HYPERTENSION

Repetitive arousals from sleep that follow episodes of obstructive apnea and hypopnea are associated with an acute systemic blood pressure rise that eventually persists during daytime. Repetitive bouts of hypoxia/hypercapnia and wide changes in intrathoracic pressures result in increased sympathetic activity that in turn contributes to insulin resistance and modulates leptin release. Due to leptin resistance, patients enter a downward spiral from weight gain to worsening of OSA. Up to 50% of patients with OSA do not experience the normal 10-20% decrease in blood pressure while asleep. The precise mechanisms that mediate the progression from nocturnal repetitive acute blood pressure elevations to chronic systemic hypertension are not well understood. Repetitive bouts of hypoxia/reoxygenation and sleep fragmentation result in a build-up of oxidative stress and vascular endothelial inflammation/activation that are the pathophysiological underpinnings of most cardiovascular conditions and particularly hypertension.

Large cross-sectional studies demonstrated a significant correlation between the severity of OSA and hypertension. An increase in AHI by 10 increases the risk of having hypertension by 11%, and each 10% decrease in nocturnal oxyhemoglobin saturation increases the odds of having hypertension by 13%. The association between AHI and hypertension is not as strong in elderly OSA patients partly due to survival biases. The Wisconsin Sleep Cohort, a population-based prospective 8-year longitudinal study, clearly demonstrated a significant relationship between sleep-disordered breathing at baseline and the presence of hypertension 4 years later. Results were adjusted for baseline hypertension status, body mass index (BMI), waist and neck circumference, gender, and weekly alcohol and cigarette consumption. The risk of developing hypertension increased with baseline AHI (baseline AHI = 5-14.9/h, OR for hypertension 95% CI = 2.03, 1.29 to 3.17; baseline AHI ≥15/h, OR for hypertension

# 17

# Critical Care for the Cardiologist

Jason N. Katz and Richard C. Becker

## PRACTICAL POINTS

- Early application of hypothermia may improve neurologic outcomes as well as rates of death after cardiac arrest.

- Exclusion criteria (though not absolute) for therapeutic hypothermia include recent major surgery, sepsis, and active ongoing bleeding, as hypothermia has been shown to increase the risk of bleeding, infection, and coagulopathy.

- Recommended speed of blood pressure reduction in hypertensive emergencies is arguable, though most authorities agree that blood pressure goals in acute aortic dissection should be reached within the first 5-10 minutes.

- In ischemic strokes, most cardiologists recommend lowering blood pressure only if it exceeds 220/120 mm Hg, while intracerebral hemorrhage blood pressure targets vary considerably within the literature.

- Continuous renal replacement therapy is ideal for renal support in critically ill patients.

## INTRODUCTION

The field of cardiovascular medicine has evolved considerably over the past several decades. With a novel arsenal of pharmacotherapeutics, interventional devices, and diagnostic tools, today's cardiologist is well-equipped to handle what were once universally considered fatal conditions. As a result, we are now challenged by an enlarging population of patients with advancing age, greater comorbidities, and higher risk—in particular, an increased susceptibility to critical illness.

Contemporary cardiologists must be adept at evaluating and managing patients from a critical care perspective. Our ability to now favorably alter the natural history of such conditions as myocardial infarction, acute heart failure, and cardiogenic shock has led to a more complex and more unstable group of patients currently occupying our cardiac care units (CCU). This chapter will focus on some of the key critical care topics now facing the cardiovascular community. It is imperative that we be able to comprehend and execute these important diagnostic and management strategies in order to care for our growing critically ill patient base. At the same time, we should be compelled to share our expertise on cardiovascular concepts which now influence the pathogenesis of other critical illnesses, in order to improve the care of an expanding population of patients with high resource use and unparalleled mortality.

## SEPSIS AND SEPTIC SHOCK

Observational data suggest that there is greater prevalence of sepsis among critically ill patients with cardiovascular disease. One might postulate that this epidemiologic finding is multifactorial. As previously mentioned, the increasing age and advancing comorbidities likely make our patients more susceptible to systemic infection. Furthermore, our increasing use of invasive and interventional strategies, including the implantation of pacemakers, defibrillators, and ventricular assist devices, surely provides a ripe milieu for provocation of the sepsis process.

### Definition

*Sepsis* is considered present when there is evidence of or highly suspected infection in the setting of the *systemic inflammatory response syndrome* (SIRS) (**Table 17-1**). The continuum of sepsis also includes the more critical subsets of *severe sepsis* (sepsis with acute end-organ dysfunction)

| Table 17-1 • Components of the Systemic Inflammatory Response Syndrome (SIRS) |
| --- |
| • Heart rate >90 beats/min |
| • Body temperature <36 or >38°C |
| • Respiratory rate >20 breaths/min or blood gas $PaCO_2$ <32 mm Hg |
| • White blood cell count <4000 cells/mm$^3$ or >12000 cells/mm$^3$, or the presence of >10% immature neutrophils. |

and *septic shock* (sepsis with refractory hypotension). Examples of acute end-organ injury patterns are shown in **Table 17-2**.

## Epidemiology

Sepsis is a seemingly ubiquitous diagnosis within U.S. intensive care units (ICUs). It is especially common among the elderly and immunocompromised. Worldwide, sepsis, and in particular septic shock, accounts for the majority of ICU resource utilization and mortality.

## Diagnosis

The diagnosis of sepsis is a clinical one, but a variety of laboratory-based and imaging studies can provide important clues to the presence and severity of disease. These include chest x-ray, computed tomography, urinalysis, cardiac markers, serum lactate, and lumbar puncture, to name a few. Identification of a causative microbiologic organism requires culturing from suspected sites of infection, such as the urine culture, sputum culture, and blood culture. Sterile technique in the acquisition of cultures is imperative, as contamination is common and may complicate therapeutic decision-making.

| Table 17-2 • Acute End-Organ Injury Patterns in Sepsis |
| --- |
| • Neurologic |
|    Encephalopathy |
| • Gastrointestinal |
|    Hyperbilirubinemia |
|    Hepatic synthetic dysfunction/coagulopathy |
|    Bowel ischemia/infarction |
| • Renal |
|    Acute kidney injury—oliguria, anuria |
|    Electrolyte abnormalities |
|    Volume overload |
| • Cardiac |
|    Systolic and diastolic heart failure |
|    Myocardial ischemia/infarction |
| • Pulmonary |
|    Acute lung injury (ALI), acute respiratory distress syndrome (ARDS) |
| • Endocrine |
|    Adrenal insufficiency |
|    Thyroid dysfunction— hypothyroidism, hyperthyroidism |
|    Hyperglycemia, hypoglycemia |

## Management

Treatment for sepsis, and especially septic shock, relies upon early and aggressive volume resuscitation, infection source control, and antimicrobial therapy. For years, marred by the lack of a systematic approach for treating afflicted patients, the development of an *early goal-directed therapy* (EGDT) protocol has produced an evidence-based and validated platform for directing resuscitative efforts. In EGDT, crystalloid is administered until the patient's central venous pressure reaches 8-12 mm Hg. Inadequate mean arterial pressure (<65 mm Hg) is then corrected with vasopressor support, followed by optimization of oxygen delivery through blood transfusion and/or inotropic therapy to target a mixed central venous oxygen saturation >70%. A more formal protocol, to be commenced within 6 hours of hospital presentation, can be seen in **Figure 17-1**. Its implementation has been associated with a marked decline in patient mortality.

Other adjunctive therapies to be considered in the treatment of sepsis include intravenous hydrocortisone for fluid and vasopressor-refractory shock, recombinant human-activated protein C for those with organ dysfunction and high risk of death (APACHE II > 25 or multiorgan failure), intensive glucose control, stress ulcer prophylaxis, and deep vein thrombosis prophylaxis.

# NONINVASIVE AND INVASIVE MECHANICAL VENTILATION

A broad understanding of the concepts of both noninvasive and invasive mechanical ventilation has become increasingly more important for cardiologists who treat patients with critical illness. Patients presenting with pulmonary edema, for example, may require emergent ventilatory support in order to reverse their respiratory failure. Those with septic shock complicating infective endocarditis may develop life-threatening acute lung injury or the acute respiratory distress syndrome (ARDS).

## Noninvasive Ventilation

This type of mechanical ventilation is administered without an invasive artificial airway—most commonly as positive pressure ventilation (PPV) via a nasal or full-face mask. It is believed that avoidance of endotracheal intubation may limit the risks of traumatic and infectious complications associated with more invasive techniques, yet still provide reliable delivery of oxygenated, pressurized gas to the distal airways sufficient to improve gas exchange. Careful patient selection is essential in order to maximize the benefits of noninvasive ventilation, and should only be employed for those individuals with rapidly reversible pulmonary

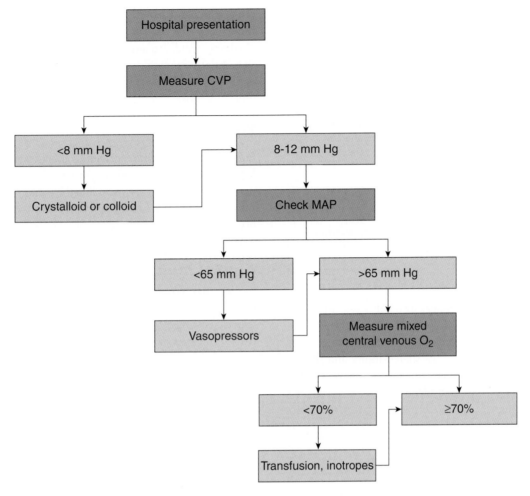

CVP = central venous pressure; MAP = mean arterial pressure

**Figure 17-1.** Early goal-directed therapy for severe sepsis and septic shock.

pathologies, those who can protect their airways, and those with a sustained ventilatory drive.

Perhaps no disease process has been better validated as a target for noninvasive ventilation than acute cardiogenic pulmonary edema. The resulting increase in functional residual capacity buttresses collapsible alveoli and can rapidly improve oxygenation. Furthermore, the increased intrathoracic pressure reduces transmyocardial pressure, resulting in beneficial decreases in both ventricular preload and afterload. Given a growing body of evidence supporting the use of noninvasive ventilation, in particular continuous positive airway pressure (CPAP), for patients with acute heart failure, the procedure should be considered first-line therapy for those with respiratory failure in the critical care setting.

## Invasive Ventilation

In cases of respiratory failure where the patient is not a candidate for noninvasive therapy, invasive mechanical ventilation should be employed. Most often delivered through an endotracheal tube, pressurized oxygen-rich gas is provided to support adequate gas exchange for the critically ill patient. There are numerous ventilator models and modes, the descriptions of which are beyond the scope of this chapter. Conventional strategies, however, focus upon gas delivery through either a volume-targeted or pressure-targeted approach. There is compelling data to support low tidal-volume (6 mL/kg) ventilation (especially in those with ARDS), avoidance of oxygen toxicity by rapidly titrating to a fraction of inspired oxygen ($F_IO_2$) <60%, and the application of positive end-expiratory pressure (PEEP) to avoid sheering trauma that may accompany repetitive alveolar unit opening and closing (ventilator-associated lung injury).

## The Ventilator Bundle

No matter what technique of mechanical ventilation is used, duration of therapy should be minimized in an effort to avoid potentially catastrophic complications which may affect the ventilated patient; these include ventilator-associated pneumonias, venous thromboembolic disease,

| Table 17-3 • Components of the Ventilator Bundle | |
| --- | --- |
| **Component** | **Rationale** |
| Elevate head of bed 30-45 degrees | Reduce risk for aspiration |
| Daily interruption of sedation | Avoid prolonged mechanical ventilation and daily assessment of "weaning" potential (spontaneous breathing trial where appropriate) |
| Thromboembolic prophylaxis | Avoid DVT, PE |
| Peptic ulcer disease prophylaxis | Avoid stress ulcer, gastrointestinal hemorrhage |

*DVT, deep venous thrombosis; PE, pulmonary embolism*

and gastrointestinal hemorrhage, to name a few. Most authorities recommend addressing these concerns through the systematic utilization of a "ventilator bundle," the goals of which are to limit ventilator-associated injury and illness. **Table 17-3** lists key components of the ventilator bundle, and the rationale for their consideration.

# VENTILATOR-ASSOCIATED PNEUMONIA

Pneumonia may complicate mechanical ventilation in up to 50% of patients, and is a primary cause for ICU morbidity and mortality. Selected risk factors pertaining to a CCU patient population include male sex, greater disease-severity at admission, the presence of multiple central venous catheters, cardiothoracic surgery, and the need for reintubation. Blood transfusion has also been suggested as a risk factor for ventilator-associated pneumonia (VAP).

## Pathogenesis

VAP is thought to occur via aspiration of pathogens colonizing the upper airways. Once a sufficient amount of pathogen has reached the distal airways, pneumonia develops when host defenses are overwhelmed. Gram negative bacilli are the most common offending organisms, followed by *Staphylococcus aureus*. Clinicians should be aware of increasing resistance patterns in most contemporary critical care units, and this should be considered particularly when one selects empiric antimicrobial therapy.

## Diagnosis

A high index of suspicion is required in mechanically ventilated patients so as not to miss the diagnosis. VAP should be considered in patients with fever, increased secretions (especially purulent samples), leukocytosis, hypoxemia, and those with new infiltrates found on radiographic studies. Qualitative and/or quantitative specimens should be sent either through sputum sampling or bronchoscopically guided bronchoalveolar lavage (BAL), prior to the initiation of empiric antibiotics.

## Therapy

Empiric, broad-spectrum antibiotics should be initiated once VAP is considered. Selection of antimicrobial therapy is based upon a number of factors, including the patient's immune status, allergy status, prior antibiotic use, patient risk factors, and hospital resistance patterns. In general, for immunocompetent hosts, monotherapy with a second- or third-generation cephalosporin, a beta-lactam/beta-lactamase inhibitor combination, or quinolone is often acceptable. For patients at risk for drug-resistant organisms, or at sites where resistance patterns dictate more aggressive therapy, one should consider empiric coverage of *methicillin-resistant Staphylococcus aureus* (MRSA), *Pseudomonas aeruginosa*, *Acinetobacter* species, and even extended spectrum beta-lactamase producing *Klebsiella*.

Once microbiologic data are available, antibiotic therapy should be appropriately narrowed. While optimal duration of therapy is unknown, most authorities now recommend a 7-day course if good response is noted. More prolonged durations of therapy should be considered for highly resistant organisms, although the data are inconclusive and increased concerns for further resistance may be warranted. The burden of evidence does suggest, however, that adherence to the aforementioned "ventilator bundle" indeed decreases the occurrence of VAP and should be employed as a preventative strategy.

# THERAPEUTIC HYPOTHERMIA

One marked evolutionary change in the way cardiologists now manage critically ill patients is that our focus of care has broadened to not only include the in-hospital setting, but to the out-of-hospital arena as well. In acute myocardial infarction, for instance, we have begun to institute elaborate systems-of-care processes, which now streamline reperfusion therapy. This includes wireless transmission of electrocardiograms from emergency medical services (EMS) teams and the rapid transfer of patients to facilities with interventional cardiology capabilities. Another key out-of-hospital event that contributes to marked cardiovascular morbidity and mortality, and has been the focus of intense investigation from both clinical and public health perspectives, is that of sudden cardiac death.

Outside of advanced cardiac life support (ACLS), electrical defibrillation, and antiarrhythmic therapy, little has been available in the clinician's armory to significantly improve outcomes for these critically ill, high-risk individuals. As a result, there has been no substantial decline in the marked mortality for this patient population over the past several decades. In the last several years, however, there has been a growing and influential body of evidence supporting the use of therapeutic induced *hypothermia* for unconscious adult patients who have a return of spontaneous circulation after out-of-hospital cardiac arrest—in particular, arrest secondary to ventricular tachycardia (VT) or ventricular fibrillation (VF). It is believed that the early application of hypothermia may improve neurologic outcomes as well as rates of death in this group.

## Eligibility

Currently, it is suggested that therapeutic hypothermia (to 32-34°C) be applied to eligible patients for 12-24 hours following return of spontaneous circulation. Eligibility criteria may be expanded to include patients with non-VF arrest or those whose arrest occurs in the in-hospital setting, though the current evidence is much less robust for these patient groups. Exclusion criteria (though not absolute) include recent major surgery, sepsis, and active ongoing bleeding, as hypothermia has been shown to increase the risk of bleeding, infection, and coagulopathy. The application of therapeutic hypothermia requires planning, education, and multidisciplinary integration from physician, hospital, and systems-of-care perspectives. The most effective use of this therapeutic modality seems to occur when established clinical protocols are developed, and when hypothermia is instituted early.

## Cooling and Rewarming Strategies

Multiple cooling techniques have been used with success and, currently, no particular style is advocated above others. Patients may be cooled externally using cooling blankets, strategically-placed ice, or using surface heat-exchange. Novel devices for external cooling continue to be developed, boasting rapid and easily induced hypothermia. Internal cooling may also be performed using catheter-based technologies. It has been suggested that endovascular cooling is more rapid and easier to titrate, though no randomized data exist to support these claims. Commercially available devices are generally placed in the femoral vein, though internal cooling may be performed through any intravenous access with the use of cold saline infusion.

During therapeutic hypothermia, supportive/adjunctive therapies are often required. These include vasopressors for the treatment of refractory hypotension, antiarrhythmic therapy, and tight glycemic control, to name a few. Shivering often occurs as a body's desperate attempt to maintain temperature homeostasis. Unfortunately, shivering can often impede aggressive therapeutic hypothermia, and usually

requires treatment. With endovascular techniques, it is thought that shivering may be controlled with sedation and analgesia alone, but in many cases, if refractory, necessitates systemic paralytic therapy.

Rewarming begins approximately 24 hours after the initiation of therapeutic hypothermia. Patients should be rewarmed slowly (0.3-0.5°C per hour) over 8-10 hours, and careful hemodynamic monitoring should continue to assess for hypotension resulting from sudden vascular dilatation.

An example of the therapeutic hypothermia protocol at one institution can be seen in **Figure 17-2**. The use of hypothermia in clinical medicine is likely to be seen in much broader patient populations over time. An understanding of its physiologic mechanism and its application as a therapeutic tool, therefore, will be increasingly important for cardiologists who will be caring for those with critical illnesses.

## HYPERTENSIVE CRISES

Hypertension affects over one billion people worldwide and over 50 million in the United States alone. As a result, great attention has been given to the basic science, translational and clinical investigation of this morbid disease. At the same time, there is a unique subset of patients with hypertension who present to the hospital with acute, severe episodes of blood pressure elevation. Classically defined as hypertensive emergencies or urgencies, depending upon the presence or absence of target organ injury, the study of these clinical conditions has been relegated largely to small observational series, case reports, and opinion pieces. Despite the suggestion that hypertensive crises may result in substantial morbidity and mortality, as well as marked resource use, there is very limited data available to guide clinicians in the diagnostic evaluation and management of these individuals.

Manifestations of end-organ injury associated with acute, severe hypertension include aortic dissection, acute heart failure, myocardial ischemia or infarction, acute kidney injury, encephalopathy, stroke, eclampsia, and symptomatic microangiopathic hemolytic anemia. Available data indicate that central nervous system sequelae, including encephalopathy, cerebral infarction, and intracerebral hemorrhage, are the most commonly encountered injury patterns.

### Epidemiology and Risk Factors

Epidemiologic estimates suggest that most patients who present with hypertensive crises have been previously diagnosed with chronic hypertension. Commonly, these individuals have been prescribed antihypertensive therapies, but have high rates of nonadherence. In addition, patients are more likely male, African American, and have high rates of illicit drug use.

Inclusion criteria

Cardiopulmonary arrest with return of spontaneous circulation
Patients 18 years of age or older
Unresponsive after return of spontaneous circulation (GCS ≤ 9)
Endotracheal intubation with mechanical ventilation
Hemodynamic stability: SBP > 90 mm Hg or mean arterial blood pressure > 60
Ability to initiate cooling within 6 hours of arrest

Exclusion criteria

Time to ACLS > 30 minutes
Time since arrest > 6 hours
Temperature < 30°C after arrest
Ongoing severe shock
Conscious with GCS > 9
Pregnant
Patients < 18 years of age
Recent major surgery within the last 14 days
Known bleeding diathesis or active ongoing bleeding
Systemic infection or sepsis
Do not resuscitate (DNR) or do not intubate (DNI) status

Protocol

1. Obtain baseline rectal temperature
2. Remove clothing and expose patient to ambient room temperature
3. Ensure at least 2 peripheral IV catheters (18-gauge) are in place and patent
4. Insert urinary catheter with in-line temperature monitoring capability
5. Sedate and paralyze as necessary
6. Administer cooled normal saline 30 mL/kg at a rapid rate
7. Place ice packs to neck, axilla, groin, and along sides of torso and thighs
8. Draw baseline labs, obtain necessary diagnostic studies
9. Initiate cooling with either an external or internal method
10. Monitor and document vital signs every 15 minutes x 4, then every 30 minutes until patient reaches goal temperature, then at least every 1 hour thereafter
11. Draw and monitor basic metabolic profile (BMP), complete blood count (CBC), prothrombin time (PT), partial thromboplastin time (PTT), and arterial blood gas (ABG) every 8 hours
12. Obtain blood cultures x 2, urine culture, and sputum culture 12 hours after initiation of cooling
13. After cooling for 24 hours, allow the patient to passively rewarm over 8–12 hours to the designated target temperature (at a rate no faster than 0.5°C per hour)
14. Draw and monitor BMP, PT, and PTT every 4 hours
15. Monitor and document temperatures every 30 minutes until normothermic
16. Wean paralytics and sedation, assess neurologic status
17. Monitor for rebound hypothermia

**Figure 17-2.** Duke University Hospital therapeutic hypothermia protocol.

## Mechanisms of End-Organ Injury

The pathophysiology of injury is largely speculative. Some suggest that the acute rise in blood pressure triggers a cascade of neurohormonal, vasoactive, and cellular events. The compensatory smooth muscle contraction and vasoconstriction of the larger arteries and arterioles, in an effort to preserve distal cellular activity, leads to endothelial dysfunction, inhibition of nitric oxide synthesis, and marked increases in peripheral vascular resistance. Concomitantly, mechanical stress serves as a potent stimulus for the release of inflammatory cytokines and endothelial adhesion molecules, also amplifying the renin-angiotensin-aldosterone system. These events, in aggregate, support the deleterious endothelial dysfunction, fibrinoid necrosis, vascular injury, impaired fibrinolysis, and ischemia that are causes of target-organ damage.

## Goals of Antihypertensive Therapy

Patients presenting with hypertensive emergencies should generally be managed with immediate blood pressure control using parenteral therapy. Those patients with hypertensive urgencies, on the other hand, may be managed with oral antihypertensives with a goal of blood pressure reduction over several days. It is important to note, however, that no consensus exists regarding the magnitude and rapidity of treatment for these acutely hypertensive patients. Some target a reduction in diastolic blood pressure of ten to fifteen percent, others argue for an absolute reduction in diastolic pressure to a value of 100 or 110 mm Hg, while still others believe that therapy should be aimed at lowering the mean arterial pressure by 20 or 25%. At the same time, the recommended speed of blood pressure reduction is arguable, though most authorities agree that blood pressure goals in acute aortic dissection should be reached within the first 5-10 minutes. In ischemic strokes, most recommend lowering blood pressure only if it exceeds 220/120 mm Hg, while intracerebral hemorrhage blood pressure targets vary considerably within the literature.

One should remember, however, that several studies have consistently highlighted significant morbidity associated with rapid reductions of blood pressure in chronically hypertensive individuals. These patients have a right-ward shift in their pressure-flow autoregulation curves; as a result, aggressively decreasing blood pressure to normal levels can result in marked tissue hypoperfusion and organ ischemia. Thus, hemodynamic targets should be defined prior to initiating antihypertensive therapies and careful attention directed towards avoiding any overshooting of blood pressure goals.

Commonly used parenteral agents for the treatment of hypertensive emergencies are shown in **Table 17-4**.

| Table 17-4 • Commonly Used Parenteral Antihypertensives for Hypertensive Emergencies ||
|---|---|
| **End-Organ Injury Pattern** | **Suggested Pharmacologic Agents** |
| Acute heart failure/ pulmonary edema | IV nitroglycerin, IV diuretics, IV nitroprusside |
| Myocardial ischemia/ infarction | IV nitroglycerin, IV beta blocker |
| Aortic dissection | IV beta-blocker + IV nitroprusside, IV labetalol, IV CCB + IV beta-blocker |
| Hypertensive encephalopathy | IV CCB, IV beta-blocker, IV nitroprusside |
| Hemorrhagic Stroke | IV CCB, IV beta-blocker, IV nitroprusside, |
| Acute renal failure | IV CCB, IV beta-blocker, IV fenoldopam |
| Hemolytic anemia | IV CCB, IV beta-blocker, IV fenoldopam |
| Eclampsia | IV labetalol, IV nicardipine, IV hydralazine |

*IV, intravenous; CCB, calcium channel blocker*

# CONTINUOUS RENAL REPLACEMENT THERAPY (CRRT)

CRRT is ideal for renal support in critically ill patients. Acute renal failure is common in the ICU and CCU settings—a prevalent target organ injury resulting from hemodynamic perturbations, shock states, and nephrotoxic agents (e.g., contrast during coronary angiography). The goal of CRRT is to support the kidneys and enhance renal recovery with prevention of profound electrolyte disturbance (e.g., hyperkalemia), severe metabolic acidosis, and refractory uremia, while rapidly correcting volume overload through gradual but consistent removal of excessive body fluid. Unlike conventional, intermittent hemodialysis, volume control with CRRT is continuous and immediately adaptable to patient-specific hemodynamic changes; furthermore, the avoidance of episodic circulating changes in intravascular volume with CRRT may prevent further treatment-associated renal injury.

There are several different modes of CRRT, which are illustrated in **Figure 17-3**. Most commonly, continuous venovenous hemodialysis or hemofiltration is employed. In this case, a double lumen cannula is inserted into a large vein, while a roller-pump mechanism serves to drive the blood into the filter/dialyzer.

## Nomenclature

*Diffusion* is the process by which solutes move across a semipermeable membrane depending upon its concentration gradient, molecular weight, and velocity size. Ultrafiltration, on the other hand, involves the movement of water by hydrostatic or osmotic forces across a semipermeable membrane, with concomitant solute drag occurring even in the absence of a significant concentration gradient. Increased ultrafiltration can usually be achieved by increasing the transmembrane pressure via increased negative pressure in the dialysate compartment, increasing the blood flow rate, or by increasing venous resistance.

## Advantages and Disadvantages of CRRT

As mentioned, CRRT is advantageous in the critical care setting because of the minimized hemodynamic perturbations it causes in comparison to conventional, intermittent hemodialysis. It limits uremia effectively and controls electrolyte and acid-base homeostasis quite well. Furthermore, it is efficacious in the removal of volume in the hypervolemic patient. It can also remove potential toxins and has been associated with reductions in proinflammatory cytokines.

However, CRRT is not without its challenges. There is a need for continuous anticoagulation in order to keep the

**Slow continuous ultrafiltration (SCUF)**

- Uses machine to remove fluid from patient by applying pressure to the hemofilters

**Continuous venovenous hemofiltration (CVVH)**

- Uses machine to remove fluid and toxins by applying pressure to the hemofilters; physiologic substitution fluid is infused to patient to maintain intravascular volume and chemical homeostasis; relies on *ultrafiltration* and *convection*

**Continuous venovenous hemodialysis (CVVHD)**

- Uses machine to remove fluid and toxins by applying pressure to the hemofilters and using a dialysate; dialysiate allows toxin removal via *diffusion*, with fluid removal via *ultrafiltration*

**Continuous venovenous hemodiafiltration (CVVHDF)**

- Uses machine to remove fluid and toxins by applying pressure to the hemofilters, using a dialysate, and also infusion of a substitution solution; uses *ultrafiltration*, *convection*, and *diffusion*

**Figure 17-3.** Modes of continuous renal replacement therapy.

CRRT circuit from clotting; this can lead to increased risks of bleeding and thrombocytopenia. CRRT is also a labor-intensive therapy, requiring constant attention to the dialysis circuit as well as close hemodynamic patient monitoring. Additionally, there is also an increased risk of infection, largely stemming from the necessary intravascular access.

# FUTURE OF CARDIAC CRITICAL CARE

With an aging population, advancing comorbidities, and our ability to now favorably alter the course of cardiovascular maladies once thought to be untreatable, cardiologists will undoubtedly be faced with an increasingly complex patient base. In particular, the burden of critical illness has and should continue to grow, forcing today's cardiologists to be adept at diagnosing and managing a growing number of morbid conditions in the CCU. We have a lot to gain and, at the same time, a lot to add to the care of critically ill patients. By embracing the management of these individuals, we can be certain that our patients with advanced cardiovascular illnesses continue to get the best evidence-based care.

## Recommended Readings

1. Rivers E, Nguyen B, Havstad S, et al. Early goal-directed therapy in the treatment of severe sepsis and septic shock. *N Engl J Med.* 2001;345:1368–1377.

2. Nava S, Carbone G, DiBattista N, et al. Noninvasive ventilation in cardiogenic pulmonary edema: a multicenter randomized trial. *Am J Respir Crit Care Med.* 2003;168:1432–1437.

3. Chastre J, Fagon JY. Ventilator-associated pneumonia. *Am J Respir Crit Care Med.* 2002;165:867–903.

4. Mehta RL. Continuous renal replacement therapy in the critically ill patient. *Kidney Int.* 2005;67:781–795.

5. Kaplan NM. Management of hypertensive emergencies. *Lancet.* 1994;344:1335–1338.

# Pulmonary Embolism

RALUCA ARIMIE

---

# 18

● **PRACTICAL POINTS**

- Acute pulmonary embolism (PE) could double the pulmonary arterial pressures, and mean PAP is usually >40 mm Hg. Sometimes it presents as acute elevation in right atrial pressure.

- ECG patterns are nonspecific.

- D-dimer normal levels have a high negative predictive value for PE.

- IVC filters are indicated if there is absolute contraindication for anticoagulation, massive PE, and recurrent PE despite adequate previous anticoagulation.

- Embolectomy is indicated in patients with massive PE with cardiogenic shock or hypotension that have a contraindication for thrombolytics.

## INTRODUCTION

Pulmonary embolism (PE) most commonly originates from deep venous thrombosis (DVT) of the legs (79% of patients with PE have evidence of DVT in their legs; if DVT is not detected, is likely that the whole thrombus has already detached and embolized). Presentation ranges from asymptomatic, incidentally discovered emboli to massive embolism causing immediate death. Chronic sequelae of DVT and PE include postthrombotic syndrome and chronic thromboembolic pulmonary hypertension.

## EPIDEMIOLOGY

- Common
- Incidence in United States >1/1000

- Mortality >15% in the first 3 months after the diagnosis—as deadly as myocardial infarction
- 300,000 people per year in U.S. die from acute PE.

## ETIOLOGY

Virchow's triad of stasis, venous endothelial dysfunction/injury, and hypercoagulable state (acquired or inherited) are relevant in assessing patients. The following are considered risk factors for pulmonary embolism:

- Reversible causes:
  ○ Obesity
  ○ Smoking
  ○ Hypertension
  ○ Long air and ground travel
  ○ Sedentary lifestyle
- In the context of illness, medication, or physiologic states:
  ○ Surgery: orthopedic, cancer surgery
  ○ Trauma and spinal injury
  ○ Immobilization
  ○ Cancer: Procoagulant effect of particular tumors, chemotherapy, venous obstruction by tumor, reduced mobility, central venous catheter
  ○ Acute medical illness: Pneumonia, congestive heart failure
  ○ Oral contraception
  ○ Postmenopausal hormone replacement therapy
  ○ Pregnancy
- Atherosclerotic disease and spontaneous venous thrombosis
- Genetic predisposition
  ○ Twin studies have demonstrated the contribution of an inherited prothrombotic state: increased levels of clotting factors and activation peptides
  ○ Deficiencies of anticoagulant factors also increase thrombotic risk
- Advanced age—risk increases after age of 40 years.

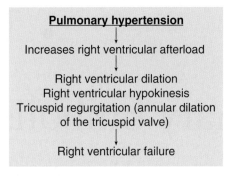

**Figure 18-1.** Pathophysiology of RV failure in pulmonary embolism.

## PATHOPHYSIOLOGY

Thrombi commonly form in deep veins in the calf and then propagate into proximal veins, including and above popliteal veins, then travel through the right side of the heart and embolize the lung.

### Hemodynamics

Acute obstruction causes hypoxemic vasoconstriction, leading to increased pulmonary vascular resistance and resulting in pulmonary hypertension. Most patients maintain a normal systemic arterial pressure for 12-48 hours and give the impression of hemodynamic stability. Then, often abruptly, pressor-resistant systemic arterial hypotension

and cardiac arrest can ensue (**Figures 18-1** and **18-2**). Pulmonary embolism could present as isolated elevated right atrial pressure. Hemodynamic response and decompensation in patients with pulmonary embolism depends on:

- Size of the embolus; responsible for the physical obstruction of the blood flow
- Coexistent cardiopulmonary disease
  ○ Patients without prior cardiopulmonary disease; mean pulmonary arterial pressure (PAP) can increase to 40 mm Hg
  ○ Patients with prior pulmonary hypertension; mean PAP can double
  ○ Patients with chronic thromboembolic pulmonary hypertension; PAP can exceed the system arterial pressure
- Neurohumoral effects—release of serotonin from platelets, thrombin from plasma, histamine from tissue (vasoactive and bronchoactive agents)
- Pulmonary infarction—usually not present due to dual pulmonary circulation from pulmonary and bronchial arteries.

### Gas Exchange

Normally, ventilation and perfusion in the lungs are well matched. The ratio of ventilation to the gas exchange structures and blood flow to the pulmonary capillaries is approximately 1.0. Acute PE impairs the efficient transfer of oxygen and carbon dioxide across the lung (**Figures 18-3** and **18-4**),

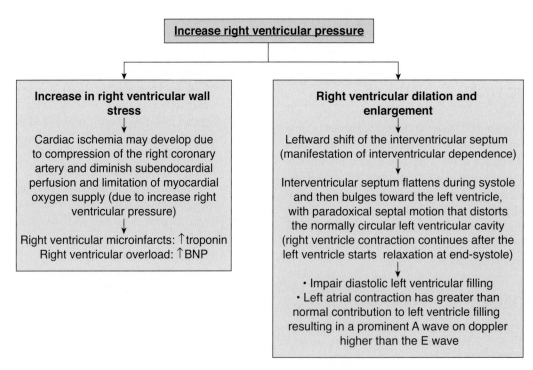

**Figure 18-2.** Pulmonary embolism-associated RV hemodynamic changes.

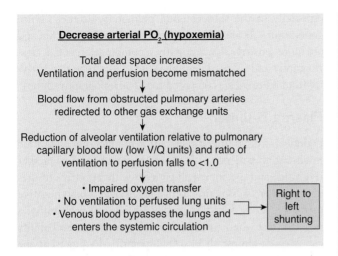

**Figure 18-3.** Causes of hypoxemia in pulmonary embolism.

resulting in decreased arterial $PO_2$ (hypoxemia) and increased alveolar-arterial oxygen tension gradient. Hypoxemia is a result of the following mechanisms:

- Mismatch of ventilation and perfusion—most common cause
  - PE produces redistribution of blood flow so that some lung gas exchange units have low ratio of ventilation/perfusion, whereas other lung units have excessively high ratio of ventilation/perfusion (**Figure 18-5**).
  - Gas exchange units have a low ratio of ventilation/perfusion secondary to the presence of atelectasis due to loss of surfactant and alveolar hemorrhage
- Shunting of the venous blood directly to the systemic arterial system without passing through ventilated gas exchange lung units. Right to left shunt can occur in the lung, heart ,or both (reflected by failure of supplemental oxygen to correct arterial hypoxemia)
  - Intrapulmonary shunt occurs due to ventilation/perfusion mismatch
  - Intracardiac shunt occurs due to opening of the foramen ovale when right atrial pressure exceeds left atrial pressure (even if both pressures are normal)
  - Positive airway pressure (positive end-expiratory pressure and continuous positive airway pressure)

**Increase in the Alveolar-arterial Oxygen Tension Gradient**

Decreased ratio of ventilation relative to perfusion in the gas exchange units

↓

Inefficiency of oxygen transfer across the lungs

↓

Increase gradient

**Figure 18-4.** Causes of increase in alveolar-arterial oxygen tension gradient.

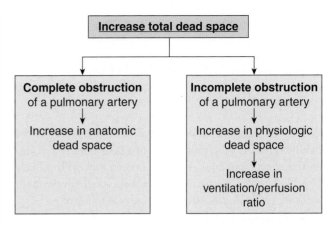

**Figure 18-5.** Causes of increased dead space after pulmonary embolism.

may worsen intracardiac shunting by increasing alveolar pressure, compressing pulmonary vessels, and increasing pulmonary vascular resistance

- Low pressure of oxygen in the venous blood—when PE causes right ventricular failure, resulting in low cardiac output, it amplifies the effect of low ventilation/perfusion ratio (this process is not present when lung is normal, with a normal ratio of 1.0 of ventilation/perfusion).

During acute PE, total dead space increases as lung units continue to be ventilated despite absent or diminished perfusion, which produces decreased elimination of carbon dioxide. Increase in arterial $PCO_2$ stimulates medullary chemoreceptors, which increases total minute ventilation. Subsequently, arterial $PCO_2$ decreases to normal and often below normal values. Most patients with PE present with low arterial $PCO_2$ and respiratory alkalosis. If the patient presents with high arterial $PCO_2$ or hypercapnia, the differential diagnosis includes a massive PE, with marked increase in anatomical and physiological dead space, or muscle fatigue due to marked increase of minute ventilation needed to maintain normal arterial $PCO_2$. Treatment with positive pressure ventilation and paralysis allows for a definitive treatment to relieve the thromboembolic obstruction (dead space) and increase in the alveolar volume of each tidal breath.

## DIAGNOSIS

### History and Physical Exam

- DVT—leg pain, warmth, swelling
- Acute PE—dyspnea, chest pain, either sudden in onset or evolving over days to weeks. Pleuritic chest pain and hemoptysis are more frequent if there is pulmonary infarction.
- Respiratory exam—tachypnea, pleural rub

- Cardiovascular exam—tachycardia, elevated jugular venous pressure, loud P2, right-sided gallop, right ventricular lift
- Symptoms and signs of DVP and PE are highly suggestive but not sensitive or specific, and further testing is needed.

Wells et al. developed a simple clinical model to predict the likelihood of PE. A scoring system of a maximum 12.5 points and based on 7 variables. A score <2 points makes PE unlikely (2% likelihood). A score >6 points suggests a high probability of PE (50% likelihood). The score is as following:

- 3 points each for:
  - Clinical evidence of deep venous thrombosis
  - An alternative diagnosis being less likely than PE
- 1.5 points each for:
  - Heart rate >100 bpm
  - Immobilization/surgery within 4 weeks
  - Previous deep venous thrombosis/PE
- 1 point each for:
  - Hemoptysis
  - Cancer.

## ECG and Chest X-ray

ECG and chest X-ray help clinician identify alternative diagnoses (myocardial infarction and pneumonia ). The typical ECG pattern is: tachycardia, S1Q3T3 pattern, RBBB, P wave pulmonale, right axis deviation. Right axis deviation is especially seen with massive PE. ECG patterns are nonspecific.

## Arterial Blood Gas

This test is disappointing toward assisting diagnosis, as normal values do not exclude PE and hypoxemia is a nonspecific finding.

## Ventilation Perfusion Lung Scan

Lung scanning is not commonly use due to often equivocal results; however, it remains the recommended first-line approach for imaging for patients with:

- Anaphylaxis to contrast agent
- Renal failure
- Pregnancy
- Patients with prior PE diagnosed by lung scan.

## Chest CT

Chest CT scan is the preferred imaging modality for diagnosis of PE. In addition, it assists in ruling out other pathologies, like pneumonia, pulmonary edema, pleural effusion, and coronary obstruction. Is important one know the type of chest CT scanner utilized. First generation CTs have a 5-mm resolution and fail to detect one-third of cases of PE, especially in the subsegmental pulmonary arteries. Third generation CTs are better as they have 1-mm resolution and are more sensitive. Occasionally, a combination of CT arteriography and CT venography is used to increased sensitivity from 83 to 90% (compared to CT arteriography alone).

## Plasma D-dimer

D-dimer is a cross-linked degradation product that is elevated in almost all patients with PE, as this test has a low predictive value and specificity, all patients with a positive test require further assessment. Normal levels have a high negative predictive value for PE, regardless of clinical probability; a negative test when combined with a low pretest probability can exclude almost all PEs. Incorporating D-dimer enzyme linked immunosorbent assay (ELISA) into the diagnostic algorithm allows for fewer chest CT scans, improved diagnostic efficiency, and reduced cost. When the pretest probability is high (e.g cancer patients), a negative D-dimer test has no utility because it does not have adequate negative predictive value for excluding the presence of a PE.

## RISK STRATIFICATION

Pulmonary embolism has a wide clinical presentation, from asymptomatic small PE to life-threatening major PE with hypotension and cardiogenic shock. Right ventricular dysfunction is a marker of high risk and increased major adverse clinical events. Right heart failure is suggested by:

- Clinical evaluation—Jugular venous distention, tricuspid regurgitation murmur, and accentuated pulmonic heart sound suggesting elevated right atrial and pulmonary arterial pressures.
- Electrocardiogram—Classic changes are S1Q3T3; in addition, T wave inversion can be seen in lead V1-V4 and new incomplete/complete right bundle branch block suggest right ventricular strain.
- Chest CT—Right ventricular enlargement can be seen relative to left ventricular size.
- Echocardiogram—Useful in acutely ill patients; it can demonstrate degree of right ventricular dysfunction, calculate an estimated systolic PAP, and show impaired left ventricular filling with leftward displacement of the interventricular septum suggestive of right ventricular pressure and volume overload. It could also show a free-floating right heart thrombus, and it can assist evaluation of the differential diagnosis (includes pericardial effusion with tamponade, aortic dissection and acute myocardial infarction with left ventricular dysfunction).
- Biomarkers—most recent development in prognostication:
  - Troponin elevation—indicates high right ventricular end diastolic pressure and impaired subendo-

# 19

# Cardiopulmonary Stress Testing

Amrut V. Ambardekar and Eugene E. Wolfel

## ● PRACTICAL POINTS

- Peak $VO_2$ < 14 mL/kg/min is used in most centers as the cutoff for eligibility criteria for cardiac transplant. Any value of peak $VO_2$ less than 85% predicted is considered abnormal.

- The $VO_2$ at the ventilatory threshold has been reported to be a better predictor of high risk for early mortality when compared to peak $VO_2$. Patients with a $VO_2$ < 11 mL/kg/min at the ventilatory threshold had a fivefold increased risk of early death.

- The breathing reserve is the most useful measurement to determine the cause of dyspnea. A low breathing reserve (<20%) suggests a pulmonary cause for the dyspnea.

- If the RER value is less than 1.10, and especially <1.0, the exercise effort is probably submaximal and the peak $VO_2$ would be falsely low.

- A high $V_E/VCO_2$ slope is associated with reduced cardiac output, increased wedge pressures, and worse survival. Patients with a $V_E/VCO_2$ slope >34 have worse prognosis.

- Would reverse order of comments about Peak $VO_2$. Thus, would start with "Any value of peak $VO_2$ less than 85% predicted is considered abnormal." Then would follow with the statement: Peak $VO_2$ < 14 ml/kg/min is used in most centers as the cutoff for eligibility for cardiac transplant."

## NATURE OF TEST AND GENERAL DEFINITIONS

Cardiopulmonary stress testing (CPET) involves the addition of expired gas analysis and determination of ventilation to standard exercise testing in patients with cardiopulmonary diseases. Cardiologists have become knowledgeable in the area of gas exchange during exercise, as these measurements provide important functional and prognostic information on patients with heart failure and other cardiovascular diseases. The information obtained from CPET has also been useful in tracking responses to various forms of therapeutic interventions, including pharmacologic therapy, pacemakers, surgical procedures, and exercise training and rehabilitation.

## Functional Capacity

Most exercise testing performed in the United States involves the use of graded treadmill exercise; the speed and grade of the treadmill have been used to estimate functional capacity in metabolic equivalents (or METs, not to be confused with MetS, the metabolic syndrome). The unit MET is defined as resting oxygen consumption ($VO_2$) of 3.5 mL/kg/min. Physical activity is then quantified by multiples of this resting $O_2$ consumption, which approximates the caloric expenditure of that activity. However, the validity and reproducibility of these estimations, when compared to directly measured $VO_2$ by gas exchange methods, have been shown to be suboptimal. Various factors influencing the relationship between measured and estimated $VO_2$ include habituation or training effect, fitness level, the presence of cardiac disease, handrail holding on the treadmill, and the nature of the exercise protocol. Thus, there are major limitations in predicting an accurate and reproducible measurement of functional capacity based on exercise duration or workload using standard clinical exercise testing and sophisticated measurements that rely on expired gas analysis for measuring $VO_2$ and other respiratory variables are frequently used in the management of patients with cardiovascular diseases.

## Physiology of Exercise: The Interdependence of Circulatory, Respiratory and Skeletal Muscle Function on Exercise Capacity

The utilization of oxygen from inspired air and the elimination of carbon dioxide ($CO_2$) from cellular respiration and buffering action is influenced by the activity of the heart and peripheral circulation, ventilation and gas exchange in the lungs, and the utilization of oxygen and elimination of $CO_2$ in exercising muscle. The cardiovascular system plays a major role in this process as it determines the flow component of delivery and elimination of these internal gases. But how does the measurement of expired gases and ventilation relate to cardiovascular function? The important link is the *Fick equation*, where cardiac output (L/min) is determined by $O_2$ consumption ($VO_2$, ml/min) divided by arteriovenous $O_2$ content difference. Rearranging this equation shows that

$$VO_2 = \text{cardiac output} \times \text{arteriovenous } O_2 \\ \text{content difference.}$$

$VO_2$ during exercise is directly related to blood flow or cardiac output and the ability of the peripheral tissues to extract $O_2$. In most subjects, $VO_2$ during exercise is primarily related to cardiac output, since stroke volume and heart rate (the components of cardiac output) increase with progressive exercise, while peripheral $O_2$ extraction occurs to a similar degree in most patients at peak exercise. Thus, $VO_2$, measured at the mouth, is a surrogate for cardiac output changes during exercise, and it becomes a useful measurement in the evaluation of patients with cardiovascular disease. Cardiac output closely matches ventilation in the lung in order to deliver $O_2$ to working skeletal muscle during exercise. *Minute ventilation* ($V_E$) is the total volume, in liters, of gas exhaled from the lungs per minute. $V_E$ increases with exercise as a result of increased blood flow to the lung, activation of the carotid bodies, and activation of ergoreceptors in the exercising skeletal muscle. Ventilation tracks changes in $VO_2$ during exercise; with the development of excessive lactate production at higher levels of exercise, ventilation increases out of proportion to $VO_2$, but still tracks $VCO_2$ up to near-maximal exercise, when a further increase due to the development of metabolic acidosis occurs. However, patients with cardiopulmonary diseases have alterations in cardiac output, ventilation-perfusion mismatch in the lung, abnormal cardiopulmonary receptor function, abnormal skeletal muscle function, and heightened sympathetic activity. All of these can lead to excessive ventilation during both submaximal and maximal exercise. Therefore, changes in ventilation—a primary respiratory variable—can be related to alterations in cardiovascular function, and relationships between $V_E$ and both $VO_2$ and $VCO_2$ have been shown to have diagnostic and prognostic value in patients with cardiovascular disease, especially heart failure.

# MECHANICS OF CARDIOPULMONARY STRESS TESTING (CPET)

## Conduct of the Test: Device and Protocol

The basic aspects of CPET incorporate similar principles related to standard cardiac stress testing with appropriate screening, ECG monitoring, and assessment of heart rate, blood pressure, and symptoms during the test. Pulse oximetry is often used to evaluate hypoxemia as a potential cause of excessive ventilation and dyspnea during exercise in patients with cardiovascular disease. Most tests are performed with a treadmill. If a cycle ergometer is used, the peak exercise $VO_2$ is usually about 10-20% lower than on a treadmill, despite a similar peak heart rate, as the patients do not have to support their weight and less muscle mass is recruited during this exercise. Ramp testing, with a gradual and continuous increase in workload, is the preferred protocol for the cycle ergometer. The usual ramp is 10 watts per minute in patients limited by cardiovascular disease. If the treadmill is used, a more gradual protocol such as the modified Naughton is preferred for functionally limited patients. Ramp protocols are available for the treadmill but they are more difficult to program and use in standard clinical practice. For most patients the total exercise duration should be between 8 and 12 minutes for an adequate but not prolonged test.

## Instrumentation

There are three basic measurements obtained during CPET: *minute ventilation*, which is the product of tidal volume and respiratory frequency; the *fraction of $O_2$ in expired air*; and the *fraction of $CO_2$ in expired air*. The "true $O_2$" is the difference between inspired fractional inspired oxygen concentration ($FiO_2$) and fractional expired oxygen concentration ($FeO_2$). With most automated systems, it is difficult to accurately measure the $FiO_2$ during a test; therefore, a CPET is usually not performed on a patient using supplemental oxygen. The $FiCO_2$ is assumed to be 0% under most conditions. The $O_2$ concentration is measured with a gas analyzer that is either an electrochemical or paramagnetic system. $CO_2$ concentration is usually measured with an infrared analyzer. Prior to testing, these analyzers require calibration with room air and special mixtures of gases with different concentrations of $O_2$ and $CO_2$. Ventilation is usually measured with expired air by means of a pneumotachometer, turbine, or anemometer, with the pneumotachometer being the most commonly used device. Sampling at rest and during exercise is obtained at the mouth and most automated systems have breath-by-breath capability. The patient uses a mouthpiece and nose clip to insure a closed system. A one-way valve allows room air to enter the system during inspiration and closes during expiration, thereby allowing sampling of expired air for gas exchange and ventilation. Small sample intervals have resulted in excessive variability in the measurements, thus an average of data at 20- to 30-second intervals have been found to give optimal results.

## Reproducibility and Variability

Serial CPET studies have been performed in both coronary artery disease and chronic heart failure patients to determine reproducibility and variability of peak exercise $VO_2$. There was minimal variation between three tests performed over a short period of time in both groups. Thus, the reproducibility with CPET is far superior to the "training effect" observed with exercise duration during non-CPET exercise testing for determination of functional capacity.

## Potential Limitations

Cardiopulmonary stress testing requires a skilled staff that possesses a high degree of knowledge in the setup and operation of the automated expired gas analyzer system, as well as knowledge of the various respiratory variables obtained during testing. In addition, a patient must be encouraged to give his or her best effort so that an accurate assessment of maximal function capacity (peak $VO_2$) may be obtained. Many patients require some familiarization with the equipment before the test. This can often be accomplished during the collection of resting data in most patients. Finally, these tests require more time than a routine stress test and there is increased cost associated with the expired gas analyzer.

# INFORMATION OBTAINED FROM GAS EXCHANGE DURING EXERCISE

## Important Physiologic Variables

There are a number of measured and derived physiologic variables from CPET that have been shown to have physiologic, diagnostic, and prognostic value in patients with cardiovascular diseases (**Table 19-1**).

### Maximal (Peak) $VO_2$

*Maximal* $VO_2$ was the classic parameter for describing exercise capacity, and the value achieved depends on age, gender, degree of fitness, genetic influences, altitude, medication, and presence of cardiovascular disease. $VO_2$ is directly related to both cardiac output and peripheral $O_2$ extraction by the Fick equation, but in most situations it is more a reflection of cardiac output than peripheral factors. The original definition of $VO_2$ max required that there was no further increase in $VO_2$ (150 mL/min or 2.1 mL/Kg/min) despite an increase in workload at high intensity exercise. However, this criterion was established with interrupted exercise protocols and a plateau in $VO_2$ has been demonstrated to be less common with graded exercise protocols. In addition, most patients are unable to maintain high intensity exercise of sufficient duration for a plateau to occur. Thus, this term has been replaced by *peak* $VO_2$ in most clinical situations, which refers to the highest attained $VO_2$ during the last 30 seconds of exercise.

| Table 19-1 • Measured and Derived Variables from CPET |
| --- |
| **Maximal oxygen uptake (VO$_2$)** Highest attainable $VO_2$ with no further increase despite increase in workload (expressed as mL/kg/min or mL/min) |
| **Peak oxygen uptake (peak VO$_2$)** Highest attainable $VO_2$ in last 20-30 sec of exercise (mL/kg/min) |
| **Respiratory exchange ratio (RER)** Ratio of $VCO_2/VO_2$; indicator of intensity of exercise at peak |
| **Oxygen pulse** Amount of oxygen consumed per volume of blood delivered to by each heartbeat; surrogate of stroke volume (expressed as mL $O_2$/beat) |
| **Circulatory power** Peak $VO_2 \times$ Systolic BP; surrogate of cardiac power; noninvasive estimate of cardiac work at peak exercise; (expressed as mm Hg $\cdot$ mLO$_2$/kg/min |
| **Ventilatory threshold** $VO_2$ at which there is a nonlinear increase in ventilation with progressive workloads; indicates imbalance between lactate production and removal; (expressed as mL/kg/min; % peak $VO_2$) |
| **V$_E$/VCO$_2$ slope** Indicator of ventilatory efficiency for removal of $CO_2$; reflects, respiratory control and determines excess ventilation; measured during submaximal exercise (expressed as integer for ratio) |
| **Oxygen uptake efficiency slope** OUES; ventilatory equivalent for $VO_2$; logarithmic relationship between ventilation and $VO_2$; integrates cardiac and respiratory function during submaximal exercise (expressed as integer) |
| **Breathing reserve** Reserve capacity of the respiratory system at peak exercise; (1 − peak $V_E$ − MVV) (expressed in percent); normal >30% |

An example of the behavior of $VO_2$ during exercise and recovery is demonstrated in **Figure 19-1(A)**. It is usually expressed relative to body weight as mL/kg/min. However, *absolute* $VO_2$, expressed in mL/min, is more representative of actual work performed than $VO_2$ and is directly related to cardiac output and arteriovenous $O_2$ content difference in the Fick equation. In very obese patients, the weight-corrected peak $VO_2$ may be misleading, as adipose tissue usually doesn't contribute to $O_2$ consumption during exercise. Several studies have reported peak $VO_2$ adjusted for lean body mass, as determined by body fat analysis, as a more accurate descriptor of exercise capacity, with potential clinical applicability for prognosis in heart failure patients. Peak $VO_2$ declines by 8-10% per decade of age in unfit and 5% in fit subjects. Peak $VO_2$ is about 10% higher in men than in women. Thus, age and gender are important factors in peak $VO_2$ evaluation in a clinical setting. Several formulas have been developed, based on age, gender, weight, and

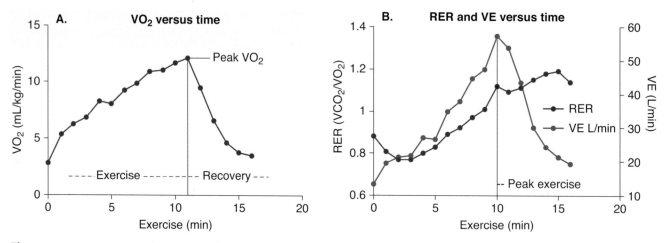

**Figure 19-1.** (A) Response of VO$_2$ over time during exercise and in recovery in a patient with left ventricular systolic dysfunction. Note the absence of a plateau in VO$_2$ at peak exercise. (B) Response of minute ventilation (V$_E$) and respiratory exchange ratio (RER) during exercise and in recovery in the same patient.

height, for helping researchers obtain a *normal predicted value* of peak VO$_2$ in a given population (**Table 19-2**). Usually, peak VO$_2$ is considered to be abnormal if it is less than 85% of the predicted normal value.

### Respiratory Exchange Ratio (RER)

Respiratory exchange ratio is the ratio of VCO$_2$ to VO$_2$, and at peak exercise it serves as an indicator of exercise intensity. Usually, the RER at peak exercise is 1.20 ± 0.1; however, there is no actual value that indicates maximal exercise. At rest, the RER is usually 0.70 to 0.85. Higher values can be

related to hyperventilation or decompensated heart failure. A very low value of <0.50 may indicate a problem with calibration of one of the gas analyzers used in a particular case. Early during exercise, the RER often decreases below the resting value and then gradually increases during incremental exercise (**Figure 19-1(B)**). The RER exceeds 1.0 when ventilation and thus VCO$_2$ exceeds VO$_2$ at a given workload, and it reflects buffering of lactate at higher intensity exercise. In the recovery period after exercise, the RER often rises further due to continued respiratory removal of CO$_2$, especially after vigorous, high intensity exercise.

| Table 19-2 • Normal Values for Peak Oxygen Uptake and Ventilatory Parameters during CPET | | |
|---|---|---|
| **Peak VO$_2$** | **Normal values (regression equations)** | |
| Treadmill: Bruce protocol[1] | Male: | 58.33 − 0.457 × age |
| | Female: | 41.3 − 0.333 × age |
| Treadmill: average body wt[2] | Male: | wt × (56.36 − 0.413 × age) |
| | Female: | wt × (44.37 − 0.413 × age) |
| Treadmill: overweight[2] | Male: | 0.79(ht − 60.7)(56.36 − 0.413 × age) |
| | Female: | 0.79(ht − 68.7)(44.37 − 0.413 × age) |
| Cycle: average body wt[2] | Male: | wt × (50.72 − 0.372 × age) |
| | Female: | (42 + wt)(22.78 − 0.17 × age) |
| Cycle: overweight[2] | Male: | [0.79 (ht − 60.7] × [50.72 − 0.372 × age] |
| | Female: | [0.79 (ht − 68.2)] × [44.37 − 0.413 × age] |
| **Ventilatory parameters** | | |
| VO$_2$ at ventilatory threshold[3] | | 40-80% peak VO$_2$ |
| V$_E$/VCO$_2$ slope[4] | | 26.3 + 4.1(SD) |
| OUES[5] | Male: | 1320 − (26.7 × age) + (1394 × BSA) |
| | Female: | 1175 − (15.8 × age) + (841 × BSA) |

*Wt, weight in kg; Ht, height in cm; BSA, body surface area; SD, standard deviation.*
[1]*Hossack and Bruce, 1980, 1981*
[2]*Hansen and Wasserman, 1984, 2005*
[3]*Wasserman et al., 2005*
[4]*Chua et al., 1997*
[5]*Hollenburg et al., 2000*

## Oxygen Pulse

Oxygen pulse is the ratio of $VO_2$ to heart rate and is expressed as mL $O_2$ /beat and not ml/min. It is derived from the Fick equation and is equal to the product of stroke volume with arteriovenous $O_2$ content difference. Arteriovenous $O_2$ content difference as a reflection of peripheral $O_2$ extraction is usually maximal and constant at peak exercise; therefore, oxygen pulse is a surrogate for stroke volume. Oxygen pulse will be lower in any condition with a reduced stroke volume or with a reduced arterial $O_2$ content, such as hypoxemia or anemia.

## Circulatory Power

Circulatory power is the product of peak $VO_2$ and systolic blood pressure and is a noninvasive surrogate of cardiac power, which is the product of cardiac output and mean arterial pressure. Invasive hemodynamic exercise testing in heart failure patients has demonstrated enhanced prognostic value with both left ventricular stroke work index [(mean arterial pressure – PWCP) × SVI × 0.0136] and cardiac power. (PWCP is pulmonary capillary wedge pressure.) Thus circulatory power is being investigated in heart failure patients as an outcome with certain therapies and as a prognostic tool. It combines expired gas measurement with noninvasive hemodynamic information to enhance the determination of cardiac function during exercise.

## Ventilatory Threshold

Ventilatory threshold is the highest attained $VO_2$ during progressive exercise without a significant rise in blood lactate concentration. This has also been described as the anaerobic threshold, although recent physiologic information indicates that the cell does not have to be under anaerobic conditions for this threshold to occur. At this threshold there is an increase in both $V_E$ (minute ventilation) and $VCO_2$ ($CO_2$ production) due to the need for buffering of hydrogen ion associated with an imbalance between lactate production and removal. Thus, $VCO_2$ and $V_E$ increase out of proportion to $VO_2$. Exercise performed significantly above this workload does not result in a physiologic steady state, and there are progressive increases in hemodynamic, metabolic, and sympathetic factors that lead to fatigue and cessation of exercise.

The most consistent determination of the $VO_2$ at the ventilatory threshold is the utilization for the V-slope method developed by Beaver, Wasserman, and Whipp (**Figure 19-2(A)**). $VCO_2$ is plotted on the y-axis and $VO_2$ on the x-axis. The point where this relationship is no longer linear represents the threshold. An alternative method involves the use of the *ventilatory equivalents* for $VO_2$ and $VCO_2$ ($V_E/VO_2$; $V_E/VCO_2$). These ventilatory equivalents increase in parallel throughout exercise until the ventilatory threshold, when $V_E/VO_2$ is increased with no change in $V_E/VCO_2$ (**Figure 19-2(B)**). This represents excessive ventilation due to increased $CO_2$ production and is no longer solely related to the rise in ventilation with progressive exercise. This method has more variability than the V-slope method and is often used as a secondary, confirmatory method. The software on most automated CPET equipment allows the determination of the ventilatory threshold without offline analysis.

## $V_E/VCO_2$ (Ventilatory Equivalent for $CO_2$)

*Ventilatory equivalent for* $CO_2$ is the relationship between minute ventilation and $CO_2$ production by metabolically active tissues. In certain conditions, such as heart failure, this ratio is elevated, indicating excessive ventilation for a given amount of $CO_2$. Factors such as chemoreceptor sensitivity, ventilation-perfusion mismatch in the lung, sympathetic activity, and acid-base status may affect this ratio. This ratio usually decreases from resting values at the beginning of exercise and does not significantly change until near maximal exercise, when additional ventilation is required to compensate for metabolic acidosis (respiratory compensation point). $T_h$ is termed the *respiratory compensation point*. The slope of the ventilatory equivalent for $CO_2$ ($V_E/VCO_2$ slope) can be determined from the onset of exercise to the respiratory compensation point. It is quite linear and has a high correlation coefficient. It is obtained by plotting the $V_E$ in L/min on the y-axis and $VCO_2$ in mL/min on the x-axis (**Figure 19-2(C)**). This slope is increased in patients with heart failure and congenital heart disease and has been shown to have significant prognostic value in these patient groups. A reduction of less than 10% in the $V_E/VCO_2$ with early exercise has also been shown to be associated with poor functional capacity in heart failure patients. The advantage of this ventilatory parameter is the ability to obtain this information without requiring near-maximal exercise performance in patients with cardiovascular disease.

## Oxygen Uptake Efficiency Slope (OEUS)

$V_E/VO_2$, the *ventilatory equivalent for* $O_2$, represents the ventilatory requirement for a given amount of $VO_2$ or workload. It is a measure of ventilatory efficiency: a high value indicates excessive ventilation. This relationship is nonlinear during exercise, since ventilation increases disproportionately to $VO_2$ at higher levels of work due to buffering of $CO_2$. The determination of this slope does not require attaining near maximal exercise; however, there is a strong correlation between OUES and peak $VO_2$ in the determination of exercise capacity.

$$VO_2 = a \log_{10} V_E + b,$$

where $a$ is the *oxygen uptake efficiency slope (OUES)*. This can be plotted on a graph with $VO_2$ in mL/min on the y-axis and $\log_{10}V_E$ on the x-axis (**Figure 19-2(D)**). This relationship is affected by the ratio of dead space to tidal volume in the lung, metabolic $CO_2$ production, and the arterial $CO_2$ set point. It has the advantage of not requiring maximal exercise; however, there is a strong correlation with peak $VO_2$.

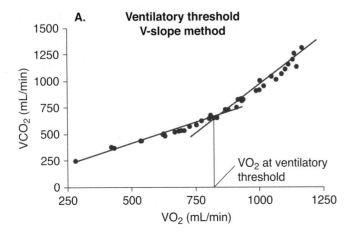

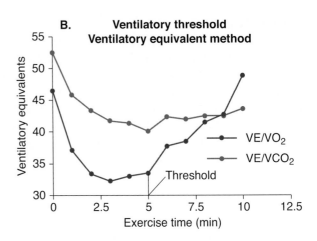

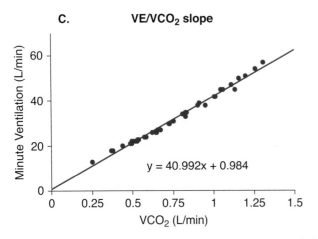

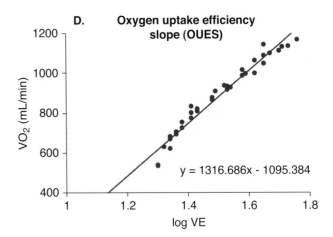

**Figure 19-2.** (A) Determination of VO₂ at the ventilatory threshold in a patient with LV systolic dysfunction using the V-slope method of Beaver, Wasserman, and Whipp. (B). Determination of the ventilatory threshold using the ventilatory equivalents of VO₂ and VCO₂ in the same patient with LV systolic dysfunction. The VO₂ at the designated exercise time from the x-axis of this graph is the VO₂ at the ventilatory threshold. (C) Determination of the $V_E/VCO_2$ slope using exercise data only in a patient with LV systolic dysfunction. In this patient there was no respiratory compensation point and all the exercise values of VCO₂ and $V_E$ were used. The slope is 40.99 using the enclosed regression equation. (D) Determination of the oxygen uptake efficiency slope (OUES) in a patient with LV systolic dysfunction. All exercise data for VO₂ and $V_E$ were used in this analysis. The slope is 1317 mL/min or 1.32 L/min.

The OUES has been shown to have good diagnostic and prognostic value in several studies of heart failure patients. Currently, this measurement requires offline analysis on most automated CPET systems.

### Breathing Reserve

*Breathing reserve* indicates the ventilatory reserve that remains at peak exercise. It is determined by subtracting the minute ventilation at peak exercise from the *maximal voluntary ventilation* (MVV) determined on a resting pulmonary function test. Breathing reserve is determined as $(1 - \text{peak exercise } V_E - MVV)$. Normally the breathing reserve should be 20-30% as most patients only achieve 60-80% of their maximal voluntary ventilation during exercise and are limited primarily by cardiovascular factors. Since MVV is often

not determined on routine pulmonary function tests, it can be approximated by $FEV_1 \times 41$.

### Normal Values

In order to interpret the results of CPET, some reference to normal values in the population are required to determine the magnitude of functional impairment. Most information is available on peak VO₂. Age, gender, and the exercise testing device are most important in assessing any variation from normal. The weight and height of a patient are also important, especially when there is a significant deviation from average anthromorphic features. **Table 19-2** contains the regression equations derived from several exercise laboratories for prediction of peak VO₂. The studies by Hossack and Bruce involved the

*Bruce treadmill protocol*, which is commonly used in cardiac testing laboratories. The other regression equations were derived by Hanson and Wasserman in normal and overweight men and women exercising on either a treadmill or cycle ergometer. Any value of peak $VO_2$ less than 85% predicted is usually considered abnormal. Normal values for several ventilatory parameters are also included; however, there are fewer studies available in normal subjects for these measurements.

# INDICATIONS FOR CPET

## American Heart Association/American College of Cardiology Guidelines

The 2002 AHA/ACC Guidelines further define the potential usefulness of CPET in the evaluation and treatment of patients with cardiovascular diseases (**Table 19-3**). These guidelines are based on available scientific evidence and not just theoretical principles. In practical terms, the initial clinical workup of patients with many of the indications for CPET starts with routine diagnostic

| Table 19-3 • ACC/AHA Guidelines Summary for Exercise Testing with Ventilatory Gas Analysis* ||
| --- | --- |
| **Strength of Indication** | **Indications** |
| Class I (Good evidence) | 1. Evaluation of exercise capacity and response to therapy in patients with heart failure who are being considered for heart transplantation<br>2. Assistance in the differentiation of cardiac versus pulmonary limitations as a cause of exercise-induced dyspnea or impaired exercise capacity when the cause is uncertain |
| Class IIa (Weight of evidence/opinion is in favor) | 1. Evaluation of exercise capacity when indicated for medical response in patients in whom the estimates of exercise capacity from exercise test time or work rate are unreliable |
| Class IIb (Efficacy less established) | 1. Evaluation of the patient's response to specific therapeutic intervention in which improvement of exercise tolerance is an important goal or endpoint<br>2. Determination of the intensity for exercise training as part of comprehensive cardiac rehabilitation |
| Class III (Not recommended) | 1. Routine use to evaluate exercise capacity |

*From Gibbons RJ, Balady GJ, Bricker JT, et al. ACC/AHA 2002 Guideline Update for Exercise Testing.*

approaches—history, physical examination, radiologic studies, electrocardiograms, and echocardiograms. The use of CPET as a diagnostic tool is limited when unanswered questions remain in these areas. The ACC/AHA guidelines for CPET highlight the necessity of basic clinical data.

# CLINICAL APPLICATIONS

## Evaluation of Dyspnea

Dyspnea on exertion is a common symptom with both cardiac and respiratory diseases. Although resting studies of pulmonary and cardiac function are useful in determining the cause of exertional dyspnea, many patients have both cardiac and pulmonary disease. In these patients a determination of the major cause of dyspnea will define the more appropriate therapy to alleviate symptoms. In addition, factors such as obesity, deconditioning, anxiety, and anemia can also cause exertional dyspnea with no evidence of underlying cardiopulmonary disease. Several measurements obtained during CPET can be useful in the evaluation of dyspnea occurring with either cardiac or pulmonary disease (**Table 19-4**).

Usually the peak $VO_2$ is reduced by at least 15-20% with either disorder, although it is important to evaluate RER at peak exercise. If the RER value is <1.10, and especially <1.0, the exercise effort is probably submaximal and the peak $VO_2$ would be falsely low. If the peak $VO_2$ is normal, then other causes for exertional dyspnea, such as anxiety, obesity, or mild disease, may be present. In a very obese patient, the $VO_2$ relative to body weight will be falsely low. In that case using either a regression formula for obese subjects or correcting the $VO_2$ for lean body mass as determined by the three-site skinfold method, will ascertain whether peak exercise capacity is reduced. Measurement of the ventilatory threshold is also important in the determination of the cause of dyspnea, although the $VO_2$ at the ventilatory threshold can be low (<40% peak $VO_2$) with either disorder. If the ventilatory threshold is normal, the cause for

| Table 19-4 • Cardiac versus Respiratory Causes of Dyspnea: CPET Findings |||
| --- | --- | --- |
| **Measurement** | **Cardiac** | **Respiratory** |
| Peak $VO_2$ | low | low |
| Ventilatory threshold | low | normal/low |
| Breathing reserve | normal | low |
| $V_E/VCO_2$ slope | increased | increased |
| OUES | decreased | decreased |
| Oxygen saturation | normal | decreased |

dyspnea is more likely to be pulmonary or a noncardiopulmonary condition. Those patients who are unable to attain a measurable ventilatory threshold usually have a noncardiac cause for their dyspnea.

The breathing reserve is the most useful measurement for determining the cause of dyspnea. A low breathing reserve (<20%) suggests a pulmonary cause for the dyspnea. In patients with a low ventilatory threshold and a low breathing reserve, often both cardiac and pulmonary causes are present. Patients with a primary cardiac cause for dyspnea, or those with noncardiopulmonary causes, usually have a normal breathing reserve. Finally, the determination of arterial oxygen saturation by pulse oximetry during exercise provides important information adjunctive to the expired gas analysis results. Most patients with cardiac disease do not develop oxygen desaturation with exercise, except with decompensated heart failure or an intracardiac right to left shunt. Even patients with advanced heart failure secondary to severe LV systolic dysfunction usually do not develop oxygen desaturation during exercise unless they are significantly volume overloaded. Arterial oxygen desaturation during exercise in a stable heart failure patient taking amiodarone should prompt an evaluation for drug toxicity.

## Chronic Heart Failure

Patients with heart failure clearly have limitations in their exercise capacity, with exertional dyspnea and fatigue being prominent symptoms. Resting measurements of cardiac systolic dysfunction are not predictive of exercise capacity. Weber's 1982 landmark study demonstrated that patients with greater functional limitations had lower cardiac outputs, lower stroke volumes, and higher wedge pressures. $VO_2$ max was used to stratify patients into four functional classes and the response of $VO_2$ correlated closely with alterations in cardiac output and filling pressures. Most of the change in peak $VO_2$ could be explained by changes in cardiac output with good separation of the four functional groups by the cardiac output response to exercise (**Table 19-5**). Thus, by application of the Fick principle, $VO_2$ measured during exercise

closely correlated to the cardiac output response, and this respiratory measurement became an important surrogate of cardiac responses during exercise in heart failure patients.

CPET was used in the first two Veterans Administration Heart Failure Trials (V-HeFT), and patients with a peak $VO_2 < 14.5$ mL/kg/min had twice the mortality of those with greater values. The prognostic value of CPET became clear with Mancini's 1991 study of 114 patients referred for cardiac transplantation. Patients with a peak $VO_2 < 14$ mL/kg/min had a poorer survival rate. With multivariate analysis, peak $VO_2$ was an independent predictor of outcome, and the authors suggested that this exercise measurement could be used to decide which patients were too well for transplant. This study subsequently led to the widespread use of CPET in heart failure centers, with many centers using a peak $VO_2 < 14$ mL/kg/min as one of the eligibility criteria for cardiac transplant. In addition, peak $VO_2$ has been used in combination with the variables of coronary disease, resting heart rate, left ventricular ejection fraction (LVEF), mean arterial pressure, QRS widening, and serum sodium as part of a heart failure survival score to determine prognosis in patients with severe HF.

Additional studies have confirmed the value of peak $VO_2$ in determining prognosis in patients with heart failure secondary to LV systolic dysfunction. However, an absolute value of peak $VO_2$ in determining prognosis has been found to have several limitations. Clearly a near maximal effort is required to obtain a valid determination. Peak $VO_2$ is also influenced by gender and may be falsely low in obese patients. Peak $VO_2$ has been corrected for lean body mass (LBM) in obese patients and a value of <19 mL/kg/min LBM has been shown to be a prognostic threshold. In a study of 594 patients with advanced heart failure, female patients had a lower peak $VO_2$, but a higher one-year transplant-free survival (94 vs. 81%). Since gender, age, body composition, and degree of physical conditioning of patients can affect peak $VO_2$, equations for determining the predicted peak $VO_2$ based on these parameters have been reported (**Table 19-2**). Using these prediction tools, the percent achieved of predicted peak $VO_2$ has been proposed

| **Table 19-5 • Weber Functional Classification of Heart Failure by CPET Parameters** | | | | |
|---|---|---|---|---|
| Severity | Class | Peak $VO_2$ | $VO_2$ at Vt | Peak Cardiac Index |
| None to mild | A | >20 | >14 | >8 |
| Mild to moderate | B | 16–20 | 11–14 | 6–8 |
| Moderate to severe | C | 10–16 | 8–11 | 4–6 |
| Severe | D | <10 | 5–8 | 2–4 |
| Very severe | E | <6 | <4 | <2 |

*$VO_2$ in mL/kg/min; cardiac index in L/min/m²*
*Data derived from Weber and Janicki, 1986.*

as an alternative index to equate the effect of these factors on the value of peak $VO_2$. In a retrospective study of 181 patients with advanced heart failure a peak $VO_2 \leq 50\%$ predicted $VO_2$ max had a lower 1-year and 2-year survival rate compared to patients with >50% predicted peak $VO_2$. Multivariate analysis suggested percent predicted peak $VO_2$ was the most significant predictor of cardiac death or status 1 (urgent) transplant priority.

Noncardiac factors, such as patient motivation, muscle deconditioning, gait instability, and arthritis, can also reduce exercise capacity. Reduced peak $VO_2$ in such patients may lead to the overestimation of severity of heart failure. In a study of 64 patients with severe heart failure severity, indicating eligibility for cardiac transplant, CPET was combined with invasive hemodynamic exercise testing to determine the relationship between peak $VO_2$ and peak exercise PWCP and cardiac output. Some patients with a low peak $VO_2$ had a near-normal hemodynamic response to exercise, while other patients with a favorable peak $VO_2$ (>14 mL/kg/min) had abnormal hemodynamic responses, indicating more severe cardiac dysfunction. These data and others have led to the development of equipment to noninvasively measure cardiac output during exercise to potentially improve the prognostic value of expired gas data at peak exercise. Inert gas rebreathing is currently being investigated in this regard in chronic heart failure patients.

Given the limitations of peak $VO_2$ in assessing prognosis in heart failure patients, there are a number of additional parameters that are derived from CPET that provide important additional prognostic information (**Table 19-6**).

### Table 19-6 • Prognostic Variables of CPET that Predict Poor Prognosis in Heart Failure

| Prognostic Variable | Cut-Point for Poor Prognosis |
| --- | --- |
| Peak $VO_2$ prior to use of beta-blockers | <14 mL/kg/min |
| Peak $VO_2$ on beta-blockers (?) | <10 mL/kg/min |
| Peak $VO_2$ adjusted for lean body mass (LBM) | <19 mL/kg/min LBM |
| Percent predicted peak $VO_2$ | <50% |
| $VO_2$ at ventilatory threshold | <11 mL/kg/min |
| $V_E/VCO_2$ slope | >34 |
| Peak exercise $PaCO_2$ | <35 mm Hg |
| Vd/Vt | >0.22 |
| $PETCO_2$ at ventilatory threshold | <36 mm Hg |
| Oxygen uptake efficiency slope (OUES) | <1.47 L/min |
| Exertional oscillatory ventilation | >60% of exercise with amplitude >15% |

The $VO_2$ at the ventilatory threshold has been reported to be a better predictor of high risk for early mortality compared to peak $VO_2$. Patients with a $VO_2 < 11$ mL/kg/min at the ventilatory threshold had a fivefold increased risk of early death. Patients with heart failure also have an increased ventilatory response to exercise. The exact mechanisms for this abnormal response are still unclear, but may include hemodynamic abnormalities causing reduced pulmonary perfusion and subsequent ventilation-perfusion mismatching and heightened sympathetic nervous system activity resulting in altered control of ventilation by enhanced sensitivity and activation of chemoreceptors and ergoreceptors. During CPET, the ventilatory response to exercise can by characterized by the minute ventilation/carbon dioxide output slope ($V_E/VCO_2$ slope). Patients with heart failure and no pulmonary disease had an elevated $V_E/VCO_2$ slope, compared to normal subjects. This elevated value of the $V_E/VCO_2$ slope was associated with reduced cardiac output, increased wedge pressures, and worse survival. Patients with a $V_E/VCO_2$ slope <34 had an 18-month event-free survival of 98% compared with 73% for those with a $V_E/VCO_2$ slope >34. One advantage of measuring the $V_E/VCO_2$ slope is that it can be assessed at submaximal exercise, which is valuable as patients with advanced heart failure are often unable to achieve peak exercise to determine a peak $VO_2$. The $V_E/VCO_2$ slope is related to the physiologic dead space (Vd) to tidal volume (Vt) ratio and arterial $CO_2$ partial pressure ($PaCO_2$). A low peak exercise $PaCO_2$ (<35 mm Hg) and a high Vd/Vt ratio (>0.22) have been shown to be predictors of poor outcomes in heart failure. In patients without significant pulmonary disease, a noninvasive estimate of $PaCO_2$ can be obtained by a measurement of the partial pressure of *end-tidal* $CO_2$ ($P_{ET}CO_2$). Low $P_{ET}CO_2$ values at rest and with exercise ($P_{ET}CO_2 < 36$ mm Hg at the ventilatory threshold) have been found to be predictors of cardiac-related events. Another prognostic indicator derived from the abnormal ventilatory response to exercise in patients with heart failure is the oxygen uptake efficiency slope (OUES). The OUES is derived from $VO_2$ and minute ventilation and a value of <1.47 L/min is a reliable indicator of poor prognosis in patients during submaximal exercise.

Finally, *exertional oscillatory ventilation (EOV)*, or periodic breathing, is sometimes witnessed in patients with heart failure during exercise. This spectrum of disordered breathing seen in patients with heart failure is associated with increased sympathetic activity and sudden death. Specific defining criteria for EOV have not been established. One study defined EOV as cyclic fluctuations in minute ventilation at rest that lasted more than 60% of exercise duration with amplitude of more 15% of average resting value. Using this definition of EOV in 323 patients with chronic heart failure who underwent CPET, EOV was found to be an independent predictor of major cardiac events. Thus, there are a number of ventilatory parameters obtained with CPET that imply poor prognosis in heart failure patients (**Table 19-6**).

The initial peak $VO_2$ and CPET data on prognosis in heart failure are limited since many studies were conducted before the routine use of beta-blockers in heart failure. Beta-blockers increase systolic function, reverse ventricular remodeling, improve quality of life, and decrease hospitalization. Despite these positive endpoints, a number of studies have shown no improvement in peak $VO_2$ with beta-blocker therapy. The precise mechanism for this lack of improvement in peak $VO_2$ with chronic beta-blockade in heart failure patients has not been determined. As beta-blockers are clearly standard of care in the treatment of heart failure, the prognostic value of peak $VO_2$ has come into question in the current era. Several studies investigating the effect of beta-blockade on the prognostic value of peak $VO_2$ in heart failure patients have demonstrated that outcome is improved with these drugs even when peak $VO_2$ is <14 mL/kg/min, the prior cutoff for poor prognosis. A study of patients receiving beta-blockers and undergoing CPET compared patients with a peak $VO_2$ > 14 mL/kg/min to those with a peak $VO_2 \leq$ 14 mL/kg/min groups. The patients in the low peak $VO_2$ group had lower ejection fractions, but no difference in event-free survival. The largest prospective study of the effect of beta-blockade on the prognostic value of peak $VO_2$ or percent predicted peak $VO_2$ was performed on 2105 patients at the Cleveland Clinic. There were no differences in peak $VO_2$ and peak $V_E/VCO_2$ values between patients on or off beta-blockers. Patients on beta-blockers had better outcomes even with peak $VO_2 \leq$ 14 mL/kg/min or at $\leq$50% predicted peak $VO_2$, but decreases in peak $VO_2$ were still predictive of death or transplantation in the beta-blocked group. Interestingly, the protective effect of beta-blockade was not evident at peak $VO_2 \leq$ 10 mL/kg/min, suggesting that this level may be the new threshold for referral for cardiac transplantation. Thus, current data suggest that peak $VO_2$ still has a role in prognosis, though perhaps lower cutoff values are needed.

The effects of beta-blockade on $V_E/VCO_2$ slope during exercise are uncertain, based on limited data. There may be a differential effect of beta-blockade on this ventilatory slope, based on clinical characteristics of the patients as one study demonstrated a reduction in the slope only in those patients with lower baseline ejection fractions and higher baseline brain naturetic peptide (BNP) levels. The largest study to date, on 614 patients with heart failure, indicated that patients receiving beta-blockers had improved $V_E/VCO_2$ slopes at both submaximal and maximal

exercise compared to those patients not receiving beta-blocker therapy. Further investigations are required to confirm these initial findings in order to determine if the measurement of $V_E/VCO_2$ slope may have important implications in gauging response to therapy and prognosis in patients with heart failure on beta-blockers, especially with the limited effects of this therapy on peak $VO_2$. To date, the effect of beta-blockade on other CPET variables, previously shown to have prognostic value, have not been evaluated.

*Cardiac resynchronization therapy* (CRT) has been shown to improve exercise capacity and reduce the risk of death or hospitalization in patients with chronic heart failure. CPET may have a prognostic role in these patients, as well. Among patients enrolled in the COMPANION trial exercise substudy who received CRT, a baseline peak $VO_2$ < 12.5 mL/kg/min predicted the clinical events of time to death, time to first hospitalization, and time to first heart failure hospitalization. Of note, 76% of these patients were being treated with beta-blockers, further illustrating the likely continued role for peak $VO_2$ in assessing prognosis in patients with heart failure utilizing current available therapy.

The vast majority of evidence with the use of CPET is related to patients with LV systolic dysfunction and resultant heart failure. Very little is known about the use of CPET in patients with heart failure with preserved systolic function. Recent data suggest that $V_E/VCO_2$ slope may have prognostic value in these patients, but further studies are needed.

## SUMMARY

Cardiopulmonary exercise testing is an important addition to the current diagnostic tests available to the cardiologist in the management of patients with cardiovascular disease. It allows a more precise and accurate determination of functional capacity, and it can provide useful information toward determining the cause of dyspnea in these patients. Its greatest utility has been in the area of heart failure, where several CPET variables have been used to determine prognosis and guide therapy. Use of this testing requires a more detailed knowledge of the physiology of exercise and the principles of gas exchange and respiration as it relates to the cardiovascular system. It is an integrated approach that considers the various components of oxygen transport during exercise, including circulation, respiration, and skeletal muscle function. This testing enhances the clinician's ability to evaluate functional capacity, natural history, and response to therapy in patients with cardiovascular diseases.

## Suggested Readings

1.  Arena R, Myers J, Williams MA, Gulati M, et al. Assessment of functional capacity in clinical and research settings: a scientific statement from the American Heart Association Committee on Exercise, Rehabilitation, and Prevention of the Council of Clinical Cardiology and the Council on Cardiovascular Nursing. *Circulation.* 2007;116:329–343.

2.  Gibbons RJ, et al. for the ACC/AHA Task Force on Practice Guidelines (Committee to update the 1997 Exercise Testing Guidelines). ACC/AHA 2002 guideline update for exercise testing: summary article: a report of the ACC/AHA Task Force on Practice Guidelines (Committee to Update the 1997 Exercise Testing Guidelines). *Circulation.* 2002;106:1883–1892.

3.  Mancini DM, Eisen H, Kussmaul W, et al. Value of peak exercise oxygen consumption for optimal timing of cardiac transplantation in ambulatory patients with heart failure. *Circulation.* 1991;83:778–786.

4.  Wasserman K, Hansen JE, Sue DY, et al. *Principles of Exercise Testing and Interpretation.* 4th ed. Philadelphia, Pa: Lippincott Williams & Wilkins; 2005.

5.  Weber KT, Kinasewitz GT, Janicki JS, et al. Oxygen utilization and ventilation during exercise in patients with chronic heart failure. *Circulation.* 1982;65:1213–1223.

# Preventive Cardiology

# 20

# Dyslipidemia

Keattiyoat Wattanakit and Amit Khera

## ● PRACTICAL POINTS

- Lipoproteins circulate in association with proteins called apolipoproteins; endogenous and exogenous metabolic lipid pathways control plasma lipid levels. Liver exports fat principally as VLDL.

- apo-B containing lipoprotein particles (LDL, small, dense LDL, IDL, VLDL, remnants) are atherogenic. HDL mediates "reverse cholesterol transport."

- Insulin-resistant states (obesity, prediabetes, and diabetes) are associated with "atherogenic" dyslipidemia: elevated TG, low HDL-C, and small, dense LDL predominance.

- Familial clustering of dyslipidemia is usually polygenic. Monogenic disorders do exist.

- Type III hyperlipoproteinemia is associated with elevated cholesterol and TG and is manifest by palmar (pathognomonic) or tuberoeruptive xanthomas.

- Types I and V hyperlipoproteinemia (very high TG levels) are associated with lipemia and increased incidence of pancreatitis.

- Therapeutic lifestyle changes have beneficial effects on all dyslipidemic patients: TG lowering and modest elevations in HDL-C are observed.

- ATP III endorse limiting dietary cholesterol to <200 mg/day, saturated fatty acids to <7%, and total fat to 25-35% of total daily calories.

- Statins predominantly lower LDL cholesterol; niacin lowers LDL-C, TG, and VLDL and is the most potent HDL-raising agent currently available; doubling statin dose usually results in an additional 6% LDL-C lowering.

- Fibric acid derivates, high dose fish oil supplements and niacin are effective in TG lowering.

## INTRODUCTION

Cardiovascular disease (CVD) has now emerged as the dominant chronic disease in many parts of the world. By 2020 it is predicted that CVD will surpass communicable diseases as the world's leading cause of morbidity and mortality. Over the past century, a series of observational and laboratory studies have implicated dyslipidemia as one of major risk factors for the development of atherosclerosis, and these findings have been confirmed by many large population-based studies. In the United States more than half of the adult population has elevated total cholesterol, and more than a quarter of adults have low HDL. A series of randomized controlled trials have demonstrated that lipid lowering therapies are beneficial in both primary and secondary prevention of CVD. This chapter will review the biology of lipids and lipoproteins and their role in atherosclerosis with emphasis on treatment strategies based on the current National Cholesterol Education Program, Adult Treatment Panel III Guidelines (NCEP-ATP III).

## LIPOPROTEIN METABOLISM

Lipids are a diverse group of fat soluble molecules that have structural and biochemical roles in the body and include cholesterol, cholesterol esters, triglycerides and phospholipids. They are packaged and transported in lipoproteins, which are spherical molecules consisting of a phospholipid shell and a core containing varying concentrations of cholesterol and triglycerides. There are five major lipoproteins and each serves a specific function and carries a variety of

| Lipoprotein Class | Major Lipid Component(s) | Apolipoprotein(s) |
|---|---|---|
| Chylomicron | TG | B-48, E, Cs |
| Chylomicron remnant | CE, TG | B-48, E |
| VLDL | TG | B-100, E, Cs |
| LDL | CE | B-100 |
| HDL | CE, PL | A-I, A-II |

**Table 20-1 • Classification of Lipoproteins and their Components**

VLDL, very low density lipoprotein; LDL, low density lipoprotein; HDL, high density lipoprotein; CE, cholesteryl-ester; TG, triglycerides; PL, phospholipid.

proteins (known as apolipoproteins) on its surface, which serve as regulatory agents, mediating lipoprotein trafficking and metabolism. These lipoproteins include high density lipoproteins (HDL), low density lipoproteins (LDL), intermediate density lipoproteins (IDL), very low density lipoproteins (VLDL), and chylomicrons. **Table 20-1** lists major lipid components and associated apolipoproteins for each lipoprotein class.

The metabolic pathways of plasma lipids can be divided into the exogenous and endogenous pathways. For the exogenous pathway, cholesterol and free fatty acids (FFA) are incorporated into chylomicrons in the gut. These particles are then delivered to skeletal muscle, adipose tissue, and other organs where apo C-II activates lipoprotein lipase to hydrolyze triglycerides of chylomicrons and release FFA for energy production and storage (**Figure 20-1**). After hydrolysis, residual cholesterol containing particles known as chylomicron remnants are returned to the liver. Smaller chylomicron remnants can also penetrate the vascular endothelium and may contribute to atherogenesis.

In the endogenous pathway, FFA and cholesterol synthesized and packaged in the liver are secreted as triglyceride-rich VLDL into the circulation (**Figure 20-2**). VLDL particles then acquire several apolipoproteins necessary for their function and metabolism, including apo C and apo E. Once at the surface of endothelium, VLDL undergoes hydrolysis by lipoprotein lipase to release FFA, resulting in a progressively increasing concentration of cholesterol. After hydrolysis, VLDL remnants (also known as IDL) can be taken up directly by liver through binding of apo E to the VLDL receptor. Alternatively, they can undergo further delipidation to form LDL particles with highly concentrated cholesterol esters, which are subsequently removed by the liver after binding to the LDL receptor. The hepatic uptake of LDL particles is determined by the cholesterol content in the liver. When hepatic

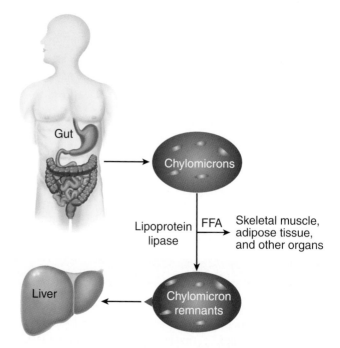

**Figure 20-1.** Exogenous pathway of lipid transport. Dietary cholesterol and free fatty acids (FFA) are incorporated into chylomicrons in the gut. Triglycerides are hydrolyzed by lipoprotein lipase in the capillaries to release FFA into several tissues, particularly adipose tissue. Chylomicron remnants are then removed from the circulation by the liver. (Adapted from *Textbook of Cardiovascular Medicine*. 3rd ed. London:Springer;2007.)

cholesterol content is high, the synthesis of the LDL receptor is suppressed, and hence less LDL cholesterol is internalized. The converse occurs when hepatic cholesterol content is low.

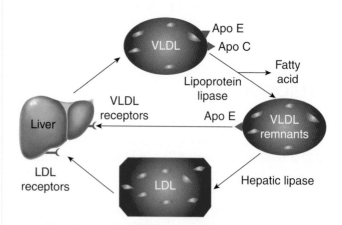

**Figure 20-2.** Endogenous pathway of lipid transport. Liver-derived cholesterol and free fatty acids are packed and secreted as triglyceride-rich VLDL. Hydrolysis of VLDL triglycerides by lipoprotein lipase liberates free fatty acids, leaving behind VLDL remnants. These remnants can either undergo further triglyceride hydrolysis to become the more dense LDL particles, or be taken up by apo E and LDL receptors in the liver. (Adapted from *Textbook of Cardiovascular Medicine*. 3rd ed.)

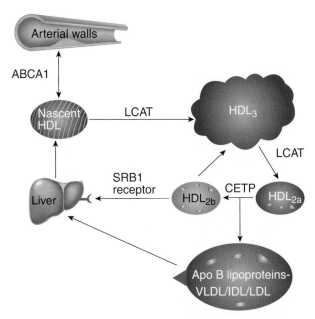

**Figure 20-3.** HDL metabolism and reverse cholesterol transport. Apolipoprotein A-1 synthesized in the liver and gut acquires phospholipid to become nascent HDL. Free cholesterol is then esterified by lecithin cholesterol acyl transferase (LCAT) to form mature HDL particles. Further cholesterol accumulation and esterification converts HDL$_3$ to HDL$_{2a}$. Cholesterol esters from HDL can either return to the liver via apo B containing lipoproteins after exchanges for triglycerides by the action of cholesterol-ester transfer protein (CETP) or by direct binding of HDL to the scavenger receptor type B1 (SRBI) on the liver. (Adapted from *Textbook of Cardiovascular Medicine*. 3rd ed.)

HDL metabolism intersects with the endogenous pathway in a process known as reverse cholesterol transport (**Figure 20-3**). Apo A-1 is synthesized by the liver and gut and acquires phospholipids to become a nascent, discoidal HDL. These particles scavenge free cholesterols from peripheral tissues and atherosclerotic plaques via the ATP-binding cassette transporter A1 (ABCA1), and the cholesterol is then esterified by lecithin cholesterol acyl transferase (LCAT) to form mature spherical HDL. Through the action of cholesterol-ester transport protein (CETP), the larger HDL particles, known as HDL$_2$, exchange cholesterol esters for triglycerides with apo B-containing lipoproteins (VLDL, IDL, and LDL). The net effect of removing and transferring cholesterol from peripheral cells to apo B-containing lipoproteins confers part of the antiatherogenic effect of HDL. These apo B-containing lipoproteins then deliver cholesterol back to the liver. HDL itself can also directly return cholesterol back to the liver by binding to the hepatic scavenger receptor type B1 (SRB1). CETP modified HDL$_2$ molecules are also converted to smaller HDL$_3$ through hydrolysis of triglyceride particles by hepatic lipase.

## ROLE OF LIPOPROTEINS IN ATHEROSCLEROSIS

LDL particles play a pivotal role in the initiation and propagation of atherosclerosis. Circulating LDL can infiltrate across the endothelium and undergo oxidation, subsequently promoting atherosclerosis in many ways. Oxidized LDL can attract circulating monocytes to enter the intima and convert them to activated macrophages. These activated macrophages then uptake oxidized LDL to become foam cells. When ruptured, foam cells release a variety of inflammatory factors, cytokines, and growth factors that promote smooth muscle cell proliferation and impair endothelial function and the integrity of the vessel wall. Furthermore, oxidized LDL can promote increased platelet aggregation, resulting in thrombus formation, and may play a role in plaque instability. LDL levels have consistently been shown to correlate with atherosclerosis risk and burden.

### LDL

VLDL mainly consists of endogenous triglycerides and, to a lesser degree, cholesterol. The contribution of hypertriglyceridemia in the development of atherosclerosis is uncertain. This is because hypertriglyceridemia is often associated with insulin resistance, low HDL, and obesity as well as other characteristics that make dissecting out the independent contribution of hypertriglyceridemia to atherosclerosis challenging. Indeed, genetic disorders resulting in markedly elevated levels of triglycerides only modestly increase cardiovascular risk. Nevertheless, a meta-analysis of population-based studies reported that hypertriglyceridemia was a modest risk factor for CHD after adjustment for HDL and other factors.

Hypertriglyceridemia alone may not be sufficient to promote atherosclerosis, but requires the presence of VLDL, which elevates to a variable degree in this setting. Several studies have demonstrated that VLDL and its remnants are related to atherosclerosis, and the added assessment of VLDL in the form of non-HDL cholesterol or total apo B may be superior to measurements of LDL cholesterol (LDL-C). In addition, recent studies have suggested that postprandial triglyceride measurements may correlate more closely with cardiovascular risk than fasting measures.

### HDL

In contrast to LDL and VLDL, HDL confers antiatherosclerotic properties. As described previously, the antiatherosclerotic effect of HDL comes from its ability to remove cholesterol from peripheral tissues and atherosclerotic plaques via reverse cholesterol transport. Moreover, HDL has ability to inhibit vascular inflammation, lipid oxidation, and plaque growth and thrombosis, further limiting progression of atherosclerosis. Epidemiologic studies have demonstrated a robust association between lower HDL cholesterol (HDL-C) levels and a higher risk of CV events such that a 1mg/dL decrease in HDL-C levels corresponds to a 3-4% absolute increase in CV outcomes. However, quantification of serum HDL-C levels does not capture the complexity of HDL biology including qualitative aspects such as HDL function, biochemical modification, and kinetics, which impact the use of HDL as a therapeutic target for CV risk reduction.

## Atherogenic Dyslipidemia

Insulin resistance states including diabetes and the metabolic syndrome are often accompanied by a characteristic lipid profile known as atherogenic dyslipidemia consisting of high triglyceride and low HDL-C levels, as well as a predominance of small, dense LDL particles. In such patients, many of whom are obese, adipose tissue releases FFA into the systemic circulation. In addition, in the setting of insulin resistance, lipoprotein lipase activity is reduced and there is decreased uptake of FFA by striated muscles, resulting in increased FFA levels delivered to the liver. The increased flux of FFA leads to increased hepatic production of triglyceride-rich VLDL. Via the action of CETP, high VLDL levels promote the exchange of triglycerides of VLDL for cholesterols from $HDL_2$, with subsequent hydrolysis of HDL triglycerides and metabolism of the remaining small, dense $HDL_3$ particles. Similar CETP-mediated exchanges occur between VLDL and LDL particles, resulting in small, dense LDL. Small, dense LDL particles are more atherogenic than large buoyant LDL as they can more easily infiltrate the arterial wall and promote atherosclerosis and are more readily oxidized. In such patients, traditional measures of serum LDL-C concentrations often underestimate the total number of LDL particles. Advanced lipoprotein measurements using nuclear magnetic resonance spectroscopy and other techniques may better quantify LDL particle concentration in such instances, but their value for clinical decision-making, especially relative to simpler measures such as non-HDL-C and apo B, are unproven (see Diagnosis of Dyslipidemia below).

# GENETIC CAUSES OF DYSLIPIDEMIA

Dyslipidemia can result from lifestyle factors and many secondary causes, although a familial predilection is quite common. Familial clustering of dyslipidemia is usually due to polygenic mechanism, but rarer, single-gene disorders also result in well-characterized forms of lipid disorders, the most common of which is *familial hypercholesterolemia* (FH) (Type II hyperlipidemia) (**Table 20-2**). This autosomal dominant disorder results from one of many mutations in the gene encoding the LDL receptor and manifests as elevated total cholesterol levels (350 to 500 mg/dL) with LDL-C levels >95th percentile in the heterozygote form affecting 1 in every 500 persons. Patients with this disorder experience premature CHD and have evidence of cholesterol deposits on exam, including tendinous xanthomas on extensor tendons, including the Achilles; corneal arcus; and xanthelasma, or soft fleshy cholesterol deposits near the eyelids. A rare, severe homozygous form affects 1 in 1,000,000 persons with resultant severe hypercholesterolemia (600 to 1000 mg/dL) and CHD developing in childhood. Treatment for FH involves dietary interventions as well as combination lipid-lowering therapies, but LDL apheresis is required in drug refractory cases, especially with malignant CHD. A related condition known as *familial defective apo B* can also result in markedly elevated levels of LDL-C and premature CHD, but such patients often lack xanthoma formation.

*Familial hypercholesterolemia* must also be differentiated from *familial combined hyperlipidemia*, which is a polygenic disorder affecting 1-2% of the population characterized by increased levels of total cholesterol and triglycerides. This disorder results from increased hepatic production of apo B and is present in 10-20% of patients with premature CHD.

| Table 20-2 • Fredrickson Classification of Hyperlipidemias | | | | |
|------|------|------|------|------|
| Type | Lipoprotein Elevations | Representative Disorder* | Lipid Levels | Atherogenicity |
| I | Chylomicrons | Familial chylomicronemia | ↑↑↑↑ TG | +/− |
| IIa | LDL | Familial hypercholesterolemia | ↑↑ TC | +++ |
| IIb | LDL and VLDL | Familial combined hyperlipidemia | ↑↑ TC, ↑↑ TG | +++ |
| III | VLDL remnants and chylomicrons | Dysbetalipoproteinemia | ↑↑ TC, ↑↑↑TG | +++ |
| IV | VLDL | Familial hypertriglyceridemia | ↑ TC, ↑↑TG | + |
| V | Chylomicrons and VLDL | | ↑ TC, ↑↑↑↑ TG | + |

*Representative disorders are provided; additional disorders may result in similar patterns of hyperlipidemia.*

A more rare but malignant condition, *familial dysbetalipoproteinemia*, also known as *broad beta disease* or *Type III hyperlipidemia*, is also characterized by elevated total cholesterol and triglycerides but is due to a defect in apo E. Patients with this disorder carry two copies of the E2 allele of the apo E gene, with decreased binding of VLDL remnants to the apo E receptor on the liver and premature atherosclerosis. On exam, these patients have characteristic tuberoeruptive xanthomas, or raised circular, fleshy lesions on extensor surfaces, and palmar striae or yellow streaked xanthomas in the palmar creases. Such patients can be identified by a VLDL-C to triglyceride ratio of >0.3.

Another more common disorder resulting in elevated triglyceride levels is *familial hypertriglyceridemia*, or Type IV hyperlipidemia, characterized by triglyceride levels between 200-500 mg/dL due to increased production of VLDL, and only a modest increase risk for CVD. This disorder has significant heterogeneity in presentation with a strong environmental component, including precipitating factors for hypertriglyceridemia such as metabolic syndrome, alcohol intake, and dietary factors. More severe elevations in triglyceride levels (>1000 mg/dL) can be found in *familial chylomicronemia* (Type I hyperlipidemia), which is caused by defective or absent lipoprotein lipase or apo C-II, or Type V hyperlipidemia, caused by overproduction and decreased lipolysis of VLDL and chylomicrons in association with insulin resistance states, obesity, and high fat diets. Patients with markedly elevated triglyceride levels often have lipemic serum due to increased chylomicrons, as well as eruptive xanthomas on extensor surfaces of the skin exam.

Low levels of HDL-C have been consistently associated with increased CHD rates and are commonly found in disorders of elevated triglycerides. Familial hypoalphalipoproteinemia is a genetically heterogenous disorder of primary low HDL levels which is caused by mutations in apo AI or in ABCA1. Homozygous mutations in ABCA1 result in a rare disorder known as *Tangier disease*, whose hallmarks are near absent HDL and enhanced cholesterol deposition resulting in enlarged orange tonsils, hepatosplenomegaly, peripheral neuropathy, and premature CHD. LCAT deficiency can also result in markedly low HDL levels as well as corneal deposits and anemia in an entity known as fish eye disease, but without a predisposition for premature CHD.

## DIAGNOSIS OF DYSLIPIDEMIA

Except for those with severe lipid disorders (i.e., familial hypercholesterolemia or Type I dyslipidemia), most patients presenting for evaluation for lipoprotein disorders lack symptoms. Nevertheless, they should undergo a comprehensive evaluation focusing on assessing global risk for CVD events, uncovering familial lipoprotein disorders, and

| Table 20-3 • Effects of Secondary Causes and Drugs on Lipoproteins ||
| --- | --- |
| **Secondary Causes** | **Effects on Lipoproteins** |
| Nephrotic syndrome | ↑ TC, TG and LDL |
| Diabetes | ↑ TG, ↓ HDL |
| Hypothyroidism | ↑ TC, TG and LDL |
| Hepatobiliary disease | ↑ TC, TG, and LDL |
| Alcoholism | ↑↑ TG, ↑ HDL |
| **Drugs** | |
| Thiazide diuretics | ↑ TC and TG |
| Beta-blockers | ↑ TG, ↓ HDL, no effect on LDL |
| Estrogens | ↑ TG and HDL, ↓ LDL |
| Anabolic steroids | ↑ TC, ↓ TG, ↓↓ HDL |
| Glucocorticoids | ↑ TC, TG and HDL |
| Antiretroviral therapy | ↑ TC and LDL, ↑↑TG, but effects are variable depending on agents used |
| Cyclosporine | ↑ TC and LDL, no effect on TG and HDL |

*TC, total cholesterol; LDL, low density lipoprotein; HDL, high density lipoprotein; TG, triglycerides*

evaluating for secondary causes. The clinical evaluation should include the following:

*History:* Clinicians should probe for a history of CHD, stroke/transient ischemic attack (TIA), and peripheral arterial disease (PAD), including carotid atherosclerosis, abdominal aneurysm, and intermittent claudication. Secondary causes, including nephrotic syndrome, diabetes, hypothyroidism, and hepatobiliary disease, should be excluded or suspected in patients who have developed refractory hyperlipidemia (**Table 20-3**).

*Medication history:* Various medications that can impact lipoprotein levels include thiazide diuretics, hormone replacement, glucocorticoids, oral contraceptive pills, and antiretroviral therapy (**Table 20-3**).

*Family history:* History of CHD, stroke/TIA, PAD, and sudden death, diabetes, and hypertension are relevant.

*Lifestyle history:* Excessive use of alcohol and tobacco use, sedentary lifestyle, and diet.

*Physical exam findings:* Physical examination should include a search for xanthomas (cholesterol deposits) in hands, elbows, knees, and Achilles tendons, xanthelasmas (cholesterol deposits in palpebral fissures), corneal arcus, and corneal opacification. If identified, primary disorders of LDL metabolism such as familial hypercholesterolemia and familial defective apolipoprotein B100 should be considered.

Body mass index (BMI), weight, waist circumference, and blood pressure should be recorded, and signs of vascular compromise should be evaluated, including carotid and renal artery bruits, and diminished peripheral pulses.

*Laboratory testing:* A standard serum lipid profile is generally sufficient for a diagnosis of lipoprotein disorders and is recommended at least every 5 years in all adults over 20 years of age. The lipid profile should be performed after 9-12 hours of fasting to minimize the influence of postprandial hypertriglyceridemia. Serum total and HDL-C can be measured in either fasting or nonfasting state. Once the total cholesterol, triglycerides, and HDL-C are known, the LDL-C can be calculated using the Friedwald formula:

$$LDL\text{-}C = \text{total cholesterol} - VLDL\text{-}C - HDL\text{-}C.$$

VLDL-C is assumed to be one-fifth of the total triglyceride concentration. This formula is valid only if the total triglyceride concentration is less than 400 mg/dL; otherwise, direct LDL-C measurements can be performed.

As mentioned, in patients with atherogenic dyslipidemia, measurement of LDL-C may underestimate the number of atherogenic lipoproteins. In this case, a more accurate marker for estimation of the atherogenic potential is to measure either serum total apo-B or to calculate non-HDL-C (this is equal to total cholesterol minus HDL-C), which accounts for all atherogenic lipoproteins, including VLDL-C and IDL, not just LDL. The acute phase response in the setting of an acute myocardial infarction (MI), surgical trauma, and infection is known to decrease serum concentrations of total cholesterol, HDL-C, LDL-C, and apo B-containing lipoproteins, and increase concentrations of triglycerides within several hours to days after the event. Thus, serum lipids should be measured several weeks after such stressors to provide more accurate values. Other tests that are recommended to exclude secondary causes of dyslipidemia include thyroid-stimulating hormone, creatinine, and liver function tests.

# TREATMENT STRATEGIES

Once secondary causes are excluded, the mainstay of treatment for dyslipidemia consists of *therapeutic lifestyle changes* (TLC) and *pharmacologic therapy*. Although challenging to implement, all patients with dyslipidemia are encouraged to participate in all aspects of TLC, including smoking cessation, dietary restriction, exercise, and weight loss. In motivated lower risk patients whose lipid levels are not markedly elevated, TLC can be attempted first. If goal LDL is not reached within 3 months, pharmacologic treatment should be considered. In higher risk patients such as those with established atherosclerotic disease or diabetes, concomitant early initiation of pharmacologic treatment is warranted. **Table 20-4** outlines the recommendations and effects of TLC on lipids.

## Therapeutic Lifestyle Changes

### Dietary Modification
In patients with dyslipidemia or atherosclerotic disease, the American Heart Association (AHA) and NCEP ATP III

| Table 20-4 • Effects of Therapeutic Lifestyle Changes on Lipids | | |
|---|---|---|
| **Components** | **Recommendation** | **Expected Change in Lipids** |
| Diet | | |
|   Saturated fat | <7% of total calories | ↓ LDL 8-10% |
|   Dietary cholesterol | <200 mg/day | ↓ LDL 3-5% |
|   Total fat | 25-35% of total calories | |
|   Carbohydrate | 50-60% of total calories | |
|   Dietary fiber | 20-30 g/day | |
|   Plant stanols/sterols | 2-3 g/day | ↓ LDL 6-15% |
|   Increased soluble fiber | 5-10 g/day | ↓ LDL 5% |
| Physical Activity | 200 kcal/day | ↓ TG 5-15% |
| | | ↓ TC 0-5% |
| | | ↓ LDL 0-3% |
| | | ↑ HDL 3-5% |
| Weight Loss | BMI <25 kg/m² | ↓ TG 7% |
| | | ↓ LDL 6% |
| | | ↓ TC 10% |
| | | ↑ HDL 8% |
| Smoking | Immediate cessation via counseling or pharmacologic treatment | ↑ HDL 5% |

*Adapted from the Third Report of the National Cholesterol Education Program (NCEP) Expert Panel on the Detection, Evaluation, and Treatment of High Blood Cholesterol in Adults (ATP III), 2001.*
*TC, total cholesterol; LDL, low density lipoprotein cholesterol; HDL, high density lipoprotein cholesterol; TG, triglycerides.*

endorse a low cholesterol and low saturated fat diet, with the goal of limiting dietary cholesterol to <200 mg/day, saturated fatty acids to <7%, and total fat to 25-35% of total daily calories, as well as limiting trans fatty acids to a minimum. The major sources of dietary cholesterol are egg yolks, animal fats, and meat, and saturated fatty acids are butter fat, animal fat, and tropical oils. Beyond these dietary restrictions, consuming 2 g/day of supplemental plant sterols/stanols preparations (see next section) and increasing viscous (soluble) fibers 5-10 g/day can reduce LDL 6-15% and 5%, respectively. In addition, foods rich in complex carbohydrates such as whole grains, fruits, and vegetables are preferred to those containing simple carbohydrates, especially for those with elevated triglyceride levels and insulin resistance.

### Exercise and Weight Loss

A regular exercise program can reduce the risk of CHD, and all adults should engage in a minimum of 30 minutes of moderately intense aerobic exercise (e.g., brisk walking) 5 times a week, or 150 minutes per week. Exercise alone in the absence of dietary changes or weight loss has modest effects on standard lipid parameters, predominantly increasing HDL-C and reducing triglycerides. However, physical activity may be more beneficial for atherogenic dyslipidemia, reducing small, dense LDL particles and increasing mean LDL particle size.

Weight loss can modestly lower LDL-C, and, by improving insulin resistance it lower triglyceride levels and raise HDL-C. In addition, other CVD risk factors such as hypertension, diabetes, and obstructive sleep apnea are improved. In a patient with morbid obesity, bariatric surgery and pharmacologic intervention such as orlistat, and sibutramine may be indicated. The long term goal of weight control is to achieve a body mass index (BMI) less than 25 kg/m².

## Pharmacologic Treatment

The six major classes of lipid lowering medications are:

1. 3-hydroxy-3-methyl-glutaryl-coenzyme (HMG-CoA) reductase inhibitor or statins,
2. bile acid sequestrants (or resins),
3. fibric acid derivatives,
4. nicotinic acid or niacin,
5. cholesterol absorption inhibitor,
6. omega-3 fatty acids.

The impact of various lipid-lowering medications on lipid levels is illustrated in **Table 20-5**.

### Statins

HMG-CoA reductase inhibitors, or *statins*, are the most commonly prescribed medications for the treatment of dyslipidemia. They are highly effective in lowering total and LDL cholesterol and can also lower triglycerides and

**Table 20-5 • Effects of Various Classes of Cholesterol Lowering Agents on Lipoprotein Metabolism**

| Drug Class | Lipoprotein Effects | |
|---|---|---|
| HMG CoA reductase inhibitors | LDL | ↓ 18-55% |
| | HDL | ↑ 5-15% |
| | TG | ↓ 7-30% |
| Ezetimibe | LDL | ↓ 17% |
| Fibric acids | LDL | ↓ 5-20% |
| | HDL | ↑ 10-20% |
| | TG | ↓ 20-50% |
| Bile acid sequestrants | LDL | ↓ 15-30% |
| | HDL | ↑ 3-5% |
| | TG | no change or increase |
| Nicotinic acids | LDL | ↓ 5-25% |
| | HDL | ↑ 15-35% |
| | TG | ↓ 20-50% |
| Omega-3 fatty acids* | LDL | variable effect |
| | Non-HDL | ↓ 9% |
| | TG | ↓ 29% |

*When combined simvastatin with omega-3 fatty acid 3-4 g/day LDL, low density cholesterol; HDL, high density cholesterol; TG, triglycerides.*

modestly raise HDL-C. The primary mechanism of statins is to inhibit hepatic HMG-CoA reductase, a rate-limiting enzyme in the production of cholesterol. Reduced hepatic cholesterol levels stimulate the synthesis of LDL receptors, resulting in increased removal of LDL and VLDL cholesterol from the circulation. Among the statins, rosuvastatin is the most potent, and fluvastatin is the least potent; knowledge of statin potency can aid in determining initial prescriptions based upon desired LDL lowering to achieve goals (**Figure 20-4**). As a rule of thumb, for every doubling of a statin dose, LDL is further reduced by 6%. This class of medications is generally very safe, with the most commonly encountered side effects of myopathy and elevation of liver function test, both of which are reversible with discontinuation of statins. In a patient with predisposing conditions to severe myopathy (**Table 20-6**), statins should be used with caution, or the dose modified, as the risk of myopathy is increased.

The benefits of statins are well documented in the primary and secondary prevention of CAD, including in high-risk populations such as those with acute coronary syndrome (ACS) and/or with diabetes. Details of the key clinical trials with primary outcomes and risk reduction are summarized in **Table 20-7**. The landmark trials for primary prevention are the West of Scotland Coronary Prevention Study (WOSCOP) and the Air Force/Texas Coronary Atherosclerosis Prevention Study (AFCAPS/TexCAPS). In the WOSCOP study, nearly 6600 middle-aged men with high LDL-C (mean 192 mg/dL) were randomized

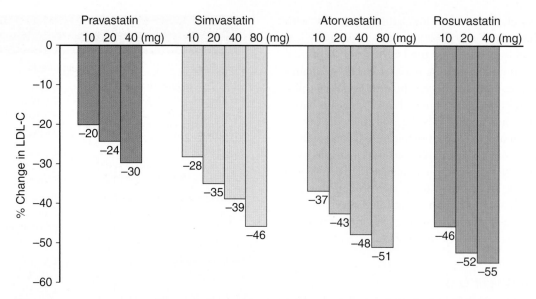

**Figure 20-4.** Comparative efficacy of various statins and doses on LDL-C reduction. (Adapted from Jones PH. *Am J Cardio.* 2003;92.)

to pravastatin 40 mg/day versus placebo. Compared with placebo, pravastatin significantly reduced the risk of coronary events (nonfatal MI or CHD death) by 31% and the need for coronary artery bypass grafting (CABG) or percutaneous transluminal coronary angioplasty by 37%. The AFCAPS/TexCAPS study extended the benefit of primary prevention to additional groups, including women and subjects >65 years of age, with "usual" average LDL-C (mean

150 mg/dL). Lovastatin (20-40 mg/day over 5.2 years) decreased the risk of first major coronary event (unstable angina, MI, or sudden death), fatal or nonfatal MI, and coronary revascularization. Taken together, both trials established the benefits of statins in the primary prevention of CHD in both men and women, even in subjects with average LDL.

The key statin trials for the secondary prevention of CHD include the Scandinavian Simvastatin Survival Study (4S), the Cholesterol and Recurrent Events (CARE), and the Long-Term Intervention with Pravastatin in Ischemic Disease (LIPID). All of these trials tested the hypothesis that statins would decrease hard clinical endpoints in men and women with known CHD, but they differed in the mean entry lipid values. The 4S trial enrolled subjects with higher lipid levels (mean LDL-C 188 mg/dL) than either CARE (mean LDL-C 139 mg/dL) or LIPID (median LDL-C150 mg/dL). Similar to the primary prevention trials, the findings from these trials demonstrated clear morbidity and mortality (except for CARE study) benefits of statins for secondary prevention, even in subjects with average LDL-C (CARE study) and in subjects who were on contemporary medications, including aspirin, beta-blockers, and antihypertensive medications (the LIPID study). The benefits of statins were seen in most if not all subgroups, including men and women, older and younger subjects, smokers and nonsmokers, hypertensive and normotensive subjects, and diabetic and nondiabetic subjects. It is important to note that these trials excluded high risk subjects such as those with symptomatic heart failure and those with low ejection fraction <25%. Of special note is the Heart Protection Study (HPS) of approximately 20,000 high risk adults with either

| Table 20-6 • Predisposing Conditions for Myopathy with Statin Therapy |
| --- |
| Very old (especially >80 years) patients |
| Small body frame and frailty |
| Multisystem disease |
| Multiple medications |
| Perioperative period |
| Fibrates |
| Nicotinic acid |
| Cyclosporine |
| Azole antifungals: itraconazole and ketoconazole* |
| Macrolide antibiotics: erythromycin and clarithromycin* |
| HIV protease inhibitors* |
| Verapamil* |
| Amiodarone* |
| Large quantities of grapefruit juice (usually >1 quart per day) |
| Alcohol abuse (independently predisposes to myopathy) |

*These drugs interact with statins metabolized by the cytochrome p450 3A4 system (lovastatin>simvastatin>atorvastatin).*
*Adapted from Pasternak, et al.. Circulation. 2002;106.*

## Table 20-7 • Landmark Statin Clinical Trials with Clinical Outcomes

| Trial | N; Yr | Drug, dose | Baseline LDL | Treated LDL 1° | Outcomes, RR% |
|---|---|---|---|---|---|
| **Primary prevention trials** | | | | | |
| WOSCOPS | 6595; 4.9 | Prava, 40 | 192 | 159 | NFMI, CHD death, ↓ 31% |
| AFCAPS/TexCAPS | 6605; 5.2 | Lova, 20-40 | 150 | 115 | NFMI, FMI, USA, SCD, ↓ 37% |
| **Secondary prevention trials** | | | | | |
| 4S | 4444; 5.4 | Simva, 20-40 | 188 | 122 | All-cause mortality, ↓ 30% |
| CARE | 4159; 5 | Prava, 40 | 139 | 98 | NFMI, FMI, ↓ 24%, no difference in all-cause mortality |
| LIPID | 9014; 6.1 | Prava, 40 | 150 | 110 | CHD death, ↓ 24% |
| **Recent clinical trials** | | | | | |
| HPS | 20,536; 6 | Simva, 40 | 128, M; 135, F | 89 | All-cause mortality, ↓ 18% |
| PROVE-IT | 4162; 2 | Atorva, 80 vs Prava, 40 | 133 | 62 vs 95 | All-cause mortality, MI, USA, revasc, CVA, ↓ 16% |
| A to Z | 4497; 2 | Simva, 40/80 vs placebo/20 | 112 | 63 vs 77 | CV death, NFMI, ACS, CVA, ↓ 11% (p = 0.14) |
| TNT | 10,001; 4.9 | Atorva, 80 vs Atorva, 10 | 98 | 80 vs 101 | CHD death, NFMI, SCD, CVA, ↓ 22% |
| CARDS | 2838; 3.9 | Atorva, 10 | 122 | 111 | ACS, revasc, CVA, ↓ 37% |
| ASCOT-LLA | 10,305; 3.3 | Atorva, 10 | 133 | 87 | FMI and CHD death, ↓ 36% |

*N, number; Yrs, duration of study; RR%, percent relative risk reduction; NFMI, nonfatal myocardial infarction; CHD, coronary heart disease; FMI, fatal myocardial infarction; USA, unstable angina; revasc, revascularization; CVA, stroke; ACS, acute coronary syndrome; SCD, sudden cardiac death.*

known atherosclerotic vascular disease or diabetes that were randomized to simvastatin 40 mg or placebo. After 5 years of therapy, simvastatin-treated subjects had a 13% reduction in mortality and 25% reduction in first vascular event. Importantly, these benefits were observed in all subgroups, including in those with LDL-C level of <100 mg/dL at baseline.

Extending the findings of HPS, recent statin trials have attempted to determine whether more aggressive lipid-lowering confers greater clinical benefits in patients with ACS, in patients with stable CHD, and in diabetic patients without significant elevation of LDL-C. The Pravastatin or Atorvastatin Evaluation and Infection (PROVE-IT) study, which randomized patients who had been hospitalized for ACS within the previous 10 days to intensive therapy (atorvastatin 80 mg/day, achieved median LDL 62 mg/dL) or standard therapy (pravastatin 40 mg/day, achieved median LDL 95 mg/dL), reported greater protection against death or major CV events in the intensive therapy arm than in the standard therapy arm. A similar trend for reduced CV events with aggressive lipid-lowering using high dose simvastatin after ACS was observed in the Aggrastat to Zocor (A to Z) study. Additionally, the Treating to New Targets (TNT) study randomized patients with stable CHD and LDL <130 mg/dL to high dose (atorvastatin 80 mg/day, achieved mean LDL 77 mg/dL) or low dose (atorvastatin 10 mg/day, achieved mean LDL 101 mg/dL) atorvastatin

groups. High dose atorvastatin significantly lowered the occurrence of any major CV event, but it did not lower total mortality.

Two recent primary prevention trials specifically assessed the value of statins in patients with diabetes and hypertension, but without significantly elevated LDL-C. The Collaborative Atorvastatin Diabetes Study (CARDS), enrolled diabetic patients without CHD and fasting LDL-C <160 mg/dL (mean LDL-C 117 mg/dL), and confirmed benefits of statins (atorvastatin 10 mg) in lowering the first major CV events in this population, defined as acute coronary events, coronary revascularization, or stroke. Similarly, the Anglo-Scandinavian Cardiac Outcomes Trial-Lipid Lowering Arm (ASCOT-LLA) demonstrated a significant reduction in the primary endpoint of fatal MI and nonfatal CHD in hypertensive patients with additional CV risk factors and mean LDL-C of 131 mg/dL assigned atorvastatin 10 mg.

### Bile Acid Sequestrants, or Resins
*Bile acid sequestrants*, also known as *bile acid resins*, are a class of medication that includes cholestyramine, colestipol, and colesevelam. These agents inhibit intestinal absorption of bile acids, reducing their enterohepatic recirculation. This in turn results in greater conversion of hepatic cholesterol into bile acids—reducing hepatic cholesterol content—and increases the synthesis of LDL receptors for LDL-binding.

Bile acid sequestrants modestly lower LDL-C levels, typically by approximately 15-20%, but have no significant effect on HDL-C and may increase triglyceride levels, making them relatively contraindicated in patients with significant hypertriglyceridemia. Intolerance to side effects, which include bloating, constipation, nausea, and esophageal reflux, is common with older preparations but less frequent with colesevelam. If given concomitantly, bile acid sequestrants can interfere with absorption of vitamin K, digoxin, warfarin, thyroxine, statins, and diuretics. Despite these side effects and drug interactions, sequestrants are useful adjunctive agent to statins or nicotinic acid in treatment of severe hyperlipidemia or as montherapy in statin-intolerant patients with elevated cholesterol levels. Indeed, the Lipid Research Clinics Coronary Primary Prevention Trial (LRC-CPPT) was one of the first randomized trials to confirm the CV benefits of cholesterol-reducing therapies, with a 19% reduction in CHD death and nonfatal MI in men with primary hypercholesterolemia receiving cholestyramine.

### Fibric Acid Derivatives

This class of medication includes fenofibrate and gemfibrozil. Their primary mechanism of action is activation of the nuclear transcription factor peroxisome proliferator-activated receptor-$\alpha$ (PPAR-$\alpha$). Together with the cofactor RXR, PPAR-$\alpha$ promotes transcription of several lipid-regulating proteins, resulting in moderate reductions in triglycerides of 20-50%. They also increase HDL-C, and transform small, dense LDL into larger, more buoyant particles, but have lesser effects on LDL-C levels compared with statins, occasionally increasing levels. Fibrates are generally safe with major side effects of gallstones, hepatotoxicity, and cholelithiasis. In addition, they can increase the risk of myopathy when used in combination with statins, in which case fenofibrate is preferred over gemfibrozil because of a lower incidence of this side effect with concomitant statin use. These drugs require dose adjustment in those with moderate renal impairment and are contraindicated in those with severe impairment (creatinine clearance <20 mL/min).

Fibrates are useful in treatment of hypertriglyceridemia and low HDL. Indeed, the Veteran Affairs Cooperative Studies Program High Density Lipoprotein Cholesterol Intervention Trial (VA-HIT) showed that patients with known CAD and low levels of HDL-C (mean 32 mg/dL) and LDL-C (mean 112 mg/dL) who were treated with gemfibrozil 1200 mg/day had a 24% risk reduction of the combined nonfatal MI, CHD death, or stroke compared with those treated with placebo. These cardiovascular benefits were also observed in the primary prevention Helsinki Heart Study (HHS) trial of approximately 4000 men with elevated non-HDL-C. However, both the secondary prevention Bezofibrate Infarction Prevention (BIP) trial, and the

Fenofibrate Intervention and Event Lowering in Diabetes (FIELD) trial of patients with diabetes failed to demonstrate reductions in their primary CV endpoints with fibrate therapy. Subanalyses from the BIP and HHS studies suggest that fibrates may be most effective in subjects with triglyceride levels >200 mg/dL and low HDL-C.

In patients with mixed hyperlipidemia, the combination of statin and fibrate therapy is an attractive option, since the addition of fibrate therapy can further reduce triglycerides by an additional 20%, modestly raise HDL-C, and possibly slightly lower LDL-C by 5%. A conclusion regarding whether combination fibrate and statin therapy is superior to statin monotherapy for clinical CV endpoints awaits the completion of the ongoing Action to Control Cardiovascular Risk in Diabetes (ACCORD) trial.

### Nicotinic Acid (Niacin)

This medication is widely used, inexpensive, and available over the counter. Although the precise mechanism is not unknown, nicotinic acid probably works by inhibiting the formation of apo-B containing lipoproteins, thereby moderately lowering total cholesterol, LDL-C, and non-HDL-C. It can also inhibit FFA mobilization in the periphery, thereby reducing triglyceride levels, and it also markedly increases HDL-C. As such, it is particularly useful in treatment of atherogenic dyslipidemia. However, this medication has numerous side effects, namely flushing, as well as pruritus, gastrointestinal intolerance, gout flare, impaired glucose tolerance, and hepatotoxicity. To minimize flushing, aspirin can be taken 30 minutes prior to the niacin dose to reduce prostaglandin release, and the medication can be taken at night after a small snack. Intermediate release nicotinic acid, Niaspan, also has better tolerability than shorter-acting preparation and a low incidence of hepatotoxicity, improving its adherence.

The only large scale clinical outcomes trial with niacin performed, the Coronary Drug Project, took place several decades ago and demonstrated a reduction in nonfatal MI, and also a reduction in all-cause mortality after 15 years in men with previous MI. Niacin has also shown favorable effects on atherosclerosis progression in combination with statins in smaller randomized trials, with ongoing studies to assess clinical endpoints.

### Cholesterol Absorption Inhibitors

The first drug in this class is ezetimibe, which works by selectively blocking intestinal absorption of cholesterol by binding to the Niemann-Pick C1-Like 1 (NPC1L1) receptor. As a result, less cholesterol returns to the liver for VLDL synthesis, and LDL receptor production is upregulated, resulting in increased clearance of LDL and VLDL from the systemic circulation. Ezetimibe can be used either as monotherapy in conjunction with diet or as combination therapy with statins (including a combination pill with simvastatin) to enhance lipid-lowering effects. Used in monotherapy, it can be expected to decrease LDL-C by 18%, while the combination of ezetimibe 10 mg with 10 mg, 20 mg, 40 mg, and 80 mg of simvastatin reduces LDL-C by 44%, 45%, 53%, and 57%, respectively. This medication is systemically absorbed and does undergo hepatic metabolism and recirculation. Consequently, it can rarely cause liver function test abnormalities, particularly with concomitant statin use.

While several studies have confirmed the LDL-C lowering effects of this agent, there are currently no published large scale trials assessing its efficacy for cardiovascular endpoints. The recently published ENHANCE trial compared the efficacy of simvastatin plus ezetimibe versus simvastatin alone on change in mean carotid intima-media thickness in 720 patients with heterozygous familial hypercholesterolemia. Despite significantly lower LDL-C levels in those receiving simvastatin plus ezetimibe (56 versus 39%), no difference in changes in carotid intima-media thickness (IMT) was observed between the two groups. However, the majority of study participants had been on long-standing statin therapy and had low values of carotid IMT at the beginning of the study. The ongoing IMPROVE-IT trial of approximately 18,000 patients assessing clinical endpoints will better define the role of ezetimibe in reducing cardiovascular events.

### Omega 3 Fatty Acids

Omega-3 fatty acids are polyunsaturated fatty acids that include the long chain docosahexaenoic acid (DHA) and eicosapentaenoic acid (EPA), which are also found in fish. From an epidemiologic perspective, populations with higher consumption of omega-3 fatty acids have a lower risk of CV events. The randomized, open label GISSI Prevenzione trial also demonstrated that 1 gram of EPA supplementation given subsequent to a recent MI reduced the risk of all-cause and CV death by 14% and 17%, respectively. In addition, the recent Japan EPA Lipid Intervention Study (JELIS) of hypercholesterolemic Japanese patients revealed a reduction in composite CV outcomes when 1.8 grams of EPA was combined with low dose statin therapy, compared with statin therapy alone. The mechanisms of these salutary effects of EPA and DHA are not known but are possibly related to antiarrhythmic effects, decreased platelet aggregation, and improved arterial and endothelial function.

Higher doses of EPA and DHA (3-4 g/day) can effectively lower triglyceride levels in those with significant hypertriglyceridemia (≥500 mg/dL) by as much as 50%, but with a variable increase in LDL-C, resulting in a net slight decrease in non-HDL-C and total cholesterol. The current AHA guidelines recommend 1 gram of omega-3 fatty acid supplementation daily for secondary prevention of CHD, and 3-4 grams daily for triglyceride lowering. The omega-3 fatty acid supplements are generally safe, with common side effects including nausea, gastrointestinal upset, and a "fishy burp," which can be minimized by ingestion at bedtime or with meals. High doses of omega-3 fatty acids may prolong bleeding time, requiring periodic monitoring of patients taking anticoagulants. Importantly, many over the counter preparations contain approximately only 300-400 mg of EPA and DHA per 1 gram capsule, while a purified prescription formulation, Lovaza, contains approximately 900 mg per 1 gram capsule.

## NCEP TREATMENT GUIDELINES FOR DYSLIPIDEMIA

The treatment guidelines for dyslipidemia are based upon the National Cholesterol Education Program's Adult Treatment Panel III. The full set of guidelines was initially published in 2001 and revised in 2004 to include findings from the five major clinical trials published in the interim.

### Risk Assessment

The guidelines state that everyone in the population would optimally have an LDL-C level less than 100 mg/dL or even <70 mg/dL, but not all patients' conditions warrant aggressive pharmacologic interventions in attempts to achieve these goals. The fundamental principle of cholesterol management is to match the intensity of lipid-lowering therapy to the absolute CHD risk of the patient, maximizing the risk-to-benefit ratio. Patients can be categorized into four risk groups:

1. high risk,
2. moderately high risk,
3. moderate risk,
4. low risk.

The algorithm in assessing CHD risk according to ATP III is as follows (**Figure 20-5**):

- Identify the presence of CHD and CHD risk equivalents (symptomatic carotid artery disease or stenosis >50%, peripheral arterial disease, abdominal aortic aneurysm, and diabetes). Patients with CHD or CHD risk equivalents are assigned to the high risk group. Very high risk patients include those with 1) recent acute coronary syndromes, or 2) CHD and either diabetes, multiple uncontrolled risk factors including smoking, or the metabolic syndrome.
- In patients without CHD or CHD risk equivalents, the next step is to count the number of CHD risk factors (**Table 20-8**). If two or more CHD risk factors are present, the patient is at least moderate risk, and the Framingham risk score (available

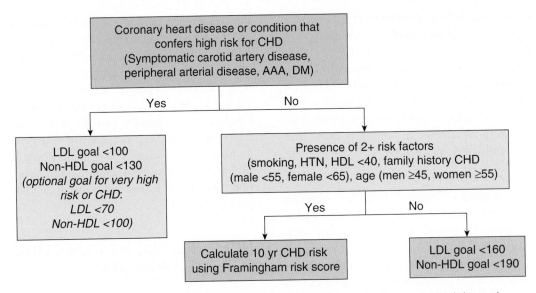

**Figure 20-5.** NCEP ATP III algorithm for determining LDL-C and non HDL-C goals. AAA, abdominal aortic aneurysm; DM, diabetes mellitus; HTN, hypertension; CHD, coronary heart disease.

online at http://hp2010.nhlbihin.net/atpiii/calculator.asp?usertype=pub) (**Figures 20-6** and **20-7**) is then calculated using age, total cholesterol, HDL-C, systolic blood pressure, and smoking history to further refine risk category. The risk score estimates the 10-year risk of hard CHD events (nonfatal MI and CHD death) and can stratify patients into the following groups: >20% 10-year risk = high risk; 10-20% = moderately high risk; <10% = moderate risk.

- Moderately high risk patients may undergo additional testing to identify individuals that should be elevated to the high risk group. Such tests include assessment of ankle-brachial index, carotid intima-media thickness, coronary artery calcium, C-reactive protein, and exercise treadmill testing.
- When 0-1 risk factors are present, Framingham risk scoring is not necessary, and these patients are assigned to the low risk group.

| Table 20-8 • Major Risk Factors (Exclusive of LDL) that Modify LDL Goals |
|---|
| Cigarette smoking |
| Hypertension (BP ≥140/90 mm Hg or on antihypertensive therapy) |
| Low HDL cholesterol (<40 mg/dL) |
| Family history of premature CHD (first degree relative, male <55 years, female <65 years) |
| Age (men ≥45 years, women ≥55 years) |

*Adapted from the Third Report of the National Cholesterol Education Program (NCEP) Expert Panel on the Detection, Evaluation, and Treatment of High Blood Cholesterol in Adults (ATP III), 2001.*

## LDL-C Lowering

The *primary goal* of therapy per ATPIII is LDL-C lowering. **Table 20-9** summarizes the LDL cutpoints for considering TLC and statin treatment for each group. New to the updated guidelines is that clinicians now have an option of reducing LDL to <70 mg/dL in very high risk patients. Furthermore, the guidelines provide an option of reducing LDL <100 mg/dL in moderately high risk patients. Factors that influence more intensive statin therapy in this group include advanced age, multiple or severe risk factors, and metabolic syndrome. Statin drugs should be the initial agents used for LDL-C lowering, and when employed, a dose sufficient to lower LDL-C by at least 30-40% should be used. The efficacy of LDL-C-lowering should be monitored every 6 weeks until the goal is reached.

## Hypertriglyceridemia and Non-HDL-C

After LDL-C goals are achieved, triglyceride levels are then evaluated. Several conditions are associated with hypertriglyceridemia, including obesity, physical inactivity, excess alcohol intake, high carbohydrate intake, insulin resistance (diabetes, metabolic syndrome), certain drugs (corticosteroids, estrogens, beta-blockers), and genetic disorders (familial combined hyperlipidemia, familial hypertriglyceridemia, and familial dysbetalipoproteinemia). The initial treatment priority is to target the underlying cause of elevated triglycerides when possible. Thereafter, specific management strategies for hypertriglyceridemia are outlined as follows:

- Borderline high triglycerides (150-199 mg/dL): Emphasis is on weight reduction and increased physical activity.

Step 1: Age

| Years | Points |
|-------|--------|
| 20–34 | –9 |
| 35–39 | –4 |
| 40–44 | 0 |
| 45–49 | 3 |
| 50–54 | 6 |
| 55–59 | 8 |
| 60–64 | 10 |
| 65–69 | 11 |
| 70–74 | 12 |
| 75–79 | 13 |

Step 4: Systolic blood pressure

| Systolic BP (mm Hg) | Points if untreated | Points if treated |
|---------------------|---------------------|-------------------|
| <120 | 0 | 0 |
| 120–129 | 0 | 1 |
| 130–139 | 1 | 2 |
| 140–159 | 1 | 2 |
| ≥160 | 2 | 3 |

Step 5: Smoking status

|  | Points at age 20–39 | Points at age 40–49 | Points at age 50–59 | Points at age 60–69 | Points at age 70–79 |
|--|--------------------|--------------------|--------------------|--------------------|--------------------|
| Nonsmoker | 0 | 0 | 0 | 0 | 0 |
| Smoker | 8 | 5 | 3 | 1 | 1 |

Step 2: Total cholesterol

| TC (mg/dL) | Points at age 20–39 | Points at age 40–49 | Points at age 50–59 | Points at age 60–69 | Points at age 70–79 |
|-----------|--------------------|--------------------|--------------------|--------------------|--------------------|
| <160 | 0 | 0 | 0 | 0 | 0 |
| 160–199 | 4 | 3 | 2 | 1 | 0 |
| 200–239 | 7 | 5 | 3 | 1 | 0 |
| 240–279 | 9 | 6 | 4 | 2 | 1 |
| ≥280 | 11 | 8 | 5 | 3 | 1 |

Step 3: HDL-cholesterol

| HDL-C (mg/dL) | Points |
|---------------|--------|
| ≥60 | –1 |
| 50–59 | 0 |
| 40–49 | 1 |
| <40 | 2 |

Step 6: Adding up the points

| Age | — |
|-----|---|
| Total cholesterol | — |
| HDL-cholesterol | — |
| Systolic blood pressure | — |
| Smoking status | — |
| Point total | |

Step 7: CHD risk

| Point total | 10-year risk |
|-------------|--------------|
| <0 | <1% |
| 0 | 1% |
| 1 | 1% |
| 2 | 1% |
| 3 | 1% |
| 4 | 1% |
| 5 | 2% |
| 6 | 2% |
| 7 | 3% |
| 8 | 4% |
| 9 | 5% |
| 10 | 6% |
| 11 | 8% |
| 12 | 10% |
| 13 | 12% |
| 14 | 16% |
| 15 | 20% |
| 16 | 25% |
| ≥17 | ≥30% |

Absolute 10-year risk of CHD death or MI

**Figure 20-6.** Framingham Risk Score algorithm for men. NCEP-ATPIII version of the Framingham Risk Score. 10-year risk of coronary heart disease death or myocardial infarction is calculated by adding points for age, total cholesterol, HDL-cholesterol, systolic blood pressure and smoking status and comparing the summed point total to the 10-year risk %. CHD, coronary heart disease; MI, myocardial infarction.

- High triglycerides (200-499 mg/dL): Non-HDL-C (equal to total cholesterol – HDL) should be calculated, as it encompasses triglyceride-rich VLDL and becomes the secondary target of dyslipidemia management. The recommended non-HDL-C goal is 30 mg/dL higher than the LDL-C goal. For example, if the LDL-C goal is <100 mg/dL, the non-HDL-C goal should be <130 mg/dL. Aside from weight reduction and increased physical activity, pharmacologic therapy is recommended. This can be achieved by increasing the dose of statin, or adding fibrates or nicotinic acid as adjunctive therapy.

- Very high triglycerides (≥500 mg/dL): The first treatment goal is to lower triglycerides to prevent acute pancreatitis. This is accomplished by a very low fat diet (≤15% of calorie intake), weight reduction, increased physical activity, and the addition of fibrates, nicotinic acid, or omega-3 fatty acids. After triglyceride levels decrease to <500 mg/dL, LDL-C lowering therapy can be initiated.

## Patients with Low HDL

Low HDL is defined as HDL-C<40 mg/dL and is often associated with metabolic syndrome, smoking, obesity, very low fat diets, drugs (anabolic steroids), and genetic causes (familial hypoalphalipoproteinemia). At this time, the ATPIII guidelines have not specified a goal level for HDL-C. In patients with LDL-C and non-HDL-C at goal and residual low HDL-C, a fibrate or nicotinic acid can be added, especially in those with CHD or CHD risk equivalents.

## SPECIAL POPULATIONS

### Older Persons

Although the association between high cholesterol and CHD events is of lesser magnitude in older than in younger persons, findings from subgroup analyses of clinical trials including HPS consistently suggest that older patients with established CVD or CVD risk factors still derive benefits

Step 1: Age

| Years | Points |
|-------|--------|
| 20–34 | –7 |
| 35–39 | –3 |
| 40–44 | 0 |
| 45–49 | 3 |
| 50–54 | 6 |
| 55–59 | 8 |
| 60–64 | 10 |
| 65–69 | 12 |
| 70–74 | 14 |
| 75–79 | 16 |

Step 4: Systolic blood pressure

| Systolic BP (mm Hg) | Points if untreated | Points if treated |
|---------------------|---------------------|-------------------|
| <120 | 0 | 0 |
| 120–129 | 1 | 3 |
| 130–139 | 2 | 4 |
| 140–159 | 3 | 5 |
| ≥160 | 4 | 6 |

Step 5: Smoking status

| | Points at age 20–39 | Points at age 40–49 | Points at age 50–59 | Points at age 60–69 | Points at age 70–79 |
|---|---|---|---|---|---|
| Nonsmoker | 0 | 0 | 0 | 0 | 0 |
| Smoker | 9 | 7 | 4 | 2 | 1 |

Step 2: Total cholesterol

| TC (mg/dL) | Points at age 20–39 | Points at age 40–49 | Points at age 50–59 | Points at age 60–69 | Points at age 70–79 |
|------------|---------------------|---------------------|---------------------|---------------------|---------------------|
| <160 | 0 | 0 | 0 | 0 | 0 |
| 160–199 | 4 | 3 | 2 | 1 | 1 |
| 200–239 | 8 | 6 | 4 | 1 | 1 |
| 240–279 | 11 | 8 | 5 | 3 | 2 |
| ≥280 | 13 | 10 | 7 | 4 | 2 |

Step 3: HDL-cholesterol

| HDL-C (mg/dL) | Points |
|---------------|--------|
| ≥60 | –1 |
| 50–59 | 0 |
| 40–49 | 1 |
| <40 | 2 |

Step 6: Adding up the points

| Age | — |
|-----|---|
| Total cholesterol | — |
| HDL-cholesterol | — |
| Systolic blood pressure | — |
| Smoking status | — |
| Point total | |

Step 7: CHD risk

| Point Total | 10-year risk |
|-------------|--------------|
| <9 | <1% |
| 9 | 1% |
| 10 | 1% |
| 11 | 1% |
| 12 | 1% |
| 13 | 2% |
| 14 | 2% |
| 15 | 3% |
| 16 | 4% |
| 17 | 5% |
| 18 | 6% |
| 19 | 8% |
| 20 | 11% |
| 21 | 14% |
| 22 | 17% |
| 23 | 22% |
| 24 | 27% |
| ≥25 | ≥30% |

Absolute 10-year risk of CHD death or MI

**Figure 20-7.** Framingham Risk Score algorithm for women. NCEP-ATPIII version of the Framingham Risk Score. 10-year risk of coronary heart disease death or myocardial infarction is calculated by adding points for age, total cholesterol, HDL-cholesterol, systolic blood pressure and smoking status and comparing the summed point total to the 10-year risk %. CHD, coronary heart disease; MI, myocardial infarction.

| Table 20-9 • ATP III Update LDL Goals and Cutpoints for TLC and Drug Therapy in Different Risk Categories | | | |
|---|---|---|---|
| **Risk Category** | **LDL Goal** | **Initiate TLC** | **Consider Drug Therapy** |
| High risk:<br>CHD or CHD risk equivalents (10-yr risk >20%) | <100 mg/dL (optional goal: ≤70 mg/dL) | ≥100 mg/dL | ≥100 mg/dL (<100 mg/dL: consider drug options) |
| Moderately high risk:<br>2+ risk factors (10-yr risk 10-20%) | <130 mg/dL (optional goal: ≤100 mg/dL) | ≥130 mg/dL | ≥130 mg/dL (100-129 mg/dL: consider drug options) |
| Moderate risk:<br>2+ risk factors (10-yr risk <10%) | <130 mg/dL | ≥130 mg/dL | ≥160 mg/dL |
| Low risk:<br>0-1 risk factor | <160 mg/dL | ≥160 mg/dL | ≥190 mg/dL (160-189 mg/dL: consider drug options) |

*Adapted from the Third Report of the National Cholesterol Education Program (NCEP) Expert Panel on the Detection, Evaluation, and Treatment of High Blood Cholesterol in Adults (ATP III) updated guidelines. Circulation. 2004;110. TLC, therapeutic lifestyle changes.*

from lipid-lowering therapy. In the Prospective Study of Pravastatin in the Elderly at Risk (PROSPER) study, of 5800 men ages 70-82 years with CVD or CVD risk factors, pravastatin 40 mg reduced the risk of CVD endpoints and coronary death by 15% and 24%, respectively, compared with placebo. Importantly, although the relative risk reduction of lipid-lowering therapy is lower in elderly compared with younger subjects, the absolute risk reduction is often greater given the higher baseline risk for CVD events with age.

## Patients with Diabetes

It is clear that patients with diabetes with or without CVD are at high risk for developing CV events and warrant aggressive risk reduction strategies. Subanalyses from several statin trials have demonstrated improved CV outcomes with statin therapy in diabetic cohorts. As previously stated, the CARDS trial clearly established that atorvastatin 10 mg daily was safe and effective in reducing the risk of first CV event in diabetic patients with fasting LDL-C <160 mg/dL (mean 117 mg/dL). Hence, the ATP III guidelines recommend LDL-C goals of <70 mg/dL for diabetic patients with a history of CVD, and <100 mg/dL for diabetic patients without history of CVD. The American Diabetes Association recommendations go a step further and call for statin therapy in all patients with diabetes over the age of 40 with one additional CVD risk factor, regardless of baseline LDL-C level. Areas of uncertainty regarding lipid-lowering therapy in patients with diabetes include those who are young or have no CVD risk factors.

## Patients with Acute Coronary Syndromes

Patients with recent ACS are at markedly high risk of recurrent CV events, approximately 25% at two years. The Myocardial Ischemia Reduction with Aggressive Cholesterol Lowering (MIRACL) reported that early initiation of intensive statin therapy reduced recurrent CV events by 16% relative to placebo in the 4-month follow-up period. These findings were extended by the PROVE-IT study in which intensive statin therapy accompanied by LDL-C levels <70 mg/dL further reduced recurrent CV events compared with standard dose statin therapy and LDL-C levels <100 mg/dL. Due to these findings along with supportive evidence from the A to Z trial, intensive statin therapy should now be considered for all patients admitted with ACS.

## References

1. Executive Summary of the Third Report of the National Cholesterol Education Program (NCEP) Expert Panel on Detection, Evaluation, and Treatment of High Blood Cholesterol in Adults (Adult Treatment Panel III). JAMA. 2001;285(19):2486–2497.

2. Durrington P. Dyslipidaemia. *Lancet.* 2003;362(9385): 717–731.

3. Grundy SM, Cleeman JI, Merz CN, et al. Implications of recent clinical trials for the National Cholesterol Education Program Adult Treatment Panel III guidelines. *Circulation.* 2004;110(2):227–239.

# 21

# Hypertension

SCOTT R. YODER AND JOHN D. BISOGNANO

## ● PRACTICAL POINTS

- "Hypertension" is the most common outpatient diagnosis (1 billion patients worldwide) and contributes directly to 7.1 million deaths annually.

- JNC-VII defines normal blood pressure as <120/80, prehypertension as 120-139/80-89, hypertension as >140/90.

- A more stringent goal of <120/80 is reserved for patients with CAD and LV dysfunction—generally an EF of <40%.

- BP measurement must conform to recommended standards.

- Good lifestyle behaviors are core to the treatment of hypertension. In overweight and obese patients, weight loss results in significant blood pressure reduction.

- Choice of drugs depends on the severity of hypertension and presence of comorbid illnesses (diabetes, nephropathy, etc.).

- African Americans have a higher prevalence of hypertension, develop hypertension at a younger age, and tend to have proportionally more morbidity and mortality associated with hypertension.

- Preeclampsia is a new-onset hypertension which occurs after the 20th week of gestation and is characterized by proteinuria (1+ dipstick, >300 mg/24 h); occurs in approximately 7% of all pregnancies, but is more common in women with chronic hypertension (25%)

- Hypertensive urgency and emergency warrant inpatient admission for evaluation and treatment. In both cases there is evidence of end-organ damage due to hypertension. The distinction between the two is based on the clinical severity and risk of significant morbidity and mortality if the blood pressure is not corrected.

- Patients with resistant hypertension (lack of blood pressure control with three or more antihypertensive medications), and very young patients with hypertension must be investigated for secondary causes: primary hyperaldosteronism, pheochromocytoma, renal artery stenosis, coarctation of aorta, etc.

## INTRODUCTION

Hypertension may well be the most important public health issue facing society. It is the most common outpatient diagnosis (1 billion patients worldwide) and contributes directly to 7.1 million deaths annually. Suboptimal blood pressure control is likely to reduce 50% of ischemic heart disease and 60% of strokes, the second and third leading causes of death in the United States. Much of the morbidity and mortality associated with hypertension can be reduced with appropriate medical therapy."

Multiple genetic and environmental factors interact in the development of hypertension. This chapter discusses the epidemiology of hypertension, diagnosis and initial therapy, as well as approaches to refractory hypertension.

### Classification of Hypertension

Optimal blood pressures and stages of hypertension were redefined in the Seventh Report of the Joint National Committee on Prevention, Detection, Evaluation and Treatment of High Blood Pressure (JNC 7) (**Table 21-1**).

| Table 21-1 • JNC 7 Classification of Blood Pressure | |
|---|---|
| **BP Classification** | **BP Measurement** |
| Normal | <120/80 |
| Prehypertension | 120-139/80-89 |
| Hypertension | >140/90 |
| Stage I | 140-159/90-99 |
| Stage II | >160/100 |

Finding its origins in previous JNC reports, the stages of hypertension are convenient guides for relative risk but are only a part of the risk evaluation for the patient. For every 20 mm Hg systolic or 10 mm Hg diastolic increase in blood pressure there is a doubling of the risk of death from cardiovascular disease or stroke, and this trend is incorporated in the JNC 7 stages. An equivalent reduction in risk is noted with blood pressure control, yet rates of target blood pressure control remain at less than 40%.

In addition to JNC7 recommendations there are additional considerations for patients with certain comorbidities. Although a goal of <140/90 is recommended for most patients, those with diabetes or renal dysfunction are given a lower target of <130/80. Recent recommendations by the American Heart Association also recommend treatment of patients with known coronary artery disease and other vascular disease to a level of <130/80. A more stringent goal of <120/80 is reserved for patients with coronary disease and left ventricular dysfunction—generally an ejection fraction of <40%. Patients with diabetes should be treated to a blood pressure level of <130/80 due to the significant interaction of hypertension and diabetes in end-organ diseases (coronary disease, nephropathy, stroke, retinopathy, etc.). Patients with evidence of chronic renal impairment should be treated to a blood pressure level of <130/80 in order to prevent progression to kidney failure, and there are some data suggesting benefit of a 125/75 goal in these patients.

## Epidemiology

Prevalence of hypertension increases with age. Ninety percent of patients who are normotensive at 55-69 years of age will develop hypertension if they reach the age of 80 years. One-half of people 60-69 years of age and 75% of people over 70 years of age will be hypertensive.

Approximately 90-95% of people with hypertension have primary (essential) hypertension. This elevation of blood pressure is multifactorial in origin and represents a complex interaction of genetic traits with lifestyle factors (weight, sodium intake/excretion, and emotional stress). In contrast, secondary hypertension has a specific cause and may improve with correction of the underlying defect. This will be addressed later in this chapter.

# MEASUREMENT OF BLOOD PRESSURE

Appropriate technique for blood pressure measurement is essential for appropriate diagnosis and management. Equipment used to measure blood pressure must be accurate and should be recalibrated on a regular basis. Blood pressure should be measured in the sitting position with the arm resting at heart level. The patient should be sitting comfortably for 5 minutes prior to blood pressure measurement. An appropriate selected cuff bladder should encompass 80% of the arm circumference, the sphygmomanonometer inflated to 20 mm Hg above the auscultated heart sounds and deflated at a rate of 2 mm Hg per second measuring the first and second Karotkoff sounds. Numerous automated devices are now available and provide excellent readings in most patients, providing great assistance in the management of outpatients with regards to blood pressure.

# PATIENT ASSESSMENT

The goal of patient assessment is to evaluate degree of hypertension, identify additional risk factors for morbid sequelae, initiate therapy, and educate the patient. Initial evaluation should include past medical history, social history, family history, current medications, and physical exam. Specific attention should be paid to common secondary causes or comorbid conditions associated with hypertension (**Figure 21-1**).

Physical exam should include bilateral blood pressures, weight, body mass index, carotid auscultation, thyroid evaluation, and palpation of aortic and peripheral pulses. Diagnostic evaluation with an ECG, basic metabolic profile, and thyroid function testing should be performed. Additional diagnostic studies may be warranted on an individual basis.

| |
|---|
| **Comorbid conditions that require more aggressive blood pressure control:**<br>Diabetes<br>Stroke (ischemic or hemorrhagic)<br>Coronary artery disease<br>Chronic heart failure<br>Chronic kidney disease |
| **Common, easily screened causes of secondary hypertension:**<br>Sleep apnea<br>Drug-induced (OCP, antidepressants, etc.)<br>Hyperaldosteronism<br>Aortic coarctation<br>White coat hypertension<br>Pseudohypertension |

**Figure 21-1.** Comorbid and secondary conditions of hypertension.

| Table 21-4 • Presentation of Hypertensive Emergency |
| --- |
| Hypertensive encephalopathy |
| Intracerebral hemorrhage |
| Acute heart failure |
| Aortic dissection |
| Acute renal failure |
| Unstable angina |

24-36 hours but oral therapy requires twice or three time daily dosing. Nitroglycerine can be symptomatically beneficial in cases of congestive heart failure but generally the degree of blood pressure effect is not as satisfying as other medications.

Hypertensive emergency has been defined as a blood pressure is >220/140 mm Hg and/or the presence of severe end organ dysfunction related to ongoing hypertension (**Table 21-4**). Therapy should be initiated immediately. Many of these patients are in a hyper-adrenergic state leading to extreme vasoconstriction in the setting of a relatively low total body volume; consequently significant shifts in blood pressure can be noted with initiation of vasodilators. Intravenous medications should be initiated early, have a rapid onset and short half life allowing easy titration. A goal of reducing the blood pressure by 25% from presentation or to 160/100 mm Hg is recommended but must be tempered based on the clinical scenario. Although the risk of hypoperfusion with sudden drops in blood pressure is present, the ongoing damage from hypertension must also be effectively ameliorated. These patients can be extremely ill and become quite complicated. Often invasive blood pressure monitoring and admission to a medical or CV ICU is warranted.

Sodium nitroprusside has been the classic medication for treatment of hypertensive urgency. It has a short half life, rapid onset of action and is easily titrated. Unfortunately, it also produces cyanide as a break-down product and toxicity becomes an issue after 24-48 hours. Intravenous nicardipine is extremely effective: It has pharmacokinetic properties similar to sodium nitroprusside but no significant toxicity. In cases related to hyperadrenergic activity, phentolamine, esmolol, or labetalol may be more appropriate/efficacious first-line agents. Labetalol should be used cautiously since its half-life is considerably longer than other medications.

## SECONDARY HYPERTENSION

Resistant hypertension is defined as sub-optimal blood pressure control with three or more antihypertensive medications, one being a diuretic. Common causes of resistant hypertension include inaccurate measurement of blood pressure, underdosing of diuretics and fluid overload, patient noncompliance/ nonadherence, and drug-drug interaction. If these simple causes are remedied and the blood pressure elevation persists then a concerted effort to evaluate for specific underlying causes (secondary hypertension) is warranted. The three-drug guideline was developed when drug therapy for hypertension was fraught with side effects and triple drug therapy was considered maximal medical therapy. Although generally reasonable, the three-drug guideline is likely to yield a high proportion of negative workups for secondary hypertension and may lead to delays in evaluation of patients at higher risk for secondary causes of hypertension. Evaluation for secondary hypertension may be appropriate regardless of blood pressure level or intensity of therapy, for specific groups such as the young, those with specific symptoms suggesting a specific cause of hypertension, and those with a history of hypertensive emergencies or severe target organ damage.

The remainder of this chapter describes the most common causes of secondary hypertension, with additional discussion of evaluation and management. It is important to note that most people with secondary hypertension also have primary hypertension and that addressing the secondary cause of hypertension rarely provides a cure. Addressing the secondary causes of hypertension may reduce but not necessarily eliminate the need for other blood pressure-lowering therapy. However, appropriate diagnosis and treatment of secondary causes of hypertension may allow a decrease in the number of medications needed to achieve blood pressure goal.

## Clinical Approach to Secondary Hypertension

Before instituting an extensive evaluation for secondary causes of hypertension, the clinician must be certain that the blood pressure readings obtained are indicative of the patient's actual blood pressure throughout most of the day. Blood pressures measured in the physician's office serve this purpose for most patients. However, a sizeable subset of patients, 20-50% by several studies, present with significant hypertension only in the physician's office ("white-coat" hypertension) due to anxiety and stress related to the visit. Additionally, patients presenting with white-coat hypertension who also have generally stressful lifestyles, may report normal blood pressure measurements at home, which are taken at opportune and stress-free periods and may give a false sense of reassurance to the patient and physician. Such labile hypertension carries an increased risk of cardiovascular events and generally warrants some treatment. Home blood pressure reading or 24-hour ambulatory blood pressure monitoring can be important in distinguishing a patient with severe hypertension from one who simply has a controlled hypertension that is significantly augmented in the physician's office. A workup for secondary causes in a patient with near-normal home blood pressure readings is likely to be unrevealing, and the cost of home blood pressure monitoring is low in comparison with most secondary evaluations. Moreover, home blood pressure readings can prevent overtreatment in patients with labile blood pressure, decrease drug side effects, and increase the patient's ability to adhere to therapy.

The evaluation of pseudohypertension in elderly patients is important because measurement in calcified and non-compressible brachial arteries of these patients can falsely elevate cuff readings and lead to overtreatment. In these patients, alternative blood pressure measuring devices such as wrist and finger monitors or even arterial lines can be useful when a calcified brachial artery is palpated.

Medical compliance must also be assessed before a clinician embarks on an extensive patient workup for secondary causes of hypertension. Moderate to severe hypertension is often treated with multiple, expensive drugs with adverse side effect profiles. Because of their power in lowering blood pressure, drugs such as clonidine, hydralazine, and minoxidil are often prescribed without regard for the patient's ability to tolerate their side effects. In short, patients are often not eager to spend money each month in order to feel miserable, particularly when they generally feel well despite their elevated blood pressure. Many clinically established medications for hypertension are now generic and have low side effect profiles. Several of these are currently available for $4 per month (of $10 for three months) through large national pharmacies. The advent of this low cost medication program, with a wide variety of effective medications, affords the practitioner an opportunity to tailor affordable and tolerable regiment for almost any patient.

Finally, all numerical and physical data from a patient should be consistent before secondary evaluation is considered. A patient with years of extremely elevated blood pressure but no evidence of any target organ damage (microalbuminuria, left ventricular hypertrophy, retinal abnormalities) is unlikely to have sustained levels of blood pressure elevation out of the physician's office and would likely have an unrevealing workup for secondary causes of hypertension. Conversely, a patient with modestly elevated readings in the physician's office but evidence of target organ damage should be evaluated more aggressively.

Once the accuracy of the blood pressure measurements is confirmed and medical compliance is reasonably documented, an evaluation for secondary causes of hypertension can proceed. Evaluation and treatment of the more common secondary causes of hypertension is discussed here (**Table 21-5**).

## EXOGENOUS DRUG USE

Exogenous drug use (illicit, prescribed, and over-the-counter) is an important, and potentially reversible, cause of hypertension. Some of the more common drugs used by patients include oral contraceptives and other estrogen-

**Table 21-5 • Initial Approach to Suspected Secondary Hypertension**

| Possible Cause of Secondary Hypertension | Initial Diagnostic Study |
|---|---|
| Labile (white coat) hypertension | Home 24-hr blood pressure monitoring |
| Noncompliance | Focused history including financial assessment, cost of medications, detailed review of side effects |
| Pseudohypertension | Wrist or finger pressures; invasive blood pressure monitoring |
| Exogenous drug use | Focused history including over-the-counter, herbal medications, and dietary supplements |
| Renal parenchymal disease | General chemistry, urinalysis, urine for microalbuminuria |
| Renal artery stenosis | Renal artery imaging: MRI, ultrasonography, angiography |
| Primary aldosteronisim | Serum potassium, aldosterone, renin, and ratio. |
| Pheocrhomocytoma | Urine VMA, catecholamines, metanephrines, or serum metanephrines |
| Cushing's syndrome | 24-hour urine for free cortisol |
| Thyroid disease | TSH for free thyroxine |
| Parathyroid disease | Serum calcium and ionized calcium levels |
| Obstructive sleep apnea | Sleep study |
| Aortic coarctation | Chest radiograph or CT |

CT, commuted tomography; MRI, magnetic resonance imaging; TSH, thyroid stimulating hormone; VMA, vanillylmandelic acid

containing compounds, sympathomimetic drugs for weight loss and sinusitis, alcohol and cocaine, immunosuppressive drugs, anabolic steroids, and nonsteroidal antiinflammatory medications.

A relatively large proportion of young women use oral contraceptive medications. Although these medications produce only small increases of blood pressure in most patients, a subset of patients experiences significant increases in systolic blood pressure, sometimes as great as 22 mm Hg. Some studies have linked the degree of hypertension with increased age (older than 35 years), duration of antiovulatory therapy, and alcohol intake. The hypertensive effect of oral contraceptives is reversible in approximately 50% of patients 3 to 6 months after discontinuation. The residual elevation in blood pressure is usually attributable to underlying primary hypertension. Postmenopausal estrogen replacement therapy does not appear to have similar hypertensive effect. Women at highest risk for renal artery fibromuscular dysplasia include a relatively high percentage that use oral contraceptives. If blood pressure elevations are modest and there is no evidence of end-organ damage, it may be worthwhile to consider discontinuation of oral contraceptives for 3 to 6 months before an evaluation for renal artery fibromuscular dysplasia (see below: Renal Artery Stenosis).

Numerous sympathomimetic medications can be purchased over the counter and at health food stores for the treatment of sinusitis (pseudoephedrine and phenylephrine) or obesity (pheylpropanolamine and others). These drugs can produce profound increases in blood pressure. Because many hypertensive patients are also overweight, it is useful to ask patients specifically during evaluation of their hypertension whether they use Over the counter weight loss drugs. The health gains associated with weight loss and the utility of continuing these medications will have to be considered in relation to the severity of and ability to successfully treat the hypertension. Inquiry should also be made about food supplements, because sympathomimetics may be included and because some products that originate outside the continental U.S. may not be labeled in English.

Recreational use of cocaine can cause transient spikes in blood pressure and hypertensive urgency. Care must be taken in this setting to avoid selective beta-blockers, which may worsen hypertensive crisis due to unopposed alpha-adrenergic activity. The transient spikes in blood pressure and coronary spasm may cause significant myocardial ischemia, but generally do not cause chronic elevations in blood pressure. Alcohol intake of more than 2 ounces per day can be associated with severe hypertension resistant to medical therapy. Social history on initial examination should include evaluation of alcohol intake. In such patients the issue of compliance with medical regimen should also be definitively evaluated before one embarks on an extensive workup for other secondary causes of hypertension.

Each year, more patients receive solid organ transplants, and a greater proportion of these patients are surviving longer. Many of these patients have underlying primary hypertension responsive to sodium restriction. However, the immunosuppressive medications cyclosporine and tacrolimus produce hypertension directly through activation of the sympathetic nervous system and nephrotoxicity. These virtually un-avoidable side effects are necessary to permit adequate immunosuppression and minimize use of steroids. (which can also cause hypertension through volume increase). Because most patients' survival depends on adequate dosing with these drugs, blood pressure must often be addressed with multiple medications (often to low target levels of 125/75 mm Hg dictated by underlying renal insufficiency) with the usual armory of antihypertensive drugs. Israpidine is frequently the favored calcium channel blocker because of its lack of effect on cyclosporine metabolism.

Some transplant groups are using diltiazem because it inhibits cytochrome p450 3A4, allowing reductions in tacrolimus while maintaining therapeutic levels.

As mentioned, the use of anabolic steroid medications medically, but more commonly for bodybuilding, can lead to mild increases in blood pressure as a result of sodium retention. It may be important to counsel hypertensive patients who participate in bodybuilding to avoid exogenous steroid usage and also to inform them that bodybuilding itself can exacerbate hypertension.

Finally, the increasing use of nonsteroidal antiinflammatory drugs can cause hypertension both acutely and chronically through analgesic nephropathy. This class of drugs generally produces small, if any, elevation in blood pressure in most patients, but certain patients have marked increase in blood pressure. Cyclooxygenase-2 (COX-2) inhibitors are generally felt to be safer compared to traditional NSAIDS, but likely have similar hypertensive effects, especially in patients with significant salt sensitivity. The initiation of either class of medication carries additional cardiovascular risk and the physician should seriously deliberate initiation of them in patients with known hypertension and/ or cardiovascular disease. It is important to consider these medications as a cause of increased blood pressure, particularly in the elderly patients, who often use these drugs at high doses. Simply withholding these medications for a few weeks may result in normalization of blood pressure and eliminate the need for a workup for other secondary causes of high blood pressure.

## RENAL PARENCHYMAL DISEASE

Disease of the renal parenchyma can be responsible for acute and chronic hypertension. In patients presenting with hypertensive crisis, it is mandatory one evaluate renal function through a general chemistry profile and a urinalysis. Although abnormalities may be the result of hypertension itself, evaluation for acute renal processes such as acute glomerulonephritis, bilateral renal artery embolism, and bilateral ureteral obstruction should be considered. Other processes, such as vasculitis and high doses nonsteroidal drug ingestion, can also lead to acute renal failure and hypertension. Prompt consultation with a nephrologist or, if indicated, a vascular surgeon or urologist, should be made in these cases.

More commonly, chronic hypertension begets chronic renal insufficiency, which in turn begets hypertension in a vicious circle unless interrupted through medical treatment. Long-standing diabetic nephropathy and chronic pyelonephritis, for example, can result in decreases in glomerular filtration rate, sodium retention, and worsening hypertension. In patients with stable renal dysfunction the careful application of angiotensin-converting enzyme inhibition or angiotensin receptor blockade can result in decreased blood pressure as well as preservation of renal function. ACEI and ARB therapy should not be withheld in the presence of stable renal insufficiency and the creatinine is never "too high" to initiate an angiotensive converting enzyme inhibitor or angiotensin receptor blocker if the GFR is stable. Medical therapy may be able to delay or halt the progression to renal replacement therapy. Those patients who are likely to proceed to dialysis or renal transplantation should receive prompt referral to a nephrologist. Aggressive cardiovascular risk modification is also warranted in these patients with end-stage renal disease, in whom the primary cause of death is cardiovascular in origin.

# RENAL ARTERY STENOSIS

Renal artery disease can result from either of two entirely separate entities: atherosclerotic renal artery stenosis and renal artery fibromuscular dysplasia. Both can cause hypertension, but they can also exist in patients without significant elevations of blood pressure. Great strides have been made since 1990 in percutaneous revascularization, including renal artery stent placement. The greatest challenge however, remains in selecting the patients more likely to benefit from percutaneous interventions, and clinical trials are presently underway to investigate this.

Atherosclerotic renal artery stenosis is primarily a disease of the renal artery ostium and the proximal one-third of the renal artery. Because atherosclerosis is a systemic disease, renal arty stenosis occurs in patients with other cardiovascular risk factors, and a high proportion of patients with atherosclerotic renal artery disease also have coronary disease, an important consideration when renal revascularization is contemplated. Patients who experience subacute onset of severe hypertension at a late age or rapid deterioration of hypertension control should be considered for renal artery evaluation, particularly if they have other atherogenic risk factors. Noninvasive imaging with renal magnetic resonance angiography, Doppler ultrasonography, or computed tomography (CT) can be helpful in screening patients prior to invasive angiography and revascularization. Other tests such as selective renal vein renin and captopril renogram can further guide the decision of whether to perform revascularization. There is some evidence that renal artery resistive indices and fractional flow reserve may be useful in predicting responsiveness to renal artery revascularization. The sensitivity and specificity of these studies vary widely by the experience level of the technicians performing and physicians reading the imaging studies. Also, not all modalities may be available in a given area. Consequently, it is most important for the clinician to explore a particular institution's area of expertise when ordering renal artery imaging.

Invasive arteriography remains the gold standard for determining the degree of stenosis and also enables the operator to evaluate the hemodynamic significance of a lesion. Several studies have demonstrated significant reductions in blood pressure with percutaneous and surgical interventions, but the results vary widely from patient to patient. Selection of patients most likely to benefit from renal artery revascularization remains an area of controversy and active research. In rare instances patients with unilateral renal artery stenosis, severe hypertension, poor response to medication, and failure of an invasive intervention (surgically or percutaneously) may require surgical nephrectomy to achieve blood pressure control.

Patients with renal artery fibromuscular dysplasia have abnormalities in the renal arterial media, leading to weblike stenosis in the distal two-thirds of the renal artery. The disease occurs in both sexes and at all ages, but young women are most frequently affected by this disease. Most noninvasive imaging studies do not provide an adequate assessment of the distal two-thirds of renal arteries and, consequently, it is often necessary to perform arteriography when fibromuscular dysplasia is suspected. This disease is worth finding because a significant improvement in hypertension can be accomplished in 60 to 70% of patients with simple balloon angioplasty, without stent placement.

# ADRENAL DISEASE

Adrenal hormonal excesses are responsible for a variety of causes of secondary hypertension. This section describes the evaluation and treatment of the three most common causes.

## Hyperaldosteronism

Primary aldosteronism, or oversecretion of aldosterone unregulated by angiotensin II, classically presents as syndrome of hypertension and hypokalemia or an exaggerated potassium loss with small doses of diuretic. Currently, many cases of subclinical hyperaldosteronism are uncovered through routine screening of aldosterone and plasma renin activity. Patients with suspected primary aldosteronism can be further evaluated with a ratio of plasma aldosterone to renin activity: a ratio of greater than 10 is abnormal, and a ratio exceeding 20 is highly suggestive of hyperaldosteronism.

Once a screening has identified a patient as having aldosteronism, the next step is to determine whether the aldosterone level can be suppressed by either saline infusion or captopril. This testing often requires referral to an endocrinologist or a hypertension specialist. Most antihypertensive medications have an effect either on plasma renin or on serum aldosterone levels, but taking a patient off all drugs before testing may increase the risk of cardiovascular complications, particularly in patients with severe elevations of their blood pressure. Once primary aldosteronism is confirmed with biochemical testing, the key diagnostic decision is whether a patient with primary aldosteronism is suffering from a benign solitary adenoma, an adrenocarcinoma, or bilateral adrenal hyperplasia. Adrenal CT or magnetic resonance imaging (MRI) can suggest this diagnosis, and solitary lesions can be further characterized with NP-59 scintigraphy after dexamethasone suppression. Benign lesions take up the isotope, adenomas unilaterally and hyperplasia bilaterally, whereas malignant lesions generally do not. Lesions thought to be malignant on the basis of either NP-59 scans or size (larger than 4 cm suggests malignancy) should be removed. Smaller, presumably benign, lesions can be monitored expectantly. Improvement in blood pressure is expected after resection of solitary adrenal adenomas. With the development of laparoscopic techniques, adrenalectomy is an increasingly attractive alternative. Patients with bilaterally adrenal hyperplasia are treated with spironolactone, but can also be treated effectively with other antihypertensive medications.

## Pheochromocytoma

The diagnosis of pheochromocytoma can be made primarily from the patient's history, but the symptoms of pheochromocytoma overlap considerably with those of numerous other diseases, including panic attacks, atrial tachyarrhythmia, alcohol withdrawal, and perimenopausal hot flashes, as well as intermittent medical compliance. The classic patient with a pheochromocytoma has wide, almost rhythmic, unprovoked fluctuations in blood pressure accompanied by tachycardia, pallor, sweating, headaches, and sometimes cardiac failure caused by progressive catecholamine-induced left ventricular failure.

In patients with an appropriate history, the most widely used screening test is a 24-hour urine collection for metanepherine, normetanephrine, and vanillylmandelic acid. Labetalol can interfere with older fluormetric assays, but the now more commonly used high performance liquid chromatography determination is not similarly affected. Another screening test is random plasma metanephrine level, which has 99% sensitivity for diagnosis.

If there is biochemical evidence for a pheochromocytoma, the next step is to localize the tumor for resection. Eighty-five percent of pheochromocytoma occurs in the adrenal glands and can be demonstrated by CT or MRI. In patients without obvious adrenal masses, metaiodobenzylguanidine (MIBG) scanning with I 131-labeled benzylguanidine can localize the tumor, which is usually found along the sympathetic chain or in the bladder.

Once localized, pheochromocytoma should be resected with careful perioperative blood pressure control, usually with phenoxybenzamine and other medications. Beta-blockers should be used cautiously until alpha-blockade is established, to prevent further increases in blood pressure. Malignant pheochromocytoma can be treated with various agents such as metyrosine and treptozocin.

## Cushing's Syndrome

Cushing's syndrome, and excess glucocorticoid secretion, is an unusual cause of secondary hypertension. One clue to this diagnosis is the lack of normal nocturnal decline in blood pressure and abnormal diurnal variation in glucocorticoid levels. This syndrome should be suspected in patients with depression and physical features of Cushing's syndrome, such as central obesity, purple striae, moon facies, etc. When Cushing's syndrome is suspected, a 24-hour urine collection for free cortisol yields nearly 100% sensitivity. A dexamethasone suppression test should help determine the site of the adenoma. If hypercortisolism is independent of adrenocorticotropic hormone (ACTH), the adrenal glands are the most likely site and should be imaged by CT or MRI. If the hormonal tests suggest that the disease is ACTH-dependent, then the pituitary gland is the likely location of the tumor. Hypertensive patients with hypercortisolism are likely to benefit from referral to an endocrinologist for evaluation, including evaluation of rarer causes of cortisol excess.

## THYROID AND PARATHYROID ABNORMALITIES

Patients with symptoms of hyperthyroidism or hypothyroidism should be screened by thyroid stimulating hormone (TSH) measurement. However, since the symptoms of hypo- and hyperthyroidism may be vague or nonspecific, routine screening with TSH may be helpful to rule out these diagnoses. Additionally, elderly patients often have atypical manifestations of thyroid dysfunction, and it is therefore prudent to screen all elderly hypertensive patients with TSH measurement. Patients with hypothyroidism often have a depressed cardiac output with a markedly increased peripheral vascular resistance, which results in hypertension. Similarly, patients with hyperthyroidism have tachycardia and increased inotropism and can be hypertensive for those reasons. Treatment of these patents can yield improvement in blood pressure, both systolic and diastolic.

Hyperparathyroidism can lead to hypertension due to increased vascular reactivity to catecholamines and/or renal parenchymal disease from chronic calcium deposition in the kidneys. Hyperparathyroidism should be considered in hypertensive patients with elevated serum calcium levels.

## OBSTRUCTIVE SLEEP APNEA

Obstructive sleep apnea may occur in as many as 30% of hypertensive patients, although some investigators have noted no daytime hypertension among patients with obstructive sleep apnea. Observational studies have shown that systemic and pulmonary pressures rise during apneic episodes, which have also been associated with increased sympathetic activity. Screening patients with clinical signs of obstructive sleep apnea and treatment with weight loss and continuous positive airway pressure ventilation may yield significant reductions in blood pressure. Diet, weight loss, and lifestyle modifications should be stressed heavily to these patients, especially as weight loss is likely to produce significant benefits.

## AORTIC COARCTATION

Significant aortic coarctation is generally diagnosed in childhood and is often amenable to balloon dilation, but does occasionally require surgical correction. Attendant lesions are often focal but can be diffuse and extend down large lengths of the aorta. Patients with less severe coarctation often survive quietly into adulthood and develop hypertension as a result of a post obstructive vasoconstriction. Coarctation causes activation of the renin-angiotensin system and excessive catecholamine elevation during exercise. Adult patients with aortic coarctation often present with heart failure, aortic rupture, bacterial endocarditis, or intracranial hemorrhage. The diagnosis can sometimes be made by evaluating the aortic contour on plain chest radiography, but it is more definitively made by CT, MRI, or transesophageal echocardiography. The prevalence of hypertension among adults with coarctation approaches 33%. Evaluation of young patients with hypertension should include consideration of aortic coarctation, because repair of the coarctation can improve the hypertension and, more important, sequelae of the coarctation can be minimized or prevented.

## CONCLUSIONS

Hypertension is a significant contributor of death and morbidity. Much of the health effects of hypertension can be prevented or delayed with appropriate diagnosis, education, and treatment. At the core of treatment is lifestyle modification: diet, exercise, and weight loss. Medical therapy, when recommended, should be initiated at all age groups. There are many medications that are effective, affordable, and easily tolerated. In patients with refractory hypertension, evaluation for secondary causes of hypertension may be warranted. It is important to realize that the overwhelming majority of patients with hypertension, even those with severe or secondary causes of hypertension, have primary (essential) hypertension. The patient's medical regimen should be reevaluated with a special focus on its cost and the patient's ability to adhere to the regimen before labeling a patient's hypertension as "refractory to treatment." In addition, it is essential to look for exogenous causes of a patient's blood pressure elevation, because attention to these causes can result in reversal of much of a patient's hypertension, and, in many ways, these causes are among the most treatable "secondary" causes of hypertension. Once it has been established that a patient's hypertension is truly refractory to treatment or has characteristics (either laboratory or clinical) suggestive of other secondary causes, prompt and complete evaluation can lead to marked improvement or even complete resolution of hypertension. Most important, an evaluation for hypertension is not simply a reason for the physician to treat the elevated numbers, it is also an opportunity—perhaps one that will not occur again before a decade passes—for examination of the patient's overall cardiovascular risk profile, with attention to modifiable risk factors and for interventions that will provide significant reduction of cardiovascular risk.

## Suggested Readings

1. Calhoun DA, Jones D, Textor S, et al. Resistant hypertension: diagnosis, evaluation and treatment. *Hypertension*. 2008; 51:1493–1419.

2. Chobanian AV, Bakris GL, Black HR, et al. Seventh Report of the Joint National Committee on Prevention, Detection, Evaluation, and Treatment of High Blood Pressure. *Hypertension*. 2003;42:1206–1252.

3. Izzo JL, Black HR, eds. Council on High Blood Pressure Research AHA. *AHA Hypertension Primer*. 4th ed. Philadelphia Pennsylvania: Lippincott, Williams and Wilkins. 2008.

4. Rosendorff C, Black HR, Cannon CP, et al. Treatment of hypertension in the prevention and management of ischemic heart disease: a scientific statement from the American Heart Association Council for High Blood Pressure Research and the Councils on Clinical Cardiology and Epidemiology and Prevention. *Circulation*. 2007;115:2761–2788.

5. Wal-Mart $4 co-pay medication list: http://i.walmart.com/i/if/hmp/fusion/four _dollar_drug_list.pdf

# 22

# Diabetes and Cardiovascular Disease

GARY E. SANDER, HOSSEIN DEHGHANI, AND THOMAS D. GILES

## • PRACTICAL POINTS

- Macrovascular disease is the most common cause of mortality in DM. CV risk begins *below* the threshold for clinical diagnosis of DM.

- Severity of hyperglycemia correlates *more strongly* with microvascular than macrovascular outcomes.

- Macrovascular disease in DM is typically multifactorial.

- 75% of diabetic patients eventually develop hypertension.

- Clustering of hyperglycemia, hypertension, obesity, dyslipidemia, and atherosclerosis may lead to "diabetic cardiomyopathy"/heart failure

- Silent myocardial ischemia is found in 10-20% of the diabetic population as compared to 1 to 4% of non-diabetics.

- Dysautonomia (25% of type 1 and 33% of type 2 diabetic patients) often results in significant CV morbidity and mortality.

- Diabetes mellitus is considered a CAD risk equivalent and merits stringent risk factor modification.

- In those with T2DM and ≥1 risk factor (cigarette smoking, hypertension, or family history of premature CAD), the LDL-C target should be <70 mg/dL; otherwise, the LDL-C target is <100 mg.

- Multiple risk factor reduction strategies can result in significant mortality benefits in those with T2DM.

## INTRODUCTION

Clinical manifestations of diabetic heart disease include atherosclerosis leading to ischemic cardiomyopathy, diabetic cardiomyopathy (DCM), and diabetic autonomic neuropathy (DAN); the complex pathophysiologic processes include macrovascular disease, microvascular disease, myocellular hypertrophy and fibrosis, and autonomic nerve fiber degeneration, as further described in **Table 22-1**. While the macrovascular component—atherosclerosis—generally receives the greatest attention, it represents only one component of the cardiovascular disease process caused by diabetes mellitus (DM). Cardiovascular disease, including coronary artery disease (CAD), cerebrovascular disease, and peripheral vascular disease, is the most common cause of death in diabetic patients; the majority of deaths result from CAD.

## ROLE OF HYPERGLYCEMIA

Increasing blood glucose concentration is an independent and continuous risk factor for cardiovascular disease; risk begins below the glucose threshold required for a clinical diagnosis of diabetes; the risk of heart failure increases by 10-15% per 1% increase in HgbA1c in individuals both with and without known diabetes. The blood glucose level during acute myocardial infarction (AMI) predicts long-term mortality in patients both with known and with previously

| Table 22-1 • Diabetic Heart Disease: Pathophysiological Process | |
|---|---|
| Macrovascular Disease | Not clearly related to glycemic control<br>↑ Incidence and severity of obstructive epicardial disease<br>Associated dyslipidemia<br>Hypercoagulable state<br>↑ Platelet aggregation (↑ glycoprotein Ib and IIb/IIIa)<br>↑ PAI-1<br>↑ Coagulation factors (TF, VII, thrombin)<br>↓ Thrombomodulin, protein C<br>↓ Bioavailability of nitric oxide (NO)<br>↓ $PGI_2$, ↑ endothelin-1 |
| Microvascular Disease | Related to degree of glycemic control<br>Intimal thickening<br>Microaneurysms<br>Thickened capillary basement membranes<br>Decreased coronary flow reserve |
| Myocellular Hypertrophy/Fibrosis | Cellular hypertrophy<br>Interstitial and myco-cytolytic necrosis<br>Accumulation of glycoproteins and collagen<br>Perimysial fibrosis |
| Diabetic Autonomic Neuropathy | Parasympathetic, followed by sympathetic, denervation, causing initial exaggerated sympathetic imbalance<br>Absent heart rate variability due to DAN is predictive of both LV failure and increased mortality<br>Loss of afferent reflex sensitivity |
| Biochemical Abnormalities | Decrease in myosin ATPase with a shift from the faster $V_1$ isoform to the slower $V_2$, leading to a decreased speed of muscle shortening<br>Reduced rate of $Ca^{2+}$ binding and uptake by sarcoplasmic reticulum<br>Reduced $Na^+/Ca^{2+}$ exchanger activity, associated with Increased protein kinase C activity and altered cell signaling<br>↑ Superoxide anion and oxidative stress<br>↓ Mitochondrial activity leading to ↓ ATP production and cardiac contractility |

undiagnosed diabetes; an increase in glucose of 18 mg/dL is associated with 4% increase in mortality in nondiabetic and 5% in diabetic patients. The relative risk of in-hospital death in nondiabetic patients with AMI with admission glucose ≥ 110 mg/dL is 3.9 compared with normoglycemic nondiabetic patients. Among AMI patients with diabetes, those with admission glucose ≥ 180 mg/dL have a 70% relative increase in the risk of in-hospital death compared with diabetic patients with normal admission glucose values.

Hyperglycemia has been associated with elevated catecholamine levels, elevated systolic blood pressure (SRD) and diastolic blood pressure (DBP), QT prolongation, a prothrombotic state with lower tissue plasminogen activator (tPA) and higher plasminogen activator inhibitor-1 (PAI-1) levels, increased platelet aggregation, reduced fibrinogen survival, and increased markers of vascular inflammation. Higher glucose levels in patients presenting with ACS have been associated with higher free fatty acid (FFA) concentrations, insulin resistance, and impaired myocardial glucose utilization, thereby increasing $O_2$ consumption and negatively impacting ischemia. When FFA availability exceeds fatty acid oxidation rates, intramyocardial lipids will accumulate, causing lipotoxicity, which plays a role in the development of contractile dysfunction; FFA may increase the incidence of malignant ventricular arrhythmias.

# CORONARY ARTERY DISEASE (CAD)

## Epidemiology

Cardiovascular mortality among patients with type 2 diabetes mellitus(T2DM) but without prior MI has been reported to be as high as that in nondiabetic patients with previous infarction in a 7-year follow-up. Diabetic patients have an AMI mortality rate approximately twice as high as that observed in nondiabetic patients. Use of fibrinolytic agents does not reduce excessive morbidity and mortality. This finding is not related to the ability of fibrinolytic agents to restore complete reperfusion or increased risk of reocclusion of the infarct-related artery, but rather the degree of hyperglycemia, impaired ventricular performance at the noninfarct areas, and metabolic derangements during the acute phase of MI.

Despite the premature occurrence of CAD, the more extensive the disease at diagnosis, the greater morbidity and mortality after infarction, and the reduced success with revascularization, histopathological studies have indicated similarity in plaque composition and structure between diabetic and nondiabetic individuals. However, diabetic atherosclerotic plaques are often more diffuse and distal in distribution; small vessel disease and endothelial dysfunction with resultant blunted vasodilatory responses are present as well. Further, CAD is frequently silent in diabetes. Silent myocardial ischemia is found in 10-20% of the diabetic population as compared to 1-4% of nondiabetics.

"Symptomatic" cardiac disease has been reported in over 15% of T2DM patients over age 65. Atypical symptoms include dyspnea, fatigue, and gastrointestinal complaints with exertion, and such complaints require further evaluation to determine etiology of symptoms and type of cardiac disease which may be present, the need for invasive testing, and the most appropriate therapeutic intervention. Unexplained congestive heart failure (CHF), particularly when resulting from systolic left ventricular (LV) dysfunction, requires testing to exclude asymptomatic CAD.

## Testing

Atypical symptoms and asymptomatic ischemia, coupled with the poor outcome in diabetic patients following AMI, mandate effective means of early identification of CAD. However, echocardiographic and nuclear testing images must be interpreted carefully due to the high prevalence of false positive tests that result from the effects of diabetes on myocardial function. Among the confounding issues are: LVH (false positive ST segment changes and nuclear perfusion defects), DCM (wall motion abnormalities, blunted adrenergic enhancement of contractility, nuclear perfusion defects), concomitant renal disease (increased adenosine concentration resulting in decreased maximal flow reserve following dipyridamole, in turn leading to decreased SPECT sensitivity), DAN (decreased chronotropic response to exercise, decreased coronary vasodilator capacity, dissociation of cardiac from external work), and endothelial dysfunction (decreased coronary vasodilator capacity).

General indications for cardiac testing as recommended by the ADA/ACC Consensus Conference are listed in **Table 22-2,** and **Table 22-3** for symptomatic diabetic patients with risk factors. **Table 22-4** lists recommended follow-up after initial use of ECG treadmill testing; even in the presence of a moderately positive test, a normal to near single photon emission computed tomography (SPECT) perfusion study indicates a very good prognosis (<2% annual cardiac event rate). The selection of initial screening tests should be governed by the intent of testing: to detect occult disease or to estimate prognosis and provide risk stratification.

The ECG itself should not be overlooked; a normal ECG virtually precludes the presence of significant systolic

### Table 22-2 • Indications for Exercise Testing in Patients with Diabetes

**ADA-ACC indications**

Typical or atypical cardiac symptoms
Resting ECG suggestive of ischemia or infarction
Peripheral or carotid occlusive arterial disease
Sedentary lifestyle, age ≥ 35 years, and plans to begin vigorous exercise program
Two or more of the following risk factors in addition to diabetes:
• Total cholesterol ≥ 240 mg/dL, LDL ≥ 160 mg/dL, or HDL < 35 mg/dL
• Blood pressure > 140/90 mm Hg
• Smoking
• Family history of premature CAD
• Nephropathy, manifested as micro/macroalbuminuria
• Unexplained systolic dysfunction

**ACC/AHA/ADA indications prior to vigorous exercise training**

Known or suspected CAD
T1DM for >15 years
T2DM for >10 years or age ≥ 35 years
Additional atherosclerotic risk factors, or
Evidence of microvascular disease, PAD, or autonomic neuropathy.

dysfunction. On the other hand, ST-T abnormalities represent a significant risk factor in both men and women for the subsequent demonstration of asymptomatic CAD by exercise ECG and SPECT imaging. For diabetic patients who are able to exercise with a normal or near normal ECG, a simple treadmill or bicycle exercise test, evaluating exercise capacity, ventricular reserve, and ST segment changes will detect almost all who have left main and significant 3-vessel disease. A normal test indicates a good prognosis. Peak treadmill heart rate is perhaps the single most important prognostic indicator; a treadmill result that was either abnormal or inconclusive due to failure to achieve 90% of the predicted maximal heart rate predicts poor outcomes. In the presence

### Table 22-3 • Cardiac Testing of Symptomatic Diabetic Patients

| Symptom | Appropriate Next Test |
|---|---|
| Unstable or moderately severe angina<br>Mild angina and MI<br>Definite ischemia on ECG<br>Mild angina and CHF | Possible angiography |
| Mild angina and normal/near normal ECG<br>Atypical chest pain and abnormal ECG | Stress perfusion imaging or stress echo (treadmill exercise preferred to pharmacological stress) |
| Atypical chest pain with normal ECG | Exercise stress test alone (if ≥2 risk factors, then stress imaging) |

### Table 22-4 • Appropriate Follow-Up after Initial Stress Testing

| Pretest Risk | ETT Results | | | |
|---|---|---|---|---|
| | Normal | Mildly | Moderately | Markedly |
| High (>RF) | 2 | 3 | 4 | 4 |
| Moderate (2-3 RF) | 1 | 3 | 3 | 4 |
| Low (<1 RF) | 1 | 3 | 3 | 4 |

1 = routine follow-up: yearly ECG, repeat ETT in 3-5 years
2 = close follow-up: repeat ETT in 1-2 years
3 = nuclear or echocardiographic imaging study
4 = coronary angiogram
(Risk factors are those listed in Table 22-1)
"Mildly" positive is defined by such observations as 1-1.5 mm ST segment depression at a moderate to high exercise level; "markedly" positive is defined by such features as hypotension during exercise, a positive test at heart rate <110 bpm, exercise capacity <6 min, ST segment depression in >5 leads, or >2 mm maximum ST segment depression.

of suspected CAD, sensitivity and specificity for maximal ECG exercise test is approximately 75% and 77%, respectively, for significant CAD ($\geq$ 70% occlusion of at least one coronary artery), compared with sensitivity and specificity of 80% and 87%, respectively, for thallium-201 ($^{201}$Tl) myocardial scintigraphy.

Perfusion imaging with $^{201}$Tl or technicium-99m ($^{99m}$Tc) sestamibi, preferably with exercise but also effective with pharmacological vasodilation, allows quantification of the extent of perfusion abnormalities, which is important in both identifying the presence of disease and providing prognostic information. Multiple perfusion defects, large defects or areas of reversibility, reduced ventricular function, increased isotope uptake in the lung, and transient left ventricular dilation are all predictive of future cardiac events. In patients with angiographically "normal" coronary arteries, abnormal perfusion scans may indicate diffuse coronary disease or endothelial dysfunction and an increased event rate relative to individuals with normal perfusion scans.

Stress echocardiography is a reasonable alternative to stress perfusion imaging in the presence of appropriate echocardiographic expertise. SPECT imaging is superior to SE in the detection of single vessel disease and in detecting ischemia; the techniques are similarly able to detect multivessel disease. The role of DSE testing appears very limited at this time due to dissociation between myocardial oxidative metabolism (demonstrated by $^{11}$C-acetate clearance by PET scanning) and cardiac work (rate-pressure product) demonstrated in T2DM with normal stress perfusion SPECT; this defect in myocardial oxidative metabolism becomes apparent during dobutamine stress. The sensitivity, specificity, positive, and negative predictive values of DSE for detection of asymptomatic CAD in T2DM are reported as 82%, 54%, 84%, and 50%, respectively.

Test selection in the symptomatic patient is determined by the severity of symptoms and presence and extent of ECG abnormalities, which could either limit the ability to interpret a routine exercise stress test or indicate more extensive heart disease, such as prior MI, than suggested clinically. Those patients with symptoms suggestive of moderate or more severe angina or ECG evidence of CAD, particularly if associated with heart failure, will in most cases benefit from cardiac catheterization without prior screening; this will quickly establish the presence and extent of atherosclerosis and allow prompt initiation of appropriate treatment. However, once asymptomatic patients with CAD have been identified, there are no data to demonstrate that treatment interventions improve their subsequent outcomes. If all diabetic patients are treated to aggressive BP, lipid, and glucose secondary prevention targets with regimens including aspirin, renin-angiotensin-aldosterone system (RAAS) inhibition, and statins, medical management alone may prove adequate; the challenge is to identify asymptomatic patients most likely to benefit from revascularization.

### Dyslipidemia

The most prevalent lipid pattern in T2DM is that of elevated triglycerides and decreased HDL-C; there is a preponderance of small, dense LDL-C (high apoB); HDL-C may be best predictor of coronary disease (inverse correlation). LDL-C-lowering is beneficial in clinical trials but is not a significant predictor in observational studies; elevated triglycerides may be a better predictor of coronary disease that elevated LDL-C because triglycerides are more closely correlated with other components of the insulin resistance syndrome.

## DIABETIC CARDIOMYOPATHY

Heart failure is not a diagnosis but rather a clinical syndrome resulting from progression of cardiomyopathy, a term defined simply as "disease of heart muscle." Diabetes produces both adaptive and maladaptive myocardial responses; altered metabolism and impaired insulin action in heart and skeletal muscle are both cause and consequence of altered cardiac function. Hyperglycemia may promote the progression of heart failure by accelerating atherosclerosis and excessive interstitial myocardial collagen accumulation, protein kinase C (PKC) activity, increasing oxidative stress, and upregulating renin-angiotensin-aldosterone system (RAAS) activity. The combination of hyperglycemia, hypertension, obesity, dyslipidemia, and atherosclerosis commonly seen with diabetes mellitus produces structural damage in the heart that manifests as both systolic and diastolic LV dysfunction and ultimately as HF, explaining the more common occurrence of this syndrome in diabetic patients. In the united kingdom prospective diabetes study (UKPDS), each 1% increase in HgbA$_{1c}$ levels was associated with a 12% increase in heart failure risk. Diabetes is a risk factor for the development of coronary atherosclerosis with resultant myocardial ischemia and infarction, is frequently associated with hypertension (a factor in the pathogenesis of approximately 70% of all HF cases), and causes the development of a specific DCM independent of CAD. Conversely, HF patients have an increased risk of developing diabetes.

## Pathophysiology

Dilated cardiomyopathy (DCM), defined as myocardial dysfunction in the absence of obstructive epicardial CAD, is characterized pathophysiologically by diastolic LV dysfunction and myocardial fibrosis. Data from animal models suggest that prediabetic metabolic derangements, such as insulin resistance, may produce abnormalities in collagen deposition and LV fibrosis prior to the development of overt DM. Myocardial fibrosis underlies the pathologic hypertrophy and dysfunction observed in HF. In vivo studies indicate that circulating and tissue RAAS are involved in the structural remodeling of the myocardial collagen matrix, resulting in fibrosis that disrupts the electrical and mechanical behavior of the hypertrophied myocardium. Subclinical vascular involvement in the form of impaired endothelial function and increased carotid intimal-medial thickness have been demonstrated in young diabetic subjects. The critical importance of this fibrosis is highlighted by the observation that pharmacological inhibition of PKC-(epsilon) attenuates cardiac fibrosis and dysfunction in hypertension-induced HF.

## Inflammation

Data appear to demonstrate that CRP levels predict cardiac risk independent of diabetic status. However, the fact that diabetics tend to have higher CRP levels and that, in some clinical studies, diabetes still remained a significant independent predictor, suggests that inflammation and metabolic derangements may represent two different aspects of the same process and thus both could be considered as independent predictors of cardiac risk.

## Insulin Resistance

Insulin resistance is commonly present in HF even in the absence of diabetes; the exact mechanisms for such insulin resistance is unknown, but hypotheses include: (1) an increased adrenergic drive leading to increases in FFA oxidation and subsequent insulin resistance; (2) elevated levels of circulating TNF-$\alpha$ exerting direct negative effects on insulin sensitive cells and also leading to elevated plasma FFA concentrations; and (3) some mechanism of HF itself that is possibly secondary to circulatory changes or as part of the overall neurohormonal and metabolic response to HF. The failing heart metabolizes carbohydrates and FFAs for energy production; insulin resistance compromises these mechanisms.

## Microcirculation

The concordant effects of the metabolic derangements of diabetes and the vascular abnormalities associated with hypertension may lead to microvascular-induced tissue injury, which then leads to HF, as suggested by the observation that patients with overt albuminuria develop higher and earlier occurrence of HF hospitalizations than those with micro- or normoalbuminuria; SBP, but not DBP, contributes to heart failure. After adjustment for age and sex, diabetics have higher SBP, pulse pressures, and heart rates, lower DBP, and longer durations of hypertension than nondiabetics (HGEN study). LV mass and relative wall thickness are higher in diabetic than nondiabetic subjects independent of covariates. Compared with nondiabetic hypertensives, diabetics had lower stress-corrected midwall shortening without any difference in LVEF. Insulin levels and insulin resistance were higher in non-insulin-treated diabetics than nondiabetic subjects. Insulin resistance is positively but weakly related to LV mass and relative wall thickness.

## Hypertension

Approximately 75% of adults with T2DM are hypertensive, resulting in a 7.2-fold increase in mortality; in the presence of nephropathy, hypertension is associated with a 37-fold increase in mortality. The pathogenesis of hypertension in diabetes is multifactorial; a relationship has been noted to both high and low renin levels, together with changes associated with abnormal free water clearance in damaged kidneys, and a possible association with increased glycoprotein and connective tissue infiltration in the walls of resistance vessels, causing a reduction in vascular compliance. Diabetic retinopathy and nephropathy are more frequent in the presence of hypertension, and an elevated serum creatinine is an independent risk factor for the development of HF. Hypertensive T2DM patients have less regression of LVH with antihypertensive therapy than do nondiabetics, and thus regression becomes a less useful surrogate marker of outcomes in these patients.

## Systolic and Diastolic Cardiac Abnormalities

The signs and symptoms of HF are the same whether or not LVEF is preserved. The existence of DCM, independent of atherosclerotic and hypertensive heart disease, has been firmly established in the adult population; its presence in younger patients with insulin-dependent diabetes mellitus is less established. Most studies have found normal resting cardiac function in young patients, but have been limited by the assessment of LV performance by ejection-phase indexes that are dependent not only on myocardial contractility but also on loading conditions. Therefore, the specific level of cardiac contractility has not been determined in this patient population. More detailed evaluation has associated the early onset of diabetes with increased LV mass, performance (shortening fraction, velocity of circumferential fiber shortening, stroke volume, and cardiac index), contractility, and BP, and it has correlated these findings with increased creatinine clearance and microalbuminuria, in turn suggesting that alterations in cardiovascular and renal function may occur in parallel. Tissue Doppler imaging can detect diastolic dysfunction more often than any other echocardiographic approach and thus would appear to markedly improve echocardiographic detection. Diastolic abnormalities occur in as many as two-thirds of insulin-dependent asymptomatic diabetic patients, are associated with higher glucose and HbgA$_{1c}$ levels, and may predict subsequent development of overt HF. Diastolic dysfunction is twice as common as systolic dysfunction; of those diabetic subjects with systolic dysfunction, 83% have impaired diastolic function, whereas only 30% of diabetic patients with diastolic dysfunction have systolic abnormalities. Clinically apparent systolic dysfunction most commonly results from associated myocardial ischemia and hypertension. Altered myocardial energy metabolism, as assessed by magnetic resonance imaging and $^{31}$P nuclear magnetic resonance spectroscopy, may contribute to LV diastolic functional changes in patients with recently diagnosed, even well-controlled and uncomplicated, T2DM.

# DIABETIC AUTONOMIC NEUROPATHY

Dysautonomia results in altered myocardial blood flow, electrical instability, and sudden death. DAN can be detected in 25% of type 1 and 33% of type 2 diabetic patients, is associated with increased mortality, and may result in severe orthostasis, postural hypotension, exercise intolerance, enhanced intraoperative instability, and an increased incidence of silent ischemia and infarction. In T1DM, DAN is associated with the HLA-DR3/4 phenotype. It does appear that prolonged hyperglycemia is a major contributor to development and progression, and that aggressive diabetes management may slow progression. The presence of DAN can be documented by $^{131}$I-metaiodobenzylguanine (MIBG) nuclear scanning or C$^{11}$ hydroxyephedrine PET imaging. Abnormalities of adrenergic cardiac innervation are related to adrenergic cardiac denervation and are characterized by cardiac sympathetic dysinnervation with proximal hyperinnervation complicating distal denervation, causing exaggerated sympathetic imbalance. The result is parasympathetic, followed by sympathetic, denervation, with loss of afferent reflex sensitivity. Subclinical autonomic neuropathy can be detected early using these autonomic function tests:

- supine resting (for 15 min) HR >100 bpm;
- lack of beat-to-beat heart rate variability;
- ratio of longest to shortest RR ≤1.10 during Valsalva;
- ratio of RR of 30th beat to 15th beat after standing ≤1.0;
- fall in systolic BP >30 mm Hg after 1 min standing, and;
- prolonged QT, at rest and particularly after exercise.

Assessment of heart rate variability by 24-hour monitoring may be more sensitive and reliable in detecting DAN than single tests, and it may provide further detection of abnormal circadian rhythms. The absent heart rate variability due to parasympathetic denervation is predictive of both LV failure and increased mortality. The presence of DAN has been associated with the presence of diabetic nephropathy, and this association contributes to the high mortality rate. Furthermore, the presence of DAN may alter the sensitivity, specificity, and interpretation of noninvasive testing by reducing chronotropic response to exercise, reducing coronary vasodilator capacity, and dissociating cardiac from external work.

# MANAGEMENT

## Glycemic Control

Although intensive glycemic control may not alter indices of systolic function, UKPDS data have clearly demonstrated that intensive BP reduction (mean = 144/88 mm Hg) and glucose control (mean HgbA1c = 7.0%) reduce stroke, microvascular outcomes, death, and all diabetes endpoints. Although BP control (even with pressure reduction significantly less than that recommended by JNC 7 and ADA standards) had a greater impact than did glycemic control in this study, glycemic control proved to be very important: Each 1% reduction in HgbA1c was correlated with reductions of 21% in risk for any endpoint or deaths related to diabetes, 14% for AMI, and 37% for microvascular complications. Metformin does have activity as a peripheral insulin sensitizer, but its main mechanism is the inhibition of hepatic gluconeogenesis; it is the only drug thus far demonstrated to decrease cardiovascular events in patients with T2DM independently of glycemic control. While the thiazolidinediones offer attractive properties (reduction in insulin resistance and decrease plasma insulin concentration), they may cause fluid accumulation and weight gain; these effects are more common during combination therapy with sulfonylureas or insulin. Data now suggest that rosiglitazone does not reduce the cardiovascular event rate despite its reducing HgbA1c; pioglitazone does not appear detrimental and may reduce cardiovascular events. The possibility that sulfonylureas may increase cardiovascular mortality has been debated since release of the UGDP results over 25 years ago. It is now established that sulfonylureas act by inhibiting the ATP-sensitive potassium channel (K$_{ATP}$); this inhibition in the pancreas induces insulin release, but in the heart blocks ischemic preconditioning and may lead to enhanced cell death and arrhythmias resulting from delayed after-depolarizations. Furthermore, sulfonylureas are vasoconstrictors, worsen vascular reactivity, and appear to adversely affect outcome after PTCA.

The ACCORD and ADVANCE trials, both designed to evaluate the effects of intensive glycemic control on vascular outcomes using intensive but differing blood-glucose-control strategies in high risk T2DM patients, provided different and confusing results. ADVANCE reported that intensive treatment produced a relative reduction of 10% in the primary composite outcome of major macrovascular and microvascular events, primarily as a consequence of a reduction in nephropathy. In ACCORD, the intensive-therapy group had an increased rate of death from any cause within 2 years that persisted throughout follow-up. Both trials showed that targeting HgbA1c to levels that are below currently accepted standards in high risk T2DM patients did not reduce the cardiovascular disease event rate. Until the availability of further information defining both targets and drug regimens for glycemic control, a target HgbA1c level of approximately 7% appears appropriate for high risk populations.

The AHA, recognizing the adverse impact of hyperglycemia in ACS, has issued a scientific statement with the following recommendations:

- Glucose level should be a part of the initial evaluation in all patients with suspected or confirmed ACS.
- In patients admitted to an ICU with ACS, glucose levels should be monitored closely and intensive glucose control initiated in patients with plasma glucose >180 mg/dL. Approximation of normoglycemia (plasma glucose 90 to 140 mg/dL) and avoidance of hypoglycemia appears to be a reasonable goal.
- Insulin, administered as an intravenous infusion, is currently the most effective means of controlling glucose.
- Treatment should be instituted as soon as feasible, without compromising the administration of established treatments.
- In patients hospitalized in the non-ICU setting, efforts should be directed at maintaining plasma glucose levels <180 mg/dL with subcutaneous insulin regimens.
- ACS patients with hyperglycemia but without prior history of diabetes should have predischarge evaluation to determine the severity of their metabolic derangements.
- Before discharge, plans for optimal outpatient glucose control should be determined in those patients with established diabetes, newly diagnosed diabetes, or evidence of insulin resistance.

## Blood Pressure

In the UKPDS epidemiological study, each 10-mm Hg decrease in mean SBP was associated with risk reductions of 12% for any complication related to diabetes, 15% for deaths related to diabetes, 11% for MI, and 13% for microvascular complications. No threshold of risk was observed for any endpoint; improvement in cardiovascular outcomes continued down to a SBP of 110 mm Hg.

The HOT trial demonstrated that more aggressive treatment (DBP at trial end = 81.1 mm Hg) reduced the risk of major cardiovascular events by approximately 50% relative to a less aggressively treated group (DBP 85.2 mm Hg). The ADA, NKF, and JNC 7 advocate lowering blood pressure to <130/80 mm Hg. The difficulty in achieving target, particularly for SBP, has been well documented; the majority of patients will require in excess of three antihypertensive agents from different antihypertensive classes. Treatment regimens should include RAAS inhibition, preferably with an ACE inhibitor or an ARB, whenever possible to delay or prevent macro- and microvascular complications. The most aggressive trials have been successful in achieving SBP targets in approximately two-thirds of subjects, and DBP targets in greater than 90%. It does appear from these trials that regimens that include a thiazide diuretic do result in an increase the incidence of new diabetes and worsen the control of existing diabetes relative to regimens that avoid thiazides.

## Dyslipidemia

The MRC/BHF HPS demonstrated that cholesterol reduction was beneficial for diabetic patients even in the absence of manifest CAD-elevated cholesterol levels, suggesting that use of a statin regimen could prevent about 5% of diabetic patients without occlusive vascular disease from having at least one major vascular event over a 5-year period. In CARDS, the first large HMG-CoA reductase inhibitor study to enroll only patients with T2DM, atorvastatin reduced cardiovascular events by 37% compared with placebo. Diabetes is now defined as a CAD equivalent by NCEP-ATP III guidelines, and statin therapy should be considered routine. Recent ACC/ADA Consensus guidelines recommend that in the presence of T2DM and ≥1 risk factor (cigarette smoking, hypertension, or family history of premature CAD), the LDL-C target should be <70 mg/dL, non-HDL-C <100 mg/dL, and apoB < 80mg/dL. In the absence of these factors, the LDL-C target becomes <100 mg/dL, non-HDL-C <130 mg/dL, and apoB <90 mg/dL. It is important to remember that the residual major vascular event rate in diabetic patients treated with statins is still higher than that of untreated patients without diabetes.

Fibric acid derivatives (fibrates) are PPAR-α agonists and alter the transcription of genes-encoding proteins that control lipoprotein metabolism; fibrates reduce plasma triglyceride levels by 30-50%, increase HDL-C levels by 10-15%, and shift the distribution of LDL-C subfractions towards larger, less atherogenic particles (lower apoB). DAIS, conducted exclusively in patients with T2DM, found that fenofibrate reduced the progression of angiographic CAD; the VA-HIT showed that gemfibrozil reduced cardiovascular events in subgroups of diabetic patients. In the FIELD trial, fenofibrate did not significantly reduce the risk of the primary outcome of coronary events, but it did reduce total cardiovascular events, mainly due to fewer nonfatal myocardial infarctions and revascularizations. Fenofibrate also reduced microvascular events: less albuminuria progression and less retinopathy needing laser treatment. Overall benefit was most apparent in patients concomitantly treated with statins.

## Coronary Artery Disease

The initial BARI trial indicated that 5 and 7 years after randomization, patients with treated DM had significantly higher overall and cardiac mortality compared to nondiabetic subjects, regardless of the initial revascularization strategy assigned. Those diabetic subjects assigned to an initial PCI strategy had significantly higher 5-year mortality than did patients randomized to CABG. Further follow-up indicated that, despite its association with smaller distal and poorer quality vessels, the presence of diabetes did not appear to adversely affect patency of internal mammary or vein grafts over the initial 4-year follow-up, suggesting that the survival differences may have resulted from noncardiac causes. However, the relevance of such trials becomes questionable in the era of drug eluting stents. A meta-analysis of over 11,000 diabetic patients with either paclitaxel or sirolimus-eluting stents has demonstrated a revascularization rate of less than 10% and major adverse cardiovascular events rate (death, MI, repeat revascularization) of 10-12%. However, the efficacy of PCI procedures for treatment of AMI requires further evaluation. The use of GpIIb/IIIa inhibitors at the time of stent placement reduces acute ischemic events and the 6-month risk of death, MI, and target vessel revascularization among diabetic patients to an extent similar to that in nondiabetic patients. Whether there are quantitative differences in this treatment effect among the available GpIIb/IIIa inhibitors remains controversial. In diabetic patients with ACS, bivalirudin monotherapy, as compared with treatment with heparin plus GpIIb/IIIa inhibitor, provided similar protection from ischemic events with less major bleeding and thus a significant reduction in net adverse 30-day clinical outcomes (ACUITY). Enteric aspirin in a dose between 81 and 325 mg daily is recommended for secondary prevention in patients with documented vascular disease and as primary prevention for high risk patients.

## Heart Failure

Functional, biochemical, and morphological myocardial abnormalities independent of atherosclerosis, particularly when associated with hypertension and LVH, may result in impaired LV diastolic function, contributing to the clinical syndrome of HF with preserved systolic function. Meta-analysis of six studies (CONSENSUS, SAVE, two SOLVD studies, SMILE, and TRACE) confirmed that treatment of patients with or without diabetes produce similar reductions in mortality (15%) with ACE inhibitor therapy. The relative risk reductions for beta-blocker trials (CIBIS, COPERNICUS, MERIT-HF) were 35% for nondiabetic patients and 23% for diabetic patients; this difference was not significant. Although the relative reduction in mortality may be less for diabetics, because the absolute risk of mortality is greater, the absolute risk reduction is certainly equal or greater for diabetic than nondiabetic HF treated with beta-blockers. Beta-blocker treatment improves outcome by decreasing the incidence of both sudden death and pump failure and is of particular benefit in AMI complicated by systolic dysfunction. Although it has been suggested that beta-blocking agents with vasodilating properties may provide additional benefit because of possible improved insulin sensitivity and vasorelaxation, this hypothesis remains unproven. The ARB candesartan has been demonstrated to reduce mortality alone and in combination with ACE inhibitors; in patients without a diagnosis of diabetes at baseline, the number of patients in the candesartan group who developed diabetes was significantly lower than that in the placebo group. In EPHESUS, treatment with the specific aldosterone receptor antagonist eplerenone resulted in a 15% reduction in overall mortality and cardiovascular mortality and hospitalization; however, this did not achieve statistical significance. If spironolactone or eplerenone is administered to diabetic patients, careful monitoring of serum potassium is absolutely essential. Although tight glycemic control decreases the risk of HF in diabetes, the effects of different diabetic treatment regimens on diastolic HF remain unproven.

## Usual Treatments

There are now data indicating that target-driven, long-term, intensified intervention aimed at multiple risk factors in patients with T2DM and microalbuminuria may reduce the risk of macrovascular and microvascular complications by about 50%. SANDS, a randomized, open-label, 3-year trial, reported the effects of aggressive LDL-C (goal < 70 mg/dL) and BP (goal < 115/75 mm Hg) reduction versus the standard goals of LDL-C < 100 mg/dL and BP < 130/85 mm Hg on the progression of subclinical atherosclerosis in over 500 American Indian men and women over 40 years of age, with T2DM. Mean target LDL-C and SBP levels for both groups were reached and maintained; the lower targets resulted in regression of carotid intimal medial thickness and greater decrease in LV mass.

Multiple studies have demonstrated the benefits of ARB and ACE inhibitors on macrovascular and microvascular outcomes in patients with both T1DM and T2DM patients

## Abbreviations and Acronyms

| | | | |
|---|---|---|---|
| (A)MI | (Acute) myocardial infarction | HOT | Hypertension optimal treatment |
| ACC | American College of Cardiology | JNC-7 | Joint National Committee - 7 |
| ACCORD | Action to Control Cardiovascular Risk in Diabetes | LV(H) | Left ventricle (hypertrophy) |
| ACE | Angiotensin-converting enzyme | LVEF | Left Ventricular Ejection Faction |
| ACS | Acute coronary syndrome | MERIT-HF | Metoprolol Controlled Release/Extended Release Randomized Intervention Trial in Chronic Heart Failure |
| ACUITY | Acute Catheterization and Urgent Intervention Triage Strategy | | |
| ADA | American Diabetes Association | MRC/BHF HPS | Medical Research Council/British Heart Foundation |
| ADVANCE | Action in Diabetes and Vascular Disease: Preterax and Diamicron Modified Release Controlled Evaluation | NCEP-ATP | National Cholesterol Education Program – Adult Treatment Program |
| AHA | American Heart Association | NKF | National Kidney Foundation |
| ARB | Angiotensin-receptor blocker | ON-TARGET | Ongoing Telmisartan Alone and in Combination with Ramipril Global Endpoint Trial |
| BARI | Bypass Angioplasty Revascularization Investigation | | |
| (S/D)BP | (Systolic/diastolic) blood pressure | PAI-1 | Plasminogen activator inhibitor-1 |
| CABG | Coronary artery bypass graft | PCI | Percutaneous coronary intervention |
| CARDS | Collaborative Atorvastatin Diabetes Study | PG | Prostaglandin |
| (C)HF | (Congestive) heart failure | PKC | Protein kinase C |
| CIBIS | Cardiac Insufficiency Bisoprolol Survival Study | PPAR-α | Peroxisome proliferator-activated alpha receptor agonists |
| CONSENSUS | Cooperative Northern Scandinavian Enalapril Survival Study | RAAS | renin-angiotensin-aldosterone system |
| COPERNICUS | Carvedilol Prospective Randomized Cumulative Survival | SANDS | Stop Atherosclerosis in Native Diabetics Study |
| CRP | C-reactive protein (cardiospecific) | SAVE | Survival and Ventricular Enlargement Trial |
| DAIS | Diabetes Atherosclerosis Intervention Study | SMILE | Survival of Myocardial Infarction Long-term Evaluation Trial |
| DAN | Diabetic autonomic neuropathy | | |
| DCM | Dilated cardiomyopathy | SOLVD | Studies of Left Ventricular Dysfunction Trial |
| DM | Diabetes mellitus | SPECT | Single photon emission computed tomography |
| DSE | Dobutamine stress echocardiography | | |
| EPHESUS | Epleronone Post-Acute Myocardial Infarction Trial | T1(2)DM | Type 1 (Type 2) diabetes mellitus |
| | | tPA | Tissue plasminogen activator |
| FFA | Free fatty acids | TRACE | Trandolapril Cardiac Evaluation Study |
| FIELD | Fenofibrate Intervention and Event Lowering in Diabetes Study | UGDP | University Group Diabetes Program |
| | | UKPDS | United Kingdom Prospective Diabetic Study |
| HGEN | Hypertension Genetic Epidemiology Network (HyperGEN) Study | VA-HIT | Veterans Affairs Cooperative Studies Program HDL-C Intervention Trial |

with either mild or more severe hypertension. In patients with microalbuminuria or clinical nephropathy, both ACE inhibitors (T1DM and T2DM) and ARB (T2DM) are considered first-line therapy for both prevention of and progression of nephropathy. There are suggestive data that RAAS inhibition may delay the progression of nephropathy by mechanisms beyond that offered by reduction of blood pressure. However, the ON-TARGET trial has suggested an adverse renal effect with the high-dose combination of telmisartan and ramipril. Although beta-blockade is generally considered less effective that RAAS inhibition in preventing diabetic complications, atenolol was equally effective as captopril in reducing blood pressure and the risk of microvascular and macrovascular endpoints in the UKPDS; similar proportions of patients in the two groups showed deterioration in retinopathy by

two grades after nine years. Intensive treatment, with a stepwise implementation of behavior modification and pharmacologic therapy that targeted hyperglycemia, hypertension, dyslipidemia, and microalbuminuria, along with secondary prevention of cardiovascular disease with aspirin has been reported to significantly lower the risk of cardiovascular disease by 53%, nephropathy by 61%, retinopathy by 58%, and DAN by 63%.

## Suggested Readings

1. American Diabetes Association. Consensus development conference on the diagnosis of coronary heart disease in people with diabetes. *Diabetes Care.* 1998;21:1551–59.

2. Creager MA, LüscherTF, Cosentino F, et al. Diabetes and vascular disease: pathophysiology, clinical consequencesand medical therapy: part I. *Circulation.* 2003;108:1527–1532.

3. Deedwania P, Kosiborod M, Barrett E, et al. Hyperglycemia and acute coronary syndrome: a scientific statement from the American Heart Association Diabetes Committee of the Council on Nutrition, Physical Activity, and Metabolism. *Circulation.*, Mar 2008; 117:1610–1619.

4. Giles TD, Sander GE. Diabetes mellitus and heart failure: basic mechanisms, clinical features and therapeutic considerations. *Cardiol Clin.* 2004;22:553–568.

5. Sowers JR, Haffner S. Treatment of cardiovascular and renal risk factors in the diabetic hypertensive. *Hypertension.* 2002;40:781–788.

6. Vinik AI, Ziegler D. Diabetic cardiovascular autonomic neuropathy. *Circulation.* 2007;115:387–397.

# 23

# Endothelial Dysfunction

PAUL E. SZMITKO AND SUBODH VERMA

## ● PRACTICAL POINTS

- Balanced release of bioactive factors from the vascular endothelium facilitates vascular homeostasis. The normal endothelium consists of a monolayer of endothelial cells that form an active barrier between the blood and the underlying tissues.

- Nitric oxide (NO), the key endothelium-derived vasorelaxing factor, plays a crucial role in the maintenance of vascular tone and reactivity.

- NO is generated from the conversion of L-arginine to L-citrulline mediated by the enzyme endothelial NO synthase (eNOS), in the presence of cofactors such as tetrahydrobiopterin (BH4).

- The endothelium secretes vasoconstrictors as well; endothelin-1 (ET-1), released in response to hypoxia, ischemia, inflammatory cytokines, and oxidized LDL, is one of the most potent vasoconstrictors.

- Ang II is a potent vasoconstrictor that increases blood pressure, stimulates aldosterone secretion, and has a proinflammatory effect resulting in endothelial dysfunction and atherosclerosis.

- Endothelial dysfunction implies diminished production or availability of NO and/or and imbalance in the relative contribution of endothelium-derived relaxing and contracting factors.

- Endothelial activation results in increased expression of selectins, VCAM-1, and intercellular adhesion molecule-1 (ICAM-1), thereby promoting monocyte adherence.

- The assessment of endothelial dysfunction depends upon the measurement of the endothelial cell response to stimulation from vasoactive (either physiologic or pharmacologic) substances.

- Strain-gauge venous impedance plethysmography assesses resistance vessel function in the forearm by examining the change in forearm blood flow in response to direct intra-arterial (brachial artery) administration of agonists.

- Brachial artery flow-mediated dilation (FMD) has emerged as the most common assessment tool of endothelial function. Flow-mediated vasodilation is the phenomenon by which blood vessels respond to an increase in flow or shear stress, by dilatation.

## WHAT IS THE ENDOTHELIUM?

The endothelium functions as a protective barrier between all tissues and the circulating blood. The single layer of continuous endothelium lining all blood vessels is strategically located to sense changes in hemodynamic forces and blood-borne signals and respond by releasing a number of autocrine and paracrine substances. The balanced release of these bioactive factors facilitates vascular homeostasis.

## The Endothelium as a Barrier

The normal endothelium consists of a monolayer of endothelial cells that form an active barrier between the blood and the underlying tissues. Intercellular junctions, cell-surface-binding proteins, electrostatic charges of the endothelial cell membranes, and transmembrane proteins regulate the integrity and permeability of the endothelium. This highly dynamic system, which may be modulated in response to selected mediators, regulates cellular and nutrient trafficking from the circulation to the underlying tissues.

## The Endothelium as a Regulator of Vascular Tone

The endothelium secretes numerous mediators that influence vascular hemodynamics, blood pressure and blood flow in various vascular beds. Under basal conditions, the endothelium functions to maintain blood vessels in a relatively dilated state. Responses to various physical and chemical stimuli depend upon the rapid synthesis and release of both vasodilators and vasoconstrictors.

Nitric oxide (NO), the key endothelium-derived vasorelaxing factor, plays a crucial role in the maintenance of vascular tone and reactivity. Furchgott and Zawadzki first demonstrated the presence of an endothelium-derived relaxing factor, which was later shown to be nitric oxide. Nitric oxide is generated from the conversion of L-arginine to L-citrulline mediated by the enzyme endothelial NO synthase (eNOS), in the presence of cofactors such as tetrahydrobiopterin (BH4). Nitric oxide, which has a half-life of 3-5 seconds, diffuses to the vascular smooth muscle cells, increasing cyclic guanosine monophosphate (cGMP) formation, leading to vasodilation. Nitric oxide release into the bloodstream may serve to inhibit leukocyte adhesion to the endothelium, augment fibrinolysis, inhibit platelet adhesion and limit smooth muscle cell (SMC) migration and proliferation. Thus, the loss of endothelium-dependent NO-mediated vasodilation sets the stage for endothelial dysfunction. Key activators of eNOS include physical stimuli such as shear stress, signaling molecules such as bradykinin, adenosine, and various cytokines.

Prostacyclin, another endothelial product that possesses vasorelaxing and antiplatelet properties, acts independently of NO. It is produced from arachidonic acid by the action of the cyclooxygenase system, also in response to shear stress. Prostacyclin's biologic effects are mediated via the activation of adenylyl cyclase, and the subsequent increase in cyclic adenosine monophosphate (cAMP). Though it does possess vasodilatory properties, it appears to play only a small role in regulating vasomotor tone in humans.

To maintain vasodilator tone, the endothelium also mediates the hyperpolarization of vascular SMCs via a nitric oxide- and prostacyclin-independent pathway. The identity and chemical structure of this endothelium-derived hyperpolarizing factor (EDHF) remains undetermined, though EDHF appears to play a more important role in smaller arteries rather than the large arterial conduits, especially in circumstances where NO bioavailability is reduced. It, too, is released in response to shear stress and bradykinin.

In addition to the release of vasodilator substances, the endothelium modulates vascular tone via the generation of vasoconstrictors. Endothelin-1 (ET-1), released by endothelial cells in response to hypoxia, ischemia, inflammatory cytokines, and oxidized low density lipoprotein (ox-LDL), is one of the most potent vasoconstrictors. It exerts its biologic effects by stimulating the G-protein-coupled receptors $ET_A$ and $ET_B$. Vascular SMCs primarily express $ET_A$ receptors, the stimulation of which induces vasoconstriction and vascular SMC proliferation. The maximal vasoconstrictive response to ET-1 takes up to an hour in vivo, and thus, ET-1 likely contributes to prolonged changes in basal vascular tone rather than to minute-by-minute regulation mediated by the shorter-acting NO. Endothelial cells express $ET_B$ receptors. Stimulation of $ET_B$ receptors leads to the formation of NO and prostacyclin, serving as a feedback mechanism in an effort to restore normal vascular tone. Angiotensin-converting enzyme (ACE), localized to the surface of the endothelium, further influences vasoregulation. ACE, as part of the renin-angiotensin-aldosterone system, cleaves angiotensin I to form angiotensin II (Ang II). Ang II is a potent vasoconstrictor that increases blood pressure, stimulates aldosterone secretion and promotes a proinflammatory effect on the endothelium resulting in the development of endothelial dysfunction and atherosclerosis. Furthermore, ACE deranges the balance between vasodilation and vasoconstriction by degrading and inactivating bradykinin, which induces NO, prostacyclin, and EDHF release.

## The Endothelium as a Controller of Hemostasis

Under normal physiologic conditions, the healthy endothelium exerts antiplatelet, anticoagulant, and fibrinolytic properties. Due to the release of NO and prostacyclin, the intact endothelial surface is resistant to platelet adhesion, activation, secretion, and aggregation. The constitutive expression of ecto-ADPase/CD39 on the endothelial cells catabolizes ADP, a potent platelet proaggregatory mediator, further inhibiting platelet function. To limit the generation and activity of thrombin, the endothelium contains surface heparin sulfate and other glycosaminoglycans, which promote intrinsic antithrombin III activity and thrombin inactivation. Endothelial cells also express tissue factor pathway inhibitor (TFPI), which binds to factor Xa, limiting thrombin formation. Furthermore, the thrombomodulin-protein C anticoagulant system limits thrombin's procoagulant activity. Once thrombomodulin, synthesized by endothelial cells, binds to thrombin, thrombin is inactivated and the complex becomes an activator of the anticoagulant protein, protein C. In the inflammatory state, thrombomodulin expression is reduced, and thus, the anticoagulant properties of the endothelium may be undermined. A distinct subpopulation of endothelial cells have been demonstrated to secrete tissue-type plasminogen activator (tPA), which stimulates the generation of the active protease plasmin from its precursor, plasminogen. However, this endothelial regulation of fibrinolysis is impaired upon exposure to an inflammatory stimulus, which in turn promotes the synthesis and release of plasminogen activator inhibitor (PAI) -1, which functions to limit plasmin generation.

## ENDOTHELIAL DYSFUNCTION

Under normal physiologic conditions, NO plays a key role in maintaining the vascular wall in a healthy state, inhibiting vascular inflammation, regulating vascular tone, limiting platelet activation and aggregation and protecting against vascular thrombosis. However, upon repeated exposure to traditional and emerging cardiovascular risk factors, the vasculature loses its intrinsic capacity for repair. The net effect of these damaging insults results in endothelial dysfunction which is marked by endothelial activation. In broad terms, endothelial dysfunction implies diminished production or availability of NO and/or imbalance in the relative contribution of endothelium-derived relaxing and contracting factors, such as ET-1 and Ang II. This represents the earliest stage of atherogenesis.

### Endothelial Activation: Setting the Stage for Atherosclerosis

As previously discussed, in addition to its vasodilatory effect, NO also protects against vascular injury, inflammation, and thrombosis. It inhibits leukocyte adhesion to the endothelium, maintains vascular smooth muscle in a non-proliferative state, and limits platelet aggregation. However, in response to the traditional cardiovascular risk factors, such as hypertension, diabetes, and hypercholesterolemia, the endogenous defenses of the vascular endothelium begin to break down. Hypercholesterolemia promotes attachment of blood leukocytes to the endothelium, a cell layer that under ordinary conditions is resistant to firm leukocyte adhesion. Ox-LDL causes endothelial activation and changes its biological characteristics in part by reducing the intracellular concentration of NO. Ang II, a vasoconstrictor, opposes NO action. Ang II can elicit the production of reactive oxygen species (ROS), increase the expression of the proinflammatory cytokines interleukin (IL)-6 and monocyte chemoattractant protein-1 (MCP-1), and up-regulate vascular cell adhesion molecule-1 (VCAM-1) on endothelial cells. Elevated C-reactive protein (CRP) levels can also promote endothelial dysfunction by quenching the production of NO and diminishing its bioactivity. These endothelial modifications promote inflammation within the vessel wall, setting the stage for the initiation and progression of an atherosclerotic lesion.

When endothelial cells undergo inflammatory activation, the increased expression of selectins, VCAM-1 and intercellular adhesion molecule-1 (ICAM-1), promotes the adherence of monocytes. Adhesion molecule expression is induced by proinflammatory cytokines such as IL-1β and tumor necrosis factor-α (TNF-α), by the acute phase protein CRP, by protease-activated receptor (PAR) signaling, by oxLDL uptake via oxidized low-density lipoprotein receptor-1 (LOX-1), and by CD40/CD40 ligand (CD40L, CD154) interactions. Once adherent, the monocytes transmigrate along a concentration gradient of MCP-1, into the tunica intima, the innermost layer of the arterial wall, passing between the endothelial cells. Once within the arterial intima, the monocytes develop into macrophages and begin to express scavenger receptors, such as SR-A, CD36 and LOX-1, that internalize modified lipoproteins, giving rise to lipid-laden macrophages or foam cells, which characterize early atherosclerotic lesions. Within the developing atheroma, the foam cells begin to secrete proinflammatory cytokines that maintain endothelial activation and a chemotactic stimulus for adherent leukocytes, augment expression of scavenger receptors, and promote macrophage replication. T cells, dendritic cells, and mast cells are also recruited into atheromatous plaques and contribute to the perpetuation of the inflammatory response and impaired endothelial function.

The fatty streak then evolves toward a complex lesion, typified by the proliferation of SMCs, their migration toward the intima, and their synthesis of collagen. Lipid accumulation within the atheroma continues, eventually leading to destabilization of the plaque. The inflammatory milieu promotes matrix metalloproteinase activity leading to fibrous cap thinning and increased plaque vulnerability. With a dysfunctional endothelium and reduced NO bioavailability, areas of endothelial cell desquamation develop, exposing subendothelial collagen, tissue factor, and von Willebrand factor. With decreased NO and prostacyclin levels, unopposed platelet activation and aggregation ensue. Combined with higher levels of PAI-1, this results in a clinically apparent thrombotic event. Thus, endothelial dysfunction and endothelial activation, resulting from vascular inflammation, are the first indications of evolving cardiovascular disease.

## ASSESSMENT OF ENDOTHELIAL FUNCTION/DYSFUNCTION

As endothelial dysfunction represents the earliest stages of atherogenesis, assessment of endothelial function prior to the onset of overt cardiovascular disease may serve as a technique to improve cardiac risk evaluation. The rationale for endothelial function testing, either directly or indirectly, to serve as an indicator of vascular disease stems from the observations that the healthy endothelium is non-thrombogenic; endothelial dysfunction occurs in response to vascular risk factors and precedes structural atherosclerosis; interventions that improve endothelial function also decrease cardiovascular events in patients with stable coronary disease; and reproducible assessments of endothelial function exist. The assessment of endothelial dysfunction depends upon the measurement of the endothelial cell response to stimulation from vasoactive (either physiologic or pharmacologic) substances. The endothelium-dependent vasomotor changes observed are compared to baseline, control conditions or the effect of endothelium-independent dilators.

## Coronary Circulation—Cardiac Catheterization

Quantitative coronary angiography, used in the initial clinical studies of endothelial function, examines the changes in vascular diameter in response to an infusion of an endothelium-dependent vasodilator such as acetylcholine (Ach). In healthy vessels with an intact endothelium, Ach evokes a NO-mediated vasodilatory response; however, in patients with endothelial dysfunction, this effect is blunted, or paradoxical vasoconstriction may occur secondarily to a direct muscarinic SMC vasoconstrictor effect. Furthermore, endothelial function of the coronary microvasculature may be assessed using intracoronary Doppler techniques to measure coronary blood flow in response to pharmacologic or physiologic stimuli. Although the study of the coronary circulation is considered by many to be the gold standard for the assessment of endothelial function, this technique is limited by its invasive nature, expense, and relative inaccessibility.

## Peripheral Circulation—Venous Occlusion Plethysmography and Ultrasound Flow-Mediated Dilation

Strain-gauge venous impedance plethysmography assesses resistance vessel function in the forearm by examining the change in forearm blood flow in response to direct intra-arterial (brachial artery) administration of agonists. Resistance vessels participate in the regulation of blood flow in response to changes in metabolic needs. Forearm blood flow and mean blood pressure provide an estimate of the forearm vascular resistance. Generally, a cuff around the wrist is inflated to suprasystolic pressure to separate the forearm from the circulation. A second cuff on the upper arm is inflated intermittently to supravenous pressures but below arterial pressures, interrupting venous

outflow but not arterial inflow to the forearm. During this occlusive phase, the accumulation of blood per unit time in the forearm is assessed, reflecting the forearm blood flow. Sensitive detectors are placed around the forearm to assess its increase in size. The rate of increase in limb size is proportional to the vasodilation of resistance vessels in the forearm. The limb size is measured under baseline conditions with an inactive solution infused in the brachial artery through a small cannula, after the infusion of an endothelium-dependent vasodilator such as Ach, and again after the infusion of an endothelium-independent dilator such as nitroprusside. Changes in limb size in response to the different stimuli reflect the extent of endothelial function/dysfunction. This technique is excellent for acute interventions with repeated measurements. The major drawbacks are its reproducibility and its rather invasive nature.

Brachial artery *flow-mediated dilation* (FMD) has emerged as the most common assessment tool of endothelial function. Flow-mediated vasodilation is the phenomenon by which blood vessels respond to an increase in flow or shear stress by dilating. The principal mediator of this is endothelium-derived NO. Several factors are responsible for its widespread use, including that: the response is NO-dependent; FMD is abnormal early in the course of atherosclerotic disease and in response to various cardiovascular risk factors; it improves with interventions known to improve cardiovascular outcomes; and it is relatively inexpensive, noninvasive, and reproducible. In this technique the brachial artery diameter is measured before and after an increase in shear stress that is induced by reactive hyperemia using ultrasound. The forearm blood flow is occluded for 5 minutes using a blood pressure cuff placed distal to the brachial artery inflated to at least 50 mm Hg above systolic pressure. Subsequent cuff deflation induces a brief high-flow state through the brachial artery, the reactive hyperemia, to accommodate the dilated resistance vessels. The resulting increase in shear stress leads to local endothelial release of NO causing the brachial artery to dilate (FMD). The longitudinal image of the artery is recorded continuously from 30 seconds before to 2 minutes after cuff deflation. This technique has the advantage of being noninvasive and can readily identify populations with attenuated endothelial function/impaired FMD response. Limitations include: the requirement of expensive equipment and offline analysis; the technique of FMD acquisition is highly operator-dependent; the lack of established normal values; and the need to minimize the effect of physiological influences such as exercise, caffeine ingestion, and the use of vasomotor medications such as nitrates, calcium channel blockers, ACE inhibitors and angiotensin receptor blockers (ARBs). (See **Table 23-1**.)

| Table 23-1 • Current Methods of Assessing Endothelial Function | | |
| --- | --- | --- |
| **Method** | **Advantages** | **Disadvantages** |
| Quantitative coronary angiography | Direct visualization of response to vasodilator in coronary circulation<br><br>May measure change in coronary blood flow directly<br><br>Remains the gold standard | Invasive<br><br>Expensive<br><br>Relatively inaccessible |
| Strain-gauge venous impedance plethysmography | May perform repeated measurements to different stimuli | Relatively invasive<br><br>Indirect measure of coronary circulation using forearm blood flow as a surrogate<br><br>Reproducibility |
| Brachial artery flow-mediated dilation | Response primarily nitric oxide-dependent<br><br>Not invasive<br><br>Fairly good reproducibility | Requires special ultrasound equipment<br><br>Operator-dependent and normal established values lacking<br><br>Influenced by the use of vasomotor medications, exercise |

# CLINICAL UTILITY OF ASSESSING ENDOTHELIAL FUNCTION/DYSFUNCTION

Endothelial cell dysfunction likely marks the earliest event in the process of lesion formation, and hence, assessing endothelial function may serve as an early, useful prognostic tool for coronary artery disease. It may be detected in children and adults many years before the development of clinically apparent disease, thereby allowing for early intervention. Heterogeneity of vascular dysfunction must be appreciated. Nonetheless, coronary endothelial cell perturbations often are reflected in peripheral vasodilator abnormalities, thereby allowing the assessment of peripheral endothelial function as a measure of coronary vasomotion. Endothelial-dependent vascular biology is not only important in the initiation of atherosclerotic disease but may also mark the transition from stable to unstable disease states.

## Cardiac Risk Factors and Endothelial Dysfunction

Traditional and emerging cardiovascular risk factors are associated with endothelial dysfunction. Hypercholesterolemia, in both apparently healthy children and adults, is associated with abnormal endothelium-dependent dilation in the absence of coronary atherosclerosis. Oxidized LDL has a deleterious effect on endothelial NO production, it interferes with normal signal transduction in endothelial cells, it promotes the generation of reactive oxygen species, perpetuates an inflammatory milieu in the vasculature, and may lead to the accumulation of competitive inhibitors of

eNOS. Both active and passive smoking appear to cause dose-dependent impairment of endothelium-dependent vasodilation, which is believed to be secondary to increases in oxidative stress leading to inactivation of NO and the oxidative modification of lipoproteins. Patients with diabetes demonstrate a loss of endothelium-dependent dilation in both coronary and peripheral circulations compared to nondiabetic controls. These detrimental changes have been associated with the reduced basal release of NO and a diminished vasodilatory response to acetylcholine. The pathogenesis of impaired endothelial function in the setting of diabetes is not completely understood, though likely is secondary to a combination of hyperglycemia, which results in endothelial cell activation and increased oxidative stress that may degrade NO, and the formation of advanced glycation end products, which promote vascular inflammation. Hyperinsulinemia, as may occur in prediabetic states with impaired glucose tolerance, is also associated with impaired endothelial function. Insulin stimulates the release of both endothelial NO and ET-1, and the imbalance between these counter regulatory molecules may favor vascular changes that promote vasoconstriction. Hypertensive and prehypertensive patients have impaired endothelium-dependent dilation, and the degree of dysfunction predicts adverse clinical outcomes. Vascular NO activity is reduced in essential hypertension, whereas ET-1 activity is increased in hypertensive patients. Therefore, the increased basal vasoconstrictive tone in hypertensive patients appears to be secondary to increased ET-1 production and increased sensitivity of vascular SMCs to ET-1. Finally, both increasing age and male gender are associated with diminishing endothelial-dependent dilation. As the number of vascular risk factors increases among individuals without overt cardiovascular disease, the extent of FMD and thus endothelial vasodilatory capacity decreases.

## Cardiovascular Events and Endothelial Dysfunction

Since endothelial dysfunction occurs early in the disease process, it is not unexpected that it is associated with cardiovascular events. A multivariant analysis including close to 2500 patients illustrated that endothelial dysfunction is strongly and independently associated with major cardiovascular events such as cardiac death, myocardial infarction, and need for revascularization. Coronary and peripheral endothelial dysfunction demonstrated similar power in their ability to predict cardiovascular events. More importantly, cardiovascular events were observed to occur remotely from the site endothelial dysfunction was detected, highlighting the systemic nature of impaired endothelial function. The presence of endothelial dysfunction among patients with cardiovascular risk factors has a high sensitivity for coronary heart disease, while its absence has a high negative predictive value. Brachial FMD predicts incident cardiovascular events in older adults, as illustrated in the Cardiovascular Health Study. FMD was measured in 2792 adults aged 72-98 years in the United States, who were followed for a period of 5 years. Event-free survival rate for cardiovascular events was significantly higher in subjects with FMD greater than the sex-specific medians than it was in subjects with FMD less than or equal to sex-specific medians (78.3% versus 73.6%, P = 0.006). After adjustment for age, gender, diabetes, cigarette smoking, blood pressure, baseline cardiovascular disease status, and total cholesterol, FMD remained a significant predictor of cardiovascular events, though, it did not add a great extent to the prognostic accuracy of traditional cardiac risk scores in this population.

Aside from serving as an independent risk factor for cardiovascular disease, assessment of endothelial function by brachial ultrasound demonstrated efficacy for preoperative risk stratification in patients undergoing vascular surgery. Low flow-mediated dilation was determined to be an independent predictor of both postoperative cardiac events at 30 days and late cardiac events at over 1 year of follow-up. In post heart transplant patients the presence of endothelial dysfunction was associated with the development of transplant vasculopathy. Patients who had a normal vasodilator response to Ach immediately following transplantation developed atherosclerosis at a rate one-third that of those with endothelial dysfunction during the first year of follow-up. Also, the presence of endothelial dysfunction in this transplant population group tended to predict the development of angiographic vasculopathy and cardiac death, either graft failure or sudden death.

## SURROGATE MARKERS OF ENDOTHELIAL DYSFUNCTION

Indirect tests used to gain information on the status of the endothelium depend upon the measurement of peripheral markers that are associated with endothelial dysfunction and the progression of inflammation and atherosclerosis. Direct products of endothelial cell activation, such as measures of NO, adhesion molecules, inflammatory cytokines or markers of endothelial damage and repair may be assessed; however, many of these remain difficult and expensive to measure and primarily have been used only in the research setting. For example, circulating levels of nitrites and nitrosylated proteins reflect endothelial NO generation though they are difficult to measure and may be confounded by other sources of NO. Endothelial adhesion molecules such as VCAM-1, ICAM-1, and E-selectin may be measured in the circulation, though these molecules may arise from multiple sources. CRP, a general marker of vascular inflammation and thus endothelial activation, and circulating endothelial progenitor cells (EPCs), markers of endothelial injury and repair, have emerged as two potential surrogate markers for overall endothelial health.

## High Sensitivity C-Reactive Protein

High sensitivity CRP has emerged as one of the most important inflammatory markers of cardiovascular disease. CRP is a powerful independent predictor of myocardial infarction, stroke, and vascular death in a variety of settings, and appears to be a better predictor of cardiovascular events than LDL-cholesterol. Furthermore, CRP at concentrations known to predict vascular disease is not only an inflammatory marker but also a mediator of atherosclerosis by contributing to endothelial dysfunction and activation, atherosclerotic lesion formation, plaque rupture, and thrombosis. CRP directly stimulates the expression of endothelial cell adhesion molecules, chemoattractant chemokines, and macrophage LDL uptake. It promotes endothelial dysfunction by modulating the production of endothelium-derived vasoactive factors, downregulating eNOS-derived NO, while augmenting production of ET-1. Additionally, CRP has been demonstrated to promote the release of PAI-1 from endothelial cells, upregulate angiotensin-mediated neointimal formation, facilitate endothelial cell apoptosis, attenuate compensatory angiogenesis, and alter EPC survival and differentiation. Patients with elevated levels of CRP elicit impaired endothelium-dependent vasodilation. Levels of CRP appear to be inversely correlated with endothelial function, as individuals with higher CRP levels demonstrate greater degrees of endothelial dysfunction.

## Endothelial Progenitor Cells

Circulating endothelial progenitor cells (EPCs) are bone marrow-derived stem cells that have the ability to differentiate into mature endothelial cells. EPCs circulate in the blood and home preferentially to sites of vascular or tissue injury, contributing significantly to both reendothelialization and neovascularization. The identification of circulating EPCs relies on their expression of characteristic cell surface markers, which may be identified using flow cytometry, and by their potential to differentiate to and function as endothelial cells. The level of circulating EPCs may serve as a reflection of the vasculature's ability to repair itself in response to injury, and thus reflects its overall health. Clinical studies suggest that traditional risk factors for coronary atherosclerosis are associated with lower levels of circulating EPCs and that the number of these progenitor cells in the circulation can be used to predict the occurrence of cardiovascular events and death. Furthermore, low EPC number and impaired EPC function correlate closely with endothelial function. A lower number of EPCs predicts severe endothelial dysfunction independent of classical cardiovascular risk factors. Therefore, the measurement of EPCs from a blood sample may reflect the extent of endothelial dysfunction as assessed by brachial FMD or quantitative coronary angiography.

## STRATEGIES TO MODIFY ENDOTHELIAL DYSFUNCTION

Strategies known to reduce cardiovascular events tend to decrease the extent of endothelial dysfunction, supporting the concept that restoration of endothelial function can stabilize atherogenesis. Smoking cessation reduces the extent of oxidative stress imparted on the vasculature. Treatment with aspirin improves endothelial dysfunction possibly via the inhibition of one or more cyclooxygenase-dependent vasoconstrictors. Correction of hyperlipidemia by diet or by statin therapy results in improved endothelial-dependent vasorelaxation likely secondary to a combination of increased NO bioavailability and a reduction in vascular inflammation. The management of hypertension via the inhibition of the renin-angiotensin system with either an ACE inhibitor or an ARB attenuates the degree of endothelial dysfunction in patients with coronary disease likely through their antagonistic effect on the potent vasoconstrictor Ang II. Obesity is associated with impaired endothelial vasorelaxation most likely mediated by elevated levels of inflammatory adipokines such as IL-6 and TNF-$\alpha$, and decreased levels of the vasculoprotective adipokine, adiponectin. Weight loss, regular aerobic exercise, and a low fat or Mediterranean diet have all been shown to improve overall endothelial function.

## SUMMARY

Endothelial dysfunction is apparent in the preclinical stage of atherosclerosis. NO bioavailability and the overall balance between vasodilator and vasoconstrictor mediators are of paramount importance. Endothelial function reflects the health of the vasculature and its ability to respond to and to resist vascular insults. Assessment of endothelial function provides a measure of vascular disease burden prior to the onset of clinically apparent cardiovascular disease and may serve as an independent marker of cardiovascular risk. Endothelial dysfunction responds to interventions currently utilized for cardiovascular disease and may be used to monitor disease activity. However, the tests currently available to assess endothelial function are costly, require expertise, and are too variable for routine clinical use. Thus, more easily measured biomarkers such as circulating levels of EPCs or CRP may emerge as useful surrogate markers of endothelial function. Clinical guidelines regarding the assessment of endothelial dysfunction are lacking. Nevertheless, endothelial function assessment and testing will likely be incorporated into diagnostic algorithms, serving as an early marker of impending cardiovascular disease.

### Suggested Readings

1. Deanfield JE, Halcox JP, Rabelink TJ. Endothelial function and dysfunction. Testing and clinical relevance. *Circulation.* 2007;115:1285–1295.

2. De Caterina R and Libby P, eds. *Endothelial Dysfunction and Vascular Disease.* Malden, MA: Blackwell Publishing; 2007.

3. Verma S, Buchanan MR, Anderson TJ. Endothelial function testing as a biomarker of vascular disease. *Circulation.* 2003;108:2054–2059.

are cumbersome and seldom used, and mathematical manipulations of fasting plasma glucose and insulin, such as Homeostasis Model Assessment of Insulin Resistance (HOMA-IR) and Quantitative Insulin Sensitivity Check Index (QUICKI), yield estimates that correlate well with clamp estimates of IR. In the Verona Diabetes Complications Study of 1326 patients with T2DM, HOMA-IR was an independent predictor of both prevalent and incident CVD. A 1-unit increase in (log) HOMA-IR value was associated with an odds ratio for prevalent CVD at baseline of 1.31 (95% CI 1.10-1.56, P = 0.002) and for incident CVD during follow-up of 1.56 (95% CI 1.14-2.12, P < 0.001). The Botnia study group reported similar results. In yet another study, plasma TG to HDL-C ratio >3.5 was the best surrogate predictor of insulin resistance (steady-state plasma glucose concentration during the insulin suppression test), with a sensitivity and specificity of 47 and 88%, respectively. However, one must bear in mind that HOMA-IR has never been validated for single-patient use, and clinical markers for IR, such as acanthosis nigricans, have poor sensitivity, making clinical confirmation of IR somewhat difficult.

The American Diabetes Association (ADA) has recently combined IGT and IFG into a separate nosologic entity, called "prediabetes". (**Figure 24-2**) although, the NCEP, ADA, and IDF have lowered the threshold for diagnosing IFG from 110 mg/dL to 100 mg/dL, there is some reluctance, especially amongst European investigators, in accepting this definition, because of the purported increase in the "at-risk" population at large, despite minimal demonstrable increase in health risks and complications attributable to the new cut-off.

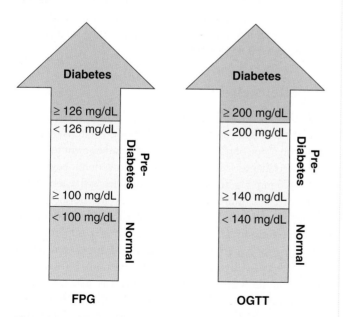

**Figure 24-2.** Prediabetes: diagnostic criteria. (Copyright 2010 American Diabetes Association from http://www.diabetes.org. Reprinted with permission from The American Diabetes Association.)

## Dyslipidemia in the Setting of the Metabolic Syndrome

The lipid abnormality in obesity/MetS is largely driven by the underlying obesity/insulin resistance. Not all obese individuals have dyslipidemia, and, in part, ethnic factors may play a role in the observed differences. Visceral adiposity may be more important pathogenetically, as compared to subcutaneous fat, and may serve to explain why some obese individuals (with predominant subcutaneous adiposity) do not have the biochemical correlates of MetS.

Elevated serum TG and low high-density lipoprotein cholesterol (HDL-C) are considered the main lipid abnormalities in MetS. It is important to realize that CVD risk increases with increasing insulin resistance, and dyslipidemia and dysglycemia are evident long before onset of clinical diabetes—the so called "ticking clock" hypothesis. This hypothesis is based partly on 8-year follow-up observations in the San Antonio Heart Study. Patients who were nondiabetic at baseline examination but went on to develop T2DM had substantially higher total cholesterol, triglycerides, BMI, and BP, accompanied by lower levels of HDL-C, compared with subjects who did not develop T2DM.

Altered metabolism of triglyceride-rich lipoproteins (TGRL) is an integral part of the atherogenic dyslipidemia seen in prediabetes and diabetes, and is observed in many patients with the METS. Many patients have elevated non-HDL cholesterol (equal to total cholesterol – HDL cholesterol), which is valid in the nonfasting state and bears a positive correlation with apo B, the principle apolipoprotein in the atherogenic lipoproteins, namely, LDL, IDL, VLDL, VLDL remnants and small, dense LDL. Obesity results in increased fat mass, and insulin resistance promotes lipolysis and generation of excess free fatty acids (FFA) (nonesterified) from adipose tissue. Increased hepatic uptake of FFA ensues, resulting in increased hepatic synthesis and export of very low-density lipoprotein (VLDL). Diminished clearance of VLDL and intestinally derived chylomicrons (CM) result in prolonged plasma retention of these particles and accumulation of highly atherogenic partially lipolyzed cholesterol-enriched intermediate-density lipoprotein (IDL) remnants (**Figure 24-3**). In the insulin-resistant patient, levels of Apo C-III, an inhibitor of the enzyme lipoprotein lipase, increases, while that of apo C-II, an activator of lipoprotein lipase, decreases with net diminished activity of the enzyme, thus impacting hydrolysis/delipidation of VLDL and causing hypertriglyceridemia. Increased hepatic production and/or diminished plasma clearance of large VLDL also results in increased production of precursors of small, dense LDL particles. Current evidence suggests that LDL particle concentrations, specifically levels of small, dense LDL are predictive of coronary events, independent of other coronary

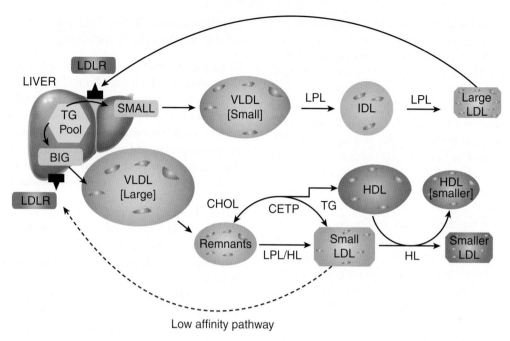

**Figure 24-3.** Lipid pathways in those with the metabolic syndrome and prediabetes/insulin resistance.

disease risk factors. Seven distinct LDL subspecies differing in their metabolic behavior and pathological roles have been identified (**Table 24-4**). Plasma VLDL levels correlate with increased density and decreased size of LDL. Small, dense LDL particles appear to arise from the progressive intravascular processing of specific larger VLDL precursors through a series of steps, including lipolysis (**Figure 24-3**).

| Lipoprotein Subclass | Pattern Seen in Diabetes Mellitus | Particle Density (g/mL) |
|---|---|---|
| LDL₁ | ↓ | 1.019-1.023 |
| LDL₂ₐ | ↓ | 1.023-1.028 |
| LDL₂ᵦ | ↓ | 1.028-1.034 |
| LDL₃ₐ | ↑ | 1.034-1.041 |
| LDL₃ᵦ | ↑ | 1.041-1.044 |
| LDL₄ₐ | variable | 1.044-1.051 |
| LDL₄ᵦ | variable | 1.051-1.063 |
| HDL₂ᵦ | ↓ | 1.1063-1.1 |
| HDL₂ₐ | variable | 1.1-1.125 |
| HDL₃ₐ | variable | 1.125-1.147 |
| HDL₃ᵦ | ↑ | 1.147-1.167 |
| HDL₃c | ↑ | 1.167-1.2 |

**Table 24-4 • LDL and HDL Subparticle Changes in Prediabetes and Diabetes (Atherogenic Dyslipidemia)**

*Adapted from Krauss RM. Lipids and lipoproteins in patients with type 2 diabetes. Diabetes Care. 27(6);2004.*

Cholesterol ester transfer protein (CETP)-mediated TG enrichment of lipolytic products and hepatic lipase mediated hydrolysis of TG and phospholipids result in increased production of small, dense LDL particles. The reduction in HDL-C seen in MetS and T2DM is multifactorial, but an important factor is the increased transfer of cholesterol from HDL to apo B-containing TGRL (VLDL, IDL, and LDL), with reciprocal transfer of TG to HDL. Hydrolysis of TG-rich HDL particles by hepatic lipase results in its rapid catabolism and clearance from plasma. The usual pattern is one of low HDL₂ᵦ, and relative increases in the small, dense subfractions HDL₃ᵦ and HDL₃c.

## Hypertension

The NCEP and IDF definitions of MetS use a BP cut off 130/85 mm Hg. A detailed discussion on hypertension is beyond the scope of this chapter, but is found elsewhere in this volume (Chapter 21, Hypertension). In general, beginning at 115/75 mm Hg, the risk of CVD doubles with each increment of 20/10 mm Hg. Individuals who are normotensive at age 55 still have a 90 percent lifetime risk for developing hypertension. Current recommendations support active screening for hypertension by routine BP measurements in all individuals 18 years or older. Hypertension affects more than 50 million Americans. Annually, it is associated with approximately 500,000 strokes and 1,250,000 heart attacks. It is a major risk factor for coronary artery disease, congestive heart failure, renal disease, retinopathy, ruptured aortic aneurysm, and stroke. Current data have shown that only 27% of adults are controlled at <140/90 mm Hg. Almost 50%

of hypertensive patients are either unaware (13 million) or aware and untreated (7 million). Of those treated, 58% are uncontrolled.

## METABOLIC SYNDROME: TREATMENT CONSIDERATIONS

### Prevention of CVD and Diabetes

A large number of studies have shown that treating dyslipidemia and hypertension prevents CVD events, as reviewed in national cholesterol and blood pressure guidelines. Multiple studies have also provided conclusive evidence that lifestyle modification with moderate weight loss can prevent or delay the onset of diabetes in patients who are at high risk for developing diabetes, including the Da Qing IGT and Diabetes Study, the Oslo Diet and Exercise Study, and the Diabetes Prevention Program. In addition, pharmacological therapies such as Metformin and acarbose have been shown to prevent/postpone diabetes.

In the Diabetes Prevention Program, in which 3234 nondiabetic individuals who had elevated fasting and post load plasma glucose concentrations were randomized to Metformin (850 mg twice daily), a lifestyle modification program (goals of 7% weight loss and 150 min physical activity per week), or placebo for an average follow-up of 2.8 years, the lifestyle modification group had the greatest reduction in the incidence of diabetes (58%), whereas the Metformin group had a 31% decrease, compared with placebo. A subsequent analysis from the Diabetes Prevention Program found that both intensive lifestyle intervention and Metformin therapy were also effective in reducing incidence of metabolic syndrome (NCEP/ATP III definition), which occurred in 53% of participants at baseline and was reduced by 41% in the lifestyle group (P <0.001) and by 17% in the Metformin group (P = 0.03) compared with placebo.

Despite the impressive evidence that DM can be prevented in individuals who are at increased risk, epidemiological statistics suggest a marked increase in the incidence and prevalence of obesity and DM globally. This portends a steep increase in morbidity and mortality attributable to CVD as well.

While therapeutic lifestyle modifications in the form of diet and exercise remain the mainstay of therapy in those with the metabolic syndrome, many patients will potentially benefit by the judicious use of pharmacological agents for the treatment of hypertension (see Chapter 21) and dyslipidemia (see Chapter 20), and in select cases, for obesity and dysglycemia. In particular, combination therapy may be required in the treatment of both hypertension and dyslipidemia with a view to reaching therapeutic targets, while minimizing side effects due to larger doses of the individual agents.

### Current Approaches to Risk Assessment for CVD and Diabetes for Metabolic Syndrome

Why are we failing in clinical practice to prevent DM despite convincing clinical trial data? A successful prevention program in clinical practice requires (1) effective screening and risk assessment to identify high risk individuals, and (2) effective implementation of therapies in high-risk individuals, which prevent the development of the disease. The current poor success in prevention of DM may be related to both lack of effective risk assessment strategies and lack of effective office-based therapeutic interventions.

Unfortunately, the current guidelines for risk assessment provided to physicians by medical societies and national organizations are not only numerous and confusing but also inconsistent in the basic approach to identifying high risk patients. The NCEP/ATP III guidelines for the prevention of CVD are based on the fundamental concept that the intensity of therapy should be determined by the absolute risk for development of CHD. Risk is initially assessed by counting the number of major risk factors; if an individual has two or more major risk factors, the absolute risk for CHD should be calculated using the Framingham risk algorithm. This approach has evolved from the initial concept of "primary" versus "secondary" prevention, as the dichotomous classification, although simple, may not be the best approach when there is a continuum of risk. The approach taken by the American Diabetes Association has been to identify those with "prediabetes," as alluded to earlier. Although most clinical trials examining the prevention of diabetes have enrolled individuals based upon OGTT results, the OGTT is not routinely performed in clinical practice and is not recommended by the American Diabetes Association for routine risk assessment for "prediabetes." An alternative approach to the dichotomous classification of presence or absence of "prediabetes" would be to assess the absolute risk for development of diabetes with an equation or risk algorithm, and to this end, several risk "engines" are available on the Internet. The UKPDS risk engine (http://www.dtu.ox.ac.uk/index.php?maindoc=/riskengine/) and the ADA risk calculator (http://www.diabetes.org/risk-test.jsp) are two such examples. Risk for diabetes can be assessed through information from clinical variables and routine clinical laboratory tests (fasting glucose and lipids) that provide similar predictive value concerning sensitivity and specificity compared with an OGTT. More importantly, the use of a risk equation or algorithm routinely to assess the absolute risk for developing diabetes over time would provide physicians with critical information to match the intensity of therapy with the risk for developing diabetes. In the ARIC study, individuals in the 9th and 10th deciles of risk as calculated by risk equations had respective observed frequencies for development of diabetes of 30 and 50% over 9 years, and individuals in the 9th and 10th deciles of risk accounted for more than 50% of all new cases of diabetes in ARIC. In contrast, for individuals who were in the lower five deciles of risk, the observed rates for developing diabetes over 9 years ranged from 1 to 9%.

Quantitative risk assessment to identify individuals at the highest risk for development of diabetes would also optimize resource allocation to identify which individuals may benefit the most from more intensive and more expensive lifestyle modification programs and/or pharmacotherapy. This approach has been used extensively to determine which patients merit drug therapy for hyperlipidemia and is the basis of reimbursement of drug therapy for hyperlipidemia in many countries.

# FUTURE DIRECTIONS

In the first half of the twentieth century, an alarming increase in the development of CVD led to intensive research on the epidemiology and pathogenesis of CVD, with development of national approaches for routine screening of blood pressure and lipids to identify individuals with increased CVD risk; development of successive guidelines recommending early and more intensive interventions for risk factor reduction; and development of many new and more effective therapies to treat elevated BP and lipid disorders. These approaches along with dramatic improvements in treatment of acute coronary syndromes, revascularization procedures for coronary artery disease, and reduced smoking have led to marked improvements in the age-adjusted incidence of cardiovascular events. In the beginning of the twenty-first century, an alarming increase in the incidence and prevalence of overweight, obesity, and diabetes, in both children and adults portends a significant increase in complications such as CVD. Extending routine systematic assessment from cardiovascular risk to cardiometabolic risk—i.e., risk for developing CVD and/or diabetes—and improved understanding of the basic mechanisms that regulate energy balance and metabolic risk factors, combined with more effective lifestyle modification and development of improved therapies, will be necessary to address this impending epidemic of diabetes, which will challenge our health care system.

## Suggested Readings

1. Grundy SM, Cleeman JI, Daniels SR, et al. Diagnosis and management of the metabolic syndrome. An American Heart Association/National Heart, Lung, and Blood Institute Scientific Statement. Executive summary. American Heart Association; National Heart, Lung, and Blood Institute, *Cardiol Rev.* 2005;13(6):322–327.

2. Klein S, Burke LE, Bray GA, et al. Clinical implications of obesity with specific focus on cardiovascular disease: a statement for professionals from the American Heart Association Council on Nutrition, Physical Activity, and Metabolism: endorsed by the American College of Cardiology Foundation. *Circulation.* 2004;110(18):2952–2967.

3. Vasudevan AR, Garber AJ. Diabetic dyslipidemia and the heart. *Heart Fail Clin.* 2006;2(1):37–52.

4. Grundy SM, Cleeman JI, Merz CN, et al. National Heart, Lung, and Blood Institute; American College of Cardiology Foundation; American Heart Association. Implications of recent clinical trials for the National Cholesterol Education Program Adult Treatment Panel III guidelines. *Circulation.* 2004;110(2):227–239. Erratum in *Circulation.* 2004;110(6):763.

5. Abuissa H, Bel DS, O'Keefe JH Jr. Strategies to prevent type 2 diabetes. *Curr Med Res Opin.* 2005;21(7):1107–1114.

# · 25

# Erectile Dysfunction and Cardiovascular Disease

CHRISTOPHER V. CHIEN AND ERNST R. SCHWARZ

## ● PRACTICAL POINTS

- Prevalence of ED can be as high as 31-52% in population studies.

- ED is highly prevalent in those with CVD; in patients with ED, the prevalence of hypertension and dyslipidemia is greater than 40% and that of DM greater than 20%.

- A major mechanism that links ED, atherosclerosis, and CV risk factors together is dysfunction of NO-releasing endothelial cells.

- Management of ED begins with a comprehensive assessment of cardiac risk and risk stratification.

- In high risk cases, cardiologic evaluation, testing, and management should be optimized before recommending restarting sexual activity.

- Sedentary lifestyle is a potentially modifiable risk factor for ED.

- Phosphodiesterase-5 (PDE-5) inhibitors have become first-line therapy for erectile dysfunction in many patients; these agents inhibit the metabolism of nitric oxide by PDE-5, thus facilitating the c-GMP-mediated relaxation of penile arteriolar smooth muscle.

- PDE-5 inhibitors may cause hypotension in those with hypotension, aortic stenosis, left ventricular outflow obstruction, and hypovolemia; concomitant usage of nitrates and PDE-5 inhibitors is absolutely contraindicated.

- Where drugs cannot be used, invasive injections, mechanical devices, and surgical implants may be indicated.

- A multidisciplinary approach involving primary care physicians, cardiologists, urologists, and psychiatrists is recommended to treat high risk patients and complex cases of ED.

## INTRODUCTION

Sexual dysfunction is defined as any problem during any aspect of sexual response which prevents satisfaction from sexual activity. Sexual dysfunction is a wide-ranging set of common disease processes that includes both female sexual dysfunction and erectile dysfunction (ED). Erectile dysfunction is a highly prevalent disease with dramatic impact on patients' quality of life. The mechanism of ED is multifactorial, with involvement of psychosocial, neurological, humoral-hormonal, and vascular processes. Historically, ED has been evaluated primarily by urologists and psychiatrists.

However, there is an increased role of cardiovascular (CV) specialists in the assessment and safe treatment of ED. This is driven by both research elucidating the relationship between ED and CV disease and the expansion of pharmacologic treatment options.

## EPIDEMIOLOGY

Male erectile dysfunction is defined by the US National Institute of Health as "an inability to achieve an erect penis as part of the overall multifaceted process of male sexual function." It is a widely prevalent condition in the general population. Large studies have reported the prevalence of ED to be 31-52% in a general population. The estimated incidence in the US is 25.9 cases per 1000 patient-years, which translates to an annual incidence of >600,000 new cases per year.

However, the prevalence of ED varies depending on the comorbidities of the population. The prevalence and incidence of ED is significantly higher in patients with known cardiovascular disease, including both patients with coronary artery disease and patients with heart failure. Several "traditional" cardiovascular risk factors are also associated with an increased prevalence of ED, including diabetes, hypertension, dyslipidemia, advanced age, tobacco use, and metabolic syndrome. Diabetes mellitus has a particularly strong association with ED. The prevalence of ED in diabetic populations has been reported to be 71-86%, and the incidence is as high as 50.7 cases per 1000 patient-years (relative risk = 1.83 compared to a general population). Erectile dysfunction is certainly an extremely common phenomenon and is even more prevalent in patients with cardiovascular disease and risk factors.

# ERECTILE DYSFUNCTION AND CARDIOVASCULAR RISK

Erectile dysfunction commonly coexists with traditional cardiovascular risk factors. In patients with ED the prevalence of hypertension and dyslipidemia is greater than 40%. The prevalence of diabetes in patients with ED is greater than 20%. This is useful information, as these diseases often lack obvious clinical symptoms. Patients with erectile dysfunction are also more likely to have metabolic syndrome, lead sedentary lifestyles, or have a history of smoking. Erectile dysfunction and cardiovascular disease share risk factors, and additionally, patients with ED are more likely to have concomitant coronary atherosclerosis. This is manifest by an increased likelihood of having a positive stress test, significant coronary artery calcification, or angiographically proven coronary artery disease. There is also prospective data that suggest ED is an independent predictor of the onset of incident coronary artery disease in diabetic patients.

Furthermore, ED is a predictor of future cardiovascular events. In a study of >9000 male patients, incident or prevalent ED was associated with a hazard ratio of 1.45 (95% confidence interval (CI) 1.25-1.69) for subsequent cardiovascular events (including angina, myocardial infarction (MI), cerebrovascular accident, transient ischemic attack, congestive heart failure (HF), or cardiac arrhythmia) at 7 years follow-up. For reference, the relationship of ED and cardiovascular events is in the range of risk associated with certain traditional cardiovascular risk factors, such as current smoking and family history of MI. Incident ED itself has been associated with a statistically significant hazard ratio of 1.25 (95% CI 1.02-1.53) for future cardiovascular events. The risk of adverse cardiovascular events in higher risk populations is even more profound. In diabetic patients with erectile dysfunction and asymptomatic coronary artery disease, the hazard ratio for incidence of major adverse cardiovascular events is 2.1 (95% CI 1.6-2.6). This is particularly remarkable, considering the absence of angina in this population. Symptoms of ED often precede diagnosis, events, or symptoms of cardiovascular disease. These symptoms may suggest cardiovascular disease in otherwise asymptomatic patients with silent ischemia, a population with a high rate of concomitant ED. Erectile dysfunction may be a precursor to the diagnosis of underlying and menacing, but largely unrecognized, cardiovascular disease and cardiovascular risk.

Erectile dysfunction is a harbinger of cardiovascular disease and cardiovascular events. Presentation of new-incident erectile dysfunction should prompt an evaluation for potentially modifiable cardiovascular risk factors and disease regardless of the presence of absence of other cardiac symptoms. The Second Princeton Consensus recommends measurement of blood pressure, blood glucose, lipids, and screening for vascular disease in all men with erectile dysfunction that lacks an obvious cause (such as trauma).

## Physiology of Erectile Dysfunction

Erection is initiated by neurological stimulation and impulses that ultimately lead to the release of nitric oxide (NO) from endothelial cells in the penis. NO, which is the principal regulating biochemical factor in penile erection, activates a cyclic guanosine monophosphate (c-GMP)-mediated process on smooth muscle that reduces intracellular calcium levels. This subsequently results in relaxation of arterial and trabecular smooth muscle, allowing for increased blood flow into the penile sinusoids. The filling of the sinusoids causes compression of the venous plexuses that drain the penis, thereby greatly reducing outflow. This combines to increase the intracavernous pressure within the penis, leading to tumescence.

The major underlying mechanism that links ED, atherosclerosis, and cardiovascular risk factors together is dysfunction of NO-releasing endothelial cells. Hypertension, dyslipidemia, obesity, and tobacco use have all been shown to be associated with endothelial dysfunction by various inflammatory and humoral-hormonal processes. Diabetes also has been shown to cause endothelial dysfunction and, additionally, may cause ED through neurogenic factors. Endothelial dysfunction is a key contributor to the development and progression of atherosclerosis itself and is correlated with myocardial ischemia and cardiovascular events. Furthermore, it has been shown that there is a significant reduction in the endothelium-dependent NO-mediated relaxation of smooth muscle in patients with ED. Endothelial dysfunction is a mechanism of systemic vascular disease— and penile vasculature is not spared.

## RISK ASSESSMENT OF SEXUAL ACTIVITY IN THE CARDIAC PATIENT

Management of ED begins with assessment of cardiac risk. A full history and physical as well as screening laboratory tests provide data necessary for proper evaluation of risk. All cardiovascular risk factors should be assessed and appropriately managed during this initial evaluation. While there is insufficient data to encompass all cardiac diseases, most patients can be stratified into one of three major graded categories of cardiac risk defined by the Second Princeton Consensus: low-risk, intermediate risk, and high risk (**Tables 25-1** to **25-3**).

The low risk group includes the following patient populations (**Table 25-1**):

1. asymptomatic patients with <3 risk factors for coronary artery disease (**Table 25-4**),
2. controlled hypertension,
3. mild, stable angina,
4. post successful coronary revascularization,
5. uncomplicated past MI (>6-8 weeks),
6. mild valvular disease,
7. HF or LVD (New York Heart Association functional class I).

Low-risk patients are generally at insignificant risk for cardiac complications from sexual activity. However, further evaluation, including noninvasive testing, may be recommended so that the risk of sexual activity may be more judiciously investigated (**Table 25-1**). However, patients at low risk may safely engage in sexual activity and may be treated for erectile dysfunction. First-line therapies should be considered on an individual basis, and it is recommended that patients be reassessed every 6-12 months for change in clinical status.

The intermediate risk group includes the following patient populations:

1. ≥3 major risk factors for coronary artery disease (**Table 25-4**),
2. moderate, stable angina,
3. recent MI (2-6 weeks),
4. HF or LVD (NYHA II),
5. noncardiac sequelae of atherosclerotic disease (such as cerebrovascular accident, peripheral vascular disease).

| Table 25-1 • Low Cardiovascular Risk Group (from Second Princeton Consensus) and Management Recommendations | |
| --- | --- |
| **Patent Categories** | **Management Recommendations** |
| Asymptomatic, <3 risk factors | • Low risk for cardiac complications<br>• Good candidates for pharmacologic and nonpharmacologic therapy for ED |
| Controlled hypertension | • Patients on beta-blockers or thiazide diuretics may be predisposed to ED<br>• Neither BP control nor change in medication class has been shown to improve symptoms of ED. Specific therapy for ED is often required but generally safe |
| Mild, stable angina pectoris | • Generally, the functional reserve for these patients is greater than the metabolic requirement of sexual activity<br>• However, the burden of coronary artery disease should be evaluated via noninvasive evaluation (such as exercise stress test) prior to engaging in sexual activity<br>• Antianginal regiments may require modification prior to using phosphodiesterase inhibitors |
| Post-revascularization | • Risk is relative to the adequacy of revascularization<br>• Exercise stress testing can be used to evaluate for residual ischemia after revascularization procedure |
| Post-MI (>6-8 weeks) | • It has been traditionally recommended that sexual activity be avoided for 6-8 weeks post-myocardial infarction. However, sexual activity may safe in as little as 3-4 weeks post-MI in asymptomatic, revascularized patients with non-ischemic treadmill tests<br>• Exercise training and cardiac rehabilitation may be helpful in reducing coital symptoms and coital heart rates |
| Mild valvular disease | • Patients with mild mitral disease are not at higher risk due to sexual activity<br>• This is also likely true in patients with mild aortic valve disease |
| LVD (NYHA Class I) | • With proper medical management, such patients do not typically have coital symptoms and can be safely managed for ED |

*MI, myocardial infarction; LVD, left ventricular dysfunction; NYHA, New York Heart Association*

**Table 25-2 • Intermediate Cardiovascular Risk Group (from Second Princeton Consensus) and Management Recommendations**

| Patient Categories | Management Recommendations |
| --- | --- |
| Asymptomatic, ≥3 risk factors | • Cardiovascular assessment such as noninvasive stress testing is recommended to stratify risk. Nonischemic stress test would be reassuring and justify assignment to low-risk group |
| Moderate, stable angina | • Myocardial ischemia can often be produced from increase in heart rate and blood pressure associated with sexual activity<br>• Exercise stress testing is recommended to further stratify patient risk |
| Recent MI (>2, <6 weeks) | • History of myocardial infarction in this time period may be at increased risk of ischemia, re-infarction, and malignant arrhythmias<br>• Risk may be reassessed with exercise stress testing |
| LVD or HF (NYHA Class II) | • Such patients may be at increased risk for exacerbation of symptoms due to left ventricular dysfunction while undergoing sexual activity<br>• Cardiovascular assessment and rehabilitation may allow for reduction of risk and subsequent restratification |
| Noncardiac sequelae of atherosclerotic disease | • Patients with clinically evident history of peripheral arterial disease, transient ischemic attacks, or stroke are at high risk due to the diffuse nature of atherosclerosis<br>• Cardiovascular assessment, including stress testing is recommended |

*MI, myocardial infarction; LVD, left ventricular dysfunction; HF, heart failure; NYHA, New York Heart Association*

Intermediate-risk patients are at indeterminate or uncertain risk of cardiac complications from sexual activity, and further testing or cardiologic evaluation is needed so patients may be restratified into high or low risk groups. Proper management of these diseases may allow patients to be restratified into the low risk group. Management recommendations are summarized in **Table 25-2**.

The high risk group includes the following patient populations:

1. unstable or refractory angina,
2. uncontrolled hypertension,
3. CHF or LVD (NYHA III or IV),
4. recent MI (<2 weeks) or CVA,
5. high risk arrhythmia,
6. hypertrophic obstructive cardiomyopathy or other cardiomyopathy,
7. moderate/severe valvular disease.

High risk patients have sufficiently severe cardiac conditions and are at significant risk of cardiac symptoms and complications from any physical activity, including sexual activity. Furthermore, common medications used in treatment of erectile dysfunction may be inappropriate

**Table 25-3 • High Cardiovascular Risk Patients (from Second Princeton Consensus) and Management Considerations**

| Patient Categories | Management Considerations |
| --- | --- |
| Unstable or refractory angina | • Patients are at high risk for coital MI<br>• Prompt cardiac evaluation should be prioritized |
| Uncontrolled hypertension | • Patients are at risk for acute cardiac events as well as other vascular events, such as strokes |
| HF (NYHA Class III or IV) | • Sexual activity may cause symptomatic, decompensated heart failure<br>• Maximal medical management including cardiac rehabilitation should be considere |
| Recent MI (<2 weeks) | • Patients are at risk for reinfarction, arrhythmias, and cardiac rupture<br>• Maximum risk is in the first 2 weeks and sexual activity should be avoided |
| High risk arrhythmias | • Sexual activity may cause malignant arrhythmias and sudden cardiac death<br>• Risk may be diminished by implantable defibrillator or pacemaker |
| Hypertrophic obstructive and other cardiomyopathies | • While there is little known about the cardiovascular risk of sexual activity in these patients, usage of vasodilators that increase the intraventricular gradient should be avoided<br>• Exercise stress testing and echocardiography may help guide management |
| Moderate-to-severe valvular disease | • Specific risk is unclear, but vasoactive drugs that decrease perfusion of coronary and cerebral vasculature should be used with caution |

*MI, myocardial infarction; NYHA = New York Heart Association; HF, heart failure*

| Table 25-4 • Major Risk Factors for Coronary Artery Disease |
| --- |
| 1. Age |
| 2. Hypertension |
| 3. Diabetes mellitus |
| 4. Obesity |
| 5. Cigarette smoking |
| 6. Dyslipidemia |
| 7. Sedentary lifestyle |
| 8. Male, postmenopausal female* |
| *Gender is excluded from cardiovascular risk assessment |

for patients with these potentially unstable conditions. Cardiologic evaluation, testing, and management should be prioritized before recommending resumption of any sexual activity. Patients should be strongly encouraged to abstain from sexual activity until cardiac condition has been stabilized and their healthcare provider deems the risk to be appropriately low. Management recommendations are summarized in **Table 25-3**.

Evaluation and co-management of heart failure and ED is a unique challenge. Epidemiological data suggests that ED is even more prevalent in patients with heart failure compared to patients with known vascular disease. There are many mechanisms that may contribute to this relationship, including atherosclerosis, loss of exercise tolerance, concomitant depression, altered endothelial function, and medications commonly used in treatment of heart failure. In particular, beta-adrenergic blockers, digoxin, and diuretics have all been associated with sexual dysfunction. Stabilization of intermediate and high risk heart failure patients with ED relies on proper usage of these medications. However, the presence of unaddressed sexual dysfunction may lead to medication noncompliance due to patients' efforts to retain sexual function. Thus, careful counseling should be done in all patients who are being treated with these agents. Even in the low risk heart failure population, addressing sexual function and frequent counseling is critical to ensure compliance with medications that have shown to improve cardiovascular outcomes.

Regardless of cardiac risk, all patients with erectile dysfunction require close monitoring and follow up of cardiovascular disease and risks. Erectile dysfunction shares risk factors with atherosclerotic disease, and it may be the sole symptom in patients with otherwise subclinical cardiovascular disease. Repeat evaluation of risk factors should be done routinely in patients with ED, and coexisting risk factors should be appropriately managed for erectile dysfunction.

## Physiology of Sexual Activity

The physiologic effect of sexual arousal and sexual activity is somewhat variable. However, sexual activity is associated with sympathetic activation, which may elevate blood pressure and may induce arrhythmias ranging from premature complexes to ventricular tachyarrhythmias. Furthermore, there is a metabolic requirement from sexual activity. The preorgasmic phase is associated with a metabolic equivalent (MET) range of 2 to 3. The orgasmic phase is associated with a range of 3 to 4 METs, and in younger individuals, the upper range of metabolic demand is approximately 5-6 METs. The physiologic response may be greater than with exercises of similar metabolic demand as sexual arousal may also augment the sympathetic response of sexual activity. While cardiac complications of sexual activity are rare, it is critical to assess cardiac risk prior to treating erectile dysfunction due to the consequences of sexual activity on cardiac physiology.

## TREATMENT OF ERECTILE DYSFUNCTION

### Lifestyle Modification

Lifestyle modifications should be considered for all patients seeking evaluation for ED. Sedentary lifestyle is a potentially modifiable risk factor for erectile dysfunction. There is some evidence that exercise and weight loss may improve symptoms of ED, and the Second Princeton Consensus supports the role of increasing exercise to improve erectile function. There is minimal evidence to support the role of dietary intervention in the treatment of erectile dysfunction. However, a small trial has suggested that a Mediterranean diet may reduce the prevalence of ED in patients with metabolic syndrome. Still, dietary recommendations should be focused towards the management of underlying cardiac disease and cardiac risk factors.

### Phosphodiesterase Inhibitors

Phosphodiesterase-5 (PDE-5) inhibitors have become first-line therapy for erectile dysfunction in many patients. These agents inhibit the metabolism of nitric oxide by PDE-5, thus facilitating the cyclic-GMP-mediated relaxation of penile arteriolar smooth muscle. This in turn leads to increased penile blood flow and subsequent penile tumescence. To date, there are three FDA-approved agents in this pharmacologic class being marketed in the United States: sildenafil (Viagra®), vardenafil (Levitra®), and tadalafil (Cialis®). Each agent differs slightly in pharmacokinetics, dosing, and PDE-5 selectivity. However, they have each been shown to be relatively efficacious in improving sexual function and may be used in most patients as first-line pharmacologic option. PDE-5 inhibitors have also been studied in the treatment of pulmonary hypertension. PDE-5 receptors are also present in lung smooth muscle, and PDE-5 inhibitors may decrease pulmonary vascular resistance, which in turn may ease symptoms of right heart failure and improve exercise capacity. To date, only sildenafil (marked as Revatio®) has been FDA-approved for the treatment of pulmonary hypertension.

The safety of PDE-5 inhibitors has been well studied and reported in both controlled and postmarketing trials. PDE-5 inhibitors do not increase rates of myocardial infarction or death. They do not cause ischemia or hemodynamic compromise in patients with known coronary artery disease or heart failure. There may be a slight decrease in blood pressure associated with PDE-5 inhibitors, but this is considered clinically insignificant in most patients. However, this response may be clinically relevant in patients with hypotension, aortic stenosis, left ventricular outflow obstruction, and hypovolemia. PDE-5 inhibitors are also generally well tolerated. Common reported side effects include headaches, flushing, and dyspepsia. Still, the safety of PDE-5 inhibitors is limited by several critical drug-drug interactions that must be investigated and avoided by clinicians (**Table 25-5**).

Nitrates including nitroglycerin, isosorbide mononitrate, and isosorbide dinitrate are commonly used to treat angina and heart failure, but concomitant usage of nitrates and PDE-5 inhibitors is absolutely contraindicated. Nitrates inhibit the breakdown of cyclic-GMP, and PDE-5 inhibitors facilitate their action by inhibiting nitric oxide metabolism. The result is an overly robust vasodilatation, which can cause significant and unpredictable reduction of blood pressure, as well as symptomatic hypotension. Hypotension may be treated with intravenous fluids and vasopressors as needed. For refractory hypotension, intra-aortic balloon pump can also be considered.

Providers should be judicious in medication review prior to prescribing PDE-5 inhibitors. It is reasonable to use PDE-5 inhibitors beginning 2 weeks after cessation of using nitrates. Patients who experience angina soon after usage of PDE-5 inhibitors should be encouraged to cease all sexual activity, and if the angina persists, they should seek emergency care. Patients should be instructed to inform emergency providers of recent PDE-5 inhibitor use. Patients who have taken sildenafil or vardenafil should not receive nitrates within the first 24 hours of use and visa versa. Tadalafil has a longer half-life than the other two drugs, and nitrates should be avoided within the first 48 hours of its use. All other usual therapy (other than nitrates) may be used in emergency treatment of angina and acute coronary syndromes.

Several other medications also interact with PDE-5 inhibitors (**Table 25-5**). Vardenafil has a mild effect on QT duration its use not recommended in patients on type 1A or type 3 antiarrhythmics, as well as patients with congenital

| Table 25-5 • Drug Interactions of Phosphodiesterase-5 Inhibitors | | |
|---|---|---|
| **Drug Class** | **Examples** | **Effect** |
| Nitrates | Nitroglycerin Isosorbide mononitrate Isosorbide dinitrate | Vasodilation, hypotension ABSOLUTE CONTRAINDICATION |
| Alpha-blockers | Terazosin Doxazosin Prazosin Tamsulosin | Vasodilation, hypotension |
| Type 1a antiarrhythmics | Quinidine Procainamide | May prolong QT interval when used with vardenafil* |
| Type 3 antiarrhythmics | Amiodarone Sotalol Bretylium | May prolong QT interval when used with vardenafil* |
| CYP3A4 inducers | Rifampin Phenytoin NNRTI Barbituates TZDs | Decrease bioavailability of PDE-5 inhibitors |
| CYP3A4 inhibitors | Fluconazole, ketoconazole Protease inhibitors Macrolide antibiotics Grapefruit juice Amiodarone Diltiazem | Increase bioavailability of PDE-5 inhibitors |

NNRTI, non-nucleoside reverse transcriptase inhibitors; TZDs, thiazoladinediones; PDE-5, phosphodiesterase-5
*Sildenafil and tadalafil not shown to prolong QT interval.

long-QT syndrome. Alpha-blockers also cause vasodilation, and when used in combination with PDE-5 inhibitors, may cause hypotension. While concomitant use of alpha-blockers and PDE-5 inhibitors is not a contraindication, caution must be taken and dosage may require adjustment. Finally, PDE-5 inhibitors are metabolized by the CYP3A4 pathway. Drugs such as azole antifungals and protease inhibitors may decrease metabolism, while agents such as rifamin and phenytoin, which induce CYP3A4, may increase metabolism of PDE-5 inhibitors. Dose adjustments should be strongly considered.

## Other Therapies for ED

Several other pharmacologic agents have been used to treat erectile dysfunction. However, neither their efficacy nor their cardiovascular safety has been well studied or established. Yohimbine is an alpha-blocker that has been used for erectile dysfunction for decades. However, its efficacy is unclear and adverse cardiovascular events have been reported. L-arginine may improve erectile function in patients with mild ED. It is a precursor of nitric oxide, which induces penile arterial vasodilation. Apomorphine is a dopamine receptor antagonist that is available only in Europe for treatment of mild ED. Its safety profile appears to be favorable, although there is a rare risk of vasovagal syncope. Finally, treatment of hypogonadism with testosterone may also improve symptoms of ED in patients who have failed PDE-5 inhibitor monotherapy. The impact of testosterone on the cardiovascular system is unclear. Patients on testosterone therapy should be monitored for elevations in prostate-specific antigen and for polycythemia (especially in patients with heart failure).

Invasive injections, mechanical devices, and surgical implants have been used for treatment of ED. Penile injections of vasoactive agents such as alprostadil are commonly used in patients who do not respond to PDE-5 inhibitors. The overall risk of these agents appears to be low, and there is no cardiovascular contraindication to their use. However, caution should be taken in all patients on anticoagulation. Intraurethral alprostadil suppositories may spare patients from injections, but they are less efficacious than invasive injections. There is also a risk of vasovagal syncope associated with intraurethral alprostadil use. Vacuum devices have been used to create negative pressure around the penis, which in turn increases blood flow to the corpus cavernosum. Lastly, surgical implantation is a final option, reserved for men who have failed other modalities for treatment of ED. Although implantation is generally successful, the procedure puts patients at operative risk from anesthesia and the surgery itself. Thus, this treatment is generally not recommended for patients with high risk cardiovascular disease. There is also a risk of infection and device failure associated with surgical implantation. Treatment of ED should also involve treatment of any coexisting mental health diseases, such as depression, which is strongly associated with ED. Erectile dysfunction is a complex disease with numerous mechanisms and comorbidities. Thus, a multidisciplinary approach involving primary care physicians, cardiologists, urologists, and psychiatrists is recommended to treat high risk patients and complex cases of ED.

# SUMMARY

Erectile dysfunction is a common condition and is increasingly frequently seen in clinical practice. While the etiology of ED is polyfactorial, the close relationship amongst ED, cardiovascular risk factors, and occult cardiovascular disease suggests that ED itself may be an early manifestation of cardiovascular disease. Female sexual dysfunction in women is a growing field of research. However, it remains poorly understood at this time, and it is unclear if female sexual dysfunction carries the same cardiovascular risk as ED. All patients with ED should be screened for modifiable cardiovascular risk factors, and the opportunity to treat them vigilantly should not be missed. The first step in treatment of ED is cardiovascular risk assessment and stabilization of any coexisting disease. Once the risk of sexual activity is minimized, PDE-5 inhibitors can be used judiciously. However, all patients on PDE-5 inhibitors must be educated on the potentially dangerous interaction with nitrates. Other pharmacologic and nonpharmacologic options are available, but their safety and efficacy are not well understood. Erectile dysfunction should be managed actively in a multidisciplinary fashion by providers to improve quality of life, to increase patient satisfaction, and to potentially reduce the risk of cardiovascular events by treatment of comorbid disease.

## Suggested Readings

1. Thompson IM, Tangen CM, Goodman PJ, et al. Erectile dysfunction and subsequent cardiovascular disease. JAMA. 2005;294:2996–3002.

2. DeBusk R, Drory Y, Goldstein I, et al. Management of sexual dysfunction in patients with cardiovascular disease: recommendations of the Princeton Consensus Panel. *Am J Cardiol.* 2000; 86:175–181.

3. Kostis JB, Jackson G, Rosen R, et al. Sexual dysfunction and cardiac risk (The Second Princeton Consensus Conference). *Am J Cardiol.* 2005;96:313–321.

4. Schwarz ER, Rastogi S, Kapur V, et al. Erectile dysfunction in heart failure patients. *J Am Coll Cardiol.* 2006;48:1111–1119.

5. Schwarz ER, Rastogi S, Rodriguez JJ, et al. A multidisciplinary approach to assess erectile dysfunction in high-risk cardiovascular patients. *Int J Impot Res.* 2005;Suppl 1:S37-43.

# Coronary Artery Disease

# 26

# The Pathophysiology of Atherosclerosis

Leon M. Ptaszek and Shawn A. Gregory

---

## ● PRACTICAL POINTS

- Nonmodifiable risk factors for atherosclerosis include male sex, family history of early-onset coronary artery disease, and age over 50 (for men) or 60 (for women).

- Cigarette smoking, the metabolic syndrome (MetS), and associated conditions (hyperlipidemia, diabetes mellitus, hypertension, obesity) are the most commonly encountered modifiable risk factors for atherosclerosis development.

- Formation and growth of atherosclerotic plaque involves interplay between accumulation of lipid material in the subendothelial compartment of arteries and other inflammatory cells, such as macrophages and lymphocytes.

- Smooth muscle cells, when activated by the presence of oxidized lipid, will secrete extracellular matrix, which comprises the "fibrous cap" of an atherosclerotic lesion.

- Increase in inflammation can lead to increase in release of matrix metalloproteinases during digestion; it can also thin the "fibrous cap" potentially leading to plaque instability.

- The Glagov phenomenon describes the relative preservation of the endoluminal diameter of the vessel in the area of a plaque in its early stages of growth. This process is not well understood, but appears to involve dilatation of uninvolved areas of vessel wall.

- Atherosclerotic lesion progression is staged: a Type I lesion involves the build-up of lipid in the intima, just beneath the vascular endothelial cells, and a Type II lesion, often referred to as a "fatty streak," is a more advanced form of a Type I lesion that does not contain activated lymphocytes. Type III lesions contain a more significant amount of lipid and also contain activated lymphocytes. Type IV and V lesions are considered "advanced" lesions. Type IV lesions are distinguished from Type III lesions by the presence of a large lipid core (~25% of the lesion volume or greater). If a fibrous cap is present, the lesion is Type V.

- A "high-risk" plaque is an advanced plaque whose fibrous cap has been thinned and is, therefore, more susceptible to rupture.

- Treatment of atherosclerosis is generally targeted at the treatment of the underlying causes (cessation of tobacco use, weight loss for overweight individuals, medical management of relevant conditions). Statins and ACE inhibitors/ARBs are particularly beneficial.

---

## INTRODUCTION

Myocardial infarction (MI) and stroke, among the most significant causes of morbidity and mortality in industrialized countries, typically occur in the context of atherosclerotic disease. In general, atherosclerotic plaques first form early in life and remain clinically silent for long periods of time. The clinical sequelae associated with atherosclerosis tend to occur many years after plaques start to form. Given the pervasiveness of atherosclerosis and the severe consequences of its sequelae, early identification of at-risk individuals is extremely important. Therefore, a working understanding of the pathophysiology and treatment of atherosclerosis is important to all cardiologists. Recent years have witnessed large strides in our understanding of the molecular mechanisms that govern the development of atherosclerotic plaques and their progression to clinically evident disease. We review here the basic pathophysiology of plaque formation, including the salient molecular interactions between the cellular players in atherosclerotic lesions. We also review risk assessment parameters, currently available points of therapeutic intervention, and accepted therapeutic strategies for atherosclerosis.

# EPIDEMIOLOGY

## Incidence

Atherosclerotic disease is exceedingly common in industrialized countries. Atherosclerosis leads to coronary artery disease and cerebrovascular disease, which are together responsible for nearly 700,000 deaths in the United States each year. The typical progression of atherosclerosis is characterized by a very long indolent period during which no symptoms are evident. For example, up to 17% of Americans have evidence of arterial thickening with fatty streaks as early as the second decade of life. While initially asymptomatic, this thickening progresses over time. Clinical manifestations of advanced atherosclerosis, such as angina, myocardial ischemia/infarction, transient ischemic attack/stroke, or limb claudication, tend to occur many years later, typically in the sixth decade and beyond. In women, atherosclerosis-related conditions typically occur even later in life.

## Risk Factors and Genetics

In most cases, the development of atherosclerosis appears to represent a complex interplay between genetic predisposition and environmental/lifestyle factors. Our ability to predict the presence of coronary atherosclerosis in an individual is limited, but a number of risk factors have been validated on a population level. Currently known risk factors can be broadly categorized according to whether or not they are based on modifiable risk factors (See **Table 26-1**).

Nonmodifiable risk factors include age greater than 45 years for men or greater than 55 for women. In addition, several genetic risk factors have been associated with atherosclerosis. The most prominent genetic factor is male sex. Most other genetic factors, such as family history of early-onset coronary artery disease (age at time of diagnosis 55 years or younger for men, 65 years or younger for women) in first-degree relatives, appear to involve multiple genes. In the case of family history, the heritability rate of atherosclerosis is

high, often measured to be in excess of 50%. Dyslipidemias, many of which have strong genetic components, are also associated with an increase in atherosclerotic risk. The classic example of low-density lipoprotein (LDL) receptor deficiency, which leads to elevated blood LDL levels and early-onset atherosclerosis, is due to a single-gene defect; however, this condition is rare, and most cases of hyperlipidemia appear to be due to defects in multiple genes.

The most common modifiable risk factor for atherosclerotic disease is a high-fat diet. A sedentary lifestyle, associated with lack of exercise is similarly associated with increase in atherosclerotic risk. Population studies have revealed that migration to a Western country confers an increase in atherosclerotic risk above heritable risk, further underscoring the influence of lifestyle. Cigarette smoking is also known to dramatically increase the risk for atherosclerotic disease; conversely, smoking cessation has also been shown to reduce the risk of atherosclerosis.

The presence of the aforementioned risk factors is also associated with several readily observable clinical phenomena, such as hypertension and hyperlipidemia, both of which are independent risk factors for the development of atherosclerosis. Clinical studies have revealed that reversal of both hypertension and hyperlipidemia can reduce the risk of atherosclerosis. Several other conditions, including diabetes mellitus, the metabolic syndrome, and obesity, also confer an increase in risk.

| Table 26-1 • Risk Factors Associated with Atherosclerosis and Coronary Heart Disease | |
|---|---|
| **Modifiable Risk Factors** | **Nonmodifiable Risk Factors** |
| Elevated LDL level | Age (>45 for men, >55 for women) |
| Depressed HDL level* | Male gender |
| Elevated Lp(a) level | Family history |
| Elevated triglyceride level | |
| Elevated homocysteine level** | |
| Cigarette smoking | |
| Diabetes mellitus | |
| Obesity/metabolic syndrome | |
| Hypertension | |
| Sedentary lifestyle and high-fat diet | |
| Elevated CRP level, systemic inflammation | |

*While HDL levels <40 are associated with an increase in risk of coronary events, increase in HDL level with lifestyle and medical interventions has not yet been shown to be associated with a reduction in risk.
** Elevated homocysteine levels are associated with an increase in risk of coronary events, but treatment has not yet been shown to reduce risk.

other materials in the plaque contact circulating platelets and clotting factors. This contact may occur after plaque rupture, erosion, or fracture. The first step in thrombus formation involves the layering of platelets on the exposed plaque surface. Along with platelets, fibrin and extracellular matrix materials are deposited. Not all ruptured plaques lead to total occlusion of the blood vessel. In fact, it should be noted that many plaque-associated thromboses are not associated with clinically apparent events. Many of these thrombi organize, and some even resolve over time. The remnants of these subclinical events are calcium deposits, as described above.

It is thought that the fibrous cap is compromised most frequently in its "shoulder" region, or the edge of the lesion, proximate to the non-affected vascular endothelium. It should be noted that the location of rupture and predilection of a particular lesion for rupture is also determined by other properties of that lesion, such as cap thickness and the presence of destabilizing microcalcifications caused by apoptotic macrophages. Neutophils, which are rare in unruptured plaques, are found quite frequently after rupture. It is thought that these neutrophils are recruited to the site as a result of thrombus formation.

## TREATMENT

The treatment of atherosclerosis is typically aimed at reversible underlying causes, notably hyperlipidemia, hypertension, and diabetes mellitus. Behavior modification through exercise, adherence to a low-fat diet, and smoking cessation is also critical. These modifications are especially important for those patients with the metabolic syndrome or obesity. The favorable effects of these interventions have been well documented and are reviewed here (see **Table 26-4**).

Recent studies reveal that a subset of lipoproteins and the renin-angiogtensin-aldosterone pathway both have direct effects on plaque progression. Targeting of these molecules with statins and angiotensin-converting enzyme (ACE) inhibitors, respectively, may therefore produce a benefit due to multiple effects.

### Hyperlipidemia

Aggressive reduction of LDL levels (20-40% as compared with baseline) with statin therapy has been shown to reduce coronary heart disease events by up to 30%. Current guidelines recommend decreasing LDL levels to 100mg/dL or lower for individuals with atherosclerotic disease. In certain individuals it is reasonable to consider a goal LDL level of 70 mg/dL or lower. While low HDL levels (below 40 mg/dL) have been associated with an increase in risk for coronary heart disease-related events, aggressive therapy for

| Table 26-4 • Summary of Treatment Strategies to Reduce Risk of Events Related to Atherosclerosis | |
|---|---|
| **Medical Therapy** | |
| Condition | Treatment goal |
| Hypertension | BP <140/90, or BP <130/80 for patients with documented coronary artery disease, chronic kidney disease, or diabetes mellitus |
| Hyperlipidemia | LDL-lowering with statin according to ATP III guidelines |
| Diabetes mellitus | HbA1c <7, avoidance of hyperglycemic episodes |
| **Nonmedical Therapy Condition** | |
| Condition | Treatment goal |
| Cigarette smoking | Cessation |
| Sedentary lifestyle | Increased exercise, low-fat diet |

increasing HDL levels has not shown significant benefit. Similarly, the treatment of other metabolites, such as attempted lowering of elevated homocysteine levels, has not been correlated with benefit.

### Hypertension

The effects of hypertension on the risk of death due to atherosclerosis-related diseases are well known. For every 20 mm Hg increase in systolic blood pressure above normal of 120 mm Hg (or a 10 mm Hg increase in diastolic blood pressure above normal of 80 mm Hg), the risk of death from myocardial infarction or stroke doubles. Treatment of hypertension has a strong effect: currently, the goal of treatment for uncomplicated patients is to maintain blood pressure less than 140/90. For patients with diabetes mellitus, chronic kidney disease (CKD), or documented coronary artery disease, the goal is less than 130/80 mm Hg. Maintenance of blood pressure at a goal level is associated with a 16% coronary heart disease mortality reduction.

### Diabetes Mellitus

Patients with diabetes have a markedly increased risk for atherosclerosis-related diseases as compared with risk factor-matched patients without diabetes. A large body of evidence suggests that reduction of hyperglycemia reduces the risk of diabetes-related microvascular disease. In type 1 diabetes, glucose control appears to produce a risk reduction for macrovascular disease progression. A similar correlation is not present for type 2 diabetes. While the bulk of evidence supports continuing treatment of diabetes mellitus, recently published reports cast some doubt on the safety of highly aggressive medical reduction of blood glucose levels.

## Cigarette Smoking and Other Lifestyle Factors

Smoking cessation produces greater coronary risk reduction than all of the other interventions listed here. The risk of coronary event increases at least twofold for every pack of cigarettes smoked per day. Smoking-associated risks are compounded in women who are simultaneously using oral contraceptive pills.

Other risk factors associated with atherosclerosis include obesity (defined as body mass index (BMI) >30) and the metabolic syndrome (MetS) (defined as being present when a person has three of the following five components: hypertriglyceridemia, low HDL, fasting hyperglycemia, hypertension, waist circumference >102cm in men and >88cm in women). This topic is discussed in detail in Chapter 24. In the United States, it is estimated that one-third of the population is obese, and an additional one-third is overweight (25<BMI<30). Therefore, patients with obesity/MetS represent a large population indeed. Treatment of the metabolic syndrome has potential for marked coronary risk reduction, especially in diabetics: for example, the estimated prevalence of coronary artery disease in diabetics is 8%, compared with nearly 20% in diabetics with the metabolic syndrome.

## Suggested Readings

1. Falk E. Pathogenesis of atherosclerosis. *J Am Coll Cardiol.* 2006;47: C7–12.

2. Lusis AJ. Atherosclerosis. *Nature.* 2000;407:233–241.

3. Yeghiazarians Y, Braunstein JB, Askar A, et al. Unstable angina pectoris. *N Engl J Med.* 2000;342:101–114.

4. Smith SC, Allen J, Blair SN, et al. AHA/ACC guidelines for secondary prevention for patients with coronary and other atherosclerotic vascular disease: 2006 update. *J Am Coll Cardiol.* 2006;47:2130–2139.

# 27

# Coronary Artery Disease: Demographics and Prevalence

### Krishnaswami Vijayaraghavan

## • PRACTICAL POINTS

- Coronary heart disease caused 425,425 deaths in 2006 and is the single leading cause of death in America today.

- Although death rates from CVD declined 29.2% between 1995 and 2006, mortality data for 2006 show that CVD accounted for 34.3% of all 2,425,900 deaths in 2006.

- Over 151,000 Americans who died due to CVD in 2006 were under age 65.

- In 2006, final death rates from CVD were 306.6 for white males and 422.8 for black males; 215.5 for white females and 298.2 for black females. (Death rates are per 100,000 population.)

- There are about 295,000 EMS-assessed out-of-hospital cardiac arrests annually in the United States.

- From 1965 to 2006, smoking in the United States declined by 50.4% among people ≥18 years of age. In 2007, among Americans ≥18 years of age, 22.0% of men and 17.5% of women were cigarette smokers, putting them at increased risk of heart attack and stroke.

- A 10% (population-wide) decrease in total cholesterol levels may result in an estimated 30% reduction in the incidence of CHD. Data from National Health and Nutrition Examination Survey (NHANES) 1999-2002 (NCHS) showed that overall, 63.3% of participants had high cholesterol.

- Prevalence of diagnosed DM in adults ≥65 years of age is 15.3%. and undiagnosed DM is 6.9%. The total number of people with DM is projected to rise from 171 million in 2000 to 366 million in 2030. The largest increase is predicted to be among blacks by 600% among those >75 years of age.

- A higher percentage of men than women have HBP until 45 years of age. From 45 to 64, the percentages of men and women with HBP are similar. After that, a much higher percentage of women have HBP than men. Compared with normal BP (<120/80 mm Hg), prehypertension was associated with a 1.5- to 2-fold risk for major CVD events in those <60, 60-79, and ≥80 years of age.

- Reduction and eradication of disparities in cardiovascular outcomes require education and advocacy programs that are population-wide, utilizing multipronged educational and cost-effective interventional strategies across all geographical and ethnic boundaries.

## GLOBAL BURDEN OF DISEASE

Cardiovascular disease (CVD) is the number one cause of death globally; more people die annually from CVD than from any other cause. An estimated 17.5 million people died from CVD in 2005, representing 30% of all global deaths (**Figure 27-1**).

Of these deaths, an estimated 7.6 million were due to coronary heart disease and 5.7 million were due to stroke. Over 80% of CVD deaths occur in low and middle income countries and

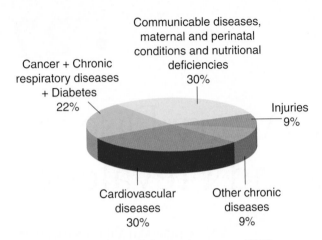

**Figure 27-1.** Prevalence of chronic diseases per WHO.

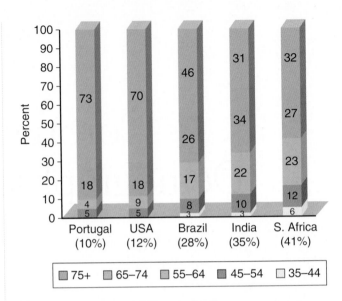

**Figure 27-2.** Projected CVD mortality (from 2000–2030.)

almost equally in men and women. By 2015 almost 20 million people will die from CVD, mainly from heart disease and stroke. According to World Health Organization statistics, total global deaths in 2005 amounted to 58 million, of which 35 million were a result of chronic diseases. Chronic diseases accounted for 6 of 10 deaths, 80% of which occurred in low- and middle-income countries. CVD, with a mortality of 17.5 million, is the leading cause of death globally. In comparison, 2.8 million deaths occurred from HIV/AIDS, 1.6 million from tuberculosis, and 0.8 million from malaria. CVD causes 3.3 times more deaths than these infectious diseases combined. Thus, cardiovascular and other chronic diseases are the leading cause of death in every part of the world except the lowest income countries, the majority of which are in sub-Saharan Africa. In low and middle income countries, there is an increase in rates of smoking and obesity, affecting younger people of working age, which portends a clear negative impact on economic growth while simultaneously threatening children. Mortality from CVD among working-age people in India, South Africa, and Brazil has been found to be 1.5 to 2 times as high as that of the United States. In South Africa 41% of all deaths from heart disease from 2000 to 2003 occurred in people 35 to 64 years of age, with a similar high figure (35%) in India. In North America, New Zealand, Australia, and parts of Europe, only 10% of those deaths occurred among individuals <65 years of age (**Figure 27-2**).

## PREVALENCE OF CARDIOVASCULAR DISEASE IN THE UNITED STATES

Overall death rate from cardiovascular disease (CVD) (International Classification of Diseases) in 2005 per 100,000 was 278.9. The rates were 324.7 per 100,000 for white males, 438.4 for black males, 230.4 for white females, and 319.7 for black females. From 1995 to 2005 death rates from CVD declined 26.4%. Mortality data for 2006 show that CHD accounted for 34.2% of all 2,425,900 deaths in 2006 (**Table 27-1**).

On the basis of 2005 mortality rate data, nearly 2400 Americans die of CVD each day: an average of 1 death every 37 seconds. The 2006 overall preliminary death rate from CVD was 262.9. More than 150,000 deaths in the US from CVD in 2005 were less than 65 years of age. In 2005, 32% of deaths from CVD occurred in persons below the age of 75 years, which is well before the average life expectancy of 77.9 years.[1] Coronary heart disease (CHD) constitutes 52% of all CVDs and caused about 1 of every 5 deaths in the United States in 2005. (**Figure 27-3**).

CHD mortality in 2005 was 445,687. It is estimated that 785,000 Americans will have a new coronary attack in 2009 and about 470,000 will have a recurrent attack. It is estimated that an additional 195,000 silent first MIs occur each year. About every 25 seconds an American will have a coronary event, and about every minute, someone will die from one. On the basis of the National Heart, Lung and Blood Institute (NHLBI)-sponsored Framingham Heart Study (FHS), CHD makes up more than half of all cardiovascular events in men and women <75 years of age. The lifetime risk of developing CHD after 40 years of age is 49% for men and 32% for women.[2] The incidence of CHD in women lags behind men by 10 years for total CHD and by 20 years for more serious clinical events such as MI and sudden death (**Figure 27-4**).

The percentage of CHD out-of-hospital deaths in 2005 was 69%. According to NCHS Data Warehouse mortality data, 309,000 CHD deaths occur out of hospital or in hospital emergency departments (EDs) annually. An analysis of FHS data (NHLBI) from 1950 to 1999 showed that overall CHD death rates decreased by 59%. Nonsudden CHD death decreased by 64% and sudden cardiac death fell by 49%. These trends were seen in men and women, in subjects with and without a prior history of CHD, and in smokers and non-smokers.[3] From 1995 to 2005, the annual death rate from

### Table 27-1 • Prevalence of Coronary Heart Disease

| Population Group | Prevalence, CHD, 2006 Age ≥ 20 yr | Prevalence, MI, 2006 Age ≥ 20 yr | New and Recurrent MI and Fatal CHD Age ≥ 35 yr | New and Recurrent MI Age ≥ 35 yr | Mortality,* CHD, 2005 All Ages | Mortality,* MI, 2005 All Ages | Hospital Discharges, CHD, 2006 All Ages | Cost, CHD, 2009 |
|---|---|---|---|---|---|---|---|---|
| Both sexes | 16,800,000 (7.6%) | 7,900,000 (3.6%) | 1 255,000 | 935,000 | 445,687 | 151,004 | 1,760,000 | $165.4 billion |
| Males | 8,700,000 (8.6%) | 4,700,000 (4.7%) | 740,000 | 565,000 | 232,115 (52.1%)‡ | 80,079 (53.0%)‡ | 1 056,000 | ... |
| Females | 8,100,000 (6.8%) | 3,200,000 (2.7%) | 515,000 | 370,000 | 213,572 (47.9%)‡ | 70,925 (47.0%)‡ | 704,000 | ... |
| NH white males | 8.8% | 4.9% | 675,000§ | ... | 203,924 | 70,791 | ... | ... |
| NH white females | 6.6% | 3.0% | 445,000§ | ... | 186,497 | 61,573 | ... | ... |
| NH black males | 9.6% | 5.1% | 70,000§ | ... | 22,933 | 7527 | ... | ... |
| NH black females | 9.0% | 2.2% | 65,000§ | ... | 23,094 | 8009 | ... | ... |
| Mexican American males | 5.4% | 2.5% | ... | ... | ... | ... | ... | ... |
| Mexican American females | 6.3% | 1.1% | ... | ... | ... | ... | ... | ... |
| Hispanic or Latino,† age ≥18 yr | 5.7% | ... | ... | ... | ... | ... | ... | ... |
| Asian,† age ≥18 yr | 4.3% | ... | ... | ... | ... | ... | ... | ... |
| American Indian/ Alaska Native, age ≥ 18 yr | 5.6% | ... | ... | ... | ... | ... | ... | ... |

CHD includes acute MI (I21, I22), other acute ischemic (coronary) heart disease (I24), AP (I20), atherosclerotic CVD (I25.0), and all other forms of ischemic CHD (I25.1-I25.9). Ellipses indicate data not available. Sources: Prevalence: NHANES 2005-2006 (NCHS) and NHLBI. Total data are for Americans ≥20 years of age; percentages for racial/ethnic groups are age adjusted for ≥20 years of age. Data are based on self-reports. Estimates from NHANES 2005-2006 (NCHS) applied to 2006 population estimates (≥20 years of age). Incidence: ARIC (1987-2004), NHLBI. Mortality: NCHS (data represent underlying cause of death only). Hospital discharges: NHDS, NCHS (data include those inpatients discharged alive, dead, or status unknown). Cost: NHLBI; data include estimated direct and indirect costs for 2009.
*Mortality data are for whites and blacks, and include Hispanics.
†NHIS, NCHS 2007—data are weighted percentages for Americans ≥18 years of age. Estimates for American Indians/Alaska Natives are considered unreliable.¹
‡These percentages represent the portion of total CHD mortality for males vs females.
§Estimates include Hispanics and non-Hispanics. Estimates for whites include other nonblack races.

CHD declined 34.3%, but the actual number of deaths declined only 19.4%. In 2005 the overall CHD death rate was 144.4 per 100,000 population. The death rates were 187.7 for white males and 213.9 for black males; for white females, the rate was 110.0, and for black females it was 140.9.³ Fifty percent of men and 64% of women who die suddenly of CHD have no previous symptoms of this disease. Between 70 and 89% of sudden cardiac deaths occur in men, and the annual incidence is 3 to 4 times higher in men than in women. However, this disparity decreases with advancing age. People who have had an MI have a sudden death rate 4 to 6 times that of the general population. According to data from the National Registry of Myocardial Infarction⁴ from 1990 to 1999, in-hospital AMI mortality declined from 11.2% to 9.4%. Mortality rate increases for every 30 minutes that elapse before a patient with ST-segment elevation is recognized and treated.

## FALL IN CHD DEATH RATES

CHD death rates have fallen from 1968 to the present. Analysis of NHANES (NCHS) data compared CHD death rates between 1980 and 2000 to determine how much of the decline in deaths from CHD over that period could be explained by the use of medical and surgical treatments

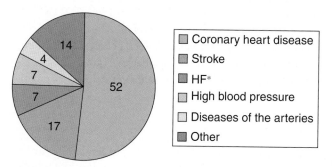

Coronary heart disease — 52
Stroke — 17
HF* — 7
High blood pressure — 7
Diseases of the arteries — 4
Other — 14

**Figure 27-3.** Percentage breakdown of deaths due to CVD (United States: 2006).

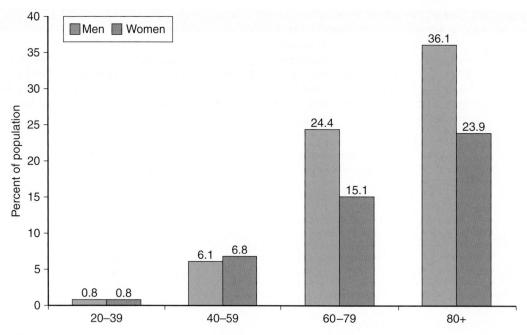

**Figure 27-4.** Prevalence of CHD by age and sex (NHANES: 2005–2006).

versus changes in CVD risk factors (resulting from lifestyle/behavior). After 1980 and 2000 data were compared, it was estimated that ~47% of the decrease in CHD deaths was attributable to treatments, including secondary preventive therapies after MI or revascularization (11%), initial treatments for AMI or unstable angina (10%), treatments for HF (9%), revascularization for chronic angina (5%), and other therapies (12%), including antihypertensive and lipid-lowering primary prevention therapies. It was also estimated that a similar amount of the reduction in CHD deaths, ~44%, was attributable to changes in risk factors, including lowering total cholesterol (24%), lowering systolic BP (20%), lowering smoking prevalence (12%), and increasing physical inactivity (5%). Nevertheless, these favorable improvements in risk factors were partially offset by increases in BMI and in diabetes prevalence, which accounted for an increased number of deaths (8 and 10%, respectively). Analysis of CHD mortality data among US adults 35 to 54 years of age showed that the annual percent change in (age-adjusted) mortality slowed markedly from 1980 to 2002 in both men and women. It is important to note, however, that the mortality rate among women 35 to 44 years of age has been increasing on average by 1.3% per year since 1997.

## ATHEROSCLEROSIS RISK IN COMMUNITIES (ARIC) STUDY

In the NHLBI-sponsored ARIC study, in participants 45 to 64 years of age, the average age-adjusted CHD incidence rates per 1000 person-years were as follows: white men, 12.5;

black men, 10.6; white women, 4.0; and black women, 5.1. Incidence rates excluding revascularization procedures were as follows: white men, 7.9; black men, 9.2; white women, 2.9; and black women, 4.9. In a multivariable analysis, hypertension was a particularly strong risk factor in black women, with hazard rate ratios (95% CI) as follows: black women, 4.8 (2.5 to 9.0); white women, 2.1 (1.6 to 2.9); black men, 2.0 (1.3 to 3.0); and white men, 1.6 (1.3 to 1.9). Diabetes mellitus was somewhat more predictive in white women than in other groups. Hazard rate ratios were as follows: black women, 1.8 (1.2 to 2.8); white women, 3.3 (2.4 to 4.6); black men, 1.6 (1.1 to 2.5); and white men, 2.0 (1.6 to 2.6)[2] (**Figure 27-5**).

The annual age-adjusted rates per 1000 population of first MI (1987-2001) in ARIC Surveillance (NHLBI) were 4.2 in black men, 3.9 in white men, 2.8 in black women, and 1.7 in white women. Among American Indians 65 to 74 years of age, the annual rates per 1000 population of new and recurrent MIs were 7.6 for men and 4.9 for women. However, analysis of data from NHANES III and NHANES 1999-2002 (NCHS) showed that in adults 20 to 74 years of age, the overall distribution of 10-year risk of developing CHD changed little during this time. Among the three racial/ethnic groups, blacks had the highest proportion of participants in the high risk group.

## RISK FACTORS

Major risk factors for CAD include age, gender, family history of premature CAD, elevated total and/or LDL cholesterol, reduced HDL cholesterol, tobacco use, hypertension,

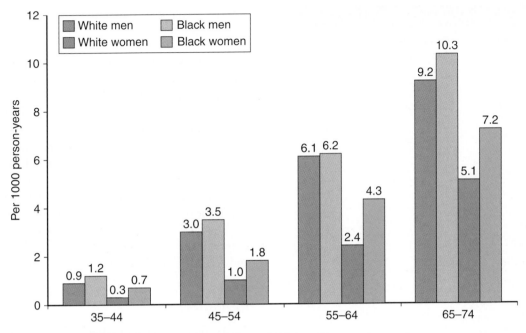

**Figure 27-5.** Incidence of MI* by age, race, and sex (ARIC Surveillance, 1987-2004).

diabetes, obesity, and physical inactivity. In three prospective cohort studies, antecedent major CHD risk factor exposures were very common among those who developed CHD. Approximately 90% of the CHD patients had prior exposure to at least one of these major risk factors, which include high total blood cholesterol levels or medication for dyslipidemia, hypertension, or medication use to lower blood pressure, current cigarette use, and clinical report of diabetes. According to a case-control study of 52 countries (INTERHEART), modifying 9 risk factors could result in a 90% reduction in the risk of an initial AMI. The effect of these risk factors is consistent in men and women across different geographic regions and by ethnic group, which makes the study applicable worldwide. These 9 risk factors include: cigarette smoking, abnormal blood lipid levels, hypertension, diabetes, abdominal obesity, a lack of physical activity, low daily fruit and vegetable consumption, alcohol over consumption, and psychosocial index.[5]

## PREVALENCE OF SMOKING

### In Youth

In 2007, 21.3% of male students and 18.7% of female students in grades 9 through 12 reported current tobacco use; 19.4% of male students and 7.6% of female students reported current cigar use; and 13.4% of male students and 2.3% of female students reported current smokeless tobacco use. Overall, 30.3% of male students and 21% of female students reported any current tobacco use. From 1980 to 2006 the percentage of high school seniors who reported smoking in the previous month decreased 29.2%. Smoking decreased by 16.4% in male students, 39.8% in female students, 20.3% in whites, and 56.3% in blacks. Among youths 12 to 17 years of age in 2006, 3.3 million (12.9%) used a tobacco product in the past month, and 2.6 million (10.4%) used cigarettes. The rate of cigarette use in the past month declined from 13.0% in 2002 to 10.4% in 2006. Cigar use in the past month declined to 4.1% in 2006 from 4.8% in 2004. Smokeless tobacco use was reported by 2.4% of youths in 2006, higher than any estimates since 2002. Results from the 2007. Monitoring the Future survey of the NIH showed a considerable drop in lifetime, past-month, and daily smoking among eighth graders. From 2006 to 2007 it dropped from 4% to 3%, down from its 10.4% peak in 1996.

### In Adults

**Table 27-2** summarizes the prevalence of smoking in multiple ethnic groups. From 1965 to 2006 smoking in the United States declined by 50.4% among people ≥18 years of age (NCHS). In 2007, among Americans ≥18 years of age, 22.0% of men and 17.5% of women were cigarette smokers, putting them at increased risk of heart attack and stroke. Rates of use of any tobacco product in 2005, among persons ≥12 years of age, were 31.2% for non-Hispanic whites only, 28.4% for non-Hispanic blacks only, 41.7% for non-Hispanic American Indians or Alaska Natives, 14.6% for non-Hispanic Asians, and 24.5% for Hispanics or Latinos of any race (NCHS). In 2006, non-Hispanic American Indian or Alaska Native adults ≥18 years of age were more likely (32.4%) to be current smokers than were

| Table 27-2 • Cigarette Smoking | | |
|---|---|---|
| **Population Group** | **Prevalence, 2006 Age ≥ 18 yr** | **Cost** |
| Both sexes | 47,100,000 (20.8%)* | $193 billion/ yr |
| Males | 26,200,000 (23.5%)* | ... |
| Females | 20,900,000 (18.1%)* | ... |
| White males | 23.5% | ... |
| White females | 18.8% | ... |
| Black males | 26.1% | ... |
| Black females | 18.5% | ... |
| Hispanic males | 20.1% | ... |
| Hispanic females | 10.1% | ... |
| NH Asian-only males | 16.8% | ... |
| NH Asian-only females | 4.6% | ... |
| NH American Indian/ Alaska Native males | 35.6% | ... |
| NH American Indian/ Alaska Native females | 29.0% | |

*Ellipses indicate data are not available.*
*\*Data are for 2006 for Americans ≥18 years of age. NHIS/NCHS percentages applied to 2006 population estimates.*

non-Hispanic white adults (21.9%), non-Hispanic black adults (23.0%), and non-Hispanic Asian adults (10.4%). According to combined data from 2005-2006, among women 15 to 44 years of age, rates of past-month cigarette smoking were lower for pregnant (16.5%) women than for nonpregnant (29.5%) women; however, among those 15 to 17 years of age, the smoking rate for pregnant women was higher than for nonpregnant women (23.1% versus 17.1%). In 2004-2005, 28% of women and 49% of men ≥65 years of age (age-adjusted) had previously smoked cigarettes. According to 2004-2006 data, most Asian adults had never smoked, with rates ranging from 65% of Korean adults to 84% of Chinese adults. Korean adults (22%) were 2 to 3 times as likely to be current smokers as were Japanese (12%), Asian Indian (7%), or Chinese (7%) adults.[6]

## PREVALENCE OF ABNORMAL CHOLESTEROL

### In Youth

Among children 4 to 11 years of age, the mean total blood cholesterol level is 165.8 mg/dL. For boys, it is 165.4 mg/dL; for girls, it is 166.3 mg/dL. The racial/ethnic breakdown is as follows (NHANES 2005-2006, NCHS and

NHLBI; unpublished analysis): for non-Hispanic whites, 166.5 mg/dL for boys and 165.9 mg/dL for girls; for non-Hispanic blacks, 166.5 mg/dL for boys and 165.1 mg/dL for girls; for Mexican Americans, 162.3 mg/dL for boys and 160.8 mg/dL for girls. Among adolescents 12 to 19 years of age, the mean total blood cholesterol level is 160.4 mg/dL. For boys, it is 156.8 mg/dL; for girls, it is 164.2 mg/dL. The racial/ethnic breakdown is as follows (NHANES 2005-2006, NCHS and NHLBI; unpublished analysis): For non-Hispanic whites, 154.5 mg/dL for boys and 165.0 mg/dL for girls; for non-Hispanic blacks, 161.7 mg/dL for boys and 162.8 mg/dL for girls; and for Mexican Americans, 158.2 mg/dL for boys and 163.1 mg/dL for girls. Approximately 9.6% of adolescents 12 to 19 years of age have total cholesterol levels ≥200 mg/dL (NHANES 2005-2006, NCHS and NHLBI.[7] (**Table 27-3**).

### In Adults

A 10% (population-wide) decrease in total cholesterol levels may result in an estimated 30% reduction in the incidence of CHD. Data from NHANES 1999-2002 (NCHS) showed that, overall, 63.3% of participants whose test results indicated high blood cholesterol or who were taking a cholesterol-lowering medication had been told by a professional that they had high cholesterol. Women were less likely than men to be aware of their condition; blacks and Mexican Americans were less likely to be aware of their condition than were whites. Fewer than half of Mexican Americans with high cholesterol were aware of their condition. Between the periods 1988-1994 and 1999-2002 (NHANES/NCHS), the age-adjusted mean total serum cholesterol level of adults ≥20 years of age decreased from 206 to 203 mg/dL, HDL levels increased from 50.7 to 51.3 mg/dL, and LDL cholesterol levels decreased from 129 to 123 mg/dL. Data from NHANES 2001-2004 (NCHS) showed the serum total crude mean cholesterol level in adults ≥20 years of age was 201 mg/dL for men and 203 mg/dL for women (**Figure 27-6**). Lipid-lowering drug use rose significantly for both sexes between 35 and 74 years of age. Awareness, treatment, and control of hypercholesterolemia have increased; however, more than half of those at borderline high risk remain unaware of their condition.[3] According to data from NHANES 2005-2006, between the periods 1999-2000 and 2005-2006, mean serum total cholesterol levels in adults ≥20 years of age declined from 204 to 199 mg/dL. This decline was observed for men ≥40 years of age and for women ≥60 years of age. There was little change over this time period for other sex/age groups. In 2005-2006 approximately 65% of men and 70% of women had been screened for high cholesterol in the past 5 years, and 16% of adults had serum total cholesterol levels of 240 mg/dL or higher. A 10-year CHD risk according to the number of risk factors per Framingham study is depicted in **Figure 27-7**.

| Population Group | Prevalence of Total Cholesterol ≥200 mg/dL, 2006 Age ≥20 yr | Prevalence of Total Cholesterol ≥240 mg/dL, 2006 Age ≥20 yr | Prevalence of LDL–C ≥130 mg/dL, 2006 Age ≥20 yr | Prevalence of HDL-C <40 mg/dL, 2006 Age ≥20 yr |
|---|---|---|---|---|
| Both sexes* | 98,600,000 (45.1%) | 34,400,000 (15.7%) | 71,800,000 (32.8%) | 33,900,000 (15.5%) |
| Males* | 45,000,000 (42.6%) | 14,600,000 (13.8%) | 35,800,000 (33.8%) | 26,300,000 (24.9%) |
| Females* | 53,600,000 (47.1%) | 19,800,000 (17.3%) | 36,000,000 (31.7%) | 7,500,000 (6.7%) |
| NH white males, % | 42.1 | 14.3 | 31.0 | 24.9 |
| NH white females, % | 47.7 | 18.1 | 33.7 | 6.5 |
| NH black males, % | 35.6 | 7.9 | 36.2 | 13.5 |
| NH black females, % | 41.4 | 13.4 | 27.4 | 6.1 |
| Mexican American males, % | 52.1 | 17.5 | 45.0 | 30.6 |
| Mexican American females, % | 48.0 | 14.5 | 30.3 | 10.5 |
| Total Hispanics† ≥20 y of age, % | ... | 29.9 | ... | ... |
| Total Asian/Pacific Islanders† ≥20 yr of age, % | ... | 29.2 | ... | ... |
| Total American Indians/Alaska Natives ≥20 yr of age,% | ... | 31.2 | ... | ... |

*Table 27-3 • High Total and LDL Cholesterol and Low HDL Cholesterol*

NH indicates non-Hispanic. Ellipses (...) indicate data not available. Prevalence of total cholesterol ≥200 mg/dL includes people with total cholesterol ≥240 mg/dL. In adults, levels of 200 to 239 mg/dL are considered borderline high. Levels of ≥240 mg/dL are considered high.
*Total data for total cholesterol are for Americans ≥20 years of age. Data for LDL cholesterol, HDL cholesterol, and all racial/ethnic groups are age adjusted for age ≥20 years.
†BRFSS (1991-2003, CDC), MMWR; data are self-reported data for Americans ≥20 years of age.
Source for total cholesterol ≥200 mg/dL, ≥240 mg/dL, LDL, and HDL: NHANES (2005-2006), NCHS, and NHLBI. Estimates from NHANES 2005-2006 (NCHS) applied to 2006 population estimates.

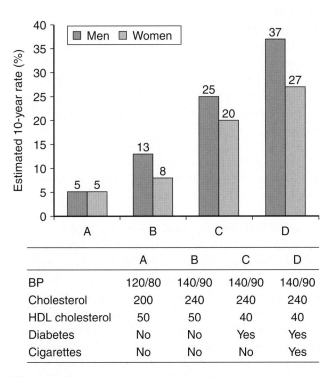

**Figure 27-6.** Estimated 10-year CHD risk in adults 55 years of age according to levels of various risk factors (Framingham Heart Study). (Source: Wilson et al.)

## PREVALENCE OF DIABETES

### In Youth

In the Search for Diabetes in Youth Study (SEARCH), the prevalence of diabetes mellitus (DM) in youths <20 years of age in 2001 in the U.S. was 1.82 cases per 1000 youths (0.79 per 1000 among youths 0 to 9 years of age and 2.80 per 1000 among youths 10 to 19 years of age). Non-Hispanic white youths had the highest prevalence (1.06 per 1000) in the younger group. Among youths 10 to 19 years of age, black youths (3.22 per 1000) and non-Hispanic white youths (3.18 per 1000) had the highest rates, followed by American Indian youths (2.28 per 1000), Hispanic youths (2.18 per 1000), and Asian/Pacific Islander youths (1.34 per 1000). Among younger children, type 1 DM accounted for ≥80% of DM; among older youths, the proportion of type 2 DM ranged from 6% (0.19 per 1000 for non-Hispanic white youths) to 76% (1.74 per 1000 for American Indian youths). This represents 154,369 youths with physician-diagnosed DM in 2001 in the United States, for an overall prevalence estimate for DM in children and adolescents of approximately 0.18%. Approximately 186,000 people <20 years of age have diabetes. Each year, about 15,000 people <20 years of age are diagnosed with type 1 diabetes. Healthcare

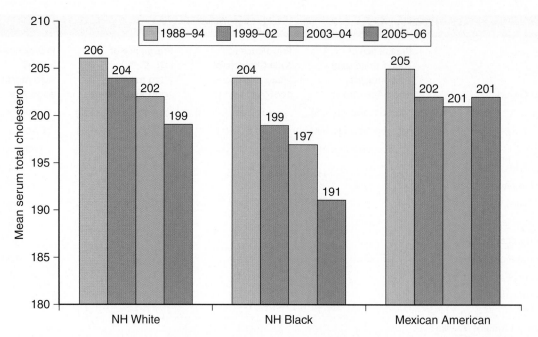

**Figure 27-7.** Trends in mean total serum cholesterol among adults by race and survey (NHANES: 1988-1994, 1999-2002, 2003-2004, and 2005-2006). (Source: NCHS and NHLBI. NH indicates non-Hispanic.)

providers are finding more and more children with type 2 diabetes. Children who develop type 2 diabetes are typically overweight or obese and have a family history of the disease. Most are American Indian, black, Asian, or Hispanic/Latino. Among adolescents 10 to 19 years of age diagnosed with diabetes, 57.8% of blacks were diagnosed with type 2 versus type 1 diabetes compared with 46.1% of Hispanic and 14.9% of white youths with type 2 versus type 1 diabetes.

## In Adults

Data from NHANES 1999-2002 (NCHS) showed the prevalence of diagnosed DM in adults ≥65 years of age to be 15.3%. The prevalence of undiagnosed DM was 6.9% (**Table 27-4**). This represents ~5.4 million and 2.4 million older individuals, respectively. Among Americans ≥20 years of age, 9.6% have DM, and among those ≥60 years of age, 21% have DM. Men ≥20 years of age have a slightly higher prevalence (11%) than women (9%). Among non-Hispanic whites ≥20 years of age, 9% have DM; the prevalence of DM among non-Hispanic blacks in this age range is 1.8 times higher; among Mexican Americans it is 1.7 times higher; and among American Indians and Alaska Natives it is 1.5 to 2.2 times higher. Data from NHANES (NCHS) show a disproportionately high prevalence of DM in non-Hispanic blacks and Mexican Americans compared with non-Hispanic whites, as shown in **Table 27-4**. The prevalence of diabetes was more than twice as high for Asian Indian adults (14%) as for Chinese (6%) or Japanese (5%) adults.[3] (**Figure 27-8**) Type 2 DM accounts for 90 to 95%

of all diagnosed cases of DM in adults In the Framingham study, 99% of DM is type 2. The prevalence of DM increased by 8.2% from 2000 to 2001. From 1990 to 2001, the prevalence of those diagnosed with DM increased 61%. On the basis of 2007 CDC data, the prevalence of adults who reported ever having been told by a doctor that they had DM ranged from 5.7% in Minnesota to 11.9% in Tennessee. The median percentage among states was 8.0%. The CDC analyzed data from 1994 to 2004 collected by the Indian Health Service that indicated that the age-adjusted prevalence per 1000 population of DM increased 101.2% among American Indian/Alaska Native adults <35 years of age (from 8.5% to 17.1%). During this time period the prevalence of diagnosed DM was greater among females than males in all age groups. The prevalence of DM for all age groups worldwide was estimated to be 2.8% in 2000 and is projected to be 4.4% in 2030. The total number of people with DM is projected to rise from 171 million in 2000 to 366 million in 2030.[4] On the basis of projections from NHANES/NCHS studies between 1984 and 2004, the total prevalence of DM in the United States is expected to more than double from 2005 to 2050 (from 5.6 to 12.0%) in all age, sex, and race/ethnicity groups. Increases are projected to be largest for the oldest age groups (for instance, increasing by 220% among those 65 to 74 years of age and by 449% among those 75 years of age or older). Diabetes mellitus prevalence is projected to increase by 99% among non-Hispanic whites, by 107% among non-Hispanic blacks, and by 127% among Hispanics. The age/race/ethnicity group with the largest increase is expected to be blacks ≥75 years of age (increase of 606%).

## Table 27-4 • Diabetes Prevalence

| Population Group | Prevalence of Physician-Diagnosed DM, 2006 Age ≥20 yr | Prevalence of Undiagnosed DM, 2006 Age ≥20 yr | Prevalence of Prediabetes, 2006 Age ≥20 yr | Incidence of Diagnosed DM 2005 Age ≥20 yr | Mortality (DM), 2005 All Ages | Hospital Discharges, 2006 All Ages | Cost, 2007 |
|---|---|---|---|---|---|---|---|
| Both sexes | 17,000,000 (7.7%) | 6,400,000 (2.9%) | 57,000,000 (25.9%) | 1,600,000§ | 75,119 | 584,000 | $174 billion |
| Males | 7,500,000 (7.4%) | 3,900,000 (3.8%) | 34,000,000 (31.7%) | ... | 36,538 (48.6%)* | 283,000 | ... |
| Females | 9,500,000 (8.0%) | 2,500,000 (2.1%) | 23,000,000 (19.9%) | ... | 38,581 (51.4%)* | 301,000 | ... |
| NH white males | 5.8% | 3.6% | 32.0% | ... | 29 628 | ... | ... |
| NH white females | 6.1% | 2.2% | 18.7% | ... | 30,127 | ... | ... |
| NH black males | 14.9% | 4.7% | 22.9% | ... | 5730 | ... | ... |
| NH black females | 13.1% | 3.1% | 19.0% | ... | 7240 | ... | ... |
| Mexican American males | 11.3% | 6.0% | 28.5% | ... | ... | ... | ... |
| Mexican American females | 14.2% | 1.9% | 23.6% | ... | ... | ... | ... |
| Hispanic or Latino,† age ≥18 yr | 11.1% | ... | ... | ... | ... | ... | ... |
| Asian,† age ≥ 18 yr | 8.9% | ... | ... | ... | ... | .. | ... |
| AI/AN, age ≥18 yr Asian Indian | 17.2% 14% | ... | ... | ... | ... | ... | ... |

Ellipses (…) indicate data not available; NH, non-Hispanic; AI/AN, American Indian/Alaska Native.
Undiagnosed DM is defined here as those whose fasting glucose is ≥126 mg/dL but who did not report being told by a healthcare provider that they had DM. Prediabetes is a fasting blood glucose of 100 to <126 mg/dL (impaired fasting glucose). Prediabetes includes impaired glucose tolerance.
*These percentages represent the portion of total DM mortality that is for males vs females.
†NHIS. Data are age-adjusted estimates for Americans ≥18 years of age.
‡Mortality data are for whites and blacks and include Hispanics.
§CDC; National Diabetes Fact Sheet, 2007. Accessed June 24, 2008.
Sources: Prevalence: Prevalence of diagnosed and undiagnosed diabetes: NHLBI computations from NHANES 2003-2006; extrapolation to the 2006 US population. Prevalence of prediabetes: CDC Fact Sheet. CDC computations are from NHANES 2003-2006; extrapolation to the 2007 U.S. population. Percentages for racial/ethnic groups are age adjusted for Americans ≥20 years of age. Incidence: NIDDK estimates. Mortality: NCHS. These data represent underlying cause of death only. Hospital discharges: NHDS, NCHS; data include those inpatients discharged alive, dead, or status unknown.

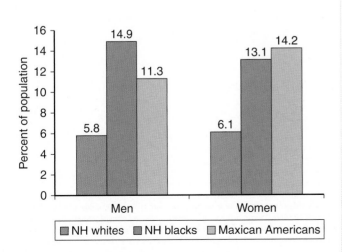

**Figure 27-8.** Prevalence of Diabetes by ethnicity.

## HYPERTENSION

A hypertensive person, i.e., diagnosed with high blood pressure (HBP), is one who has systolic blood pressure (SBP) ≥140 mm Hg or diastolic blood pressure (DBP) ≥90 mm Hg; or who takes antihypertensive medicine; or who has been told at least twice by a physician or other health professional that he or she has HBP. One in three U.S. adults has HBP. A higher percentage of men than women have HBP up to 45 years of age. From 45 to 54 years and 55 to 64 years of age, the percentages of men and women with HBP are similar. Beyond these age ranges, a much higher percentage of women have HBP than men. HBP is 2 to 3 times more common in women taking oral contraceptives, especially in obese and older women, than in women not taking them.[9] Data from NHANES 2005-2006 found that 29% of US adults ≥18 years of age were hypertensive. The prevalence of hypertension was nearly equal between men and women. An additional 37% of U.S. adults

**Table 27-5 • Hypertension Awareness, Treatment, and Control: NHANES 1988-1994 and 1999-2004, by Race**[36]

|  | Awareness | | Treatment | | Control | |
|---|---|---|---|---|---|---|
|  | 1988-94 | 1999-2004 | 1988-94 | 1999-2004 | 1988-94 | 1999-2004 |
| NH white male | 63.0% | 70.4% | 46.2% | 60.0% | 22.0% | 39.3% |
| NH white female | 74.7% | 73.4% | 61.6% | 64.0% | 32.2% | 34.5% |
| NH black male | 62.5% | 67.8% | 42.3% | 56.4% | 16.6% | 29.9% |
| NH black female | 77.8% | 81.8% | 64.6% | 71.7% | 30.0% | 36.0% |
| Mexican American male | 47.8% | 55.9% | 30.9% | 40.4% | 13.5% | 21.4% |
| Mexican American female | 69.3% | 66.9% | 47.8% | 54.9% | 19.4% | 27.4% |

had prehypertension, and 7% of adults with hypertension had never been told that they had hypertension. Among hypertensive adults, 78% were aware of their condition, 68% were using antihypertensive medication, and >64% of those treated were controlled. (**Table 27-5**)

## Older Adults

Age-adjusted estimates show that in 2004-2005, diagnosed chronic conditions that were more prevalent among older women than men included hypertension (51% for women, 45% for men). The age-adjusted prevalence of hypertension (both diagnosed and undiagnosed) in 1999-2002 was 78% for older women and 64% for older men on the basis of data from NHANES/NCHS. (**Table 27-6**)

## Children and Adolescents

Analysis of NHES, HHANES, and NHANES/NCHS surveys of the NCHS (1963-2002) found that the BP, pre-HBP, and HBP trends in children and adolescents 8 to 17 years of age moved downward from 1963 to 1988 and upward thereafter. Pre-HBP and HBP increased 2.3% and 1%, respectively, between 1988 and 1999. Increased obesity (more so

**Table 27-6 • Prevalence of High Blood Pressure**

| Population Group | Prevalence, 2006 Age ≥ 20 yr | Mortality,* 2005 All Ages | Hospital Discharges, 2006 All Ages | Estimated Cost, 2009 |
|---|---|---|---|---|
| Both sexes | 73,600,000 (33.3%) | 57,356 | 514 000 | $73.4 billion |
| Males | 35,300 000 (34.1%) | 24,046 (41.9%)[†] | 204,000 | ... |
| Females | 38,300 000 (32.1%) | 33,310 (58.1%)[†] | 309,000 | ... |
| NH white males | 34.1% | 17,312 | ... | ... |
| NH white females | 30.3% | 25,814 | ... | ... |
| NH black males | 44.4% | 6019 | ... | ... |
| NH black females | 43.9% | 6746 | ... | ... |
| Mexican American males | 23.1% | ... | ... | ... |
| Mexican American females | 30.4% | ... | ... | ... |
| Hispanic or Latino[‡] ≥18 yr | 20.6% | ... | ... | ... |
| Asian[‡] ≥18 yr | 19.5% | ... | ... | ... |
| American Indians/Alaska Natives[‡] ≥18 yr | 25.5% | ... | ... | ... |

*Ellipses (...) indicate data not available.*
*\*Mortality data are for whites and blacks and include Hispanics.*
*†These percentages represent the portion of total HBP mortality that is for males vs females.*
*‡NHIS (2007), NCHS; data are weighted percentages for Americans ≥18 years of age.*[12]
*Sources: Prevalence: NHANES (2005-2006, NCHS) and NHLBI; percentages for racial/ethnic groups are age adjusted for Americans ≥20 years of age. Estimates from NHANES 2005-2006 (NCHS) applied to 2006 population estimates ≥20 years of age. Mortality: NCHS. These data represent underlying cause of death only. Hospital discharges: NHDS, NCHS; data include those discharged alive, dead, or status unknown. Cost: NHLBI; data include estimated direct and indirect costs for 2009.*
*Note: Hypertension is defined in a person who has SBP ≥140 mm Hg or DBP ≥90 mm Hg, or who takes antihypertensive medication, or being told twice by a physician or other professional that one has hypertension. The NHLBI computed the numbers and rates on the basis of NHANES 2005-2006 (NCHS). Many studies define hypertension as present in a person who has BP ≥140/90 mm Hg or who takes antihypertensive medication. Under this definition, extrapolation of NHANES 2005-2006 (NCHS) data to the U.S. population in 2006 gives an estimated prevalence of 65.6 million. That is 30% of the population ≥20 years of age, compared with 33%, according to the more complete definition, a difference of 8 million persons.*

# 28

# Novel Risk Factors for Atherosclerosis

ASIMUL H. ANSARI, NAJAMUL H. ANSARI, AND JYOTHY PUTHUMANA

## ● PRACTICAL POINTS

- Of patients that experience cardiovascular events, 20% do not have a "traditional" risk factor for CAD and 50% have normal cholesterol levels.

- It has been recognized that inflammation plays a significant role in the development of atherosclerosis, leading to the study of several newer "novel" risk factors.

- It is important to recognize that these novel risk factors are markers of inflammation and not the mechanism leading to atherosclerosis.

- Hs-CRP is the most validated marker, and has received significant attention since the JUPITER study was released, potentially expandng the role for statin therapy.

- Important cutoff values for hs-CRP are <1, indicative of low risk; and >3, indicative of higher risk.

- Other (non hs-CRP) markers for inflammation and/or oxidation, as well as cardiac and renal dysfunction are less validated for purposes of primary prevention.

## INTRODUCTION

### Overview

Cardiovascular disease (CVD), defined variously as coronary artery disease (CAD), cerebrovascular disease, or peripheral arterial disease (PAD), is a major cause of death in developed countries. Atherosclerosis, the predominant underlying etiology of CVD, is responsible for approximately 20% of all deaths annually in the United States, with direct and indirect costs of $150 billion in 2007.

Traditional risk factors have been derived from the landmark Framingham Heart Study; they are blood pressure, smoking status, dyslipidemia, and the presence of diabetes mellitus. Worldwide validation of the Framingham study as well is the effect age and gender impact cardiovascular risk led to the development of the Framingham Risk Score, which is widely utilized to estimate 10-year risk. Additionally, significant emphasis has been placed on the assessment, treatment, and monitoring of these risk factors in the form of research investigation, AHA/ACC guidelines, and measures of physician and hospital performance.

While great strides have been made in realizing the goals of reducing clinical events with treatment and prevention programs, it is widely recognized that 20% of individuals with cardiovascular events do not have a traditional risk factor, and that 50% of individuals presenting with acute coronary syndrome (ACS) have normal levels of serum cholesterol.

In recognition of the limitations presented by utilizing traditional risk factors, and due to newer insights into the role inflammatory mechanisms play in the pathogenesis of atherosclerosis, extensive interest has developed in using "novel risk factors" to improve risk prediction. This biomarker strategy for estimating risk is attractive, since it is readily available for screening purposes via a simple blood test, unlike the newer applications of imaging techniques.

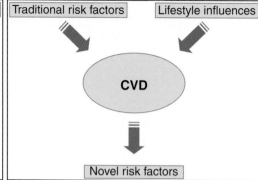

**Figure 28-1.** The two proposed models for the interaction of "novel risk factors" and cardiovascular disease ("CVD"). In the risk mechanism model, novel risk factors are contributing to the deveeopment of CVD whereas in the risk marker model, novel risk markers are associated with CVD but not causative of atherosclerosis.

It must be noted, however, that some argue that these novel risk factors are not the *mechanism* of the inflammatory cascade, but rather *markers* of the injurious process leading to cardiovascular disease (**Figure 28-1**). It has been shown that prediction of events for individual patients is difficult and the addition of novel risk factors only incrementally add to risk stratification. Additionally, the importance of nonbiomarker factors such as those related to lifestyle is gaining appreciation among health researchers. Therefore, approaches that combine novel risk markers or calculate a risk score based upon multiple risk markers have been developed and are being considered for estimating cardiovascular risk in individuals.

## Atherosclerosis and Inflammation

As the principle underlying cause of CVD, atherosclerosis consists of a complex interaction between lipids, smooth muscle cells, and macrophages within the arterial wall, regulated by inflammatory cytokines and other blood elements. Atherosclerosis is a process often starting early in life and progressing insidiously and silently, until plaque rupture and subsequent thrombosis causes transient complete or partial arterial occlusion within a particular vascular territory in the form of unstable angina (USA), acute myocardial infarction (NSTEMI/STEMI), stroke, or transient ischemic attack (TIA), or limb ischemia, depending upon whether the vascular bed is in the coronary, cerebral, or peripheral circulation.

It has been well established that inflammatory pathways play a role in all stages of atherosclerosis, from atherogenic plaque development to plaque rupture at the shoulder region, a process initiated by insult/injury to the vascular endothelium by traditional risk factors such as elevated blood pressure, hyperglycemia, and tobacco and modulated by noxious inflammatory proteins.

Pathophysiological insights into role that inflammatory risk factors contribute to the progression of atherosclerosis provide potential targets for measurement at several points in the inflammatory cascade. These "novel" inflammatory risk factors include oxidized low-density lipoproteins, cytokines (e.g., IL-1, IL-6, IL-18, and TNF-α), vascular markers (e.g., sICAM-1, selectins), liver proteins, such as C-reactive protein (CRP), and fibrinogen, and a host of other acute-phase reactants (**Tables 28-1** and **28-2**).

## NOVEL RISK FACTORS

### Inflammatory Proteins

#### hs-CRP
C-reactive protein (CRP, high sensitivity (hs)-CRP) is an acute phase reactant produced by the liver that has been

| Table 28-1 • Proposed Novel Risk Factors |
| --- |
| **Liver Proteins/Acute Phase Reactants** |
| • C-reactive protein (CRP and hs-CRP) |
| • Fibrinogen |
| • Serum amyloid A (SAA) |
| **Other Proteins** |
| • Homocysteine |
| • von Willebrand factor (vWF) |
| **Markers of Renal Dysfunction** |
| • Cystatin C |
| • Urinary albumin/creatinine ratio (ACR) |
| **Cardiac Markers** |
| • Troponin |
| • BNP and N-Pro-BNP |
| • Lipoproteins |
| • Lipoprotein-associated phospholipase A2 (Lp-PLA2) |
| • Lipoprotein (a) |
| **Cytokines** |
| • Interleukin-18 |
| • Interleukin-6 |
| **Lifestyle Risk Factors** |
| • Soft drink consumption |
| • Sleep loss |

| Table 28-2 • Summary of Proposed Novel Risk Factors | | | |
|---|---|---|---|
| **Novel Risk Factor** | **Values of Interest** | **Category** | **Treatment** |
| hs-CRP | <1 mg/L<br>1-3 mg/L<br>>3 mg/L | Inflammatory | Probably statin |
| Fibrinogen | >1 | Hemostatic | None |
| Homocysteine | >30 µmol/L<br>>100 µmol/L | Oxidant stress/<br>endothelial dysfunction | Folate and B vitamins<br>(not effective) |
| Cystatin C | >1.0 mg/L | Renal dysfunction | ACEI, ARB |
| U Alb/Cr | ≥30 µg/mg | Renal dysfunction/endothelial<br>dysfunction | ACEI, ARB |
| Troponin | >0.035 µg/L | Cardiac damage | ASA, BB, statins |
| BNP | 100 ng/L | Cardiac damage | ASA, BB, statins |
| Pro-BNP | 125 ng/L | Cardiac damage | ASA, BB, statins |
| Lp-PLA2 | >400-450 g/L | Inflammatory | Lp-PLA2 inhibitors (being developed) |
| Lp(a) | >30 mg/dL | Lipoprotein | Statins, niacin, estrogen |
| IL-6 | Not standardized | Inflammatory | Aspirin, statin, estrogen |
| IL-18 | Not standardized | Inflammatory | Aspirin, statin, estrogen |

extensively studied in connection to CVD, with a large body of literature supporting its use as a biomarker for future CVD events. hs-CRP has been studied as a surrogate of other inflammatory mediators, such as the cytokines IL-6 and TNF-a, and it has been implicated in multiple aspects of atherogenesis and plaque vulnerability, including expression of adhesion molecules, alteration of nitric oxide, modulation of complement function, inhibition of fibrinolysis, and induction of apoptosis of vascular smooth muscle cells, thereby essentially acting as a final end product of multiple various and converging pathways of inflammation in atherosclerosis and acute ischemic syndromes. The highly anticipated JUPITER trial, a study designed to assess directly whether statin therapy should be given to apparently healthy individuals with low LDL-cholesterol (LDL-C) levels but elevated hs-CRP levels, was recently halted early due to beneficial effects of statin therapy towards cardiovascular morbidity and mortality. CRP has been shown to be influenced by many cardiovascular risk factors including age, gender, body size, exposure to tobacco and lipid levels.

CRP has been studied in both the primary and secondary prevention population of individuals, and has been demonstrated to independently predict future myocardial infarction, stroke, cardiovascular death, and ischemic PAD. Numerous prospective and retrospective studies have demonstrated the additive value of hs-CRP to the Framingham Risk Score. The largest U.S. prospective studies that included hs-CRP assessment were the Physicians Health Study (PHS), the Women's Health Study (WHS), the Atherosclerosis Risk in Communities (ARIC) Study and the Air Force/Texas Atherosclerosis Prevention (AFCAPS/TexCAPs) studies, as well as the European Monitoring of Trends and Determinants of Cardiovascular Disease (MONICA) and

Reykjavik studies. In fact, in the PHS and WHS, hs-CRP had a higher predictive value than traditional cholesterol risk factors (TC, HDL, LDL) and other novel risk factors (lipoprotein (a) and homocysteine) that were obtained (**Figure 28-2**). In regards to individuals with established CVD, levels of hs-CRP have been strongly linked with recurrent ischemic cardiovascular events as well as prognosis in patients presenting with ACS, regardless of troponin status.

While initial work with CRP divided patients into tertiles or quartiles of risk, more recent work with hs-CRP and guideline recommendations by the CDC/AHA suggests the

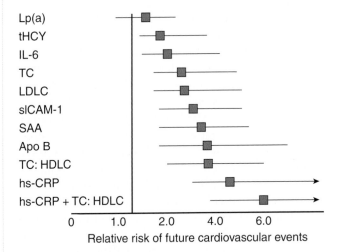

**Figure 28-2.** In an analysis of the WHS, hs-CRP was found to have a higher predictive value than other novel risk factors and traditional factors such as TC. (Reprinted with permission from Ridker PM. Clinical application of C-reactive protein for cardiovascular disease detection and prevention. *Circulation.* 2003;107:363.)

following cutoff values: <1 mg/L, 1-3 mg/L, and >3 mg/L for low, intermediate, and high risk, respectively; also, there is the suggestion (from further analysis of the WHS) that further subdivision be made of the hs-CRP concentrations into five categories ($\leq$0.5, 0.5-1, 1-3, 3-10, $\geq$10 mg/L), with an extremely low ($\leq$0.5 mg/L) and extremely high ($\geq$10 mg/L) category for providing additional predictive risk. Recent studies have also revealed potential evidence for the hypothesis that extremely low levels of hs-CRP may be protective and that extremely high levels of hs-CRP, from any source of inflammation, may affect both atherogenesis and acute thrombotic events, as supported by results of the Dutch Echographic Cardiac Risk Evaluation Applying Stress Echo III (DECREASE III) Study. DECREASE demonstrated a mortality benefit of statin in vascular surgery patients postoperatively and also a marked decrease in postoperative levels of hs-CRP, as well as WHS data that aspirin prevented vascular events amongst patients with the highest levels of hs-CRP.

Although clearly a predictor of vascular events, the levels of hs-CRP do not correlate with overall atherosclerotic burden, as measured by cardiac catheterization, coronary calcification, carotid intimal-medial thickness, or anklebrachial index, reflecting the fact that hs-CRP provides additive and complementary data to other testing modalities, with an important measure of the inflammatory component of the atherosclerotic disease process, and hence, the risk of plaque instability or rupture. In regard to testing, the current CDC/AHA/ACC guidelines recommend testing in intermediate- and high- Framingham Risk individuals, with two separate measurements made at least several weeks apart, and that those individuals with an hs-CRP >3 mg/L be placed into a higher risk group and considered for a more aggressive treatment regimen. In fact, when this approach is utilized, approximately 30% of individuals of "intermediate Framingham risk" can be reclassified into another risk category. Although there is no "CRP lowering agent" in the sense of LDL lowering with statin or other agents, there has been an association of lower hs-CRP levels with statin use as seen in the Cholesterol and Recurrent Events (CARE), AFCAPS/TexCAPS trials, lending further support of the pliotropic effects of statins, while other nonstatin cholesterol-lowering agents, such as ezetimibe, have shown no capacity to decrease CRP when used as monotherapy. Interestingly, lower levels of hs-CRP are noted, in general, in individuals who are receiving aspirin and thiazolidines, while higher levels are noted in those who have a chronic inflammatory state, smoke, are obese, and are receiving estrogens. Currently, a CRP inhibitor is undergoing animal testing, which, if approved and efficacious in lowering CRP, could potentially solve the "mechanism versus marker" debate in addition to lowering individual risk for CVD.

## Fibrinogen

Fibrinogen, a hemostatic factor and the precursor for fibrin, is the major coagulation protein in the blood and an important determiner of blood viscosity and platelet aggregation. Due to its role in the coagulation cascade, and the role that systemic or local low-grade inflammation may play in the atherosclerosis, fibrinogen has been associated with increased cardiovascular risk. However, fibrinogen has been found to affect smooth muscle cells and plaque stability, in addition to the critical role it plays in formation of the fibrin clot in the event of plaque rupture.

Plasma fibrinogen levels vary widely in the population and have been shown to vary by season, smoking, aging, and atherosclerosis burden; they differ according to sex and race. In the hemostatic factors in the Coronary Artery Risk Development in Young Adults (CARDIA) Study, a 13-year analysis of several markers in the coagulation cascade and progression of subclinical surrogates for atherosclerosis were compared in young adults aged 25-37. While levels of **Factors** VI, VII and von Willebrand factor (vWF) did not correlate with changes in coronary artery calcification (CAC) **or** carotid intimal/medial thickness (CIMT), the age-, race-, and gender-adjusted prevalences of CAC and CIMT with increasing quartiles of fibrinogen were significant, even after adjusting for body mass index (BMI), smoking, systolic blood pressure (SBP), diabetes, antihypertensive medication use, total and high-density lipoprotein (HDL) cholesterol, and CRP. Further evidence comes from the Fibrinogen Studies Collaboration, a meta-analysis of 154,000 individuals and 31 clinical studies that prospectively evaluated plasma fibrinogen levels and the risk of CHD or stroke at minimum 1 year of follow-up. In this meta-analysis, each 1-g/L elevation of fibrinogen carried a relative risk of 1.8 for future CHD or stroke in a large population demographic, with multiple comorbid conditions and risk factors for CVD such as diabetes, hypertension, smoking status, SBP, and cholesterol levels. Interestingly, additive value of hs-CRP in individuals in which both fibrinogen and hs-CRP were measured did not add incremental gain in prognostic significance in this analysis. In the secondary prevention population, recent evidence from the AIRGENE Study has shown the role that genetic polymorphisms play in fibrinogen levels, and hence, elucidates the fact that there is a genetic basis for inter- and intra-individual variability of fibrinogen levels.

## Lipoprotein-Associated Phospholipase A2 (Lp-PLA2)

Lipoprotein-associated phospholipase A2 (Lp-PLA2) is an enzyme synthesized by macrophages and platelets that is believed to be involved in the formation of vulnerable plaque. It circulates in the blood attached to LDL cholesterol and is expressed by macrophages within the core and the fibrous cap of these advanced plaques. Lp-PLA2's primary enzymatic role is to hydrolyze oxidized phospholipids, which yield proinflammatory and proatherogenic products.

Daniels et al., in the Rancho Bernardo Study, found Lp-PLA2 to be a strong and independent predictor of fatal and nonfatal CHD events above other traditional risk factors in healthy older men without a known history of CAD, a population where Lp-PLA2 might not contribute anything to risk prediction on account of age already being a strong predictor of risk.

Previous studies, such as the West of Scotland Coronary Prevention Study (WOSCOPS) and MONICA, have shown that higher levels of Lp-PLA2 levels were associated with an increased risk of coronary disease, even after adjustment for traditional risk factors and CRP levels. The ARIC study reported a similar positive association between Lp-PLA2 and events: the investigators found that patients with LDL levels below the study median of 130 mg/dL were nearly twice as likely to have CHD if they were in the second or third tertile of Lp-PLA2 as if they were in the lowest tertile. Lp-PLA2 levels do not appear to be reliably useful for risk assessment during hospitalization for ACS. However, when measured later, Lp-PLA2 can offer prognostic information incremental to that provided by traditional risk markers, including LDL. However, an analysis in the Women's Health Study found no association after adjustment for other risk factors, suggesting that perhaps Lp-PLA2 is not predictive of CHD in women.

An inhibitor of Lp-PLA2 is currently undergoing clinical trial evaluation.

## Oxidation

### Homocysteine

Homocysteine has been proven a risk marker and not a true risk factor in atherosclerotic cardiac disease. An amino acid produced in methionine metabolism, homocysteine can be elevated due to several factors, including genetic, dietary (deficiency of folic acid, vitamin B12, vitamin B6, methionine), and lifestyle (smoking, alcohol, and coffee intake). Homocysteine is also secondary to medical conditions such as advanced diabetes and renal failure and medications (methotrexate, sulfonamides). Serum homocystiene normally ranges between 5 and 15 umol/L when measured in the fasting State. Levels of >100 umol/L are severely elevated. Many possible mechanisms have been proposed, including endothelial and platelet dysfunction, activation of clotting or inflammatory factors, or alteration of lipid metabolism and oxidation.

While initial observational studies linked hyperhomocysteinemia to arteriosclerosis and that treatment favorably altered surrogate outcomes, randomized trials such as NORVIT, WAFACS, and HOPE-2 all consistently showed that there was no causal relationship and that treatment with folic acid and B vitamin supplements was without benefit. While folic acid and B vitamins significantly reduced homocysteine levels, when combined the treatments showed a trend to be potentially harmful in terms of the combined endpoint of MI and stroke in NORVIT.

Because of these findings, routine screening of homocysteine levels for CVD prevention purposes is not recommended.

## Markers of Renal Dysfunction

### Cystatin C

Renal dysfunction has been recognized as a significant risk factor for the development of CVD. Cystatin C is a low molecular weight protein that is a member of the cystatin family of cysteine protease inhibitors and plays an important role in the regulation of proteolytic degradation. While both creatinine and cystatin C are cleared by the glomerulus, cystatin C levels are not related to muscle mass or protein intake and do not appear to be as influenced as creatinine by age, gender, or race. Therefore, cystatin C is believed to be a more precise reflection of kidney function, signaling a state of preclinical renal dysfunction when elevated, termed the "creatinine-blind" range. Furthermore, cystatin C has a stable production rate even in the setting of an inflammatory response.

Numerous outcome studies measuring levels of cystatin C involving stable outpatients with various disease entities have been performed. In a recent study funded by the NHLBI, Shlipak et al. published a report using data from the Cardiovascular Health Study (CHS) showing that after adjustment for traditional risk factors, stroke, heart failure, coronary heart disease, and C-reactive protein levels, individuals without chronic kidney disease and high cystatin C levels had statistically significantly increased risk for MACE compared with the individuals without chronic kidney disease and low cystatin C levels. These individuals had approximately 50% higher overall mortality and double the risk of cardiovascular death. In addition, they had statistically significant increased risks for heart failure, stroke, and myocardial infarction. Cystatin C levels >1.0 mg/L were considered abnormal.

Moreover, Lassus et al. studied a population of patients admitted for acute heart failure in Finland as part of the multicenter FINN-AKVA study. About one-half of the patients were newly diagnosed on admission and approximately one third had an ejection fraction ≥45% that could be classified as diastolic heart failure. Lassus et al. analyzed a variety of biomarkers, including BNP, troponin T, and serum creatinine, and found that cystatin C was the strongest predictor of mortality at 6 months.

Measurement of cystatin C levels may be appropriate in the evaluation of patients who appear to have a normal creatinine-based renal function, but because of other comorbid conditions or age might be expected to be at higher risk for chronic kidney disease. Testing is available on a national basis, however, at almost 10 times the cost of serum creatinine measurement.

### Urinary Albumin/Creatinine Ratio (ACR)

The normal rate of albumin excretion is <20 mg/day, whereas albumin excretion between 30 and 300 mg/day is referred to as microalbuminuria. This level of proteinuria is inaccurately detected by urine dipstick, yet the gold standard of 24-hour urine measurement is itself cumbersome and prone to errors. The ACR has been used to compensate for variations in urine concentration, and microalbuminuria currently is defined as an ACR value >30 µg/mg. It should be noted that this single value does not take into account muscle mass differences that are observed among gender and racial lines.

Microalbuminuria was originally found to be an early indicator of glomerular dysfunction in renal and diabetic patients and directly correlated with future adverse outcomes. Additionally, it may also represent a marker of endothelial cell dysfunction throughout the body preceding hypertension. In high risk individuals studied in the HOPE and LIFE trials, ranges of microalbuminuria in the high normal range were associated with increased risk. In lower risk patients, data from Framingham and the Nurses' Health study show higher levels of albumin excretion, also within the normal range, were associated with near twice the risk of a person developing hypertension, particularly older women. The PEACE trial found that a high ACR even in the normal range was associated with increased risk for all-cause mortality as well as cardiovascular death in a low risk population with stable CAD. Therefore, it appears that microalbuminuria at any level appears to be an independent predictor of unfavorable outcomes.

Interestingly, race and ethnicity have been independently associated with microalbuminuria. Mattix et al. found that when a sex-specific ACR was used (>17 µg/mg in men and >25 µg/mg in women), African American race remained significantly associated with microalbuminuria, whereas gender did not. The significant association between race and microalbuminuria found highlighted it as a possible risk factor for both kidney and cardiovascular disease.

Therefore, ACR levels can be monitored in individuals with stable CHD, diabetes, hypertension, and family history of kidney disease. Racial considerations may also be made. Serial measurements of ACR may be followed, as a metric of therapy efficacy. Treatment is with inhibitors of the renin angiotensin system, such as ACEI or ARB.

## Cardiac Markers

### Troponin

The troponins are very sensitive and specific indicators of myocardial injury and infarction and have been endorsed as the preferred biomarkers when cardiac ischemia is suspected. Elevation carries prognostic significance in a variety of acute cardiac disease states ranging from the acute coronary syndromes, demand ischemia, and acute and chronic heart failure; as well as noncardiac conditions such as end-stage renal disease (ESRD), pulmonary embolism, and sepsis. Measurement of troponin in the stable outpatient setting for long term risk assessment has only recently been investigated.

The historical normal range for troponin consisted of patients who had both very low levels and those who had mild elevations probably related to comorbidities. The first such study to provide data in this important area was published by the group from Uppsala, which noted a difference between the 99th percentile values of younger compared to older individuals. They evaluated the outcomes of these patients and found that over time these minor elevations were associated with a substantial increase in the frequency of adverse events such as stroke, myocardial infarction, and death.

Two other studies from the same group suggest that minor increases in troponin can occur from structural abnormalities alone and recent data from the Dallas Heart Study extends these observations to the general population. They reported that 0.7% of the general population had an increased cardiac troponin T. Elevations were associated with substantial comorbidities, such as LV mass, heart failure, or renal dysfunction. When one had all three of those factors, the incidence of elevations was over 30%. Thus, structural abnormalities, or target organ damage, can lead to detectable levels of troponin.

### BNP and N-Pro-BNP

BNP is a neurohormone indicator secreted by the ventricles in response to excessive stretching of heart muscle cells. Its primary functions are to decrease systemic vascular resistance and increase natriuresis. BNP is cleaved from the C-terminal end of its prohormone, with the resultant residual protein termed NT-proBNP. Immunoassays exist to detect both. Under "normal" situations, BNP and NT-proBNP levels are approximately equal. However, NT-proBNP rises to a level approximately fourfold higher than BNP in patients with LV dysfunction. Also, while BNP is, primarily, cleared by a specific clearance receptor and neutral endopeptidase, NT-proBNP is cleared by the kidney. There are theoretical benefits to NT-proBNP; for example, it has better in vitro stability and its higher value may make it a more sensitive marker.

Irrespective of hemodynamic considerations, elevated BNP and NT-proBNP are also now known to identify patients with LVH and ischemia. It is theorized that hypoxia from either condition results in myocyte stress, which causes the secretion of a small amount of BNP and NT-proBNP. This process therefore identifies true forms of cardiac target organ damage. This could change the asymptomatic patient into a secondary prevention target, and lead to greater use of proven strategies, such as antihypertensive medications and statins.

## Lipoproteins

### Lipoprotein (a) (Lp(a))

Lp(a) is a lipoprotein that consists of an LDL-like particle bound covalently with apolipoprotein (a). Many studies have identified Lp(a) as an independent risk factor for atherosclerotic disease. Lp(a) levels vary markedly (<0.1 mg/dL to >200 mg/dL) between individuals, with levels <15 mg/dL felt to be ideal, and levels >30 mg/dL associated with higher cardiovascular risk. Unlike the other cholesterol components, Lp(a) levels are largely almost entirely genetically determined, and patients generally have the same level from birth. A noted exception is during acute MI, when levels are increased. African Americans tend to have comparatively higher Lp(a) levels.

Lp(a) appears to have some function in the repair of blood vessels by the way they enable the deposition of cholesterol in the arterial wall. It may therefore promote atherosclerosis in this manner. In addition, Lp(a) is similar in structure to plasminogen, which is a fibrinolytic in the coagulation cascade. It is hypothesized that Lp(a) competes for receptor-binding with plasminogen, and therefore favors clotting.

Measurement of Lp(a) level seems to be appropriate in patients who have established heart disease and normal lipids or a strong family history of heart disease with normal lipids.

Niacin, and perhaps fish oil, may lower Lp(a) levels at high doses, however neither is very effective. Estrogen appears to be a more effective therapy and may be used in postmenopausal women. In extreme situations, apheresis can be performed, however no study has shown that lowering Lp(a) levels is beneficial. Therefore, in patients with elevated Lp(a), a strategy of aggressive treatment of lipids and traditional risk factors is most often employed.

## Cytokines

### Interleukin-6 (IL-6)

IL-6 is an inflammatory cytokine that functions upstream and stimulates eventual production of CRP and fibrinogen. As an acute phase reactant, levels fluctuate depending on the clinical scenario. It has been less extensively studied than some of the other inflammatory markers due to its short plasma half-life, and evaluation of a true baseline to determine long term cardiac risk has been difficult due to variable levels within the same individual.

Two recent prospective studies, the Reykjavik Study and the British Regional Heart Study, analyzed long term baseline levels of IL-6 in patients who had previously experienced a coronary event. Analysis of the results revealed that IL-6 levels over time, correcting for fluctuations, were associated with long term CHD risk in a linear manner, similar in magnitude to traditional risk factors. Previous studies have shown a relationship between IL-6 levels and smoking, presence of hypertension, and adiposity. Finally, IL-6 has been shown to have association with future cardiovascular events and mortality among healthy men and women independently of CRP levels.

### Interleukin-18 (IL-18)

IL-18 is a key cytokine involved in the inflammatory response that contributes to atherosclerosis, with increased levels associated with plaque instability in animal models. Unlike the other inflammatory markers (CRP, fibrinogen and IL-6), IL-18 is independent of traditional risk factors such as smoking status, age, or hypertension.

Blankenberg and Tiret initially showed baseline IL-18 levels to be predictive of future cardiovascular mortality in patients with known CAD in the AtheroGene prospective cohort. These findings were then extended to primary events with the results from the European Prospective Epidemiological Study of Myocardial Infarction (PRIME), which suggested IL-18 accurately predicts coronary events in healthy men (with levels significantly higher in those who developed a coronary event independent of traditional risk factors as well as CRP and IL-6). However, the opposite observation was made in initially healthy, middle-aged men and women from the MONICA/KORA Augsburg studies, which found elevated concentrations of CRP and IL-6, but not IL-18, were independently associated with risk of CHD in a heterogeneous group of patients with moderate risk. Moreover, after the initial strongly positive findings from AtheroGene were made, the study period was extended and baseline IL-18 levels appeared no longer predictive of outcome after 4 years of follow-up.

## Lifestyle Risk Factors

### Soft Drink Consumption

A recent prospective evaluation of the Framingham Offspring Study has evaluated cola soft drink consumers against infrequent or nondrinkers for the risk of developing component markers consistent with metabolic syndrome (MetS). Metabolic syndrome is defined to be present in an individual displaying three or more of the following: obesity, increased waist circumference, hypertension, elevated fasting glucose, hypertriglyceridemia, and low HDL. Individuals consuming ≥1 soft drink per day had approximately 50% greater incidence of developing MetS, compared with those who consumed <1 cola beverage per week. The authors reasoned that both physiological mechanisms, such as weight gain and insulin resistance from fructose corn syrup, as well as associated behavioral patterns in individuals who consume soft drinks, such as poor diet and exercise, contributed to the metabolic derangements.

Additionally, analysis was performed to determine if consumption of "diet" rather than "regular" cola lessened this risk. In this subanalysis, both types of cola posed similar metabolic hazards.

### Sleep Loss

Voluntary bedtime restriction and the resultant sleep deprivation is frequently observed in industrialized countries. The sleep/wake cycle modulates glucose metabolism, and now recent data reveals that the act of curtailing sleep is associated with development of diabetes and obesity. However, even small reductions in sleep resulted in decreased heart rate variability (HRV). Prior evidence has shown that decreased HRV has been associated with hypertension as well as increased mortality after acute myocardial infarction.

Sleep disordered breathing due to obstructive sleep apnea (OSA) has been independently associated with cardiovascular diseases such as CAD, cardiac arrhythmias, and stroke. Central sleep apnea (CSA), as observed in patients with congestive heart failure (CHF), is also linked with increased mortality; however, a causal role has not yet been definitively established. Treatment strategies for OSA with positive airway pressure, weight loss, and surgery have been established, whereas with CSA no therapy has been demonstrated to improve survival.

## CONCLUSIONS

Inflammation has clearly been shown to play a prominent role in atherosclerosis, and novel biomarkers offer an attractive additional method of assessing an individual's risk of developing CVD beyond traditional risk factors. Given the large amount of, at times, conflicting data regarding the utility of these markers, great care must be taken in order to effectively understand the additive information obtained from these serum tests, as well as in determining which individual would benefit from the additional testing. Additionally, a multimarker approach may be beneficial, as specific biomarkers may point to different and perhaps nonoverlapping, perturbations of the inflammatory cascade, and may play more or less of a role in the development of atherosclerosis. The biomarker with the greatest strength of literature supportive to its use is hs-CRP, even though it is a nonspecific marker of inflammation and is prognostic of future cardiac and vascular ischemic events in both primary and secondary prevention. However, the utilization of other biomarkers, especially the cardiac biomarkers, is attractive in that there is a wide spectrum of patient types for these agents, from stable patients with congestive heart failure to patients presenting with ACS, and both primary care physicians and specialists in cardiovascular disease typically have a breadth of experience and familiarity. A risk calculator using multiple novel risk factors is currently not been published. However, data utilizing hs-CRP combined with the Framingham Risk Score has been published by Ridker and colleagues (**Figure 28-3**), and several authors have

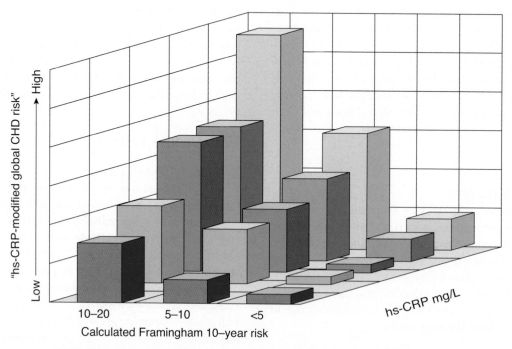

**Figure 28-3.** Moving toward an hs-CRP-modified CHD risk score. Relative risks of future vascular disease using baseline levels of hsCRP in addition to calculated 10-year Framingham risk.

combined hs-CRP with markers such as with BNP, TNF-a, WBC, and/or troponin to demonstrate an increased relative risk with increased numbers or levels of markers. In primary prevention, a "test everyone for everything" strategy would fail the cost/benefit analysis, and lead to increased overall burden to the health care system. However, as recommended by the AHA/ACC guidelines for utilization of inflammatory biomarkers, a "selective screening" process of intermediate risk individuals is recommended at this time. Given the growing data available, it is plausible that a risk calculator combining traditional and novel risk factors will become available.

## Suggested Readings

1. Wang TJ, Gona P, Larson MG, et al. Multiple biomarkers for the prediction of first major cardiovascular events and death. *N Engl J Med.* 2006; 355:2631–2639.

2. Zethelius B, Berglund L, Sundstrom J, et al. Use of multiple biomarkers to improve the prediction of death from cardiovascular causes. *N Engl J Med.* 2008;358:2107–2116.

3. Danesh J, Wheeler JG, Hirschfield GM, et al. C-reactive protein and other circulating markers of inflammation in the prediction of coronary heart disease. *N Engl J Med.* 2004;350:1387–1397.

4. Pearson TA, Mensah GA, Alexander RW, et al. AHA/CDC Scientific Statement: Markers of inflammation and cardiovascular disease. Application to clinical and public health practice. *Circulation.* 2003;107:499–511.

5. Mozaffarian D, Wilson PF, Kannel WB. Beyond established and novel risk factors: lifestyle risk factors for cardiovascular disease. *Circulation.* 2008;117;3031–3038.

# 29

# Chronic Stable Angina

Shawn A. Gregory

## • PRACTICAL POINTS

- The most common form of ischemic heart disease is chronic stable angina.

- Angina is a clinically defined syndrome of discomfort in the chest, jaw, arm, back, or epigastric area associated with suspected ischemic heart disease.

- Ischemia is most often caused by epicardial coronary artery stenoses, typically obstructing greater than 70% of the luminal diameter of the affected artery.

- Historical features suggestive of higher risk of progression to myocardial infarction or death include: ongoing chest pain at rest (typically greater than 20 minutes duration), nocturnal angina, and/or a change in angina frequency, severity, or duration.

- High risk physical examination findings are those suggestive of congestive heart failure (pulmonary rales, S3 gallop) and hypotension.

- Therapeutic strategies for the management of stable angina rely on producing a favorable balance in the relationship between myocardial consumption and demand while preventing the progression of atherosclerosis.

- Guidelines recommend the "ABCDE" strategy for managing chronic stable angina.

- There are two well-established methods of coronary revascularization available for patients with coronary artery disease: percutaneous coronary intervention and coronary artery bypass grafting.

- Both forms of revascularization are effective in the treatment of symptoms. However, coronary artery bypass grafting is the only one to have proven mortality benefit in patients with chronic stable angina.

## INTRODUCTION

Ischemic heart disease is the leading cause of death in the Unites States, and its most common form is chronic stable angina. Chronic stable angina is the initial presentation of ischemic heart disease for approximately 50% of patients, and it is estimated that there are 30 patients with chronic stable angina for every 1 patient hospitalized with myocardial infarction. Current treatment guidelines for chronic stable angina recognize adult patients with stable chest pain syndromes associated with known or suspected ischemic heart disease. Further, patients with other symptoms attributable to ischemic heart disease, the so-called "anginal equivalents" occurring with exertion (including arm, jaw, or epigastric discomfort as well as dyspnea), also fall under the recommendations set forth in the treatment guidelines.

Many of the recommendations are also applied to patients whose ischemic heart disease is presently or has always been asymptomatic (e.g., those with angina successfully treated with medications and/or revascularization, and those who are asymptomatic but found to have evidence of ischemic heart disease on diagnostic studies).

## SIGNS AND SYMPTOMS

### Angina: Definitions and Classification

Angina is a clinically defined syndrome of discomfort in the chest, jaw, arm, back, or epigastric area associated with suspected ischemic heart disease. It is important to use the term "discomfort" when questioning patients, as many

| Table 29-1 • The "PQRST" of Anginal Symptoms | |
|---|---|
| P | Precipitants/position exertion or emotional stress/anywhere from umbilicus to ears |
| Q | Quality tightness, squeezing, heaviness |
| R | Radiation to the jaw, arm (especially left) |
| S | Severity gradually builds |
| T | Timing longer than a few seconds, >20 minutes |

with angina will deny any frank "pain." Typical angina is substernal in location and described as a tightness, heaviness, or squeezing sensation. It is precipitated and magnified by physical exertion or emotional stress and relieved by rest and/or nitroglycerin. The discomfort does not peak at its onset but is gradually progressive. It typically lasts longer than a few seconds and ≤20 minutes (unless it is progressing to myocardial infarction (MI)). Body position and respiration do not usually affect its intensity. The "PQRST" system is a useful mnemonic describing the typical presentation of angina (**Table 29-1**). However, variants in this presentation are not uncommon, especially in female patients. The clinician is wise to remember that angina and its equivalents can be localized anywhere between the umbilicus and the ears. Further, angina can be manifest as dyspnea, nausea, or other symptoms that may be attributed to gastrointestinal causes. Again, an association of such symptoms in a patient at risk for ischemic heart disease should raise the possibility of an "anginal equivalent," especially if the syndrome is provoked by exertion or emotional stress.

Angina is graded using the Canadian Cardiovascular Society Classification System. This system provides a standardized system for communication between health care providers and for use in clinical studies. It classifies patients based on the level of exertion required to precipitate their symptoms (**Table 29-2**). Patients who have symptoms while at rest,

| Table 29-2 • Canadian Cardiovascular Classification of Angina | |
|---|---|
| Class I | Angina with strenuous exertion |
| Class II | Angina that limits ordinary activity slightly (more than 2 city blocks of level ground walking, and greater than one flight of stairs) |
| Class III | Angina that limits ordinary activity markedly (less than 2 city blocks of level ground walking, and less than one flight of stairs) |
| Class IV | Angina with any activity or at rest |

| Table 29-3 • Potential Causes of Ischemia |
|---|
| **Increased Oxygen Demand** |
| • Hypertrophic cardiomyopathy |
| • Aortic stenosis |
| • Dilated cardiomyopathy |
| • Tachycardia |
| • Hyperthyroidism |
| • Hyperthermia |
| • Sympathomimetic use |
| • Uncontrolled hypertension |
| • Arteriovenous fistulae |
| **Decreased Oxygen Supply** |
| • Hypertrophic cardiomyopathy |
| • Aortic stenosis |
| • Anemia |
| • Hypoxemia |
| • Hemoglobinopathies |
| • Hyperviscosity |
| • Sympathomimetic use |

severe new onset symptoms, or progression of symptoms are classified as having unstable angina. These patients can carry a much higher short term risk of death or MI related to their underlying pathophysiology (i.e., unstable plaque) and are therefore managed using separate, albeit overlapping, guidelines.

## Differential Diagnosis

Ischemia is most often caused by epicardial coronary artery stenoses, typically obstructing greater than 70% of the luminal diameter of the affected artery. However, ischemia and resultant angina can occur in association with no or less significant epicardial coronary artery disease (CAD). Such conditions cause ischemia due to alterations in the balance of myocardial oxygen supply and consumption. Examples include hypertension, hypertrophic cardiomyopathy, valvular aortic stenosis, tachycardia, and systemic hypoxemia (**Table 29-3**).

There are many other conditions which may cause chest pain in the adult. It is important to first evaluate the patient for dangerous and/or life-threatening conditions prior to working through the rest of this extensive differential. Such potentially life threatening conditions include pulmonary embolism, aortic dissection, pneumonia, pneumothorax, esophageal perforation, and peptic ulcer disease. These and the other conditions in the differential diagnosis are best organized by their structure of origin (**Table 29-4**). Chest pain may result from disorders of the chest wall (musculoskeletal and skin), lungs and pleura, gastrointestinal tract, or those portions of the peripheral and central nervous system related to pain perception in the chest (including the patient's central perception of pain).

to balance the risk of bleeding and antiplatelet efficacy. Aspirin is continued indefinitely.

Ticlopidine and clopidogrel are alternatives to aspirin. The latter is typically recommended, as it offers the convenience of once daily dosing and has a lower risk of causing neutropenia. Further, there are more data supporting clopidogrel directly reducing adverse cardiovascular outcomes than there is for ticlopidine. Both inhibit platelet aggregation by preventing adenosine diphosphate (ADP)-mediated platelet activation by blocking its interaction with platelet receptors. Clopidogrel can be used by those in whom aspirin is contraindicated. It may also be used in combination with aspirin in certain situations (e.g., soon after coronary stent implantation and longer term with drug-eluting stents). However, if used in combination, the dose of aspirin should be reduced below 325 mg a day.

*Antianginal Agents* Antianginal agents target the rate-pressure product with the aim of decreasing myocardial oxygen demand and relieving ischemia with its associated symptoms. Beta-blockers have additional advantages with respect to the prevention of MI and dysrhythmias, including life-threatening ventricular rhythms. Therefore, guidelines recommend beta-blockers as initial therapy in those with CAD. The agents are more specifically recommended for those with a history of MI, and the duration of therapy is indefinite. Heart rate goals on beta-blockade are resting rates of approximately 60 beats per minute and/or 75% of the heart rate which causes angina/ischemia. The duration of therapy is indefinite, but these agents are particularly useful during and in the first 6 to 12 months after an acute coronary syndrome.

Nondihydropyridine calcium channel blockers (e.g., diltiazem or verapamil) also reduce myocardial oxygen demand by lowering the heart rate. They are recommended as add-on therapy when beta-blockers have not proven successful or as a substitute for these agents when they are either contraindicated or not tolerated.

Nitrates are endothelium-independent vasodilators which tend to reduce preload more than afterload. However, they are thought to decrease ventricular wall tension through their affects on preload and do have some effect on systemic blood pressure. These factors result in a decrease in myocardial oxygen demand. They also increase myocardial oxygen supply by dilating coronaries and increasing collateral flow. Their ability to vasodilate the coronary arteries in the presence of atherosclerosis (which normally disrupts endothelial dilatation) is due in large part to their endothelium-independent mechanism of action. Further, nitrates have some antithrombotic properties. In sublingual and spray form they are highly effective for the immediate relief of angina. They are also available in long-acting formulations

for maintenance therapy. However, tachyphylaxis can occur if an adequate "nitrate free" interval is not allowed. The short-acting formulations are considered first-line therapy to be used on an as needed basis. Daily use of long-acting preparations is recommended as add-on therapy when beta-blockers have not proven sufficient or when beta-blockers are contraindicated or not tolerated.

The dihydropyridine calcium channel antagonists (e.g., nifedipine, amlodipine, felodipine) are vasodilators that can be used as antianginal agents. Immediate release formulations are contraindicated due to a potential risk of precipitating stroke and myocardial infarction. However, longer-acting formulations have been effective in decreasing systemic vascular resistance (and myocardial oxygen demand) as well as promoting increased coronary flow (and myocardial oxygen supply). They are typically employed as add-on therapies or when the patient cannot take beta-blockers and/or nitrates.

### Beta-blockers and Blood Pressure

While all antihypertensive agents have the ability to assist in the relief of angina due to their affects on the rate-pressure product (lowering systolic blood pressure), certain agents have additional benefits, which make them first-line therapy for patients with CAD. For example, as mentioned previously, beta-blockers are indicated in patients with CAD for reasons beyond their antiischemic properties. Another such group of drugs are those that affect the renin-angiotensin aldosterone system (angiotensin-converting enzyme inhibitors, angiotensin receptor blockers, and aldosterone receptor blockers).

Angiotensin-converting enzyme inhibitors are recommended for all patients with coronary artery disease who also have diabetes and/or left ventricular dysfunction (ejection fraction ≤40%). Newer modifications to the guidelines also suggest that they should be used as first-line therapy for anyone with CAD and hypertension, diabetes, and/or chronic kidney disease. Further, they have been recommended in patients with any form of atherosclerotic vascular disease alone (including CAD without associated risk factors).

Angiotensin receptor blockers are used when angiotensin-converting enzyme inhibitors are not tolerated (typically due to cough). They have shown similar benefits in large clinical trials, and can also be used in combination with angiotensin-converting enzyme inhibitors for treatment of those with congestive heart failure. Aldosterone blockade (e.g., spironolactone and eplerenone) are indicated as add-on therapy (in addition to angiotensin-converting enzyme inhibitors or angiotensin receptor blockers and beta-blockers) for patients post-MI with normal serum creatinine and potassium levels, diabetes or congestive heart failure, and an ejection fraction ≤40%.

The goal blood pressure for those with CAD is ≤140/90 mm Hg and preferably lower. If the patient is diabetic or has chronic kidney disease, that goal if further intensified to levels below 130/80 mm Hg. If the patient's hypertension is not under adequate control on first-line agents such as beta-blockers and angiotensin-converting enzyme inhibitors, additional medications should be added. It is often useful to choose agents such as long-acting nitrates or calcium channel blockers in patients with angina as these drugs have antiischemic properties, as discussed previously.

### Cholesterol and Cigarettes

Treatment of dyslipidemia has been associated with substantial improvements in cardiovascular outcomes. Statin therapy in particular with the aim of reducing LDL-C levels has shown the greatest benefit. Further, statin therapy has been shown to reduce adverse cardiovascular events even in the absence of what are thought to be elevated LDL-C levels (e.g., levels <100 mg/dL). This effect is not completely understood, but may be related to plaque stabilization and/or antiinflammatory properties. Therefore, statin therapy should be used in all patients with known or suspected coronary artery disease with a goal low density lipoprotein level below 100 mg/dL and perhaps lower (guidelines suggest that levels below 70 mg/dL are reasonable in certain patient populations, including those with prior revascularization).

Cigarette smoking is one of the most important and devastating risk factors for CAD. United States Surgeon General estimates conclude that smoking increases the risk of cardiovascular mortality by 50%, and the effect is dose-dependent. Smoking cessation is associated with significant reductions in the risk of adverse cardiovascular outcomes.

### Diet and Diabetes

Diet is also an essential component in the management of those with stable angina and in those with CAD. Weight reduction plays a key role in preventing and reversing metabolic syndrome, diabetes, hypertension, and dyslipidemia. Moderation of alcohol consumption, reduced sodium diets, and diets rich in fruits, vegetables, and low fat dairy products have been beneficial in the treatment of hypertension. Diets low in saturated fat and cholesterol (<7% saturated fat and <200 mg cholesterol), supplemented by plant sterols and fiber as well as omega-3 fatty acids (e.g., fish oil) have been helpful in managing dyslipidemia.

Diabetes is an extremely important risk factor for CAD and is now treated as equivalent to having already suffered a myocardial infarction with respect to secondary treatment guidelines for coronary artery disease. The goal of treating diabetes is to get the patient's blood sugar as close to normal levels as possible. The recommended goal hemoglobin A1c is <7%.

### Education and Exercise

In order to accomplish the goals prescribed by the guidelines (smoking cessation, weight/dietary management, diabetes control, and use of appropriate medications), the patient must obviously agree to and work to achieve these aims with their physician. This makes patient education about the benefits of these strategies paramount, as many require significant lifestyle modifications.

Exercise has an important role to play in achieving many of the recommended goals. Guidelines encourage patients to increase their daily activities (e.g., walk whenever possible, take stairs, do gardening and housework) and exercise for 30 minutes or more at least three times per week. The exercises preferred are aerobic activities such as jogging, cycling, walking, or swimming. Medically supervised programs (such as cardiac rehabilitation programs) are advised for patients with moderate to high risk of adverse cardiac outcomes. Along with diet, exercise helps the patient achieve the weight management goals of a body mass index between 18.5 and 24.9 kg/m². A reasonable first step is for the patient to aim for a 10% loss in body weight.

## Other Therapies

Influenza vaccination has been associated with a reduction in adverse cardiovascular outcomes in the year after its administration. Therefore, the guidelines recommend influenza vaccine for all patients with cardiovascular disease. Chelation therapy can be complicated by hypocalcemia and is not recommended under the current guidelines due to unproven efficacy. Data are also lacking for spinal cord stimulation and enhanced external counterpulsation as treatments for refractory angina. A new class of antianginal drug, ranolazine, has shown some promise in treating refractory angina. Its mechanism of action involves shifting myocardial cell metabolism to decrease lactate production. Side effects of ranolazine include QT prolongation.

## Revascularization

There are two well-established methods of coronary revascularization available for patients with CAD: percutaneous coronary intervention and coronary artery bypass grafting. The general theme is that both are effective in the treatment of symptoms. However, coronary artery bypass grafting is the only one to have proven mortality benefit in patients with chronic stable angina. Further, this mortality benefit is only seen in subsets of patients with certain combinations of severe disease, left ventricular dysfunction, and diabetes.

Those most likely to attain survival benefit from coronary artery bypass grafting are those at highest risk of cardiac death. As survival rates for patients with chronic stable angina are largely dependent on the extent and severity of their coronary artery disease, their left ventricular function, and whether or not they suffer from diabetes, these are important variables to use for consideration of an individual for surgical revascularization. Coronary artery bypass grafting has been shown to yield mortality benefit in patients with left main CAD, 3-vessel CAD with abnormal LVF (ejection fraction ≤50%), 2- or 3-vessel disease, which includes a significant (>70% stenosis) lesion of the proximal left anterior descending coronary artery, and diabetic patients with multivessel CAD. There are some data to suggest a mortality benefit for surgical revascularization of significant proximal left anterior descending coronary artery disease alone. Therefore, patients with chronic stable angina and these characteristics can be considered for surgical revascularization in hopes of mortality benefit.

Both coronary artery bypass grafting and percutaneous coronary intervention are effective and indicated for the treatment of anginal symptoms not sufficiently relieved by medical therapy. Percutaneous coronary intervention offers lower periprocedure morbidity and mortality than cardiac surgery, but problems with restenosis and/or incomplete revascularization leads to higher rates of recurrent angina than in patients undergoing cardiac surgery, as well as more repeat procedures. Further, there are no clear data supporting a mortality benefit for percutaneous intervention in chronic stable angina. However, it should be noted that improvements in catheter-based technology, such as drug-eluting stents, and increased operator experience have led to reductions in restenosis rates as well as procedural complications.

Transmyocardial revascularization involves using a laser to create channels in the myocardium in a hope of creating a network of connections between the left ventricular cavity (with its oxygenated blood) and areas of ischemia. This has been accomplished via thoracotomy and through percutaneous means. There have been conflicting reports as to its efficacy, and its role in the therapy of refractory angina in individuals who are not candidates for percutaneous or surgical revascularization, remains unclear.

## Suggested Readings

1. Gibbons RJ, Abrams J, Chatterjee K, et al. ACC/AHA 2002 guideline update for the management of patients with chronic stable angina: a report of the American College of Cardiology/American Heart Association Task Force on Practice Guidelines (Committee to Update the 1999 Guidelines for the Management of Patients with Chronic Stable Angina). 2002. Available at www.acc.org/clinical/guidelines/stable/stable.pdf.

2. Fraker TD Jr., Fihn SD, for the 2002 Chronic Stable Angina Writing Committee. American College of Cardiology/American Heart Association Task Force on Practice Guidelines, Writing Group to Develop the Focused Update of the 2002 guidelines for the management of patients with chronic stable angina. *Circulation.* 2007;116:2672–2772. Available at www.acc.org.

3. Smith SC Jr., Allen J, Blair SN, et al. AHA/ACC guidelines for secondary prevention for patients with coronary and other atherosclerotic vascular disease. 2006 update: endorsed by the National Heart, Lung, and Blood Institute. *Circulation.* 2006;113:2363–2372.

4. Gibbons RJ, Balady GJ, Bricker JT, et al. ACC/AHA 2002 guideline update for exercise testing: summary article. A report of the American College of Cardiology/American Heart Association Task Force on Practice Guidelines (Committee on Exercise Testing). *J Am Coll Cardiol.* 2002;40:1531–1540.

5. Grundy SM, Cleeman JI, Merz CN, et al. Implications of recent clinical trials for the National Cholesterol Education Program Adult Treatment Panel III guidelines. *Circulation.* 2004;110:227–239.

# Acute Coronary Syndromes

Section VI

# Acute Coronary Syndromes

# 30

# Unstable Coronary Syndromes: Important Updates in the 2007 ACC/AHA Guidelines for UA/NSTEMI

CHARLES D. SEARLES JR. AND NANETTE K. WENGER

## ● PRACTICAL POINTS

- Current guidelines emphasize risk stratification of unstable angina/non-STEMI patients with respect to selecting a conservative versus an early invasive approach.

- High risk features in patients with unstable coronary syndromes are predicted by recurrent ischemia on treatment, hemodynamic and electrical instability, previous revascularization, ST-segment depression, advanced age, elevated biomarkers, reduced left ventricular function (ejection fraction less than 40%), and high risk score using TIMI, and GRACE criteria.

- Patients with unstable angina/non-STEMI who remain unstable despite adequate treatment and stabilized patients who are at high risk should undergo an invasive strategy.

- The use of GPIIb/IIIa inhibitors has been established for patients undergoing an invasive strategy. The use of such agents in a conservative strategy has not yet been established and is associated with an increased bleeding risk.

- In patients undergoing initial conservative strategy, echocardiography, stress testing, and BNP analysis may provide useful information regarding future diagnostic studies and treatment.

## INTRODUCTION

Coronary heart disease (CHD) is a major public health problem worldwide, particularly in Western societies. In the United States it is the single largest cause of mortality, responsible for 1 of every 5 deaths (AHA Heart Disease and Stroke Statistics, 2008). The estimated prevalence of CHD among U.S. adults aged 20 and older is 16 million (8.7 million men and 7.3 million women), and, in 2007, an estimated 1.57 million Americans experienced an acute coronary syndrome (ACS). ACS is an umbrella term for any group of clinical presentations compatible with acute myocardial ischemia. ACS encompasses the diagnoses of myocardial infarction (MI) and unstable angina (UA), both of which are the result of decreased coronary blood flow. This blood flow decrease is most commonly caused by acute thrombosis consequent to a ruptured atherosclerotic plaque. Other causes of ACS include nonplaque-associated coronary thromboembolism, vasospasm, progressive mechanical obstruction, arterial inflammation, secondary UA (conditions causing increased myocardial oxygen requirements), and coronary artery dissection.

The extent to which a thrombus obstructs coronary blood flow in ACS patients determines the severity of the clinical syndrome and the nature of ST-segment changes on the ECG. Patients with total coronary occlusion typically present with ST-segment elevation myocardial infarction (STEMI), and those with sub-total occlusion present with non-ST-segment elevation myocardial infarction (NSTEMI) or UA. In the clinical spectrum of ACS, UA and NSTEMI are more frequent: of the 1.57 million Americans who experience ACS yearly, approximately 1.24 million are diagnosed with UA or NSTEMI, and 0.33 million are diagnosed with ST-elevation MI. It is worthy to note that 99% of all plaque ruptures are believed to be clinically silent; these silent ruptures are small and subsequently form small clots, which heal but lead to lesion progression.

Pathophysiologically, UA and NSTEMI are closely related conditions and clinically are defined by ST-segment depression or prominent T wave inversion. Elevation of serum biomarkers (troponin I, troponin T, or CK-MB) distinguishes NSTEMI from UA, although these markers may not be elevated at the time of presentation. The most common ECG presentation in non-ST-elevation ACS is ST-depression, a finding particularly important to recognize because of its association with increased risk. Compared to patients with ST-elevation, ACS patients with ST-depression are more likely to have had previous cardiovascular events (MI, PCI, CABG, or CHF), more likely to have 3-vessel disease, and more likely to die within 6 months of their event.

This review highlights the significant changes in the American College of Cardiology/American Heart Association recommendations for management of patients with UA/NSTEMI since 2002. It will focus on the choice between early invasive and early conservative strategies, more intensive antithrombotic and antiplatelet therapy, and secondary prevention. This review uses the guidelines' classification system:

- Class I: Indicates a procedure/treatment should be performed or administered; there is evidence or general agreement as to its usefulness and efficacy.
- Class IIa: Indicates it is reasonable to perform procedure or administer treatment, but there is some controversy about usefulness and efficacy. The weight of evidence and opinion indicate that benefit of the therapy is greater than its risk.
- Class IIb: The procedure or treatment may be considered; the usefulness and efficacy of the treatment or procedure are less well established by evidence or opinion.
- Class III: The procedure or treatment should not be performed or administered; there is evidence or general agreement that the procedure or treatment is not useful and effective, and/or actually may be harmful.

In addition, the management recommendations are qualified by the level of evidence supporting their clinical effect:

- Level A: Recommendation is supported by evidence from multiple randomized trials or meta-analysis.
- Level B: Recommendation is supported by limited evidence from single randomized trial or nonrandomized studies.
- Level C: Recommendation is supported only by expert opinion, case studies, or standard-of-care.

# RISK STRATIFICATION AND MANAGEMENT STRATEGY SELECTION

## Risk Stratification

Patients with UA/NSTEMI are diverse in their risk for adverse cardiovascular outcomes. Therefore, a crucial first step in their management is to estimate their risk for death or MI based on history, physical examination, ECG, and cardiac biomarker findings. Features associated with poorer prognosis include acceleration of angina symptoms in the preceding 48 hours, prolonged angina at rest (>20 minutes), signs of heart failure or worsening mitral regurgitation, hemodynamic or arrhythmic instability, age >75 years old, new ST-segment depression (>0.5 mm), and elevated cardiac biomarkers. Several risk-predictive tools have been devised that assist in assigning patients to different risk categories (low, intermediate, or high), but clinical estimation of risk is a multivariable problem and the predictive ability of these risk assessment tools is only moderate.

The most validated and commonly used risk assessment tool is the TIMI risk score, composed of seven (1-point) indicators: age, ECG changes, clinical characteristics and cardiac biomarkers (STAARBUCs, **ST**-segment deviation, **A**ge, **A**spirin use, ≥3 **R**isk factors, elevated **B**iomarkers, **U**nstable angina—2 anginal events ≤24 hours, known **C**oronary stenosis >50%). The risk of death, recurrent MI, or recurrent ischemia prompting urgent revascularization within 14 days of presentation increase as TIMI risk score increases. The PURSUIT risk model uses age, heart rate, systolic blood pressure, ST-segment depression, signs of heart failure, and cardiac biomarkers to predict death or myocardial (re)infarction at 30 days. Similarly, the GRACE risk model predicts mortality from hospital discharge to 6 months and incorporates age, Killip class, systolic blood pressure, ST-segment deviation, cardiac arrest during presentation, serum creatinine level, biomarkers, and heart rate into its risk score. All three risk scores have shown good predictive accuracy for death and MI at 1 year and therefore are helpful in identifying patients who may benefit from more aggressive therapies.

## Selection of Initially Invasive or Conservative Strategies

The initial major decision in the management of patients with UA/NSTEMI is whether an early invasive strategy or an early conservative strategy should be used. The 2002 ACC/AHA guideline favored the routine use of an early invasive strategy (i.e., diagnostic angiography with intent to perform revascularization within 4 to 24 hours of admission),

| Table 30-1 • Clinical Features Guiding Initally Invasive Versus Conservative Strategy for Patients with UA/NSTEMI. (Adapted from 2007 ACC/AHA UA/NSTEMI Guidelines) ||
| --- | --- |
| **Invasive** | **Conservative** |
| Recurrent ischemia at rest despite intensive medical therapy | Low risk score (e.g., TIMI) |
| Elevated cardiac biomarkers (TnT or TnI) | Stabilized patient with high risk features and patient/ physician preference |
| ST-segment depression | |
| Heart failure or worsening mitral regurgitation | |
| High risk findings from noninvasive testing | |
| Hemodynamic instability | |
| Sustained ventricular tachycardia | |
| PCI within 6 months | |
| Prior CABG | |
| High risk score (e.g., TIMI, GRACE) | |
| Reduced LV function (<40%) | |

but more recent data indicate that there can be more flexibility in the selection of the early invasive versus early conservative strategies. While patients with refractory angina, hemodynamic instability, or electrical instability who otherwise do not have clinical contraindications to angiography and revascularization (percutaneous or surgical) benefit from an early invasive strategy (Class I, Level B indication), it is less clear which strategy is optimal for the patient with ACS who is immediately stabilized. The ACC/AHA 2007 guideline emphasizes that subsequent management should be based on an estimation of the patient's global risk, using the features described above and in **Table 30-1**. An early invasive strategy is indicated in initially stabilized UA/NSTEMI patients who have an elevated risk for clinical events (Class I, Level A). However, the guideline also gives the option for an initially conservative strategy (i.e., selectively invasive) in higher risk patients (Class IIb, Level B) who are troponin-positive, especially if it is the preference of the physician and patient (Class IIb, Level C). Also, because ACS is a dynamic physiologic process, risk estimation should be modified as dictated by changes in the patient's status. Thus, an initially stabilized patient who subsequently develops ischemic symptoms or ECG changes should be transferred to the cardiac catheterization laboratory for angiography and possible intervention.

In TACTICS-TIMI-18 trial (see text box before the suggested readings for full names of acronyms used in this review) of 2220 patients with UA/NSTEMI, an early invasive strategy was associated with decreased death, MI, and rehospitalization for ACS at 6 months. This benefit was observed in both medium and high risk patients, as defined by elevated troponin, ST-segment deviation, and TIMI risk score >3; benefit was particularly apparent for older adults. Of note, patients lacking high risk features did not benefit from the early invasive strategy, and low risk female patients actually had worse outcomes when managed with an invasive strategy, a phenomenon related to increased bleeding complications in these patients. However, high risk female patients did benefit from the invasive strategy. This study, together with data from the GRACE registry, highlights the importance of strongly considering an invasive strategy in elderly patients. Elderly patients are typically high risk at baseline and likely receive the most benefit from aggressive therapies.

The benefit of an early invasive strategy for intermediate to high risk patients is also supported by data from several smaller studies, including the ISAR-COOL, FRISC-2, RITA-3, and VINO trials, although the latter study had a high crossover rate (40%) from the initial conservative arm by 6 months. Interestingly, high crossover rates from an early conservative strategy at time points remote from presentation appear to be a recurrent theme in many of these studies. In both FRISC-2 and RITA-3, the benefit of the invasive strategy was confined to men with high risk status; there was no benefit for women, regardless of risk. This finding led to the Class I recommendation (level of evidence: B) for an early conservative strategy for women with ACS who were otherwise at low risk. For women with ACS at higher risk, the Class I recommendation (level of evidence: B) is similar to that for men: An invasive strategy should be used unless the patient has contraindications to coronary angiography and/or revascularization.

The routine use of an early invasive strategy is challenged by the results of the TIMI IIIB trial, where no benefit was observed for this strategy in endpoints of death or MI. However, this study preceded the routine use of stents, GP IIb/IIIa inhibitors, and thienopyridines. A later study in which thienopyridines and GP IIb/IIIa inhibitors were regularly used, the ICTUS trial, similarly demonstrated no difference in death or MI when an invasive strategy was routinely used. Although these findings suggest that an early conservative (selectively invasive) strategy may be considered in high risk patients, enthusiasm for this approach is tempered by the high crossover rate for the initially conservative arm and the fact that patients enrolled in this study were overall lower risk compared to other studies. Nonetheless, the results of these studies have led to the Class IIb, Level C recommendation for an early conservative or selectively invasive approach for stabilized high risk patients, including those who have elevated troponin levels (level of evidence B).

## Medical Therapy for Initially Invasive Strategy

All patients who present with UA/NSTEMI should receive aspirin (or clopidogrel if aspirin-intolerant). When the invasive strategy is selected, anticoagulant therapy with enoxaparin, unfractionated heparin (UFH), bivalirudin, or fondaparinux should be used as soon as possible after presentation (Class I, Level A recommendation for enoxaparin or UFH; Class I, Level B recommendation for bivalirudin or fondaparinux). Prior to angiography, these patients should also receive one (Class I, Level A recommendation) or both (Class IIa, Level B recommendation) clopidogrel or an IV GP IIb/IIIa inhibitor. In particular, the use of both agents should be considered if there is a delay to angiography, the patient has high risk features, or the patient demonstrates early recurrent ischemic symptoms. Although the recommendations for anticoagulant and antiplatelet therapy are supported by several recent studies, application of the trial data to clinical practice is somewhat challenging because no single trial addresses the spectrum of therapeutic possibilities.

In general, the evidence supporting the use of enoxaparin over UFH for UA/NSTEMI is inconsistent, but enoxaparin appears to be at least noninferior to UFH. The ESSENCE trial enrolled 3171 patients with UA/NSTEMI and demonstrated a benefit for enoxaparin versus UFH in reducing death, MI, or recurrent MI, but this benefit occurred at the cost of more minor bleeding complications. An association between enoxaparin and increased bleeding risk (minor, major, or both) has been observed in several studies, including the TIMI IIB, INTERACT, SYNERGY, and A to Z trials. The TIMI IIB trial (3910 patients) demonstrated less death, MI, or urgent revascularization in the enoxaparin arm, but enoxaparin was associated with increased major and minor bleeding. In the INTERACT trial (746 patients), high risk patients treated with enoxaparin had less death or MI, an increase in minor bleeding, and a decrease in major bleeding. The SYNERGY trial (9978 patients) was designed to prove that enoxaparin was not inferior to UFH in patients undergoing an early invasive strategy. In SYNERGY, enoxaparin was noninferior to UFH in terms of death and MI, but there was an increase in major bleeding events in patients who received enoxaparin, a finding in part attributed to the crossover to UFH in patients who underwent early PCI. In a more recent study of patients with UA/NSTEMI, ACUTE II, there was no difference in the rate of death or MI for patients treated with enoxaparin compared to those treated with UFH, and there was no difference in major or minor bleeding complications. Similarly, in the A to Z trial (3987 patients), there was no benefit in the use of enoxaparin compared to UFH, but there was an increase in major bleeding associated with enoxaparin.

The data in support of the use of bivalirudin, a direct thrombin inhibitor, in patients with UA/NSTEMI largely derives from two trials, ACUITY and REPLACE-2, which demonstrated noninferiority of bivalirudin compared to heparin in terms of clinical outcomes and an association between bivalirudin and fewer bleeding complications. ACUITY was a complex study that compared three anticoagulation strategies: UFH or enoxaparin with and without a GP IIb/IIIa inhibitor; bivalirudin with and without a GP IIb/IIIa inhibitor; and bivalirudin with possible GP IIb/IIIa inhibitor use. Compared to heparin plus GP IIb/IIIa inhibitor, bivalirudin plus GP IIb/IIIa inhibitor was noninferior in terms of ischemia, major bleeding, and net clinical outcomes. Bivalirudin alone compared to heparin plus GP IIb/IIIa inhibitor resulted in noninferior rates of ischemia, reduced major bleeding, and superior 30-day net clinical outcomes, but the clinical benefit appeared to be limited to those patients who received a thienopyridine before angiography or PCI. These findings led to the recommendation that, whether a bivalirudin- or heparin-based strategy is used, patients should also receive a GP IIb/IIIa inhibitor or thienopyridine before angiography or PCI. In the REPLACE-2 trial, bivalirudin plus provisional GP IIb/IIIa inhibitor was compared to heparin plus planned GP IIb/IIIa inhibitor. Similar to the results of ACUITY, the bivalirudin-based therapy was noninferior to the heparin-based therapy, and bivalirudin-based therapy was associated with fewer bleeding complications.

The OASIS-5 trial (20,078 patients) provides the strongest evidence for the use of fondaparinux, a Factor Xa inhibitor, in patients with UA/NSTEMI. Fondaparinux was compared to enoxaparin in patients undergoing PCI; concomitant therapy with ASA, clopidogrel, and GP IIb/IIIa was at the discretion of the investigator. Nine days after randomization, there was no difference in death, MI, or refractory angina in the two arms, but at 30 and 180 days there were significant differences in these outcomes that favored fondaparinux. Importantly, fondaparinux was associated with significantly less major bleeding compared to enoxaparin.

Thienopyridines are adenosine diphosphate antagonists that inhibit platelet activation. Because their antiplatelet mechanism is different from that of aspirin, the combination exerts an additive effect. The recommendation for the addition of clopidogrel to ASA therapy as part of the initial medical management of patients with UA/NSTEMI is based on several studies, some of which involved patients who did not have ACS. The CURE trial enrolled 12,562 patients with UA/NSTEMI and compared clopidogrel to placebo, against a background of ASA therapy. Compared to ASA alone, the combination of clopidogrel and ASA decreased the primary combined endpoint of cardiovascular death, nonfatal MI, or stroke, and decreased the rate of recurrent ischemia and revascularization. Clopidogrel therapy was associated with a 1% absolute risk of major bleeding complications. This study, reported in 2001, was notable for the relatively infrequent use of an invasive strategy and GP IIb/IIIa inhibitors, which contrasts with today's practice patterns and may have had an impact on bleeding risk. More recently, the ISAR-REACT-2 trial (2022 patients) examined high risk UA/NSTEMI patients treated with either combinations of ASA, clopidogrel and abciximab, or ASA and clopidogrel. The addition of abciximab to ASA and clopidogrel decreased death, MI, or urgent target vessel revascularization at 30 days after presentation. This benefit was limited to patients who had elevated troponin, and there was no difference between the groups in major or minor bleeding complications. The findings of this study led to the Class IIa, Level B recommendation for the use of both a GP IIb/IIIa inhibitor and clopidogrel in high-risk patients undergoing an invasive strategy.

Further information regarding GP IIb/IIIa inhibitor therapy in patients with UA/NSTEMI is provided by the PURSUIT (10,948 patients), PRISM, and PRISM-PLUS trials. In PURSUIT, patients received low-dose or high-dose eptifibatide or placebo against of a background of ASA and heparin therapy. Compared to placebo, eptifibatide was associated with a decrease in death and MI but an increase in major bleeding. Importantly, an increased event rate was observed in patients not receiving heparin concomitantly. The PRISM investigators enrolled 3232 patients within 24 hours of presentation for UA/NSTEMI and compared therapy with tirofiban versus UFH against a background of ASA therapy. There was a decrease in death, MI, or refractory ischemia in patients treated with tirofiban. In PRISM-PLUS, 1915 patients were enrolled within 12 hours of presentation for UA/NSTEMI and treated with tirofiban alone, UFH alone, or both. There was a high rate of angiography in this trial. The tirofiban alone arm was discontinued prematurely because of its association with increased mortality. However, the tirofiban plus UFH arm was associated with a decrease in death, MI, and refractory ischemia. Together, these studies highlight the importance of the combination of a GP IIb/IIIa inhibitor and heparin in UA/NSTEMI patients, whether treated with an initial invasive or conservative strategy.

## Medical Therapy for Initially Conservative Strategy

The patient managed with an early conservative strategy should receive ASA (or clopidogrel if ASA-intolerant) as soon as possible after presentation (Class I, Level A recommendation) as well as anticoagulation with heparin (enoxaparin or UFH) or fondaparinux (Class I recommendation; level of evidence A for enoxaparin/UFH and B for fondaparinux). Enoxaparin or fondaparinux are considered preferable to UFH (Class IIa, Level B). Also, the patient should receive a loading dose of clopidogrel and subsequently be given maintenance therapy (Class I, Level A recommendation), and consideration should be given for administering eptifibatide or tirofiban (Class IIb, Level B recommendation).

The evidence for use of aspirin in high risk patients is well established; in a meta-analysis of 195 trials involving more than 143,000 patients, ASA therapy was associated a 22% decrease in risk of vascular death, MI, or stroke across a broad spectrum of clinical presentations that included UA/NSTEMI. Although the benefit of ASA therapy was similar for doses of 75 to 1500 mg daily, the bleeding risk is dose-dependent. In addition the full antithrombotic effect of low-dose ASA takes up to 2 days to manifest, whereas standard doses of ASA are effective within hours. Therefore, an initial dose of 160 to 325 mg ASA, nonenteric formulation is recommended, followed by 75 to 325 mg/day of enteric or nonenteric formulation. The basis for the recommendation of clopidogrel in patients intolerant to ASA stems from the CAPRIE trial, which enrolled 19,185 patients who had recent stroke, MI, or symptomatic peripheral arterial disease (PAD) and compared ASA to clopidogrel therapy. Clopidogrel was associated with a decrease in the incidence of stroke, MI, or vascular death, a benefit that was greatest for patients with PAD. The ARMYDA-2 trial addressed the question of optimal clopidogrel loading dose, 600 mg versus 300 mg. The 600 mg dose appeared to be better in terms of death, MI, or target vessel revascularization, but this benefit appeared to be driven by a decrease in periprocedural MI. The challenges to this latter study are its small size, the relatively low risk patients enrolled, and the low use of GP IIb/IIIa inhibitors.

GP IIb/IIIa antagonists block platelet aggregation, resulting in a potent antithrombotic effect. In general, the ACC/AHA recommendations regarding GP IIb/IIIa antagonists are based on the results of several trials that tested different agents in patients with UA/NSTEMI, some of whom were undergoing PCI. For example, in PRISM-PLUS, 30% of patients underwent PCI, and in PURSUIT, 13% of patients underwent PCI. Although the use of a GP IIb/IIIa antagonist in patients scheduled for an initial invasive strategy is established, the administration of GP IIb/IIIa antagonists in patients not scheduled for an initial invasive strategy is less clear. A meta-analysis of GP IIb/IIIa antagonists in all trials of this strategy showed a relatively small benefit for the use of GP IIb/IIIa antagonists in terms of death or MI, but also showed that these agents are associated with an increased risk of major bleeding. The GUSTO IV-ACS trial studied the effect of abciximab administration in 7800 patients with NSTEMI not scheduled to undergo revascularization and found no benefit with abciximab therapy, even in the subgroup of patients who had troponin elevation. Notably, the use of abciximab is a Class III, Level A recommendation for NSTEMI patients in whom PCI is not planned.

## Initial Hospital Care for Conservative Strategy

For patients in whom an initial conservative strategy has been selected, certain diagnostic studies may assist in further management, particularly the assessment of whether the patient is at high enough risk to go to the cardiac catheterization laboratory. One of these studies is echocardiography, because left ventricular ejection fraction (LVEF) ≤0.40 is a high risk feature in patients with UA/NSTEMI, and it is reasonable to perform diagnostic angiography solely on the basis of low LVEF (Class IIa, Level B recommendation). A stress test should be performed for the assessment of ischemia in the patient who is not initially going to the catheterization laboratory (Class I, Level B recommendation). Although not explicit in the guideline, this study should be performed during the hospitalization or immediately thereafter. If the stress test is classified as other than low risk, diagnostic angiography should be performed (Class I, Level A recommendation). Finally, measurement of BNP or NT-pro-BNP may be considered to supplement assessment of global risk in patients with suspected ACS (Class IIb, Level B recommendation). This recommendation is based on evidence that natriuretic peptides are strong predictors of both short- and long-term mortality in patients with STEMI and UA/NSTEMI.

The current recommendations for beta-blocker therapy in patients with UA/NSTEMI differ from those in the 2002 ACC/AHA guideline, and differ from those for STEMI. It is recommended that patients with UA/NSTEMI be given oral beta-blocker therapy; it should be started within the first 24 hours of presentation, unless the patient has heart failure, low cardiac output state, increased risk for cardiogenic shock, or relative contraindications (Class I, Level B recommendation). Beta-blocker therapy may be given IV in the setting of uncontrolled hypertension and no contraindications (Class IIa, Level B recommendation). However, in the absence of uncontrolled hypertension, IV beta-blocker therapy is probably unwise because of its association with an increased risk of cardiogenic shock. In fact, IV therapy is a Class III recommendation in UA/NSTEMI patients with signs of heart failure or low-output state, or other risk factors for cardiogenic shock (level of evidence: A). This Class III recommendation is based on data from the COMMIT trial, which enrolled 45,852 patients within 24 hours of acute MI (NSTEMI and STEMI). The investigators assessed the effect of IV beta-blocker therapy (up to 15 mg IV, transitioned to 500 mg po metoprolol daily versus placebo) on the outcome of death, reinfarction, or cardiac arrest, as well as death from any cause during hospitalization. Beta-blocker therapy did not provide benefit

for either outcome, and IV beta-blocker therapy actually increased the risk of cardiogenic shock, particularly during the initial period of presentation. Therefore, it is recommended that beta-blocker be started po and only when the patient is hemodynamically stable.

Patients with UA/NSTEMI should have a fasting lipid profile obtained within the first 24 hours (Class I, level C recommendation), and, in the absence of contraindications, a statin should be started predischarge, regardless of baseline LDL-C (Class I, Level A recommendation). Patients with pulmonary congestion or LVEF ≤0.40 should receive oral ACE inhibitor therapy, provided they are not hypotensive (SBP <100 mm Hg or <30 mm Hg below baseline) or have known contraindications (Class I, Level A recommendation). An ARB should be prescribed in those patients who are ACEI-intolerant (Class I, Level A recommendation). ACEI or ARB therapy may be useful in UA/NSTEMI patients without pulmonary congestion or low EF and has a Class IIa classification (level of evidence: B) in this setting. Intravenous ACEI therapy in the first 24 hours from the time of presentation has a Class III classification (level of evidence: B) because of increased risk of hypotension.

The ACC/AHA recommendation for statin therapy is based on data from several studies, including the PROVE-IT TIMI 22 trial, which enrolled 4162 patients within 10 days of their ACS. This study examined the efficacy of pravastatin, 40 mg, compared to atorvastatin, 80 mg, in preventing death, MI, UA requiring hospitalization, revascularization, and stroke. Only atorvastatin was beneficial, and the difference in efficacy between the two drugs was attributed to the degree by which each drug lowered LDL-C. The HPS enrolled 20,536 patients with CHD, none of whom had ACS, and compared the effect of simvastatin (40 mg) versus placebo in reducing mortality, stroke, and revascularization. Simvastatin was beneficial in these patients, irrespective of their initial cholesterol level and baseline comorbidities. In addition, the benefit of statin therapy appeared to increase over time. Thus, it is recommended that statin therapy be initiated in all UA/NSTEMI patients prior to discharge, regardless of baseline LDL-C level.

## LONG-TERM MEDICAL THERAPY IN PATIENTS WITH UA/NSTEMI

### Antiplatelet Therapy

The recommendations regarding long-term antiplatelet therapy in patients with UA/NSTEMI have been significantly modified since the publication of the 2002 ACC/AHA guideline. For patients who do not receive PCI with coronary stent, the current recommendation is ASA 75-162 mg/d indefinitely (Class I, Level A recommendation) and clopidogrel 75 mg/d for at least 1 month (Class I, Level A recommendation), but ideally up to 1 year (Class I, Level B recommendation). The "ideally" term relates to the relatively high cost of this drug and the fact that its benefit after 1 month is modest. Patients who receive bare metal stents should be prescribed ASA 162-325 mg/d for at least 1 month and 75-162 mg/d indefinitely thereafter (Class I, Level A recommendation). These patients should also be prescribed clopidogrel 75 mg/d for at least 1 month (Class IA recommendation), but ideally for up to 1 year (Class IB recommendation). The Class I recommendation (level of evidence: A) for patients who receive drug-eluting stents is ASA 162-325 mg/d for either 3 months (if their stent elutes sirolimus) or 6 months (if their stent elutes paclitaxel). Thereafter, these patients should be prescribed ASA 75-162 mg/d indefinitely (Class I, Level A recommendation). Importantly, patients with drug-eluting stents should also receive clopidogrel 75 mg/d for at least 1 year (Class I, Level B recommendation). Recommendation for clopidogrel in patients selected for an initial conservative strategy is that clopidogrel be taken for at least 1 month, but ideally continued for up to 1 year (Class I, Level A).

## Renin-Angiotensin-Aldosterone System Blockade in Patients with UA/NSTEMI

Patients with heart failure, LVEF <0.40, hypertension, or diabetes should be on ACEI therapy indefinitely (Class I, Level A recommendation). It is reasonable to prescribe ACEI to patients with atherothrombotic disease who do not have LV dysfunction, hypertension or diabetes (Class IIa, Level A recommendation). Similarly, ACEI therapy could be considered for UA/NSTEMI patients who have had heart failure but have a fairly normal LVEF (Class IIa, Level A). For patients with a low EF and persistent HF despite conventional therapy, consideration for treating with an ACEI/ARB combination is a Class IIb recommendation (level of evidence: B). ARB should be administered at discharge (Class I, Level A recommendation) and long-term (Class IIa, Level B) to HF patients with low EF who are intolerant to ACEI and have signs of HF and low LVEF (Class I, Level A recommendation). The recommendations are based on data from the HOPE (9297 patients), EUROPA (12,218 patients), and TRACE (1749 patients) trials. Although only one of these trials enrolled patients with ACS (TRACE), all had patients with coronary artery disease, and together these studies indicate that the benefit of ACEI is directly related to the patient's global risk.

Aldosterone receptor blockade is recommended as a long-term therapy for patients on ACEIs who have low EF (<0.40) and either symptomatic heart failure or diabetes (Class I, Level A). Significant renal dysfunction or hyperkalemia are contraindications to aldosterone receptor blockade.

Regarding lipid management, the recommendation of initiating statin therapy prior to discharge, regardless of baseline LDL-C, was mentioned previously (Class I, Level A recommendation). The target LDL-C for UA/NSTEMI patients is <100 mg/dL (Class I, Level A recommendation), but a goal of <70 mg/dL is reasonable for the high risk patient (Class IIa, Level A recommendation). Triglycerides and non-HDL-C should be addressed; when the TG is 200-499 mg/dL, the non-HDL target is <130 mg/dL (Class I, Level B recommendation). If the TG are >500 mg/dL, fibrate or niacin should be started before LDL-C-lowering agents to prevent pancreatitis (Class I, Level C recommendation).

## Discharge Planning: Other Secondary Prevention Recommendations

Overall, the blood pressure target is <140/90 mm Hg (Class I, Level A), but the target is slightly lower (<130/80 mm Hg) in patients with diabetes and chronic kidney disease (Class I, Level A recommendation). Smoking cessation and avoidance of exposure to environmental tobacco is recommended (Class I, Level B recommendation). This may be accomplished by education, pharmacotherapy, and referrals to smoking cessation programs. Discharge education should include medication, diet, exercise, smoking cessation, and cardiac rehabilitation (Class I, Level C recommendation). Patients who are higher risk need to return to clinic within 14 days of discharge, while lower risk medically treated or revascularized patients can return in 2-6 weeks (Class I recommendation).

The UA/NSTEMI current guidelines also contain Class III recommendations for a few strategies that have proven to be nonbeneficial or harmful. Menopausal hormone therapy (estrogen plus progestin or estrogen alone) should not be given de novo for secondary prevention of coronary events (Class III, Level A recommendation for hormone replacement therapy). Likewise, antioxidant vitamin supplements (vitamin C, E, or beta carotene) and folic acid should not be given for secondary prevention (Class III, Level A recommendation for antioxidant vitamin supplements). NSAIDS should be discontinued at presentation (Class I, Level C recommendation). NSAIDs, nonselective or COX-2 selective (except ASA) inhibitors should not be given to patients hospitalized for UA/NSTEMI, because of their associated risk of mortality, reinfarction, blood pressure elevation, heart failure, and myocardial rupture (Class III, Level C recommendation). At discharge, patients with chronic musculoskeletal pain should be tried on acetaminophen, small-dose narcotics, or nonacetylated salicylates (Class I, Level A recommendation), but a nonselective NSAID is reasonable if there is still a need for pain control (Class IIa, Level C recommendation). For those patients

| **Abbreviations Used in This Review** | | | |
|---|---|---|---|
| ACC | American College of Cardiology | ISAR-COOL | Intracoronary Stenting with Antithrombotic Regimen Cooling-Off Study |
| A to Z | Aggrastat to Zocor trial | ISAR-REACT-2 | Intracoronary Stenting and Antithrombotic Regimen-Rapid Early Action for Coronary Treatment 2 |
| ACS | Acute coronary syndrome | | |
| ACUITY | Acute Catheterization and Urgent Intervention Triage Strategy trial | | |
| | | OASIS-5 | Organization to Assess Strategies for Ischemic Syndromes |
| ACUTE II | Antithrombotic Combination Using Tirofiban and Enoxaparin trial | PRISM | Platelet Receptor Inhibition in Ischemic Syndrome Management |
| AHA | American Heart Association | | |
| ARMYDA-2 | Antiplatelet therapy for Reduction of Myocardial Damage during Angioplasty-2 trial | PRISM-PLUS | Platelet Receptor Inhibition in Ischemic Syndrome Management in Patients Limited by Unstable Signs and Symptoms |
| CAPRIE | Clopidogrel versus Aspirin in Patients at Risk of Ischemic Events | PROVE-IT TIMI 22 | Pravastatin or Atorvastatin Evaluation and Infection Therapy-Thrombolysis in Myocardial Infarction 22 |
| COMMIT | Clopidogrel and Metoprolol in Myocardial Infarction Trial | | |
| CURE | Clopidogrel in Unstable angina to prevent Recurrent ischemic Events trial | PURSUIT | Platelet Glycoprotein IIB/IIIA in Unstable Angina: Receptor Suppression Using Integrilin Therapy |
| ESSENCE | Efficacy and Safety of Subcutaneous Enoxaparin in Non-Q-Wave Coronary Events trial | REPLACE-2 | Randomized Evaluation of PCI Linking Angiomax to Reduced Clinical Events |
| EUROPA | European Trial on Reduction of Cardiac Events with Perindopril in Patients with Stable Coronary Artery Disease | RITA-3 | Third Randomized Intervention of Angina |
| | | SYNERGY | Superior Yield of the New strategy of Enoxaparin, Revascularization and Glycoprotein IIb/IIIA Inhibitors trial |
| FRISC-2 | Fragmin during Instability in Coronary Artery Disease 2 trial | | |
| GRACE | Global Registry of Acute Coronary Events | TACTICS-TIMI-18 | Treat Angina with Aggrastat and Determine Cost of Therapy with an Invasive or Conservative Strategy TIMI-18 trial |
| GUSTO IV-ACS | Global Utilization of Strategies to Open Occluded Coronary Arteries Trial IV in Acute Coronary Syndromes | | |
| | | TIMI | Thrombolysis in Myocardial Infarction |
| | | TRACE | Trandolapril Cardiac Evaluation Study |
| HOPE | Heart Outcomes Prevention Evaluation | VINO | Value of First Day Angiography/Angioplasty in Evolving Non-ST-Segment Elevation Myocardial Infarction: Open Multicenter Randomized Trial |
| HPS | Heart Protection Study | | |
| ICTUS | Invasive versus Conservative Treatment in Unstable Coronary Syndromes trial | | |
| INTERACT | Integrilin and Enoxaparin Randomized Assessment of Acute Coronary Syndrome Treatment | | |

who still have intolerable symptoms, a selective COX-2 inhibitor may be given, but it is recommended that the lowest dose be used for the shortest period of time (Class IIb, Level C).

## SUMMARY

Since 2002, new data from several clinical trials of ACS patients have led to a greater understanding of how various strategies and therapies impact clinical outcomes. This has led to a revision of the ACC/AHA Guidelines for UA/NSTEMI, but the current version of these guidelines is not dramatically different from the 2002 version. Rather, the current version "fine tunes" many of the 2002 recommendations and endorses a few new therapies. One of the overarching themes of the 2007 guidelines is greater recognition of the value of an initially conservative strategy. The 2007 update emphasizes the importance of risk stratifying UA/

NSTEMI patients and selecting an early invasive or conservative (i.e., selectively invasive) strategy based on this risk. Importantly, an initially conservative strategy may be considered for high risk patients who have been stabilized. Other important revisions in the 2007 update describe the optimal use of anticoagulant and antiplatelet therapies, both during hospitalization and long term. Future guidelines will likely refine these recommendations further, as well as provide greater detail on the utility of newer imaging modalities (e.g., multislice CT angiography and cardiac MRI) for risk stratification.

### Suggested Readings

1. Anderson JL, Adams CD, Antman EM, et al. ACC/AHA 2007 Guidelines for the Management of Patients with Unstable Angina/Non ST-Elevation Myocardial Infarction: a report of the American College of Cardiology/American Heart Association Task Force on Practice Guidelines (Writing Committee to Revise the 2002 Guidelines for the Manage-

ment of Patients with Unstable Angina/Non ST-Elevation Myocardial Infarction): developed in collaboration with the American College of Emergency Physicians, the Society for Cardiovascular Angiography and Interventions, and the Society of Thoracic Surgeons: endorsed by the American Association of Cardiovascular and Pulmonary Rehabilitation and the Society for Academic Emergency Medicine. *Circulation.* 2007;116(7):e148–e304.

2. Savonitto S, Ardissino D, Granger CB, et al. Prognostic value of the admission electrocardiogram in acute coronary syndromes. *JAMA.* 1999;281(8):707–713.

3. Cannon CP, Weintraub WS, Demopoulos LA, et al. Comparison of early invasive and conservative strategies in patients with unstable coronary syndromes treated with the glycoprotein IIb/IIIa inhibitor tirofiban. *New Engd J Med.* 2001;344(25):1879–1887.

4. de Winter RJ, Windhausen F, Cornel JH, et al. Early invasive versus selectively invasive management for acute coronary syndromes. *New Engd J Med.* 2005;353(11):1095–1104.

5. Giugliano RP, Braunwald E. The year in non-ST-segment elevation acute coronary syndromes. *J Amer Coll Card.* 2005;46(5):906–919.

# ST-Segment Elevation Myocardial Infarction (STEMI)

Josh Todd and Sidney C. Smith, Jr.

## ● PRACTICAL POINTS

- Prompt recognition of the symptoms and signs of STEMI with timely diagnosis and early treatment is the most important determination of successful long-term outcome in patients with STEMI.

- Unfortunately, delay in recognition and treatment represents the most significant obstacle in the treatment of this disease.

- Both fibrinolytic therapy and percutaneous intervention are beneficial in treating patients with STEMI; however, percutaneous intervention is the preferred method of treatment, provided there is no significant delay in transporting the patient to the catheterization lab.

- ST-segment elevation of 1 mm or more in 2 contiguous leads and new LBBB in patients with chest pain constitute a diagnosis of STEMI, in which case treatment should be instituted immediately.

- Medical treatment for STEMI includes chewable aspirin, nitrates in the absence of hypotension, oxygen, morphine sulfate with severe chest pain, oral beta-blockers in the absence of contraindications, ACE inhibitors in the absence of hypotension, and the use of aldosterone antagonist in patients with Class II and III heart failure, provided that reasonably good renal function is present.

- Complications of STEMI include recurrent ischemia, arrhythmias, and hemodynamic disturbances. The latter comprise the leading cause of mortality in STEMI after the infarction occurs.

- ICD is indicated in patients who have sustained VT and who at 40 days are New York Heart Association Class II and III and have ejection fractions of less than 35%; and in patients with New York Heart Association Class I with ejection fractions of less than 30%.

## INTRODUCTION

This chapter will focus on the recognition, pre-hospital issues, management, and secondary prevention strategies of ST-segment myocardial infarction (STEMI) with particular focus on the major ACC/AHA recommendations and the evidence leading to the Class I and Class III guidelines.[1,2] In the continuum described as acute coronary syndrome (ACS), STEMI has highest in-hospital mortality rates, ranging from 7 to 13%, and a yearly incidence estimated at 500,000.[3-5] Unlike Non-ST-segment elevation myocardial infarction (NSTEMI) or unstable angina (UA), STEMI is a result of acute plaque rupture that results in epicardial coronary artery thrombus formation with total occlusion in nearly 90% of patients at time of angiography.[6,7] Based upon the understanding of this pathophysiology, advances have been made in the treatment of STEMI that have reduced mortality and morbidity due to timely reperfusion strategies, adjunctive therapies, and secondary prevention at discharge. Despite these advances, prompt recognition of symptoms and rapid transfer to hospital facilities with a timely diagnosis remains the most significant obstacle in the treatment of this disease.

## PRE-HOSPITAL ISSUES

Since many patients may be asymptomatic prior to presentation, the goal of the primary care provider is to first identify patients at higher risk for myocardial infarction and then implement comprehensive prevention strategies. Additionally, primary care providers should focus on the education of the patient regarding the symptoms of angina. If nitroglycerin is prescribed for stable angina symptoms, the patient should be instructed to seek medical attention and preferably call 9-1-1 if chest pain worsens or is unimproved 5 minutes after only 1 nitroglycerin dose has been taken. Evidence from the Global Registry of Acute Coronary Events (GRACE) has demonstrated the average delay for patients with STEMI from onset of symptoms is a mean of 4.7 hours, with only 41% of patients presenting within 2 hours of symptom onset.[8]

If the patient is initially evaluated outside the hospital by EMS first responders, then aspirin (ASA, 162-325 mg, chewed) is to be given and early risk stratification by EMS should be considered with 12-lead ECG. Particular attention should be given to high risk patients with STEMI. These are defined as those in cardiogenic shock who are less than 75 years of age, or patients who have contraindications to fibrinolytic therapy. These high risk populations should be preferentially transported immediately to a facility capable of performing percutaneous coronary intervention (PCI) or coronary artery bypass grafting (CABG) if revascularization can be performed within 18 hours of onset of symptoms regardless of transport time.[9] This recommendation is based on the SHOCK (Should We Emergently Revascularize Occluded Coronaries for Cardiogenic Shock) Trial, which demonstrated at 1 year follow-up a 13.2% absolute risk reduction in all-cause mortality for nonelderly patients (defined as less than 75 years of age) who received early revascularization (PCI or CABG) versus those who received initial medical stabilization (which included thrombolysis and/or IABP placement). Outside of this high risk group of patients, it is reasonable to transport all other patients with STEMI to any hospital capable of fibrinolysis (within 30 minutes) if PCI is not available within 90 minutes of the EMS diagnosis. There is less evidence supporting the notion that pre-hospital fibrinolysis by EMS has a significant benefit, and therefore carries a Class IIa recommendation by ACC/AHA guidelines.

## EMERGENCY DEPARTMENT DIAGNOSIS

Prompt recognition by the emergency department is essential for the efficient management of patients presenting with STEMI. In patients who are suspected of having an ACS, a targeted history and physical should be performed to evaluate for signs and symptoms of cardiac ischemia, cardiovascular risk factors, and evidence of noncardiac causes of symptoms that suggest an alternative diagnosis including aortic dissection, esophageal rupture, and pulmonary embolism. If fibrinolytics are considered, the physical examination should include a brief neurological exam to evaluate for a cerebrovascular accident. An electrocardiogram (ECG) should be performed within 10 minutes of arrival to the emergency department.

The ECG changes in patients with epicardial coronary artery occlusion typically follow the initial pattern of a prominent peaked T wave (termed "hyperacute") which progress to convex ST-segment elevations. The sine qua non of a STEMI is either ST-segment elevations of more than 1 mm in two or more contiguous leads or a new left bundle branch block (LBBB) in the context of symptoms consistent with myocardial ischemia. If the ECG is consistent with an inferior STEMI, then a right-sided ECG should be performed to evaluate for right ventricular involvement. If the initial ECG is not diagnostic of a STEMI and the patient remains symptomatic with a high clinical suspicion, serial ECGs should be performed in 5-10-minute intervals.

Emergency department laboratory evaluation should not delay the implementation of reperfusion strategy in the STEMI patient. In addition to basic laboratory evaluation (**Table 31-1**), cardiac specific troponins are considered the optimum biomarkers for myocardial injury. Point of care qualitative assays can be used in the initial evaluation, but subsequent sets should be quantitative.

Radiological imaging plays an important role in the management of patients presenting with a STEMI; these patients should have a chest X-ray. Further imaging such as a CT or MRI may be considered if aortic dissection is a consideration. SPECT imaging should not be used as a modality for risk stratification when the ECG is considered diagnostic for STEMI.

---

**Table 31-1 • Laboratory Evaluations for Management of ST-Elevation Myocardial Infarction\***

Serum biomarkers for cardiac damage
(do not wait for results before implementing reperfusion strategy)
CBC with platelet count
INR
aPTT
Electrolytes and magnesium
BUN
Creatinine
Glucose
Serum lipids

*\*Adapted from Antman et al. J Am Coll Cardiol. 2004.*

# EMERGENCY DEPARTMENT MANAGEMENT

Emergency room management of the patient with ACS should incorporate initial antiplatelet therapy with an aspirin (162-325 mg), which is chewed–nonenteric coated, as coated tablets may impair absorption. Sublingual nitroglycerin is to be considered for patients with ongoing chest discomfort, 3 total doses before one assesses the need for intravenous nitroglycerin. Additional clinical situations for which nitroglycerin is indicated in patients with STEMI are control of refractory hypertension and management of pulmonary congestion. However, nitrates should not be administered to patients with hypotension (defined at systolic less than 90 mm Hg, or 30 mm Hg below baseline) or severe bradycardia (<50 bpm); patients who received a phosphodiesterase type 5 inhibitor within 24 hours; or patients suspected of having a right ventricular infarction. Supplemental oxygen should be administered to those patients with evidence of arterial desaturation (defined as $SaO_2$ of less than 90%). The analgesic of choice for continued angina chest pain in the patient awaiting revascularization is morphine sulfate. Current recommendations are to give 2-4 mg intravenously, repeated at 5-15 minute intervals as needed for pain relief.

Oral beta-blocker therapy should be administered to patients with STEMI who do not have signs of heart failure, evidence of cardiogenic shock, increased risk of cardiogenic shock (signified by age >70 years, systolic blood pressure <120 mm Hg, sinus tachycardia >110 bpm or heart rate <60 bpm, and increased time since onset of symptoms of STEMI); or to patients who have relative contraindications to beta blockade therapy. Importantly, it is a new recommendation that intravenous beta-blocker therapy not be given to patients with these risk factors for hypotension. These recommendations for beta-blocker therapy have been updated by the 2007 AHA/ACC STEMI guidelines based upon the results of the COMMIT/CCS-2 (Clopidogrel and Metoprolol in Myocardial Infarction Trial/Second Chinese Cardiac Study), which was a randomized controlled trial in 45,852 Chinese patients with suspected myocardial infarction.[10] In this large, prospective, randomized controlled trial, patients received intravenous metoprolol up to 3 doses of 5 mg within the first 15 minutes of onset and then 200 mg per day orally versus placebo. For the primary combined outcome of death, reinfarction, and cardiac arrest there was no significant difference. In the subgroup analysis there was benefit in reinfarction rates and ventricular fibrillation favoring the metoprolol arm. However, there was also a significant increase among higher risk patients of cardiogenic shock within the first day of hospitalization if they received early intravenous beta-blocker therapy. Current guidelines now reflect the adverse hemodynamic effects from early intravenous beta-blockade given to higher risk patients.

# REPERFUSION STRATEGIES

Once the diagnosis and initial medical management of patients with a STEMI have been performed, attention is directed towards rapid reperfusion strategies. This restoration of coronary blood flow can be by fibrinolysis, PCI, or surgical revascularization. Much appears in the literature concerning attempts to find the optimal reperfusion treatment in various patient populations presenting with STEMI. One key point found in all studies is that prompt reperfusion is important in saving myocardium, and therefore decisions are based upon the timing associated with options available.

In general, the evidence supports PCI over fibrinolysis for patients with STEMI. A large meta-analysis comparing PCI to fibrinolytic therapies, with 7500 patients, demonstrated a statistically significant reduction in both short- and long-term outcomes for death, recurrent ischemia, and recurrent infarction.[11] In this analysis, the PCI group received stents in 12 of the trials and GP IIb/IIIa inhibitors in 8 trials. Time to treatment was 6 hours or less in 9 of the trials, and 12 hours in 13 of the trials. Specifically PCI offers an absolute reduction in a combined endpoint of death, myocardial infarction, and a reduction of cerebrovascular accident of 5% in the short term (4-6 weeks) and 7% in the long term (6-18 months). (**Figure 31-1**) Current ACC/AHA guidelines recommend that, if available, primary PCI should be performed in all patients with STEMI, posterior MI, or new LBBB, experiencing less than 12 hours of symptoms. However, in the U.S. only 20% of hospitals have a cardiac catheterization laboratory, and less have the ability to perform primary PCI.

## Fibrinolytics

Patients presenting to a facility with chest pain symptoms of less than 3 hours, ST elevation of >1 mV in 2 or more contiguous leads, or new complete LBBB and without the ability for primary PCI within 90 minutes of presentation should undergo fibrinolysis. The evidence supporting this statement comes from a meta-analysis of 13 randomized controlled trials comparing fibrinolysis and PCI.[12] Based on these studies, PCI is favored up to 60 minutes from the estimated fibrinolytic door to needle time, which is assumed to be 30 minutes (**Figure 31-2**).

If the decision has been made to give fibrinolytics, absolute and relative contraindications must first be reviewed. (**Table 31-2**) In the absence of contraindications, the fibrinolytic agent choice has less evidence and no

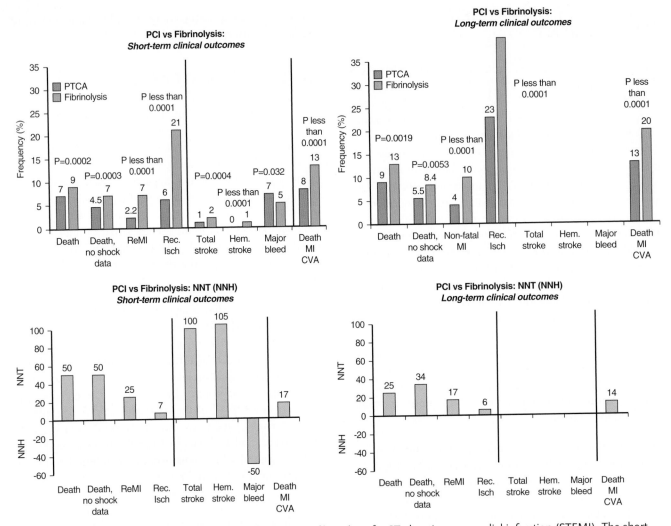

**Figure 31-1.** Percutaneous coronary intervention (PCI) versus fibrinolysis for ST-elevation myocardial infarction (STEMI). The short term (4-6 week) (top left) and long term (top right) outcomes for the various endpoints shown are plotted for patients with STEMI randomized to percutaneous coronary intervention (PCI) or fibrinolysis for reperfusion in 23 trials (N = 7739). Based on the frequency of events for each endpoints in the two treatment groups the number needed to treat (NNT) or number needed to harm (NNH) are shown for the short term (bottom left) and long term (bottom right) outcomes. The magnitude of the treatment differences for death, non-fatal reinfarction, and stroke vary depending on whether PCI is compared with streptokinase or a fibrin-specific lytic. For example, when primary PCI is compared with alteplase (tPA) and the SHOCK trial is excluded, the mortality rate is 5.5% versus 6.7% (OR 0.81, 95% CI 0.64-1.03, P = 0.081) (421a). See references (40,421a) for additional discussion. PTCA = percutaneous transluminal coronary angioplasty; ReMI = recurrent MI; Rec. Isch = recurrent ischemia; Hem. Stroke = hemorrhagic stroke; MI = myocardial infarction; and CVA = cerebrovascular accident. (Reprinted from Antman EM, et al. ACC/AHA guidelines for the management of patients with ST-elevation myocardial infarction: a report of the American College of Cardiology/American Heart Association Task Force on Practice Guidelines (Committee to Revise the 1999 Guidelines for the Management of Patients With Acute Myocardial Infarction). *J Am Coll Cardiol.* 2004;44(3):e42, with permission from Elsevier.)

formal recommendations for clinical practice. Two studies (GUSTO I, GUSTO III) in particular did demonstrate higher coronary patency rates with alteplase and reteplase over streptokinase, although this was at the expense of slightly higher rates of intracranial hemorrhage.[13,14] Additionally, there is some evidence that tenecteplase over alteplase may have lower incidence of noncerebral mild to moderate bleeding complications and reduced frequency of blood transfusions, with similar rates of mortality and intracranial hemorrhage[15] (**Table 31-3**).

## Facilitated PCI

There is only limited evidence regarding a strategy of facilitated PCI (defined as a planned immediate intervention, after administration of an initial pharmacological regimen intended to improve coronary artery patency), and this strategy when other than full dose fibrinolytic therapy is used currently has only a IIb recommendation from 2007 guidelines.[2] The majority of evidence to date has failed to identify a pharmacologic reperfusion strategy for facilitated PCI that will improve outcomes. Based upon the results of ASSENT-4 (primary versus

## Table 31-4 • Secondary Prevention for Patients with Coronary and Other Vascular Diseases*

**Blood pressure control**

*Goal: < 140/90 mm Hg, or < 130/80 mm Hg if the patient has diabetes or chronic kidney disease*
- For patients with blood pressure ≥140/90 mm Hg (or ≥130/80 mm Hg for patients with diabetes or chronic kidney disease), it is recommended that patient initiate or maintain lifestyle modification (weight control, increased physical activity, alcohol moderation, sodium reduction, and emphasis on increased consumption of fresh fruits, vegetables, and low-fat dairy products). It is useful, as tolerated, to add blood pressure medication, treating initially with beta-blockers and/or ACE inhibitors, with the addition of other drugs, such as thiazides, as needed to achieve goal blood pressure.

**Beta-blockers**

- It is beneficial to start and continue beta-blocker therapy indefinitely in all patients who have had MI, acute coronary syndrome, or LV dysfunction with or without HF symptoms, unless contraindicated.

**Renin-angiotensin aldosterone system blockers: ACEI and ARBs**

- ACEIs should be started and continued indefinitely in all patients recovering from STEMI with LVEF ≤40% and for those with hypertension, diabetes, or chronic kidney disease, unless contraindicated.
- ACEIs should be started and continued indefinitely in patients recovering from STEMI who are not lower risk ("lower risk" defined as referring to those with normal LVEF in whom cardiovascular risk factors are well controlled and revascularization has been performed), unless contraindicated.
- Use of angiotensin receptor blockers is recommended in patients who are intolerant of ACEIs and have HF or have had an MI with LVEF <40%.
- It is beneficial to use angiotensin receptor blocker therapy in other patients who are ACEI-intolerant and have hypertension.

**Renin-angiotensin aldosterone system blockers: Aldosterone blockers**

- Use of aldosterone blockade in post-MI patients without significant renal dysfunction (creatinine should be <2.5 mg/dL in men and <2.0 mg/dL in women) or hyperkalemia (potassium should be <5.0 mEq/L) is recommended in patients who are already receiving therapeutic doses of an ACEI and beta-blocker, have an LVEF ≤ 40%, and have either diabetes or HF.

**Lipid management**

*Goal: LDL-C substantially < 100 mg/dL (if triglycerides are ≥200 mg/dL, non-HDL-C should be <130 mg/dL).*
- Starting dietary therapy is recommended for all patients. Reduce intake of saturated fats (to <7% of total calories), transfatty acids and cholesterol (to <200 mg/day)
- Promotion of daily physical activity and weight management is recommended.
- A fasting lipid profile should be assessed in all patients and within 24 hours of hospitalization for those with an acute cardiovascular or coronary event. For hospitalized patients, initiation of lipid-lowering medication is indicated as recommended above, before discharge.
- If triglycerides >150 mg/dL or HDL-C <40 mg/dL, then weight management, physical activity and smoking cessation should be emphasized. If triglycerides are 200-499 mg/dL, then non-HDL-C target should be <130 mg/dL. Therapy to reduce non-HDL-C should include more intense lowering of LDL-C
- If triglycerides ≥ 500 mg/dL, therapeutic options indicated and useful to prevent pancreatitis are a fibrate or niacin before LDL therapy, and treatment of LDL-C to goal after triglyceride-lowering therapy. Achieving non-HDL-C <130 mg/dL is recommended.

**Diabetes management**

*Goal: HbA1c < 7%.*
- It is recommended the patient initiate lifestyle and pharmacotherapy to achieve near-normal HbA1c.
- Beginning vigorous modification of other risk factors (e.g., physical activity, weight management, blood pressure control, and cholesterol management as recommended above) is beneficial.

**Anticoagulants: Aspirin and clopidogrel**

- For all post-PCI STEMI stented patients without aspirin resistance, allergy, or increased risk of bleeding, ASA 162-325 mg daily should be given for at least 1 month after BMS implantation, 3 months after sirolimus-eluting stent implantation, and 6 months after paclitaxel-eluting stent implantation, after which long-term aspirin use should be continued indefinitely at a dose of 75-162 mg daily.
- All post-PCI patients who receive a DES, clopidogrel 75 mg daily should be given for at least 12 months if not at high risk of bleeding. For post-PCI patients receiving a BMS, clopidogrel should be given for a minimum of 1 month and ideally up to 12 months (unless the patient is at increased risk of bleeding; then, it should be given for a minimum of 2 weeks).
- For all STEMI patients not undergoing stenting (medical therapy alone or PTCA without stenting), treatment with clopidogrel should continue for at least 14 days.

**Anticoagulants: Warfarin**

- Managing warfarin to an INR equal to 2.0-3.0 for paroxysmal or chronic atrial fibrillation or flutter is recommended, and in post-MI patients when clinically indicated (e.g., atrial fibrillation, left ventricular thrombus).

*(continued)*

| Table 31-4 • (continued) |
|---|

- Use of warfarin in conjunction with aspirin and/or clopidogrel is associated with an increased risk of bleeding and should be monitored closely.
- In patients requiring warfarin, clopidogrel, and aspirin therapy, an INR of 2.0-2.5 is recommended with low dose aspirin (75-81 mg) and a 75-mg dose of clopidogrel.

**Smoking**

*Goal: Complete cessation, no exposure to environmental tobacco smoke.*
- Status of tobacco use should be asked about at every visit. Strongly encourage patient and family to stop smoking and to avoid secondhand smoke.
- Every tobacco user and family member who smoke should be advised to quit at every visit.
- The tobacco user's willingness to quit should be assessed.
- Provide counseling, pharmacological therapy (including nicotine replacement and bupropion), and formal smoking cessation programs as appropriate.
- The tobacco user should be assisted by counseling and develop a plan for quitting.
- Follow-up, referral to special programs, or pharmacotherapy (including nicotine replacement and pharmacological treatment) should be arranged.
- Exposure to environmental tobacco smoke at work and home should be avoided

**Physical activity**

*Goal: 30 minutes, 7 days per week (minimum 5 days per week).*
- Advising medically supervised programs (cardiac rehabilitation) for high risk patients (e.g., recent ACS or revascularization, HF) is recommended.
- For all patients, it is recommended that risk be assessed with a physical activity history and/or an exercise test to guide prescription.
- For all patients, encouraging 30-60 min of moderate-intensity aerobic activity is recommended, such as brisk walking on most–preferably all–days of the week, supplemented by an increase in daily lifestyle activities (e.g., walking breaks at work, gardening, and household work).

**Weight management**

*Goals: BMI–18.5 to 24.9 kg/m²; waist circumference–men <40 inches (102 cm), women <35 in. (89 cm).*
- It is useful to assess BMI and/or waist circumference on each visit and consistently encourage weight maintenance/reduction through an appropriate balance of physical activity, caloric intake, and formal behavioral programs when indicated to maintain/achieve a BMI between 18.5 and 24.9 kg/m².
- The initial goal of weight loss therapy should be to reduce body weight by approximately 10% from baseline. With success, further weight loss can be attempted if indicated through further assessment.
- If waist circumference (measured horizontally at the iliac crest) is 35 in. (89 cm) or greater in women and 40 in. (102 cm) or greater in men, it is useful to initiate lifestyle changes and consider treatment strategies for metabolic syndrome as indicated.

*\*Modified from Antman et al Circulation. 2008;117(2):316–319.*

an assessment of left ventricular function; however, reassessment by echocardiography prior to discharge of a patient without change in clinical status or revascularization procedure is a Class III indication.

# CONCLUSIONS

ST-segment myocardial infarction (STEMI) is a unique, high risk disease process that requires prompt identification and efficient transfer to hospital facilities. Once the diagnosis of STEMI has been made, prompt intervention with PCI (if the patient is initially triaged to a PCI capable facility or can be rapidly transferred within 60 minutes) is the preferred strategy; fibrinolytics is preferred if PCI is not available. Once reperfusion has been established, the patient should be cared for in a critical care unit with close monitoring of the post infarct mechanical complications

and rhythm disturbances. Medical therapy should included appropriate antiplatelet agents and antithrombin therapy, along with adjunctive therapies to reduce myocardial work load and afterload and lipid reduction to recommended LDL-C goals. Patients with a post infarct decreased left ventricular systolic function should be seen after 40 days of infarct with repeat evaluation of left ventricular ejection fraction and NYHA classification to determine if ICD therapy is necessary. Most importantly, the patient needs adequate follow-up and long-term management of secondary prevention measures, with enrollment in cardiac rehabilitation programs when possible.

## References

1. Antman EM, Anbe DT, Armstrong PW, et al. ACC/AHA Guidelines for the Management of Patients with ST-Elevation Myocardial Infarction: A Report of the American College of

Cardiology/American Heart Association Task Force on Practice Guidelines (Committee to Revise the 1999 Guidelines for the Management of Patients with Acute Myocardial Infarction). *J Am Coll Cardiol.* 2004;44(3):e1–e211.

2. Antman EM, Hand M, Armstrong PW, et al. 2007 Focused Update of the ACC/AHA 2004 Guidelines for the Management of Patients with ST-Elevation Myocardial Infarction: A Report of the American College of Cardiology/American Heart Association Task Force on Practice Guidelines: developed in collaboration with the Canadian Cardiovascular Society endorsed by the American Academy of Family Physicians: 2007 Writing Group to Review New Evidence and Update the ACC/AHA 2004 Guidelines for the Management of Patients with ST-Elevation Myocardial Infarction, writing on behalf of the 2004 Writing Committee. *Circulation.* 2008;117(2):296–329.

3. Hasdai D, Behar S, Wallentin L, et al. A prospective survey of the characteristics, treatments and outcomes of patients with acute coronary syndromes in Europe and the Mediterranean basin; the Euro Heart Survey of Acute Coronary Syndromes (Euro Heart Survey ACS). *Eur Heart J.* 2002;23(15):1190–1201.

4. Law MR, Watt HC, Wald NJ. The underlying risk of death after myocardial infarction in the absence of treatment. *Arch Intern Med.* 2002;162(21):2405–2410.

5. Steg PG, Goldberg RJ, Gore JM, et al. Baseline characteristics, management practices, and in-hospital outcomes of patients hospitalized with acute coronary syndromes in the Global Registry of Acute Coronary Events (GRACE). *Am J Cardiol.* 2002;90(4):358–363.

6. Boersma E, Mercado N, Poldermans D, et al. Acute myocardial infarction. *Lancet.* 2003;361(9360):847–858.

7. DeWood MA, Spores J, Notske R, et al. Prevalence of total coronary occlusion during the early hours of transmural myocardial infarction. *N Engl J Med.* 1980;303(16):897–902.

8. Goldberg RJ, Steg PG, Sadiq I, et al. Extent of, and factors associated with, delay to hospital presentation in patients with acute coronary disease (the GRACE registry). *Am J Cardiol.* Apr 1 2002;89(7):791–796.

9. Hochman JS, Sleeper LA, White HD, et al. One-year survival following early revascularization for cardiogenic shock. *JAMA.* 2001;285(2):190–192.

10. Chen ZM, Pan HC, Chen YP, et al. Early intravenous then oral metoprolol in 45,852 patients with acute myocardial infarction: randomised placebo-controlled trial. *Lancet.* 2005;366(9497):1622–1632.

11. Keeley EC, Boura JA, Grines CL. Primary angioplasty versus intravenous thrombolytic therapy for acute myocardial infarction: a quantitative review of 23 randomised trials. *Lancet.* 2003;361(9351):13–20.

12. Nallamothu BK, Bates ER. Percutaneous coronary intervention versus fibrinolytic therapy in acute myocardial infarction: is timing (almost) everything? *Am J Cardiol.* 2003;92(7):824–826.

13. The Global Use of Strategies to Open Occluded Coronary Arteries (GUSTO) Investigators. An international randomized trial comparing four thrombolytic strategies for acute myocardial infarction. *N Engl J Med.* 1993;329(10):673–682.

14. The Global Use of Strategies to Open Occluded Coronary Arteries (GUSTO III) Investigators. A comparison of reteplase with alteplase for acute myocardial infarction. *N Engl J Med.* 1997;337(16):1118–1123.

15. Van De Werf F, Adgey J, Ardissino D, et al. Single-bolus tenecteplase compared with front-loaded alteplase in acute myocardial infarction: the ASSENT-2 double-blind randomised trial. *Lancet.* 1999;354(9180):716–722.

16. Primary versus tenecteplase-facilitated percutaneous coronary intervention in patients with ST-segment elevation acute myocardial infarction (ASSENT-4 PCI): randomised trial. *Lancet.* 2006;367(9510):569–578.

17. Ellis SG, da Silva ER, Heyndrickx G, et al. Randomized comparison of rescue angioplasty with conservative management of patients with early failure of thrombolysis for acute anterior myocardial infarction. *Circulation.* 1994;90(5):2280–2284.

18. Wijeysundera HC, Vijayaraghavan R, Nallamothu BK, et al. Rescue angioplasty or repeat fibrinolysis after failed fibrinolytic therapy for ST-segment myocardial infarction: a meta-analysis of randomized trials. *J Am Coll Cardiol.* 2007;49(4):422–430.

19. Sutton AG, Campbell PG, Graham R, et al. A randomized trial of rescue angioplasty versus a conservative approach for failed fibrinolysis in ST-segment elevation myocardial infarction: the Middlesbrough Early Revascularization to Limit INfarction (MERLIN) trial. *J Am Coll Cardiol.* 2004;44(2):287–296.

20. Madsen JK, Grande P, Saunamaki K, et al. Danish multicenter randomized study of invasive versus conservative treatment in patients with inducible ischemia after thrombolysis in acute myocardial infarction (DANAMI). DANish trial in Acute Myocardial Infarction. *Circulation.* 1997;96(3):748–755.

21. SWIFT (Should We Intervene Following Thrombolysis?) Trial Study Group. SWIFT trial of delayed elective intervention v conservative treatment after thrombolysis with anistreplase in acute myocardial infarction. *BMJ.* 1991;302(6776):555–560.

22. Hochman JS, Buller CE, Sleeper LA, et al. Cardiogenic shock complicating acute myocardial infarction–etiologies, management and outcome: a report from the SHOCK Trial Registry. SHould we emergently revascularize Occluded Coronaries for cardiogenic shocK? *J Am Coll Cardiol.* 2000;36(3 Suppl A):1063–1070.

23. Holmes DR, Jr, Bates ER, Kleiman NS, et al. Contemporary reperfusion therapy for cardiogenic shock: the GUSTO-I trial experience. The GUSTO-I Investigators. Global Utilization of Streptokinase and Tissue Plasminogen Activator for Occluded Coronary Arteries. *J Am Coll Cardiol.* 1995;26(3):668–674.

24. Latini R, Maggioni AP, Flather M, et al. ACE inhibitor use in patients with myocardial infarction. Summary of evidence from clinical trials. *Circulation.* 1995;92(10):3132–3137.

25. Pitt B, Remme W, Zannad F, et al. Eplerenone, a selective aldosterone blocker, in patients with left ventricular dysfunction after myocardial infarction. *N Engl J Med.* 2003;348(14):1309–1321.

26. Gislason GH, Jacobsen S, Rasmussen JN, et al. Risk of death or reinfarction associated with the use of selective cyclooxygenase-2 inhibitors and nonselective nonsteroidal antiinflammatory drugs after acute myocardial infarction. *Circulation.* 2006;113(25):2906–2913.

27. Braat SH, de Zwaan C, Brugada P, et al. Right ventricular involvement with acute inferior wall myocardial infarction identifies high risk of developing atrioventricular nodal conduction disturbances. *Am Heart J.* 1984;107(6):1183–1187.

28. Campbell RW, Murray A, Julian DG. Ventricular arrhythmias in first 12 hours of acute myocardial infarction. Natural history study. *Br Heart J.* 1981;46(4):351–357.

29. Alexander JH, Granger CB, Sadowski Z, et al. Prophylactic lidocaine use in acute myocardial infarction: incidence and outcomes from two international trials. The GUSTO-I and GUSTO-IIb Investigators. *Am Heart J.* 1999;137(5):799–805.

30. MacMahon S, Collins R, Peto R, et al. Effects of prophylactic lidocaine in suspected acute myocardial infarction. An overview of results from the randomized, controlled trials. *JAMA.* 1988;260(13):1910–1916.

31. The Antiarrhythmics versus Implantable Defibrillators (AVID) Investigators. A comparison of antiarrhythmic-drug therapy with implantable defibrillators in patients resuscitated from near-fatal ventricular arrhythmias. The Antiarrhythmics versus Implantable Defibrillators (AVID) Investigators. *N Engl J Med.* 1997;337(22):1576–1583.

32. Connolly SJ, Gent M, Roberts RS, et al. Canadian implantable defibrillator study (CIDS): a randomized trial of the implantable cardioverter defibrillator against amiodarone. *Circulation.* 2000;101(11):1297–1302.

33. Siebels J, Kuck KH. Implantable cardioverter defibrillator compared with antiarrhythmic drug treatment in cardiac arrest survivors (the Cardiac Arrest Study Hamburg). *Am Heart J.* 1994;127(4 Pt 2):1139–1144.

34. Buxton AE, Lee KL, Fisher JD, et al. A randomized study of the prevention of sudden death in patients with coronary artery disease. Multicenter Unsustained Tachycardia Trial Investigators. *N Engl J Med.* 1999;341(25):1882–1890.

35. Moss AJ, Hall WJ, Cannom DS, et al. Improved survival with an implanted defibrillator in patients with coronary disease at high risk for ventricular arrhythmia. Multicenter Automatic Defibrillator Implantation Trial Investigators. *N Engl J Med.* 1996;335(26):1933–1940.

36. Moss AJ, Zareba W, Hall WJ, et al. Prophylactic implantation of a defibrillator in patients with myocardial infarction and reduced ejection fraction. *N Engl J Med.* 2002;346(12):877–883.

37. Epstein AE, DiMarco JP, Ellenbogen KA, et al. ACC/AHA/HRS 2008 Guidelines for Device-Based Therapy of Cardiac Rhythm Abnormalities: A Report of the American College of Cardiology/American Heart Association Task Force on Practice Guidelines (Writing Committee to Revise the ACC/AHA/NASPE 2002 Guideline Update for Implantation of Cardiac Pacemakers and Antiarrhythmia Devices) developed in collaboration with the American Association for Thoracic Surgery and Society of Thoracic Surgeons. *J Am Coll Cardiol.* 2008;51(21):e1–62.

38. Pedersen OD, Bagger H, Kober L, et al. The occurrence and prognostic significance of atrial fibrillation/-flutter following acute myocardial infarction. TRACE Study group. TRAndolapril Cardiac Evalution. *Eur Heart J.* 1999;20(10):748–754.

39. Wong CK, White HD, Wilcox RG, et al. New atrial fibrillation after acute myocardial infarction independently predicts death: the GUSTO-III experience. *Am Heart J.* 2000;140(6):878–885.

40. Fuster V. *Hurst's The heart.* 12th ed. New York: McGraw-Hill Medical; 2008.

41. Tofler GH, Muller JE, Stone PH, et al. Pericarditis in acute myocardial infarction: characterization and clinical significance. *Am Heart J.* 1989;117(1):86–92.

# Right Ventricular Myocardial Infarction

Paul B. Yu

## • PRACTICAL POINTS

- RVMI should always be considered in patients who present with inferior posterior myocardial infarction, particularly if signs of cardiogenic shock are present.

- High degree atrioventricular block with inferior infarction significantly increases the probability of RVMI.

- Right side chest leads and echocardiograms can provide useful information for diagnosis of RVMI and should always be performed in patients with hemodynamic instability with inferior STEMI.

- Volume resuscitation for hemodynamic instability should be instituted immediately followed by a reperfusion strategy as soon as possible. Should high-grade AV block exist, immediate pacemaker placement is indicated.

- Standard treatment modalities employed for acute infarction may often be detrimental in patients with RVMI. Such modalities include nitroglycerin and Lasix, which should be avoided in hemodynamically unstable patients. Beta-blockers also should be avoided in patients with bradycardia and high-degree AV block.

Acute right ventricular myocardial infarction (RVMI) results from substantial ischemic injury of the right ventricular free wall and septum manifesting with hemodynamic instability and impaired cardiac output. RVMI and its associated physiology are thought to be present in more than one-third of cases of acute inferior MI, adding unique layers to the morbidity and management of acute coronary syndromes. RVMI occurs most frequently with proximal occlusion of the right coronary artery, complicating an infero-posterior MI, but it occurs occasionally from occlusion of a large dominant circumflex with IPMI, and rarely with large anterior MIs extending to the anterior RV free wall. RVMI is defined electrocardiographically by significant right ventricular epicardial injury (>1 mm elevation in right-sided leads $V_3R$-$V_6R$, particularly $V_4R$, sensitivity >80%, **Figure 32-1**) or echocardiographically with demonstrated right ventricular

dilatation or dysfunction or associated findings in the setting of an acute MI (sensitivity >80%). Other evidence of elevated right-sided filling pressures in the setting of ACS, including IVC engorgement or invasive measurement demonstrating elevation beyond 10 mm Hg, helps corroborate this diagnosis.

The occurrence of shock and low output with RVMI is likely multifactorial, but occurs principally from diminished capacity of the RV for generating adequate LV preload, a problem that is complicated by the effect of a dysknetic and/or dilated RV free wall and/or septum compressing upon the LV while being constrained by the pericardium (**Figure 32-2**). In support of this model, significant RVMI is associated with near-equalization of left- and right-heart filling pressures (RAP:PCWP ≥ 0.8 with normal being

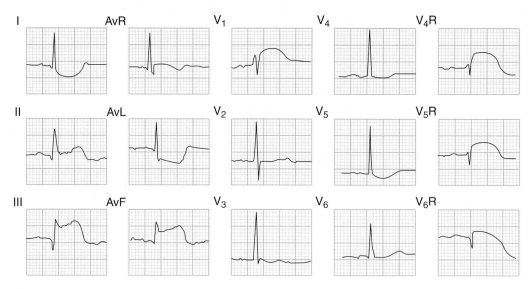

**Figure 32-1.** Sample ECG demonstrating ST elevation in $V_3R$-$V_6R$ in the context of an inferior ST elevation MI. (Courtesy of Dr. Christian Witzke, Massachusetts General Hospital.)

<0.6). The low-output state can be exacerbated further by bradyarrhythmias and AV conduction system block occurring at high frequency with RVMI as compared to non-RV MI. In fact, at least 50% of inferior MIs exhibiting new or intermittent high grade AV block are found to right ventricular involvement. Bradyarrhythmias can be attributed to infarction of sinus node or the atria, or can result simply from reflex vagal hypertonicity with RV dysfunction, both in the setting of acute ischemia and with ischemia-reperfusion injury following successful PCI or thrombolysis. High degree

AV conduction abnormalities are present in 48% of RVMI versus 13% of IMIs lacking significant RV infarction. Both bradyarrhythmias and AV conduction system disturbances must be anticipated and corrected quickly in the setting of RVMI.

Early reperfusion, volume resuscitation, correction of dysrhythmias, and inotropic support are keys for the management of acute MI involving the RV (see **inset box**). Once the diagnosis of RVMI is made, volume resuscitation should

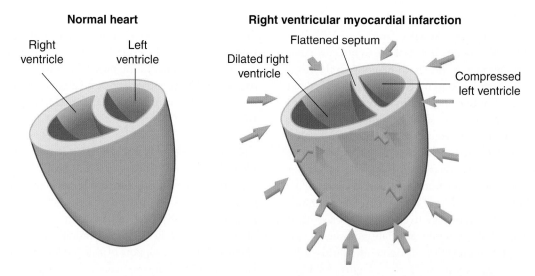

**Figure 32-2.** Pathophysiologic effect of dilated and dyskinetic RV upon LV function. The low-output state is mediated by ventricular interaction (resulting in a flattened septum) and the restraining effect of the pericardium (arrows) during acute right ventricular distention. (Adapted figure from Dell'Italia LJ, *NEJM.* 1998.)

| Table 33-3 • Fibrinolytic Agents | | | | |
|---|---|---|---|---|
| | Reperfusion | Allergies | Heparin | Application |
| **Streptokinase (SK)** | 50% | Yes | In high risk | 30-60 min |
| **Tissue Plasminogen Activator (tPA) (Alteplase)** | 80% | None | Essential | 30 min bolus, then 60 min infusion |
| **Recombinant Plasminogen Activator (rPA) (Reteplase)** | 80% | None | Essential | IV bolus over 2 min, repeat ×1 in 30 min |
| **TNK-tPA (Tenecteplase)** | 80% | None | Essential | Single weight adjusted IV bolus over 5 min |

*Although thrombolysis is the commonest form of treatment for acute MI, it also has important limitations: a rate of recanalization (restoring normal flow) in 90 minutes of only 55% with streptokinase or 60% with accelerated alteplase; a 5-15% risk of early or late reocclusion leading to AMI, worsening ventricular function, or death; a 1-2% risk of intracranial hemorrhage, with 40% mortality; and 15-20% of patients with a contraindication to thrombolysis (From Antman et al., 2004; Pollack Jr et al., 2008).*

degrades fibrin-rich clots. However, plasmin is also a very potent inducer of platelet aggregation. Several clinical trials have demonstrated the beneficial effects of these therapies in reducing mortality rates in patients with suspected acute myocardial infarction. Alteplase is administered as an intravenous infusion. The relatively long half-lives of reteplase and tenecteplase enable bolus administration, which is less time-consuming. Reteplase is administered as a double bolus, and dosing does not depend on the patient's weight; tenecteplase is administered as a single, weight-based bolus. Notably, the ASSENT-2 trial has demonstrated the equality of alteplase and tenecteplase with no difference in mortality between the two agents (Van de Werf et al., 1999) (**Table 33-3**).

## Complications of Fibrinolysis

The main complication of fibrinolysis is the occurrence of bleeding. The most devastating is the development of an intracranial hemorrhage (ICH) carrying a more than 50% mortality and significant morbidity leading to residual neurological symptoms in nearly all survivors of ICH during fibrinolysis. The risk of ICH increases with age, in particular, in those >75 years, in patients with low body weight, and in patients with uncontrolled hypertension (HTN). It is highest with the combined use of fibrinolysis with adjunct therapy (e.g., TNK with low molecular weight heparin). The occurrence of ICH increased from streptokinase to t-PA and TNK to r-PA.

The diagnosis of ICH is usually a clinical and confirmed by imaging such as non-contrast enhanced computed tomography. There is, unfortunately, no treatment for ICH in the setting of fibrinolytic therapy (**Table 33-4**).

## Adjunctive Therapy for Fibrinolysis

### Aspirin (ASA)
As shown early during the investigations on reperfusion therapies in patients with acute MI, aspirin lowers mortality by 20% alone and by around 40% when added to thrombolytic therapy (SK) (ISIS-2, 1988).

### Clopidogrel
The recent COMMIT and CLARITY trials have demonstrated the role of clopidogrel for an improved patency of coronary vessels post-STEMI (Chen et al., 2005; Sabatine et al., 2005). The addition of clopidogrel (300 mg loading dose followed by 75 mg/day) to aspirin (150-325 mg loading dose on the first day followed by 75-162 mg/day) plus a standard fibrinolytic regimen resulted in a 36% reduction in the occurrence of an occluded infarct-related artery or death or recurrent myocardial infarction before angiography in the Clopidogrel as Adjunctive Reperfusion Therapy-Thrombolysis in Myocardial Infarction 28 (CLARITY-TIMI 28) study (Sabatine et al., 2005).

### Low Molecular Weight Heparin (LMWH)
When compared to UFH, treatment with LMWH (enoxaparin) is superior in patients receiving fibrinolysis for STEMI, but it is also associated with an increase in major bleeding episodes (Antman et al., 2006). Since the occurrence of both minor and major bleeding increases, LMWH has a controversial role in the treatment of patients with STEMI. It is contraindicated in patients older than 75 years.

| Table 33-4 • Contraindications to Lysis | |
|---|---|
| **Absolute Contraindication** | **Relative Contraindication** |
| Prior intracranial hemorrhage | Oral anticoagulation (e.g., Coumadin or warfarin) |
| Structural intracranial vascular disease | Pregnancy |
| Known intracranial neoplasm | CVA >3 months |
| Ischemic CVA <3 months | Uncontrolled HTN >180/110 mm Hg |
| Aortic dissection | Recent trauma 2-4 months |
| Significant head/facial trauma <3 months | Recent internal bleeding 2-4 months |

*No contraindications are diabetic retinopathy and menses! (From Antman et al., 2004; Pollack Jr et al., 2008)*

**Table 33-5 • Thrombolysis In Myocardial Infarction (TIMI) Coronary Blood Flow Classification**

| | |
|---|---|
| TIMI 0 flow | Total occlusion, no coronary flow |
| TIMI 1 flow | Penetration of obstruction with no distal perfusion |
| TIMI 2 flow | Slow flow, perfusion only with delayed flow |
| TIMI 3 flow | Normal flow with full perfusion |

*(Reprinted from Antman EM, Anbe DT, Armstrong PW et al. 2004 ACC/AHA guidelines for the management of patients with ST-elevation myocardial infarction: a report of the American College of Cardiology/American Heart Association Task Force on Practice Guidelines (Committee to Revise the 1999 Guidelines for the Management of Patients with Acute Myocardial Infarction). J Am Coll Cardiol. 2004;44:e1–e211 with permission from Elsevier.)*

A Class IIb indication exists for patients <75 years without impaired renal function as an alternative to unfractionated heparin (Antman et al., 2006).

### Gp IIb/IIIa Inhibitors

While Gp IIb/IIIa inhibitors have a clear role in PCI, no benefit has been found in patients with STEMI undergoing fibrinolysis, either as a substitute or as an adjunctive agent to this therapy (Pollack Jr et al., 2008).

## Reperfusion Criteria for Successful Fibrinolysis

Coronary blood flow criteria after successful fibrinolysis have been established by the Thrombolyis in Myocardial Infarction (TIMI) study group (**Table 33-5**).

Criteria for successful reperfusion after fibrinolysis are resolution of ST elevation and/or resolution of chest pain. Potential events after successful reperfusion are reperfusion arrhythmias (ventricular tachycardias, ventricular fibrillation, accelerated idioventricular rhythms, or bradyarrhythmias in up to 50% of patients).

## Pre-hospital Lysis

A pre-hospital use of fibrinolysis can be administered in the ambulance if the transport time to the hospital is longer than 60 minutes in high volume emergency medical service systems (Antman et al., 2004; Pollack Jr et al., 2008). Other factors to consider include the ability to transmit and interpret ECGs and the level of expertise in the management of STEMI. A meta-analysis of six randomized trials comparing pre-hospital versus in-hospital fibrinolysis demonstrated a 17% reduction in all-cause hospital mortality among patients who received pre-hospital fibrinolytic therapy (Morrison et al., 2000). The decreased mortality is explained by a reduction in time to thrombolysis through pre-hospital administration strategy.

## Timing of PCI After Fibrinolysis

### Facilitated PCI

Facilitated PCI, defined as elective PCI after successful fibrinolysis, could provide the advantage of early pharmacologic reperfusion to increase the benefit and use of mechanical reperfusion. Facilitated PCI is a Class IIb recommendation and may be performed in high risk patients under circumstances when immediate PCI is not available and risk of bleeding from pharmacologic treatment is low (Antman et al., 2004; Pollack Jr et al., 2008). Pharmacologic regimens include a full-dose or half-dose fibrinolytic; a glycoprotein (GP) IIb-IIIa inhibitor; or a combination of a reduced-dose fibrinolytic and a GP IIb-IIIa inhibitor. However, a recent meta-analysis of 17 trials involving patients with STEMI who were assigned to either facilitated or primary PCI showed higher mortality and nonfatal reinfarction rates with facilitated PCI (Keeley et al., 2006). In contrast, a recent prospective study involving 254 patients with STEMI reported a significant reduction in the rate of major adverse cardiac endpoints (p = 0.021) and higher TIMI 3 flow rates among patients treated with facilitated PCI compared with primary PCI (Coleman et al., 2006). Patients received either a half dose of reteplase (62.2%), a full dose of reteplase (7.9%), another fibrinolytic agent (6.3%), and/or a GP IIb-IIIa inhibitor (76.4%) followed by facilitated PCI or primary PCI without drug treatment. Overall, the study concluded greater treatment effectiveness and cost savings with facilitated PCI versus primary PCI. These findings require large, multicenter, randomized trials in order to be confirmed.

The recently published Facilitated Intervention with Enhanced Reperfusion Speed to Stop Events (FINESSE) study investigated half-dose reteplase (two 5-U injections given 30 minutes apart) in combination with abciximab in facilitated PCI versus primary PCI to study the benefits of facilitated PCI. The study included 3000 patients arriving for treatment within 6 hours of onset of symptoms of acute myocardial infarction. Neither facilitation of PCI with reteplase plus abciximab nor facilitation with abciximab alone significantly improved the clinical outcomes, as compared with abciximab given at the time of PCI (Ellis et al., 2008).

### Rescue PCI After Failed Fibrinolysis

Rescue PCI, defined as PCI performed within 12 hours after failure of fibrinolytic therapy for patients with ongoing or recurrent STEMI, may provide significant benefit in improving reperfusion and survival after ineffective reperfusion with fibrinolytics (Gershlick et al., 2005). No significant differences were reported in procedural success rates for patients treated with rescue PCI versus primary PCI in a study of 659 patients with STEMI arriving within 12 hours of symptom onset. In addition, rescue PCI also did not increase the risk of major bleeding complications or major adverse cardiac endpoints compared with primary PCI (Ellis et al., 2005). Finally, the REACT trial demonstrated that event-free survival after failed thrombolytic therapy was significantly higher with rescue PCI than with repeated thrombolysis or conservative treatment (Gershlick et al., 2005).

## Suggested Readings

1. Ellis SG, Tendera M, de Belder MA, et al. Facilitated PCI in patients with ST-elevation myocardial infarction. *N Engl J Med.* 2008;358:2205–2217.

2. Gershlick AH, Stephens-Lloyd A, Hughes S et al. Rescue angioplasty after failed thrombolytic therapy for acute myocardial infarction. *N Engl J Med.* 2005;353:2758–2768.

3. Keeley EC, Boura JA, Grines CL. Primary angioplasty versus intravenous thrombolytic therapy for acute myocardial infarction: a quantitative review of 23 randomised trials. *Lancet.* 2003;361:13–20.

4. Pinto DS, Kirtane AJ, Nallamothu BK, et al. Hospital delays in reperfusion for ST-elevation myocardial infarction: implications when selecting a reperfusion strategy. *Circulation.* 2006;114:2019–2025.

5. Pollack CV Jr, Antman EM, Hollander JE. 2007 Focused Update to the ACC/AHA Guidelines for the Management of Patients with ST-Segment Elevation Myocardial Infarction: Implications for Emergency Department Practice. *Ann Emerg Med.* 2008.

# Risk Stratification and Post-Myocardial Infarction Therapy

ERIC S. DAVIDSON AND GEORGE J. PHILIPPIDES

## ● PRACTICAL POINTS

- The short-term risk of major adverse cardiac events in patients with unstable angina and non-STEMI can best be determined by clinician assessment of characteristics of chest pain and previous history of coronary artery disease, presence or absence of abnormal hemodynamic factors, electrocardiographic patterns of ischemia, and cardiac markers.

- Post-myocardial infarction patients who develop clinical manifestations of recurrent ischemia, complex ventricular arrhythmias, and congestive heart failure represent high risk patients requiring aggressive management to help clinicians further define the most appropriate treatment.

- Post-myocardial infarction patients deemed to be low risk on the basis of clinical findings may benefit from additional risk assessment with stress testing.

- Resting left ventricular function should be assessed in all patients with acute myocardial infarction, as this is one of the most accurate predictors of future cardiovascular events.

- Complex ventricular ectopy occurring greater than 48 hours after infarction is much more predictive of future cardiac death than similar arrhythmias occurring within 48 hours of infarction.

## INTRODUCTION

Risk stratification after acute myocardial infarction (AMI) is an integral step toward identifying those patients at higher risk for recurrent cardiovascular events and death. Post-myocardial infarction (post-MI) patients have varying risk for recurrent ischemic events and numerous tools are available to identify higher risk patients who may benefit from therapies that can lessen risk and reduce mortality. The overall prognosis of acute coronary syndromes has improved with increasing use of primary percutaneous intervention (PCI), more aggressive antiplatelet therapy and secondary risk factor modification. However, recurrent ischemia, reinfarction, congestive heart failure (CHF), and sudden cardiac death (SCD) still pose significant risk to the post-MI patient. Post-MI risk stratification is a continuous process that begins with the initial emergency triage and continues throughout the hospital course and into the post-hospital period. Mortality in all acute coronary syndromes remains highest during the index event and within the first month. The in-hospital mortality increases across the spectrum from unstable angina to ST elevation myocardial infarction (STEMI). Interestingly non-ST elevation myocardial infarction (NSTEMI) has been demonstrated to have higher mortality rates further out from the index event (6 months and 1 year). This has been attributed to a higher likelihood of residual ischemia.

## APPROACH TO RISK STRATIFICATION

The approach to post-MI risk assessment can be categorized into five major areas of assessment: (1) clinical risk factors, (2) left ventricular function, (3) stress testing, (4) catheterization, and (5) risk for arrhythmic death.

## Clinical Risk Factors

Myocardial ischemia results from the disruption of a vulnerable plaque and manifests as a broad spectrum of clinical presentations ranging from unstable angina, NSTEMI, and STEMI. Both STEMI and NSTEMI represent ischemic coronary disease of similar etiology and have analogous post infarct risk assessment and treatment strategies with subtle differences. However, unlike patients with STEMI who are typically triaged to a revascularization strategy, NSTEMI patients undergo an early risk stratification process, which helps the clinician decide between early invasive strategy (diagnostic angiography within 4 to 48 hours with intent to perform revascularization) versus early conservative strategy. At the time of an MI, patients often have prior data (i.e., LV function, stress test, or catheterization) that aids in the risk stratification process in the acute infarct setting. However, the assessment of current clinical risk factors is a rapid and easy process that guides the very early management of a myocardial infarction.

### Early NSTEMI Risk Stratification by Clinical Risk Factors

The early risk categorization process with NSTEMI is based on independently associated clinical factors (the medical history, physical exam, ECG, and cardiac biomarkers (**Table 34-1**)) that are associated with a worse short-term

| **Table 34-1 • Short-Term Risk of Death or Nonfatal MI in Patients with UA/NSTEMI*** | | | |
|---|---|---|---|
| **Feature** | **High Risk** *At least 1 of the following features must be present:* | **Intermediate Risk** *No high-risk feature, but must have 1 of the following:* | **Low Risk** *No high- or intermediate-risk feature but may have any of the following features:* |
| History | Accelerating tempo of ischemic symptoms in preceding 48 h | Prior MI, peripheral or cerebrovascular disease, or CABG; prior aspirin use | |
| Character of pain | Prolonged ongoing (greater than 20 min) rest pain | Prolonged (greater than 20 min) rest angina, now resolved, with moderate or high likelihood of CAD Rest angina (greater than 20 min) or relieved with rest or sublingual NTG Nocturnal angina New-onset or progressive CCS class III or IV angina in the past 2 weeks without prolonged (greater than 20 min) rest pain but with intermediate or high likelihood of CAD (see Table 6) | Increased angina frequency, severity, or duration Angina provoked at a lower threshold New onset angina with onset 2 weeks to 2 months prior to presentation |
| Clinical findings | Pulmonary edema, most likely due to ischemia New or worsening MR murmur S3 or new/worsening rates Hypotension, bradycardia, tachycardia Age greater than 75 years | Age greater than 70 years | |
| ECG | Angina at rest with translent ST-segment changes greater than 0.5 mm Bundle-branch block, new or presumed new Sustained ventricular tachycardia | T-wave changes Pathological Q waves or resting ST-depression less than 1 mm in multiple lead groups (anterior, inferior, lateral) | Normal or unchanged ECG |
| Cardiac markers | Elevated cardiac TnT, TnI, or CK-MB (e.g., TnT or TnI greater than 0.1 ng per mL) | Slightly elevated cardiac TnT, TnI, or CK-MB (e.g., TnT greater than 0.01 but less than 0.1 ng per mL) | Normal |

*Estimation of the short-term risks of death and nonfatal cardiac ischemia events in UA (or NSTEMI) is a complex multivariable problem that cannot be fully specified in a table such as this: therefore, this table is meant to offer general guidance and illustration rather than right algorithms. Adapted from AHCPR Clinical Practice Guidelines No. 10. Unstable Angina: Diagnosis and Management, May 1994 (124).

CABG = coronary artery bypass graft surgery; CAD = coronary artery disease; CCS = Canadian Cardiovascular Society; CK-MB = creatine kinase, MB fraction; ECG = electrocardiogram; MI = myocardial infarction; MR = mitral regurgitation; NTG = nitroglycerine; TnI = troponin I; TnT = troponin T; UA/NSTEMI = unstable angina/non-ST-elevation myocardial infarction.

(Reprinted with permission from: Anderson, J, Adams, C, Antman, E, et al. ACC/AHA 2007 guidelines for the management of patients with unstable angina/non-ST-elevation myocardial infarction. J Am Coll Cardiol. 2007; 116:803–877.)

outcome. This early risk stratification step relies on these basic clinical variables and enables the swift triage of high risk NSTEMI patients to an invasive strategy. Risk is highest during the acute phase of MI, and these simple clinical variables can identify the category for patients early and rapidly. A history of present illness (HPI) suggestive of an accelerating course of ischemic symptoms and pain characterized as prolonged (greater than 20 minutes) puts patients at high short-term risk and typically warrants an early invasive strategy. Additionally, clinical findings such as pulmonary edema, jugular venous distinction, S3 gallop, peripheral hypo-perfusion, hypotension, bradycardia, or tachycardia place patients at high short-term risk. Many of these physical exam features correlate with intermediate to advanced Killip class and highlight active heart failure as a poor prognostic marker.

## 12-Lead ECG

The 12-lead ECG should be done within 10 minutes of patient arrival to the emergency department if there is suspicion of acute coronary syndrome. The ECG provides important information regarding location, size, and presence of ongoing ischemia and conduction abnormalities. The magnitude, location, extent, and nature (recurrent or persistent) of ST segment changes relate to worse prognosis. ST depressions greater than or equal to 0.5 mm that are associated with symptoms at rest suggest severe CAD.

Various findings on ECG relate to increased cardiovascular risk; these include: multiple leads showing ST-segment elevation, a high degree of ST-segment elevation, persistent horizontal or down-sloping ST-segment depression, persistent or advanced heart block, Q waves in multiple leads, RV infarct pattern accompanied with inferior infarction, and ST-segment depressions in anterior leads in patients with inferior infarction. When corrected for infarct size, mortality is higher in patients experiencing an anterior wall MI compared to an inferior wall MI. It is important to recognize that roughly 4% of MI patients may present with isolated ST elevations in the posterior (leads V7-V9). These patients should be managed as ST-elevation MI even though ST elevations are not present on the standard 12-lead ECG.

### Cardiac Biomarkers

Conventional markers for myocardial damage today include troponin-I or T, creatine kinase (CK), and CK-MB. A cardiac-specific troponin is the preferred biomarker. Patients with a negative biomarker test within 6 hours of the onset of symptoms should have markers remeasured within 8-12 hours of symptom onset. Although these laboratory tests should be performed, they should not delay implementation of a reperfusion therapy if other clinical factors (medical history, character of pain, clinical findings, ECG) indicate high short-term risk. Cardiac-specific troponin levels have a linear predicative nature of mortality rates at roughly 40 days post infarct (**Figure 34-1**).

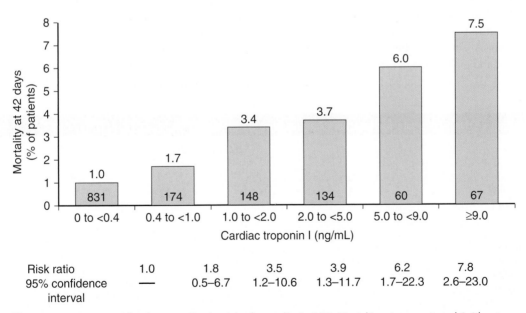

| Risk ratio | 1.0 | 1.8 | 3.5 | 3.9 | 6.2 | 7.8 |
| 95% confidence interval | — | 0.5–6.7 | 1.2–10.6 | 1.3–11.7 | 1.7–22.3 | 2.6–23.0 |

**Figure 34-1.** Troponin I levels to predict the risk of mortality in ACS. Mortality rates are at 42 d (without adjustment for baseline characteristics) in patients with acute coronary syndrome. The numbers at the bottom of each bar are the numbers of patients with cardiac troponin I levels in each range, and the numbers above the bars are percentages. p less than 0.001 for the increase in the mortality rate (and the risk ratio for mortality) with increasing levels of cardiac troponin I at enrollment. (Reprinted with permission from Antman EM, Tanasijevic MJ, Thompson B, et al. Cardiac-specific troponin I levels to predict the risk of mortality in patients with acute coronary syndromes. *N Engl J Med.* 1996;335:1342–1349(201). Copyright © 1996 Massachusetts Medical Society. All rights reserved. From Anderson J, et al. *J Am Coll Cardiol.* 2007.)

## Risk Stratification Scores

In addition to the very early assessment of short-term risk with clinical factors as outlined in **Table 34-1**, there are multiple risk stratification models developed from multivariate analysis that have been validated in large cohorts of patients. These integrated risk tools incorporate the most effective predictive variables for patient risk-stratification; they are designed to estimate the risk of death and nonfatal cardiac events in the short term and beyond. These risk scores are multifaceted and are useful to guide management (i.e., help the clinician decide which patients would benefit most from the early invasive versus conservative strategy in the NSTEMI setting). Additionally, the risk scores can help identify lower risk patients in order to allow for an early discharge, and they can calculate future risk of cardiovascular events and death. The most widely utilized models—Thrombolysis in Myocardial Infarction (TIMI) and Global Registry of Acute Coronary Events (GRACE)—use basic clinical variables to categorize patients into low risk, intermediate-risk and high risk groups.

*TIMI Score* The TIMI risk score is designed for NSTEMI and STEMI and is based on scales ranging from 0-7 and 0-14, respectively (**Table 34-2**). The 7-point scale applied to the NSTEMI patient consists of 7 (1-point) risk indicators which predict all-cause mortality, new or recurrent MI, or severe recurrent ischemia. One point is given for each of the following variables; age (>65 years), at least 3 CAD risk factors, prior coronary stenosis >50%, ST-segment deviation on ECG, at least 2 anginal events in prior 24 hours, use of aspirin within 7 days, and elevated serum cardiac biomarkers. A TIMI risk score of <2-3 constitutes a lower risk patient and makes up more than 50% of patients presenting with AMI. A higher TIMI risk score correlates

with increased cardiovascular events and all-cause mortality at 14 days and 6 weeks.

*GRACE Score* The GRACE risk model has been validated for in-hospital and 6-month outcomes in the setting of NSTEMI (**Figure 34-2**). The prediction score is based on 9 variables, which include: age, history of congestive heart failure, history of MI, resting heart rate, systolic blood pressure, ST-segment depression, initial serum creatinine, elevated cardiac biomarkers, and whether in-hospital percutaneous coronary intervention (PCI) is utilized. The sum of 9 scores is applied to a reference nomogram, which predicts all-cause mortality from hospital discharge to 6 months.

All the above mentioned clinical variables and models help predict future risk, but age alone strongly correlates with risk of death in the setting of myocardial infarction and is the most well-reproduced clinical variable. Older patients are more likely to have a prior history of MI, advanced CAD, and develop CHF and cardiogenic shock.

## Early Management of NSTEMI Using Clinical Risk Factors

Typically, when high risk clinical factors are identified in the very early risk stratification process (**Table 34-1**) patients undergo an early invasive strategy, absent any contraindications (**Figure 34-3**). In addition to these high risk clinical findings of **Table 34-1**, other factors—including sustained ventricular tachycardia, PCI within 6 months, prior coronary artery bypass grafting (CABG), reduced LV function, and a high risk score (e.g., TIMI or GRACE)—contribute to the decision to pursue an early invasive strategy (**Table 34-3**). Additionally, high-risk

| Table 34-2 • TIMI Risk Score for Unstable Angina/Non-ST-Elevation MI | | | | | | |
|---|---|---|---|---|---|---|
| | **TIMI Risk Score** | | | | | |
| | **0–1** | **2** | **3** | **4** | **5** | **6–7** |
| **All-Cause Mortality, New or Recurrent MI, or Severe Recurrent Ischemia Requiring Urgent Revascularization Through 14 d after Randomization, %** | 4.7 | 8.3 | 13.2 | 19.9 | 26.2 | 40.9 |
| **TIMI Risk Factors** | Age (>65 years) | At least 3 CAD risk factors | Prior coronary stenosis > 50%, ST segment deviation on ECG factors | At least 2 anginal events in prior 24 hours | Use of aspirin within 7 days | Elevated serum cardiac biomarkers |

The TIMI risk score is determined by the sum of the presence of 7 variables at admission; 1 point is given for each of the following variables; age 65 y or older; at least 3 risk factors for CAD; prior coronary stenosis of 50% or more; ST-segment deviation on ECG presentation; at least 2 anginal events in prior 24 h; use of aspirin in prior 7 d; elevated serum cardiac biomarkers. Prior coronary stenosis of 50% or more remained relatively insensitive to missing information and remained a significant predictor of events. CAD, coronary artery disease; ECG, electrocardiogram; MI, myocardial infarction; y, year.

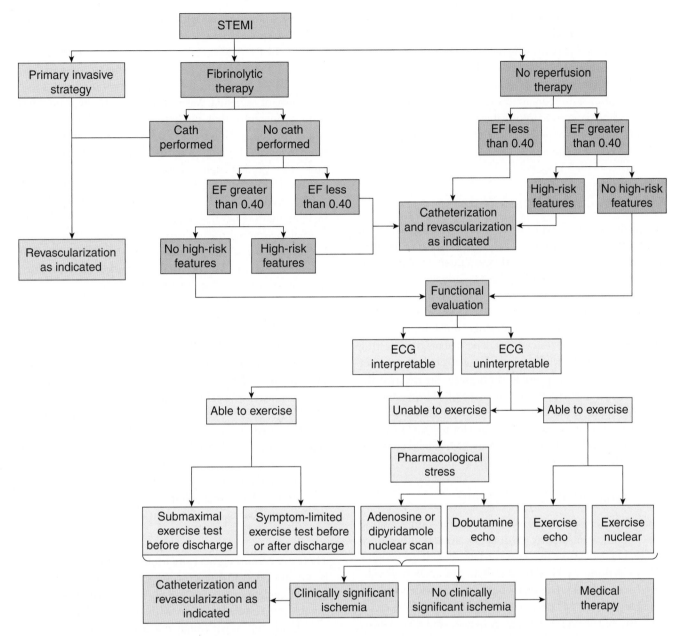

**Figure 34-5.** Evidence-based approach to need for catheterization (cath) and revascularization after STEMI. The algorithm treatment paths for patients who initially undergo a primary invasive strategy, receive fibrinolytic therapy, or do not undergo reperfusion therapy for STEMI. Patients who have not undergone a primary invasive strategy and have no high-risk features should undergo functional evaluation with one of the noninvasive tests shown. When clinically significant ischemia is detected, patients should undergo catheterization and revascularization as indicated; if no clinically significant ischemia is detected, medical therapy is prescribed after STEMI. (From: Antman, EM et al. ACC/AHA Guidelines for the Management of Patients with ST-Elevation Myocardial Infarction. *Circulation.* 2004.)

stress with imaging (typically nuclear and echocardiography). For the clinician considering stress testing, the ACC/AHA guidelines recommend the exercise ECG as the primary noninvasive stress testing tool if the patient is able to exercise and the 12-lead ECG is interpretable. In patients with baseline ECG abnormalities that compromise interpretation, echocardiography or myocardial perfusion imaging should be added to standard exercise testing. However, the incremental value of adding imaging to a regular exercise test after AMI has not been established. There is no indication for a pharmacological stress test if the patient is able to exercise, unless concerns are raised regarding the presence of viable myocardium in which other modalities can be utilized (dobutamine, rest-redistribution thallium, positron emission tomography (PET) and magnetic resonance imaging (MRI)).

Stress testing (with or without imaging) in the post-infarction time period can be useful in: (1) risk stratification of post-infarction patients who have not undergone an invasive strategy (both NSTEMI and STEMI); (2) assessment of partially revascularized myocardium for ischemia; (3) establishment of exercise parameters for cardiac rehabilitation; (4) providing prognostic information and reassurance to the patient; and (5) evaluation of the efficacy of the patients, current medical regimen.

## Submaximal and Symptom-limited Stress Tests

Submaximal testing, typically defined as 70% of maximum heart rate, can be performed safely at 4-6 days after an AMI if patients are symptom-free with respect to heart failure, angina, or arrhythmias for 12-24 hours. Early after discharge, symptom-limited exercise testing can be performed at 14-21 days for prognostic assessment, activity prescription, evaluation of medical therapy, and for cardiac rehabilitation if the predischarge exercise test was not done. Submaximal testing in the predischarge window has adequate predictive power compared to what is possible if one waits in the postdischarge time frame to perform a more maximal level of stress. Exercise testing is not utilized if severe comorbidities likely limit life expectancy and/or candidacy for revascularization. Patients taking beta-blockers after an AMI should continue them at the time of exercise testing.

## Key Variables of Stress Testing

Post-MI patients who are unable to undergo stress testing due to clinical instability or disabling comorbidities have the highest adverse cardiac event rate. For those patients able to perform exercise testing there are many well-validated exercise test predictors. The three most widely utilized variables in post-MI exercise testing include: (1) exercise capacity, (2) exercise-induced ischemia, and (3) systolic blood pressure. One of the strongest and most consistent prognostic markers is maximum exercise capacity. Exercise duration or workload expressed as metabolic equivalent unit (MET) provides a standard measurement of exercise capacity. A functional capacity <5 METs is a poor prognostic indicator. Exercise-induced ischemia is measured by the 12-lead ECG. ST-segment depression greater than or equal to 1 mm in leads (without pathological Q waves and not in lead aVR), particularly if in conjunction with symptoms at a low level of exercise or in the presence of controlled heart failure, is a poor prognostic indicator. A failure to increase systolic blood pressure by 30 mm Hg, peak systolic blood pressure <110 mm Hg, or exercise-induced hypotension are also poor prognostic indicators.

Patients who cannot achieve a 4-5 MET workload or develop ischemia at a low level of exercise or have an abnormal

blood pressure response with exercise should not have any further stress testing and should undergo catheterization. (**Figure 34-6**) Additionally, if imaging is indicated various findings confer high risk, and in general these include (**Table 34-4**) significant LV dysfunction or moderate to severe areas of ischemia. More specifically, findings on stress echocardiography that predict high risk for adverse outcomes include: resting LVEF of 35% or less and wall motion score index >1. Findings on stress radionuclide ventriculography that predict high risk for adverse outcomes include: exercise LVEF <50%, resting LVEF <35%, or a fall in LVEF ≥10%. Findings on stress radionuclide myocardial perfusion imaging that predict high risk for adverse event include: abnormal myocardial tracer distribution in more than 1 coronary region at rest or with stress a large anterior defect that reperfuses; abnormal myocardial distribution with increased lung uptake; and cardiac enlargement.

## Indications for Stress Testing

For NSTEMI and STEMI patients initially deemed to be low or intermediate risk during the post-MI phase by clinical markers and/or who have not undergone diagnostic catheterization, the results of an exercise test at 4-7 days, 14-21 days, or 3-6 weeks helps determine whether further imaging-based stress testing or catheterization is indicated (**Figures 34-4** and **34-5**). The ACC/AHA Guideline Update for Exercise Testing (**Figure 34-6**) indicates that if clinically significant ischemia is detected on any type of stress test (submaximal, symptom-limited, exercise alone, imaging, or pharmacologic), then catheterization with intent to revascularize is warranted.

There are certain clinical situations in which stress testing is not indicated in the post-MI setting. The ACC/AHA STEMI guidelines recommend all STEMI patients that are suitable for revascularization with LVEF <40% and those with LVEF >40% with high risk features undergo angiography without stress testing. The ACC/AHA NSTEMI guidelines recommend that the NSTEMI patient with high risk features or any clinically significant subsequent events during an initial conservative strategy undergo diagnostic angiography without stress testing (**Figure 34-4**).

Stress testing is indicated in the STEMI patient that has not undergone catheterization, with an LVEF >40% and without high-risk features (**Figure 34-5**). The initial conservative NSTEMI patient (without high risk features or without subsequent significant events) can either undergo assessment LVEF or a stress test for further risk stratification (**Figure 34-4**). In this setting if a stress test is not low risk or LVEF is <40%, diagnostic angiography is indicated.

Another subset of AMI patients with indications for stress testing includes those who were partially revascularized and

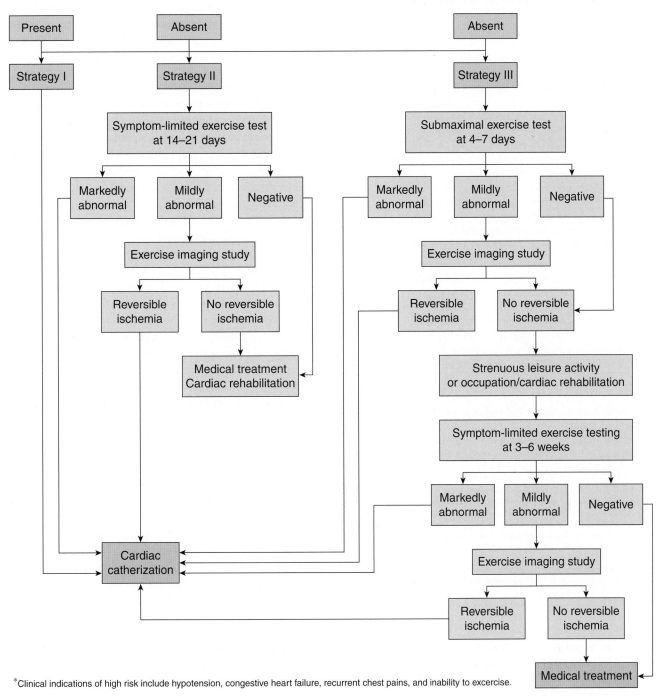

Clinical indications of high risk at predischarge*

*Clinical indications of high risk include hypotension, congestive heart failure, recurrent chest pains, and inability to excercise.

**Figure 34-6.** Strategies for exercise test evaluation soon after myocardial infarction. If patients are at high risk for ischemic events, base on clinical criteria, they should undergo invasive evaluation to determine if they are candidates for coronary revascularization procedures (strategy I). For patients initially deemed to be at low risk at the time of discharge after myocardial infarction, two strategies for performing exercise testing can be used. One is a symptom-limited exercise test at 14 to 21 days (strategy II). If the patient is on digoxin or if the baseline electrocardiogram precludes accurate interpretation of ST-segment changes (eg, baseline left bundle branch block or left ventricular hypertrophy), then an initial exercise imaging study could be performed. The results of exercise testing should be stratified to determine the need for additional invasive or exercise perfusion studies. Another strategy (strategy III) is to perform a submaximal exercise test at 4 to 7 days after myocardial infarction or just before hospital discharge. The exercise test results could be stratified using the guidelines in strategy I. If the exercise test studies are negative, a second symptom-limited exercise test could be repeated at 3 to 6 weeks for patients undergoing vigorous activity during leisure time activities, at work, or exercise training as part of cardiac rehabilitation. The extent of reversible ischemia on the exercise imaging study should be considered before proceeding to cardiac catheterization. A small area contiguous to the infarct zone may not necessarily require catheterization.

**Table 34-4 • Noninvasive Risk Stratification**

High risk (greater than 3% annual mortality rate)
  Severe resting LV dysfunction (LVEF less than 0.35)
  High risk treadmill score (score −11 or less)
  Severe exercise LV dysfunction (exercise LVEF less than 0.35)
  Stress-induced large perfusion defect (particularly if anterior)
  Stress-induced multiple perfusion defects of moderate size
  Large fixed perfusion defect with LV dilation or increased lung uptake (thallium-201)
  Stress-induced moderate perfusion defect with LV dilation or increased lung uptake (thallium-201)
  Echocardiographic wall-motion abnormality (involving more than 2 segments) developing at low dose of dobutamine (10 mcg per kg per min or less) or at a low heart rate (less than 120 beats per min)
  Stress echocardiographic evidence of extensive ischemia

Intermediate risk (1% to 3% annual mortality rate)
  Mild/moderate resting LV dysfunction (LVEF = 0.35 to 0.49)
  Intermediate-risk treadmill score (−11 to 5)
  Stress-induced moderate perfusion defect without LV dilation or increased lung intake (thallium-201)
  Limited stress echocardiographic ischemia with a wall-motion abnormality only at higher doses of dobutamine involving less than or equal to 2 segments

Low risk (less than 1% annual mortality rate)
  Low-risk treadmill score (score 5 or greater)
  Normal or small myocardial perfusion defect at rest or with stress*
  Normal stress echocardiographic wall motion or no change of limited resting wall-motion abnormalities during stress*

*Although the published data are limited, patients with these findings will probably not be at low risk in the presence of either a high-risk treadmill score or severe resting LV dysfunction (LVEF less than 0.35). Reproduced from Table 23 in Gibbons RJ. Abrams J. Chatterjee K. et al. ACC/AHA 2002 guidelines update fro the management of patients with chronic stable angina: a report of the American College of Cardiology/American Heart Association Task Force on Practice Guidelines (Committee to Update the 1999 Guidelines for the Management of Patients with Chronic Stable Angina). 2002, Available at: www.acc.org/qualityandscience/clinicalstatements.hm(4). LV = left ventricular; LVEF = left ventricular ejection fraction.

warrant an ischemic evaluation of a coronary lesion with questionable severity. This particular situation requires an imaging modality (preferable with exercise) or a pharmacologic stress (dipyridamole, adenosine, or dobutamine) if these patients are unable to exercise. Similar to exercise testing, pharmacologically stressed patients must be symptom-free with respect to heart failure, angina, or arrhythmias for 12-24 hours prior to testing.

## CATHETERIZATION

Cardiac catheterization serves as a risk stratification tool for patients who have not undergone angiography during the early infarction time frame. Not every AMI patient is a candidate for catheterization based on other comorbidities agrees to an invasive procedure or requires it. The ACC/AHA NSTEMI guidelines state a patient appropriately triaged to an initial conservative strategy with a low risk stress test can be treated with maximum medical therapy (**Figure 34-4**).

Coronary angiography is considered the traditional gold standard for the assessment of obstructive coronary disease. Although there are limitations with respect this test's ability to determine the functional significance of a coronary stenosis and inability to predict which plaques are more likely to cause an acute coronary syndrome, the extent and severity of coronary disease is a powerful clinical predictor of long-term outcome. The acute coronary syndrome patient that is triaged to an early invasive strategy allows for further risk stratification based upon the degree of coronary stenosis. Higher risk patients are categorized as having more severe coronary artery disease (CAD) such as left main, proximal left anterior descending artery or 3-vessel disease. These patients may have concomitant depressed left ventricular systolic function. The invasive strategy can identify up to 20% of patients with no significant coronary stenosis and 20% who gain survival benefit from coronary artery bypass grafting (CABG) such as those with 3-vessel disease and LV dysfunction or left main CAD. The other 60-70% of patients who obtain PCI of a culprit lesion have reduction of subsequent hospitalizations and need for multiple antiangina medications, but gain no clear mortality benefit.

The most widely accepted classification of CAD categorizes patients into 1-vessel, 2-vessel, 3-vessel, or left main, CAD. In the Coronary Artery Surgical Study (CASS) group of medically treated patients, the 12-year survival rate of patients with normal coronary arteries was 91% compared to 74% for those with 1-vessel disease, 59% for those with 2-vessel disease, and 40% for those with 3-vessel disease. Recent angiographic studies indicate that severe coronary stenosis may correlate with more angiographic insignificant plaque elsewhere in the coronary tree, and the higher mortality rate in patients with multivessel CAD may correlate with more potential sites for acute coronary syndrome in these mildly stenotic areas.

## RISK FOR ARRHYTHMIC DEATH

All post-MI patients are at increased risk for sudden cardiac death (SCD) due to ventricular tachyarrhythmias (morphologically referred to as ventricular fibrillation, polymorphic VT, or monomorphic VT). Approximately one-half of arrhythmic deaths occur within the first year after an AMI. In general the risk for arrhythmic death associated with myocardial infarction relates to the degree of resultant left ventricular dysfunction and occurrence of ventricular arrhythmias. LV dysfunction is a major entry criterion in all

# · 35

# Cardiogenic Shock

AMAR R. CHADAGA AND TIMOTHY A. SANBORN

---

## ● PRACTICAL POINTS

- Mortality from cardiogenic shock remains high (50%) despite improved therapeutic attempts with intra-aortic balloon pump (IABP) supported primary PCI.

- Mortality predictors for cardiogenic shock include age, prior myocardial infarction, physical findings of shock, oliguria, and echocardiographic findings of a low ejection fraction (less than 28%) and mitral regurgitation.

- Severe left ventricular failure is the most common cause of cardiogenic shock (78.5%). Other causes include acute mitral regurgitation, ruptured ventricular septum, right ventricular failure, and pericardial tamponade.

- Acute myocardial infarction complicated by severe left ventricular failure results in findings of pulmonary congestion, signs of systemic hypoperfusion,

- and severe systemic hypotension, all of which are classic signs of cardiogenic shock. However, these findings are not common at time of admission but frequently develop within 24 hours of admission.

- Early revascularization with coronary artery bypass grafting or percutaneous intervention is a Class I indication for treatment of cardiogenic shock in patients <75 years of age.

- Fibrinolytic therapy is recommended for cardiogenic shock when patients are unsuitable for invasive approach, when a cardiac catheterization laboratory is not immediately available, and when there is no contraindication for fibrinolysis.

- Recommended therapy for cardiogenic shock includes pressors, intra-aortic balloon pump, and revascularization.

---

## INTRODUCTION

Cardiogenic shock represents the most ominous challenge in acute myocardial infarction (MI), with historic mortality rates approaching 90%. Although the pathophysiology varies, this chapter will address cardiogenic shock as a complication of acute MI with subsequent left ventricular failure leading to refractory hypotension and hypoperfusion. Historically, the frequency with which cardiogenic shock complicates acute MI has remained unchanged at approximately 8-9%.

An encouraging trend toward decreased incidence and mortality from cardiogenic shock has been demonstrated in recent investigations. Increased use of intra-aortic balloon pump (IABP) counterpulsation and emergent coronary

reperfusion strategies are thought to be the basis for these improvements in incidence and mortality. Thus, in cardiogenic shock, primary percutaneous coronary intervention (PCI) and placement of an IABP are currently American College of Cardiology (ACC)/American Heart Association (AHA) Class I recommendations in young patients. Recently, data from 775 hospitals with revascularization capability revealed mortality rates in cardiogenic shock decreased dramatically from 60.3% in 1995 to 47.9% in 2004, according to the Second, Third, and Fourth National Registry of Myocardial Infarction (NRMI-2, NRMI-3, NRMI-4).

Cardiogenic shock continues to cause unacceptably high mortality rates, despite the aforementioned trends in mortality and incidence. The Should We Emergently Revascularize Occluded Coronaries for Cardiogenic Shock (SHOCK)

Trial conducted by Dr. Judith Hochman and colleagues and the corresponding SHOCK registry have provided a myriad of opportunities to study this destructive entity more closely. A description of cardiogenic shock and a review of the current medical and percutaneous interventions are presented in this chapter.

## PREDICTORS OF MORTALITY AND ETIOLOGY

Notwithstanding the aforementioned survival benefits correlated with IABP and primary PCI, current in-hospital mortality for cardiogenic shock remains extremely high at around 50% for all age groups. However, there is a significantly higher mortality among patients over the age of 75 years, a group of patients who continue to suffer devastating mortality rates of 60-70% compared to younger patients in whom mortality is about 40-50%.

Age confers a strong impact on mortality in cardiogenic shock. Numerous studies have attempted to identify further risk factors for mortality in shock and an analysis from the Global Utilization of Streptokinase and Tissue Plasminogen Activator for Occluded Coronary Arteries (GUSTO-I) database identified four such predictors: increasing age (odds ratio 1.49 for each 10 year increase), prior MI, physical findings at the time of diagnosis (presence of altered sensorium and cold, clammy skin), and oliguria. Furthermore, given that most patients with cardiogenic shock complicating an acute MI have severe coronary disease, the SHOCK trial registry revealed variable mortality with the location of the culprit lesion. Mortality was found to be higher in patients with a left main or saphenous vein graft lesion than in those with a circumflex, left anterior descending, or right coronary artery lesion (79 and 70% versus 37 to 42%, respectively). Left ventricular ejection fraction (LVEF) and severity of mitral regurgitation (MR) were found to be the only independent echocardiographic predictors of outcome in a substudy from the SHOCK trial. Of 169 cardiogenic shock patients who underwent echocardiography, the survival at one year was 24% for those with an LVEF of <28% (versus 56% for those with a higher LVEF). Survival at 1 year was 31% for those patients with moderate or severe MR (versus 58% for those with mild or no MR). Lastly, although cardiogenic shock was significantly more common with ST elevation infarcts, the mortality rate in patients in cardiogenic shock did not differ significantly between those with an ST-elevation myocardial infarction (STEMI) or those with a non-ST elevation acute coronary syndrome (ACS).

Several complications of acute MI can induce cardiogenic shock. As stated above, moderate or severe MR, likely resulting from rupture of a papillary muscle or chordae tendineae or severe papillary muscle dysfunction, portends poorer survival in cardiogenic shock. However, the most frequent cause of cardiogenic shock complicating an acute MI is severe dysfunction of the left ventricle, which occurs most often with an anterior MI. Other complications of acute MI causing cardiogenic shock include ventricular septal rupture, right ventricular failure, and tamponade. In a review of 1190 patients from the SHOCK registry, the frequency of these causes was evaluated. Left ventricular failure was the predominant cause of cardiogenic shock in 78.5% patients, while severe mitral regurgitation, ventricular septal rupture, right ventricular failure, and tampondae were the causes of cardiogenic shock in 6.9%, 3.9%, 2.8%, and 1.4% of patients, respectively. Rupture of the ventricular septum post-MI resulting in cardiogenic shock was the harbinger of the worst outcome with the mortality reaching 87.3% (**Table 35-1**).

## CLINICAL MANIFESTATIONS, TIME OF ONSET, AND DIAGNOSIS

Acute MI complicated by severe left ventricular failure leads to a three classic signs: clinical signs of pulmonary congestion, signs of systemic hypoperfusion, and severe systemic hypotension. Pulmonary congestion manifests itself in roughly two-thirds of the cases of left ventricular failure post MI with resultant dyspnea, rales, and pulmonary edema. Signs of systemic hypoperfusion are the aforementioned altered sensorium, cold clammy skin, and oliguria. Hypotension is classically caused by a marked decrease in left ventricular ejection fraction due to the MI and leads to an increase in systemic vascular resistance in order to maintain blood pressure. This elevated systemic vascular resistance results in a reduction in tissue perfusion. With hypotension, perfusion is further reduced in the coronary arteries. This results in additional left ventricular dysfunction and further hypotension and hypoperfusion, leading to a vicious cycle ultimately culminating in death if not interrupted.

The signs and symptoms mentioned above are very infrequently present on hospital admission. In a report from the GUSTO-I trial of 41,000 patients with acute MI, 5.3% of the patients developed shock after hospital admission while 0.8% of patients were in cardiogenic shock on admission. However, although not present on admission, the majority of patients who develop shock after admission will do so within the first 24 hours post infarct. The SHOCK trial demonstrated that the median time from MI to the onset of cardiogenic shock was 5.5 hours, and 75% of patients who developed shock did so within 24 hours. Cardiogenic shock that develops later may be related to mechanical complications such as rupture of a papillary muscle, ventricular free wall, or ventricular septum.

**Table 35-1 • Summary of American College of Cardiology and American Heart Association Recommendations in Cardiogenic Shock**

| Recommendation | Description |
|---|---|
| Class I | • Intra-aortic balloon counterpulsation is recommended for STEMI patients when cardiogenic shock is not quickly reversed with pharmacological therapy. The IABP is a stabilizing measure for angiography and prompt revascularization. (Level of evidence: B)<br>• Intra-arterial monitoring is recommended for the management of STEMI patients with cardiogenic shock. (Level of evidence: C)<br>• Early revascularization, either PCI or CABG, is recommended for patients <75 years with ST elevation or LBBB who develop shock within 36 hours of MI and are suitable for revascularization that can be performed within 18 hours of shock, unless further support is futile because of the patient's wishes or contraindications/unsuitability for further invasive care. (Level of evidence: A)<br>• Fibrinolytic therapy should be administered to STEMI patients with cardiogenic shock who are unsuitable for further invasive care and do not have contraindications to fibrinolysis. (Level of evidence: B)<br>• Echocardiography should be used to evaluate mechanical complications unless these are assessed by invasive measures. (Level of evidence: C) |
| Class IIa | • Pulmonary artery catheter monitoring can be useful for the management of STEMI patients with cardiogenic shock. (Level of evidence: C)<br>• Early revascularization, either PCI or CABG, is reasonable for selected patients ≥75 years with ST elevation or LBBB who develop shock within 36 hours of MI and are suitable for revascularization that can be performed within 18 hours of shock. Patients with good prior functional status who agree to invasive care may be selected for such an invasive strategy. (Level of evidence: B) |

In order to rule out a mechanical etiology to cardiogenic shock, an emergency echocardiogram is warranted. Echocardiography is an ACC/AHA Class I (Level of evidence: C) recommendation in an acute MI complicated by cardiogenic shock (**Table 35-1, Figures 35-1 to 35-3**).

In addition to echocardiography, several other diagnostic modalities are recommended in the setting of cardiogenic shock. Pulmonary artery catheterization is recommended in those patients with suspected mechanical complication of ST elevation MI if an echocardiogram has not been

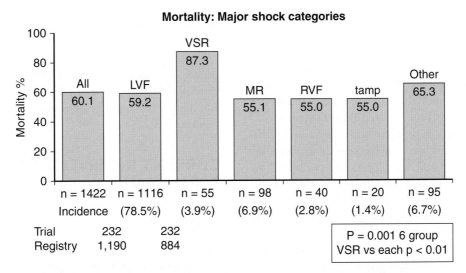

**Figure 35-1.** The complete population of all shock patients screened, including 1190 registered patients and 232 Trial patients randomized concurrent with the Registry from 4/93 to 8/97, is represented in the figure. Of the 1116 patients with LVF, 884 were Registry and 232 were Trial. The mortality rates for the 1190 Registry patients and 884 LVF Registry patients are 61.4% and 60.8%, respectively. The incidence (%, below each bar) and mortality for the major shock categories is shown. LVF, predominant LV failure; RVF, isolated RV shock; MR, acute severe mitral regurgitation; VSR, ventricular septal rupture; Tamp, cardiac tamponade/rupture. (Hochman, *J Am Coll Cardiol* 36:1063,2000.)

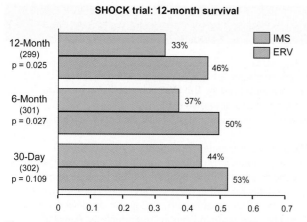

**SHOCK trial: 12-month survival**

**Figure 35-2.** Survival at 30 days, 6 months and 1 year in the SHOCK trial comparing strategies of early revascularization with either PCI or CABG (pink bars) to intensive medical therapy (green bars).

performed and in patients with progressive hypotension who are unresponsive to fluid administration or when fluid administration may be contraindicated. Pulmonary arterial catheterization is an ACC/AHA Class IIa (Level of evidence: C) recommendation, while intra-arterial pressure monitoring is an ACC/AHA Class I (Level of evidence: C) recommendation in the setting of cardiogenic shock (**Table 35-1**).

# CURRENT MEDICAL TREATMENTS

## Aspirin, Heparin, and Glycoprotein IIa/IIIb Inhibitors

Although neither aspirin nor intravenous heparin infusion has been evaluated in the setting of cardiogenic shock, both have proven to reduce mortality in acute MI and thus should be considered in acute MI complicated by cardiogenic shock. In a subgroup analysis from the Platelet Glycoprotein IIb/IIIa in Unstable Angina: Receptor Suppression Using Integrilin Therapy (PURSUIT) trial, the impact of eptifibatide on cardiogenic shock was evaluated. Although eptifibatide did not affect the incidence of shock, patients who developed shock and were treated with eptifibatide had a significantly reduced incidence of death at 30 days when compared to those patients receiving placebo. Glycoprotein IIb/IIIa inhibitors use in combination with primary PCI and stents in cardiogenic shock is discussed in further detail below.

## Sympathomimetic Inotropic and Vasopressor Agents

The two first-line agents that should be used in the setting of cardiogenic shock remain dopamine and norepinephrine. Dopamine is most often used, usually in alpha-agonist doses. Norepinephrine is also a potent vasopressor and given when the response to dopamine is inadequate. However, as discussed previously, patients in cardiogenic shock classically have an elevated systemic vascular resistance and these two medications further increase systemic vascular resistance. To avoid this, rapid institution of mechanical support devices such as IABP are preferred. In addition, possible alternatives to strict vasopressors include dobutamine or milrinone, which produce vasodilation in addition to their inotropy. Given the possibility of vasodilation and further hypotension, these medications, especially dobutamine should be reserved to those normotensive patients with low cardiac index and a high pulmonary capillary wedge pressure. Given the classic increase in systemic vascular resistance seen in cardiogenic shock, L-NMMA (tilarginine acetate)—an inhibitor of nitric oxide synthase that produces vasoconstriction—was studied in the TRIUMPH trial. Unfortunately, no statistical difference in all-cause mortality at 30 days was seen between treatment and placebo.

## Thrombolytics

Prior to augmentation of coronary perfusion pressure, thrombolysis enjoyed limited efficacy in patients who had cardiogenic shock. In a 1994 meta-analysis, thrombolysis was associated with a 7% absolute reduction (54 versus 61%) in mortality at one month in patients with a systolic blood pressure of less than 100 mm Hg and a heart rate of greater than 100 bpm. The impact of thrombolytic therapy on mortality when used in combination with medical therapy versus PCI is discussed in detail below. Fibrinolytic therapy alone is an ACC/AHA Class I recommendation (Level of evidence: B) in STEMI patients with cardiogenic shock who are unsuitable for further invasive care and have no contraindications to fibrinolysis (**Table 35-1, Figure 35-3**).

# CURRENT INTERVENTIONAL TREATMENTS

## IABP

IABP has been used in the setting of shock for 30 years and effectively solved the decreased efficacy of fibrinolysis by countering the hypotension present in cardiogenic shock. In 1994, a study by Prewitt et al. demonstrated that under moderate hypotension, IABP enhanced the rate of clot dissolution with thrombolysis in canines. IABP is almost always used in combination with fibrinolytic therapy or PCI or both. Mortality was significantly reduced with IABP use in combination with fibrinolysis (67 versus

# Interventional Cardiology

# Invasive Hemodynamics

MICHAEL J. LIM

- Invasive hemodynamic measurements form the backbone of the basic understanding of cardiac pathophysiology.

- Familiarity with interpretation of the normal cardiac waveforms is essential.

- Assessment of stenotic valves revolves around the ability to understand the pressure gradient across the valve in question and estimate the amount of blood flow traversing the valve. A simplified estimate of valve area can be derived by dividing the cardiac output by the square root of the pressure gradient.

- Valvular regurgitation results in volume overload and subsequent compensatory stages that are depicted by classic hemodynamic abnormalities.

- The evaluation of a patient with potential constrictive or restrictive physiology focuses on the understanding of the equalization of diastolic pressures throughout all of the chambers and the presence or absence of ventricular interdependence.

## INTRODUCTION

Blood within the heart or vessels exerts characteristic pressure; proper understanding of the heart chamber's pressures forms the physiologic basis of understanding the cardiovascular system. In the catheterization lab, these pressure waves are created by cardiac muscular contraction and from a vessel or chamber along a closed, fluid-filled column (catheter) to a pressure transducer, converting the mechanical pressure to an electrical signal that is displayed on a video monitor. Cardiac pressure waveforms are cyclical, repeating the pressure change from the onset of one cardiac contraction (systole) to the onset of the next contraction.

Assessment of cardiac physiology, including cardiomyopathies, valvular heart disease, and structural heart disease, mandates an ability to interpret and assimilate invasive hemodynamic waveforms. Interpretation of pressure measurements is aided by the simultaneous assessment of cardiac output by thermodilution technique or the Fick (oxygen consumption) method. The ABIM examination in cardiovascular medicine expects one to recognize and interpret basic invasive hemodynamic waveforms. This chapter reviews normal waveforms and discusses the hemodynamics associated with the most prevalent disease states.

## FUNDAMENTALS OF HEMODYNAMIC INTERPRETATION

All the necessary background for interpreting hemodynamics comes from an understanding of the Wigger's diagram (**Figure 36-1**). Hemodynamic waveforms are representative of cardiac mechanical forces occurring immediately following the electrical impulse as seen on the electrocardiogram. Every electrical activity is followed normally by a mechanical function (either contraction or relaxation) resulting in a pressure wave. The timing of mechanical events can be obtained by looking at the ECG and corresponding pressure tracing.

The electrocardiograph P wave is responsible for atrial contraction, the QRS for ventricular activation, and the T wave for ventricular relaxation. The periods between electrical activation reflect impulse transmission times to different areas of the heart. These time delays permit the mechanical

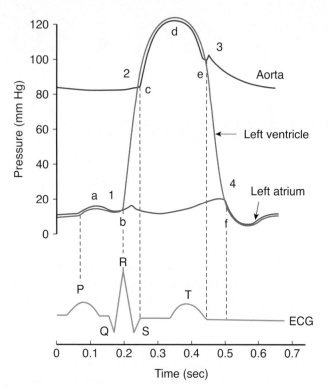

**Figure 36-1.** Wigger's diagram demonstrating simultaneous representation of left ventricular, left atrial and aortic pressures. The electrocardiogram is depicted on the bottom of the figure, with representative time scale in seconds; the vertical axis represents pressure in mm Hg.

functions to be in synchrony and generate efficient cardiac output and pressure.

Walking through a single cardiac cycle, one first sees the P wave. A vertical line drawn to the corresponding pressure waveforms demonstrates that there is an atrial pressure wave (a wave, point 1 on **Figure 36-1**) following the P wave by 30-50 msec. Following the A wave peak, the atrium relaxes and pressure falls, generating the X descent (point b). The next electrical event is the depolarization of the ventricles with the QRS (point b). The LV pressure after the A wave is called the end diastolic pressure. About 15-30 msec after the QRS, the ventricles contract and the LV (and RV) pressure increase rapidly. This period with rise in LV pressure without change in LV volume is called the isovolumetric contraction period (interval b-c). When LV pressure rises above the pressure in the aorta, the aortic valve opens and blood is ejected into the circulation (point c).

About 200-250 msec after the QRS, the T wave can be seen representing ventricular relaxation. At the end of the T wave (point e), the LV contraction has ended and LV relaxation produces a fall in the LV (and aortic pressure). When the LV pressure falls below the aortic pressure, the aortic valve closes (point e). The arterial pressure waveform exhibits a brief

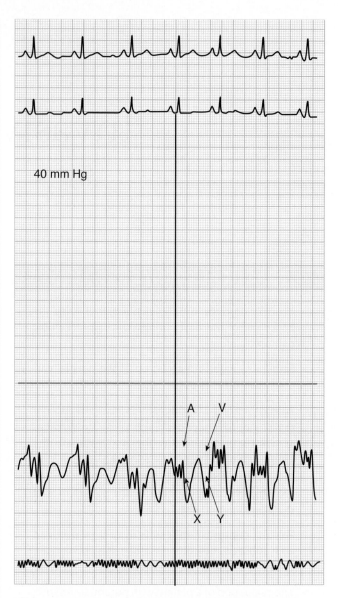

**Figure 36-2.** Normal right atrial pressure tracing recorded on 40 mm Hg. The vertical line is drawn from the end of the p-wave to demonstrate the timing of the A wave. This is followed by the X descent, V wave, and Y descent (as labeled).

"bump," termed the dicrotic notch (point 3 on **Figure 36-1**) immediately after aortic valve closure. When the LV pressure falls below the LA pressure, the mitral valve opens and the LA empties into the LV (point f). The period from aortic valve closure to mitral valve opening is call the isovolumetric relaxation period (interval e-f). The cycle then repeats itself.

## Right Atrial Pressure (RA)

Right pressure is normally composed of multiple waves and inflection points. There are discrete A and V waves (assuming sinus rhythm) with corresponding X and Y descents (**Figure 36-2**). Abnormalities in atrial pressure tracings frequently are associated with unique pathologies that should

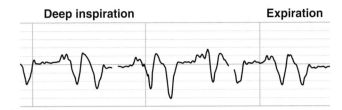

**Figure 36-3.** Right atrial pressure tracing during inspiration and expiration showing no change in the pressure, i.e., Kussmaul's sign.

be recognized. Normally, venous pressure falls with inspiration. Lack of a decrease or rise in right atrial pressure with inspiration is called Kussmaul's sign (**Figure 36-3**). This is traditionally associated with constrictive pericarditis, but can accompany advanced heart failure, right ventricular infarction, and pulmonary embolism.

## Right Ventricular Pressure (RV)

This pressure waveform (**Figure 36-4**) is characterized by a rapid rise and fall in pressure surrounding the systole. The diastolic portion of the waveform consists of an initial period

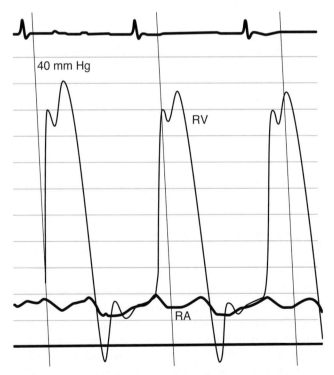

**Figure 36-4.** Right ventricular (RV) and right atrial (RA) pressures recorded simultaneously on 40 mm Hg scale. There is a slow increase in diastolic pressure of the RV, concurrent with the increase in RA pressure. This is followed by a steep upslope indicative of ventricular contraction. The dip seen one-third of the way into systole is an artifact from the pressure measurement system and is not representative of a true decrease in pressure. This is followed by a sharp descent in pressure just prior to the onset of diastole.

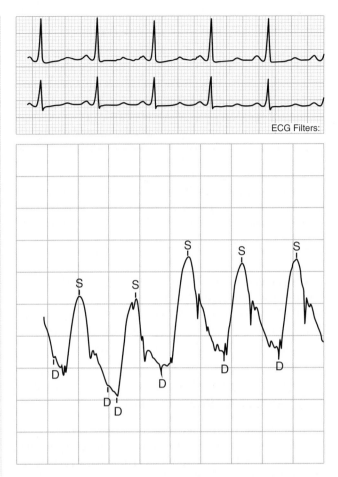

**Figure 36-5.** Recording of pulmonary arterial pressure (PA).

when the tricuspid valve opens, producing early rapid filling. The middle phase consists of a slow filling phase, followed by atrial systole which produces a reflected A wave, representing the right ventricular end-diastolic pressure.

## Pulmonary Artery Pressure (PA)

Rapid flow of blood into the pulmonary artery across the open pulmonic valve from the right ventricle produces the systolic upsloping of the pulmonary arterial pressure tracing (**Figure 36-5**). The systolic pressure is identical to that of the right ventricle without the presence of pulmonic or subpulmonic stenosis. As the right ventricular pressure falls below that of the pulmonary artery, a dicrotic notch in the PA pressure following the closure of the pulmonic valve. Diastolic PA pressure is greater than that of the RV and shows a slight decrease through the course of diastole as blood flows through the pulmonary arteries and veins to the left atrium.

## Pulmonary Capillary Wedge Pressure (PCWP) and Left Atrial Pressure (LA)

The PCWP is essentially identical to that of the LA, except for a slight delay in the transmission of the specific

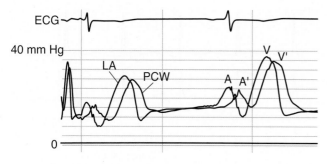

**Figure 36-6.** Simultaneous recording of the left atrial (LA) and pulmonary capillary wedge (PCW) pressures on 40 mm Hg scale and fast paper speed showing the A and V waves, as well as the time delay in each of these waves in the PCW tracing (A' and V').

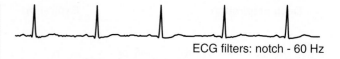

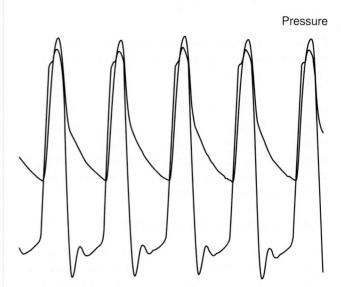

**Figure 36-7.** Recorder of left ventricular and aortic pressures on 200 mm Hg scale.

waves (**Figure 36-6**). An A wave can be identified, signifying atrial contraction, followed by an X descent from atrial relaxation. The second visible positive deflection is termed the V wave and is associated with ventricular contraction and is followed by a Y descent during left ventricular diastole.

## Left Ventricular Pressure (LV)

The LV waveform is almost identical in nature to the RV waveform except for the higher corresponding diastolic and systolic pressures that characterize the former (**Figure 36-7**).

## COMPUTATIONS FOR HEMODYNAMIC MEASUREMENTS

Once the hemodynamic data have been obtained, computations are made to clarify and enhance quantitation of cardiac function.

1. Cardiac output (CO) by Fick ($O_2$ consumption) method:

$$CO = \frac{O_2 \text{ consumption (mL/min)}}{A\,VO_2 \text{ difference(mL } O_2/100 \text{ mL blood)} \times 10}$$

Oxygen consumption can be estimated as 3 mL $O_2$/kg. $AVO_2$ (arteriovenous oxygen) difference is calculated from (arterial − mixed venous (pulmonary artery) $O_2$ content), where $O_2$ content = saturation × 1.36 × hemoglobin.

2. Cardiac index (CI, L/min/m²):

$$CI = \frac{CO(\text{mL/beat})}{BSA(\text{m}^2)}$$

where CO is cardiac output and BSA is body surface area.

3. Pulmonary arteriolar resistance (PAR, units):

$$PAR =$$
$$\frac{\text{mean pulmonary arterial pressure (or PCW)} - \text{mean LA pressure}}{CO}$$

4. Systemic vascular resistance (SVR, WOOD units):

$$SVR =$$
$$\frac{\text{mean systemic arterial pressure} - \text{mean right arterial pressure}}{CO}$$

## INTRACARDIAC SHUNTS

A shunt is an abnormal communication between the left and right heart chambers. The direction of blood flowing through the shunt is left to right, right to left, or sometimes bidirectional. In the absence of shunting, the pulmonary blood flow (right heart) is equal to the systemic blood flow (left heart). A left-to-right shunt is suggested at a chamber or vessel when a step-up of oxygen saturation in that chamber or vessel exceeds that of a proximal chamber. The desaturation of arterialized blood samples from the left heart chambers and/or the aorta suggests a right-to-left shunt.

Without shunting, mixed venous saturation is obtained in the pulmonary artery (this is why the pulmonary artery saturation is part of the Fick cardiac output calculation). If there is a left-to-right shunt, mixed venous blood is found one

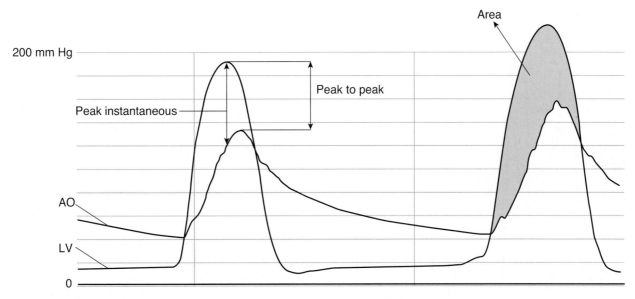

**Figure 36-8.** Simultaneous recording of left ventricular (LV) and aortic (AO) pressures on 200 mm Hg scale demonstrating the three potentially measured gradients used to assess the aortic valve in clinical practice.

chamber proximal to the step-up (e.g. an atrial septal defect with left to right shunting requires a weighted average of vena caval blood to determine the mixed venous saturation).

## Shunt Calculation (Qp:Qs)

The determination of the significance of any cardiac shunt is based on the Fick principal of blood flow. Flow through the pulmonary and systemic circuits is calculated independently to determine this ratio, as follows:

Systemic flow (L/min):

$$Q_S(L/min) = \frac{O_2 \text{ consumption}(mL/min)}{(\text{arterial} - \text{mixed venous}) \ O_2 \text{ content}}$$

Pulmonary flow (L/min)

$$Q_P(L/min) =$$

$$\frac{O_2 \text{ consumption}(mL/min)}{(\text{pulmonary venous} - \text{pulmanory arterial}) \ O_2 \text{ content}}$$

## VALVULAR HEART DISEASE

### Aortic Stenosis

The most recently published guidelines for patients with valvular heart disease strongly discourage routine invasive hemodynamic measurements to assess the severity of aortic stenosis when there is adequate echocardiographic data concordant with the patient's clinical presentation. Assessing the aortic valve gradient at the time of coronary angiography is currently reserved for those situations when noninvasive testing is inconclusive or if there is a discrepancy between noninvasive testing and clinical symptoms.

There are numerous techniques that have been utilized to determine the gradient across the aortic valve (e.g., dual lumen pigtail catheter, left ventricular and femoral artery pressures, or left ventricular and central aortic pressures). From these, many parameters can be determined and reported in the catheterization laboratory (**Figure 36-8**). The mean pressure gradient across the aortic valve is determined by planimetry of the area separating the left ventricular and aortic pressure curves. The peak instantaneous gradient is the maximum pressure difference between the left ventricle and the aorta at the same moment in the cardiac cycle, and it typically occurs in early systole. The peak-to-peak gradient is the measured difference between the peak aortic pressure and peak left ventricular pressure. The peak-to-peak gradient is often used to assess the severity of aortic stenosis, because it is the easiest to determine based upon initial visual inspection. The peak left ventricular pressure and peak aortic pressures, however, do not occur at the same time, and therefore the peak-to-peak gradient has been stated to have no true physiologic basis.

There are times when one may encounter a difference between peripheral arterial pressure and central arterial pressure. This frequently represents the presence of peripheral arterial disease and/or pressure amplification of the peripheral arterial pressure. Amplification usually is found in older patients with calcified vessels and results from the aortic pressure wave moving in a smaller diameter conduit (resulting in a greater flow velocity) with decreased arterial

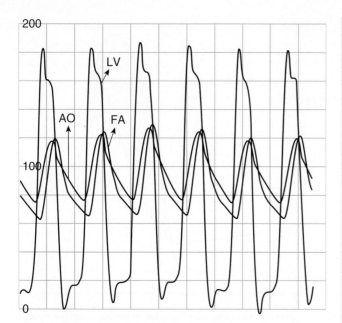

**Figure 36-9.** Recording of the left ventricular (LV), central aortic (AO), and femoral arterial (FA) pressures on 200 mm Hg scale. These recordings were made with a dual-lumen pigtail catheter (LV and AO) and from the sidearm of the femoral sheath. Note the time delay seen in the FA tracing as compared to the upstroke of the AO and LV pressures.

compliance. This situation mandates that a central aortic pressure must be used in the accurate calculation of valve area rather than a peripheral pressure.

In the absence of a central aortic to peripheral arterial pressure gradient, routine utilization of arterial sheath pressure and left ventricular pressure produces a tracing similar to **Figure 36-9**, with a time delay (usually 40-50 msec) separating the upstroke of the left ventricular pressure with the upstroke of the peripheral arterial pressure. Many operators or catheterization technicians "phase shift" the femoral artery pressure tracing to align with the left ventricular tracing prior to the determination of the gradient. Without realignment, left ventricular–femoral artery gradient overestimates the left ventricular-aortic mean gradient by approximately 9 mm Hg. When the left ventricular–femoral artery gradients were aligned, underestimation of the left ventricular–aortic mean gradient by approximately 10 mm Hg was noted, representing the fact that peak systolic (femoral) arterial pressure is higher (due to overshoot) and the upstroke faster for the peripheral arterial than central aortic pressure tracings, with a planimetered gradient smaller when using aligned left ventricular–femoral artery pressures (**Figure 36-10**).

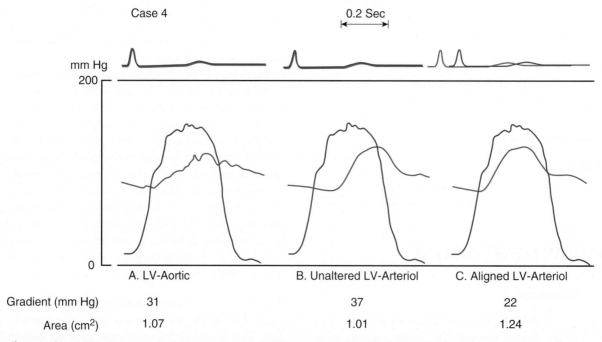

| | A. LV-Aortic | B. Unaltered LV-Arteriol | C. Aligned LV-Arteriol |
|---|---|---|---|
| Gradient (mm Hg) | 31 | 37 | 22 |
| Area (cm$^2$) | 1.07 | 1.01 | 1.24 |

**Figure 36-10.** Simultaneous tracings showing comparisons between the (A) left ventricular and central aortic pressure, (B) left ventricular and femoral arterial pressure (in green), and (C) left ventricular and "phase-shifted" femoral arterial pressure. The gradient is seen to be greater in the LV to FA (in green) comparison (B) when contrasted to that of the LV to AO comparison (A), resulting in a smaller calculated valve area. Tracing C depicts the "phase-shifted" femoral arterial / pressure tracing from B, resulting in a decrease in gradient when compared to A and a resultant larger valve area. (From Folland et al. *J Am Coll Cardiol.* 1984; 4:1207–1212.)

## Calculating Aortic Valve Area

The aortic valve area is calculated using the Gorlin equation. Gorlin and Gorlin first described this equation in 1951 as a means of calculating the mitral valve area in patients with mitral stenosis. The Gorlin equation for determining the aortic valve area (AVA) is:

$$AVA = \frac{[CO/(SEP \times HR)]}{(44.3 \times \sqrt{\text{mean Gradient}})}$$

where CO is cardiac output in L/min, SEP is systolic ejection period in seconds, HR is heart rate in beats per minute, and G is the mean pressure gradient across the obstruction in mm Hg. It should be noted, however, that although the Gorlin equation is reasonably accurate in calculating aortic valve area, it has only been validated in patients with mitral stenosis.

The Gorlin equation for calculating AVA is flow-dependent and varies directly with flow across the aortic valve—that is, the calculated AVA depends upon the patient's cardiac output. In most patients with severe AS and a large transvalvular gradient, the Gorlin equation accurately calculates a critically stenotic aortic valve. However, in the setting of reduced cardiac output (<3 L/min) and low gradients (<30 mm Hg), dobutamine infusion can be done to better stratify treatment strategies for patients with aortic valve disease (**Figure 36-11**). Typically, dobutamine infusion resulting in an increased calculated valve area represents a group of patients in whom valve replacement surgery is not helpful. However, a fixed valve area (increased gradient with increased cardiac output) represents a patient with "contractile reserve" and significant aortic stenosis in whom surgical replacement has shown improved outcomes.

A simplified formula for the estimation of aortic valve area has been adopted after having been validated by Hakke. This formula is based on the fact that the systolic ejection period, heart rate, and constant portion of the Gorlin equation approximates 1 under resting conditions. Therefore, estimated aortic valve area can be calculated as:

$$AVA = \frac{\text{cardiac output (L/min)}}{\sqrt{\text{gradient}}}$$

Aortic stenosis is graded as mild, moderate, or severe (see **Table 36-1**) with the normal aortic valve area between 3.0 to 4.0 cm². In general, patients do not develop symptoms until the valve area is less than or equal to 0.7 cm². Exceptions obviously exist, and correlation must be made between a patient's aortic valve area, gradient, and the clinical symptoms.

## LV Gradient Below the Aortic Valve

Hypertrophic cardiomyopathy is a condition in which very thick heart muscle, especially inside the LV chamber, contracts so hard that it obstructs flow out of the ventricle, and thus by its own contraction produces a pressure gradient with a normal aortic valve. **Figure 36-12a** depicts simultaneous LV and aortic pressure showing large aortic-LV gradient. On pullback of the LV catheter (multipurpose) from the distal LV to a position just beneath the aortic valve, the AO-LV gradient disappears. Obviously, care must be taken to avoid mistaking this gradient with that of true valvular stenosis. **Figure 36-12b** exhibits postextrasystolic potentiation producing an increase in left ventricular inotropy and contractility, which may result in an increase in systolic anterior motion (SAM) and outflow obstruction, and a decrease in aortic pulse pressure (also known as the Brockenbrough effect.)

## Aortic Regurgitation

**Figure 36-13** illustrates simultaneous AO and LV pressures (0 to 200 mm Hg scale) in several patients with different degrees of aortic regurgitation. The characteristic hemodynamic feature of this condition is a wide pulse pressure. The aortic (femoral) brisk pressure upstroke can be easily seen. Regurgitation of blood from the aorta into the left ventricle results in an increase in left ventricular end-diastolic volume (preload). This is manifest by a rapid fall in measured central aortic diastolic pressure. Left ventricular end-diastolic volume (LVEDV) increases and, initially, there is an augmented stroke volume. Often, this creates elevated systolic pressures and, when coupled with the reduced diastolic pressure, results in a substantial pulse pressure.

Close examination of **Figure 36-13(a)** shows that the left ventricular diastolic pressure will reveal a relatively flat slope and a prominent early A wave, which characterize mild regurgitation. Left ventricular end-diastolic pressure (LVEDP), left atrial pressure, and pulmonary capillary wedge pressure (PCWP) usually remain in the normal range during the early stages of chronic aortic insufficiency because of preserved LV wall diastolic compliance. As chronic LV overload leads to myocardial fibrosis, impaired compliance, and compromised contractility, the left ventricle begins to progressively decompensate.

The decompensated LV is marked by an elevated LV end-systolic volume, LV end-diastolic pressure, and elevated pulmonary pressures, as the progression of valvular incompetence exceeds the ability of the LV to remodel. The severity of aortic regurgitation can be estimated by evaluating the diastolic pressure difference between the aorta and left ventricle, with special attention to the slope of the

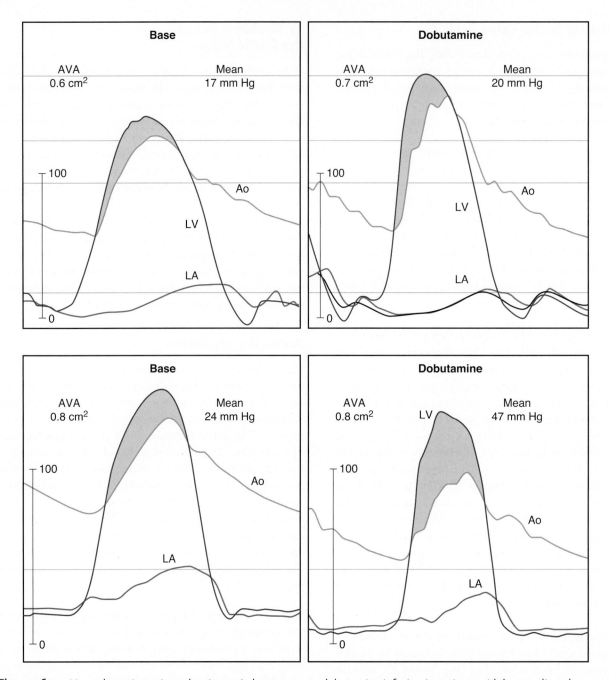

**Figure 36-11.** Hemodynamic tracings showing varied responses to dobutamine infusion in patients with low-gradient, low-output aortic stenosis. (Upper Panels) This patient had an increase in gradient from 17 to 20 mm Hg with an increase in cardiac output. Calculated valve area was increased by only 0.1 cm², and the patient was sent for surgery. At the time of operation, the valve was found to be only mildly stenotic. (Lower Panels) This patient demonstrated an increase in mean gradient from 24 to 47 mm Hg with an increase in cardiac output. Calculated valve area remained <1.0 cm². This example meets the criteria for severe aortic stenosis with potential benefit from valve replacement surgery.

| Table 36-1 • Classification of Aortic Valve Disease | | | |
|---|---|---|---|
| Indicator | Mild | Moderate | Severe |
| Mean gradient (mm Hg) | <25 | 25-40 | >40 |
| Valve area (cm²) | >1.5 | 1-1.5 | <1.0 |

*Data from the ACC/AHA 2006 Guidelines for the Management of Patients with Valvular Heart Disease.*

ventricular diastolic waveform. As the LV diastolic pressure waveform increases its rate of rise, the regurgitation through the aortic valve is more severe, leading to earlier equalization of the aortic and ventricular pressures in diastole (**Figure 36-13b**). The natural progression leads to progressive LV cavity dilatation with a subsequent reduction in stroke volume and eventual signs and symptoms of heart failure and pulmonary edema.

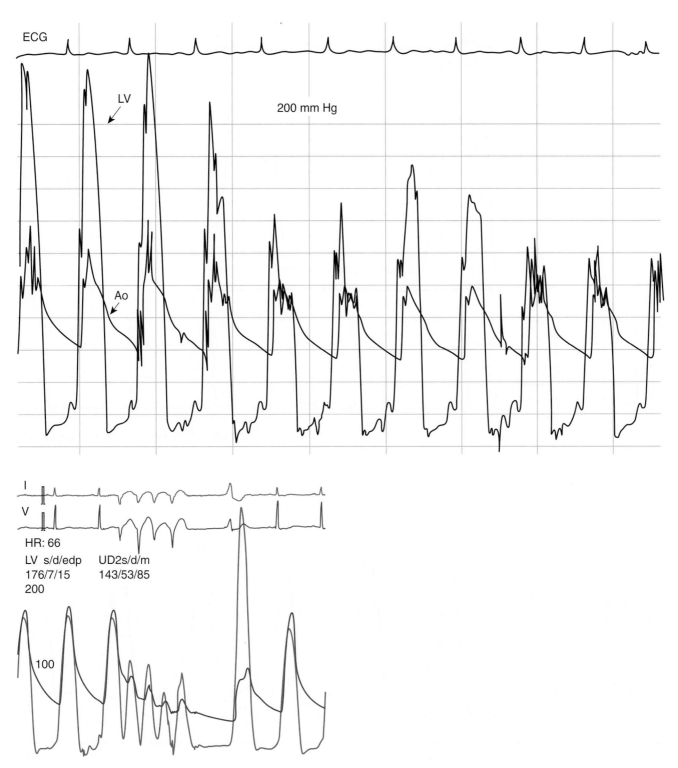

**Figure 36-12.** (Top) Simultaneous recording of central aortic and left ventricular pressures on 200 mm Hg scale. The catheter in the left ventricle is slowly pulled back from the apex (left side of figure) to just inside of the aortic valve (right side of figure) demonstrating a >100 mm Hg gradient between the pressures that is not seen upon pullback. There is a definite left ventricular waveform on the right side of the figure, proving that the gradient lies within the ventricle itself and is not valvular in origin. However, this still could represent subaortic stenosis or hypertrophic cardiomyopathy. (Bottom) Left ventricular pressure and aortic pressure on a 200 mm Hg scale. The left side of this figure shows only a small gradient between the pressures. As seen on the ECG tracing, multiple PVCs are induced with a corresponding large gradient in the postextrasystolic beat. This potentiation of gradient is termed the Brockenbrough–Braunwald–Morrow sign and is consistent with a gradient from hypertrophic cardiomyopathy and not valvular aortic stenosis.

**A**

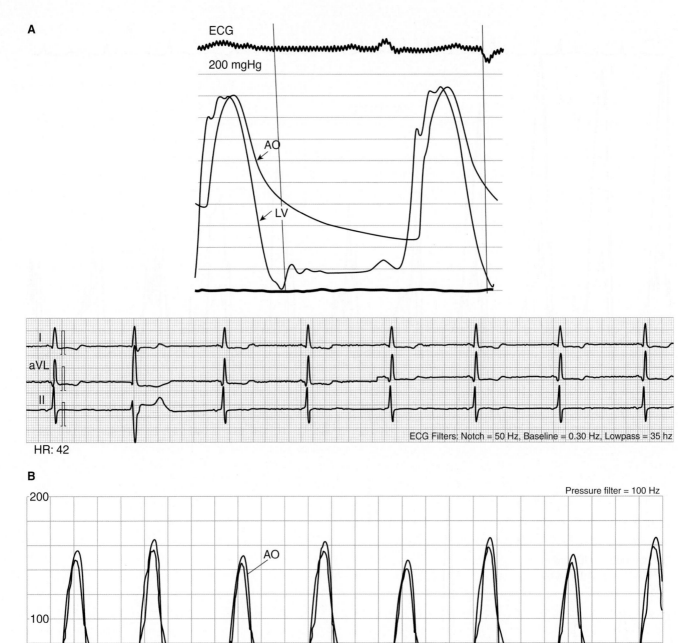

ECG

200 mgHg

AO

LV

I

aVL

II

ECG Filters: Notch = 50 Hz, Baseline = 0.30 Hz, Lowpass = 35 hz

HR: 42

**B**

Pressure filter = 100 Hz

200

AO

100

0

LV

25 mm/sec.

**Figure 36-13.** (A) Simultaneous recording of the left ventricular (LV) and aortic pressures (AO) on a 200 mm Hg scale in a patient with mild aortic insufficiency. Note the relatively flat diastolic slope of the left ventricular pressure tracing, the prominent early A wave with a relatively normal left ventricular end-diastolic pressure, and the progressive decline in the aortic diastolic pressure tracing. (B) Simultaneous pressure recording of the aortic (AO) and left ventricular (LV) pressures demonstrating significant deterioration of the aortic pressure throughout diastole. There is a reflective rapid increase in LV diastolic pressure, which equalizes the aortic pressure at end-diastole. This is indicative of severe, compensated aortic insufficiency.

| Table 36-2 • Major Hemodynamic Features of Severe Aortic Regurgitation | | |
|---|:---:|:---:|
| | **Acute** | **Chronic** |
| Left ventricular compliance | ↔ | ↑ |
| Regurgitant volume | ↑ | ↑ |
| Left ventricular end-diastolic pressure | ↑↑↑ | May be normal |
| Left ventricular diastolic pressure/diastolic tamponade | ↔ | ↑↑↑ |
| Aortic systolic pressure | ↔ | ↑ |
| Aortic diastolic pressure | ↔ to ↓ | ↓↓↓ |
| Systemic arterial pressure | ↑ to ↑↑ | ↑↑↑ |
| Ejection fraction | ↔ | ↑ |
| Effective stroke volume | ↓ | ↔ |
| Effective cardiac output | ↓ | ↔ |
| Heart rate | ↑ | ↔ |
| Peripheral vascular resistance | ↑ | ↔ |

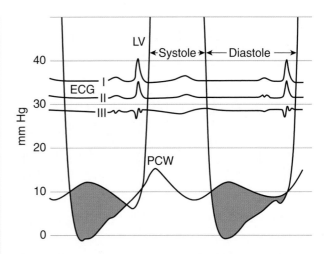

**Figure 36-14.** Left ventricular (LV) and pulmonary capillary wedge pressure (PCW) tracings shown simultaneously on 40 mm Hg scale. There is a sizeable and stable gradient that exists between these tracings, as depicted by the hashed regions, indicative of mitral stenosis.

Acute aortic insufficiency is often associated with rapid cardiovascular deterioration, necessitating early identification, evaluation, and treatment. The hemodynamic environment of acute aortic regurgitation is comparable to chronic regurgitation, except the LV does not have the time for adaptation to the large increase in diastolic blood volume. Compliance is relatively low, so the increased volume in acute regurgitation therefore results in a swift and marked increase in LVEDP. Acute aortic regurgitation exposes the unconditioned left ventricle to large diastolic volumes. The immediate and rapid increase in diastolic pressure in the left ventricle with or without a wide aortic pulse pressure is one of several findings that distinguish acute from chronic aortic regurgitation (see **Table 36-2**).

## Mitral Stenosis

**Figure 36-14** simultaneous LV and PCW pressures demonstrate a mitral valve gradient throughout diastole typical of a patient with mitral stenosis (MS). More severe mitral stenosis is associated with a normal V wave. In the following beat, atrial activity is delayed and follows the QRS, contributing to large giant V wave (36 mm Hg). More severe mitral stenosis chronically results in concomitant increases in pulmonary pressures (i.e., pulmonary hypertension). Mitral valve gradients are influenced by heart rate. When the rhythm is irregular (atrial fibrillation), calculations of gradients should be made from the average of 10 beats.

Patients with the classic findings of severe mitral stenosis that present when they are older (>45 years) have calcified annular and subvalvular structures. As with other purely valvular-related lesions, echocardiography has largely supplanted the use of cardiac catheterization for the assessment of MS severity in the majority of patients. Cardiac catheterization for hemodynamic evaluation has mainly been relegated for use prior to valvotomy when there is a discrepancy between a patient's symptoms and Doppler-derived hemodynamics. Regardless of the clinical presentation, the determination of the mitral valve gradient with its characteristic atrial and (consequently altered) pulmonary and ventricular pressure waveforms is critical to both diagnostic and therapeutic considerations.

## MITRAL VALVE AREA CALCULATION

As in calculating the aortic valve area, mitral valve area (MVA) calculation utilizes the Gorlin formula. The MVA formula is:

$$MVA = \frac{((CO / DFP) \times HR)}{(K \sqrt{MVG})}$$

where CO = cardiac output (mL/min); DFP = diastolic filling period (sec); MVA = mitral valve area; MVG = mean valve gradient (mm Hg); and K = constant from Gorlin's empiric data for mitral values (44.3 × 0.8 = 38).

The Hakke formula can also be utilized for estimation of valve area in the same way that it is used for aortic valve calculations. For example (see **Figure 36-15**), assuming the cardiac output is 3.5 L/min and heart rate 80 bpm, the valve area by available data can be estimated as $3.5/\sqrt{11}$, or $3.5/3.3 = 1.1$ cm$^2$. In mitral stenosis, the Hakke valve area

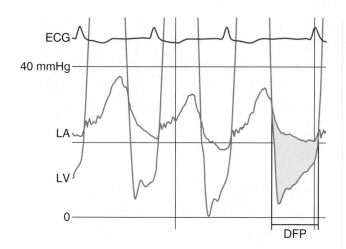

**Figure 36-15.** Example of information needed to calculate an estimation of mitral valve area from invasive hemodynamics. The computerized planimetered area (9.46 cm²), and measurement of the diastolic filling time (DFP = 3.4) are shown. This gives a mean gradient of 10.85 mm Hg that is plugged into the Gorlin formula. (From *The Cardiac Catheterization Handbook*, 4th ed. 2003.)

estimate should be used with caution, if at all, especially in patients with tachycardia.

## Mitral Regurgitation

Large V waves that can be seen in the PCW tracing represent LV pressure transmitted backward through an incompetent mitral valve. The V wave occurs on the downstroke of the LV pressure. **Figure 36-16** shows large V waves (up to 60 mm Hg) in a patient with mitral regurgitation. The morphology and magnitude of the V wave is determined principally by the pressure-volume relationship of the left atrium. Large V waves may be due to valvular mitral regurgitation or stenosis or a number of other nonvalvular conditions in which the pressure/volume relationship of the atrial chamber is altered (e.g., ventricular septal defect, left ventricular ischemia, or hypertrophy).

## RESTRICTION AND CONSTRICTION

One of the most challenging and sometimes confusing aspects of hemodynamic interpretation involves patients with restrictive and constrictive myopathies. This is because of

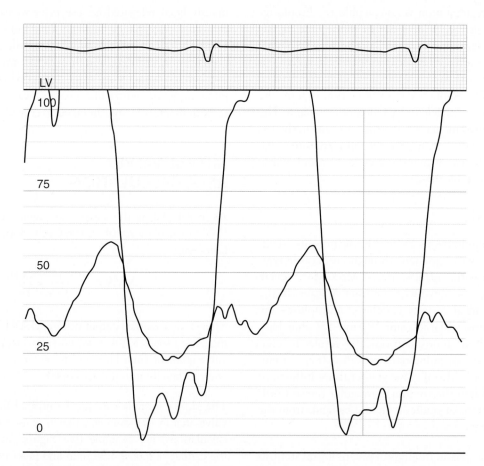

**Figure 36-16.** Simultaneous recording of left ventricular and left atrial pressures on 200 mm Hg scale demonstrating large V waves in the left atrial waveform, approaching 60 mm Hg.

the great number of similarities in the profiles of these types of patients.

## Restriction

The typical hemodynamic pattern for a restrictive cardiomyopathy shows elevation in venous pressure, with the right atrial pressure demonstrating a striking Y descent. Right ventricular pressure tracings typically show a dip and plateau (called the "square root sign") and the diastolic right ventricular pressure to systolic pressure ratio is <0.33. *Typically the left and right ventricular diastolic pressures are >5 mm Hg apart and the right ventricular systolic pressure is elevated above 50 mm Hg.*

## Constriction

The classic finding of constriction involves the equalization of pressures (i.e., right atrial, right ventricular diastolic, pulmonary arterial diastolic, pulmonary capillary wedge, and left ventricular diastolic pressure). Constrictive pericarditis is further characterized by low arterial pressure, tachycardia, Kussmaul's sign (inspiratory increase in RA pressure), M or W configuration on RA pressure, and dip and plateau of early rapid diastolic filling with abrupt cessation caused by pericardial constraint (**Figure 36-17**). Thus, **Table 36-3** demonstrates the classic hemodynamic differentiation between constriction and restriction.

Constriction and tamponade physiology are differentiated by the RA waveform (elevated and blunted in tamponade) and pulsus paradoxus (inspiratory decrease in arterial pressure in tamponade) (**Table 36-4**). Because these two entities are similar in their early stages, the RA pressures also may be similar. The diagnosis of pericardial tamponade is usually suggested by classical clinical findings such as hypotension, elevated jugular venous pressure, and clear lungs, along with the presence of pulsus paradoxus exceeding 10 mm Hg.

## Ventricular Interdependence

Normal RV and LV pressures are separated by >5 mm Hg in early and late diastole, and the RV pressure tracing is usually contained completely within the LV pressure tracing (**Figure 36-18**). The diastolic ventricular pressures normally differ in slope and end-diastolic pressure. Changes in the RV-LV pressure relationship are related to ventricular septal interaction and will occur in pulmonary hypertension, bundle branch block, myocardial infarction, RV volume overload, and, most commonly, pericardial constrictive physiology.

Thus, evaluation of simultaneous left ventricular and right ventricular pressures across multiple respiratory cycles has

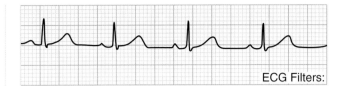

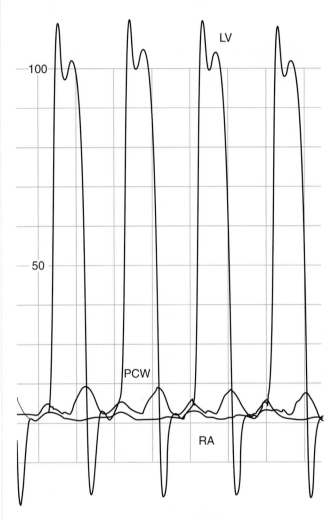

**Figure 36-17.** Pressure recording of the left ventricular (LV), right atrial (RA), and pulmonary capillary wedge (PCW) pressures in a patient with a cardiomyopathy. Note M or W configuration of the right atrial pressure. Also note the significant early diastolic dip (square root sign) seen in the RV and LV pressures. (From *Cardiac Cathet Intervent.* 1999;116:473–486.)

| Table 36-3 • Constriction vs. Restriction | | |
|---|---|---|
| | **Constriction** | **Restriction** |
| LVEDP – RVEDP | ≤5 mm Hg | >5 mm Hg |
| RV systolic pressure | ≤50 mm Hg | >50 mm Hg |
| RVEDP / RVSP | ≥0.33 | <0.3 |

| Table 36-4 • Differentiating Constriction from Tamponade | | |
|---|---|---|
| | **Tamponade** | **Constriction** |
| Paradoxical pulse | Present | Absent in 2/3 |
| RA pressure morphology | Absent Y descent | Prominent Y descent (M or W configuration) |
| Inspiratory changes in RA pressure | Decrease | Increase (Kussmaul's sign) |
| "Square root" sign | Absent | Present |

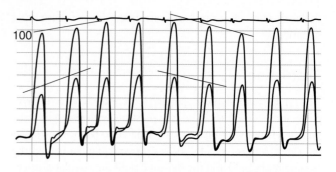

**Figure 36-18.** Simultaneous recording of left and right ventricular pressures (LV and RV) during inspiration and expiration. One can see the concordant changes in systolic pressure associated with respiration that are *not* consistent with a constrictive process. (From *Cardiac Cathet Intervent.* 1999;116:473–486.)

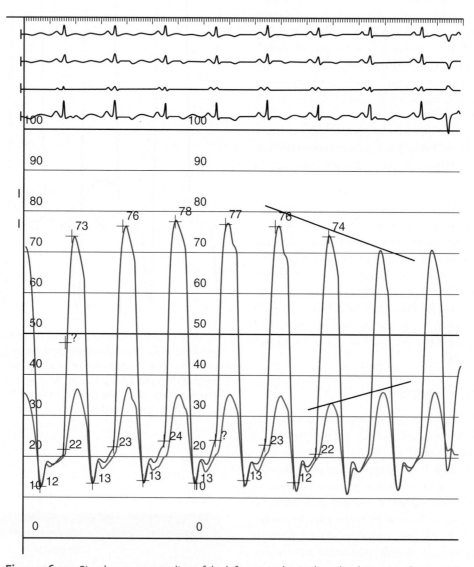

**Figure 36-19.** Simultaneous recording of the left ventricular (red) and right ventricular (green) pressures during inspiration and expiration. In this tracing, there is a decrease in LV systolic pressure and an increase in RV systolic pressure with respiration. This discordant response is classic for the diagnosis of constriction. (From *Cardiac Cathet Intervent.* 1999;116:473–486.)

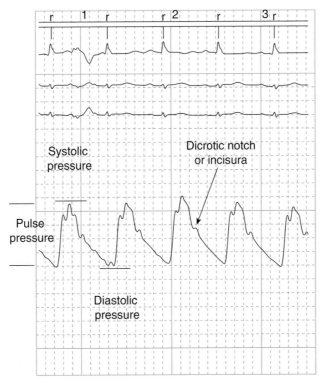

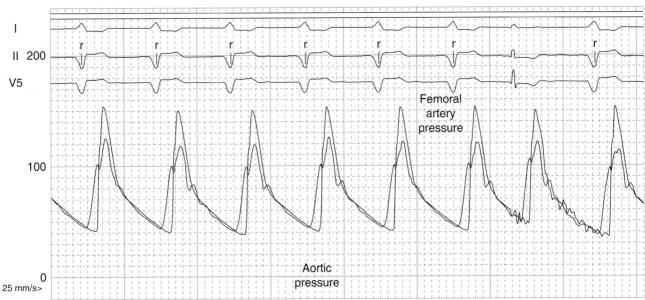

**Figure 37-2.** Pressure tracings taken from the central aorta. In panel b, femoral artery pressure is superimposed showing peripheral amplification.

The aortic pressure wave is determined both by LV ejection (a forward-traveling wave) and a pressure wave reflected from the periphery. Ejection of blood into the aorta generates a pressure wave that is propagated to other arteries throughout the body. At any discontinuity of the vascular wall, but mainly at the arteriolar branching points, the wave is reflected and comes back towards the heart. Peripheral amplification is caused by the reflected pressure waves returning to the aorta during diastole, making pulse pressure higher in peripheral (e.g., femoral or brachial) than in central arteries (mean pressures will be the same; **Figure 37-2b**).

## Cardiac Output and Intracardiac Shunts

Cardiac output is the amount of blood moved per unit time from the venous system to the arterial system. It is a dynamic process and tightly regulated so that blood flow through the heart equals perfusion needs of the body. Cardiac output is equal to the heart rate X stroke volume (in the absence of valvular regurgitation). Since accurate measurement of stroke volume is challenging, cardiac output is primarily measured at the time of right heart catheterization using either the Fick method or the indicator dilution method (e.g., thermodilution). Cardiac index is the cardiac output divided by the body surface area.

The Fick method is based on the principle that oxygen uptake in the lungs is entirely transferred to the blood and therefore cardiac output can be calculated from knowledge of oxygen consumption of the body and difference in oxygen content between arterial and mixed venous blood. Direct measurement of an individual's oxygen consumption is cumbersome and time consuming and thus, in modern practice, oxygen consumption is generally "assumed." The Fick cardiac output can be calculated using the equation:

$$\text{cardiac output} = \frac{O_2 \text{ consumption}}{(\text{arterial} - \text{venous})O_2 \times \text{hemoglobin concentration} \times 1.36 \times 10}$$

(The units of the constant 1.36 are mL $O_2$/g hemoglobin.)

The indicator dilution method involves injection of an indicator substance into the circulation followed by measurement of this substance at a distal point in the circulation. In current practice, the thermodilution method generally involves injecting saline into the RA and measuring the temperature of blood in the pulmonary artery. The thermodilution method tends to be more accurate in high-output states, whereas the Fick method is generally more accurate in low output states (because the differences in oxygen saturations between arterial and mixed venous blood are large) and when the patient's rhythm is irregular such as in atrial fibrillation or ventricular bigeminy.

Once cardiac output and pressures have been measured, systemic vascular resistance (SVR) and pulmonary vascular resistance (PVR) can be calculated:

$$\text{normal SVR} = 700 \text{ to } 1600 \text{ dyne-sec-cm}^{-5}$$

and

$$\text{PVR} = 20 \text{ to } 130 \text{ dyne-sec-cm}^{-5}.$$

$$\text{SVR (in dyne-sec-cm}^{-5}) = \frac{(\text{mean arterial pressure} - \text{RA pressure}) \times 80}{\text{cardiac output}}$$

$$\text{PVR (in dyne-sec-cm}^{-5}) = \frac{(\text{mean pulmonary artery pressure} - \text{PCWP}) \times 80}{\text{cardiac output}}$$

Intracardiac shunting of blood results when there is a connection and a pressure difference between right and left heart chambers. Because left heart pressures are generally higher than right heart pressures, most shunts are predominantly left-to-right, although right-to-left and bidirectional shunts are seen (predominantly in Eisenmenger's syndrome). Of note is that arterial to venous shunts can exist outside of the heart (e.g., intrapulmonary, intrahepatic, arterio-venous malformation) and affect oxygen saturations.

The amount of blood flowing through the shunt can be quantified by measuring oxygen saturations in various locations in the venous system and the right heart ("oxygen saturation run"). The samples need to be acquired with the patient breathing room air or a gas mixture containing no more than a maximum of 30% oxygen (to minimize the amount of dissolved oxygen in the blood). A left-to-right shunt can be quantified using the ratio of pulmonary blood flow to systemic blood flow, termed $Q_P/Q_S$, where $Q_P$ is the pulmonary blood flow and $Q_S$ is the systemic flow. $Q_P$ and $Q_S$ are calculated using the equation shown above for the Fick method of estimating cardiac output, where the only difference between the pulmonary flow equation and the systemic flow equation is the arterial and venous saturations used. A simplified formula can be used to estimate $Q_P/Q_S$:

$$\frac{Q_P}{Q_S} = \frac{(SAO_2 - MVO_2)}{(PVO_2 - PAO_2)}$$

In this equation, the mixed venous oxygen saturation ($MVO_2$) should be from the chamber proximal to the shunt. If there is an atrial septal defect (ASD), the $MVO_2$ is calculated from the superior vena cava (SVC) and the inferior vena cava (IVC). While theoretically coronary sinus blood flow contributes to mixed venous blood along with blood from IVC and SVC, the contribution is so small that it may be safely ignored. The equation most frequently used is:

$$\frac{(3 \text{ SVC} + \text{IVC})}{4}.$$

## VALVULAR HEART DISEASE

### Mitral Regurgitation

On echocardiography, left atrial (LA) enlargement may be one of the earlier signs of hemodynamically important mitral regurgitation (MR). Later, as the regurgitant volume increases, the LV dilates and pulmonary hypertension develops. Color flow Doppler can be used to quantitate the regurgitant orifice and measure the size of the regurgitant volume using proximal isovelocity surface area measurement (PISA). Regurgitant orifice area >40 mm² has been associated with a poor prognosis and is considered a strong indication for surgery.

One difference between acute and chronic MR is left atrial and pulmonary vein compliance. When MR is chronic and the LA dilated, the pressure gradient and thus flow between LV and LA persists throughout systole, resulting in a holosystolic murmur.

In acute MR, where the LA and pulmonary veins are normal in size, LA pressure rises rapidly during ventricular systole, the gradient between LV and LA diminishes earlier, and the murmur ends in mid systole. The rapid rise in LA pressure results in large V waves on the LA or PCWP tracing (**Figure 37-3**). Occasionally, large V waves can also be seen on the pulmonary arterial tracing. Doppler echocardiography showing systolic flow reversal in the pulmonary venous circulation is suggestive of severe MR, but this finding lacks sensitivity.

The hemodynamics of the LV pressure curve reflects the loading conditions of the left ventricle in response to MR. When MR is severe, the LV enlarges and LV end diastolic pressure (LVEDV) increases in order to maintain forward stroke volume. Rapid filling of the ventricle in early diastole produces a "square root" sign on LV pressure tracing. Although well tolerated initially, chronic LV dilation can result in negative remodeling and irreversible LV dysfunction. Eventually cardiac output begins to decline, resulting

in worsening functional limitation. Decreased ejection fraction (<60%) is a negative prognostic sign and is considered a strong indication for mitral valve surgery.

## Mitral Stenosis

The incidence of mitral stenosis (MS) has declined in most developed nations with the use of aggressive antibiotic therapies for rheumatic fever. However, there is an increasing frequency of degenerative and calcific MS among patients receiving chronic hemodialysis. Mild MS is rarely symptomatic and is often not detected on physical exam. As MS progresses, the development of hemodynamic sequelae become apparent on physical exam, and the findings often correlate with hemodynamic changes seen on echocardiography and in the catheterization lab. Severe MS produces a pressure gradient across the mitral valve that can be measured by Doppler echo. The continuity equation produces a reliable and accurate estimate of the mitral valve area. In the

A.

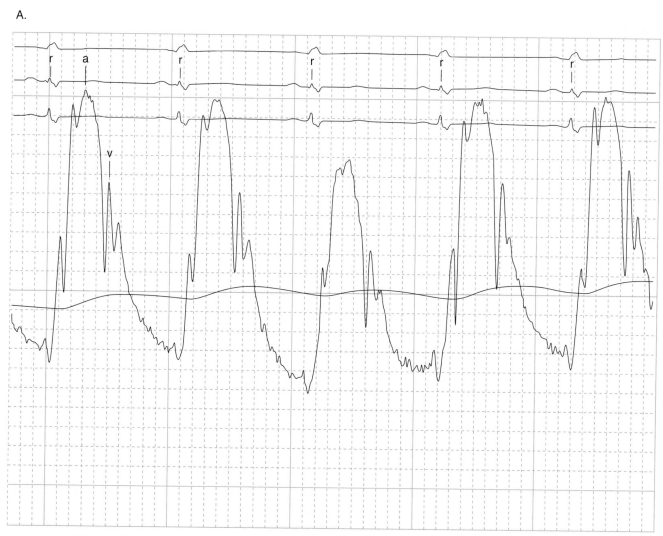

**Figure 37-3.** PCWP and PA tracings from a patient with severe MR. Large V waves are apparent in both the PA tracing (A) and in the PCWP tracing (B).

B.

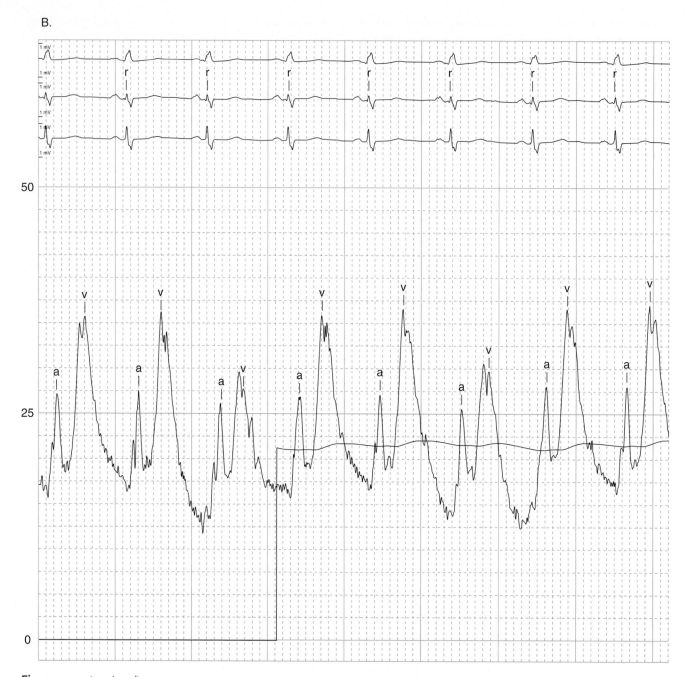

**Figure 37-3.** *(continued)*

catheterization laboratory, accurate measurement of the mi-tral valve gradient requires trans-septal puncture and simul-taneous measurement of the LV and LA pressures (PCWP can be used in place of LA pressure in certain situations). The Gorlin formula is then used to convert hemodynamic data to an estimate of the mitral valve area.

Intracardiac pressure tracings in patients with severe MS usually reveal a large A wave in the LA or PCWP tracing due to elevated LA pressure during early diastole (**Figure 37-4**). The Y descent on the LA pressure tracing will flatten due to delayed emptying of the atrium into the ventricle fol-lowing opening of the mitral valve. Early in disease course,

transmission of elevated LA pressure results in pulmonary venous hypertension. Later, chronic pulmonary venous hy-pertension can result in pulmonary arteriolar constriction and hypertrophy, which can lead to irreversible pulmonary arterial hypertension.

## Aortic Stenosis

Aortic stenosis (AS) is the second most common symptom-atic valvular lesion after mitral regurgitation. Severe AS is identified as a valve area of less than 1 cm². Moderate AS is usually not symptomatic at normal levels of exertion, and mild AS is asymptomatic in almost all cases. Hemodynamic

has been reduced to normal levels by pericardiocentesis. It is rare but can occur with all types of pericarditis. The majority of patients diagnosed with effusive-constrictive pericarditis will progress to chronic constriction, but a proportion of those with idiopathic disease may have only temporary cardiac constriction and then go on to eventual full resolution.

As in both constrictive pericarditis and cardiac tamponade, the expansion of the cardiac chambers during diastole is limited and there is elevation and equalization of diastolic pressures in the atria and ventricles. Prior to drainage of the effusion, the hemodynamic findings most resemble cardiac tamponade with a preserved X descent and an absent or attenuated Y descent on the right atrial pressure tracing. Once the effusion has been drained, constrictive physiology predominates with return and exaggeration of the Y descent leading to a classic M- or W-shaped configuration of the right atrial pressure waveform. The ventricular pressure tracings demonstrate the square root sign due to rapid ventricular filling in early diastole.

## CORONARY ARTERY DISEASE

### Right Ventricular Infarction

Acute RV infarction classically occurs in the setting of inferior myocardial infarction and can be diagnosed when ST elevations are apparent on right-sided chest leads. The acute hemodynamic significance of RV ischemia is a failure to provide adequate preload to the left ventricle, resulting in hypotension and possibly cardiogenic shock. RV infarction is considered a "preload-dependent" condition because patient survival depends on displacing enough volume into the pulmonary circulation to augment left ventricular filling. Right heart catheterization is useful in this situation, as it allows the physician to directly measure the RV preload and afterload in order to ensure RV and LV filling pressures are maintained. In patient with adequate intravascular volume, initial pressure tracings in patients with adequate RV filling pressures may show a square root sign due to rapid filling of the dilated, noncompliant ischemic right ventricle.

If the RV remains ischemic and volume is replaced appropriately, there is an increase in the RVEDP while the RV systolic pressure remains normal. This can also be accompanied by a broadening of the RV systolic pressure curve (**Figure 37-11**). Severe RV dilation can lead to physiology that is similar to constrictive pericarditis, where the RV and LV compete for limited pericardial space and demonstrate interdependence. This can result in equalization of the diastolic pressures typical of constrictive physiology.

### Fractional Flow Reserve

One major limitation of standard angiographic techniques is the inability to assess coronary physiology. Although

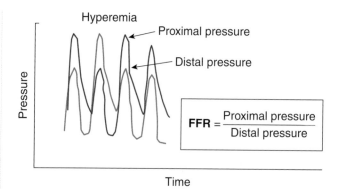

**Figure 37-12.** Fractional flow reserve (FFR) as determined by assessing coronary pressure distal and proximal to the coronary stenosis. Measurements are taken after maximal hyperemia has been achieved with the administration of intracoronary adenosine.

quantitative coronary angiography can accurately determine the percent stenosis on an epicardial vessel, it is unable to determine the hemodynamic significance of the lesion. This knowledge of coronary physiology is essential in determining whether or not to perform percutaneous coronary intervention on coronary lesions. The fractional flow reserve (FFR) can be used to assess the hemodynamics of coronary stenosis. FFR is determined with the use of an intracoronary pressure wire. This wire has a pressure sensor that is placed distal to the coronary stenosis. This pressure is then compared to the proximal (aortic pressure) during maximal hyperemia (**Figure 37-12**). The FFR is calculated with the following formula:

$$FFR = \frac{\text{pressure distal to stenosis}}{\text{pressure proximal to stenosis.}}$$

FFR should be measured both under basal conditions and during maximal hyperemia (usually accomplished by administration of intracoronary adenosine). Studies correlating FFR to nuclear stress testing results have shown that a FFR < 0.75 is hemodynamically significant.

## References

1. Faber JE, Stouffer GA. Introduction to basic hemodynamic principles. In: Stouffer GA, ed. *Cardiovascular Hemodynamics for the Clinician*. Oxford: Blackwell-Futura; 2007.

2. Cohen MV, Gorlin R. Modified orifice equation for the calculation of mitral valve area. *Am Heart J*. 1972;84:839–840.

3. Wilkinson JL. Haemodynamic calculations in the catheter laboratory. *Heart*. 2001;85:113–120.

4. Bonow RO, Carabello BA, Chatterjee K, et al. ACC/AHA 2006 Guidelines for the Management of Patients with Valvular Heart Disease: A Report of the American College of Cardiology/American Heart Association Task Force on Practice Guidelines (Writing Committee to Revise the 1998 Guidelines for the Management of Patients with Valvular Heart Disease) developed in collaboration with the Society of Cardiovascular Anesthesiologists endorsed by the Society for Cardiovascular Angiography and Interventions and the Society of Thoracic Surgeons. *J Am Coll Cardiol*. 2006;48:e1–148.

# Coronary Artery Physiology: Intracoronary Ultrasonography, Coronary Flow Velocity and Pressure Measurements

Bon-Kwon Koo, Yasuhiro Honda, and Peter J. Fitzgerald

## ● PRACTICAL POINTS

- The oxygen extraction by the myocardium is much higher than that by the other organs and reaches near maximum. The oxygen saturation of coronary sinus venous blood is only about 20~30%.

- Resting coronary blood flow can be maintained at a relatively constant level under various coronary perfusion pressures in the range of 40 to 130 mm Hg through the mechanism of autoregulation.

- Coronary angiography is the gold standard in the assessment of coronary artery disease. However, there are two major limitations: inter- and intra-observer variabilities of visual evaluation and discrepancies between the angiographic severity of the lesion and the actual degree of underlying atherosclerosis.

- Intracoronary ultrasound (IVUS) imaging is useful in clarifying situations in which angiography is equivocal or difficult to interpret, selecting appropriate catheter-based intervention, and optimizing the results of coronary procedures. The outcome of the patients in whom revascularization was deferred according to IVUS is favorable.

- Coronary flow reserve (CFR) is the ratio of maximal coronary blood flow to resting coronary blood flow and can be measured by a Doppler wire. Coronary flow reserve is reduced with epicardial artery stenosis, microvascular disease, or both.

- In patients with intermediate coronary artery stenosis, previous studies have demonstrated that a CFR < 2 was closely associated with an abnormal stress perfusion imaging and IVUS lumen area < 4mm². However, CFR is easily influenced by the hemodynamic conditions and is not an epicardial stenosis-specific index.

- In patients with acute myocardial infarction, short diastolic deceleration time, presence of systolic flow reversal, and absence of systolic anterior flow are the signs of severe and extensive microvascular damage and are associated with poor ventricular function and poor prognosis.

- Fractional flow reserve (FFR) represents the fraction of maximal myocardial flow that can be maintained in the presence of epicardial coronary stenosis. FFR is an epicardial lesion-specific index and is nearly independent of hemodynamic conditions such as heart rate, blood pressure, and contractility.

*(continued)*

---

● **PRACTICAL POINTS (continued)**

- FFR is a useful guide for decision making about the need for revascularization in intermediate stenoses. Five-year follow-up results of DEFER study showed that the event-free survival rate of deferral group was 80%. Furthermore, the rate of hard endpoint (composite of acute myocardial infarction and cardiac death) was only 3.3% in a deferral group.

- Post-procedural FFR ≥ 0.9~0.95 after bare metal stent implantation is known to be associated with good clinical outcomes. However, FFR criterion for optimal drug-eluting stent implantation is not known.

---

## CORONARY ARTERY PHYSIOLOGY

### Coronary Arterial Circulation

The coronary arterial circulation consists of large arteries, small arteries (prearterioles), and arterioles (**Figure 38-1**). Large arteries include left main trunk and three major coronary arteries and their branches. The diameter of large arteries ranges from several millimeters to 400-500 μm. As most large arteries run over the epicardial surface of the heart, these are called as epicardial arteries. These arteries do not create significant resistance to coronary blood flow and are also called as conductance vessels.

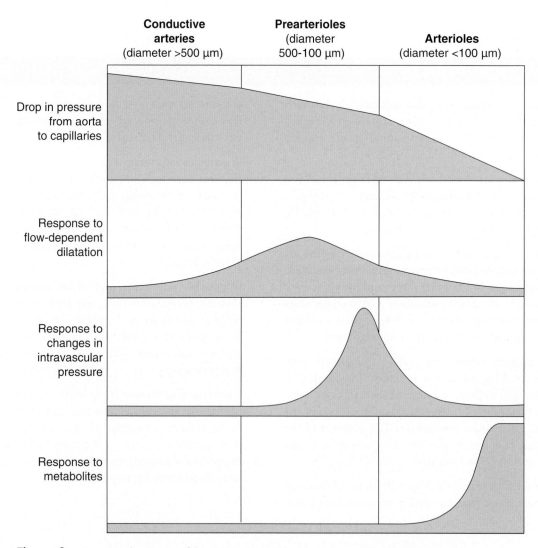

**Figure 38-1.** Functional anatomy of the coronary arterial system (From *N Engl J Med.* 2007.)

Prearterioles and arterioles cannot be clearly delineated by coronary angiography. These microvessels take most of the coronary vascular resistance, and are called as resistance vessels. They can modulate the vascular tone and resistance under various physiologic and pharmacological conditions to control the myocardial blood flow. Prearteriolar vessels (100-500 μm) are responsive to flow and pressure changes, and their function is to maintain the pressure in a narrow range at the origin of arterioles when coronary perfusion flow or pressure changes. Intramural arterioles (<100 μm) are the main part of the metabolic regulation of coronary blood flow. When oxygen consumption increases, arterioles are dilated and vascular resistance is reduced in response to myocardial metabolites. This induces the dilatation of other vessels by the increase in flow and shear stress.

## Coronary Blood Flow and Concept of Coronary Flow Reserve

Coronary arterial blood flow occurs predominantly during diastole, and the systolic component at hyperemia is less than 25% of total flow. The myocardial oxygen demand is much higher than other organs even in the resting condition, and coronary capillary density is also higher to meet the high oxygen demand. Nevertheless, the oxygen extraction by the myocardium is much higher than the other organs and reaches near maximum. The oxygen saturation of coronary sinus venous blood is only about 20-30% (renal vein: 85%). According to Fick's principle, oxygen consumption is the product of blood flow and oxygen extraction. Therefore, coronary circulation can meet the increasing oxygen demand mainly by increasing coronary blood flow.

Resting coronary blood flow can be maintained at a relatively constant level under various coronary perfusion pressures in the range of from 40 to 130 mm Hg through the mechanism of autoregulation. In contrast, when resistance is minimized by a vasodilator, the relationship between pressure and flow becomes linear (**Figure 38-2**).

The concept of coronary flow reserve was developed to describe the flow increase in response to an increase in oxygen demand. It is the ratio of maximal coronary blood flow to resting coronary blood flow:

$$\text{Coronary flow reserve} = \frac{\text{Maximal coronary blood flow}}{\text{Resting coronary blood flow}}$$

Coronary flow reserve is reduced with epicardial artery stenosis, microvascular disease and both. Although the resting coronary flow can be maintained until 80-90% diameter stenosis of the epicardial coronary artery, coronary flow reserve is reduced as the portion of vasodilatory reserve is already used to maintain normal coronary flow. In patients with microvascular disease, coronary flow reserve is decreased due to the decrease in maximal coronary blood flow.

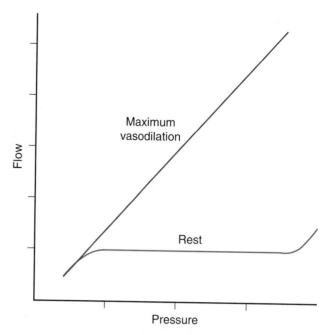

**Figure 38-2.** Schematic illustration of coronary pressure-flow relation at rest and at maximal vasodilatation.

To measure the coronary flow reserve in a catheterization laboratory, pharmacologic stimuli that can minimize the vascular resistance and induce maximal coronary blood flow are needed. Inadequate hyperemia results in underestimation of the coronary flow reserve. Various routes and drugs are currently being used to induce maximal hyperemia (**Table 38-1**). Intracoronary bolus administration of adenosine is a simple and safe way to induce maximal hyperemia. The peak effect occurs in less than 10 seconds and the duration of action is less than 20 seconds. However, this method cannot be used when the steady status of maximal hyperemia is required, and underestimation of the lesion severity is possible in patients with borderline fractional flow reserve (FFR). In general, intracoronary

| Table 38-1 • Drugs for Maximal Vasodilatation | | |
|---|---|---|
| **Drug** | **Dose** | **Time to Maximal Hyperemia** |
| **Adenosine** | | |
| Intracoronary bolus | 20-60 μg | <10 sec |
| Intravenous continuous | 140 μg/kg/min | ≤1-2 min |
| **ATP** | | |
| Intracoronary bolus | 20-50 μg | <10 sec |
| Intravenous continuous | 140 μg/kg/min | ≤1-2 min |
| **Papaverine** | | |
| Intracoronary bolus | 10-15 mg | 30-60 sec |

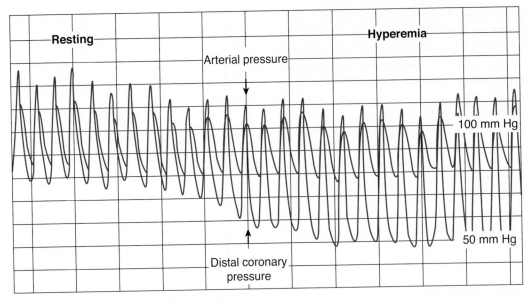

**Figure 38-3.** Arterial and distal coronary pressure changes in a patient with coronary artery disease during continuous infusion of adenosine. Maximal hyperemia corresponds with maximum trans-stenotic pressure gradient and minimal distal coronary pressure. Steady state maximum coronary hyperemia is maintained by continuous infusion of adenosine.

bolus administration of adenosine is commonly used for coronary flow velocity reserve measurement, and intravenous continuous infusion of adenosine is recommended for fractional flow reserve measurement (**Figure 38-3**). Papaverine was considered the gold standard for induction of hyperemia as this drug can induce long maximal hyperemic plateau with bolus administration. However, its use is decreasing due to the potential risk of ventricular arrhythmia.

# INTRACORONARY ULTRASUNOGRAPHY, DOPPLER, AND PRESSURE

Coronary angiography is the most respected method of assessing coronary artery disease. However, there are two major limitations: inter- and intra-observer variability of visual evaluation and discrepancies between the angiographic severity of the lesion; and the actual degree of underlying atherosclerosis. Although the quantitative coronary angiography has reduced its limitations, it cannot completely overcome the limitation of two-dimensional angiographic analysis. Therefore, additional procedures are required in lesions with ambiguous or questionable angiographic findings. Intravascular ultrasound is commonly used in such conditions and can give detailed three-dimensional information on both the lumen and vessel. Pressure- and flow-derived indexes are also frequently used to evaluate the physiologic significance of lesions in both epicardial artery and microvasculature.

ACC/AHA/SCAI practice guidelines for the use of intravascular ultrasound and physiologic evaluation are as follows:

## Intravascular Ultrasound Imaging

### Class IIa

a. Assessment of the adequacy of deployment of coronary stents. (Level of evidence: B)

b. Determination of the mechanism of stent restenosis and to enable selection of appropriate therapy. (Level of evidence: B)

c. Evaluation of coronary obstruction at a location difficult to image by angiography in a patient with a suspected flow-limiting stenosis. (Level of evidence: C)

d. Assessment of a suboptimal angiographic result after percutaneous coronary intervention. (Level of evidence: C)

e. Establishment of the presence and distribution of coronary calcium in patients for whom adjunctive rotational atherectomy is contemplated. (Level of evidence: C)

f. Determination of plaque location and circumferential distribution for guidance of directional coronary atherectomy. (Level of evidence: B)

### Class III

IVUS is not recommended when the angiographic diagnosis is clear and no interventional treatment is planned. (Level of evidence: C)

## Use of Fractional Flow Reserve and Coronary Vasodilatory Reserve

### Class IIa

It is reasonable to use intracoronary physiologic measurements (Doppler ultrasound, fractional flow reserve) in the assessment of the effects of intermediate coronary stenoses in patients with anginal symptoms. Coronary pressure or Doppler velocimetry may also be useful as an alternative to performing noninvasive functional testing to determine whether an intervention is warranted. (Level of evidence: B)

### Class III

Routine assessment with intracoronary physiologic measurements such as Doppler ultrasound or fractional flow reserve to assess the severity of angiographic disease in patients with a positive, unequivocal noninvasive functional study is not recommended. (Level of evidence: C)

## Intravascular Ultrasound

### Ultrasound Catheters and Image Acquisition

The equipment for performing intravascular ultrasound (IVUS) consists of a transducer catheter, a pullback device, and a console for reconstructing the image. High ultrasound frequencies (20-40 MHz) are used for coronary artery evaluation. Axial and lateral resolution of currently available system is 100-150 μm and 200-250 μm, respectively. Two types of transducers are available: mechanically

rotated device and solid state device. The mechanical system has a single transducer, which can rotate at the speed of 1800 rpm, while the solid state system has multiple, cylindrically arrayed transducer elements that can be activated sequentially.

During cardiac catheterization, an IVUS catheter is advanced over a guidewire beyond the target lesion, and a pullback of the transducer tip through the segment of interest is performed to obtain a series of cross-sectional images of the lumen, plaque, and vessel. When performed by an experienced operator, the risk of this invasive imaging procedure is very low. The most frequent complication is transient coronary artery spasm, but this event usually responds well to the intracoronary nitroglycerin. The rate of major complications and acute vascular complication ranges from 0.1% to 0.4%.

### Image Interpretation

When the coronary artery is imaged by IVUS, the relative echolucency of media compared with intima and adventitia creates a three-layered appearance (**Figure 38-4**). In some of the normal subjects, only a monolayer structure is observed due to very thin medial layer. Intimal thickness increases with age, and normal thickness in adults is considered to be >250-500 μm. Average thickness of media in normal coronary arteries is about 200 μm and becomes thinner with the progression of atherosclerosis. The lower ultrasound reflectance of the media is due to the lesser amount of collagen than is seen in the neighboring layers.

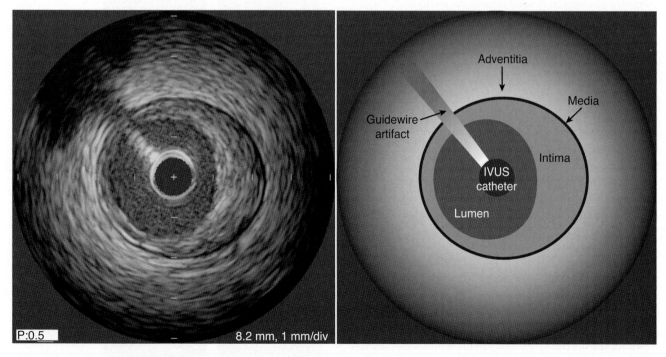

**Figure 38-4.** Intravascular ultrasound image demonstrating the classic three-layered appearance of intima (+ plaque), media, and adventitia.

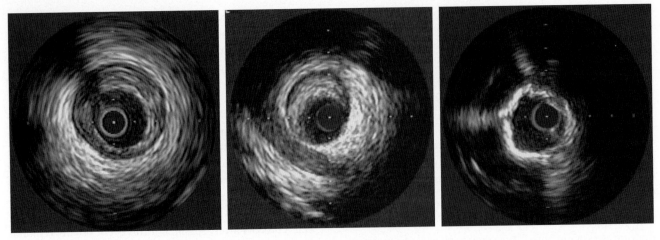

**Figure 38-5.** Example of fibrofatty (left), fibrous (middle), and calcified (right) plaques.

Coronary atherosclerotic plaques can be divided into fibro fatty, fibrous, and calcified lesion according to the IVUS characteristics (**Figure 38-5**). The brightness of the adventitia can be used as a gauge to discriminate fibrofatty from fibrous plaque. Calcified lesions create very bright echo reflections with acoustic shadowing; therefore, it is difficult to acquire information of structures behind the calcium. Although densely fibrous plaque can also induce a bright appearance with shadowing, the brightness is less intense than calcium and the beam penetrates a short distance into the tissue beyond the initial interface.

An important potential application of IVUS is the identification of atherosclerotic plaque at risk of rupture. However, currently available gray scale ultrasound technology cannot accurately evaluate the vulnerability of plaques.

## Measurements

Coronary lumen area is measured by the leading edge of the blood/intima interface. Total vessel area is usually substituted for external elastic membrane (EEM) area, as the EEM represents a reliable boundary. The plaque area is calculated as the difference between total vessel area and lumen area; therefore, this area contains both plaque and media. The percentage of the EEM area occupied by plaque is referred to as percent plaque area, plaque burden, or percent area stenosis. In a stented segment, intimal hyperplasia area can be calculated as the difference between stent area and lumen area.

Three-dimensional volumetric IVUS analysis is also possible with motorized automatic pullback recording and dedicated software. Measurements of the vessel, stent, and lumen areas are usually made at 1-mm axial intervals and volumetric data of each parameter can be calculated using Simpson's rule. To adjust for the difference in length of measured segments, the parameter of volume index is derived from each volume data using the formula of volume/measured length ($mm^3/mm$).

## Clinical Applications

IVUS imaging has proven useful in clarifying situations in which angiography is equivocal or difficult to interpret, selecting appropriate catheter-based intervention, and optimizing the results of coronary procedures (**Figure 38-6**). In lesions with intermediate angiographic stenosis (40-70% diameter stenosis), it is difficult to make a decision for revascularization by angiographic finding alone. In a study by

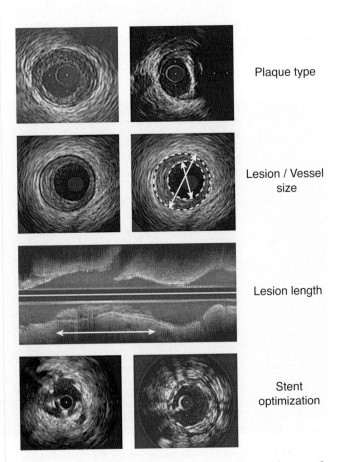

Plaque type

Lesion / Vessel size

Lesion length

Stent optimization

**Figure 38-6.** Common indications of intravascular ultrasound.

Abizaid et al., there was a strong correlation between minimum lumen area by IVUS and coronary flow reserve; → minimum lumen cross-sectional area ≥4.0 mm$^2$ had a diagnostic accuracy of 92% in identifying a CFR of ≥2.0. When compared with the results of SPECT scan, IVUS criteria of minimal lumen area <4 mm$^2$ showed sensitivity and specificity of about 90%.

The outcome of the patients in whom revascularization was deferred according to IVUS was favorable. In patients with deferred intervention after IVUS, target lesion revascularization-free survival rate was reported to be over 90% at 24 months. Therefore, lesions with lumen area <4.0 mm$^2$ in proximal epicardial arteries are considered to be flow-limiting stenoses and to require revascularization. In left main coronary artery stenosis, lesions with minimum lumen area <6 mm$^2$ are considered significant.

IVUS is also commonly used for the evaluation of the revascularization procedures. Among several morphologic findings associated with stenting, two major IVUS-detected problems are stent underexpansion and incomplete stent apposition (**Figure 38-7**). Incomplete stent apposition is defined as one or more struts clearly separated from the vessel wall with the evidence of blood speckle behind the strut. Previous studies showed that the stent implantation with low to intermediate pressures resulted in a high incidence of these problems and IVUS-guided, high pressure balloon dilatation can achieve better stent expansion. There are various IVUS criteria for optimal stent implantation. A commonly used criterion for bare-metal stents is minimal stent area ≥80% of average reference lumen area or

absolute minimum stent area ≥6.5-7.5 mm$^2$. It is controversial whether routine IVUS-guided stent implantation can improve patient outcomes. However, some studies showed that the IVUS-guided stent implantation resulted in larger stent area than angiographic guidance and subsequently reduced the need for target lesion revascularization. In the CRUISE (Can Routine Ultrasound Influence Stent Expansion) study, the IVUS-guided group had a larger minimum stent area and a lower target vessel revascularization rate at 9 months.

IVUS is also useful in identification of complications of stent implantation that require further therapy, such as dissections and intramural hematomas. Therefore, although IVUS is not required for all stent procedures, the use of IVUS in high risk patients or in complex lesions seems to be warranted.

IVUS is also commonly used for the evaluation of the efficacy of newly developed antirestenotic therapies. IVUS has become an essential part of the trials for new drug-eluting stents. Through serial IVUS evaluation, amount of neointimal hyperplasia, presence of acute and late-acquired incomplete stent apposition, edge effect, and vascular response can be assessed. IVUS is also useful in detection of the cause of the drug-eluting stent failure during follow-up. As drug-eluting stents have dramatically reduced the amount of neointimal hyperplasia, different criteria for optimal stent implantation may be needed for these devices. Recent IVUS studies in patients with Cypher sirolimus-eluting stent (Cordis Corporation, Miami Lakes, FL) implantation showed that minimum lumen area of >5-5.5 mm$^2$ was the best predictor of stent patency at follow-up. The incidence of late-acquired, incomplete stent apposition (**Figure 38-8**) is higher in drug-eluting stents than in bare-metal stents. However, it is still not clear whether this finding is linked with adverse cardiac events such as late stent thrombosis.

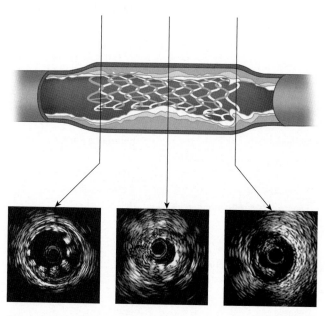

**Figure 38-7.** Intravascular ultrasound findings of stent-related problems: incomplete stent apposition (left), stent underexpansion (middle), and stent edge dissection (right).

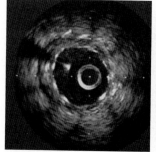
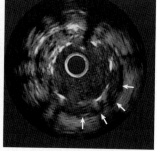

**Figure 38-8.** A case of late acquired incomplete stent apposition. Incomplete stent apposition is seen only at follow-up (right, arrows), not at post-stent implantation (left).

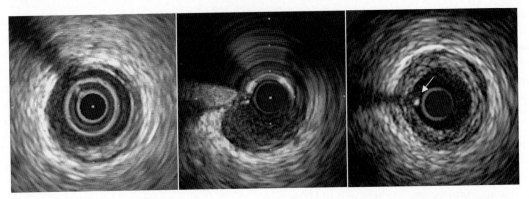

**Figure 38-9.** Common artifacts during intravascular ultrasound procedures: ring-down artifact (left), nonuniform rotational distortion (middle), and wire artifact with posterior acoustic shadowing (left).

There are several limitations in current IVUS devices. Various artifacts can adversely affect ultrasound images. Nonuniform rotational distortion arises from frictional forces to the rotating transducer in the mechanical catheters. It creates stretched or compacted portions of the images (**Figure 38-9**). Ring-down artifacts caused by transducer oscillation obscure near field imaging. They can be seen as bright halos of variable thickness surrounding the catheter (**Figure 38-9**). Due to the profile of IVUS catheter, it is sometimes difficult to get an adequate image in highly tortuous, severely calcified, or far distal lesions.

## Doppler Wire

### Doppler Wire and Coronary Flow Velocity Measurement

Coronary flow reserve (CFR) is the ratio between maximal hyperemic flow and resting flow. As the blood flow is directly proportional to the flow velocity (flow = velocity × cross-sectional area), the ratio of coronary flow velocity (coronary flow velocity reserve, CFVR) can work as a surrogate for coronary flow reserve.

Coronary flow velocity reserve =

$$\frac{\text{Hyperemic average peak velocity (hAPV)}}{\text{Baseline average peak velocity (bAPV)}}$$

Coronary blood flow velocity can be measured using the Doppler guidewire (**Table 38-2**). Current 0.014-inch Doppler guidewire has 12 MHz piezoelectric ultrasound transducer at its tip and this transducer emits ultrasound from the tip of the guidewire in a pulsed wave pattern. Doppler wire records the peak velocity at the sample volume depth of about 5 mm from the tip of the guidewire. As Doppler wire has almost the same handling characteristics as conventional guidewires, it can be easily advanced into the distal part of the coronary artery stenosis. After achieving proper and stable velocity signal, baseline and hyperemic peak velocities are sequentially recorded (**Figure 38-10**). As the measured velocity can be varied according to the position of a wire without the change

in absolute blood flow, the operator should always be careful to keep the tip of the wire at the same location during baseline and hyperemic velocity measurements.

### Clinical Applications

Doppler wire measurements can be useful in evaluation of intermediate lesion, monitoring of coronary blood flow during coronary interventions, and evaluation of microvascular disease.

In patients with intermediate coronary artery stenosis, previous studies have demonstrated that a CFVR <2 was closely associated with an abnormal stress perfusion imaging and IVUS lumen area <4 mm². The outcome of the deferral of revascularization according to CFVR was reported to be favorable. However, as CFVR is easily influenced by the hemodynamic conditions and is not an epicardial stenosis-specific index, fractional flow reserve (FFR) is more commonly used in the evaluation of intermediate stenosis.

| Table 38-2 • Doppler-derived Flow Velocity Parameters | |
|---|---|
| **Variable** | **Normal Reference Range** |
| Average peak velocity (APV) | |
| • Basal | ≥20 cm/sec |
| • Hyperemic | ≥30 cm/sec |
| Diastolic/systolic mean velocity ratio (DSVR) | |
| • Left anterior descending coronary artery | >1.7 |
| • Left circumflex coronary artery | >1.5 |
| • Right coronary artery | >1.2 |
| Coronary flow velocity reserve | ≥2.0 |
| Relative coronary flow reserve | 1.0 |

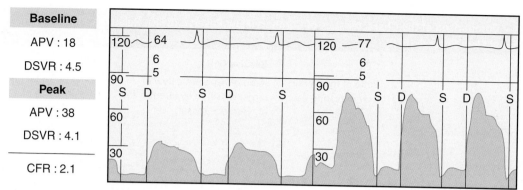

**Figure 38-10.** Example of coronary flow velocity recording at rest (baseline, left) and during hyperemia (peak, right). APV, average peak velocity; DSVR, diastolic/systolic velocity ratio; CFR, coronary flow reserve.

To overcome the limitations of CFVR, relative CFVR (CFVR of target vessel/CFVR of reference vessel) was developed. This parameter is more epicardial stenosis-specific and less sensitive to hemodynamic variation than CFVR. However, this parameter requires four measurements of coronary flow velocity and truly normal reference vessel. Several other velocity-derived parameters have been developed to overcome the shortcomings of Doppler-derived CFR but have failed to prove their clinical significance.

At present, Doppler wire is more commonly used for the assessment of microvascular dysfunction than for the evaluation of epicardial stenosis. In patients with successful primary angioplasty for acute myocardial infarction, Doppler flow velocity pattern has better prognostic importance than CFVR. Large myocardial infarction causes severe microvascular damage, and this increases vascular resistance and decreases microvascular pool. → Therefore, early systolic flow reversal or reduction in systolic flow occurs

due to increased microvascular resistance and shortening of deceleration time occurs due to the rapid reduction of flow velocity after early filling of reduced microvascular pool(**Figure 38-11**). Short diastolic deceleration time, presence of systolic flow reversal, and absence of systolic anterior flow are the signs of severe and extensive microvascular damage and are associated with poor ventricular function and poor prognosis.

## Pressure Wire

### Pressure Wire and Fractional Flow Reserve
When there is a significant epicardial coronary artery stenosis, a pressure gradient across the lesion develops due to the loss of kinetic energy (friction and separation losses). Attempts to correlate trans-stenotic pressure gradient and functional severity of a stenosis have been made since the beginning of percutaneous coronary intervention. However, these attempts were not successful, as the trans-stenotic pressure

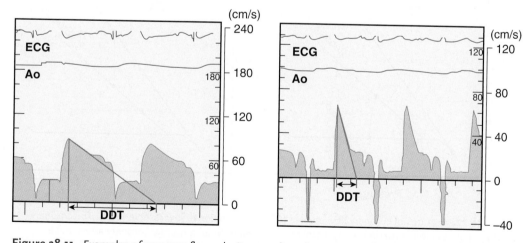

**Figure 38-11.** Examples of coronary flow velocity recordings in patients with acute myocardial infarction after successful percutaneous revascularization. Left: Coronary blood flow spectrum in a patient without severe microvascular injury. Antegrade flow is dominant during systole. The diastolic peak velocity shows a normal deceleration. Right: Coronary blood flow spectrum in a patient with severe microvascular injury. Early systolic retrograde flow is dominant, and antegrade flow is decreased. The diastolic peak velocity shows rapid deceleration. DDT; diastolic deceleration time (From *Circulation.* 2002.)

**Table 38-3 • Comparison of the Characteristics of Coronary Flow Reserve (CFR), Relative CFR, and Fractional Flow Reserve (FFR)**

| | CFR | Relative CFR | FFR |
|---|---|---|---|
| Definition | Ratio of hyperemic flow to resting flow | Ratio of hyperemic flow in target vessel to hyperemic flow in reference vessel | Ratio of hyperemic flow in the presence of a stenosis to normal hyperemic flow |
| Independent of hemodynamic condition | No | Yes | Yes |
| Independent of microvascular dysfunction | No | Yes | Yes |
| Applicable to 3-vessel disease | Yes | No | Yes |

gradient at rest is influenced by hemodynamic conditions and is not the main determinant of myocardial perfusion.

Fractional flow reserve represents the fraction of maximal myocardial flow that can be maintained in the presence of epicardial coronary stenosis.

Fractional flow reserve =

$$\frac{\text{Maximal myocardial flow in the presence of a stenosis}}{\text{Normal maximal flow}}$$

The flow is the ratio of pressure difference and resistance. Since resistances are minimal and equal under maximal hyperemia and venous pressure is negligible when compared to coronary arterial pressure, FFR can be derived from the ratio of distal coronary artery pressure to aortic pressure.

$$FFR = \frac{Q^{s}_{max}}{Q^{N}_{max}} = \frac{(Pd - Pv)/R}{(Pa - Pv)/R} = \frac{P_d}{P_a}$$

where $Q^{s}_{max}$ is hyperemic myocardial blood flow in the presence of a stenosis, $Q^{N}_{max}$ is normal hyperemic myocardial blood flow, Pd is distal coronary pressure, Pa is aortic pressure; Pv is venous pressure, and R hyperemic myocardial resistance

FFR is an epicardial lesion-specific index and is nearly independent of hemodynamic conditions such as heart rate, blood pressure, and contractility (**Table 38-3** and **Figure 38-12**). In normal coronary arteries, the distal pressure equals the aortic pressure during maximal hyperemia and, therefore, normal FFR is 1.0.

A 0.014-inch pressure, sensor-tipped coronary guidewire has been developed to measure intracoronary pressure

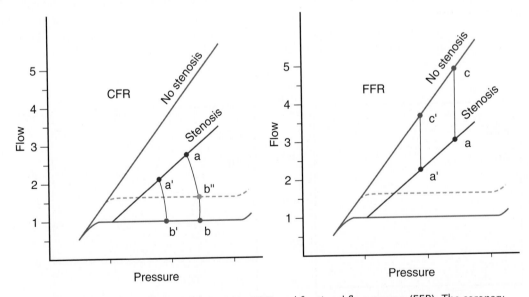

**Figure 38-12.** Features of coronary flow reserve (CFR) and fractional flow reserve (FFR). The coronary pressure–flow relation at maximum hyperemia is indicated both for a normal coronary artery and a coronary stenosis. The resting pressure–flow relation is represented by the solid horizontal line. Left: CFR is defined as the ratio of hyperemic to resting flow (a/b). It is obvious that with changing blood pressure, the value of CFR changes to a'/b'. Also, when resting flow changes as with changing heart rate or contractility, CFR changes to a/b". Right: FFR is defined as the ratio of maximum flow in the presence of a stenosis divided by normal maximum flow (a/c). This ratio remains unaffected by changes in blood pressure (a/c = a'/c') or by variations in resting flow. (From *Heart.* 1998.)

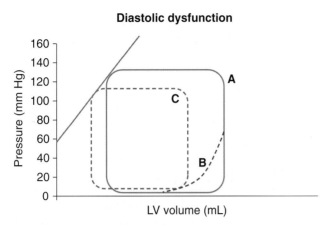

**Figure 39-2.** Diastolic dysfunction shown by increased LVEDP (dashed red line).

volume. The elevated LVEDP may result in dyspnea. The elevation in LVEDP may be more marked during tachycardia. Once treated with diuretics and other medications, the loop may change to Loop C in **Figure 39-2**, which shows reduced LVEDP and LV volumes. Diastolic dysfunction is seen in persons with hypertensive heart disease and in those of advanced age, for example.

## Systolic Dysfunction

Conditions such as dilated cardiomyopathy may represent chronic systolic dysfunction. In order to compensate for the decreased contractility, the left ventricle dilates and Starling's principle comes into play in order to maintain stroke volume. These changes result in dilatation of the left ventricle with increased diastolic volumes. The ejection fraction falls and the red dashed line (B) in **Figure 39-3** represents some of these changes. Principally, the pressure-volume loop shows increased end diastolic and end systolic volumes, resulting in shift of the whole curve to the right. There is reduced stroke

volume and the concomitant diastolic dysfunction is represented by the elevated end diastolic pressure. Systolic dysfunction occurs, for example, in idiopathic dilated cardiomyopathy, ischemic cardiomyopathy, or alcoholic cardiomyopathy.

## Volume and Pressure Overload

In a volume overload condition such as from chronic aortic regurgitation or mitral regurgitation, there is essentially an increase in the LV diastolic volume. This results in a rightward shift of the pressure-volume loop. That results in an increase in stroke volume and gradually leads to an increase in end-systolic volume (Loop B, **Figure 39-4**). Eventually, it may lead to increased end-diastolic pressure. Pressure overload, such as may be seen in chronic hypertension or in aortic stenosis, results in increased systolic pressure in the LV in the heart's effort to overcome the increased resistance (Loop C, **Figure 39-4**). This typically results in a small stiff ventricle and leads to decreased end-diastolic volume and increased end-diastolic pressure with decreased stroke volume. Examples of volume overload are conditions of chronic aortic regurgitation and chronic mitral regurgitation; pressure overload is seen in persons with hypertension and aortic stenosis.

## Acute Changes in Afterload

An increase in afterload will result in increased systolic pressure, increased diastolic pressure and reduced stroke volume (Loop B, **Figure 39-5**). Reduced afterload will result in reduced diastolic and systolic pressures (Loop C, **Figure 39-5**). Afterload changes refer to changes in peripheral vascular resistance. Vasodilators will typically result in afterload reduction and vasoconstrictors will result in increases in afterload. Increased afterload occurs, for example, during intravenous administration of norepinephrine,

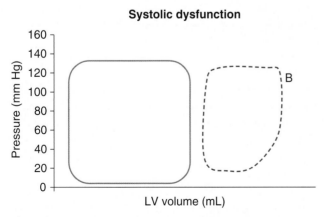

**Figure 39-3.** Systolic dysfunction (chronic) in dilated cardiomyopathy showing increased LV volumes, reduced stroke volume, and elevated LVEDP.

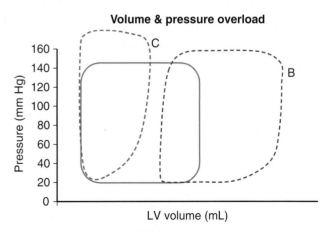

**Figure 39-4.** Pressure-volume loops seen in chronic volume and pressure overload conditions.

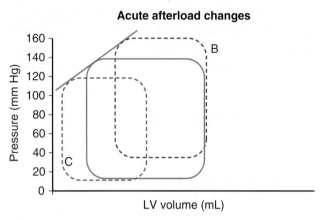

**Figure 39-5.** Pressure-volume responses in acute afterload changes.

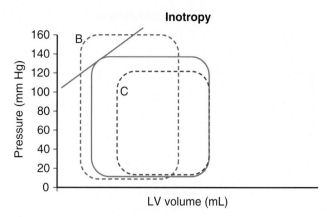

**Figure 39-7.** Changes in inotropic conditions. Increased inotropy seen in green and decreased inotropy in red.

vasopressin, or phenylephrine. Decreased afterload occurs in administration of hydralazine and ACE inhibitors.

## Changes in Preload

Preload refers to the filling volume in diastole. In an acute change, increased preload results in increased end-diastolic volume and increased stroke volume (Loop B, **Figure 39-6**), while decreased preload results in decreased pressures and volumes (Loop C, **Figure 39-6**), shifting the curve to the left and down as well as reducing stroke volume. Examples of increases in preload are those associated with administration of IV fluids; decreased preload occurs with blood loss, diarrhea, Valsalva maneuver, and administration of nitrates or diuretics.

## Inotropic Changes

Inotropy refers to force of contraction of the heart. Increased inotropy will result in increased stroke volume. It will also typically result in increased systolic pressure and reduced end-systolic volume, which reflects greater ventricular ejection and increased ejection fraction (Loop B, **Figure 39-7**). Decreased inotropic state will result in reduced LV systolic

pressure, reduced ejection, and stroke volume (Loop C, **Figure 39-7**). Examples of increased inotropy are seen after administration of digoxin or dobutamine. Decreased inotropy can occur with beta-blockers or diltiazem.

## Key Changes in Pressure Volume Loops in Various Conditions

Some key changes are represented in a tabular fashion in **Table 39-1**. Note that in advanced disease states, the

| Table 39-1 • Key components of the pressure-volume loop in various conditions. ESV, end-systolic volume; EDV, end-diastolic volume; SV, stroke volume; EF, ejection fraction; LVEDP, LV end-diastolic pressure. | | | | | |
|---|---|---|---|---|---|
| | **ESV** | **EDV** | **SV** | **EF** | **LVEDP** |
| Increased preload | o | + | + | + | o/+ |
| Decreased preload | o/− | − − | − | − | − |
| Increased afterload | + | o | − | − | o/+ |
| Decreased afterload | − | o | + | + | − |
| Aortic insufficiency | + | ++ | + | + | o/+ |
| Aortic stenosis | − | − | − | o | o/+ |
| Mitral regurgitation | + | ++ | − | + | + |
| Mitral stenosis | − | − | − − | o | − |
| Dilated cardiomyopathy | + | ++ | − | − − | + |

o = no change
− = mild decrease
− − = marked decrease
+ = mild increase
++ = marked increase

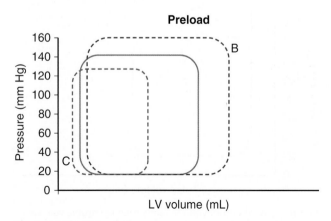

**Figure 39-6.** Preload changes.

LVEDP tends to rise in most conditions where decompensation exists, with the possible exception of mitral stenosis, in which there is a rise in the left atrial pressure causing pulmonary congestion without a rise in the LV diastolic pressure due to the gradient across the mitral valve. Interventions may cause shifts in the existing pressure-volume loops in accordance with their respective mechanisms of action. Examples of such interventions are administration of diuretics, which will cause reduced LVEDP. Afterload reduction with ACE inhibitors will cause decreased LVEDP; decreased LV systolic pressure and increased stroke volume; positive inotropes will cause increased stroke volume.

## Suggested Readings

1. Guyton AC, Hall JE. *Textbook of Medical Physiology*. 11th ed. Philedelphic. WB Saunders Co.; 2006.

2. Libby P, Bonorr Ro, Mann DL, Zipes DP, Braunwald E. eds. *Braunwald's Heart Discase*. 8th ed. Philedelphic. Elsevier Saunders.; 2008.

# 40

# ST Segment Elevation Myocardial Infarction (STEMI)

Melike Bayram, Ernest L. Mazzaferri Jr., and Richard Gumina

## ● PRACTICAL POINTS

Reperfusion in STEMI:

- Patients presenting to a non-PCI-capable hospitals, should have medical contact-to-needle time less than 30 minutes.

- Patients presenting to a PCI-capable hospitals should have medical contact-to-balloon time of 90 minutes or less.

- For patients presenting to non-PCI-capable hospitals, it is appropriate to consider interhospital transfer to a PCI-capable hospital if:

  ○ there is a contraindication to fibrinolysis;

    or

  ○ PCI can be initiated within 90 minutes of initial presentation to the receiving hospital or within 60 minutes of the time of fibrinolysis with a fibrin-specific agent that can be initiated at the receiving hospital;

    or

  ○ fibrinolysis is administered and is unsuccessful (i.e., rescue PCI).

- Initial medical management in STEMI includes oxygen, sublingual or intravenous nitroglycerin (unless contraindicated), analgesia and beta-blockade. Use of oral beta-blockers is recommended within 24 hours unless contraindicated whereas intravenous beta-blockade is only recommended in hypertensive patients.

- ASA 325 mg chewable should be given to all patients.

- Thienopyridines (clopidogrel or prasugrel) can be used for patients who will undergo primary PCI.

- For patients who have already received fibrinolytics, clopidogrel is the recommended thienopyridine. Prasugrel should not be used in patients with prior history of TIA or stroke.

- For patients undergoing primary PCI, abciximab, tirofiban, or eptifibatide may be used as the GPIIb/IIIa inhibitor at the time of PCI. The usefulness of these agents as part of a preparatory pharmacologic strategy before arrival to the cardiac catheterization lab is uncertain.

- For patients undergoing primary PCI, UFH or bivaluridin (in the presence of thienopyridine-loading) can be used as the anticoagulant agent. With fibrinolytic therapy, UFH, LMWH, or fondaparinux can be used as the anticoagulant. Fondaparinux should not be used as a sole agent to support PCI because of risk of catheter thrombosis.

- Facilitated PCI with GPIIb/IIIa inhibitors, half-dose or full-dose fibrinolytics is not recommended.

- Rescue PCI reduces mortality in high risk patients.

- Patients presenting to non-PCI-capable hospitals should be transferred to PCI capable hospitals as soon as possible regardless of the initial reperfusion strategy.

- In patients presenting with shock, either of PCI or surgical revascularization is superior to fibrinolytic therapy, showing better survival rates.

- It is reasonable to use drug-eluting stents as an alternative to bare-metal stent for primary PCI in STEMI.

# PATHOPHYSIOLOGY AND DIAGNOSIS

ST-segment elevation myocardial infarction (STEMI) results from acute occlusion of a coronary artery, most often secondary to the abrupt rupture of a nonobstructive plaque, which has a thin fibrous plaque and is rich in macrophages and other inflammatory cells. After plaque disruption, there is release of substances that promote platelet aggregation and attract more inflammatory cells, ultimately leading to thrombus formation. Acute occlusion of the infarct artery leads to injury current on the ECG (ST-elevation). More than 500,000 STEMIs per year are done in the United States (ACC/AHA Practice Guidelines 2004).

A 12-lead ECG should be performed as soon as possible on patients suspected of having acute coronary syndrome (ACS). Mortality is higher if a greater number of ECG leads show ST elevation; if there is left bundle branch block (LBBB), and/or by anterior location of the ST elevation. The current diagnostic ECG criteria for STEMI are: ≥1-mm ST elevation in 2 or more contiguous leads, or LBBB, or anterior ST depression suggesting posterior infarction with reciprocal changes in opposite leads (ACC/AHA Practice Guidelines 2004).

# INITIAL MEDICAL MANAGEMENT

## Oxygen

Oxygen administration has become a universal practice in management of acute MI. Even though some patients may need oxygen because of poor arterial oxygen saturation/secondary pulmonary edema, for patients who have pulse oximetry saturation better than 90% it is not clear whether oxygen limits myocardial injury or reduces morbidity or mortality. For patients whose oxygen saturation is normal at baseline, there is no reason to continue supplementation for more than 6 hours.

## Nitroglycerin

Nitroglycerin administration (sublingual or intravenous) causes peripheral arterial and venous vasodilation as well as endothelium-independent coronary artery dilatation. It reduces preload and afterload, and increases coronary blood flow. A pooled analysis of more than 80,000 patients in 72 trials suggests a small mortality benefit when oral or intravenous form is used in the acute MI setting, reducing mortality by 3 to 4 deaths per 1000. However, caution is advised when nitroglycerin is used in patients with acute MI as it may cause hypotension, and it is not recommended if SBP is less than 90 mm Hg or equal to more than 30 mm Hg below baseline systolic blood pressure (ACC/AHA Practice Guidelines 2004). Also, nitroglycerin reduces left ventricular preload and can cause severe hypotension in patients undergoing right ventricular infarction.

## Analgesia

In the acute phase of STEMI, there is increased sympathetic activity and pain associated with myocardial injury, which may be heightened by apprehension and anxiety. Morphine sulfate is the main analgesic recommended in this setting secondary to effects on pain and anxiety relief (ACC/AHA Practice Guidelines 2004). It causes withdrawal of catecholamines and augmentation of the vagal tone. Morphine also has peripheral venous and arterial vasodilatory effect, potentially reducing symptoms from pulmonary edema. One should exercise caution when prescribing high doses of morphine, given its potential effects on lowering blood pressure and enhancing respiratory depression.

## Beta-blockade

Use of intravenous (i.v.) beta-blockade within the first few hours of infarction has been shown, in the prefibrinolysis era, to reduce magnitude of infarction and to reduce mortality by day one, the latter shown to be a sustained benefit in ISIS-1 (International Study of Infarct Survival-1) and MIAMI trials (Metoprolol in Acute Myocardial Infarction). In the fibrinolytic therapy era, early trials show that early use of i.v. beta-blockade (within 6 hours) reduces the rate of reinfarction, recurrent ischemia, and mortality (if used within 2 hours) (Thrombolysis in Myocardial Infarction trial (TIMI)). Subsequent randomized trials, including the post hoc analysis GUSTO-1 (Global Utilization of Streptokinase and Tissue Plasminogen Activator for Occluded Coronary Arteries-1) and a systematic review of STEMI trials have challenged the benefit of early use of intravenous beta-blockade, showing no mortality benefit. Therefore, early use of i.v. beta-blockade in the reperfusion era is controversial. Most recently, COMMIT/CCS-2 Trial (Clopidogrel and Metoprolol in Myocardial Infarction Trial/Second Chinese Cardiac Study-2) studied early use of beta-blockade in 45,852 patients within 24 hours of acute MI. Patients received up to 3 doses of 5 mg of i.v. metoprolol within the first 15 minutes followed by 200 mg of metoprolol daily versus placebo. Metoprolol was shown to decrease the rate of reinfarction and ventricular fibrillation but there were increased episodes of cardiogenic shock in high risk patients. The absolute reduction in arrhythmia-related deaths was similar to the absolute increase in cardiogenic shock-related deaths with no overall mortality difference. Patients over 70 years of age, with a presenting heart rate >110 bpm, systolic BP <120, or presenting Killip class >1 were at higher risk for developing cardiogenic shock. Based on the results from COMMIT/CCS-2, the most recent ACC/AHA Practice Guidelines (2007 Update) give the following Class I recommendation:

*"Oral beta-blocker therapy should be initiated in the first 24 hours for patients who do not have any of the following:*

1. *signs of heart failure,*
2. *evidence of a low output state,*
3. *increased risk for cardiogenic shock, or*
4. *other relative contraindications to beta blockade (PR interval greater than 0.24 seconds, second- or third-degree heart block, active asthma, or reactive airway disease)."*

A Class IIa recommendation is use of i.v. beta-blockade in patients who are hypertensive if they do not have the mentioned contraindications (ACC/AHA Practice Guidelines 2007).

## Reperfusion

Time to restoration of blood flow in the obstructed infarct artery after symptom onset in STEMI patients is a key determinant of both short-term and long-term outcomes regardless of method of reperfusion (fibrinolysis or percutaneous coronary intervention (PCI). Mortality increases as the time to reperfusion increases (**Figure 40-1**). A Class I indication is that all STEMI patients undergo rapid evaluation for reperfusion therapy and have a reperfusion strategy implemented promptly after contact with the medical system (ACC/AHA Practice Guidelines 2004). The goal is to recognize STEMI as quickly as possible and decrease the medical contact-to-needle time to <30 minutes or medical contact-to-balloon time to <90 minutes. Selection of the ideal reperfusion strategy varies depending on the clinical scenario, patient characteristics, and the capabilities of the medical facility.

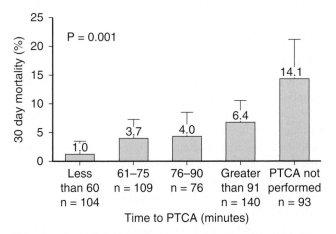

**Figure 40-1.** Relationship between 30-day mortality and time from study enrollment to first balloon inflation (intention to treat analysis: patients assigned to angioplasty in whom angioplasty was not performed are also shown). PTCA, percutaneous transluminal coronary angioplasty. (Reprinted with permission from Berger et al. *Circulation.* 1999;100:14–20.)

## Fibrinolysis versus Primary PCI

Available data from numerous trials suggest that time saved during the early hours (within the first 2 hours) of STEMI have greater impact on outcome compared to later, during symptomatic presentation. The efficacy of fibrinolytic agents in lysing the thrombus diminishes as time passes, with greatest efficacy being within the first hour (*Am Heart J* 1999;137:34–8). An overview of 9 trials shows 35-day mortality benefit of 18% from fibrinolysis in patients with ST elevation compared to control (18 deaths per 1000 patients). This survival benefit was maintained over 10 years. Mortality benefit was greatest when administered within the first hour, declining in benefit by 1.6 lives per 1000 people per 1 hour delay. Fibrinolytics almost completely lose their beneficial effects within 12 hours after symptom onset.

For facilities that can offer primary PCI, the available data show that this approach is superior to fibrinolysis (ACC/AHA Practice Guidelines 2004). However, these data compared fibrinolysis and PCI prior to the advent of most recent approaches in both fields. In these trials, the magnitude of treatment differences in death, stroke, or nonfatal reinfarction varied based on whether primary PCI was compared to streptokinase or a fibrin-specific lytic as well as the differences in the door-to-balloon and door-to-needle times. A meta-analysis of 23 trials (7739 patients combined) by Keeley et al.[1] shows that much of the superiority of primary PCI is driven by a reduction in recurrent MI. Recent trials make superiority of PCI over fibrinolysis more controversial. A meta-analysis shows that if fibrinolytics can be administered to the appropriate patients in the prehospital setting, time to treatment is reduced by 1 hour and mortality is reduced by 17%[2]. CAPTIM (The Comparison of Angioplasty and Prehospital Thrombolysis in Acute Myocardial Infarction), SWEDES (Swedish Early Decision) and WEST (Which Early ST-Elevation Myocardial Infarction Therapy) showed that when fibrinolytic therapy is administered within the first 2 hours of symptom onset, it has superior outcomes compared to primary PCI; however, it should be kept in mind that in these trials, a significant proportion of patients randomized to fibrinolytic therapy (20-25%) underwent rescue PCI. In comparison, patients in PRAGUE-2 (Long Distance Transport for Primary Angioplasty versus Immediate Thrombolysis in Acute Myocardial Infarction) who were randomized within 3 hours of symptom onset did not have any difference in mortality regardless of the reperfusion strategy (7.4% with fibrinolysis versus 7.3% if transferred for primary PCI), whereas those presenting between 3-12 hours from symptom onset showed superiority of primary PCI.

The conclusion from these trials is that when primary PCI is available with a medical contact-to-balloon time <90 minutes, it seems to be superior over fibrinolysis

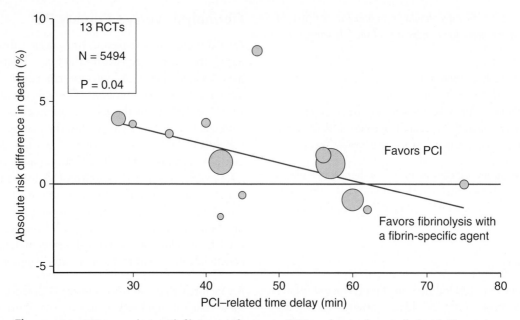

**Figure 40-2.** PCI versus lysis with fibrin-specific agents. RCT, randomized controlled trial; N, number of patients; PCI, percutaneous coronary intervention. (Modified from Nallamothu BK et al. *Am J Cardiol.* 2003;92:824–826.)

(**Figure 40-2**). For patients who present within the first 2 hours of symptoms and have access to prehospital administration of fibrinolytic agents, this approach is at least noninferior to primary PCI if not superior (ACC/AHA Practice Guidelines 2004).

However, when estimated mortality with fibrinolysis is high, as in cardiogenic shock, existing evidence supports superiority of a primary PCI strategy (low coronary flow decreases the efficacy of the fibrinolytic agent on the intracoronary thrombus). The SHOCK trial (Should We Emergently Revascularize Occluded Coronaries for Cardiogenic Shock?) showed that patients with cardiogenic shock had better 1-year survival with early coronary revascularization compared to medical therapy. Observational data from NRMI (Second National Registry of Myocardial Infarction-2) also supports superiority of PCI over fibrinolysis for patients with Killip class ≥ II (see **Table 40-1** for Killip classification).

When a STEMI patient arrives at a center without interventional cardiology facilities, fibrinolysis can usually be provided faster than primary PCI. It should be kept in mind that as the time delay to primary PCI increases, its benefit over fibrinolysis decreases. Compared to a fibrinolytic agent, primary PCI may not reduce mortality when a time delay >1 hour is anticipated compared to immediate administration of a fibrinolytic agent (fibrin-specific agent) (**Figure 40-2**)[3]. On the other hand, invasive strategy is preferred if a skilled PCI facility is available with surgical back-up with door-to-balloon time <90 minutes; if patient is high risk (cardiogenic shock and/or Killip class >II); if there is a contraindication to fibrinolysis; or if symptom onset is >3 hours previous.

## Fibrinolytic Agents

All fibrinolytic agents are direct or indirect plasminogen activators. Streptokinase is an indirect activator whereas alteplase, reteplase, and tenecteplase are direct activators. Direct activators are not antigenic and do not cause allergic reactions (unlike streptokinase, they do not cause production of neutralizing antibodies). Direct activators are more effective in achieving early reperfusion and TIMI-3 flow than streptokinase; however, they are more expensive and are associated with a slightly higher risk of intracranial hemorrhage (ICH). Of the three, tenecteplase is associated with fewer mild to moderate systemic bleeding complications with similar rates of reperfusion, 30-day mortality and incidence of ICH (ASSENT-2). Older age, female sex, black race, prior stroke, SBP ≥160 mm Hg, lower weight (<65 kg for females; <80 kg for males), INR >4 and choice of fibrinolytic agent (tPA is associated with more bleeding than streptokinase)

| Table 40-1 • Killip Classification | | |
|---|---|---|
| **Class** | **Definition** | **Mortality** |
| I | No CHF | 6% |
| II | + S3 and/or basilar rales | 17% |
| III | Pulmonary edema | 30-40% |
| IV | Cardiogenic shock | 60-80% |

*From Am J Cardiol. 1967;20:457.*
*Under the current ACC/AHA guidelines, "STEMI patients presenting to a facility without the capability for expert intervention with primary PCI within 90 minutes of first medical contact should undergo fibrinolysis unless contraindicated (Class I)" (see Table 40-2 for contraindications).*

## Table 40-2 • Advisory Contraindications/Cautions to Fibrinolysis in STEMI

| |
|---|
| **Absolute contraindications** |
| Any prior ICH |
| Known structural cerebral vascular lesion (e.g., AVMs) |
| Known intracranial neoplasm (primary or metastatic) |
| Ischemic stroke within 3 months except ischemic stroke within 3 hours |
| Suspected aortic dissection |
| Active bleeding or bleeding diathesis (excluding menses) |
| Significant closed head or facial trauma within 3 months |
| **Relative contraindications** |
| History of chronic, severe, poorly controlled hypertension |
| Severe uncontrolled hypertension on presentation (SBP > 180 mm Hg or DBP > 110 mm Hg) (can be an absolute contraindication in low risk patients with MI) |
| History of ischemic stroke >3 months previous, dementia or known intracranial pathology not mentioned under absolute contraindications |
| Traumatic or prolonged (>10 minutes) CPR or major surgery (within <3 weeks) |
| Recent (within 2-4 weeks) internal bleeding |
| Noncompressible vascular punctures |
| For streptokinase/anistreplase, prior exposure (more than 5 previous) or prior allergic reaction to these agents |
| Pregnancy |
| Active peptic ulcer |
| Current use of anticoagulants; the higher the INR, the higher the risk of bleeding |

*ACC/AHA Practice Guidelines 2004.*

abciximab. In the arm with abciximab and fibrinolytic, a reduced dose of heparin was used, unlike the full-dose in the fibrinolytic arm. In the arm with abciximab and fibrinolytic, a reduced dose of heparin was used, unlike the full-dose in the fibrinolytic arm. Both studies showed a lower reinfarction rate and less refractory ischemia in the abciximab plus half-dose fibrinolytic arm; however, the 30-day or 1-year mortality was similar in both arms. The biggest caveat was that the rate of major bleeding was higher in the combined therapy arm, with the exception of ICH, which was similar in both arms. In the subgroup analysis, those over age 75 years were at greatest risk for excess bleeding (including higher risk of ICH). It was a Class IIb recommendation to use abciximab and half-dose reteplase or tenecteplase for the prevention of reinfarction and other complications of STEMI in selected patients (those with anterior location of MI, age less than 75 years, and no risk factors for bleeding) even though in the two clinical trials, prevention of reinfarction did not translate into survival benefit at either 30 days or 1 year (ACC/AHA Practice Guidelines 2004).

Based on the recent 2009 update to ACC/AHA Practice Guidelines, the term "facilitated PCI" is no longer used.

## Primary PCI

Primary PCI (PPCI) has been compared to fibrinolysis in 22 randomized clinical trial. The SHOCK trial compared PPCI to fibrinolysis in a specific group of patients with cardiogenic shock. Review of these trials show that PPCI patients experience lower rates of short-term mortality (5% versus 7%, p = 0.0002), less nonfatal reinfarction rates (3% versus 7%, p = 0.0003) and less hemorrhagic stroke (0.05% versus 1%, p = 0.0001), but higher risk of major bleeding (7% versus 5%, p = 0.032), with the greatest mortality benefit in high risk patients. In the SHOCK trial, the reduction in 30-day mortality was 9% in the PPCI group in comparison to the medical stabilization group. In NRMI-II, patients with CHF who underwent PPCI had a 33% relative risk reduction compared with 9% in the fibrinolytic therapy group. Mortality increases significantly with each 15-minute delay in the time between arrival and restoration of TIMI-3 flow. After adjustment of baseline characteristics, time from symptom onset to balloon inflation predicts 1-year mortality with RR 1.08 for each 30-minute delay from symptom onset to balloon inflation (p = 0.04).

The following are abbreviated STEMI reperfusion recommendations by the ACC/AHA Practice Guidelines (2004),

1. *Perform primary PCI, if immediately available, in patients presenting with STEMI (including posterior MI) or MI with LBBB who can undergo PCI of the infarct artery within 12 hours of symptom onset, if performed in a timely fashion (door-to-balloon time 90 minutes) by persons skilled in the procedure (individuals who perform more than 75 PCI procedures per year). The procedure should be supported by ex-*

are factors that increase risk of bleeding (Brass LM et al., *Stroke* 2000;31:1802–11). Patients with none or 1 of these risk factors have a 0.69% risk of ICH whereas those with 5 or more risk factors have 4.1% risk of ICH.

## Fibrinolysis Combined with GPIIb/IIIa Inhibitors

GPIIb/IIIa inhibitors alone without fibrinolysis or PCI do not achieve TIMI 3 flow and are not recommended as a single pharmacological agent for reperfusion (ACC/AHA Practice Guidelines 2004). However, there have been studies looking at use of GPIIb/IIIa agents in combination with fibrinolytic agents and higher TIMI-3 flow rates have been achieved within 60 to 90 minutes. GUSTO-V (Global Utilization of Streptokinase and Tissue Plasminogen Activator for Occluded Coronary Arteries-V) and ASSENT-3 (Assessment of the Safety and Efficacy of a New Thrombolytic Regimen-3) trials compared use of full-dose fibrin-specific lytics (reteplase and tenecteplase, respectively) to half-dose fibrinolytic in combination with *perienced personnel in an appropriate laboratory environment (a laboratory that performs more than 200 PCI procedures per year, of which at least 36 are primary PCI for STEMI, and [that] has cardiac surgery capability). (Class I)*

2. *STEMI patients presenting to a hospital with PCI capability should be treated with primary PCI within 90 minutes of first medical contact as a systems goal. (Class I)*

3. *STEMI patients presenting to a facility without the capability for expert, prompt intervention with primary PCI within 90 minutes of first medical contact should undergo fibrinolytic therapy unless contraindicated. (Class I)*

4. *STEMI patients presenting to a hospital without PCI capability and who cannot be transferred to a PCI center and undergo PCI within 90 minutes of first medical contact should be treated with fibrinolytic therapy within 30 minutes of hospital presentation as a systems goal unless fibrinolytic therapy is contraindicated. (Class I)*

5. *If the symptom onset is within 3 hours and the expected door-to-balloon time minus the expected door-to-needle time is within 1 hour, primary PCI is preferred; if greater than 1 hour, fibrinolytic therapy is preferred. (Class I)*

6. *If symptom duration is greater than 3 hours, primary PCI is generally preferred and should be performed as quickly as possible (with goal door-to-balloon time less than 90 min). (Class I)*

7. *Primary PCI should be performed for patients less than 75 years old (also reasonable for selected patients 75 years or older with ST elevation or LBBB who develop shock within 36 hours of MI and are suitable for revascularization that can performed within 18 hours of shock). Also, primary PCI should be performed in patients with severe CHF and/or pulmonary edema (Killip class 3) and onset of symptoms within 12 hours. (Class IIa)*

8. *It is reasonable to perform primary PCI for patients with onset of symptoms within the prior 12 to 24 hours and severe CHF and/or hemodynamic or electrical instability and/or persistent ischemic symptoms. (Class IIa)*

9. *Perform primary PCI in hospitals without on-site cardiac surgery, provided that a proven plan for rapid transport to cardiac surgery operating room exists in a nearby hospital with appropriate hemodynamic support capability for transfer. (Class IIb)*

10. *The benefit of primary PCI for STEMI patients eligible for fibrinolysis is not well established when performed by an operator who performs fewer than 75 PCI procedures per year. (Class IIb)*

11. *PCI should not be performed in a noninfarct artery at the time of primary PCI in patients without hemodynamic compromise or in asymptomatic patients more than 12 hours after onset of STEMI if they are hemodynamically and electrically stable (Class III) nor at hospitals without on-site cardiac surgery capabilities and without a proven plan for rapid transport to a cardiac surgery operating room in a nearby hospital. (Class III)*

## Delayed Primary PCI

In the Occluded Artery Trial (OAT) trial, 2166 patients >24 hours post-MI were randomized to PCI with optimal medical therapy versus optimal medical therapy only. There was no difference in 4-year event rates (death, MI, or Class IV CHF) between the two groups (17.2% PCI versus 15.6% medical therapy, p = 0.20). However, it should be kept in mind that patients with LM or 3-vessel disease, hemodynamic or electrical instability, rest or low-threshold angina, and Class III-IV heart failure or shock were excluded in this study.

## Primary Stenting

Of the 22 randomized trials that compared primary PCI and fibrinolysis, 12 compared primary PCI with stenting and fibrinolytic therapy. PCI with primary stenting was shown to be associated with lower mortality rates (5.9% versus 7.7%, p = 0.013), lower reinfarction rates (1.6% versus 5.1%, p = 0.0001) and hemorrhagic stroke compared to fibrinolytic therapy. Primary stenting when compared with PTCA in a large meta-analysis was associated with similar mortality, reinfarction rates; however. major cardiac events were reduced, driven by a reduction in target vessel revascularization with stenting (**Figure 40-3**)[4].

In terms of comparing BMS (bare-metal stents) and DES (drug-eluting stents), there are data from three trials that became available since the last update of clinical guidelines. PASSION (Paclitaxel-Eluting Versus Uncoated Stents in Primary Percutaneous Coronary Intervention) compared paclitaxel-eluting stents (n = 309) to BMS (n = 310) among patients undergoing PCI for STEMI. Each patient received 80-100 mg daily ASA and 300 mg of clopidogrel load followed by 75 mg daily. Rate of primary endpoint of death, reinfarction, and target vessel revascularization at 1 year did not differ between the two groups (8.8% for paclitaxel versus 12.8% for BMS group, p = 0.12). There was no difference between paclitaxel-eluting and bare-metal stent groups in rates of cardiac death, MI, TVR, or stent thrombosis when analyzed separately. TYPHOON (Trial to Assess the Use of the Cypher Stent in Acute Myocardial Infarction Treated with Balloon Angioplasty) and SESAMI (Sirolimus Stent versus Bare Stent in Acute Myocardial Infarction) trials randomized STEMI patients (primary or rescue PCI) to sirolimus-eluting stents versus BMS. There were 712 patients in the TYPHOON trial and 312 patients in the SESAMI trial. Patients in both arms received ASA, and 300 mg of clopidogrel load followed by 75 mg daily. Patients, unlike those in PASSION study, also underwent angiographic follow-up at 8 months (TYPHOON) or at 1 year (SESAMI). In TYPHOON, primary endpoint of target vessel revascularization was lower in the sirolimus group (7.3% versus 14.3%, p = 0.004) driven by a reduction in TVR (5.6% versus 13.4%, p < 0.001) with no difference in

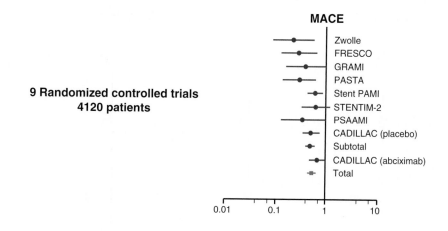

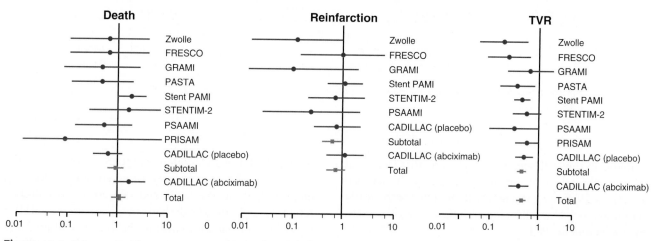

**Figure 40-3.** Primary stenting versus primary angioplasty. OR and their 95% confidence intervals for primary stenting vs. primary angioplasty for the risk of death, reinfarction, target vessel revascularization (TVR), and major adverse cardiac events (MACE) over a 6- to 12-month follow-up after ST-elevation myocardial infarction (STEMI). (Modified from Zhu MM et al. *Am J Cardiol.* 2001;88:297–301.)

death (2.3% versus 2.2%), recurrent MI (1.1% versus 1.4%), or stent thrombosis. Similarly, SESAMI trial showed lower rates of primary endpoint of binary restenosis (both clinical and angiographic), and lower rates of TVR (target vessel revascularization) (4.3% versus 11.2%) and MACE (major cardiac events) (6.8% versus 16.8%) in the sirolimus group. When results from PASSION are compared to TYPHOON and SESAMI, there are several important differences that should be noted in addition to the different type of DES that was used, including lack of angiographic follow-up in PASSION trial. This may have decreased the repeat revascularization rate in PASSION, which was very low in both arms, whereas TVR in TYPHOON and SESAMI trials, in both DES and BMS arms, was much higher.

## Facilitated PCI

Facilitated PCI is a strategy of planned immediate PCI after initial treatment with a pharmacologic agent such as GPIIb/IIIa inhibitor, high-dose heparin, GPIIb/IIIa inhibitor plus half-dose fibrinolytic agent, or full-dose fibrinolytic agent.

Uptill the most recent 2009 ACC/AHA updated guidelines, recommendations were based on the results from 17 trials comparing facilitated PCI with primary PCI alone. Of these, ASSENT-4 PCI trial is the largest and randomized 1667 patients to full-dose tenecteplase and PCI versus primary PCI. This study was terminated early because of the increased in-hospital mortality rate in the facilitated PCI group (6% versus 3%, p = 0.01). The combined primary endpoint of 90-day event rate (death, shock, or congestive heart failure) was higher (18.6% versus 13.4%, p = 0.0045) as well as a trend towards higher mortality in the facilitated PCI group. It should be kept in mind that, in ASSENT-4 PCI, patients in the facilitated PCI arm did not receive any heparin after the initial bolus nor clopidogrel load. GPIIb/IIIa was used only as a bailout creating a suboptimal antithrombotic therapy.

Similarly, a review of the 17 trials (including ASSENT-4) (**Figure 40-4**) that compared facilitated PCI with primary PCI (9 trials with GPIIb/IIIa inhibitors, 6 trials with fibrinolytic therapy, 2 trials with fibrinolytics plus GPIIb/IIIa

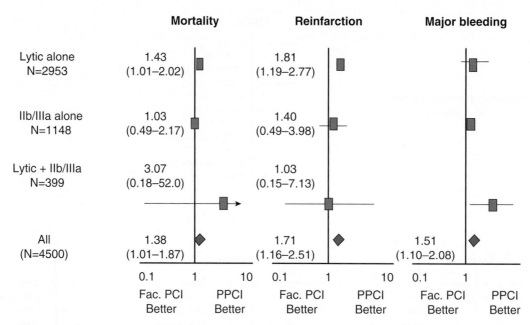

**Figure 40-4.** Meta-analysis: Facilitated PCI vs. primary PCI. (Modified from Keeley E et al. *Lancet.* 2006;367:579–588.)

inhibitors in the facilitated PCI arm) found that facilitated PCI with fibrinolytic therapy was associated with increased mortality and bleeding whereas facilitated PCI with GPIIb/IIIa inhibitors had no difference in efficacy or safety compared with primary PCI.

Based on the recent 2009 update to ACC/AHA Practice Guidelines, the term "facilitated PCI" is no longer used. Transfer to facilities capable of PCI is recommended for patients who present to facilities without PCI capabilities if they are high risk (Class IIa) or not high risk (Class IIb) regardless of the initial therapy they receive, i.e., fibrinolysis. In contrast, 2007 Guidelines recommended that *"facilitated PCI using regimens other than full-dose fibrinolytic therapy might be considered as a reperfusion strategy when all of the following are present: a. Patients are at high risk, b. PCI is not immediately available within 90 minutes, and c. Bleeding risk is low (younger age, absence of poorly controlled hypertension, normal body weight) (Class IIb). A planned reperfusion strategy using full-dose fibrinolytic therapy followed by immediate PCI may be harmful (Class III)."*

Results from FINESSE trial (Facilitated Intervention with Enhanced Reperfusion Speed to Stop Events), a study larger than ASSENT-4 PCI, were also incorporated into the 2009 guidelines. Patients with STEMI were randomized to abciximab with half-dose reteplase (n = 828), abciximab alone (n = 818), or placebo (n = 706). Patients then underwent PCI, and intravenous abciximab 0.125 μg/kg/min was administered to all patients in the catheterization laboratory and continued for 12 hours. All patients received ASA and UFH or enoxaparin. Administration

of clopidogrel or ticlodipine was at the discretion of the investigator. At arrival to the catheterization laboratory, more patients in the facilitated PCI arm with half-dose reteplase and abciximab had an open artery (TIMI-3 flow) (33%) compared with the abciximab facilitated arm (14%, p < 0.001) and primary PCI alone group (12%, p < 0.001). Resolution of ST segments was also more common in the combined facilitated PCI group compared to the other two groups. There was no difference in the primary endpoint of death, heart failure, or resuscitated ventricular fibrillation by 90 days between the three groups (9.8% of the combination facilitated PCI arm, 10.5% of the abciximab facilitated PCI arm, and 10.7% of primary PCI alone arm; p = 0.55). There was no difference in the components of the primary endpoint including mortality, heart failure, cardiogenic shock, or ventricular fibrillation. However, TIMI major or minor bleeding was higher in the combination facilitated arm 14.5%, abciximab facilitated arm 10.1%, p = 0.008; combination facilitated arm 14.5%, primary PCI arm 6.9%, p <0.001. In the FINESSE trial, unlike ASSENT-4 where few patients received GPIIb/IIIa inhibitors, all patients received abciximab in the catheterization laboratory.

## Rescue PCI

If fibrinolysis fails, rescue PCI is reasonable in high risk patients with cardiogenic shock, severe CHF, pulmonary edema, or hemodynamically compromising ventricular tachycardia, especially in patients younger than 75 years (Class I by ACC/AHA Practice Guidelines 2004). Incomplete fibrinolysis or

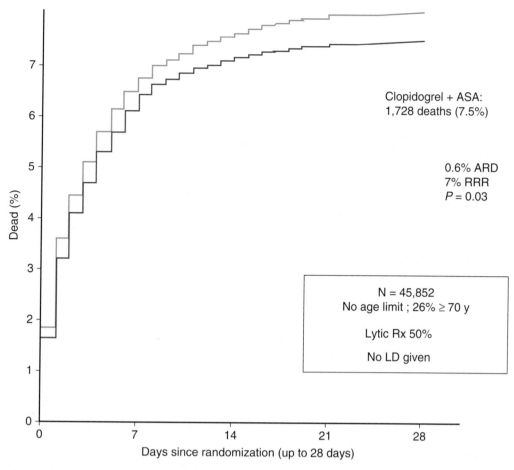

**Figure 40-7.** COMMIT: Effect of CLOPIDOGREL on death in hospital. (Adapted from Chen ZM et al. *Lancet.* 2005;366:1607.)

(a Trial to Assess Improvement in Therapeutic Outcomes by Optimizing Platelet Inhibition with Prasugrel (TRITON)–Thrombolysis in Myocardial Infarction (TIMI)-38), which enrolled 13,608 patients with moderate to high risk PCI, 3534 of whom had STEMI, to receive prasugrel or clopidogrel for an average of 14.5 months. Prasugrel was associated with a significant reduction (2.2% absolute risk reduction and 19% relative risk reduction) in the composite endpoint of cardiovascular death, nonfatal MI, or nonfatal stroke during the follow-up period. However, prasugrel was also associated with increased rate of bleeding when used in those with prior history of TIA or stroke, and a tendency towards increased bleeding in patients over age 75 and in patients with body weight of less than 60 kg. It should be avoided in patients with prior history of TIA or stroke and should be used very cautiously if not avoided in those over age 75 and/or with body weight less than 60kg.

## GPIIb/IIIa Inhibitors

The 2004 ACC/AHA Guidelines favored use of abciximab over other GPIIb/IIIa inhibitors in the setting of STEMI since more data became available that studied the use of this medication in the acute MI setting. It was Class IIa recommendation to start abciximab (Class IIb for tirofiban and eptifibatide) as early as possible prior to PCI for patients with STEMI. Based on new data from trials such as ON-TIMI 2 (Ongoing Tirofiban in Myocardial Infarction Evaluation Trial) and HORIZONS-AMI, updated 2009 Guidelines put equal weight on use of abciximab, eptifibatide, and tirofiban. It is a Class IIa recommendation to use any of the three agents in the setting of STEMI to be started at the time of primary PCI. These more recent trial used thienopyridines in addition to GPIIb/IIIa use.

In relation to the urgency of initiation of GPIIb/IIIa, there are several trials now that have shown us that early use of GPIIb/IIIa inhibitors may improve constitution of TIMI-3 flow, post-PCI myocardial blush grade, ST-segment resolution, and reduce post-PCI cardiac enzyme elevation. However, these have not been shown to improve long-term rate of major cardiac events. Therefore, their early use is still under debate.

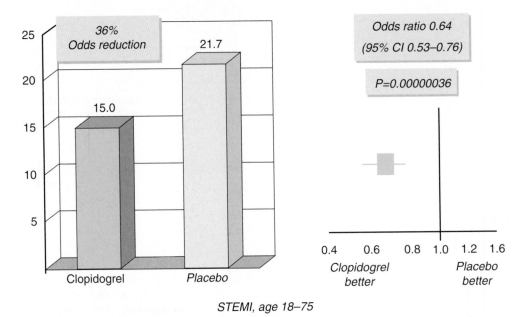

*STEMI, age 18–75*

**Figure 40-8.** CLARITY–TIMI-28 primary endpoint: Infarct artery occlusion, recurrent MI or death was reduced in the treatment group (21.7% in placebo group vs. 15.0% in clopidogrel group, p <0.001.) (Adapted from Scirica BM et al. *J Am Coll Cardiol.* 2006;48:37–42.)

## References

1. Keeley EC, Boura JA, Grines CL. Primary angioplasty versus intravenous thrombolytic therapy for acute myocardial infarction: a quantitative review of 23 randomised trials. *Lancet.* 2003;361:13–20.

2. Morrison LJ, Verbeek PR, McDonald AC, et al. Mortality and prehospital thrombolysis for acute myocardial infarction: a meta-analysis. JAMA. 2000;283:2686–2692.

3. Nallamothu BK, Bates ER. Percutaneous coronary intervention versus fibrinolytic therapy in acute myocardial infarction: is timing (almost) everything? *Am J Cardiol.* 2003;92:824–826.

4. Zhu MM, Feit A, Chadow H, et al. Primary stent implantation compared with primary balloon angioplasty for acute myocardial infarction: a meta-analysis of randomized clinical trials. *Am J Cardiol.* 2001;88:297–301.

5. Wijeysundera HC, Vijayaraghavan R, Nallamothu BK, et al. Rescue angioplasty or repeat fibrinolysis after failed fibrinolytic therapy for ST-segment myocardial infarction: a meta-analysis of randomized trials. *J Am Coll Cardiol.* 2007;49:422–430.

*ACC/AHA 2004, 2007 and 2009 guidelines can be found at www.acc.org.

# 41

# PTCA and CABG in Stable Coronary Artery Disease

Julian M. Aroesty

## ● PRACTICAL POINTS

- Revascularization should be thought of as supplementing, not replacing, a maximal medical program for stable coronary disease patients.

- Only a small proportion of coronary patients will sustain a decrease in morbidity and/or mortality following revascularization.

- In most percutaneous coronary intervention (PCI) studies, major adverse cardiac event (MACE) is defined as death, MI, CVA, or urgent revascularization.

- MACE for elective PCI is 1/1000 for MI, 1/1000 for CVA, and 1/1000 for stroke. The rate of local vascular problems is approximately 1/100 PCI with this falling somewhat with the use of small-diameter catheters currently.

- For studies that include elective revascularization as a component of a combined end point, there will obviously be increased revascularization for PCI, which is directed toward the culprit lesion only, versus CABG that is applied to all lesions amenable to bypass.

- ACE or ARB is recommended for patients with LVEF <40%, CHF, hypertension, or diabetes.

- Beta blockers are effective antianginal agents and should be given to symptomatic chronic stable angina patients or those with a history of AMI or CHF.

- Beta blockers do not improve mortality in the absence of reduced LVEF, CHF (metoprolol succinate, carvedilol), or prior MI.

- Beta 1 blocking agents are preferred for patients with bronchospasm or peripheral artery disease.

- Beta blockers should be avoided in patients with vasospastic (Prinzmetal's) or cocaine angina.

- The LDL goal for patients with stable coronary disease is now at 70 mg/dL, with the possibility that even lower levels might provide additional benefit.

- Strict glycemic control (hgb A1c 6.5) improved risk of renal (microvascular) complications but not that of macrovascular (coronary, peripheral vascular, or cerbrovascular) events.

- Post MI chronic stable angina patients with LVEF <40%, diabetes, or CHF, who are taking beta blockers and ACE, should be treated with aldosterone inhibitor.

- The Duke Treadmill Score, using minutes of exercise, degree of ST depression, and presence/character of chest pain, separates patients into low mortality (<1%/yr) and high mortality (>3%/yr) groups.

- Except for patients with large territory at risk (e.g., LMCA stenosis, 3-vessel CAD, especially with LV dysfunction, and proximal LAD involvement), PCI and CABG will have equal mortality at 10-15 yr.

- Late stent thrombosis is rare (1/1000 per year) but has a high mortality. It was associated with premature discontinuation of ASA or clopidogrel in almost half the cases.

- PCI is unfavorable in degenerated venous bypass grafts, small vessels, heavily calcified vessels, chronic total occlusions, lesions in a tortuous segment, and ostial bifurcation lesions.

# INTRODUCTION: WHEN SHOULD REVASCULARIZATION BE PERFORMED?

Revascularization of patients with chronic stable angina is performed to accomplish two goals:

1. improvement of symptoms
2. improvement in morbidity and mortality.

Coronary revascularization by either PCI (percutaneous coronary intervention) or CABG (coronary artery bypass grafting) is not a replacement for maximal medical therapy: Any patient with established coronary artery disease or with a high risk coronary profile should be treated with those agents known to provide symptom relief and to decrease morbidity and mortality. Almost all patients can expect improvement in symptoms following revascularization, but only a small proportion can expect a decrease in morbidity and mortality. Thus, it becomes very important to ensure that a maximal medical regimen has failed prior to subjecting patients to the increased risk of morbidity etc of PCI or CABG.

For elective CABG, in patients with preserved LV function, the early mortality is now 1-2%, with major morbidity (MI, CVA, prolonged intubation, etc.) approximately 3-4%.

For elective PCI, results are often reported as MACE (major adverse cardiovascular events), which is defined to be death, MI, stroke, or urgent revascularization occurring within 30 days of intervention. The rate of death, MI, and stroke is approximately 1/1000 for each event. Local vascular problems (large or retroperitoneal hematoma requiring intervention or transfusion, occlusion at puncture site, etc.) occur in approximately 1% of patients. As expected, the need for revascularization following successful PCI is much higher than it is for CABG since PCI is generally directed toward the culprit lesion producing the symptoms while CABG is performed on all lesions amenable to bypass.

# MEDICAL THERAPY

Medical therapy is the mainstay therapy for the majority of chronic stable angina patients.

## "AA BCDE SS"

> **A**spirin—post-MI, all males >50 years, transient ischemic attack (TIA)
>
> **A**ce inhibitor—s/p MI with LVEF <40%, hypertension (HTN), diabetes mellitus (DM), CHF
>
> **B**eta blocker—post-AWMI, ventricular or atrial ectopy, AF
>
> **C**holesterol control with statins to LDL in the 70s
>
> **D**iet, diabetic control—prudent coronary diet, diabetic control that avoids extremes of blood sugar
>
> **E**xercise—regular program, minimum 20-30 minutes of endurance exercise three or four times weekly.

> **S**pironolactone—post MI on ACE, beta blocker (BB) with DM or CHF and LVEF<40, without renal disease or increased K
>
> **S**moking—cessation

## Antiplatelet Therapy, Aspirin, Clopidogrel

The 2007 ACC/AHA Update on Treatment of Chronic Stable Angina recommends aspirin for all patients with multiple risk factors, or with known coronary artery disease. Clopidogrel may be used in patients intolerant of aspirin. Ticlopidine is not as well tolerated as clopidogrel but may be used for patients unable to take clopidogrel. Proton pump inhibitors are given for patients with increased risk of GI bleeding. PPI, but not raditidine (Zantac), had been suspected of interfering with the effectiveness of clopidogrel resulting in an FDA alert, but this has not been confirmed by subsequent investigations. At the time this was written (2010), this matter had not been fully resolved.

## ACE Inhibitor or ARB

The 2007 ACC/AHA Update on Treatment of Chronic Stable Angina recommends ACEI treatment for patients with acute MI, LVEF <40%, hypertension, diabetes mellitus, or chronic kidney disease. ARBs may be substituted for patients in whom the ACE inhibitors are not well tolerated.

## Beta-Blocker

2007 ACC/AHA Update on Treatment of Chronic Stable Angina recommends beta-blockade for chronic stable angina patients who have had an ACS (acute coronary syndrome) or CHF. Beta-1-blocking agents are preferred especially in patients with peripheral vascular disease or bronchospasm.

All beta-blockers seem to be equivalent at similar levels of beta-blockade although the side effect profile; cost and duration of action will vary among different agents. For patients with chronic stable angina, beta-blockers have not been shown to improve morbidity or mortality in the absence of prior myocardial infarction.

Beta-blockers should be avoided in Prizmetal's (vasospastic) or cocaine-related angina since the beta-blockade results in unopposed alpha effect, which may *increase* the tendency toward vasospasm. In general, for these patients, calcium channel blockers are preferred.

## Cholesterol Control

There are several studies documenting the improvement in morbidity and mortality accompanying the use of HMG-CoA reductase inhibitors (statins) to improve lipid levels. Over the years, the LDL goal for patients with known coronary disease has decreased progressively from 100 mg/dL to <70 mg/dL, although this appears to be a moving target. The LDL of newborns and of those living on a largely vegetarian diet is in the 30-40mg/dL range, and the incidence of premature atherosclerosis is extremely low in populations with a largely vegetarian diet.

Since the protection from instituting intensive statin therapy occurs before there is a significant change in lipid pattern, an important part of the protective effect is related to the pleotropic—that is, nonlipid—effects of this class of drugs, such as plaque stabilization and decreased inflammation.

## Diet, Diabetic Control

It is well established diabetic patients should avoid blood sugar level extremes. An important issue is the possible benefit of more rigid glucose control as compared to ordinary diabetic management for patients with type II diabetes. Three large multicenter studies (ADVANCE, ACCORD, VA), in which hgb A1c levels of 6.5 were compared with levels of 7.5, noted improvement in microvascular events such as nephropathy, but no improvement was seen in macrovascular (cardiovascular) events. There was also a trend toward increased mortality in the strict glucose control groups—perhaps related to more frequent episodes of hypoglycemia.

## Exercise

Regular exercise results in increased muscular efficiency, resulting in a decrease in the amount of myocardial oxygen requirement for a given amount of physical work. Regular exercise is a necessary part of achieving significant weight loss, with its accompaniment of improved blood pressure, lipid pattern, and diabetic control, potentially producing a decrease in morbidity and mortality. Exercise plus an aggressive medical regimen is at least equivalent to PCI and may even be superior with regard to symptoms, morbidity, and possibly mortality. Unfortunately this requires a level of compliance with a vigorous regular exercise program and a rigid diet that is difficult to achieve in Western societies.

## Spironolactone

The ACC/AHA 2007 guidelines for treating chronic stable angina recommend aldosterone inhibitors for post MI patients taking therapeutic doses of ACE or ARB and beta-blocker, with an LVEF <40% and either diabetes mellitus or CHF.

# STRATIFYING PATIENTS INTO HIGH AND LOW RISK CATEGORIES

Beyond achieving good control of ischemic symptoms it is important to identify those patients in whom revascularization is associated with an improvement in mortality. This involves stratification of chronic stable angina patients into high risk and low risk categories:

- *High risk* (mortality >3%/year) **DEFILE** – Duke **EF** Ischemia **LargE**

The acronym derives from the criteria of:
**D**uke treadmill score ≤11
LV**EF** ≤ 35%
Larg**E** area of ischemia on stress testing or combination of fixed with substantial ischemic territory (stress-induced LV dilatation, hypotension, prolonged ST depression during recovery).

- *Low risk* (mortality < 1%/year)
Duke treadmill score ≥ 5
Small or no ischemic territory with stress (but risk will be high if LVEF ≤ 35% or Duke Treadmill risk score is high).

For patients with chronic stable angina, *no studies* show a decrease in morbidity or mortality by PTCA or stent placement as opposed to CABG. There is, however, a decrease in NTG use and an improvement in symptoms, which is confirmed by an objective improvement in the exercise tolerance test. PCI for chronic stable angina is performed for symptom control alone, not for decreasing either morbidity or mortality, and this is true regardless of the patient having high risk or low risk features.

There are few reasons for *adding* revascularization to a maximal medical program

1. *Clinical high risk*: The clinical status, and/or anatomy are more safely treated by CABG. PCI for these conditions will improve symptomatic status but will not decrease morbidity or mortality.
   Left main coronary stenosis >50%
   Multivessel coronary disease in diabetic patients
   2-vessel coronary disease including proximal LAD involvement and decreased LVEF
2. *Failed maximal Rx*: A maximally tolerated medical regimen has not controlled symptoms well. In this case, the intervention is performed solely for improvement in symptoms. Unless patients are included from the high risk groups mentioned above, major morbidity (MI, CVA) and mortality of patients already on a maximal medical program is not improved by added revascularization through either PCI or CABG.
3. *Patient preference:* Some patients may elect revascularization for personal reasons of not wanting to deal with the side effects of the antianginal medications.

The rapid advancement of techniques in both PCI (introduction of short term and long term highly effective antiplatelet regimens, bare-metal tents (BMS) and drug-eluting stents (DES)) and CABG (increased use of LIMA, better myocardial protection during cardiopulmonary bypass, minimal access bypass, off pump bypass), as well as more vigorously applied and widely utilized medical regimens to control lipids, blood pressure, smoking, and heart failure,

**Table 41-1 • Summary of Class I Indications for PCI and/or CABG**

| LV | CAD#-vessel | LAD Prox Involved | Clinical | PCI | CABG | Survival Benefit Established |
|---|---|---|---|---|---|---|
| | LMCA | | | | + | yes |
| | 3 | | | | + | yes |
| abn | 2 | yes | High risk testing | | + | yes |
| nl | 2, 3 | yes | Not diabetic | + | + | no |
| | 1, 2 | no | High risk testing | + | + | no |
| | 1, 2 | no | VT or VF | | + | no |

*nl, normal; abn, abnormal; CAD, coronary artery disease; LAD, left anterior descending artery; PCI, percutaneous coronary intervention; CABG, coronary artery bypass graft surgery*

have made randomized studies completed only recently no longer fully applicable to currently applied therapy.

Further difficulty in applying studies to current therapy involves the use of troponin levels to define myocardial cell death. Increased sensitivity of troponin assays to myocardial ischemia/death have led to many more patients being classified as having sustained some degree of cell death (and thus infarction) who would not have received this diagnosis in the pre-troponin era.

This review will utilize the meta-analysis or the latest large randomized studies of revascularization for chronic stable angina. Class I (strategy supported by published large randomized investigations) and Class III (strategy not supported by published investigations) will be emphasized (**Table 41-1**, **Table 41-2**).

Class I indication for PCI

  A. LV: normal
  B. CAD: 1-vessel, 2-,3-vessel without proximal LAD
  C. Clinical: without high risk criteria on noninvasive testing; without treated diabetes mellitus

Class I indication for either PCI or CABG

  A. LVEF: mild to moderate decrease
  B. CAD: 1- or 2-vessel without proximal LAD
  C. Clinical: high risk criteria on noninvasive testing

Class I indication for CABG

  A. LMCA: Any patient with significant left main coronary disease

  B. LVEF: abnormal plus
  C. CAD: 3-vessel or left main equivalent disease (>70% proximal LAD and circumflex disease)

## CABG VS. PCI FOR CHRONIC STABLE ANGINA

For the hard endpoint of mortality, meta-analysis of several studies has consistently shown no difference in mortality at 5 years for patients with good LV function and the absence of large territories in jeopardy (left main disease, 2- or 3-vessel disease including proximal LAD), but repeat intervention is performed much more often in those patients receiving PCI.

The most important of these studies is the BARI study (Bypass Angioplasty Revascularization Investigation), which compared balloon angioplasty (without stent placement) and bypass surgery in patients with multivessel coronary disease having an anatomy that was suitable for either treatment. Except for diabetics treated with a LIMA conduit, mortality was the same following both treatments, and 10-year follow-up continues to show no significant difference in mortality or the presence of angina between CABG and PCI (*J Am Coll Cardiol.* 2007). Registry data and meta-analysis of several studies confirm the similar survival in both PCI and CABG patients out to 15 plus years post intervention, in the absence of his risk characteristics.

**Table 41-2 • Summary of Class III Indications (CABG or PCI Not Recommended)**

| LV | CAD#-vessel | LAD Prox Involved | Clinical | PCI | CABG | Survival Benefit Established |
|---|---|---|---|---|---|---|
| nl | 1, 2 | no | sx controlled | no | no | no |
| nl | 1 | yes | sx controlled | no | no | no |

## Isolated Proximal LAD Disease (so Called "*Widow Maker Lesion*")

Although this lesion is widely revascularized by either drug-eluting stent or minimally invasive LIMA bypass with a very low morbidity and mortality, there are no studies that confirm improvement in mortality with either strategy when compared to optimal medical therapy.

Initially the cost of PCI was considerably lower than that of CABG, but this differential narrowed considerably to an equal cost at 5 years for patients with 3-vessel disease and still, about 5% lower in the PCI group without 3-vessel disease.

Restenosis is related to myocyte proliferation in response to the balloon-induced injury at the angioplasty site. Clinical restenosis for balloon angioplasty (PTCA) averaged 30% at about 6 months, reduced by half to 15% by the introduction of bare-metal stents and further reduced again by half to approximately 6-7% by the introduction of drug-eluting stents. Stent thrombosis and late stent thrombosis have been well controlled by current regimen that includes long term aspirin and clopidogrel, although late stent thrombosis has been reported out to 3 years. In about half the patients, antiplatelet treatment was discontinued shortly before stent thrombosis ensued. Late stent thrombosis was associated with a significant mortality but was fortunately infrequent (3/1000 cases at 3 years follow-up). Current recommendations are to continue aspirin indefinitely and clopidogrel for at least one year, longer if tolerated in patients receiving DES.

The picture is somewhat clouded by the report of the New York State Registry Data (Hannan 2008) covering the years from 1997 through 2000 in which patients were treated often with BMS and LIMA (left internal mammary artery) implantation. As for all registry data, the choice of therapy was at the discretion of the treating physician. The analysis attempted to make the risk profiles comparable in the PCI and CABG patients. After risk adjustment, comparison of survival at approximately 5 years was as follows:

| | |
|---|---|
| Non-LAD single vessel disease | PCI superior to CABG |
| 1-vessel disease not involving proximal LAD | PCI = CABG |
| 2-vessel disease not involving LAD | PCI = CABG |
| 3-vessel disease not involving proximal LAD | ABG superior to PCI |
| 1-, 2-, or 3-vessel disease involving proximal LAD | CABG superior to PCI |

## Summary

If proximal LAD is involved, CABG resulted in a better survival than PCI. PCI was superior to CABG only in non-LAD one vessel disease, i.e., isolated right or circumflex artery disease. PCI = CABG in 1- or 2-vessel disease not involving proximal LAD, or 2-vessel non-LAD disease

A subsequent analysis by the same group looked at matched patients in the registry undergoing CABG or PCI with drug-eluting stents. In this analysis, with an 18-month follow-up, CABG was superior to PCI for survival (94.0 versus 92.7%), and for the combined endpoint of survival or MI (92.1 versus 89.7%) for patients with 2-vessel coronary disease. For patients with 3-vessel coronary disease, there was a similar benefit to CABG over PCI at 18 months for death (96.0 versus 94.6%) or for combined endpoint of death/MI (94.5 versus 92.5%). This study carries all of the disadvantages of registry data and has a short follow-up but suggests there *may* be an advantage of CABG over PCI for all patients with multivessel coronary disease. Until more data are available, proximal LAD involvement, multivessel disease, markedly depressed LV function, and the presence of treated diabetes mellitus remain prime candidates for CABG.

Overall, recurrent angina and repeat revascularization is much more frequent in PCI compared to CABG. However, in the absence of critical left main coronary disease, diabetes, and significant LV dysfunction, both CABG and PCI have similar rates of morbidity and mortality.

For chronic stable angina, PCI does not decrease morbidity or mortality while CABG is known to accomplish this result in selected patients, as shown in the table above. For all patients the likelihood of needing repeat procedures to manage recurrence of symptoms is much higher for PCI as compared to CABG, but this difference narrows considerably as the follow up analysis extends to 5-10 years by which time an increasing number of CABG patients will have recurrent symptoms due to graft closure

# PCI FOR CHRONIC STABLE ANGINA

One of the benefits of CABG over PCI for chronic stable angina is the likelihood that all vessels with significant disease will be bypassed at time of initial CABG, while PCI is typically carried out on the culprit lesion alone. PCI patients are more likely to have recurrent symptoms and require revascularization of the original treated site (TLR, target lesion revascularization), other disease in the same artery (TVR, target vessel revascularization) as well as advancement of disease in nontreated arteries (nontarget vessel revascularization). The introduction of bare-metal stents and drug-eluting stents has resulted in a dramatic decrease in the target lesion revascularization rate. (Valgimigli 2007)

The factors that result in progressive disease in target and nontarget vessel are the usual coronary disease risk factors that have not been well controlled—smoking, hypertension, diabetes, and lipid abnormality.

Lesion factors that are unfavorable for a good immediate result by PCI are:

1. lesions in diffusely degenerated saphenous vein grafts
2. lesions in vessels under 2 mm in diameter
3. heavily calcified lesions
4. diffusely diseased vessels
5. ostial bifurcation lesions
6. lesions in a segment with increased tortuosity
7. chronic total occlusions

In addition, there are factors that result in increased restenosis rate at the treated site. There are:

1. increased length of lesion
2. decreased diameter of lesion
3. increased length of stented segment
4. increased number of overlapping stents
5. treatment of bifurcation lesions
6. presence of diabetes under treatment
7. in the presence of nonjeopardized collateral vessels to the ischemic territory

# PREOPERATIVE TREATMENT OF CHRONIC STABLE ANGINA

Preoperative management of chronic stable angina patients undergoing CABG has undergone some significant changes.

Aspirin, clopidogrel: Because of the risk of increased perioperative bleeding, until recently discontinuation of aspirin and/or clopidogrel was generally advised for 8-10 days prior to the scheduled operative date.

Medical therapy to reduce CABG perioperative complications (AHA/ACC guidelines)

- ASA
- antibiotics to reduce perioperative infections
- beta-blockers
- tight glycemic control
- statins.

Aspirin: Preoperatively and postoperatively, ASA should be given not only in high risk patients, but also in all elective patients. This therapy results in improved graft patency at 1-year post CABG as well as decreased mortality. While this therapy brings an increase in bleeding, the benefit outweighs the risk in studies that have excluded patients at high risk of bleeding.

Beta-blockers—meta-analysis of various studies have confirmed the utility of preoperative beta-blockers in reducing the incidence of atrial fibrillation (AF) by 30-60%, and reducing mortality at 30 days by 30%, except for patients with severe LV dysfunction (EF < 30%), for whom there was no benefit.

Aggressive glycemic control: For both diabetic and nondiabetic patients, continuous intravenous insulin use to maintain a glucose level between 100 and 140 mg% will decrease morbidity (including, post-op ischemia and wound infection) and will decrease mortality. (Note that the improvement in morbidity noted in the preoperative period for diabetic patients with strict glucose control has not been duplicated for the outpatient treatment of diabetic patients with chronic stable angina. Strict diabetic control has not reduced morbidity or mortality and there is a suggestion that there might actually be a slight increase in mortality related to strict control of blood sugars, which is presumed to be related to increased likelihood of episodic hypoglycemia.)

Statin therapy—a meta-analysis of over 30,000 patients has compared the outcome post CABG of patients who had received statin therapy with those without statins. Patients on statins had a 35% decrease in all-cause mortality, a 15% decrease in AF, and a 25% decrease in stroke.

## Suggested Readings

1. Fraker TD Jr, Fihn SD, Goibbons RJ et al. Focused update of ACC/AHA guidelines for management of patients with chronic stable angina. *Circulation*. 2007;116:2762–2772.

2. Eagle KA, Guyton RA, Davidoff R et al. ACC/AHA guideline update for coronary artery bypass surgery. *Cuirculation*. 2004;110:1168.

3. Serruys PW, Morice MC, Kappetein AP et al. Percutaneous coronary ntervention versus coronary artery bypass grafting for severe coronary artery disease. *New Engl J Med*. 2009; 360:961–972.

4. Boden WE, O'Rourke RA, Teo KK et al. Optimal medical therapy with or without PCI for stable coronary disease. *New Engl J Med*. 2007;356:1503–1516.

5. Katritsis DG, Ioannidis JP. Percutaneous coronary intervention versus conservative therapy in nonacute coronary artery disease; a met-analysis. *Circulation*. 2005;111:2906–2912.

# 42

# Revascularization in Unstable Angina and Non-ST-Segment Elevated Myocardial Infarction

ERNEST L. MAZZAFERRI JR.

## ● PRACTICAL POINTS

- Although ST-segment elevation myocardial infarctions (STEMI) carries the highest risk of early death, according to Savonitto et al. (2005), ST-depression on the presenting ECG portends the highest risk of death at 6 months, with the degree of ST depression showing a strong relationship to outcome.

- UA/NSTEMI most commonly arises from the disruption or erosion of an atherosclerotic plaque and subsequent prothrombotic cascade in the coronary artery which ultimately leads to a supply and demand imbalance in the myocardium. The causes that lead to this imbalance are not mutually exclusive, often involving two or more of the following underlying mechanisms (Braunwauld 1998):

  ○ Thrombus or thromboembolism, usually arising on a disrupted or eroded atherosclerotic plaque (occlusive with collaterals or subtotal occlusion or distal microvascular thromboembolism).

  ○ Progressive mechanical obstruction to coronary flow

  ○ Secondary UA/NSTEMI

  ○ Non-plaque-associated thromboembolism

  ○ Dynamic obstruction (coronary vasospasm or vasoconstriction)

  ○ Coronary artery dissection or inflammation.

- Multiple prognostic factors integrated in a simultaneous fashion using algorithms such as the TIMI risk score, PURSUIT risk score, and GRACE risk model optimize early risk stratification for death and ischemic events in patients presenting with UA/NSTEMI.

- The optimal strategy to care for the UA/NSTEMI includes a combination of antiischemic therapy, antianginal therapy, antithrombotic therapy, ongoing risk stratification and consideration of invasive procedures.

- Morphine sulfate is potentially beneficial in UA/NSTEMI patients as it has potent analgesic and anxiolytic effects; however, there are no randomized trials to suggest a defined contribution to outcomes in this patient population. Caution should also be advised that in observational studies of UA/NSTEMI patients this agent has been associated with a higher mortality and has the potential to mask the need for more urgent revascularization in patients with occluded vessels that do not show ST-elevation on serial standard 12-lead ECGs.

- The aggregate of the data suggests that early beta-blockade in ACS patients may pose a substantial hazard, and the risk versus benefit must be weighed in each individual.

- Several randomized, placebo-controlled trials evaluated the efficacy of heparin in UA/NSTEMI, and two meta-analyses have shown the combination of heparin and ASA reduce the short term risk of death or MI significantly (up to 56%).

*(continued)*

- The current evidence base and expert opinion suggest that for UA/NSTEMI patients in whom an initial invasive strategy is selected, either an intravenous GP IIb/IIIa inhibitor or clopidogrel should be added to ASA and anticoagulant therapy before diagnostic angiography (upstream) for lower risk, troponin-negative patients, and that both should be given before angiography for high risk, troponin-positive patients (Class I recommendations).

- Overall, higher risk patients with elevated cardiac biomarker levels at baseline benefited more from routine intervention, with no significant benefit observed in lower risk patients with negative baseline marker levels.

- The decision to proceed from diagnostic angiography to revascularization is dependent upon multiple variables, including complexity of the coronary anatomy, amount of myocardium at risk, patient comorbidities, left ventricular function, and life expectancy. In general, the goal of revascularization is improvement in survival and a reduction in the risk of myocardial infarction and symptoms of coronary disease. However, the optimal means of providing revascularization, PCI, or bypass surgery for patients with UA/NSTEMI remains controversial, as a great deal of the evidence is outdated.

## INTRODUCTION

A subset of acute coronary syndrome (ACS), unstable angina (UA) and non-ST-segment elevated myocardial infarction (NSTEMI) constitute a clinical syndrome that is most often caused by atherosclerotic coronary artery disease (CAD). These closely related syndromes are potentially life-threatening and according to the American Heart Association accounted for approximately 1,565,000 hospital admissions in 2004, the majority being NSTEMI (896,000). In the United States alone, in 2003, there were almost 4,500,000 visits to emergency departments for the primary diagnosis of cardiovascular disease (CVD). Although ST-segment elevation myocardial infarction (STEMI) carries the highest risk of early death, according to Savonitto et al. ST-depression on the presenting ECG portends the highest risk of death at 6 months, with the degree of ST depression showing a strong relationship to outcome.

## PATHOPHYSIOLOGY

The clinical presentation and pathogenesis of UA and NSTEMI are similar, but differ primarily in whether the ischemia is severe enough to cause enough myocardial damage to cause the release of cardiac biomarkers, most commonly troponin I (TnI), troponin T (TnT), or creatine kinase MB (CK-MB). UA/NSTEMI most commonly arises from the disruption or erosion of an atherosclerotic plaque and subsequent prothrombotic cascade in the coronary artery, which ultimately leads to a supply and demand imbalance in the myocardium. The causes which lead to this imbalance are not mutually exclusive, often involving two or more of the following underlying mechanisms (Braunwauld, 1998):

- Thrombus or thromboembolism, usually arising on a disrupted or eroded atherosclerotic plaque (occlusive with collaterals or subtotal occlusion or distal microvascular thromboembolism)
- Progressive mechanical obstruction to coronary flow
- Secondary UA/NSTEMI
- Non-plaque–associated thromboembolism
- Dynamic obstruction (coronary vasospasm or vasoconstriction)
- Coronary artery dissection or inflammation.

Patients with UA/NSTEMI present with a clinical syndrome defined by chest discomfort (or anginal equivalent), electrocardiographic (ECG) ST-segment depression or T-wave inversion, and/or positive biomarkers of necrosis in the absence of ST-segment elevation. The rapid risk stratification for this continuum of patients is imperative for decisive triage and management.

## EVALUATION AND MANAGEMENT

### Early Risk Stratification

The initial evaluation of patients with suspected ACS can have substantial clinical consequences. Although the first triage decision is made by the patient's willingness or unwillingness to approach the health care system, health care professionals must make a rapid clinical determination of the likelihood of obstructive CAD in patients with symptoms suggestive of ACS.

Initial assessment should focus on the history, physical findings, ECG findings, and cardiac biomarkers. If initial ECG is nondiagnostic, however, suspicion will remain high, so serial ECGs should be performed in 15–30-minute intervals to evaluate for ST-segment abnormalities ( ACC/AHA 2007). Serial cardiac biomarkers, preferably including troponins, should be followed at 6-8-hour intervals for three sets, or until the enzymes have peaked, to allow an estimate of infarct size.

Multiple prognostic factors integrated in a simultaneous fashion using algorithms such as the TIMI risk score, PURSUIT risk score, and GRACE risk model optimize early risk stratification for death and ischemic events in patients presenting with UA/NSTEMI. An analysis by Giugliano et al. (2005) compared risk scores and concluded that all three demonstrated good predictive accuracy for death and MI at 1-year, thus identifying patients who might be likely to benefit from more aggressive therapy and possibly early revascularization. The more widely applied TIMI risk score (Antman EA et al. 2000) is determined by the sum of the presence of seven variables at admission age of 65 years or older (see **Figure 42-1**, **Table 42-1**). As the TIMI risk score increases, the 14-day composite endpoint of all-cause mortality, new or recurrent MI, or severe recurrent ischemia prompting urgent revascularization also increases.

Although only incorporated into the GRACE risk model, renal insufficiency is also recognized as a high risk variable in patients with UA/NSTEMI. Mild to moderate renal dysfunction is associated with moderately increased short and long term risks, and severe renal dysfunction is associated with severely increased short and long term mortality risks (Das 2006) (see **Figure 42-2**, **Table 42-2**). Further risk assessment can be generated by the quantitative troponin assessment. While troponin should not be used as the sole

| Table 42-1 • TIMI Risk Score Variables | |
| --- | --- |
| **TIMI Risk Score Variables** | **Score** |
| Age ≥65 | 1 |
| ≥3 risk factors for CAD | 1 |
| Prior coronary stenosis of ≥50% | 1 |
| ST-segment deviation on ECG presentation | 1 |
| ≥ anginal events in prior 24 hours | 1 |
| Use of aspirin in prior 7 days | 1 |
| Elevated serum cardiac biomarkers | 1 |

*Adapted from EM Antman et al. JAMA. 284(7); 2000.*

marker of definitive risk, a quantitative relationship exists between the amount of elevation of troponin and the risk of death (**Figure 42-3**). Thus, among patients presenting with UA/NSTEMI, those with positive troponins may warrant more aggressive therapy. Finally, a newer biomarker of considerable interest is B-type natriuretic peptide (BNP). A review of studies in ACS patients by Galvani (2004) showed that when this cardiac neurohormone is measured at first patient contact or during the index hospitalization, increasing levels are a strong predictor of both short and long term mortality increase.

## Immediate Management

Patients with symptoms suggestive of UA/NSTEMI who have positive cardiac biomarkers or ECG ST-segment abnormalities and who are hemodynamically stable require hospital admission for continuous monitoring and management with either a conservative or invasive strategy. The optimal strategy to care for the UA/NSTEMI patient includes a combination of antiischemic therapy, antianginal therapy, antithrombotic therapy, ongoing risk stratification, and consideration of invasive procedures (ACC/AHA 2007).

## Early Antiischemic and Antianginal Therapy

### Oxygen.

In the absence of signs of respiratory distress or hypoxemia, there are no data to suggest that supplemental oxygen improves outcomes in ACS patients; however, supplemental oxygen should be administered to patients with UA/NSTEMI with an arterial saturation less than 90%, respiratory distress, or other high risk features for hypoxemia (Class I, Level of evidence B) (ACC/AHA 2007).

### Nitrates

Nitroglycerin is an endothelium-independent vasodilator and reduces myocardial oxygen demand while enhancing myocardial oxygen delivery. Sublingual nitroglycerin

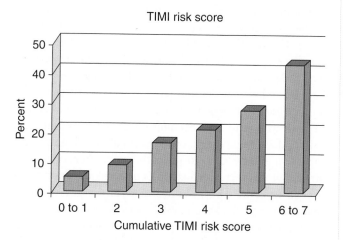

**TIMI risk score**

**Figure 42-1.** All-cause mortality, new or recurrent MI, or severe recurrent ischemia requiring urgent revascularization through 14 days after randomization, %. (Adapted from EM Antman et al. *JAMA.* 284(7); 2000.)

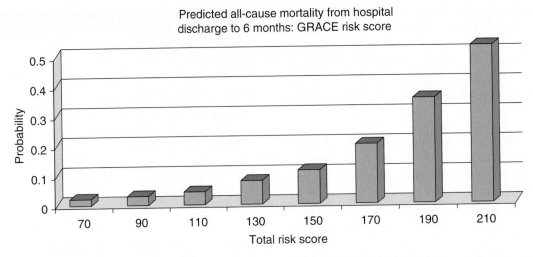

**Figure 42-2.** GRACE risk score predicted all-cause mortality from hospital discharge to six months. (Adapted from KA Eagle et al. *JAMA.* 291; 2004.)

tablets should be given to patients presenting with ischemic type chest pain, followed by intravenous nitroglycerin for continued symptoms. Caution is advised with nitroglycerin in certain patient populations such as those with suspected right ventricular infarction and those with baseline hypotension.

### Morphine

Morphine sulfate is potentially beneficial in UA/NSTEMI patients as it has potent analgesic and anxiolytic effects;

| Table 42-2 • GRACE Risk Score Variables | |
|---|---|
| **GRACE Risk Score Variables** | **Score (Points)** |
| Age<br>≤39:0 pts; 40–49: 18; 50–59: 36; 60–69: 55; 70–79: 73; 80–89: 91; ≥90: 100 | 0 to 100 |
| History of congestive heart failure | 24 |
| History of myocardial infarction | 12 |
| Resting heart rate (bpm)<br>≤49.9: 0 pts; 50–69.9: 3; 70–89.9: 9; 90–109.9: 14; 110–149.9: 23; 150–199.9: 35; ≥200: 43 | 0 to 43 |
| Systolic blood pressure<br>≤79.9: 24 pts; 80–99.9: 22; 100–119.9: 18; 120–139.9: 14; 140–159.9: 10; 160–199.9: 4; ≥200: 0 | 0 to 24 |
| ST-segment depression | 11 |
| Initial serum creatinine<br>0–0.39: 1 pt; 0.4–0.79: 3; 0.8–1.19: 5; 1.2–1.59: 7; 1.6–1.99: 9; 2–3.99: 15; ≥4: 20) | 1 to 20 |
| Elevated Cardiac Enzymes | 15 |
| No In-Hospital Percutaneous Coronary Intervention | 14 |

*Adapted from KA Eagle et al. JAMA. 291; 2004.*

however, there are no randomized trials to suggest a defined contribution to outcomes in this patient population. Caution should also be advised that in observational studies of UA/NSTEMI patients this agent has been associated with a higher mortality and has the potential to mask the need for more urgent revascularization in patients with an occluded coronary artery who do not show ST-elevation on serial standard 12-lead ECGs (*Eur Heart J.* 1991).

### Beta-blockers

Beta-blockers inhibit beta-1-adrenergic receptors in the myocardium, which results in a decrease in cardiac work and myocardial oxygen demand. Although most of the data are extrapolated from STEMI trials, traditionally, oral and intravenous (i.v.) beta-blockade has been recommended for patients with UA/NSTEMI who do not have a contraindication (ACC/AHA 2007). It is noteworthy that the benefit of routine early use has been challenged by several recent studies and retrospective reviews. The COMMIT study (N = 45,852, 93% STEMI, 7% NSTEMI) randomly allocated metoprolol, up to 15 mg i.v., then 200 mg oral, or matching placebo, and overall a modest reduction in reinfarction and ventricular fibrillation was counterbalanced by an increase in cardiogenic shock, which primarily occurred in those who were hemodynamically compromised, at high risk for developing shock, or in heart failure. There was no reduction in the composite of death, reinfarction, or cardiac arrest, nor was there a reduction of death alone for up to 28 days in hospital. Thus, the aggregate of the data suggests that early beta-blockade in ACS patients may pose a substantial hazard and the risk versus benefit must be weighed in each individual. For patients with contraindications to beta-blockers, meta-analyses combining UA/NSTEMI studies of all CCBs have suggested no overall benefit; however, those utilizing verapamil alone have reported favorable

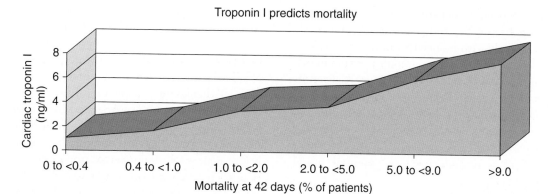

**Figure 42-3.** Troponin I levels predict the risk of mortality in acute coronary syndrome. (Adapted from EM Antman et al. *N Engl J Med*. 335; 1996.)

effects on outcomes, although in varied patient populations (ACC/AHA 2007).

### Intra-Aortic Balloon Pump (IABP) Counterpulsation

An IABP may be useful in patients with refractory ischemia despite maximal medical management or in those with hemodynamic instability until coronary angiography and revascularization can be completed. Although there is a high rate of successful placement and a low risk of complication, there are no randomized data proving efficacy in this patient population (ACC/AHA 2007).

## Antithrombotic Therapy

Based on the pathophysiology of ACS, a combination of antiplatelet therapy and anticoagulant therapy provides the cornerstone of therapy, with more aggressive therapy tailored towards higher risk patients.

### Antiplatelet Therapy: Aspirin, Clopidogrel, Ticlidopine

#### Aspirin

Aspirin (ASA) diminishes platelet aggregation by irreversibly inhibiting the cyclooxygenase-1 and 2 (COX-1 and 2) enzymes, which result in decreased formation of prostaglandin precursors. A marked benefit of ASA compared to placebo in UA/NSTEMI trials has been consistently documented irrespective of differences in study design. Based on prior randomized trial protocols, initial dose should be between 162 mg and 325 mg of the more rapidly absorbed non–enteric-coated ASA, and it should be administered as soon as the diagnosis of ACS is made or suspected (ACC/AHA 2007).

#### Thienopyridines

Ticlopidine, clopidogrel and prasugrel are adenosine diphosphate receptor (PY212) antagonists with a unique antiplatelet mechanism that, when given in combination with aspirin, has become a cornerstone of treatment for preventing thrombotic complications of ACS patients. The adverse side effects of ticlopidine (gastrointestinal problems, neutropenia in 2.4%, severe neutropenia in 0.8%, and rarely thrombotic thrombocytopenia purpura) limit its clinical use; however, it has been shown to be beneficial in the ACS patient population (ACC/AHA 2007). Clopidogrel is the most widely studied thienopyridine in ACS patients, and its efficacy has been established in several randomized trials, including CURE and PCI-CURE in both the revascularized and nonrevascularized cohorts. For patients admitted with UA/NSTEMI in whom an initial invasive strategy is selected, antiplatelet therapy with either clopidogrel or an intravenous GP IIb/IIIa inhibitor should be used in addition to aspirin (ACC/AHA 2007).

### Anticoagulant Therapy: Unfractionated Heparin, Low Molecular Weight Heparin, Direct Thrombin Inhibitors, Glycoprotein IIb/IIIa Inhibitors

#### Unfractionated Heparin (UFH)

UFH, a naturally occurring polysaccharide with molecular chains of varying lengths, prevents thrombus formation, but not thrombolysis, by accelerating the action of circulating antithrombin, a proteolytic enzyme that inactivates Factor IIa (thrombin), Factor IXa, and Factor Xa of the clotting cascade. Several randomized, placebo-controlled trials evaluated the efficacy of heparin in UA/NSTEMI and two meta-analyses have shown the combination of heparin and ASA reduce the short term risk of death or MI significantly (up to 56%) (ACC/AHA 2007).

#### Low Molecular Weight Heparin (LMWH)

LMWH has similar anticoagulant effects; however, it a synthetic short chain polysaccharide, has less of an effect on thrombin compared to heparin while maintaining the same effect on Factor Xa, and is given subcutaneously once (or twice) daily with no need for monitoring coagulation parameters. There have been multiple randomized trials comparing LMWH and UFH; however, trial results have been variable, as heterogeneous clinical design and patient populations make a direct comparison difficult. Currently, for patients with UA/NSTEMI undergoing initial conservative therapy or early invasive strategy, LMWH or UFH is recommended as potential initial strategy (ACC/AHA 2007).

### Direct Thrombin Inhibitors (DTIs)

DTIs are a class of anticoagulant that binds directly to thrombin and inhibits clot-bound thrombin. There are several DTIs; however, the most extensively studied in ACS are hirudin and bivalirudin. Early trials with hirudin had mixed results, and currently the U.S. Food and Drug Administration advocates its use only for the anticoagulation in patients with heparin-induced thrombocytopenia or for the prophylaxis of deep venous thrombosis (DVT) in patients undergoing hip replacement surgery. Bivalirudin is a synthetic analog of hirudin that binds reversibly to thrombin and has shown significant promise in UA/NSTEMI patients in REPLACE-2 and ACUITY, mostly driven by lower bleeding rates in the bivalirudin groups when compared to heparin + GP IIb/IIIa. Currently, for patients with UA/NSTEMI undergoing early invasive strategy, bivalirudin may be used in lieu heparin/glycoprotein IIb/IIIa, however, with a lesser level of evidence of recommendation (ACC/AHA 2007).

### Glycoprotein (Gp) IIb/IIIa Inhibitors

GpIIb/IIIa inhibitors bind the GpIIb/IIIa receptor on the platelet surface to block the final pathway for platelet aggregation. The efficacy of GpIIb/IIIa antagonists in prevention of the complications associated with percutaneous interventions has been documented in numerous trials, many composed largely of patients with UA. Two of the GpIIb/IIIa antagonists, tirofiban and eptifibatide, have been proven beneficial for UA/NSTEMI patients who undergo revascularization as well as those who are not revascularized (PURSUIT and PRISM-PLUS trials, respectively). Abciximab has been primarily studied in PCI trials; however, there are suitable data to support its use for treatment of UA/NSTEMI and as an adjunct for percutaneous intervention based on the CAPTURE trial. Interestingly, GUSTO-IV ACS showed no benefit to abciximab in the management of patients with UA/NSTEMI in whom an early invasive strategy was not planned. A meta-analysis of GP IIb/IIIa antagonists of all six large, randomized, placebo-controlled trials suggest that GP IIb/IIIa inhibitors are of substantial benefit in patients with UA/NSTEMI who undergo PCI, are of modest benefit in patients who

are not routinely scheduled to undergo revascularization (but who may do so), and are of questionable benefit in patients who do not undergo revascularization. The current evidence base and expert opinion suggest that for UA/NSTEMI patients in whom an initial invasive strategy is selected, either an intravenous GP IIb/IIIa inhibitor or clopidogrel, should be added to ASA and anticoagulant therapy before diagnostic angiography (upstream) for lower risk, troponin-negative patients and that both should be given before angiography for high risk, troponin-positive patients (Class I recommendations) (ACC/AHA 2007). For UA/NSTEMI patients in whom an initial conservative (i.e., noninvasive) strategy is selected, the evidence for benefit is less; for this strategy, the addition of eptifibatide or tirofiban to anticoagulant and oral antiplatelet therapy may be reasonable for high risk UA/NSTEMI patients (Class IIb recommendation).

## EARLY INVASIVE VERSUS INITIAL CONSERVATIVE THERAPY

### Definitions

Initial aggressive medical therapy is the standard of care in all ACS patients upon admission to the hospital or entrance to the Emergency Department; however, two divergent pathways have emerged for further management: the "early invasive strategy" and the "initial conservative strategy."

The *early invasive strategy* often referred to as the "invasive strategy," triages patients to undergo a cardiac catheterization without first having a noninvasive stress test or without failing medical treatment. Although these patients are treated with analgesia, antiischemic therapy, and antiplatelet therapy, they will often undergo coronary angiography within 24 hours of admission. This group of patients can be further subdivided into two groups: One group that proceeds directly to angiography due to continued pain or hemodynamic instability despite aggressive medical management; the other group proceeds to angiography at the discretion of the physician due to a perceived risk for an adverse outcome.

The *initial conservative strategy*, often referred to as "selective invasive management," triages patients to medical management first, then follows with some form of noninvasive risk stratification (i.e., stress test or coronary CT-angiography). An invasive evaluation is pursued only in patients who fail medical therapy (refractory angina, angina at rest, or newly developed hemodynamic or electrical instability) or in whom objective evidence of ischemia is identified (i.e., dynamic ECG changes or high risk stress test) (ACC/AHA 2007).

## Clinical Decision-Making Strategies

Determining the appropriate pathway for the individual ACS patient can be a difficult charge; however, risk assessment for potential adverse outcome compared to the risk of an invasive procedure is of principal importance. Although most physicians rely upon clinical intuition to make this decision, there are several validated risk stratification tools (TIMI, PURSUIT, GRACE) that may be helpful in the decision-making process. A meta-analysis of 7 trials (N = 9212 patients) demonstrated favorable long term outcomes for the early invasive strategy, identifying an impressive 18% relative reduction in death or MI, including a significant reduction in MI alone. There was also a significant decrease in severe angina after discharge and fewer readmissions with the early invasive strategy. To offset the advantages of the early invasive strategy, during initial hospitalization it was associated with a significantly higher early mortality (1.1 versus 1.8% for conservative versus early invasive, respectively; P = 0.007) and the composite of death or MI (3.8versus 5.2%; P = 0.002). Overall, higher risk patients with elevated cardiac biomarker levels at baseline benefited more from routine intervention, with no significant benefit observed in lower risk patients with negative baseline marker levels (ACC/AHA 2007).

Although there are select trials such as ICTUS (Invasive versus Conservative Treatment in Unstable Coronary Syndromes), which suggest that conservative strategy may be reasonable in ACS management, a significant number of the conservatively managed patients ultimately underwent invasive angiography and revascularization (up to 47%). Nevertheless, a meta-analysis of contemporary randomized trials in UA/NSTEMI, including ICTUS, currently support a conclusion of long term mortality and morbidity benefits of an early invasive compared with an initial conservative strategy.

## CORONARY REVASCULARIZATION

Coronary angiography is helpful to further risk-stratify patients presenting with UA/NSTEMI and for identifying those patients who may most benefit from revascularization. The decision to proceed from diagnostic angiography to revascularization is dependent upon multiple variables, including complexity of the coronary anatomy, amount of myocardium at risk, patient comorbidities, left ventricular function, and life expectancy. In general, the goal of revascularization is improvement in survival and a reduction in the risk of myocardial infarction and symptoms of coronary disease. However, the optimal means of providing revascularization, PCI, or bypass surgery for patients with UA/NSTEMI remains controversial, as a great deal of the evidence is outdated.

Predictably, the decision-making process regarding revascularization is at times very complex; however, it is noteworthy that the indications for coronary revascularization in patients with UA/NSTEMI are similar to those for patients with chronic stable angina. Although based on somewhat antiquated data, high risk patients with LV systolic dysfunction, patients with diabetes mellitus, and those with 2-vessel disease with severe proximal LAD involvement or severe 3-vessel or left main disease should be considered for CABG (ACC/AHA 2007). The contemporary Synergy between Percutaneous Coronary Intervention with Taxus and Cardiac Surgery (SYNTAX) trial randomly assigned 1800 patients with 3-vessel or left main coronary artery disease to undergo CABG or PCI (drug-eluting stents) in a noninferiority design with a combined primary endpoint of major adverse cardiac or cerebrovascular event during a 12-month period after randomization. At 12 months the rate of repeat revascularization was higher in the PCI group (13.5 versus 5.9%, p < 0.001); however, the rates of death and MI were similar and the risk of stroke was significantly higher with CABG (2.2 versus 0.6%, p = 0.003). It is important to realize that CVA in this trial was defined as focal, central neurological deficit lasting >72 hours, which resulted in irreversible brain damage or body impairment. Furthermore, clinical outcomes correlated with SYNTAX scores, which is a relatively complex scoring system designed to characterize the coronary vasculature with respect to the number of lesions and their functional impact, location, and complexity. Higher SYNTAX scores, indicative of more complex disease, are hypothesized to represent a bigger therapeutic challenge and to have potentially worse prognosis. Of importance, patients with low or intermediate SYNTAX scores in the CABG group and the PCI group had similar rates of MACE/cerebrovascular events at 12 months, while the group with high SYNTAX scores fared better with CABG. The Future Revascularization Evaluation in Patients with Diabetes Mellitus—Optimal Management of Multivessel Disease (FREEDOM) trial is currently enrolling and designed to compare PCI versus CABG in patients with multivessel disease who have diabetes mellitus. The primary endpoint will not include repeat revascularization but will be a composite of all-cause mortality, non-fatal myocardial infarction, and stroke.

The indications and justifications for revascularization are presented in greater detail elsewhere; however, **Tables 42-3** and **42-4** cover the Class I and Class III indications for revascularizations. (See ACC/AHA Guidelines for the Management of Patients with Chronic Stable Angina, ACC/AHA Guidelines for Coronary Artery Bypass Graft Surgery, 2005 ACC/AHA/SCAI Guidelines Update for Percutaneous Coronary Intervention, and ACC/AHA 2007 Guidelines for the Management of Patients with UA/NSTEMI.)

**Table 42-3 • ACC/AHA 2007 Class I Recommendations for Coronary Revascularization with PCI and CABG in Patients with UA/NSTEMI**

| PCI | Class | LOE | CABG | Class | LOE |
|---|---|---|---|---|---|
| Percutaneous coronary intervention (or CABG) is recommended for UA/NSTEMI patients with multivessel coronary disease with suitable coronary anatomy, with normal LV function, and without diabetes mellitus | I | A | SAME | | |
| Percutaneous coronary intervention (or CABG) is recommended for UA/NSTEMI patients with 1- or 2-vessel CAD with or without significant proximal left anterior descending CAD but with a large area of viable myocardium and high risk criteria on noninvasive testing | I | B | SAME | | |
| | | | CABG surgery is recommended for UA/NSTEMI patients with significant left main CAD (>50% stenosis) | I | A |
| | | | CABG surgery is recommended for UA/NSTEMI patients with 3-vessel disease; the survival benefit is greater in patients with abnormal LV function (LVEF <0.50) | I | A |
| | | | CABG surgery is recommended for UA/NSTEMI patients with 2-vessel disease with significant proximal left anterior descending CAD and either abnormal LV function (LVEF <0.50) or ischemia on noninvasive testing | I | A |
| | | | CABG surgery is recommended for UA/NSTEMI patients in whom percutaneous revascularization is not optimal or possible and who have ongoing ischemia not responsive to maximal nonsurgical therapy. (Level of evidence: B) | I | B |
| | | | CABG surgery (or PCI) is recommended for UA/NSTEMI patients with 1- or 2-vessel CAD with or without significant proximal left anterior descending CAD but with a large area of viable myocardium and high-risk criteria on noninvasive testing. (Level of evidence: B) | I | B |

*Adapted from JL Anderson JL et al. J Am Coll Cardiol. 50(7); 2007.*

**Table 42-4 • ACC/AHA 2007 Class III Recommendations for Coronary Revascularization with PCI and CABG in Patients with UA/NSTEMI**

| PCI | Class | LOE | CABG | Class | LOE |
|---|---|---|---|---|---|
| Percutaneous coronary intervention (or CABG) is not recommended for patients with 1- or 2-vessel CAD without significant proximal left anterior descending CAD with no current symptoms or symptoms that are unlikely to be due to myocardial ischemia and who have no ischemia on noninvasive testing | III | C | SAME | III | C |
| In the absence of high-risk features associated with UA/NSTEMI, PCI is not recommended for patients with UA/NSTEMI who have single-vessel or multivessel CAD and no trial of medical therapy, or who have 1 or more of the following:<br>a. Only a small area of myocardium at risk<br>b. All lesions or the culprit lesion to be dilated with morphology that convey a low likelihood of success<br>c. A high risk of procedure-related morbidity or mortality<br>d. Insignificant disease (<50% coronary stenosis)<br>e. Significant left main CAD and candidacy for CABG. | III<br><br><br><br>C<br>C<br><br>C<br>C<br>B | | CABG surgery (or PCI) is not recommended for patients with 1- or 2-vessel CAD without significant proximal left anterior descending CAD with no current symptoms or symptoms that are unlikely to be due to myocardial ischemia and who have no ischemia on noninvasive testing. | III | C |
| A PCI strategy in stable patients with persistently occluded infarct-related coronary arteries after NSTEMI is not indicated | III | B | | | |

*Adapted from JL Anderson JL et al. J Am Coll Cardiol. 50(7); 2007.*

21. Pannu N, Manns B, Lee H, et al. Systematic review of the impact of N-acetylcysteine on contrast nephropathy. *Kidney Int.* 2004;65:1366–1374.

22. Guru V, Fremes S. The role of N-acetylcysteine in preventing radiographic contrast-induced nephropathy. *Clin Nephrol.* 2004;62:77–83.

23. Bagshaw S, Ghali WA. Acetylcysteine for prevention of contrast-induced nephropathy: a systematic review and meta-analysis. *BMC Med.* 2004;2:38.

24. Misra D, Leibowitz K, Gowda R, et al. Role of N-acetylcysteine in prevention of contrast-induced nephropathy after cardiovascular procedures: a meta-analysis. *Clin Cardiol.* 2004;27:607–610.

25. Nallamothu BK, Shojania KG, Saint S, et al. Is acetylcysteine effective in preventing contrast-related nephropathy? A meta-analysis. *Am J Med.* 2004;117:938–947.

26. Liu R, Nair D, Ix J, et al. N-acetylcysteine for prevention of contrast-induced nephropathy: a systematic review and meta-analysis. *J Gen Intern Med.* 2005 20:193–200.

27. Duong M, MacKenzie T, Malenka D: N-acetylcysteine prophylaxis significantly reduces the risk of radiocontrast-induced nephropathy. *Catheter Cardiovasc Interv.* 2005 64:471–479.

28. Bagshaw SM, McAlister FA, Manns BJ, et al. Acetylcysteine in the prevention of contrast-induced nephropathy: a case study of the pitfalls in the evolution of evidence. *Arch Intern Med.* 2006;166:161–166.

29. Marenzi G, Assanelli E, Marana I, et al. N-acetylcysteine and contrast-induced nephropathy in primary angioplasty. *N Engl J Med.* 2006;354(26):2773–2782.

30. Briguori C, Airoldi F, D'Andrea D, et al. Renal Insufficiency Following Contrast Media Administration Trial (REMEDIAL): a randomized comparison of 3 preventive strategies. *Circulation.* 2007;115(10):1211–1217.

31. Khanal S, Attallah N, Smith DE, et al. Statin therapy reduces contrast-induced nephropathy: an analysis of contemporary percutaneous interventions. *Am J Med.* 2005;118(8):843–849.

32. Patti G, Nusca A, Chello M, Pasceri V, D'Ambrosio A, Vetrovec GW, Di Sciascio G. Usefulness of statin pretreatment to prevent contrast-induced nephropathy and to improve long-term outcome in patients undergoing percutaneous coronary intervention. *Am J Cardiol.* 2008 Feb 1;101(3):279–85.

33. McCullough PA, Rocher LR. Statin therapy in renal disease: harmful or protective. *Curr Atheroscler Rep.* 2007;9(1):18–24.

34. Bachorzewska-Gajewska H, Malyszko J, Sitniewska E, et al. Neutrophil-gelatinase-associated lipocalin and renal function after percutaneous coronary interventions. *Am J Nephrol.* 2006;26(3):287-292. Epub 2006 Jun 13.

35. Mishra J, Dent C, Tarabishi R, et al. Neutrophil gelatinase-associated lipocalin (NGAL) as a biomarker for acute renal injury after cardiac surgery. *Lancet.* 2005;365(9466):1231–1238.

36. McCullough PA. Contrast-induced acute kidney injury. *J Am Coll Cardiol.* 2008;51(15):1419–1428.

# 44

# Adjunctive Pharmacology for PCI

GILBERT J. ZOGHBI AND WILLIAM B. HILLEGASS

## ● PRACTICAL POINTS

- The most potent platelet agonists *in vivo* stimulated by PCI are thrombin, thromboxane A2, platelet-activating factor, and collagen.

- Platelet activation causes conformational changes in the GP IIb/IIIa receptor, leading it to bind fibrinogen and von Willebrand factor that cross-link platelets resulting in platelet aggregation.

- Thienopyridines block the adenosine diphosphate (ADP) P2Y12 receptor.

- Clopidogrel is a prodrug that must be converted in the liver to its active thiol derivative.

- At least one year of dual antiplatelet therapy is recommended after implantation of a drug-eluting stent (DES). Many authorities recommend lifetime dual antiplatelet therapy after first-generation DES implantation with a sirolimus- or paclitaxel-eluting stent.

- For patients intolerant of aspirin or thienopyridines, the intracellular phosphodiesterase inhibitor cilostazol is effective as a second-line antiplatelet agent.

- In the TRITON-TIMI 38 trial, patients receiving prasugrel had a sub-acute stent thrombosis rate (24 hours to 30 days after PCI) of 0.36% versus 1.19% with clopidogrel (p<0.0001). The major bleeding rate with prasugrel was 2.4% versus 1.9% with clopidogrel (p=0.06), which approached statistical significance.

- During PCI, the intensity of antithrombotic therapy with unfractionated intravenous heparin (IV-UFH) is monitored with the activated clotting time (ACT).

- Based on the randomized EPILOG study and other observational data, the optimal ACT during PCI with IIb/IIIa therapy and unfractionated intravenous heparin (IV-UFH) is 200 to 250 seconds.

- Direct thrombin inhibitors (DTI) such as bivalirudin bind to and inactivate thrombin directly without the need to bind to antithrombin as is the case with the heparins. Compared to IV-UFH, DTIs can inhibit clot-bound thrombin, are not inhibited by circulating inhibitors, do not bind to plasma proteins, and do not activate platelets but inhibit thrombin-mediated platelet activation.

- The ACUITY and REPLACE2 trials showed that bivalirudin monotherapy was as effective as UFH or enoxaparin plus a GPIIb/IIIa inhibitor or as bivalirudin plus a GPIIb/IIIa inhibitor with respect to ischemic complications and had significantly lower rates of major bleeding in elective and NSTEMI/ACS patients undergoing PCI.

- Nitroglycerin dilates the large coronary arteries and the arterioles >100μm in diameter, but has little effect on the microvasculature.

- No-reflow is the failure of restoration of normal myocardial blood flow despite the mechanical relief of obstruction in the target vessel. Microvascular vasodilators are the first-line therapy of no-reflow and include sodium nitroprusside, adenosine, nicardipine, and nicorandil.

- Adenosine is the commonly used vasodilator to induce maximal hyperemia during studies of coronary physiology with the pressure wire to determine fractional flow reserve (FFR) or with the flow wire to determine coronary flow reserve (CFR).

# INTRODUCTION

Adjunctive administration of pharmacological agents is critical to the success and safe performance of modern percutaneous coronary intervention (PCI). PCI has become the dominant mode of mechanical revascularization of coronary artery disease in the United States. Considerable basic and clinical research has contributed to the development of a robust array of effective and reasonably safe adjunctive medications. Since PCI treats and also causes disruption of atherosclerotic plaque, the main focus of its use has been antithrombotic therapy.

# THE COAGULATION CASCADE

Injury to the vessel such as occurs during PCI activates the coagulation cascade to achieve hemostasis. The final product of hemostasis is the generation of fibrin and formation of the cross-linked fibrin clot. The coagulation cascade occurs in overlapping stages.

## Initiation and Formation of the Platelet Plug

Vascular injury activates platelets to form the platelet plug. The process involves platelet adhesion to the subendothelial matrix, followed by platelet aggregation and secretion of granule proteins, which potentiate the platelet procoagulant activity and enhance thrombin generation.[1] During the cascade, platelets are activated by strong platelet agonists such as thrombin, thromboxane A2, platelet-activating Factor, and collagen or by the weak agonists ADP, epinephrine, and serotonin.[1] Disruption of the intact endothelium exposes subendothelial elements such as von Willebrand factor, collagen, fibronectin, laminin, and microfibrils, which serve as anchors to which platelets can adhere. Integrin glycoproteins (GP) GPIa/IIa, GPVI, GPIIb are the platelet collagen receptors, and GPIb is the platelet von Willebrand factor receptor.[1,2] High flow shear rates activate the von Willebrand factor and enhances its binding to GPIb.[1,2] Platelet adhesion contributes to the initiation of the thrombotic cascade. Platelet activation causes conformational changes in the GPIIb/IIIa receptor to bind to fibrinogen and von Willebrand factor that cross-links other platelets, resulting in platelet aggregation.[1,2] Platelet activation or stimulation causes platelet secretion of various substances from their granules such as ADP, serotonin, fibronectin, thrombospondin, fibrinogen, thromboxane A2, and platelet-derived growth Factors, creating a positive feedback loop for further platelet stimulation and activation (**Figure 44-1**).[1,2]

## Clotting Cascade

The clotting cascade involves the sequential activation of proenzymes to active enzymes that are involved in the various steps of the intrinsic and extrinsic pathways of the cascade (**Figure 44-2**).

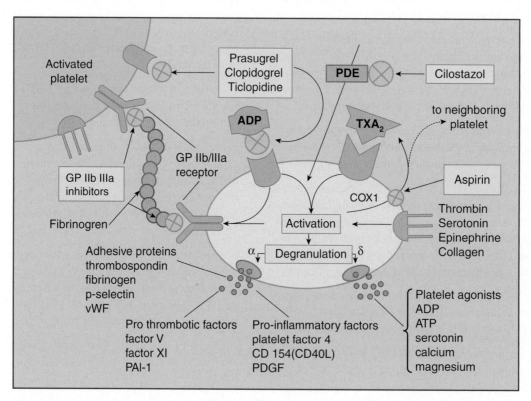

**Figure 44-1.** Platelet activation and aggregation pathways with sites of action of commonly used platelet-inhibiting medications.

# ANTITHROMBIN THERAPY

The necessity of administration of an antithrombin agent became apparent in the earliest animal models of angioplasty.[38] Abrupt vessel closure occurred frequently if balloon dilatation was performed without an antithrombin. This same phenomenon was observed in human coronary angioplasty when heparin was inadvertently not administered prior to initial device activation in the target coronary vessel.[39]

Intravenous unfractionated heparin (UFH) was the first agent employed. Typically, a fixed dose of 10,000 units was administered intravenously prior to balloon dilation or atherectomy during the first decade of PCI. In the early 1990s, the intensity of heparin anticoagulation was monitored with determination of the activated clotting time. There appeared to be a trade-off between bleeding and ischemic complications.[39,40] In addition to studies trying to define the "optimal ACT" to balance ischemic benefit and bleeding risk, intensive research focused on the development of alternative agents to UFH. The goal, of course, was to improve antithrombotic efficacy and clinical ischemic complications such as abrupt closure, emergency coronary artery bypass graft (CABG), and periprocedural myonecrosis/infarction while reducing bleeding risk.

## Unfractionated Heparin

Unfractionated heparin is a sulfated polysaccharide with a molecular weight ranging from 3000 to 30,000 Da. It produces its main anticoagulant effect through inactivation of thrombin (Factor IIa) and activated Factor X (Factor Xa). It is an indirect thrombin inhibitor since its action occurs due to binding with antithrombin (AT) through a high-affinity pentasaccharide. The heparin-AT complex then inhibits thrombin. By inactivating thrombin, heparin prevents fibrin formation. It also inhibits thrombin-induced activation of platelets as well as Factor V and Factor VIII.[41]

The major limitation of heparin is its nonspecific binding to positively charged proteins. This nonspecific binding causes considerable variability in the dosing of UFH from one patient to another. During PCI, the intensity of antithrombotic therapy with UFH is monitored with the activated clotting time. Earlier studies demonstrated a higher ACT to be associated with fewer ischemic complications of PCI.[39] More recent stent studies in the stent era with dual antiplatelet therapy, such as ESPRIT, suggest no strong relationship between ACT and the likelihood of ischemic complications.[42]

Studies have generally confirmed, however, that higher ACTs are associated with a higher clinical bleeding risk.[40] This is particularly true in the setting of concomitant administration of the parenteral IIb/IIIa antagonists abciximab, eptifibatide, and tirofiban. Based on the randomized EPILOG study and other observational data, the optimal ACT during PCI with IIb/IIIa therapy and UFH is 200-250 seconds.[35] The optimal ACT for PCI with stenting without IIb/IIIa therapy remains less well-defined but is generally accepted to be approximately 300 seconds in the stent era.[42]

## Low Molecular Weight Heparin

Low molecular heparins (LMWHs) include enoxaparin, dalteparin, nadroparin, and tinzaparin. Enoxaparin is more commonly used during PCI. LMWH is derived from unfractionated heparin that is chemically or enzymatically depolymerized into smaller polysaccharide chains of different molecular weights (2000-9000 Da), which are equal to about one-third the molecular weight of UFH.[43,44] Pentasaccharide chains containing > 18 saccharide units (which comprise 25-50% of the LMWH chains) inactivate Factor Xa directly and thrombin (Factor IIa) indirectly via antithrombin activation.[43,44] The remaining pentasaccharide chains inhibit only Factor Xa resulting in an anti Factor Xa to anti Factor IIa ratios of 1.9 to 3.8.[43,44] Subcutaneous LMWHs have predictable pharmacokinetics, with a plasma half-life of 3-6 hours, peak effect at 3-5 hours, and duration of action of around 12 hours.[44] LMWHs are metabolized in the liver and excreted renally.[44] Unlike UFH, LMWHs have dose-independent clearance, lower binding to endothelium, plasma proteins, platelets, and macrophages, and superior bioavailability. These properties all result in more predictable and sustained anticoagulation.[43-45] Additionally, LMWHs are easier to administer, don't require monitoring, cause less platelet activation, and less inactivation by platelet Factor 4, and less frequency of heparin-induced thrombocytopenia.[45,46]

The ACC/AHA 2007 Guidelines for the Management of Patients with Unstable Angina or Non-ST Elevation Myocardial Infarction consider LMWH to have established efficacy for patients in whom an invasive or conservative strategy is planned (Class I).[43] LMWH is preferred to unfractionated heparin in patients with a conservative strategy unless CABG is planned within 24 hours (Class IIa).[43] In a meta-analysis of six studies that compared enoxaparin with UFH in patients with ACS, enoxaparin showed favorable point estimates for death or nonfatal MI with a pooled odds ratio (OR) of 0.91 (CI 0.83 to 0.99).[43] **Table 44-3** lists the pivotal randomized studies of enoxaparin use compared to UFH use during PCI.

The ACC/AHA/SCAI PCI guidelines consider LMWHs a reasonable alternative to heparin in patients with ACS (Class IIa) and with STEMI (Class IIb) undergoing PCI.[46] The other LMWHs were studied mainly in ACS trials.

| Table 44-3 • Randomized Trials Comparing Enoxaparin to Unfractionated Heparin During PCI | | | | |
|---|---|---|---|---|
| Study | Patient Population | Treatment | Outcome: Bleed | Outcome: MACE |
| CRUISE[91] | 261 patients, elective or urgent PCI, all received Integrilin | Enoxaparin 0.75 mg/kg i.v. UFH (60 U/kg, ACT >200) | Bleeding index 0.8 1.1 | 48 h 8.5% 7.6 % |
| SYNERGY[50] | 10,027 patients, non-STEMI, early invasive strategy, received anticoagulant on admission | Enoxaparin 1 mg/kg S/Q q 12 h† (PCI 47%) Heparin 60 U/kg bolus, 12u/kg/h maintenance (PCI 46%) | TIMI major: GUSTO severe 2.7-9.* 2.2-7.6 | 30 days 14.0% 14.5% |
| STEEPLE[51] | 3528 patients, elective PCI, 41% received GPIIb/IIIa inhibitors | Enoxaparin 0.5 mg/kg i.v. Enoxaparin 0.75 mg/kg i.v. UFH (ACT 300-350 sec) | Major + minor 6.0%* 6.7%* 8.7% | 30 days 7.2% 7.9% 8.4% |

*p-value <0.05 versus UFH
† During PCI, if the last enoxaparin dose was given <8 h before balloon inflation, no additional enoxaparin was to be given. If the last enoxaparin dose was given ≥8 h before balloon inflation, 0.3 mg/kg of i.v. enoxaparin was given before proceeding with PCI

The FRISC trial compared Dalteparin to placebo and showed a lower rate of death or new MI (1.8 versus 4.8%) with no difference in bleeding rates.[47] The FRAXIS trial compared nadroparin to UFH and did not show an advantage in MACE compared to UFH.[48] Nadroparin had a significant increase in major bleeding (3.5 versus 1.6% for UFH).[48] The EVET trial compared enoxaparin and tinaparin. Enoxaparin was superior with significantly lower rates of persistent unstable angina at 7 days (11.8 versus 19.3%), of recurrent angina or MI at 30 days (17.8 versus 28.9%), and of death or MI, angina at 6 months (26 versus 44%).[49]

Enoxaparin dosing during PCI depends on the timing of the most recent subcutaneous (SC) dose received prior to PCI. SC enoxaparin is administered as 1mg/kg twice daily if creatinine clearance is ≥30 cc/min, and once daily if creatinine clearance <30 cc/min.[46] No additional enoxaparin is given if the last SC enoxaparin dose was given <8 hours prior to PCI.[46] A 0.3 mg/kg bolus of intravenous (i.v.) enoxaparin is given if the last SC enoxaparin dose was administered >8 hours prior to PCI.[46] A 0.75-1.0 mg/kg bolus of i.v. enoxaparin or other anticoagulant is given if the most recent SC enoxaparin dose was > 12 hours prior to PCI. The dosing of enoxaparin with GPIIb/IIIa inhibitors has not been well defined.

Patients who receive dalteparin (120 IU/kg S/Q every 12 hours) prior to PCI should receive i.v. UFH before PCI procedure.[43] Studies that compared LMWH with UFH during PCI have found bleeding and ischemic complication rates of LMWHs to be low and comparable to those observed with UFH.[46] However, the SYNERGY trial, which randomized patients with NSTEMI to treatment with either unfractionated heparin or subcutaneously administered enoxaparin, found higher rates of bleeding, especially in those patients who crossed over from one anticoagulant to the other.[46,50]

The STEEPLE trial that randomized patients undergoing elective PCI to i.v. enoxaparin (0.5 mg/kg or 0.75 mg/kg before PCI) or UFH showed higher mortality rate with the 0.5 mg/kg enoxaparin dose and a nonstatistically significant lower rate of major and minor bleeding with the 0.75 mg/kg dose compared with UFH.[51]

The anticoagulation effect of enoxaparin cannot be monitored with activated partial thromboplastin time (aPTT) and ACT. LMWH pharmacokinetics may be not as predictable in patients with impaired renal function, morbid obesity, weight <50 kg, or during pregnancy.[45] LMWH should be used with caution in such patients.[45] Antifactor Xa activity can be measured where levels of 0.8 to 1.8 IU/mL are considered therapeutic but have not been well established for PCI guidance.[43,44] A Rapidpoint ENOX point-of-care test was developed to test the anticoagulation effect of enoxaparin. An ENOX time range of 250-450 seconds corresponded with procedural anti-Xa level of 0.8-1.8 IU/m, and <200-250 seconds was the safe range for sheath removal.[52] Sheath removal and manual compression may be performed 4 hours after the most recent i.v. enoxaparin dose or 6 to 8 hours after the last SC dose.[46]

## Fondaparinux

Fondaparinux, a synthetic heparin pentasaccharide analog, has a higher binding affinity to antithrombin than UFH and LMWHs, and exclusively neutralizes Factor Xa via antithrombin activation.[53,54] Fondaparinux does not bind or interact with cellular elements, plasma proteins, or platelet factor 4 and does not induce thrombocytopenia.[55] Fondaparinux has a 100% bioavailability after SC injection and reaches peak serum levels 1.7 hours after its administration.[55] Its half-life of 17 hours permits once a day dosing.

It does affect the ACT or aPTT and has no antidote.[55] Fondaparinux is, predominantly, cleared renally.

The OASIS 5 trial randomized 20,078 patients with non-STEMI to 2.5 mg/day SC fondaparinux or 1 mg/kg twice daily of SC enoxaparin for 6 days.[53,54] In subgroup analysis of the 6238 who underwent PCI, fondaparinux had comparable 9-day rate of death, MI, or stoke (5.3 versus 5.4%), significantly lower 9-day rate of major bleeding (2.4% versus 5.1%). However, a significant increase in catheter-related thrombus (0.9 versus 0.4%) occurred. To prevent this, it is recommended that UFH be administered at the time of PCI in patients receiving fondaparinux for ACS. This approach has not been observed to increase bleeding risk.[54]

Fondaparinux is preferred in ACS patients at increased risk of bleeding (Class I) and is administered at a dose of 2.5 mg SC once daily.[43] It should be avoided in patients with a creatinine clearance <30 cc/min. As mentioned above, fondaparinux should not be used as the sole anticoagulant during PCI because of increased risk of catheter thrombosis. Again, supplemental UFH should be administered prior to PCI.[5]

## Direct Thrombin Inhibitors

Direct thrombin inhibitors (DTIs) bind to and inactivate thrombin directly without the need to bind to antithrombin as is the case with the heparins. Of the i.v. DTIs available in the U.S., bivalirudin is approved for use in ACS and PCI. Lepirudin and argatroban are approved for use in patients with heparin-induced thrombocytopenia.[56] Thrombin exocite 1 binds fibrinogen and then the active site cleaves fibrinogen via a serine protease.[56] Bivalent inhibitors such as lepirudin and bivalirudin bind to exosite site 1 and to the active site while univalent inhibitors such as argatroban bind to the active site only.[56] Bivalent inhibitors tend to be more selective and have a higher affinity for thrombin.[56]

Hirudin is a 65-amino acid polypeptide that was originally isolated from the salivary glands of the leech *Hirudo medicinalis*. Lepirudin is manufactured by recombinant DNA technology and differs from hirudin by the two amino acids at the amino terminal and by lack of the sulfate group on tyrosine at position 63.[56] Lepirudin binds to thrombin in an irreversible 1:1 stoichiometric complex and thus has no antidote.[56] Bivalirudin is a 20-amino acid polypeptide synthetic analog of hirudin. Bivalirudin binds to thrombin in a 1:1 stoichiometric fashion, but once bound, thrombin cleaves the active site of the bivalirudin molecule and allows recovery of thrombin activity.[56] This results in a weaker and short-lived thrombin inhibition.[56] Argatroban is a synthetic derivative of arginine. It binds reversibly to thrombin in a 1:1 stoichiometric complex and does not inhibit other serine proteases.[56]

Compared to UFH, DTIs can inhibit clot-bound thrombin, are not inhibited by circulating inhibitors, do not bind to plasma proteins, and do not activate platelets but inhibit thrombin-mediated platelet activation. Bivalirudin will be discussed in what follows as it is the only DTI used during PCI.

Intravenously administered bivalirudin has linear pharmacokinetics, a small volume of distribution, and rapid plasma clearance.[56] Around 80% of bivalirudin is degraded by blood peptidases. The degraded fragments and 20% of the active drug are cleared renally.[56] Bivalirudin has immediate onset of action, a half-life of 25 minutes in patients with normal renal function, and respective half-lives of 57 and 210 minutes in patients with severe renal impairment and patients on dialysis.[56] The anticoagulation effect can be monitored with ACT or aPTT and returns to normal within 1-2 hours from infusion termination.[56]

The ACC/AHA 2007 Guidelines for the Management of Patients with Unstable Angina or Non-ST Elevation Myocardial Infarction consider bivalirudin to have established efficacy for patients in whom an invasive strategy is planned (Class I).[43] In patients who have received upstream bivalirudin as initial antithrombin therapy for acute coronary syndrome, an additional 0.5 mg/kg i.v. bolus is given prior to PCI and the infusion rate is increased to 1.75 mg/kg/h.[43] In patients not receiving bivalirudin as medical therapy prior to the decision to proceed with PCI, bivalirudin is administered with an initial, 0.75 mg/kg i.v. bolus prior to PCI along with a maintenance infusion of 1.75 mg/kg/h. An additional 0.3 mg/kg i.v. bolus is administered if ACT <225 seconds, although most operators do not check ACTs since it is rarely subtherapeutic. The infusion rate should be reduced by 20% in patients with moderate renal insufficiency, by 60% in patients with severe renal insufficiency, and by 90% in patients on dialysis. The bivalirudin infusion is usually discontinued at the conclusion of the PCI.[43] However, some operators will continue the infusion for 1 to 3 hours if the patient did not receive preloading with clopidogrel.

In a meta-analysis of eleven earlier studies that compared DTI to UFH in 35,970 patients with acute coronary syndrome, DTI showed a significant reduction in 30-day death or MI.[57] The benefit was seen with hirudin and bivalirudin and not with argatroban. The risk of bleeding was higher with hirudin and lower with bivalirudin in comparison to UFH.[57] The results of pivotal studies using bivalirudin during PCI are listed in **Table 44-4**. A meta-analysis of BAT, CACHET, and REPLACE 1 trials that compared bivalirudin to UFH during PCI showed that the absolute benefit in ischemic and bleeding complications increased with decreasing creatinine clearance.[58]

**Table 44-4 • Randomized Trials Comparing Bivalirudin to Other Anticoagulants or GPIIb/IIIa Inhibitors During PCI**

| Study | Patient Population | Treatment | Outcome: Bleed | Outcome: MACE |
|---|---|---|---|---|
| BAT | 4098 patients, unstable angina, or post infarct angina | Bivalirudin bolus + 20 h infusion UFH bolus + 18-24 h infusion | All bleed 3.8%* 9.8% | In hospital 11.4% 12.2% |
| CACHET | 268 patients, elective PCI | Bivalirudin 1mg/kg bolus + inf + reopro Bivalirudin 0.5 mg/kg bolus + inf ± reopro Bivalirudin 0.75 mg/kg bolus + inf ± reopro UFH 70 u/kg bolus + reopro | Major bleed 3.3% 2.4% 0% 4.3%† | Discharge or 7 days 0% 4.7% 0% 6.4%† |
| REPLACE 1[92] | 1056 patients, elective or urgent PCI, 72% received GPIIb/IIIa inh | Bivalirudin bolus/inf UFH 70 U/kg bolus | Major bleed 2.1% 2.7% | 48 h 5.6% 6.9% |
| REPLACE 2[93] | 6010 patients, urgent or planned PCI | Bivalirudin +/– GPIIb/IIIa inh UFH + GPIIb/IIIa inh | Major bleed 2.4* 4.1 | 30 days 7.6% 7.1% |
| ACUITY[59] | 7789 of 13,819 patients, unstable angina or NSTEMI, underwent PCI | Bivalirudin Bivalirudin + GPIIb/IIIa inh Enoxaparin or UFH + GPIIb/IIIa inh | Major bleed 4% * 8% 7% | 30 days 9% 9% 8% |

*p<0.05
† p<0.05 of UFH compared to combined bivalirudin groups

The REPLACE2 and ACUITY trials showed that bivalirudin monotherapy was as effective as UFH or enoxaparin plus a GPIIb/IIIa inhibitor or bivalirudin plus a GPIIb/IIIa inhibitor in preventing ischemic complications but had significantly lower rates of major bleeding in stable PCI and NSTEMI/ACS patients, respectively.[59] Similar results were noted in the HORIZONS AMI trial, which compared bivalirudin with GPIIb/IIIa inhibitor in patients undergoing primary PCI for ST elevation MI.

## Oral Anticoagulants

Warfarin was included in the antithrombotic therapy regimen with the first generation Gianturco-Roubin 1 and Palmaz-Schatz coronary stents. Colombo et al., however, demonstrated that high pressure stent deployment was associated with a very low stent thrombosis and major bleeding rate with aspirin and 4 weeks of ticlopidine therapy. The Stent Antithrombotic Regimen Study (STARS) specifically randomized patients to three arms: aspirin alone, aspirin + warfarin, and aspirin + ticlopidine.[60] The trial showed conclusive advantage of aspirin + ticlopidine with a stent thrombosis rate of 0.5% over aspirin alone with stent thrombosis of 3.6% or aspirin and warfarin with stent thrombosis rate of 2.7% Hence, warfarin has no present role as an adjunctive medicine for PCI except in patients with other indications for long-term anticoagulation.

## OTHERS

### Intracoronary Thrombolytics

Several trials tested the intracoronary administration of thrombolytic agents for thrombus-laden lesions in the balloon angioplasty era. Agents tested included urokinase, streptokinase, and tPA. In the era prior to stenting and dual antiplatelet therapy, the intracoronary administration of thrombolytics for NSTEMI-ACS patients with thrombus-laden lesions did not demonstrate any benefit. Specifically, the UTOPIA trial administered tPA without apparent benefit.[61]

## VASODILATOR USE

### Nitroglycerin Use

Nitrates produce their vasodilatory effects by entering vascular smooth muscle cells and interacting with sulhydryl groups to form nitric oxide that stimulates guanylate cyclase to produce cGMP that causes smooth muscle relaxation. Nitrates dilate the large coronary arteries and the arterioles $>100\mu m$ in diameter. Intracoronary nitrates are used to reverse coronary artery spasm in situations of spontaneous, catheter, guide catheter, or device- (guide wire, rotablation, IVUS) related spasm. The dose ranges from 50 to 300 $\mu g$ that could be repeated if need be and if systolic blood pressure >90 mm Hg. Prophylactic administration of intracoronary nitrates is commonly used before IVUS and rotablation device activation.

## No-reflow Treatment

No-reflow is the failure of restoration of myocardial blood flow despite the mechanical relief of the stenosis. No-reflow complicates 0.5-3% of PCIs and occurs more commonly in SVG and acute MI PCIs.[62] No-reflow results from distal embolization of atherosclerotic debris, thrombi, or both that cause vasospasm of the microvascular circulation.[63] Vasodilators are the first line therapy of no-reflow and include sodium nitroprusside, adenosine, calcium channel blockers (verapamil, cardizem, nicardipine), nicorandil, or papaverine. These agents should be preferably administered via a distally placed infusion catheter or perfusion balloon. The studies that evaluated no-reflow therapy are small. The more commonly studied drugs are verapamil, adenosine, nicardipine, and nitroprusside. Intracoronary verapamil boluses of 50 to 200 $\mu g$ up to 900 $\mu g$ have been used to treat no-reflow with 60-100% success rates in different PCI settings, including SVG and rotablation interventions.[63-65] Nitroglycerin administration did not have any effect on alleviating no-reflow.[63,64] Intracoronary adenosine boluses of 10-20 $\mu g$ have used to treat no-reflow with 90% success rate in SVG PCI[66,67] Rapid and repeated boluses (>5 boluses) of 24 $\mu g$ adenosine doses alleviated no-reflow in 91% of patients compared to 33% of patients who had <5 adenosine boluses.[68] Intracoronary 50-200 $\mu gm$ nitroprusside boluses up to 1000 $\mu g$ doses to treat no-reflow improved the TIMI grade and the TIMI frame count in native and SVG PCI[69] and in PCI for acute MI.[70,71] Nicardipine (200 $\mu g$) boluses reversed no-reflow in 99% of patients in one study[72] and were beneficial in decreasing the rate of no-reflow in SVG PCI when administered prophylactically.[73] Nicorandil, an ATP-sensitive potassium channel opener, prevented the occurrence of no-reflow more effectively (2.7-4.5%) during rotablation compared to verapamil (11.8-17.4%).[74-76] The combination of sequential adenosine with nitroprusside and adenosine with nicorandil boluses improved no-reflow better than adenosine alone.[77-79]

## Fractional Flow Reserve and Coronary Flow Reserve

Adenosine is the commonly used vasodilator in the U.S. to induce maximal hyperemia during studies of coronary physiology with the pressure wire to determine fractional flow reserve (FFR ) or with the flow wire to determine coronary flow reserve (CFR). Adenosine stimulates the A2 receptor of vascular myocytes to produce microvascular dilation.[80] The peak effect of intracoronary adenosine occurs within 10 seconds of its administration and its duration of action is

around 20 seconds.[80] Optimal hyperemia is achieved with intracoronary boluses of 40 $\mu g$ in the right coronary artery and 60 $\mu g$ in the left coronary artery.[80] Higher doses (in 20-30 $\mu g$ increments) up to a maximum dose of 150 $\mu g$ have been used when the FFR was in the borderline range of 0.75-0.8.[80] Intravenous infusion of 140 $\mu g/kg/min$ of adenosine allows measuring a pullback FFR and provides a more pronounced hyperemia than high doses of intracoronary adenosine.[81] The peak effect is usually achieved within 1 to 2 minutes.[81] Side effects of adenosine include bronchospasm, chest pain, dyspnea, flushing, and AV block (more common with intracoronary administration especially in the right coronary artery). Adenosine causes modest hypotension and modest increase in heart rate. The side effects are short lived and usually well tolerated. Aminophylline (50-100 mg) can be administered to reverse severe side effects of adenosine.

Papaverine is not commonly used in the United States. Its mechanism of action is not entirely clear, but is thought to inhibit the phodiesterase enzyme, causing elevation of cyclic AMP levels and subsequent vasodilation. Intracoronary papaverine has peak effect within 10 to 30 seconds from administration and lasts for 45 to 60 seconds, allowing its use to measure pullback FFR.[80] The dose is 12-16 mg for the right coronary artery and 16-20 mg for the left coronary artery.[80] Intracoronary papaverine had comparable steady state hyperemia to 140 $\mu g/kg/min$ of intravenous adenosine.[82,83] Papaverine can prolong the QT interval, which may trigger serious ventricular arrhythmias.[83] When combined with some of the ionic contrast agents crystallization can occur.[83] Additionally, it increases coronary venous lactate production that may produce myocardial ischemia.[83]

# MISCELLANEOUS AGENTS

## Preprocedural Statins

Pre-PCI administration of statins has been shown to reduce post-PCI ischemic complications. It is thought that the pleotropic effects of statins mitigate the induced vascular injury during PCI.[84] Preprocedural statins reduced the incidence of postprocedural non Q wave MI defined by CK-MB or troponin elevations, as well as 30-day and 6-month mortality in one study.[84] The type and dose of statin were variable. Treatment duration ranged from 12 hours pre-PCI to >1 week pre-PCI.[84] There are no current recommendations regarding the optimal dosing and timing of pre-PCI treatment with statins.

## Preprocedural Beta-blockers

Beta-blocker administration during PCI is thought to protect a patient from myocardial injury resulting from distal embolization.[85] Administration of 15$\mu/kg$ of intracoronary propanolol before PCI reduced post-PCI CK-MB and troponin T elevations, as well as 30-day rates of major adverse cardiac events.[85] Pre-PCI administration of oral beta-blockers was shown to be protective in one observational study and non-protective in one observational and one randomized trial.[86]

## References

1. Shattil SJ, Kashiwagi H, Pampori N. Integrin signaling: the platelet paradigm. *Blood*. 1998;91:2645–2657.

2. Kroll MH, Schafer AI. Biochemical mechanisms of platelet activation. *Blood*. 1989;74:1181–1195.

3. Ferguson JJ, Waly HM, Wilson JM. Fundamentals of coagulation and glycoprotein IIb/IIIa receptor inhibition. *Am Heart J*. 1998;135:S35–42.

4. Holmes DR, Jr. Antiplatelet therapy after percutaneous coronary intervention. *Cerebrovasc Dis*. 2006;21 Suppl 1:25–34.

5. King SB, 3rd, Smith SC, Jr, Hirshfeld JW, Jr, et al. 2007 Focused Update of the ACC/AHA/SCAI 2005 Guideline Update for Percutaneous Coronary Intervention: A Report of the American College of Cardiology/American Heart Association Task Force on Practice guidelines. *J Am Coll Cardiol*. 2008;51:172–209.

6. Kariyazono H, Nakamura K, Arima J, et al. Evaluation of anti-platelet aggregatory effects of aspirin, cilostazol and ramatroban on platelet-rich plasma and whole blood. *Blood Coagul Fibrinol*. 2004;15:157–167.

7. Schwartz L, Bourassa MG, Lesperance J, et al. Aspirin and dipyridamole in the prevention of restenosis after percutaneous transluminal coronary angioplasty. *N Engl J Med*. 1988;318:1714–1719.

8. Balsano F, Rizzon P, Violi F, et al. Antiplatelet treatment with ticlopidine in unstable angina. A controlled multicenter clinical trial. The Studio della Ticlopidina nell'Angina Instabile Group. *Circulation*. 1990;82:17–26.

9. Godard P, Zini R, Metay A, et al. The fate of ticlopidine in the organism. II.—Distribution and elimination of ticlopidine 14C after a single oral administration in the rat. *Eur J Drug Metab Pharmacokinet*. 1979;4:133–138.

10. Savi P, Pereillo JM, Uzabiaga MF, et al. Identification and biological activity of the active metabolite of clopidogrel. *Thromb Haemost*. 2000;84:891–896.

11. Taubert D, Kastrati A, Harlfinger S, et al. Pharmacokinetics of clopidogrel after administration of a high loading dose. *Thromb Haemost*. 2004;92:311–316.

12. Cuisset T, Frere C, Quilici J, et al. Benefit of a 600-mg loading dose of clopidogrel on platelet reactivity and clinical outcomes in patients with non-ST-segment elevation acute coronary syndrome undergoing coronary stenting. *J Am Coll Cardiol*. 2006;48:1339–1345.

13. Frere C, Cuisset T, Quilici J, et al. ADP-induced platelet aggregation and platelet reactivity index VASP are good predictive markers for clinical outcomes in non-ST elevation acute coronary syndrome. *Thromb Haemost*. 2007;98:838–843.

14. Harder S, Klinkhardt U. Thrombolytics: drug interactions of clinical significance. *Drug Saf*. 2000;23:391–399.

15. White CW, Chaitman B, Lassar TA, et al. Antiplatelet agents are effective in reducing the immediate complications of PTCA: results from the ticlopidine multicenter trial (abstr). *Circulation*. 1987;76(suppl IV):IV–400.

16. Serruys PW, de Jaegere P, Kiemeneij F, et al. A comparison of balloon-expandable-stent implantation with balloon angioplasty in patients with coronary artery disease. Benestent Study Group. *N Engl J Med*. 1994;331:489–495.

17. Colombo A, Hall P, Nakamura S, et al. Intracoronary stenting without anticoagulation accomplished with intravascular ultrasound guidance. *Circulation*. 1995;91:1676–1688.

18. Lesesve JF, Callat MP, Lenormand B, et al. Hematological toxicity of ticlopidine. *Am J Hematol*. 1994;47:149–150.

19. Bennett CL, Connors JM, Carwile JM, et al. Thrombotic thrombocytopenic purpura associated with clopidogrel. *N Engl J Med*. 2000;342:1773–1777.

20. Randomised placebo-controlled and balloon-angioplasty-controlled trial to assess safety of coronary stenting with use of platelet glycoprotein-IIb/IIIa blockade. *Lancet*. 1998;352:87–92.

21. A randomised, blinded, trial of clopidogrel versus aspirin in patients at risk of ischaemic events (CAPRIE). CAPRIE Steering Committee. *Lancet*. 1996;348:1329–1339.

22. Steinhubl SR, Berger PB, Mann JT, 3rd, et al. Early and sustained dual oral antiplatelet therapy following percutaneous coronary intervention: a randomized controlled trial. *JAMA*. 2002;288:2411–2420.

23. Finn AV, Joner M, Nakazawa G, et al. Pathological correlates of late drug-eluting stent thrombosis: strut coverage as a marker of endothelialization. *Circulation*. 2007;115:2435–2441.

24. Lee SW, Park SW, Hong MK, et al. Triple versus dual antiplatelet therapy after coronary stenting: impact on stent thrombosis. *J Am Coll Cardiol*. 2005;46:1833–1837.

25. Lee SW, Park SW, Kim YH, et al. Comparison of triple versus dual antiplatelet therapy after drug-eluting stent implantation (from the DECLARE-Long trial). *Am J Cardiol*. 2007;100:1103–1108.

26. Meadows TA, Bhatt DL. Clinical aspects of platelet inhibitors and thrombus formation. *Circ Res*. 2007;100:1261–1275.

27. Lembo NJ, Black AJ, Roubin GS, et al. Effect of pretreatment with aspirin versus aspirin plus dipyridamole on frequency and type of acute complications of percutaneous transluminal coronary angioplasty. *Am J Cardiol*.1990;65:422–426.

28. Wiviott SD, Antman EM, Winters KJ, et al. Randomized comparison of prasugrel (CS-747, LY640315), a novel thienopyridine P2Y12 antagonist, with clopidogrel in percutaneous coronary intervention: results of the Joint Utilization of Medications to Block Platelets Optimally (JUMBO)-TIMI 26 trial. *Circulation*. 2005;111:3366–3373.

29. Wiviott SD, Braunwald E, McCabe CH, et al. Intensive oral antiplatelet therapy for reduction of ischaemic events

including stent thrombosis in patients with acute coronary syndromes treated with percutaneous coronary intervention and stenting in the TRITON-TIMI 38 trial: a subanalysis of a randomised trial. *Lancet.* 2008;371:1353–1363.

30. Seligsohn U. Glanzmann thrombasthenia: a model disease which paved the way to powerful therapeutic agents. *Pathophysiol Haemost Thromb.* 2002;32:216–217.

31. Coller BS. GPIIb/IIIa antagonists: pathophysiologic and therapeutic insights from studies of c7E3 Fab. *Thromb Haemost.* 1997;78:730–735.

32. Labinaz M, Ho C, Banerjee S, et al. Meta-analysis of clinical efficacy and bleeding risk with intravenous glycoprotein IIb/IIIa antagonists for percutaneous coronary intervention. *Can J Cardiol.* 2007;23:963–970.

33. Kereiakes DJ. Adjunctive pharmacotherapy before percutaneous coronary intervention in non-ST-elevation acute coronary syndromes: the role of modulating inflammation. *Circulation.* 2003;108:III22–27.

34. The EPIC Investigators. Use of a monoclonal antibody directed against the platelet glycoprotein IIb/IIIa receptor in high-risk coronary angioplasty. *New England J Med.* 1994;330:956–961.

35. The EPILOG Investigators. Platelet glycoprotein IIb/IIIa receptor blockade and low-dose heparin during percutaneous coronary revascularization. *N Engl J Med.* 1997;336:1689–1696.

36. Kastrati A, Mehilli J, Schuhlen H, et al. A clinical trial of abciximab in elective percutaneous coronary intervention after pretreatment with clopidogrel. *N Engl J Med.* 2004;350:232–238.

37. Kastrati A, Mehilli J, Neumann FJ, et al. Abciximab in patients with acute coronary syndromes undergoing percutaneous coronary intervention after clopidogrel pretreatment: the ISAR-REACT 2 randomized trial. *JAMA.* 2006;295: 1531–1538.

38. Heras M, Chesebro JH, Penny WJ, et al. Importance of adequate heparin dosage in arterial angioplasty in a porcine model. *Circulation.* 1988;78:654–660.

39. Narins CR, Hillegass WB, Jr, Nelson CL, et al. Relation between activated clotting time during angioplasty and abrupt closure. *Circulation.* 1996;93:667–671.

40. Hillegass WB, Brott BC, Chapman GD, et al. Relationship between activated clotting time during percutaneous intervention and subsequent bleeding complications. *Am Heart J.* 2002;144:501–507.

41. Chesebro JH, Rauch U, Fuster V, et al. Pathogenesis of thrombosis in coronary artery disease. *Haemostasis.* 1997;27 Suppl 1:12–18.

42. Tolleson TR, O'Shea JC, Bittl JA, et al. Relationship between heparin anticoagulation and clinical outcomes in coronary stent intervention: observations from the ESPRIT trial. *J Am Coll Cardiol.* 2003;41:386–393.

43. Anderson JL, Adams CD, Antman EM, et al. ACC/AHA 2007 Guidelines for the Management of Patients with Unstable Angina/Non-ST-Elevation Myocardial Infarction: A Report of the American College of Cardiology/American Heart Association Task Force on Practice Guidelines (Writing Committee to Revise the 2002 Guidelines for the Management of Patients With Unstable Angina/Non-ST-Elevation Myocardial Infarction) developed in collaboration with the American College of Emergency Physicians, the Society for Cardiovascular Angiography and Interventions, and the Society of Thoracic Surgeons endorsed by the American Association of Cardiovascular and Pulmonary Rehabilitation and the Society for Academic Emergency Medicine. *J Am Coll Cardiol.* 2007;50:e1–e157.

44. Hirsh J, Raschke R. Heparin and low-molecular-weight heparin: the Seventh ACCP Conference on Antithrombotic and Thrombolytic Therapy. *Chest.* 2004;126:188S–203S.

45. Graf J, Janssens U. Low-molecular weight heparins in percutaneous coronary interventions: current concepts, problems, and perspectives. *Curr Pharm Des.* 2004;10:375–386.

46. Smith SC, Jr, Feldman TE, Hirshfeld JW, Jr, et al. ACC/ AHA/SCAI 2005 Guideline Update for Percutaneous Coronary Intervention: A Report of the American College of Cardiology/American Heart Association Task Force on Practice Guidelines (ACC/AHA/SCAI Writing Committee to Update the 2001 Guidelines for Percutaneous Coronary Intervention). *J Am Coll Cardiol.* 2006;47:e1–121.

47. Lindahl B, Venge P, Wallentin L. Troponin T identifies patients with unstable coronary artery disease who benefit from long-term antithrombotic protection. Fragmin in Unstable Coronary Artery Disease (FRISC) Study Group. *J Am Coll Cardiol.* 1997;29:43–48.

48. Comparison of two treatment durations (6 days and 14 days) of a low molecular weight heparin with a 6-day treatment of unfractionated heparin in the initial management of unstable angina or non-Q wave myocardial infarction: FRAX.I.S. (FRAxiparine in Ischaemic Syndrome). *Eur Heart J.* 1999;20:1553–1562.

49. Michalis LK, Katsouras CS, Papamichael N, et al. Enoxaparin versus tinzaparin in non-ST-segment elevation acute coronary syndromes: the EVET trial. *Am Heart J.* 2003;146:304–310.

50. Ferguson JJ, Califf RM, Antman EM, et al. Enoxaparin vs unfractionated heparin in high-risk patients with non-ST-segment elevation acute coronary syndromes managed with an intended early invasive strategy: primary results of the SYNERGY randomized trial. *JAMA.* 2004;292:45–54.

51. Montalescot G, White HD, Gallo R, et al. Enoxaparin versus unfractionated heparin in elective percutaneous coronary intervention. *N Engl J Med.* 2006;355:1006–1017.

52. Moliterno DJ, Hermiller JB, Kereiakes DJ, et al. A novel point-of-care enoxaparin monitor for use during percutaneous coronary intervention. Results of the Evaluating Enoxaparin Clotting Times (ELECT) Study. *J Am Coll Cardiol.* 2003;42:1132–1139.

53. Ferguson JJ, Idelchik GM. OASIS-5: how do fondaparinux and enoxaparin compare in patients with acute coronary syndromes? *Nat Clin Pract Cardiovasc Med.* 2006;3:474–475.

54. Mehta SR, Granger CB, Eikelboom JW, et al. Efficacy and safety of fondaparinux versus enoxaparin in patients with acute coronary syndromes undergoing percutaneous coronary intervention: results from the OASIS-5 trial. *J Am Coll Cardiol.* 2007;50:1742–1751.

55. Gallus AS, Coghlan DW. Heparin pentasaccharide. *Curr Opin Hematol.* 2002;9:422–429.

56. Linkins LA, Weitz JI. Pharmacology and clinical potential of direct thrombin inhibitors. *Curr Pharm Des.* 2005;11: 3877–3884.

57. Direct thrombin inhibitors in acute coronary syndromes: principal results of a meta-analysis based on individual patients' data. *Lancet.* 2002;359:294–302.

58. Chew DP, Bhatt DL, Kimball W, et al. Bivalirudin provides increasing benefit with decreasing renal function: a meta-analysis of randomized trials. *Am J Cardiol.* 2003;92:919–923.

59. Stone GW, White HD, Ohman EM, et al. Bivalirudin in patients with acute coronary syndromes undergoing percutaneous coronary intervention: a subgroup analysis from the Acute Catheterization and Urgent Intervention Triage strategy (ACUITY) trial. *Lancet.* 2007;369:907–919.

60. Leon MB, Baim DS, Popma JJ, et al. A clinical trial comparing three antithrombotic-drug regimens after coronary-artery stenting. Stent Anticoagulation Restenosis Study Investigators. *N Engl J Med.* 1998;339:1665–1671.

61. DiSciascio G, Cowley MJ. The role of intracoronary thrombolysis and percutaneous transluminal coronary angioplasty in evolving myocardial infarction. *Cardiol Clin.* 1985;3:73–83.

62. Eeckhout E, Kern MJ. The coronary no-reflow phenomenon: a review of mechanisms and therapies. *Eur Heart J.* 2001;22: 729–739.

63. Piana RN, Paik GY, Moscucci M, et al. Incidence and treatment of 'no-reflow' after percutaneous coronary intervention. *Circulation.* 1994;89:2514–2518.

64. Kaplan BM, Benzuly KH, Kinn JW, et al. Treatment of no-reflow in degenerated saphenous vein graft interventions: comparison of intracoronary verapamil and nitroglycerin. *Cathet Cardiovasc Diagn.* 1996;39:113–118.

65. Abbo KM, Dooris M, Glazier S, et al. Features and outcome of no-reflow after percutaneous coronary intervention. Am J Cardiol 1995;75:778–782.

66. Fischell TA, Carter AJ, Foster MT, et al. Reversal of "no reflow" during vein graft stenting using high velocity boluses of intracoronary adenosine. *Cathet Cardiovasc Diagn.* 1998;45:360–365.

67. Assali AR, Sdringola S, Ghani M, et al. Intracoronary adenosine administered during percutaneous intervention in acute myocardial infarction and reduction in the incidence of "no reflow" phenomenon. *Cathet Cardiovasc Interv.* 2000;51:27–31; discussion 32.

68. Sdringola S, Assali A, Ghani M, et al. Adenosine use during aortocoronary vein graft interventions reverses but does not prevent the slow-no reflow phenomenon. *Cathet* Cardiovasc Interv 2000;51:394–399.

69. Hillegass WB, Dean NA, Liao L, et al. Treatment of no-reflow and impaired flow with the nitric oxide donor nitroprusside following percutaneous coronary interventions: initial human clinical experience. *J Am Coll Cardiol.* 2001;37:1335–1343.

70. Pasceri V, Pristipino C, Pelliccia F, et al. Effects of the nitric oxide donor nitroprusside on no-reflow phenomenon during coronary interventions for acute myocardial infarction. *Am J Cardiol.* 2005;95:1358–1361.

71. Wang HJ, Lo PH, Lin JJ, et al. Treatment of slow/no-reflow phenomenon with intracoronary nitroprusside injection in primary coronary intervention for acute myocardial infarction. *Cathet Cardiovasc Interv.* 2004;63:171–176.

72. Huang RI, Patel P, Walinsky P, et al. Efficacy of intracoronary nicardipine in the treatment of no-reflow during percutaneous coronary intervention. *Cathet Cardiovasc Interv.* 2006;68: 671–676.

73. Fischell T, Haller S, Ashraf K. Intragraft nicardipine prophylaxis to prevent no-reflow in triple-vessel saphenous vein graft intervention. *J Invasive Cardiol.* 2005;17:334–337.

74. Tsubokawa A, Ueda K, Sakamoto H, et al. Effect of intracoronary nicorandil administration on preventing no-reflow/slow flow phenomenon during rotational atherectomy. *Circ J.* 2002;66:1119–1123.

75. Matsuo H, Watanabe S, Watanabe T, et al. Prevention of no-reflow/slow-flow phenomenon during rotational atherectomy—a prospective randomized study comparing intracoronary continuous infusion of verapamil and nicorandil. *Am Heart J.* 2007;154:994 e1–6.

76. Iwasaki K, Samukawa M, Furukawa H. Comparison of the effects of nicorandil versus verapamil on the incidence of slow flow/no reflow during rotational atherectomy. *Am J Cardiol.* 2006;98:1354–1356.

77. Barcin C, Denktas AE, Lennon RJ, et al. Comparison of combination therapy of adenosine and nitroprusside with adenosine alone in the treatment of angiographic no-reflow phenomenon. *Cathet Cardiovasc Interv.* 2004;61:484–491.

78. Lim SY, Bae EH, Jeong MH, et al. Effect of combined intracoronary adenosine and nicorandil on no-reflow phenomenon during percutaneous coronary intervention. *Circ J.* 2004;68:928–932.

79. Parikh KH, Chag MC, Shah KJ, et al. Intracoronary boluses of adenosine and sodium nitroprusside in combination reverses slow/no-reflow during angioplasty: a clinical scenario of ischemic preconditioning. *Can J Physiol Pharmacol.* 2007;85: 476–482.

80. McGeoch RJ, Oldroyd KG. Pharmacological options for inducing maximal hyperaemia during studies of coronary physiology. *Cathet Cardiovasc Interv.* 2008;71:198–204.

81. Casella G, Leibig M, Schiele TM, et al. Are high doses of intracoronary adenosine an alternative to standard intravenous adenosine for the assessment of fractional flow reserve? *Am Heart J.* 2004;148:590–595.

82. van der Voort PH, van Hagen E, Hendrix G, et al. Comparison of intravenous adenosine to intracoronary papaverine for

calculation of pressure-derived fractional flow reserve. *Cathet Cardiovasc Diagn.* 1996;39:120–125.

83. De Bruyne B, Pijls NH, Barbato E, et al. Intracoronary and intravenous adenosine 5'-triphosphate, adenosine, papaverine, and contrast medium to assess fractional flow reserve in humans. *Circulation.* 2003;107:1877–1883.

84. Cahoon WD, Jr, Crouch MA. Preprocedural statin therapy in percutaneous coronary intervention. *Ann Pharmacother.* 2007;41:1687–1693.

85. Wang FW, Osman A, Otero J, et al. Distal myocardial protection during percutaneous coronary intervention with an intracoronary beta-blocker. *Circulation.* 2003;107:2914–2919.

86. Atar I, Korkmaz ME, Atar IA, et al. Effects of metoprolol therapy on cardiac troponin-I levels after elective percutaneous coronary interventions. *Eur Heart J.* 2006;27:547–552.

87. O'Shea JC, Hafley GE, Greenberg S, et al. Platelet glycoprotein IIb/IIIa integrin blockade with eptifibatide in coronary stent intervention: the ESPRIT trial: a randomized controlled trial. *JAMA.* 2001;285:2468–2473.

88. Topol EJ, Moliterno DJ, Herrmann HC, et al. Comparison of two platelet glycoprotein IIb/IIIa inhibitors, tirofiban and abciximab, for the prevention of ischemic events with percutaneous coronary revascularization. *N Engl J Med.* 2001;344:1888–1894.

89. Stone GW, Grines CL, Cox DA, et al. Comparison of angioplasty with stenting, with or without abciximab, in acute myocardial infarction. *N Engl J Med.* 2002;346:957–966.

90. Montalescot G, Barragan P, Wittenberg O, et al. Platelet glycoprotein IIb/IIIa inhibition with coronary stenting for acute myocardial infarction. *N Engl J Med.* 2001;344:1895–1903.

91. Bhatt DL, Lee BI, Casterella PJ, et al. Safety of concomitant therapy with eptifibatide and enoxaparin in patients undergoing percutaneous coronary intervention: results of the Coronary Revascularization Using Integrilin and Single bolus Enoxaparin Study. *J Am Coll Cardiol.* 2003;41:20–25.

92. Lincoff AM, Bittl JA, Kleiman NS, et al. Comparison of bivalirudin versus heparin during percutaneous coronary intervention (the Randomized Evaluation of PCI Linking Angiomax to Reduced Clinical Events [REPLACE]-1 trial). *Am J Cardiol.* 2004;93:1092–1096.

93. Lincoff AM, Bittl JA, Harrington RA, et al. Bivalirudin and provisional glycoprotein IIb/IIIa blockade compared with heparin and planned glycoprotein IIb/IIIa blockade during percutaneous coronary intervention: REPLACE-2 randomized trial. *JAMA.* 2003;289:853–863.

# 45

# Endomyocardial Biopsy

MICHAEL CRAIG AND VALERIAN FERNANDES

## ● PRACTICAL POINTS

- Endomyocardial biopsy (EMB) is diagnostic for cardiac allograft rejection and helps in management. In this setting the risk of perforation and tamponade is low.

- EMB in the cardiac nontransplant setting is controversial and has a higher risk of complications, especially perforation leading to tamponade.

- The decision to do an EMB in a non-transplant setting is dictated by the prebiopsy likelihood of the disorder and the availability of effective therapy based on the histological diagnosis.

- The 2007 AHA/ACC/ESC scientific statement includes 14 nontransplant clinical scenarios and qualifies where EMB is appropriate, reasonable or contraindicated.

- The Dallas criteria standardize histopathological interpretation of cellular myocarditis.

- The US Myocarditis Trial did not show a benefit for immunosuppressive treatment for histologically proven myocarditis.

## ENDOMYOCARDIAL BIOPSY

Endomyocardial biopsy (EMB) is a well-established procedure for evaluating allograft rejection after heart transplant. However, the role of EMB in the diagnosis of many other primary and secondary cardiovascular conditions remains controversial. Although noninvasive imaging techniques and biochemical, and serological tests have improved considerably, there are still considerable limitations to these techniques, and EMB is often needed for diagnostic, prognostic, and therapeutic monitoring purposes.

EMB was first performed by the nonsurgical route in 1958. In 1962, Sakakibara and Konno first introduced the flexible bioptome which was later modified by Caves for EMB via a transvascular approach. The present day, single-use, Stanford–Caves flexible bioptome allows pinched percutaneous right ventricle (RV) biopsies through jugular, subclavian, and femoral venous access by altering the sheath lengths. EMB is a safe, simple, and effective interventional procedure with a very low rate of morbidity and mortality when perfomred by experienced operators.

## PROCEDURE

### RV Biopsy

The interventricular septum is the preferred biopsy site because of its thickness, its continuity with the left ventricle, and its location in the natural path of blood flow, which facilitates bioptome access. The right ventricular free wall and right ventricular apex are avoided because of the risk of free wall perforation and tamponade. Fluoroscopy is the standard imaging modality for biopsy guidance, but it can also be done safely with echocardiographic (ECG) guidance, which is invaluable for native heart biopsies and for biopsies of tumors or certain locations in the heart which cannot be ascertained by fluoroscopy alone.

The right internal jugular vein is the favored access site for EMB, which is performed in a supine position under local anesthesia. Routine 3-lead ECG monitoring, noninvasive blood pressure monitoring, and oxygen saturation monitoring is done throughout the procedure. The head of the patient is placed on a flat cushion to facilitate puncture, and the table is positioned head-low or a wedge is placed under the legs to increase central venous filling and engorge the

**491**

vein for easier access. Ultrasound guidance or a Doppler "smart needle" is used for localizing the internal jugular vein in patients with difficult anatomy. The access is done by Seldinger technique. In some patients for whom the bioptome tends to "hang up" over the superior vena caval suture line or over the tricuspid valve annulus, a longer sheath is used to bypass the impeding structure, thereby limiting trauma and facilitating the biopsy.

When right internal jugular vein access is not possible, EMB can be done via the left internal jugular vein, right or left subclavian veins, or via the femoral veins. When these accesses are needed for EMB, a long sheath is mounted over a 6-Fr pigtail catheter and positioned across the tricuspid valve into the right ventricle. A flexible bioptome can then easily access the interventricular septum for biopsy. Long sheaths tend to clot easily and hence they must be flushed continuously or repeatedly between biopsies. Alternatively 1000-2000 units of heparin (i.v.) help to keep the long sheath clot-free.

## LV Biopsy

No significant differences exist between biopsies from the right or left ventricle. Sometimes, a left ventricle (LV) biopsy may be necessary for cardiomyopathic processes limited to the left ventricle or rarely for biopsies of masses. The femoral artery is the favored access site for LV biopsy. A preformed sheath is inserted over a 6-Fr pigtail catheter into the LV, and biopsies are taken with a long flexible bioptome. Arterial sheaths are maintained under constant pressurized infusion and patients are systemically anticoagulated with heparin to reduce the risk of systemic embolization.

## ANALYSIS OF EMB TISSUE

Samples should be obtained from more than one region of the RV septum and the number of samples should range from 5 to 10, depending upon the studies to be performed. At least 4-5 samples are generally submitted for light microscopic examination. Samples may be submitted for transmission electron microscopy, particularly if the clinical question is anthracycline cardiotoxicity, infiltrative disorders (e.g., amyloidosis), and occasionally viral myocarditis. Routine testing for viral genomes in EMB specimens is only recommended at centers with extensive experience in viral genome analysis. Conditions that can be diagnosed with EMB are shown in **Table 45-1**.

## COMPLICATIONS OF EMB

Before EMB, the diagnostic yield, prognostic value, and the availability of therapy for a given disorder should be considered against the risk of complications. The overall

**Table 45-1 • Conditions That Can Be Diagnosed with EMB**

| Inflammatory |
| --- |
| Cardiac allograft rejection |
| Myocarditis (lymphocytic, giant cell, hypersensitivity/eosinophilic) |
| Rheumatic myocarditis |
| Infections (bacteria, fungi, rickettsia, Chagas) |
| Collagen vascular disease |
| **Restrictive/Infiltrative heart disease** |
| Amyloidosis |
| Hemochromatosis |
| Sarcoidosis |
| Endocardial fibroelastosis |
| Hypertrophy |
| Fibrosis |
| Storage disorders—mucopolysaccharidosis |
| **Malignancy/treatment** |
| Anthracycline cardiomyopathy |
| Cytoxan |
| Radiation fibrosis |
| Carcinoid tumors |
| Malignancy (primary and metastatic tumors/lymphoma) |
| **Miscellaneous** |
| Myocardial ischemia/scar |
| TTP |

incidence of serious complications is <2% and the risk of perforation is <1%. The incidence of death in a large series is about 0.03%. The risks of perforation and tamponade are low when EMB is done for transplant rejection evaluation, because of the adherent pericardium overlying the right ventricle. ECG guidance is used along with fluoroscopic imaging to reduce the risk of perforation and tamponade in surgically naive hearts. In higher risk cases, a right ventriculogram (LAO cranial projection) with delayed phase left ventriculogram will delineate the interventricular septum and aid in the biopsy.

The risk of perforation is higher when there is ventricular dilatation, elevated RV systolic pressures, bleeding diathesis, or heparin anticoagulation. Unrecognized perforations causing tamponade cause the majority of deaths after EMB. Echocardiography should be done whenever there is a suspicion of perforation. Small perforations in transplanted hearts can usually be managed conservatively without need for pericardiocentesis. However perforation in hearts that have not been subject to pericardiotomy (previous cardiac surgery) can result in tamponade very quickly and need emergent pericardiocentesis to restore hemodynamic stability.

Cardiac transplant recipients who undergo repeated surveillance biopsies may develop significant tricuspid regurgitation from repeated tricuspid valve injury or develop

# SECTION VIII

# Imaging

# 46

# Chest Radiography: What the Cardiologist Needs to Know

AMGAD N. MAKARYUS AND LAWRENCE M. BOXT

## ● PRACTICAL POINTS

- The key to chest film evaluation lies in an organized examination of particular cardiac and pulmonary structures, recognizing the variance between observation and expected normal, and an awareness of common pathophysiologic mechanisms that can produce the observed changes.

- A successful approach to plain-film cardiac diagnosis is based upon identification of particular border forming landmarks, observation of particular changes in the contours, reflecting pathologic change, and understanding those pathophysiologic mechanisms responsible for the constellation of changes found in a particular radiograph or series of radiographs.

- An organized approach to observation is dictated by evaluation of the particular silhouette contours.

- The left heart border is formed from the aortic arch segment, the pulmonary artery segment, the left atrial appendage segment, and the left ventricular contour.

- The right heart border is composed of the superior vena cava segment, the ascending aortic segment, and the right atrial segment.

- The role of the chest film has shifted in the last half century from a central role in cardiac diagnosis and patient management to more of a measure of patient physiologic status. This change reflects the rise of more sensitive and accurate imaging modalities.

- While the role of the plain chest film may wane in the era of advancing invasive means of monitoring physiologic status and more advanced imaging techniques, continued technological advancement in cardiac imaging will provide even more reliable means of acquiring high-resolution imagery, high rates of image data transfer, and high-volume archival devices, and the plain chest film will remain the initial easily accessible, cost-effective, and effective diagnostic tool in this advancement in cardiac imaging.

## INTRODUCTION

The plain chest film contains a great deal of useful structural and physiologic information concerning the immediate condition of the patient as well as pathophysiologic mechanisms accounting for the current state of the patient's health. The key to successful chest film evaluation lies in organized evaluation of particular cardiac and pulmonary structure, recognition of the variance between observation and expected normal state, and awareness of common pathophysiologic mechanisms that can produce the observed changes.

By convention, chest radiographs are obtained in the posteroanterior projection (i.e., the patient faces the detector or film-screen combination, and the X-ray beam is transmitted from the patient's back toward the detector). However, many radiographs are obtained by portable technique and employ anteroposterior projection (i.e., the patient lies on the film, and the technologist acquires the image from a beam passing from in front-to-in back of the patient). The difference in appearance of the chest image when obtained in posteroanterior versus anteroposterior projection is less significant than the difference between an upright and a supine radiograph. Furthermore, the value of the examination is more significantly affected by patient rotation than by the projection obtained. This is because the limited contrast resolution of the plain chest film cannot differentiate among ventricular myocardium and intra- and extracardiac structures when patient rotation is present. That is, we recognize a cardiac contour because it forms a border of the heart. If rotated, either due to intrinsic cardiac or pulmonary disease or because of oblique patient position, and the expected structure forming a portion of cardiopulmonary silhouette does not rotate also, then either the X-ray cannot be evaluated, or, if such rotation is not recognized, the resulting diagnosis may be in doubt. Thus, a successful approach to plain film cardiac diagnosis is based upon identification of particular border-forming landmarks and observation of specific changes in the contours, reflecting pathologic change. In addition, the clinician must understand those pathophysiologic mechanisms responsible for the constellation of changes found in a radiograph or series of radiographs. In summary, approach to the plain film should be organized, rigorous, and complete.

## APPROACH TO THE CHEST FILM

In evaluating the chest film, it is necessary one observe everything, doing so in the same way and the same order each time. Starting with the osseous structures, look at all the ribs and the interspaces between them. Fractures and asymmetric interspaces may be the only information relating to earlier palliative or curative cardiothoracic surgery (**Figure 46-1**).

Scoliosis, kyphosis, or pectus deformity may result in cardiac displacement or rotation within the chest, giving a normal heart the appearance of abnormality. In particular, pectus deformity limits the anteroposterior dimension of the mid chest, causing the heart to be displaced toward the left, giving the impression of clockwise rotation, and right heart enlargement (**Figure 46-2**).

Rib notching, the result of dilated intercostals collateral blood flow in coarctation of the aorta, is rarely seen in individuals under 8 or 9 years of age. When rib notching is present, it typically has a wavy lucent (eroded) appearance, showing along the underside of the mid-to-upper ribs, immediately subjacent to a sclerotic, proliferative bony response to the traumatic injury of systolic expansion against bone (**Figure 46-3**). Certainly, midline sternal sutures, or mediastinal clips and sutures are important signs of previous cardiac surgery.

Identify all lines, catheters, and cannulas, and be sure to understand where they enter the chest and where their tips lie. Identify any extra anatomic devices or objects, such as sternal sutures, ventricular assist devices, pacemakers, or automated defibrillators (**Figure 46-4**). Many valvular prostheses are fabricated without the use of radio opaque materials and cannot be seen on chest exam. However, many do contain

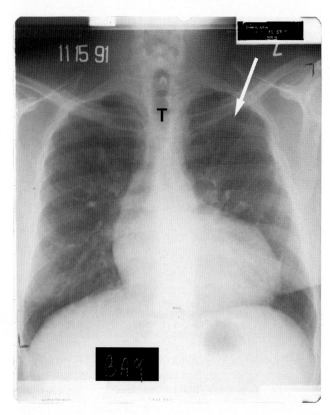

**Figure 46-1.** PA examination in a 34-year-old man with a history of previous surgery, now complaining of shortness of breath. The trachea (T) is midline, and there is no apparent aortic arch segment. Notice (arrow) the asymmetry of the left upper rib, secondary to previous surgery to repair an aortic coarctation.

metallic rings and struts, so their presence, if not model type, can be identified (**Figure 46-5**). Coronary artery stents are radio-opaque, but small, and generally placed within the proximal coronary tree, which, on frontal radiograph, is lost over the spine, toward the center of the film.

Examination of the pulmonary parenchyma, pleura, and pulmonary vasculature may be performed prior to or after evaluation of the heart. In this chapter we will suggest that either is fine, but given the relationship between cardiac function and the appearance of the lungs, and the fact that the right and left sides of the heart communicate across the pulmonary bed, we will discuss pulmonary findings in the context of the appearance of the main pulmonary artery (PA) segment and hilar pulmonary arteries.

To assist and encourage organized evaluation of the heart and great arteries, one may divide the cardiothoracic silhouette (the heart and great vessels in the middle mediastinum) into a left heart border and a right heart border (**Figure 46-6**). Then, an organized approach to observation is dictated by evaluation of the particular contours. The left heart border is formed from the aortic arch segment, the pulmonary artery segment, the left atrial appendage segment, and the left

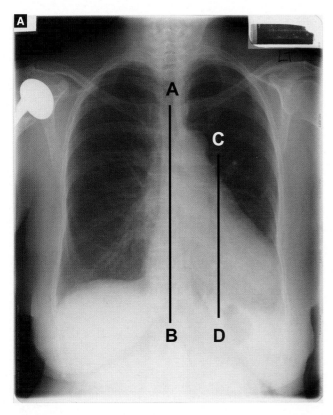

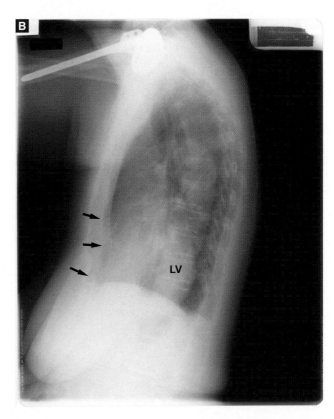

**Figure 46-2.** PA and Lateral radiographs in a 60-year-old woman with pectus excavatum. A. PA examination shows displacement of the heart toward the left. Line CD is drawn through the midportion of the heart. Notice its displacement to the left of the midline (AB). B. On lateral view, the indentation of the lower sternum (arrows) pushes the heart. The left ventricle (LV) is projected over the lower thoracic spine.

ventricular contour. The right cardiothoracic border is composed of the superior vena cava segment, the ascending aortic segment, and the right atrial segment. When observing these specific portions of the cardiothoracic silhouette, ask explicit questions about the appearance of these structures, and organize your answers in standardized, easy to convey terms. That

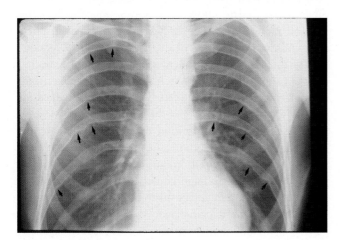

**Figure 46-3.** PA radiograph of a 52-year-old man with an unoperated aortic coarctation. The aortic arch segment is small. There are multiple erosions along the undersides of the upper and mid ribs (short arrows).

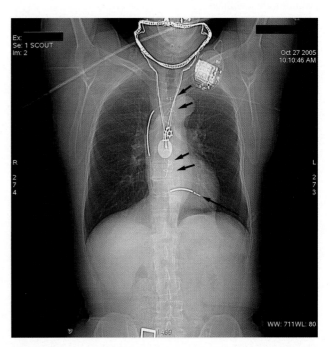

**Figure 46-4.** PA radiograph of a 56-year-old man with palpitations. The midline sternal sutures (small arrows) and the tip of the automated defibrillator (long arrow) are identified.

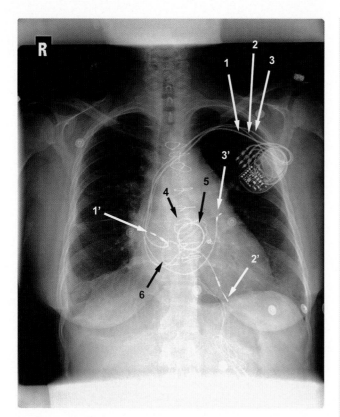

**Figure 46-5.** Enhanced AP radiograph of a 67-year-old woman. Midline sternal sutures are evident. There are 3 leads leaving the pacemaker in the subcutaneous tissues of the upper left chest (arrows 1, 2, and 3); one wire is in the right atrial append-age (arrow 1'), right ventricle (arrow 2'), and coronary sinus (arrow 3'). In addition, the rings of valvular prostheses in the aortic (arrow 4), mitral (arrow 5), and tricuspid (arrow 6) positions are identified.

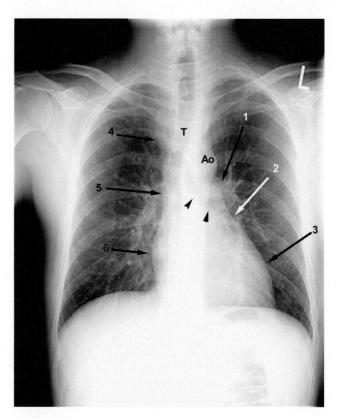

**Figure 46-6.** Normal PA examination from a 36-year-old man. The left-sided aortic arch (Ao) displaces the tracheal air shadow (T) toward the right. The main PA segment (arrow 1) passes just superior to the left main bronchus (black arrowheads) and is about the same caliber as the Ao. The left atrial appendage seg-ment (arrow 2) is concave toward the right. Notice how the left ventricular contour (arrow 3) drops gently to the diaphragm. The superior vena cava segment (arrow 4) lies to the right of the T. The ascending aortic segment (arrow 5) is normal, barely making it to the right hilum. The normal right atrial contour (arrow 6) does not extend to the descending right pulmonary artery.

is, first ask, "Can I identify this segment?" Then character-ize the structure in simple terms; i.e., Is the structure normal (no different than in comparison with what was expected)? If the answer is no, then, characterize the abnormality; i.e., Is the segment calcified or not, dilated or not, smaller than expected or not? In this way, the observer collects a series of observations that will provide the basis for generating a dif-ferential diagnosis, and from this list (with appreciation of the patient's history, physical examination, and laboratory val-ues), a first, best diagnosis.

# EVALUATION OF THE CARDIOTHORACIC SILHOUETTE

## Left Heart Border

### Aortic Arch segment

The uppermost left contour of the cardiothoracic silhouette is the aortic arch segment. Anatomically, this portion of the border is formed by the compression of the distal aortic

arch and proximal descending thoracic aorta into a two-dimensional "aortic knob." The aortic arch displaces the midline trachea. Therefore, by definition, a left-sided aortic arch will displace the trachea toward the right. The con-tour of the aortic arch segment should be sharp. Expected normal caliber of the aortic arch should be no greater than 25 mm, measured from the left border of the tracheal air shadow to the lateral border of the aorta. As the aortic arch segment represents compression of a long aortic segment into a two-dimensional profile, the appearance depends sig-nificantly on patient position during examination. That is, patient rotation has an important effect on the apparent size of this contour, and should be taken into consideration prior to suggesting a pathologic diagnosis. A common finding is partial, or circumferential, calcification of the arch segment, indicating systemic atherosclerosis (**Figure 46-7**).

Not uncommonly, arch calcification is the only outward sign of atherosclerosis on the radiograph. Since atherosclerotic

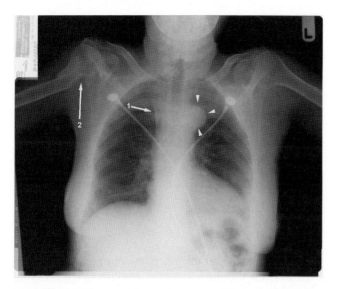

**Figure 46-7.** PA examination of a 72-year-old woman with systemic hypertension. The aortic arch is quite conspicuous, but not dilated. However, notice the circumferential arch calcification (arrowheads). The superior vena caval shadow (arrow 1) is sharp. Arrow 2 notes an incidental bony structure finding in this patient.

calcification is intimal, the distance between the calcified aortic intima, and its outer border represents the thickness of the aortic wall. Thus, an interval change in this

measurement (**Figure 46-8**), or value greater than 8 mm, may represent changes secondary to aortic hematoma or dissection (separating the intima from the rest of the aortic wall). Thus, the aortic arch segment can be characterized as normal or not. If normal, then move on to the next portion of the left heart border. If not, then characterize the abnormality. That is, determine if the aorta is calcified. Whether it is calcified or not, it may still be of normal caliber. Furthermore, determine if the aorta is smaller or greater in caliber than expected. Dilatation of the aortic arch is defined as the presence of an arch segment greater than 25 mm from trachea to left heart border (**Figure 46-9**). A small, or inconspicuous aortic arch segment is one that requires a second look to be sure that it is actually present (**Figure 46-10**). If the trachea is not displaced toward the right, then (1) the aortic arch may be small, or (2), it may not be present. The differential diagnosis of an abnormal aortic arch is given in **Table 46-1**.

## Pulmonary Artery Segment

The pulmonary valve sits atop the right ventricular infundibulum, lying in a variable plane, always nearly parallel to the body axis, and is thus not well visualized in the posteroanterior radiograph. The main pulmonary artery arises from the semilunar valve annulus, and then passes superiorly and

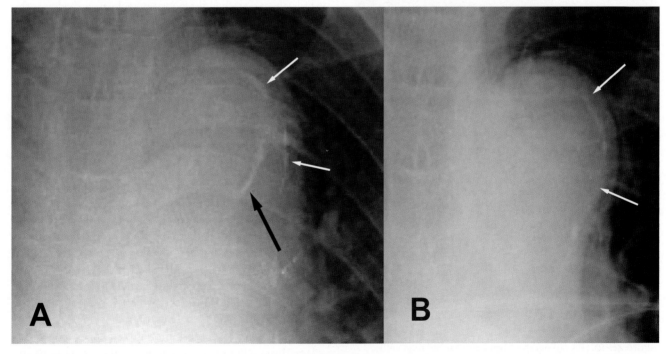

**Figure 46-8.** Cropped views from the PA chest films of a 67-year-old man presenting with upper back pain. (A) From the admitting radiograph. Thin curvilinear calcification (white arrows) is seen immediately subjacent to the lateral aspect of the aortic shadow. The distance between calcification and outer aortic edge is 4 mm. An additional calcification (black arrow) is also found, nearly 12 mm from the lateral aortic wall. (B) A previous exam, obtained 2 years prior to this admission, shows no change in the thin calcifications (white arrows), but also that the larger calcification, which is now quite apart from the aortic wall, was not present at that time. This is evidence of an acute aortic dissection.

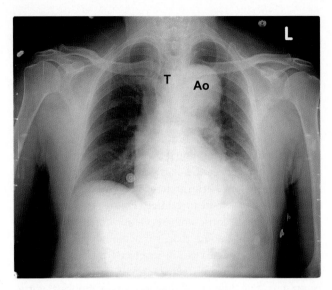

**Figure 46-9.** AP radiograph of a 73-year-old man with a cough. The aortic arch (Ao) is markedly enlarged (measuring 38 mm), representing an aneurysm. Notice the displacement of the tracheal air shadow (T) to the right, by the proximal extension into the transverse arch.

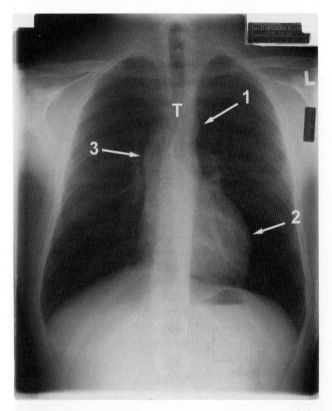

**Figure 46-10.** PA radiograph from a 24-year-old man with coarctation of the aorta and bicuspid aortic valve stenosis. The aortic arch shadow (arrow 1) is small, and barely displaces the trachea (T) to the right. Also notice the rounded contour of the hypertrophied left ventricular segment (arrow 2) and the extension of the ascending aortic shadow (arrow 3) over the right hilum, secondary to post stenotic dilatation.

| Table 46-1 • Differential Diagnosis of an Abnormal Aortic Arch Segment |
| --- |
| 1. Dilated aortic arch<br> a. Aortic aneurysm<br> b. Aortic dissection<br> c. Aortic pseudoaneurysm<br> d. Mass adjacent to aortic arch<br> e. Left upper lobe collapse |
| 2. Small or unapparent aortic arch<br> a. Coarctation of the aorta<br> b. Right aortic arch<br> c. Double aortic arch<br> d. Interrupted aortic arch |

posteriorly, and toward the left. The right pulmonary artery originates from the underside of the main PA and passes along the roof of the left atrium to enter the right hilum. The left pulmonary artery is the continuation of the main PA, after it crosses over the left main bronchus, to enter the left hilum. The main pulmonary artery segment (PA segment) of the left heart border is formed by the top of the main and the proximal portion of the left pulmonary artery. The projection of the PA segment is a round density, convex to the left (away from the heart), just above the projection of the left main bronchus. The "size" of the PA segment is nearly the same as the caliber of the aortic arch segment (i.e., right-sided cardiac output equals left-sided output) (**Figure 46-6**). In other words, the mogul that displaces the tracheal air shadow is the aortic arch segment, and the mogul that is immediately superior to the projection of the bronchus is the PA segment. An unapparent aortic arch segment should not be characterized as a dilated PA segment, and a hypoplastic, or concave, PA segment should not be interpreted as a dilated aorta.

Pulmonary artery calcification is unusual and nearly always associated with a dilated PA segment and bilateral dilated hilar PAs and pulmonary hypertension (**Figure 46-11**). Increased pulmonary artery pressure, increased flow, and the combination of increased pressure and flow all cause dilatation of the PA segment. Furthermore, these conditions are all associated with increased caliber of the hilar PAs, as well. Bilateral hilar adenopathy most commonly mimics dilated pulmonary arteries, but is not commonly associated with a dilated main PA segment. Increased PA pressure is the result of the response of the right ventricle to the elevation of pulmonary vascular resistance, which is controlled by the post hilar pulmonary bed. Thus, on radiographs of patients with pulmonary hypertension of any etiology, one expects to see the combination of dilatation of the PA segment and hilar PAs, associated with vasoconstriction of the peripheral bed. This produces a dramatic change in vessel caliber between the central and peripheral pulmonary vasculature. As vessel caliber in the periphery decreases, the smaller vessels fall beneath the spatial resolution of the imaging system and

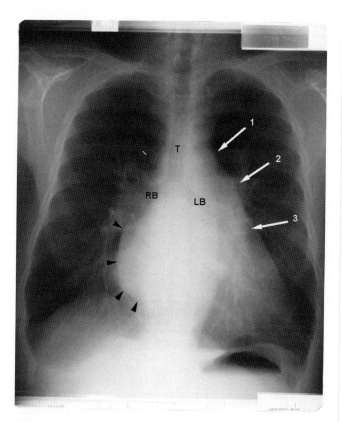

**Figure 46-19.** PA radiograph of a 67-year-old man with chronic mitral stenosis. The main pulmonary artery segment (arrow 2) is greater in caliber than the aortic arch segment (arrow 1). Notice the dilated hilar right pulmonary artery (arrow 3) seen through the rotated heart. Left atrial enlargement is indicated by the "double density" (arrowheads) seen through the heart, and the increased angle formed by the bifurcation of the trachea (T) into the left (LB) and right (RB) bronchi.

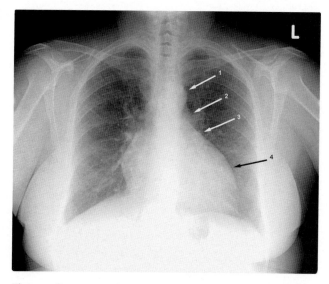

**Figure 46-20.** PA radiograph of a 50-year-old woman with chronic mitral regurgitation. The left atrial appendage segment (arrow 3) is flat, and the contour of the left ventricular segment is rounded, indicating left atrial and left ventricular enlargement. Notice that the main pulmonary artery segment (arrow 2) is not as large as the aortic arch segment (arrow 1), indicating normal pulmonary artery pressure. The lungs appear typically mild-to-moderately congested; the vessels are not sharp, and the central upper lobe vessels are greater in caliber than the lower lobe vessels. The left ventricular contour (arrow 4) extends farther toward the left (appears more rounded), and the cardiac silhouette appears enlarged, all reflecting left ventricular dilatation.

and the atrium is not judged to be enlarged. However, eventually, the left atrial myocardium can no longer hypertrophy to maintain function at normal chamber size, and the atrium begins to dilate.

The earliest radiographic sign of left atrial enlargement is posterior displacement of the left bronchus, best viewed in the lateral chest film. The earliest PA film finding in left atrial enlargement is reflected in straightening and later convexity of the left atrial appendage segment. Eventually, as the left atrium continues to enlarge, there is elevation of the left bronchus (widening of the angle of the tracheal carina), development of the so-called double density sign, and subsequently filling of the right heart border by the dilated left atrium (**Figure 46-19**).

The radiographic changes of left atrial enlargement due to left atrial volume loading cannot be differentiated those secondary to left atrial hypertension. Left atrial enlargement associated with left ventricular enlargement is commonly found in mitral regurgitation (**Figure 46-20**). However, the

pulmonary veins contain no valves, so elevation in left atrial pressure is transmitted to the pulmonary veins.

Pulmonary venous hypertension results in a series of radiographic changes, reflecting increasing severity of the abnormality. The first signs of left atrial hypertension result from the dilatation of the pulmonary venules and increasing separation of the cells of the venular wall, increasing the size of the interspaces between the cells, allowing passage of water from the vascular compartment into the perivascular sheaths surrounding these structures. When this occurs, the fluid-filled pulmonary veins are no longer surrounded by air-filled lungs (causing sharp vascular edges). Rather, they are surrounded by fluid in the perivascular sheaths. Thus, the lower lobe veins become not sharp and less apparent (**Figure 46-21**). If the process elevating left atrial pressure continues, the venular pressure rises and more fluid leaves the vascular space to enter the interstitial space, and the vessels become less and less apparent. Eventually, fluid spills into the pulmonary interstitium surrounding the veins, and they are no longer visible. Instead, there is a generalized lower lobe infiltrate.

As pulmonary venous pressure continues to rise and the parenchyma becomes more edematous, resistance to lower lobe pulmonary blood flow increases. This results in redistribution of lower lobe pulmonary blood flow to the upper

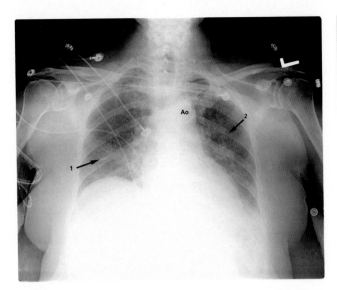

**Figure 46-21.** AP radiograph of a 64-year-old woman complaining of shortness of breath. The aortic arch (Ao) is calcified, but not dilated. None of the pulmonary vessels are especially well visualized. However, the parenchyma appears denser (i.e., edematous) in the right lower lobe (arrow 1), and left perihilar zone (arrow 2). The left diaphragm is obscured, indicating a left pleural effusion, as well.

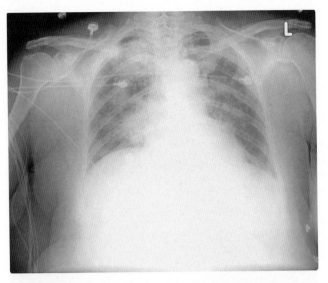

**Figure 46-22.** AP radiograph of the same patient in Figure 46-20, obtained 3 hours later. The interstitial infiltrates have become denser (while still retaining their not sharp edges), indicating progression to alveolar pulmonary edema.

lobes. When this occurs, the upper lobe arteries carry greater flow, and thus enlarge (**Figure 46-20**). Furthermore, increased upper lobe arterial flow results in increased upper lobe venous return to the heart; thus both the upper lobe arteries and veins enlarge. Dilatation of the upper lobe arteries in left-to-right shunts and the upper lobe arteries and veins may be difficult to differentiate (as one may ask, "Is an individual vascular structure an artery or vein?"). However, when the upper lobe arteries are enlarged in increased conditions associated with increased pulmonary blood flow, the main and hilar pulmonary arteries are enlarged, the lower lobe vessels are dilated, and all pulmonary vessels remain sharp. Upper lobe enlargement associated with pulmonary venous hypertension is always associated with absence of sharpness of the lower lobe veins, and depending upon the underlying disease, it may or may not be associated with dilatation of the main or hilar pulmonary arteries.

If the pulmonary venous hypertension persists and continues to rise, then overcoming colloid oncotic pressure (22 mm Hg), fluid begins to fill the alveolar spaces of the lower lobes; then frank alveolar edema and fluffy pulmonary infiltrates begin to appear (**Figure 46-22**). The nature of these infiltrates is very helpful for differentiating these lesions from the typical infiltrates of pneumonia.

The infiltrates of pneumonia are usually solitary and take a segmental, subsegmental, or lobar (anatomic) distribution (**Figure 46-23**). All the alveolar spaces are filled, so the infiltrate is dense, with sharp edges defining the anatomic distribution.

The natural course of pneumonic infiltrates is resolution with therapy. The infiltrates associated with pulmonary edema are different. First, in segments involved with the pulmonary edema, there are alveoli filled with fluid and alveoli that are not. Thus, the infiltrates are less dense than in typical pneumonia. Furthermore, the distribution of the infiltrates is not as anatomically defined as in pneumonia. Therefore the edges of the infiltrates are not sharp and fluffy. Finally, the underlying etiology of pulmonary infiltrates in pulmonary edema is local pulmonary venous pressure,

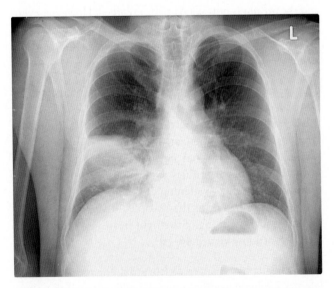

**Figure 46-23.** PA radiograph of a 24-year-old man with cough and fever. The nearly homogeneous density and anatomic distribution (right middle lobe) of this infiltrate characterize it as pneumonia.

which is very dependent upon patient position. Thus, the infiltrates of pneumonia tend to stay put. On the other hand, the infiltrates of left atrial hypertension are fleeting. As intrathoracic pressure gradients change (patient lying on back, upright, right or left side down), the distribution in the lungs changes, and the infiltrates change their distribution (so called "fleeting infiltrates").

If the cause of the left atrial hypertension is resolved, then this progression from lower lobe indistinctness (mild) to redistribution (moderate), to alveolar infiltrates (severe) radiographic abnormality reverses, and a normal chest film is to be expected. Chronic left atrial hypertension ultimately progresses to pulmonary hypertension (with the expected appearance of the pulmonary arteries) (**Figure 46-18**). Chronic mild left atrial hypertension often goes on to a pattern of interstitial fibrosis.

Right heart dilation causes cardiac rotation, which will change the appearance of the mid left heart border in the region of the expected left atrial appendage segment. In a normal heart, the right ventricular outflow tract is medial to the projection of the left atrial appendage and left ventricular contour. When the right heart dilates, clockwise rotation of the heart rotates the left atrial appendage posteriorly and brings the outflow tract to the left. The dilated right ventricular outflow tract then becomes left heart border-forming. This changes the appearance of the left heart border and gives the impression of a convex (away from the heart, i.e., dilated) left atrium (**Figures 46-11–46-13, 46-18, 46-19**). This, of course, can be confusing. Clockwise cardiac rotation affects the relationship of the projection of the left bronchus to the projection of the left heart border. Under normal circumstances, the projection of the left bronchus crosses the projection of the left heart border. In fact, we define the left atrial appendage segment of the left heart border as that portion below the projection of the left bronchus, and above the curvature of the left ventricular contour. When the right heart dilates, and the heart rotates, the left bronchus is not affected; it stays put. However, the relation between the projection of the left bronchus and altered left heart border changes. In individuals with right heart dilatation, the projection of the left bronchus appears to be parallel, or nearly so, to the projection of the left heart border (**Figure 46-24**). Although in such rotated hearts changes in left atrial appendage size cannot be monitored on the PA radiograph, all other signs of left atrial enlargement (or its absence) are still present. The differential diagnosis of left atrial appendage segment enlargement is given in **Table 46-3**.

## Left Ventricular Contour

The lowest portion of the left heart border is the left ventricular contour. Actually, this portion of the heart border is formed by the anterolateral wall of the left ventricle (**Figure 46-6**).

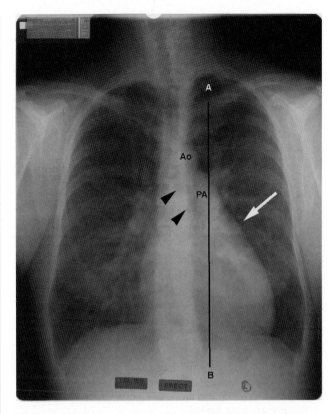

**Figure 46-24.** PA radiograph of a 24-year-old woman with a longstanding murmur. The center of the heart (line AB) lies well to the left of the spine. The main pulmonary artery segment (PA) is greater in caliber than the aortic arch segment (Ao). The superior mediastinum at the level of the Ao is very narrow, reflecting the leftward rotation of the superior vena cava over the spine. The left bronchus (arrowheads) is not elevated, and there is no double density; the left atrium is not enlarged. Furthermore, notice how the left bronchus appears to run parallel to the upper left heart border. Although there is no evidence of left atrial enlargement, the mid left heart border (arrow) is convex to the left. The left atrium is not enlarged! The right ventricular outflow has rotated toward the left to occupy a portion of the left heart border.

Thus, unless there is a global left ventricular change, or a local change in this portion of the left ventricular myocardium, an abnormality may not be apparent and diagnosable. Global changes to the appearance of the left ventricular contour result in increased roundness in the contour. In the normal heart, the left ventricular portion of the left heart border takes a nearly vertical orientation. That is, the contour just drops

| Table 46-3 • Differential Diagnosis of a Dilated LAA Segment |
|---|
| 1. Mitral stenosis, LA outflow obstruction |
| 2. Mitral regurgitation |
| 3. Ventricular septal defect |
| 4. Patent ductus arteriosus |
| 5. Congestive heart failure |

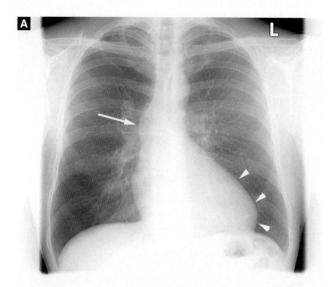

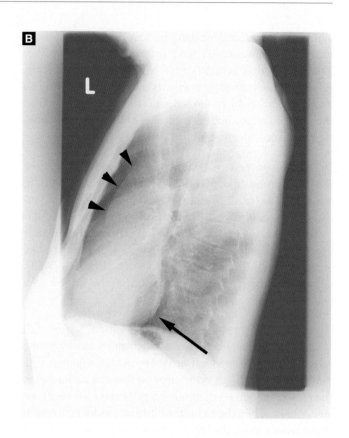

**Figure 46-25.** PA and lateral radiographs of a 36-year-old man with aortic regurgitation. (A) On PA examination the lower left heart border (arrowheads) is rounder, and extends toward the left. The ascending aortic segment (arrow) is enlarged, extending over the hilar right pulmonary artery. (B) Lateral view shows posterior extension of the left ventricular contour (arrow) into the inferior retrocardiac space, reflecting ventricular dilatation. The dilated ascending aorta (arrowheads) begins to fill the retrosternal space from behind.

to the diaphragm. Global left ventricular change results in increasing the curvature, and thus radius of the left heart border (**Figure 46-25A**). Overall heart size may not increase, but the shape of the left heart border is altered. Such global change may be found in individuals with left ventricular volume loading (dilatation), left ventricular pressure loading (hypertrophy), and abnormalities of left ventricular compliance. Therefore, differentiation between left ventricular dilatation and hypertrophy may be difficult in the PA projection. Certainly, when the left heart border approaches the lateral left chest wall, we can all agree that the ventricle is dilated. However, short of such pronounced change, this differentiation may be difficult. If a lateral view is provided, then one can make this differentiation. In cases of left ventricular dilatation, a point 18-mm cephalad to the intersection of the inferior vena cava and right diaphragm (on lateral view) will be contained within the contour of the posterior heart border (**Figure 46-25B**).

If the appearance of the left ventricular contour on PA examination appears abnormally rounded, and this point is outside the posterior left ventricular contour, (i.e., the left ventricle does not occupy the inferior retrocardiac space), then the left ventricle is hypertrophied and not dilated (**Figure 46-10, 46-26**). If, in lateral view, this point is contained by the posterior aspect of the lower heart border, then the left ventricle is dilated. Certainly, if the left ventricle is in fact dilated, then hypertrophy can be "lost" in the enlarged contour.

Focal abnormalities in the contour of the lower left heart border reflect local processes (**Figure 46-27**).

Only an abnormality along a heart border-forming portion of the left ventricle will be apparent. Thus, an abnormality located posterior or anterior to the left ventricular contour may not be identified. In such circumstances, an oblique (or lateral) view may bring these abnormalities into tangency with the projected heart border, thus making them visible. Calcification often directs the observer to an abnormality and may help characterize it as well. Peripheral, thin, or lamillated, nearly circumferential calcification that takes a "coronary distribution" (i.e., reflecting myocardial segmental anatomy) is typical of a left ventricular aneurysm (**Figure 46-28**). Central, heavy calcification may be the only radiologic evidence of an intracardiac tumor. Cysts calcify peripherally.

The differential diagnosis of an abnormal left ventricular segment contour is given in **Table 46-4**.

## Right Heart Border

### Superior Vena Caval Segment
The uppermost portion of the right cardiovascular silhouette is formed by the descent of the superior vena cava (SVC) to the right atrium. This shadow is usually seen just to the right of the spine (**Figure 46-7**), but may not

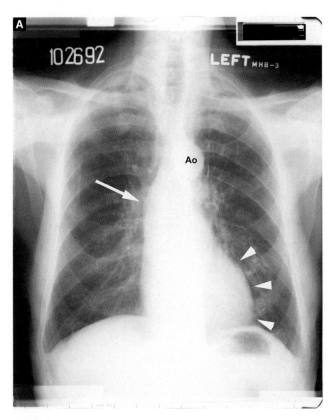

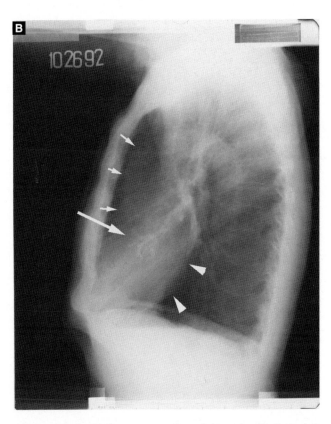

**Figure 46-26.** PA and lateral radiographs of a 67-year-old man with aortic stenosis. A. The heart is not enlarged. However, the lower left heart border (arrowheads) exhibits increased curvature and extension toward the left. Although the aortic arch (Ao) is normal, the dilated ascending aorta (arrow) extends over the hilar right pulmonary artery. B. The lateral view reveals thick aortic valve calcification in the geometric center of the heart. The posterior left ventricular border (arrowheads) does not extend into the inferior retrocardiac space, indicating that the left ventricle is not dilated. The dilated ascending aorta (small arrows) fills the retrosternal space from behind.

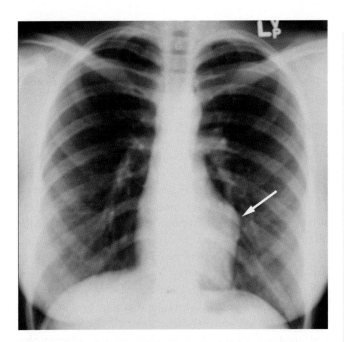

**Figure 46-27.** PA radiograph of a 26-year-old woman being worked up for a connective tissue disorder, with a cardiac lipoma. The mid left ventricular contour contains a focal contour abnormality. The bump is the same attenuation of the adjacent heart. There is no pleural or pericardial effusion.

be readily apparent in a normal individual (**Figure 46-6**). Abnormalities of this portion of the heart border can be generally described as increasing the width of the superior mediastinum, or they may be associated with decreased width of this region. Dilatation of the segment is associated with increased SVC volume or pressure. Thus, increased venous return from the head or upper extremities causes enlargement of this segment (**Figure 46-29**). In addition, superior caval obstruction (causing increased SVC pressure) widens the mediastinum as well. On the other hand, when the right heart dilates there is a clockwise (leftward) rotation of the heart, which has the effect of distorting the mid left heart border, but also causes the SVC to rotate leftward, narrowing the superior mediastinum (**Figures 46-11, 46-12, 46-17–19, 46-24**). The differential diagnosis of an abnormal superior vena cava segment is given in **Table 46-5**.

## Ascending Aortic Segment

The ascending aorta is connected to the heart by the aortic annulus, within the contour of the heart on chest film examination. The aorta then ascends, heading anteriorly

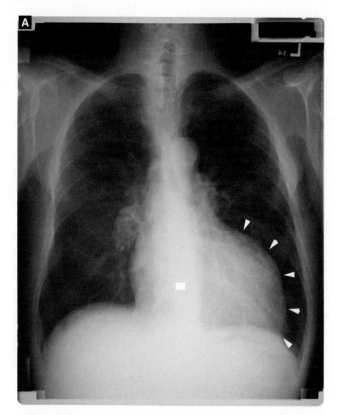
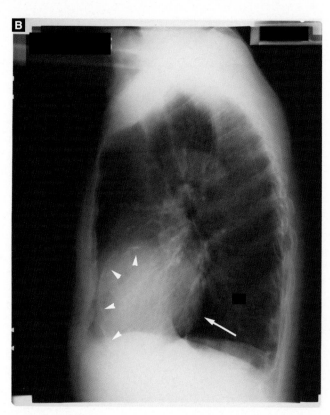

**Figure 46-28.** PA and lateral examination from a 69-year-old man with prior history of myocardial infarction. (A). The left ventricular contour (arrowheads) is characterized by prominent increase in curvature and extension toward the left chest wall. There is vague increased attenuation beneath the contour, but no discrete calcification. (B) In lateral view, the calcified myocardium of the bulging interventricular septum (arrowheads) is better seen. The posterior left ventricular contour (arrow) extends into the inferior retrocardiac space, indicating left ventricular chamber enlargement.

and toward the patient's right. The proximal portion of the ascending aorta should not extend farther to the right than the medial aspect of the right hilum and right pulmonary artery (**Figure 46-6**). If it extends farther, then dilatation of the ascending aorta should be considered. If the lateral aspect of the ascending aorta covers or obscures the right hilar structure, then the ascending aorta is dilated (**Figure 46-10, 25A, 26A**). Dilatation of this portion of the aorta may be found in volume loaded aortas or may be the result of

poststenotic dilatation secondary to aortic valve stenosis. Whenever any aortic abnormality is entertained, and especially if the ascending aorta is involved, aortic dissection is a possibility. The differential diagnosis of a dilated ascending aortic segment is given in **Table 46-6**.

## Right Atrial Contour

The right atrium forms the inferior portion of the right heart border. There is a large body of literature attesting to the limited value of changes in this cardiac contour as an indicator of cardiac or cardiac chamber abnormality. When the right heart dilates, it rotates in a clockwise manner, moving the anterior right heart toward the left. Since the right atrium is generally spherical in shape, this rotation has little effect on its appearance. When the curvature of the right heart border is markedly abnormal, then right atrial enlargement may be considered (**Figures 46-16** and **46-30**). Short of the right atrial contour approaching the right chest wall, changes in the appearance of the right heart contour are not obvious. Focal changes in the right heart border are most commonly the result of adjacent pericardial changes (such as loculated pericardial effusion or pericardial cyst) or the

| Table 46-4 • Differential Diagnosis of an Abnormal Left Ventricular Segment Contour |
| --- |
| 1. Global |
|   a. Left ventricular dilatation |
|   b. Left ventricular hypertrophy |
|   c. Left ventricular ischemia, infarction |
|   d. Cardiomyopathy |
| 2. Focal |
|   a. Pericardial cyst |
|   b. Left ventricular aneurysm |
|   c. Left ventricular pseudoaneurysm |
|   d. Cardiac tumor |

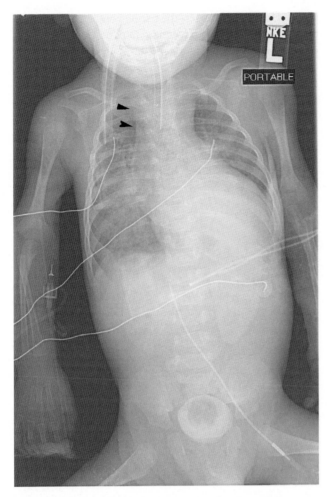

**Figure 46-29.** AP radiograph of a newborn in heart failure. An endotracheal tube is placed just proximal to the carina. The widened mediastinum (arrowheads) is bordered by the dilated superior vena cava draining a large vein of Galen aneurysm. The heart is very large.

| Table 46-5 • Differential Diagnosis of an Abnormal Superior Vena Cava Segment |
| --- |
| 1. Widened mediastinum<br>  a. Intracranial shunt<br>  b. Lower extremity venous obstruction with systemic venous return to the azygos vein<br>  c. Mediastinal tumor |
| 2. Narrow mediastinum<br>  a. Right heart dilatation |

| Table 46-6 • Differential Diagnosis of a Dilated Ascending Aortic Segment |
| --- |
| 1. Aortic stenosis<br>2. Aortic regurgitation<br>3. Aortic aneurysm<br>4. Aortic dissection (hematoma) |

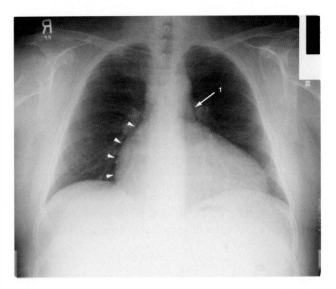

**Figure 46-30.** PA radiograph of a 30-year-old man with Ebstein malformation. The main pulmonary artery segment (arrow) is concave toward the heart. All pulmonary vascular markings are small and indistinct. The lower right heart border (arrowheads) bulges toward the right.

rare, though occasionally found on incidental examination, mass. Larger pericardial effusions (**Figure 46-31**) affect both the right and left heart borders. The differential diagnosis of an abnormal right atrial contour is shown in **Table 46-7**.

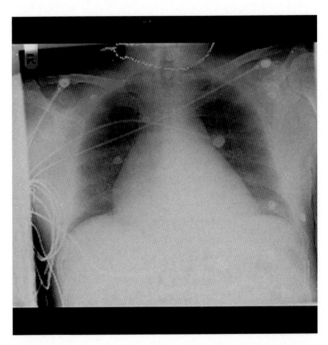

**Figure 46-31.** AP radiograph of a 23-year-old man with viral pericarditis and pericardial effusion. Both the left and right heart borders appear rounded and smooth. The expected moguls ("lumps and bumps") of the heart borders are not found. The fluid filled pericardial sac effaces the heart border forming structures.

**Table 46-7 • Differential Diagnosis of an Abnormal Right Atrial Contour**

1. Right atrial or right heart enlargement
2. Pericardial effusion
3. Pericardial cyst
4. Pericardial tumor

## CONCLUSIONS

The role of the chest film has shifted in the past half century from a central role in cardiac diagnosis and patient management to more of a measure of patient physiologic status. This change reflects the rise of more sensitive and accurate imaging modalities. In an era of advancing invasive means of monitoring physiologic status, the role of the chest film for assessment of cardiac chamber pressure may wane. However, continued technological advancement in cardiac imaging will provide even more reliable means of acquiring high resolution imagery, high rates of image data transfer, and high volume archival devices, and the plain chest film will remain the initial, easily accessible, cost-effective, and efficacious diagnostic tool in this advancement in cardiac imaging.

# 47

# Basics of Ultrasound Physics

Rajiv S. Hede

## ● PRACTICAL POINTS

- Ultrasound employs frequencies above 20,000 Hz, the normal human hearing being in the range of 20–20,000 Hz. Sound with frequency below 20 Hz is called infrasound.

- Frequency is the number of cycles per second.

- Wavelength is the length of a cycle.

- Attenuation increases with frequency and distance and is caused by absorption, reflection, and scattering. The average attenuation of soft tissue is 0.5 dB/cm per MHz of frequency.

- The speed of propagation through soft tissue is 1540 m/sec.

- Impedance is density of the medium times the propagation speed.

- Ultrasound used in clinical practice is not known to produce any significant bioeffects. However, the FDA allows for two maximum limits for Ispta for cardiac imaging. Although the bioeffects are not well studied, it is good practice to be aware of the effects and use echocardiography only where indicated and keeping the mechanical index and thermal index as low as possible to mitigate any bioeffects.

- Ultrasound transducers operate on the piezoelectric effect, where during transmission, electric energy is converted to acoustic energy and in the receiving mode the acoustic energy is changed to electric energy, which is used to display the image.

- Transducers are used in the pulsed echo mode. They have a dampening material to reduce the spatial pulse length to improve resolution. The beams produced have a near and a far zone. The lateral resolution is equal to the beam width, which can be reduced by focusing to improve resolution.

- Resolution is the capacity of the instrument to discriminate echoes from different sources close to each other and includes axial resolution (minimum reflector separation along the direction of the ultrasound) and lateral resolution (minimum separation perpendicular to the direction), and is equal to the bandwidth and elevational resolution (related to section thickness).

- Modes of image presentation include A mode (amplitude mode) and B mode (brightness mode), which includes M mode and 2D imaging. M mode displays motion in time while B mode displays anatomical sections through a plane.

- Continuous wave Doppler involves continuous transmission and reception and records all velocities along the path and hence is not subject to aliasing. It is used to record high velocities. However it does not have depth selection.

- Pulsed wave Doppler involves intermittent transmission and reception with a delay and is useful for recording velocities at a particular location. However it is subject to aliasing. It is used for recording normal intracardiac velocities.

- Color flow Doppler imaging is useful for quantification of regurgitant lesions. It is subject to the same drawbacks of pulsed wave Doppler. Aliasing will produce mosaic of colors that indicate turbulence.

- Tissue Doppler Echocardiography (TDE) is used to evaluate motion from slow reflectors such as myocardium, valves and typically measures velocities in the range of 1-20 cm/sec. It includes Tissue Doppler Imaging (TDI) and Pulsed Wave Tissue Doppler (PWTD).

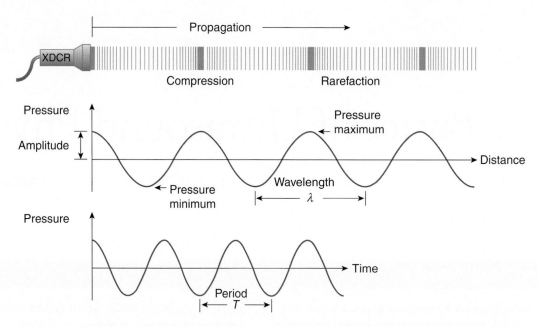

**Figure 47-1.** Diagram showing compressions and rarefactions in a medium through which a sound wave is travelling. The X axis denotes distance, and the Y axis denotes pressure. The baseline indicates a pressure of zero. The figure displays the inverse relationship between frequency and wavelength.

## PRINCIPLES OF ULTRASOUND

Sound is defined as mechanical vibrations or energy transmitted through a medium and capable of inducing rarefactions and compressions of the medium that is traversed. The compressions and rarefactions vary over time and space during the passage through the medium (**Figure 47-1**). Essentially, a sine wave is generated in a longitudinal direction, the wave traveling a straight line.

## PARAMETERS OF SOUND WAVES

The features of a sound wave are shown in (**Figure 47-2**); they are defined here.

**Frequency (C)**: Number of cycles per second, or Hertz (Hz), named after Rudolf Hertz, a nineteenth century German physicist.

**Wavelength ($\lambda$)**: Distance between corresponding areas on adjacent cycles, measured in mm. Frequency and wavelength are inversely related:

C = $\lambda$f: Wavelength is inversely dependent on density of material through which the sound is traveling (mass per unit volume) and directly dependent on the material stiffness (capacity to resist compression).

**Velocity (v)**: The rate at which sound waves travel through a medium.

**Amplitude**: The distance from the baseline to the peak of the wave. It is measured in units pressure (dB). This value is not an absolute value, but compares the logarithmic ratio of two amplitudes by the equation

$$\text{Relative amplitude (dB)} = 20 \log (A_2/A_1)$$

As a rule of thumb, a change in sound of 6 dB reflects a doubling or halving of signal amplitude.

**Power**: Rate of energy transfer, measured in watts; Directly proportional to the pressure amplitude squared.

**Intensity**: Concentration of energy within the sound beam; dependent on power and cross-sectional area of the beam.

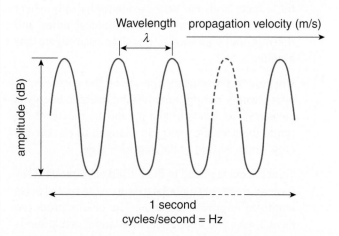

**Figure 47-2.** Schematic representation of an ultrasound wave.

$$\text{Intensity (watts/cm}^2\text{)} = \frac{\text{Power (watts)}}{\text{Beam area (cm}^2\text{)}}$$

**Period**: Time required for completion of a single wave cycle.

**Speed**: Rate of wave propagation through a medium.

Important facts related to waves:

**Normal human hearing range**: 20-20,000 Hz (audio frequencies)

**Ultrasonic frequencies**: These are wave frequencies that are above audio frequencies.

**Common echocardiographis frequencies**: 2-10 MHz (2-10 million cycles/sec)

**Velocity of propagation in blood**: approximately 1540 m/sec.

**Image resolution**: Generally no better than 1 or 2 wavelengths.

**Depth of penetration**: This is directly proportional to wavelength.

# INTERACTION OF ULTRASOUND WITH TISSUES

Generally, interaction of ultrasound with various tissues can include:

- reflection
- scattering
- refraction
- attenuation.

(See **Figure 47-3**.)

## Reflection

Reflection occurs at the boundary of two media that have different acoustic impedances (Z), expressed as Rayles. (Acoustic impedance is is the product of the density of the media and propagation velocity. The difference of propagation velocities between (soft) bodily tisues tends to be insignificant, so impedance is mainly dependent on density factor.)

The amount of reflection is constant. However, the amount received by the transducer depends on the angle between the ultrasound beam and the medium. Ideal return of the ultrasound beam occurs when the beam is perpendicular to the tissue (90°). This explains the echo "dropout," in which little reflected ultrasound reaches the tranducer due to parallel alignment between the ultrasound beam and the tissue.

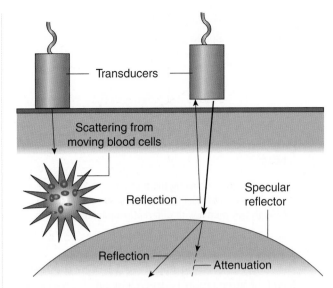

**Figure 47-3.** Diagram showing interaction of an ultrasound wave and tissue. 2D imaging is based on reflections from a specular reflector as indicated on the right side. Doppler imaging is based on scattering of ultrasound from red cells in all directions resulting in Doppler shift, as indicated on the top left of the diagram. Refraction is alteration of the path of ultrasound, resulting in artifacts. Attenuation, as indicated in the lower section, limits penetration of ultrasound.

## Scattering

This phenomenon generally occurs when the ultrasound beam interacts with a structure smaller than the wavelength of the signal (<1 wavelength). The ultrasound is reflected in all directions and only a fraction is reflected to the tranducer with the amplitude of the scattered signal being 100 to 1000 times less than a reflected signal from a specular reflector (**Figure 47-3**). *Rayleigh scattering* is diffuse scattering from a surface smaller than the ultrasound wavelength.

## Refraction

Deflection from the original path occurs when an ultrasound beam passes at an angle through two media with different impedences. This is analogous to refraction of light (Snell's law). The degree of bending depends on the relative speeds of propagation through the two, different media. (**Figure 47-4**).

Refraction can be beneficial by allowing enhancement of images. However, it can also be a source of artifacts, especially the "double image" artifact.

## Attenuation

As ultrasound travels through tissue, there is *attenuation*—progressive loss of amplitude, due to conversion of the wave's energy to heat by friction, scattering, and reflection

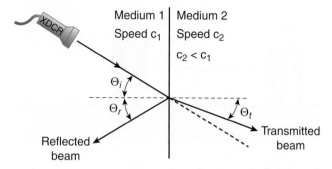

**Figure 47-4.** Diagram showing the principles of Snell's law resulting in deflection of the incident beam when ultrasound travels through two media with different propagation speeds.

from the different acoustic impedances within the tissue. The degree of attenuation is dependent on the frequency of the ultrasound. Lower frequencies will travel more deeply than higher frequencies, albeit with a loss in resolution. The *attenuation coefficient* (dB/cm) for a particular frequency in a particular tissue is the measure of attenuation (loss of amplitude) for each centimeter of travel. Typically, the depth of penetration is approximately 200 wavelengths, which corresponds to penetration depth of 30 cm for a 1-MHz transducer, 6 cm for a 5-MHz transducer and 1.5 cm for a 20-MHz transducer. Liquids (water, blood, body fluids) cause lesser attenuation than solid tissue (bone, cartilage) and air, both of which cause very high attenuation. Air-induced attenuation can be circumvented by the use of acoustic gels and employment of "acoustic windows" during acquisition of transthoracic echocardiogram (TTE).

## BIOEFFECTS OF ULTRASOUND

Diagnostic ultrasound used in clinical practice is not known to produce patient injury of any kind, although few studies have evaluated bioeffects. Ultrasound, however, has the capacity to produce bioeffects at higher intensities. These are related to:

- frequency of the ultrasound
- duration of exposure
- spatial pattern of the energy
- sensitivity of the tissue exposed
- energy at the site of interest.

### Mechanisms of Bioeffects

The bioeffect mechanisms are:

- thermal effects (heating)
- cavitation (bubble formation or liquid bubble vibration)
- mechanical effects (microstreaming, acoustic streaming, torque forces).

Heat produced in a tissue is secondary to absorption of mechanical energy of the ultrasound. This is proportional to the intensity of the ultrasound, the attenuation coefficient and the depth from the transducer. Focused transducers tend to produce more heat. However, these tend not to produce any significant bioeffects than do unfocused transducers. The heating is negated by the heat loss due to convection, conduction, and diffusion from the blood flow in the local tissue.

The rate of change of temperature dT/dt is dependent on the tissue absorption coefficient $a$, and the beam intensity I. It is inversely related to the tissue density r and the specific heat of the tissue $C_m$:

$$dT/dt = 2\alpha I/\rho C_m$$

Denser tissue like muscle tends to heat less than lower density tissue, like fat.

*Cavitation* implies formation of bubbles or vibration of existing liquid bubbles by the ultrasound beam. Bubble formation occurs with the dissolved gases in the tissues, specifically oxygen and carbon dioxide. The effect occurs with high intensity beams. Rarefaction results in decreased local pressure in the tissue, leading to "boiling" out of the dissolved gas. The microbubble formation can be either *stable* or *transient*. Stable microbubbles can resonate (expand or decrease in size) under the effects of ultrasound and convert the absorbed energy to heat. *Transient* bubble formation occurs under the influence of high intensity ultrasound, leading to cavitation during rarefaction and collapse during the compression phase. The phenomenon of cavitation is not noted with clinically used ultrasound.

*Microstreaming* implies shearing of molecules from oscillating bubbles.

The above-mentioned effects are not significant in the clinical setting. However, concern remains in fetal imaging. Fetal imaging should be as short as possible. Secondly, Doppler imaging is also recommended only if necessary due to higher energy levels in Doppler imaging.

Intensity (I) of ultrasound exposure or acoustic intensity is commonly expressed as power per cross-sectional area. That is,

$$I = \text{power/area (watts/cm}^2 \text{ or milliwatts/cm}^2)$$

acoustic power = rate of energy transfer to the tissue (watts or milliwatts)

A focused ultrasound beam will have varying intensities depending on the location within the beam. This kind of intensity is referred to as *spatial intensity* (**Figure 47-5.**)

The maximal intensity is then expressed as the highest exposure (spatial peak) averaged over the period of exposure

difficult to appreciate, but does play an important role in echocardiography.

Elevational resolution tends to the weakest in phased array systems as compared to lateral resolution, since the larger effective aperture is in the lateral direction. This can produce beam width artifacts and produce images in the center.

## IMAGING ARTIFACTS

In addition to the artifacts described in the preceding paragraphs, there are additional artifacts of note:

- Reverberation artifact—These are produced when high amplitude echo signals travel back and forth between two surfaces before returning to the transducer. These are parallel lines or shadows and are spaced equally, extending into the far field.
- Near field clutter or ring down artifacts are produced by multiple reverberations at the transducer face.
- Acoustic shadowing—These are produced by lack of transmission of ultrasound beyond a structure with high impedance like bone or a mechanical prosthesis. This causes a lack of signal beyond the structure. The closer the structure to the transducer, the larger the shadow.
- Mirror image artifact—This occurs when a strong reflector redirects a portion of the echo signal towards the transducer and the structure is thus wrongly displayed within the image; this may cause duplication of the image. Typically mirror image artifacts display opposite motion, which can be eliminated by reducing output or gain.
- Suboptimal image—This is due to interposition of tissue with high impedance in the path of the beam, resulting in a high noise-to-signal ratio.
- Range ambiguity—This occurs when echo signals return from a reflector deep to the range setting of the instrument and returns to the transducer during the listening phase for the succeeding cycle, causing that structure to be displayed as if it occurred in that particular range setting. This can be circumvented by changing the depth setting and pulse repetition frequency.

## INSTRUMENT SETTING FOR IMAGING

Many of the controls on the instrument panel perform data manipulation (preprocessing) during image acquisition, and stored data can be reviewed (postprocessing). Some of the functions of the instrument setting include:

- Power—This control adjusts energy output. Normally it is kept as minimal as possible for an optimal image quality and to reduce bioeffects and artifacts.
- Gain—This control adjusts the displayed amplitude. Gain is set high enough, while at the same time keeping the "noise" as minimal as possible.
- Time gain compensation—This panel helps to adjust the relative sensitivity of the instrument to the signals received from a particular depth. Some instruments combine this with lateral gain compensation.
- Depth—This parameter determines the pulse repetition frequency and the frame rate and is normally set to a value minimal enough to display the region of interest.
- Compression (dynamic range /greyscale)—This control adjusts the grey scale range, which helps in increasing contrast and gradation between the light and dark regions. This assists in displaying subtle variations in the image, for example, mural thrombus.
- Sector width/steer—This adjusts the angle of the sector. Reducing the angle increases the frame rate. The steer function controls the position of the sector without moving the transducer.
- Brightness, contrast, color, greyscale—These are adjusted to produce a visually optimal and meaningful image.

## PRINCIPLES OF HARMONIC IMAGING

### Tissue Harmonics

Harmonic imaging is a form of B-mode imaging wherein the pulse is emitted at the fundamental frequency $f_o$. However, the images are formed from frequencies, which are integer multiples of the fundamental frequency; e.g., $2f_o$ ($2^{nd}$ harmonic), $3f_o$ ($3^{rd}$ harmonic), etc.

Harmonic frequencies are generated due to tissue compressibility. Since the velocity of sound is related to tissue density, the peak velocity (at compression) is more the trough velocity (at rarefaction). This results in peaking of the normal sine waveform. Harmonic frequency generation increases with distance. The images generated by harmonic frequencies are significantly improved due to less distortion. They are also helpful in reducing side lobe artifacts and near field artifacts. Lateral resolution is enhanced as well, since the low energy signals are processed. Last but not least, resolution is also increased because the images are formed from higher frequency return signals.

### Contrast Harmonics

The idea behind contrast harmonics is the principle that when microbubbles in circulation interact with ultrasound, they vibrate or oscillate at a different frequency, typically twice the fundamental frequency. This occurs due to different impedances among the microbubbles, leading to compressions and rarefaction. This leads to generation of harmonic frequencies. Unlike tissue harmonic imaging, a low power is used, since the microbubbles are destroyed at higher power. The microbubbles are effective reflectors, and, when tuned, the ultrasound will preferentially display the microbubbles in range. The microbubbles currently in use are small enough ($1$-$5\mu$) to traverse the pulmonary capillary circulation into the left side of the heart. These are most commonly used for left ventricular opacification (LVO) in patients will suboptimal endocrinal definition. Other uses include myocardial perfusion imaging and visualization of left ventricular mural thrombus.

Harmonic power Doppler imaging, also called angiomode, entails Doppler reflections from microbubbles employing color B-mode imaging, which reduces tissue artifact.

## DOPPLER ECHOCARDIOGRAPHY

*Doppler shift* or frequency is the change in sound frequency from moving objects interacting with ultrasound. Essentially the frequency of the returning signal is higher when the reflecting object moves towards the transducer and lower when it moves away from the transducer. This phenomenon is named after the Austrian physicist Christian Johann Doppler, who described the effect in 1842. Hence the name *Doppler shift* ($F_d$), which is the difference between the transmitted frequency ($F_t$) and the returning frequency ($F_r$)

Normally, the Doppler shift frequencies are in the audible range. The Doppler equation is expressed as follows:

$$F_d = F_t - F_r = (2\,F_t V \cos \theta)/c,$$

where V is the velocity of the moving object, and $\theta$ is the angle between the sound wave and the direction of the moving object. The factor of 2 indicates that the Doppler shift occurs twice (from the source to the object and then back from the object to the transmitter). Hence, it is obvious that the Doppler angle will affect the Doppler shift. When the angle is zero, the beam is parallel to the flow, i.e., $\cos 0 = 1$. When the angle is 90° (perpendicular), i.e., $\cos 90 = 0$, essentially no Doppler shift results. Typically angles <20° will cause <6% change in Doppler shift, which is not significant.

## DOPPLER SPECTRAL ANALYSIS AND INSTRUMENTATION

The ultrasound machine uses a *spectrum analyzer* to determine the frequency of the returning signal and hence the Doppler shift. Two methods exist for this purpose. The *zero crossings* method is no longer used. The newer echo machines use a method called *fast Fourier transform* (FFT) (after Jean Baptiste Joseph Fourier, a nineteenth century French mathematician). The algorithm in the calculation determines the frequency content of a signal (*frequency domain analysis*). The display generated is called *spectrum analysis*. In this display, frequency shifts towards the transducer are displayed above the baseline, and shifts away from the transducer are displayed below the baseline. Because there are multiple frequencies for a given point in time, each signal will be displayed depending on its brightness (greyscale or color). Hence, the display will provide information about

- direction of blood flow
- velocity (frequency shift)
- signal amplitude.

Stronger signals emanate from specular filters, e.g., myocardial walls and blood vessel walls. These signals can overload the spectrum analyzer. A *wall filter* (high pass filter) is used to eliminate low frequency strong signals and is set at as low a level as possible, in order to prevent any information that is sought from being lost. Tissue Doppler imaging uses a *reverse wall filter* and utilizes these low frequency strong signals. Modalities used in modern Doppler echocardiography include

- continuous wave Doppler
- pulsed wave Doppler
- color Doppler flow imaging.

The essential differences of these modalities are described below:

| Continuous wave | Pulsed wave | Color |
|---|---|---|
| Continuous transmission and reception | Intermittent transmission Reception after a delay Uses 2 crystals | Color coded Uses 1 crystal |
| Records all velocities along the path | Records velocity at a particular location | Used for spatial mapping |
| Used for high velocities | Useful for low velocities | Useful for quantification of regurgitant flow |
| Smooth signal | Potential for aliasing | Color reversal with aliasing |

## Continuous Wave Doppler

Continuous wave (CW) Doppler utilizes continuous transmission and reception of signals utilizing two crystals. The spectral signal is smooth and has the narrowest frequency and the best resolution. It records signals along the entire path and there is no aliasing. There is overlap of all signals from all depths. However, CW Doppler allows precise timing and direction of flow and is valuable in high velocity lesion, such as aortic stenosis. The disadvantage is that exact location and depth cannot be assessed. Dedicated nonimaging CW probes are available that have high signal-to-noise ratio. These probes tend to be small and can be used in the narrow rib spaces.

## Pulsed Wave Doppler

As mentioned earlier, this modality employs intermittent transmission and samples velocities at a specific location of interest. It is used in conjunction with 2D imaging, termed *duplex imaging*. Typically a pulse of ultrasound is sent and after a delay, retuning signals are analyzed at specific times that would correspond to the desired depth. This sequence is repeated at intervals called *pulse repetition frequency*. The pulse repetition frequency is depth-dependent, since the wait time for the returning signal will be longer for increasing depths. Consequently, the PRF will be high for shallow depths and low for deeper tissue sites. *Sample volume* is the selected depth of interest at which the returning signals will have shifted phase and is used to generate the Doppler shift frequency.

The pulse wave signal tends to demonstrate a linear appearance as opposed to the filled-in appearance of the continuous wave Doppler. This is secondary to the limited range of frequencies within the sample volume. With increasing turbulence and complex flow, the wider range of velocities produce spectral broadening of the envelope. This will result in filling in of the display with ranges of greyscale.

The major drawback of the PW Doppler is its capacity to measure limited velocities unambiguously. Velocities outside the limits of the spectral display, also known as the Nyquist limit (called after Harry Nyquist, a physicist and engineer at Bell Laboratories), will produce the 'wrap around' phenomenon that appears at another location within the display, with a reversal of direction. This is called aliasing. This phenomenon occurs when the Doppler shift frequency exceeds one half of the PRF.

Measures used to reduce aliasing include

- using CW Doppler
- shifting baseline
- increasing PRF
- using low frequency transducer

## High Pulse Repetition Doppler

This modality uses high PRF at short intervals and hence the range ambiguity. This helps in detection of higher velocities.

## Color Flow Doppler

Color flow Doppler uses real time display of flow information superimposed on 2D or M-mode imaging. A group of pulses are emitted for each pixel in the color scan. Typically between 3 and 16 pulses (packet size, color packets or pulse packets) are emitted and the returned signals are recorded; about 100 samples are recorded along each color scan line.

A color map allows for selection of colors ranging from saturated red for velocities towards the transducer to saturated blue for velocities away from the transducer (mnemonic: BART = Blue Away, Red Towards). Color flow Doppler requires a significant amount of computation. There are a large number of sample volumes in a color flow image. Only the mean velocity is displayed in each pixel. Because of the large numbers of reflectors in blood (cells), large packet sizes are used. Three parameters are measured:

- mean phase shift (mean velocity)
- variance of the mean value (turbulence)
- amplitude (indicates number of reflectors).

Variance can be adjusted to display shades of green and yellow. Variance indicates regions with turbulence or complex flow states.

This process of acquisition is repeated for each scan line of the image plane. This process takes a finite time and is reflected in the frame rate, which signifies the rate of image update. The frame rate is determined by:

- sector depth (PRF)
- sector width (number of lines)
- number of ultrasound bursts (burst length)
- density of lines (number of lines)

Properties of color are expressed in terms of *hue*, *saturation*, and *intensity*.

Color flow Doppler being a form of pulsed Doppler is subject to the same limitations, e.g., aliasing and the wrap-around phenomenon, where the color can change from red to blue and vice versa without transitioning through the intermediate colors. This produces a mosaic of colors that signify turbulence or high velocity flows. The other major limitation of color flow Doppler is temporal and spatial resolution.

## Tissue Doppler Echocardiography

This modality evaluates motion of slow-moving reflectors, for example, valves, myocardium, etc. It measures velocities in the typical range 1-20 cm/s. Tissue Doppler is of two kinds:

- tissue Doppler imaging (TDI)
- pulsed wave tissue Doppler (PWTD.)

The difference between TDI and color flow Doppler is that the signal is not passed through a clutter filter, and low amplitude signals are rejected.

PWTD quantifies velocities of tissue motion and has an improved velocity range and temporal resolution as compared to TDI, which provides better spatial resolution. PWTD reflects true tissue motion as well as translational and rotational movements. PWTD can be used for assessing various aspects of cardiac function including diastolic function, regional systolic function, and global systolic function.

## ACKNOWLEDGMENTS

We thank Mr. Dennis E. Mathias for the artistic contribution provided in generating the figures published in this chapter.

# 48

# Essentials of Echocardiography

RAGAVENDRA R. BALIGA AND THEODORE ABRAHAM

## ● PRACTICAL POINTS

- Contrast echo: Because the ultrasound characteristics of microbubbles are distinctly different from those of the surrounding blood cells and heart tissue, the backscatter that they produce with second harmonic images enhances myocardial border delineation and the resultant echocardiographic image.

- Left atrial volume is measured in apical 4-chamber view on two-dimensional (2D) echo by tracing the inner edge of the atrial border at end-systole. It is then corrected for body surface area, normal is <28 mL/m².

- Left ventricular volume: American Society of Echocardiography (ASE) recommends that modified Simpson's rule (using the 2D biplane method of disks) be utilized for volume measurements.

- Myocardial and annular velocities: A ratio of E-mitral inflow velocity to E" is >15 mm Hg suggests elevated left ventricular end diastolic pressure (LVEDP).

- LV wall motion abnormalities: The ASE in 1989 recommended a 16-segment model (6 segments at basal and midventricular levels and 4 segments at apex) for LV segmentation, which is best used for studies assessing wall motion abnormalities. The AHA Writing Group recommended a 17-segment model, which included apical cap, and this model is best used for myocardial perfusion studies or when comparisons are made between imaging modalities

- Pressure gradients are calculated using the simplified Bernoulli equation $\delta P = 4V^2$, where $\delta P$ is the pressure gradient (in mm Hg) and V is peak blood velocity (in m/s) as measured by the Doppler across the narrowing. The equation that describes the relationship between Doppler gradient and cardiac catheterization-derived peak-to-peak gradient is:

  Peak-to-peak gradient $\simeq$ (0.84 × peak Doppler gradient) – 14 mm Hg.

- Right ventricular systolic pressure (RVSP) is given by:

  RSVP = Estimate of mean RA pr + Peak RV – RA gradient or RVSP = $4V_2$ + estimated RA pr.

  In the absence of pulmonary stenosis, pulmonary artery systolic pressure, (PASP) = peak RVSP. In the presence of pulmonary stenosis,

  PASP = RVSP – maximal pulmonary valve pressure gradient.

  The latter is derived from velocity across the pulmonary valve by continuous wave Doppler.

- Valve lesions

  ○ Aortic and mitral stenosis: Continuity equation is typically used in assessing aortic stenosis. In mitral stenosis the continuity equation is useful when the pressure half-time method is limited. Calculating valve areas using the pressure half-time method is an accurate method for determining the severity of mitral stenosis. Pressure half-time is time needed for maximal pressure gradient to decrease by half:

    Mitral valve area = 220/Pressure half-time.

  ○ Aortic regurgitation: Semiquantitative assessment of the severity is done by color flow jet area and width by Doppler echocardiography, quantitative measurement of regurgitant volume, regurgitant fraction, and regurgitant orifice area.

  ○ Mitral regurgitation: A central color flow jet with a structurally normal MV apparatus suggests the presence of functional MR, which may be due to annular dilatation from LV dilatation or tethering of the posterior leaflet because of regional LV dysfunction in patients with ischemic heart disease.

*(continued)*

529

---

**● PRACTICAL POINTS (continued)**

An eccentric color flow jet of MR with abnormalities of the MV apparatus indicates organic MR.

○ Prosthetic valve: All prosthetic valves have some "in-built" regurgitation.

• Constrictive pericarditis: There is no single echocardiographic sign diagnostic of constrictive pericarditis—a combination of echocardiographic and Doppler

studies along with clinical features usually indicates the diagnosis of constrictive pericarditis.

• Pericardial tamponade: Although right atrial collapse is a sensitive sign of increased pressure in the pericardial space, diastolic RV collapse is more specific for hemodynamic compromise in pericardial tamponade

---

## TYPES OF ECHOCARDIOGRAPHY

### M-Mode

M-Mode, or motion echo, is a graph that reflects depth and strength of reflection with time (**Figures 48-1** and **48-2**).

It is generated by transmission and reception of the ultrasound signal along only one line. The sampling rate of 1800 times per second allows it higher sensitivity than 2D echo for moving structures, e.g., valve opening or closing or movements of ventricular wall. It is important that the ultrasound beam be aligned perpendicular to the structure being assessed with this modality. M-mode measurements are used to determine size and thickness of the various chambers of the heart, valve orifices, and blood vessels.

### Two-Dimensional

Two-dimensional (2D) echocardiography is a sector of a tomographic image plane in real-time motion (**Figure 48-3** and **Table 48-1**). It involves generation of a "snapshot" in time of a cross-section of the tissue, which is followed by rapid succession of the next frame of the cross-section, resulting in real-time imaging of the chambers of the heart, valves, and blood vessels.

### Three-Dimensional

Three-dimensional echocardiography (3D) is under evolution. It currently utilizes matrix probes that consist of 2000 to 3000 imaging elements in a rectangular array. Currently, these devices have been acquiring four or more separate sub-pyramidal volumes, triggered to the electrocardiogram and then merged or "stitched" to a full volume. Limitations of capturing a full volume data include relatively low frame rates, especially with color Doppler imaging and integrating other data such tissue Doppler and M-mode.

### Doppler Echocardiography

Doppler echocardiography utilizes the reflection of ultrasound waves from moving red blood cells. The direction and velocity of blood flow influences the frequency shift of the ultrasound wave. Therefore, the hemodynamic information (**Table 48-2**) derived from Doppler is used to:

• Measure the severity of valvular stenosis
• Detect valvular regurgitation
• Detect intracardiac shunts such as VSD and ASD.

The three traditional Doppler techniques that are routine in an echocardiographic study are as follows:

1. **Pulse Wave Doppler (Figure 48-4)**—This utilizes a single crystal to transmit ultrasound and then receive the sound wave after a preset time delay. It only allows measurement of blood flow velocity from a small region. When combined with 2D imaging, a small "sample volume" can be seen on the screen from where the velocities are measured. This sample volume can be moved by the sonographer. The signals that are reflected can only be measured from a depth that corresponds to the product of half the time delay with the speed of sound in tissue, that is,

$$\frac{1}{2} \text{ (time delay} \times 1540 \text{ m/s).}$$

The time delay also limits the rate at which sampling occurs, which in turn limits the maximum velocity that can be measured—a phenomenon that is known is "*aliasing*," which occurs with velocities in excess of 2 m/s. Pulse wave Doppler is utilized to measure normal intracardiac transvalvular flow velocities.

2. **Continuous Wave Doppler (Figure 48-5)**—This utilizes two crystals—one that is transmitting continuously and another that is receiving continuously. The advantage of this technique is that it is able to measure high velocities (without signal aliasing). Also, its ability to localize a flow signal precisely can originate at any point along the length or width of the ultrasound beam. It's ability to measure high velocities makes it useful in assessing flows across stenotic and regurgitant valves.

Note both continuous and pulsed wave Doppler are referred to as "spectral" Doppler because they allow a graphical depiction of velocity and time.

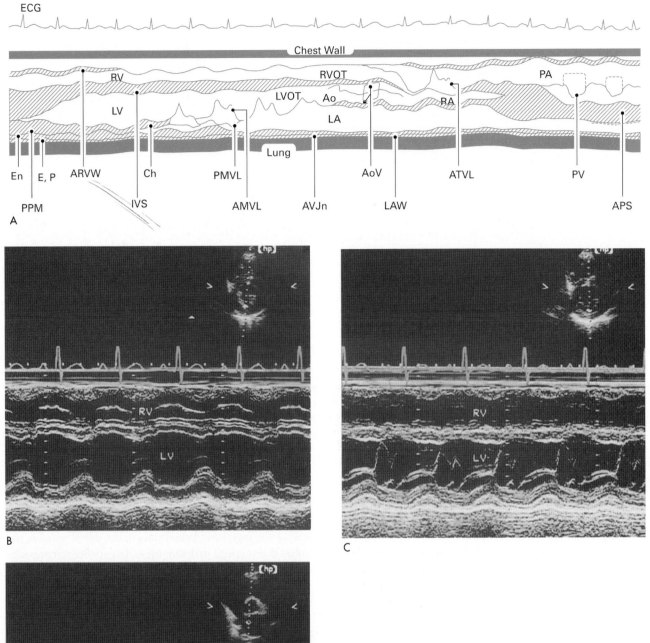

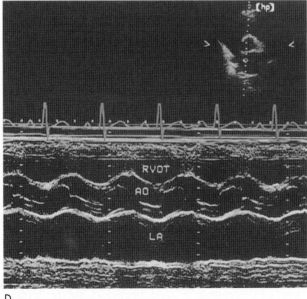

**Figure 48-1.** A. Diagram of an M-mode sweep from apex to base in a normal heart (parasternal view). B to D. M-mode sweep from apex to base in a normal individual. aMVL, anterior mitral valve leaflet; Ao, aorta; AoV, aortic valve; APS, atriopulmonic sulcus; ARVW, anterior right ventricular wall; ATVL, anterior tricuspid valve leaflet; AVJ, atrioventricular junction; Ch, chordae tendineae; EN, endocardium; E,P, epicardial/pericardial interface; IVS, interventricular septum; LA, left atrium; LAW, left atrial wall; LV, left ventricle; LVOT, left ventricular outflow tract; PA, pulmonary artery; PMVL, posterior mitral valve leaflet; PPM, posterior papillary muscle; PV, pulmonic valve; RA, right atrium; RV, right ventricle; RVOT, right ventricular outflow tract. (Source: A, from Felner JM, Schlant RC. Echocardiography: A Teaching Atlas. New York: Grune & Stratton; 1976. With permission.)

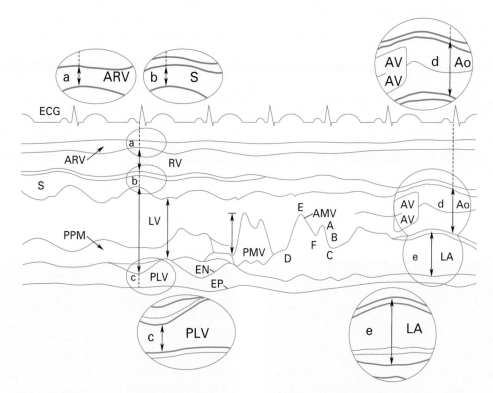

**Figure 48-2.** Recommended criteria for M-mode measurement of cardiac dimensions (see text for details). The figure and the elliptical inserts (*a, b, c, d,* and *e*) illustrate the leading-edge method. aMVL, anterior mitral valve leaflet; Ao, aorta; AoV, aortic valve; ARV, anterior right ventricular wall; EN, endocardium; EP, epicardium; LA, left atrium; LV, left ventricle; PLV, posterior left ventricular (wall); PPM, papillary muscle; PMVL, posterior mitral valve leaflet; RV, right ventricle; S, septum. (Source: Reproduced with permission from Sahn DJ, DeMaria AN, Kisslo J, Weyman AE.)

3. **Color Flow Mapping (Figure 48-6)**—This is generated by an automated 2D pulsed wave Doppler superimposed on 2D real-time image. It is used for assessment of regurgitation and shunts. Color flow mapping calculates both blood velocity and direction at several points along a number of scan lines that are superimposed on a 2D image. Color coding is used to depict the direction and velocity of blood flow. The BART convention or (blue away, red towards the transducer) is now the standard for color coding.

As the velocities increase, the shades of color become lighter progressively. "Color reversal" occurs at the threshold velocity (the Nyquist limit) due to aliasing. Regions of turbulence or high flow acceleration are depicted in green.

**Tissue Doppler** is performed in apical views to determine mitral annular velocities. Mitral annular velocities are used to draw inferences about LV relaxation and, along with mitral peak E velocity (E/e' ratio), is used to predict LV filling pressures. Primary measurements include the systolic (S), early diastolic, and late diastolic velocities. The early diastolic annular velocity has been expressed as Ea, Em, E', or e', and the late diastolic velocity as Aa, Am, A', or a'. Use of E' or e' is preferred because Ea is also commonly used to refer to arterial elastance. To determine global LV diastolic function, it is recommended one acquire and measure tissue Doppler signals at least at the septal and lateral sides of the mitral annulus and utilize their average to determine e'. In patients with myocardial disease, e' can be used to correct for the effect of LV relaxation on mitral E velocity, and the E/e' ratio can be applied for the prediction of LV filling pressures. Normal values tissue Doppler-derived velocities are influenced by age, similar to other indices of LV diastolic function. With age, e' velocity decreases, whereas a' velocity and the E/e' ratio increase. An E/e'>15 is associated with elevated LV filling pressures. The E/e' ratio, however, has limitations, and is not accurate as an index of filling pressures in normal subjects or in patients with heavy annular calcification, mitral valve (MV) disease, and constrictive pericarditis.

## Contrast Echocardiography

Contrast echocardiography involves intravenous administration of microbubbles that opacify the left or right heart (**Figure 48-7**).

Right-sided contrast is used to detect patent formen ovale, whereas left-sided contrast is used to better delineate left ventricular border when transthoracic images are suboptimal.

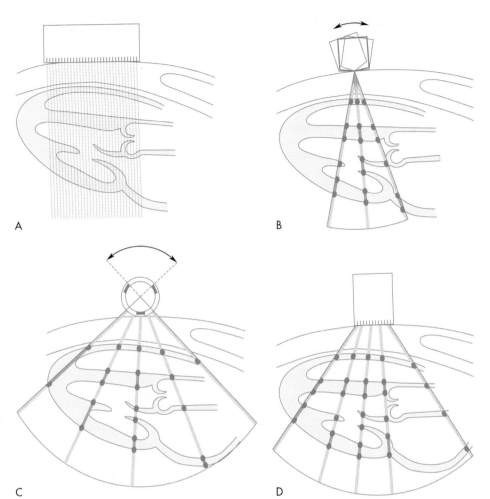

**Figure 48-3.** The four major types of ultrasonic scanners used to acquire 2D echocardiographic images. A. Linear-array scanner. B. Oscillating scanner. C. Rotating mechanical scanner. D. Phased-array scanner. (Source: From Hagan AD, DeMaria AN. Clinical Applications of Two-Dimentional Echocardiography and Cardiac Doppler. Boston: Little, Brown; 1989. With permission.)

## ASE Recommendations for Contrast Echocardiography

In difficult-to-image patients presenting for rest echocardiography with reduced image quality, the following uses of contrast echocardiography are recommended:

1. to enable improved endocardial visualization and assessment of left ventricular (LV) structure and function when ≥2 contiguous segments are not seen on noncontrast images;
2. to reduce variability and increase accuracy in LV volume and LV ejection fraction (LVEF) measurements by 2D echocardiography;
3. to increase the confidence of the interpreting physician in LV functional, structure, and volume assessments.

In difficult-to-image patients presenting for stress echocardiography with reduced image quality, the following uses of contrast echocardiography are recommended:

1. to obtain diagnostic assessment of segmental wall motion and thickening at rest and stress;
2. to increase the proportion of diagnostic studies;
3. to increase reader confidence in interpretation.

In all patients presenting for rest echocardiographic assessment of LV systolic function (not solely difficult-to-image patients), the following uses of contrast echocardiography are recommended:

1. to reduce variability in LV volume measurements through 2D echocardiography;

2. to increase the confidence of the interpreting physician in LV volume measurement.

To confirm or exclude the echocardiographic diagnosis of the following LV structural abnormalities, when nonenhanced images are suboptimal for definitive diagnosis:

1. apical variant of hypertrophic cardiomyopathy;
2. ventricular noncompaction;
3. apical thrombus;
4. complications of myocardial infarction, such as LV aneurysm, pseudoaneurysm, and myocardial rupture.

To assist in the detection and correct classification of intracardiac masses, including tumors and thrombi.

For echocardiographic imaging in the intensive care unit (ICU) when standard tissue harmonic imaging does not provide adequate cardiac structural definition

- for accurate assessment of LV volumes and LVEF;
- for exclusion of complications of myocardial infarction, such as LV aneurysm, pseudoaneurysm, and myocardial rupture.

To enhance Doppler signals when a clearly defined spectral profile is not visible and is necessary to the evaluation of diastolic and/or valvular function

## Table 48–1 • Cardiac Dimensions by Two-Dimensional Echocardiography

| Cardiac Feature | Range | Mean | Index, cm/m² |
|---|---|---|---|
| **Apicol four-chamber view** | | | |
| $LV_d$ major | 6.9–10.3 cm | 8.6 cm | 4.1–5.7 |
| $LV_d$ minor | 3.3–6.1 cm | 4.7 cm | 2.2–3.1 |
| $LV_s$ minor | 1.9–3.7 cm | 2.8 cm | 1.3–2.0 |
| $LV_d$ area | 21.2–40.2 cm² | 31.2 cm² | — |
| $LV_s$ area | 8.0–21.1 cm² | 14.2 cm² | — |
| RV major | 6.5–9.5 cm² | 8.0 cm | 3.8–5.3 |
| $RV_d$ minor | 2.2–4.4 cm² | 3.3–3.5 cm | 1.0–2.8 |
| $RV_d$ area | 12.0–22.2 cm² | 18.6–2.1 cm² | — |
| $RV_s$ area | 5.4–14.6 cm² | 9.9 cm² | — |
| LA major | 4.1–6.1 cm | 5.1 cm | 2.3–3.5 |
| LA minor | 2.8–4.3 cm | 3.5 cm | 1.6–2.4 |
| LA area | 10.2–17.8 cm² | 14.7 cm² | — |
| RA major (inf-sup) | 3.5–5.5 cm | 4.3–4.5 cm | 2.0–3.1 |
| RA minor | 2.5–4.9 cm | 3.7 cm | 1.7–2.5 |
| RA area | 11.3–16.7 cm² | 13.8–14 cm² | — |
| **Apicol two-champer view** | | | |
| $LV_d$ major | 6.8–9.4 cm | 8.0 cm | — |
| $LV_d$ minor | 3.8–5.7 cm | 4.6 cm | — |
| $LV_d$ area | 19.4–48.0 cm² | 35.6 cm² | — |
| $LV_s$ | 8.9–27.0 cm | 14.3 cm | — |
| **Parasternal long-axis view** | | | |
| $LV_d$ | 3.5–6.0 cm | 4.8 cm | 2.3–3.1 |
| $LV_s$ | 2.1–4.0 cm | 3.1 cm | 1.4–2.1 |
| RV | 1.9–3.8 cm² | 2.8 cm | 1.2–2.0 |
| LA [A-P] | 2.7–4.5 cm | 3.6 cm | 1.6–2.4 |
| LA [S-I] | 3.1–5.5 cm | 4.4 cm | — |
| LA area | 9.0–19.3 cm² | 13.8 cm² | — |
| Ao | 2.2–3.6 cm | 2.9 cm | 1.4–2.0 |
| **Parasternal short-axis view** | | | |
| Ao | 2.3–3.7 cm | 3.0–2.3 cm | 1.6–2.4 |
| RVOT | 1.9–2.2 cm | 2.7 cm | — |
| RA | 1.5–2.5 cm | 1.9–2.2 cm | — |
| LA | 2.6–4.5 cm | 3.6 cm | 1.6–2.4 |
| LA area | 7.2–13.0 cm² | 10.8 cm² | — |
| $LV_d$ (PM level) | 3.5–5.8 cm | 4.7 cm | 2.2–3.1 |
| $LV_s$ (PM level) | 2.2–4.0 cm | 3.1 cm | 1.4–2.2 |
| $LV_d$ area (PM level) | 16.0–31.2 cm² | 22.2 cm² | — |
| $LV_s$ area (PM level) | 5.2–13.4 cm² | 8.5 cm² | — |
| $LV_d$ (Ch. level) | 3.5–6.2 | 4.8 cm | 2.3–3.2 |
| $LV_s$ (Ch. level) | 2.3–4.0 | 3.2 cm | 1.5–2.2 |
| $LV_d$ area (Ch. level) | 16.4–32.3 cm² | 22.5 cm² | — |
| $LV_s$ area (Ch. level) | 6.1–16.8 cm² | 10.7 cm² | — |
| **Subcostal view**<br>IVC diameter | | 1.8 cm | — |

*Ao, aorta; Ch., chordal; IVC, inferior vena cava; LA, left atrium; LV, left ventricle; LV_d, left ventricle end diastole; LV_s, left ventricle, end systole; PA, pulmonary artery; PM, papillary muscle; RA, right atrium; RV, right ventricle, RVd, right ventricular end diastole; RVOT, right ventricle outflow tract; RV_s, right ventricle end systole*
*Source: The values shown in this table represent a compilation of data from three sources: Schnitfinger I, Gorden EP, Fitzgerold PJ, et al. Standardized intracardiac measurements of two-dimensional echocardiography. J Am Call Cardial 1983;5:934. Triulzi M, Weymon A. Normal cross-sectional measurements in adults. In: Weyman A, ed. Echocardiography, Philadelphia: Lea & Febiger; 1982;497. Hagan AD, DiSessa TG, Bloor CM, et al. Two-Dimensional Echocardiography: Clinical-Pathological Corrections in Adult and Congenital Heart Disease. Boston: Little, Brown; 1983;553.*

Newer generation of ultrasound contrast agents consists of microbubbles of a high molecular weight gas encapsulated in a shell of phospholipid or protein. Because the ultrasound characteristics of microbubbles are distinctly different from those of the surrounding blood cells and heart tissue, the backscatter that they produce with second harmonic images enhances myocardial border delineation and the resultant echocardiographic image (**Figure 48-8**).

| Table 48-2 • Normal Intracardiac Doppler Velocites | |
| --- | --- |
| | **Velocity, m/sec** |
| Right ventricle | |
|   Tricuspid flow | 0.3–0.7 |
|   Pulmonary artery | 0.6–0.9 |
| Left ventricle | |
|   Mitral flow | 0.6–1.3 |
|   Aorta | 1.0–1.7 |

*Source: Hatle L, Angelsen B. Doppler Ultrasound in Cardiology. 2nd ed. Philadelphia; Lea & Febiger; 1985*

Contrast echocardiography has made possible the assessment of myocardial perfusion, permitting simultaneous assessment of global and regional myocardial structure, function, and perfusion. This has enabled the optimal noninvasive assessment of chronic coronary artery disease (CAD) and acute coronary syndromes (ACS). The use of contrast significantly enhances imaging not only in routine echocardiography but also stress echocardiography, frequently allowing the salvage of procedures that do not provide images of diagnostic quality.

# ASSESSMENT OF CHAMBER SIZE AND WALL THICKNESS

## Left Ventricular Size

### LV Dimensions
- 2D, guided M-mode measurements of LV internal dimensions at end-diastole and end-systole are made when the M-line is oriented appropriately in the parasternal long axis view. The measurements are made perpendicular to the LV minor axis (to avoid overestimating the size that occurs at an oblique angle) and at level of mitral valve chords.

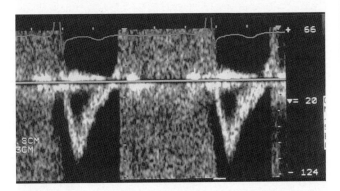

**Figure 48-4.** PW Doppler tracing from a patient with aortic regurgitation. The transducer is in the apical position and the sample volume is in the left ventricular outflow tract. A laminar envelope is seen during systole, whereas aliased flow is present during diastole because of high-velocity flow.

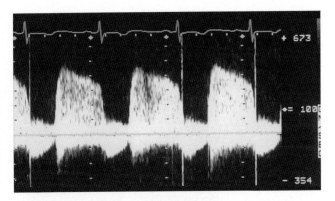

**Figure 48-5.** CW Doppler tracing through the left ventricular outflow tract (with transducer in the apical position). The maximal velocity of the aortic regurgitation is now measurable, but all other velocities along the Doppler beam are recorded as well. CW, continuous wave; PW, pulsed wave.

- The onset of QRS complex is used to make end-diastolic measurements, and end-systolic measurements are made just before the close of the aortic valve when the LV chamber size is at its minimum.
- Measurements are made, at the level of the mitral valve chords, from the leading edge of the septal endocardium to leading edge of the posterior LV wall (the latter is identified on M-mode as the steepest most continuous line).

### LV Chamber Volumes
- These are determined by tracing endocardial borders in apical 4-chamber views and end-diastole and end-systole.

## Left Ventricular Wall Thickness

LV wall thickness is determined by 2D guided M-Mode measurement of LV posterior wall and septal thickness in

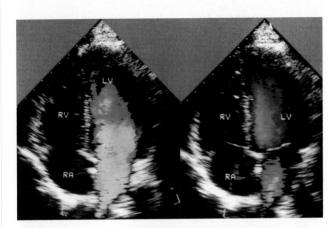

**Figure 48-6.** Apical four-chamber images with color-flow Doppler during diastole and systole. Red flow indicates movement toward the transducer (diastolic filling); blue flow indicates movement away from the transducer (systolic ejection). LV, left ventricle; RA, right atrium; RV, right ventricle.

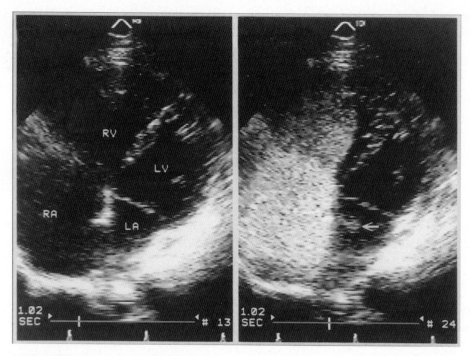

**Figure 48-7.** Contrast microbubble injection demonstrating a shunt (*arrow*) from the right atrium (*RA*). lo left atrium (*LA*) LV, left ventricle; RV, right ventricle.

the left parasternal view, at end-diastole and at the level of mitral valve chordae. LV wall thickens during systole. The normal range of thickness is 6-12 mm. Walls thinner than 6 mm may be stretched as in dilated cardiomyopathy or due to myocardial damage following a myocardial infarction. LV wall thickness >12 mm indicates left ventricular hypertrophy.

## Left Atrial Size

- M-mode measurements include anterior-posterior dimensions. It is measured in long-axis view at end of ventricular systole to obtain maximum size.
- Left atrial volume is measured in apical 4-chamber view on 2D echo by tracing the inner edge of the atrial border at end-systole. It is then corrected for body surface area,

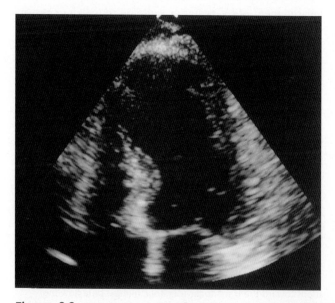
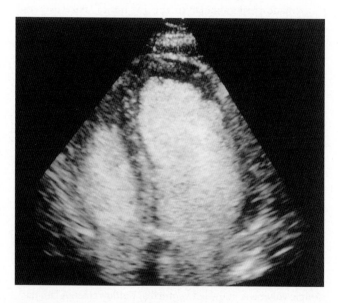

**Figure 48-8.** Harmonic imaging after intravenous injection of echocardiographic contrast. Endocardial border definition before injection is fair (*upper panel*) but is markedly improved with harmonic imaging following contrast injection (*lower panel*).

normal is <28 mL/m². It is usually increased with mitral regurgitation or when the LV filling pressure is elevated. It is recommended that volume determinations be preferred over linear dimensions because they allow accurate assessment of the asymmetric remodeling of the LA chamber and the strength of the relationship between LA volume, and cardiovascular disease is stronger than that for linear LA dimensions (Lang et al.)[2].

## Right Ventricular Size

Right ventricular size is best determined in the apical 4-chamber view tilted towards the right ventricle and the subcostal 4-chamber view. The latter view provides the most accurate estimate of the RV size because the ultrasound beam is perpendicular to the RV free wall and ventricular septum. The RV size may be overestimated in the apical 4-chamber view if it is foreshortened, particularly when the transducer is medial to the LV apex or when the free wall of the RV is not well seen. Normal mid RV diameter = 2.7 cm – 3.3 cm), RV outflow tract diameter = 2.5 cm – 2.9 cm. The size can be graded qualitatively as severely enlarged when the RV > LV, moderately enlarged RV = LV, or mildly enlarged where RV < LV.

## Right Atrial Size

Right atrial size is usually determined in the apical 4-chamber view. The minor-axis dimension should be measured in the plane perpendicular to the long axis of the right atrium. It extends from the lateral border of the right atrium to the interatrial septum. Normal values are 1.7-2.5 cm/m². A paucity of data exists for normal RA volumetric values and limited data suggest that RA volumes are similar to LA normal values in men, 21 mL/m², but they are slightly smaller in women.

## Right Ventricular Wall Thickness

Right ventricular wall thickness is determined qualitatively (i.e., RV free wall appears to be the same thickness as the LV free wall) or free wall thickness is measured (normal <5 mm).

## ASSESSMENT OF VENTRICULAR FUNCTION

### Global

#### Systolic

- Ejection fraction
  - Left ventricular ejection fraction is usually estimated visually from parasternal short axis and apical 4-chamber, 2-chamber, and long-axis views.
  - It is also calculated from the formula [(EDV– ESV)/ESV] × 100%, where EDV is end-diastolic volume

and ESV is end-systolic volume. The volume in end-diastole is estimated as (LVEDD)³ and ESV as (LVESD).³
  - When the visual estimate does not agree with the measured EF, the two are repeated and compared. If they disagree (e.g., when the endocardial borders are poorly delineated) then the visual estimate is reported using a descriptive scale.
  - Normal >55%, mildly reduced (40-55%), moderately reduced (20-40%), and severely reduced <20%.
  - Most echocardiographic laboratories have relied on M-mode measurements or linear dimensions from the 2D image for quantification. However, the previously used Teichholtz or Quiñones methods of calculating LVEF from linear dimensions often result in inaccurate measurements as a result of geometric assumptions used in the conversion of linear measurements to 3D volume. Therefore, it is recommended that, instead, modified Simpson's rule (using the 2D biplane method of disks) be utilized for volume measurements (**Figure 48-9**).
- E-point septal separation
- Fractional shortening or the % change in LV internal dimensions (not volumes) between systole and diastole. Normal range 30-45%:

$$FS = (LVEDD - LVESD)/LVEDD \times 100\%.$$

In the settings of concentric hypertrophy, it is recommended that calculation of midwall rather than

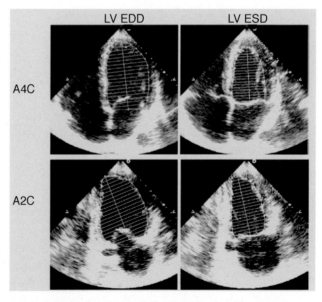

**Figure 48-9.** Two-dimensional measurements for volume calculations using biplane method of disks (modified Simpson's rule) in apical 4-chamber (A4C) and apical 2-chamber (A2C) views at end diastole (LV EDD) and at end systole (LV ESD). Papillary muscles should be excluded from the cavity in the tracing. (Permission to be obtained from Lang et al. 2005).

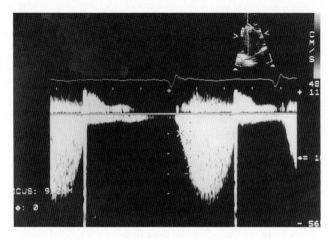

**Figure 48-10.** CW tracing of mitral regurgitation with calculation of dP/dt (apical transducer position). The time period between velocities of 1 and 3 m/sec is 0.07 sec; the calculated dP/dt is approximately 460 mm Hg/sec. See text for details. CW, continuous wave.

endocardial fractional shortening be utilized because contraction of muscle fibers in the LV midwall wall better reflects intrinsic contractility than contraction of fibers in the endocardium does. Midwall fractional shortening is calculated according the following mathematical formulas:

$$\text{Inner shell} = [(\text{LVIDd} + \text{SWTd}/2 + \text{PWTd}/2)^3 - \text{LVIDd}^3 + \text{LVIDs}^3]^{1/3} - \text{LVIDs}$$

$$\text{MWFS} = \frac{([\text{LVIDd} + \text{SWTd}/2 + \text{PWTd}/2] - [\text{LVIDs} + \text{inner shell}])}{(\text{LVIDd} + \text{SWTd}/2 + \text{PWTd}/2) \times 100}$$

Cardiac output = Stroke volume × Heart rate,

where stroke volume = EDV − ESV.

- Aortic root anterior-posterior motion
- Mitral annular apical motion
- Left ventricular dP/dt (**Figure 48-10**)
  - dP/dt is the rate of rise of ventricular pressure or change in pressure (dP) over time (dt).
  - It is a load-independent measure of LV function.
  - It is calculated from a rise in velocity of regurgitant jet of mitral valve.
  - A normal dP/dt = 1000 mm Hg/s.

## Diastolic *(Figures 48-11 and 48-12)*

The assessment of LV diastolic function includes measurement of:

- Mitral inflow velocity: These are recorded at the tips of mitral leaflets and at the mitral annulus in the apical four chamber view using pulsed Doppler with a sample volume of 2-2.5 cm. Standard measurements include E-velocity and deceleration time and A-velocity and duration.
- Pulmonary vein velocity: Left atria inflow velocities in the right superior pulmonary vein from apical four chamber view with transthoracic echocardiography

or in any pulmonary vein during TEE. Measurements include peak systolic velocity ($PV_s$), peak diastolic velocity ($PV_d$), atrial velocity peak ($PV_a$), and duration ($a_{dur}$).

- Myocardial and annular velocities: Tissue Doppler measurements at the mitral annulus in the apical 4-chamber view. The measurements of the septal side are more reproducible than the lateral wall. Usual measurements include early myocardial velocity (E') and atrial myocardial velocity ($A_M$). A ratio of E-mitral inflow velocity to E' is >15 mm Hg suggests elevated LVEDP.
- Isovolumic relaxation time (IVRT): This is measured using pulsed Doppler in the anteriorly angulated 4-chamber view. IVRT is the interval between closure of the atrial valve and opening of the mitral valve. Normal is 50-100 ms and it is prolonged with impaired relaxation but shortened with severe diastolic dysfunction and impaired compliance.

## Regional

The wall motion abnormalities and wall thickening/thinning are determined visually for each myocardial segment. Wall motion and thickening for each myocardial segment are characterized as normal, hypokinetic, akinetic, dyskinetic (i.e., movement in the wrong direction, e.g., outward movement of the LV free wall during systole) or aneurysmal

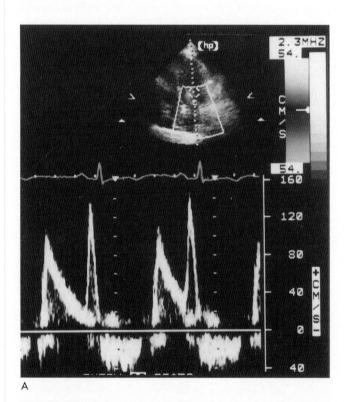

A

**Figure 48-11.** A. PWD tracing of diastolic relaxation abnormality (see text for details).

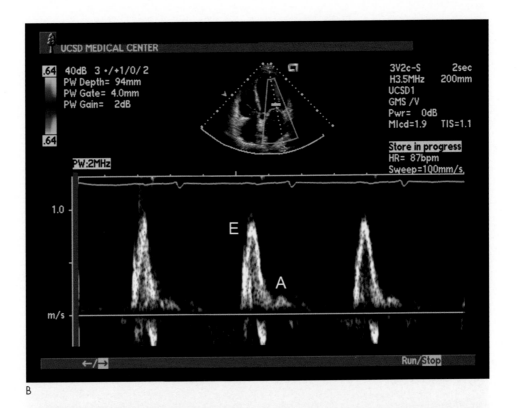

B

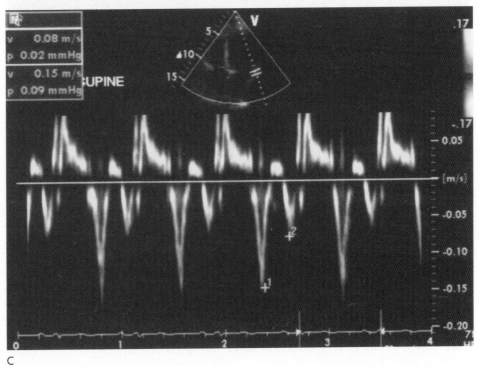

C

**Figure 48-11.** (continued)  B. PWD tracing of diastolic restrictive abnormality (see text for details) C. Tissue Doppler recording of normal lateral mitral annular motion (apical transducer position). Peak early diastolic annular velocity is 15 cm/sec.

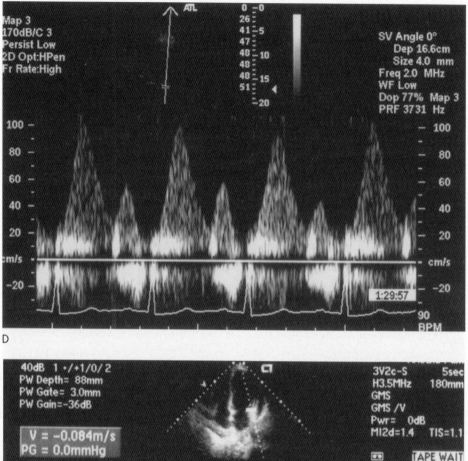

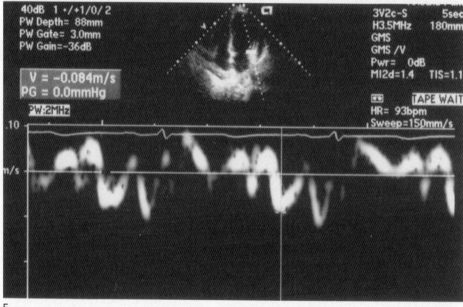

**Figure 48-11.** (continued) D. PWD recording of pulmonary venous flow in mild diastolic dysfunction (abnormal relaxation). The S wave is prominent whereas the D wave is small. E. Tissue Doppler image (lateral mitral annulus) in mild diastolic dysfunction. Early diastolic velocity is blunted (8 cm/sec).

(outpouching of all three layers of the wall). Regional or segmental ventricular abnormalities corresponding to coronary artery perfusion suggest ischemic heart disease.

The American Society of Echocardiography in 1989 recommended a 16-segment model (6 segments at both basal and midventricular levels and 4 segments at apex) (**Figure 48-13**) for LV segmentation; this model is best used for studies assessing wall motion abnormalities. The AHA Writing Group recommended a 17-segment model (**Figure 52-1**), which included apical cap, and this model is best used for myocardial perfusion studies or when comparisons are made between imaging modalities. The distribution of the coronary arteries to the various segments (although variability exists) is shown in the transthoracic echocardiography views in **Figure 48-10**.

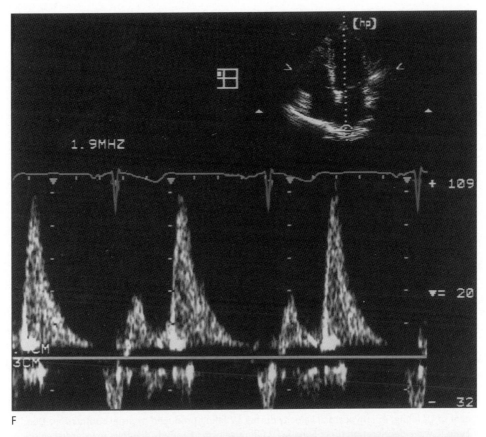

F

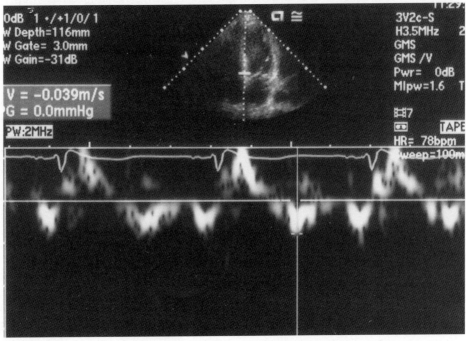

G

**Figure 48-11.** (continued) F. PWD recording of pulmonary venous flow in severe diastolic dysfunction. The S wave is small whereas the D wave is prominent. G. Tissue Doppler image in severe diastolic dysfunction. Both $E_m$ and $A_m$ velocities are abnormally low. A, atrial contraction; E, early rapid filling; PWD, pulsed-wave Doppler.

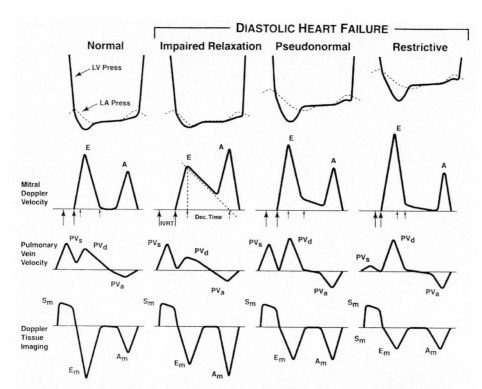

**Figure 48-12.** Doppler assessment of progressive diastolic dysfunction utilizing transmitral PWD, pulmonary venous Doppler, and mitral annular tissue Doppler imaging. A, atrial component of LV filling; $A_m$, myocardial velocity during LV filling produced by atrial contraction; Dec. Time, E wave deceleration time; E, early LV filling velocity; $E_m$, early diastolic myocardial velocity; IVRT, isovolumic relaxation time; $PV_a$, pulmonary vein velocity resulting from atrial contraction; $PV_d$, diastolic pulmonary vein velocity; $PV_s$, systolic pulmonary vein velocity; $S_m$, systolic myocardial velocity. (Source: From Zile MR, Brutsart DL.. New concepts in diastolic dysfunction and diastolic heart failure: Part I. *Circulation.* 2002;105:1387–1393. With permission.)

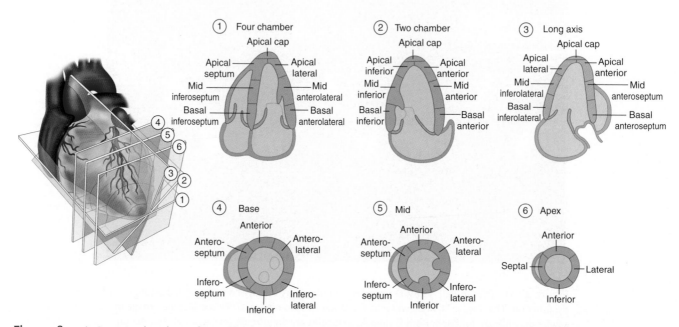

**Figure 48-13** A. Segmental analysis of LV walls based on schematic views, in a parasternal short- and long-axis orientation, at three different levels. The "apex segments" are usually visualized from apical 4-chamber, apical 2-, and 3-chamber views. The apical cap can only be appreciated on some contrast studies. A 16-segment model can be used, without the apical cap, as described in an ASE 1989 document. A 17-segment model, including the apical cap, has been suggested by the AHA Writing Group on Myocardial Segmentation and Registration for Cardiac Imaging. (Permission from Lang et al. 2005.)

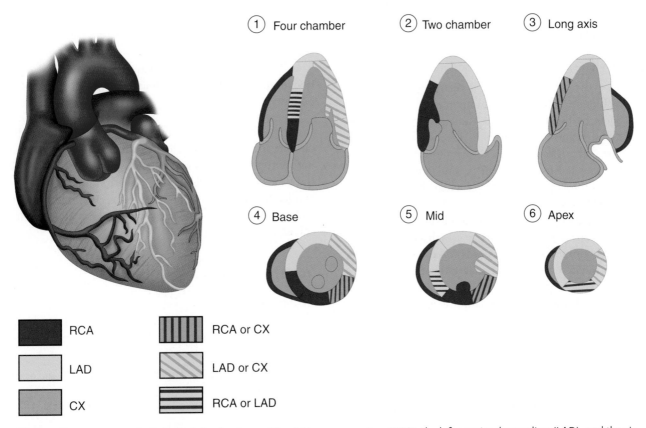

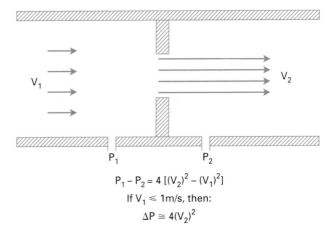

**Figure 48-13.** (continued) B. Typical distributions of the right coronary artery (RCA), the left anterior descending (LAD), and the circumflex (CX) coronary arteries. The arterial distribution varies between patients. Some segments have variable coronary perfusion.

## HEMODYNAMIC ASSESSMENT

### Pressure Gradients

When the blood is moving towards the transducer, the frequency of the ultrasound signal increases and the converse is also true. This property is used to derive severity of valvular stenosis because it is possible to correlate velocity with the pressure difference or the "pressure gradient" using the simplified Bernoulli equation

$$\delta P = 4V^2,$$

where $\delta P$ is the pressure gradient (in mm Hg) and V is peak blood velocity (in m/s) as meas3ured by the Doppler across the narrowing (**Figure 48-14**). In valve stenosis, the jet velocity can be used to determine peak instantaneous and mean pressure gradient across the valve. The mean pressure gradient is obtained by averaging the instantaneous gradients.

Advantages of this technique are:

    i. It measures instantaneous gradient, i.e., real-time, unlike the peak-to-peak gradient that is calculated from cardiac catheterization studies where the peak LV and peak aortic pressure gradients do not occur at the same time. The equation that describes the rela-

tionship between Doppler gradient and cardiac catheterization derived peak-to-peak gradient is:

$$P_1 - P_2 = 4\,[(V_2)^2 - (V_1)^2]$$

If $V_1 \leq 1\text{m/s}$, then:

$$\Delta P \cong 4(V_2)^2$$

**Figure 48-14.** The modified Bernoulli equation. Pressure drop across a small orifice can be estimated as four times the square of the peak velocity (if the proximal velocity is <1 m/sec). $V_1$ and $P_1$, proximal velocity and pressure; $V_2$ and $P_2$, distal velocity and pressure. (Source: Modified from Pearlman AS. Technique of Doppler and color flow Doppler in the evaluation of cardiac disorders and function. In: Schlant RC, Alexander RW, eds. The Heart, Arteries, and Veins, 8th ed. New York: McGraw-Hill; 1994:2229. With permission.)

Peak-to-peak gradient $\simeq$ (0.84 × peak Doppler gradient) − 14 mm Hg.

The main limitations of this technique are

i. That the blood velocity is a vector by the Doppler technique. Therefore, it is important that the transducer be lined up in such a manner that the ultrasound beam is parallel with direction of the blood flow; otherwise the peak velocity (and consequently the pressure gradient) can be underestimated. This limitation is particularly seen when the direction of blood flow is eccentric.

ii. With pulsed wave, Doppler blood velocity of <2m/s only can be examined, above which aliasing occurs and continuous Doppler needs to be used. However, continuous wave Doppler underestimates the velocity of an eccentric jet.

iii. Although the Doppler equation is fairly accurate in determining valve gradients across a tight stenosis, in aortic stenosis the phenomenon of pressure recovery may result in a larger gradient by Doppler when compared to cardiac catheterization, particularly when the distal pressure is measured several cm from valve. In clinical practice this error is not clinically significant.

Exceptions to this technique occur when:

i. velocity proximal to the stenosis is >1.5 m/s;

ii. two stenotic areas are proximal to each other, e.g., subpulmonic stenosis accompanied by valvular pulmonic stenosis;

iii. there is a tunnel-like extended stenotic lesion.

## Intracardiac Pressures

### Right-sided Pressures

When tricuspid regurgitation is present, the peak velocity of the regurgitant jet can be used to estimate the pressure gradient between the right atrium and right ventricle using the formula $4V^2$. Therefore,

$$RVSP = \text{Estimate of mean RA pressure} + \text{Peak RV} - \text{RA gradient}$$

where mean RA = magnitude of the inferior vena cava (IVC) collapse with inspiration and variation in hepatic vein velocities.

In the absence of pulmonary stenosis,

$$PASP = \text{peak RVSP.}$$

In the presence of pulmonary stenosis,

$$PASP = RVSP - \text{maximal pulmonary valve pressure gradient.}$$

The latter is derived from velocity across the pulmonary valve by continuous wave Doppler.

The PA diastolic pressure is derived using the $4V^2$ equation from the velocity of pulmonary regurgitation (when present).

In the presence of significant pulmonary hypertension, RV outflow and pulmonary velocities are often altered, including shorter acceleration times and a mid-systolic notch in the flow velocity envelope. The relationship between the acceleration time and mean PA pressures is curvilinear with wide confidence limits making accurate estimates for clinical use unreliable.

## Volumetric Flow

### Stroke Volume

The preferred sites for determining stroke volume (SV) and cardiac output in descending order of preference are:

1. Left ventricular outflow tract (LVOT) or aortic annulus
2. Mitral annulus

$$SV = CSA \times VTI$$

where CSA is cross-sectional area and VTI is velocity time integral. Cross-sectional area of the aortic annulus is calculated (using $\pi r^2$ formula for area of circle), with annulus diameter D measured in the parasternal long-axis view (the largest of 3 to 5 measurements should be taken because, typically, annulus diameters tend to be underestimated in this tomographic plane).

$$CSA = D^2 \times \pi/4 = D^2 \times 0.785$$

The LVOT velocity is recorded using apical 5-chamber or long-axis view with the sample volume positioned about 5 mm proximal to the aortic valve. To derive VTI, it is best to trace the outer edge of the densest or brightest portion of the spectral tracing and ignore the dispersion that occurs near peak velocity. In sinus rhythm, an average of 3 to 5 tracings is adequate, but in irregular rhythms such as atrial fibrillation 5 to 10 cycles may be needed to derive an accurate value.

# VALVE AREAS

## Valve Areas Using the Continuity Equation

The continuity equation (**Figure 48-15**) states that the blood flow passing through a stenotic valve is equal to the flow proximal to the stenosis.

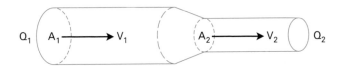

$$(A_1) = \pi r^2 = \pi \left(\frac{D}{2}\right)^2 = 0.785 \, (D^2)$$

$$(A_2)(V_2) = (A_1)(V_1) \text{ or } (A_2) = \frac{(A_1)(V_1)}{(V_2)}$$

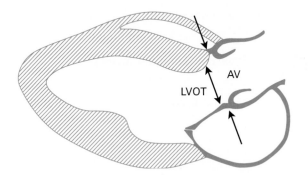

**Figure 48-15.** The continuity equation. In a closed system (top) with constant flow, $Q_1 = Q_2$. Therefore, $A_1 \times V_1$ must equal $A_2 \times V_2$. Determination of any three of the variables allows calculation of the fourth. Clinically (*bottom*), the area of the left ventricular outflow tract (*LVOT*) can be estimated and used to determine AoV area. AoV, aortic valve. (Source: From Hagan AD, DeMarial AN. Clinical Applications of Two-Dimensional Echocardiography and Cardiac Doppler. Boston: Little, Brown; 1989. With permission.)

Since flow = velocity × CSA, if the flow is known the area of stenosis can be determined using the equation

Stenotic area = Flow/Velocity across the stenosis.

The continuity equation is typically used in assessing aortic stenosis. In mitral stenosis the continuity equation is useful when the pressure half-time method is limited. However, determining flow across the mitral valve is difficult, therefore, this is measured at the aortic annulus and is used as a numerator of the equation. The denominator is the integral of mitral stenosis jet. In the absence of accompanying mitral regurgitation, this method is fairly accurate in estimating the severity of mitral stenosis

## Valve Areas Using the Pressure Half-time Method

This method is an accurate method to determine the severity of mitral stenosis (**Figure 48-16**).

Mitral valve area = 220/Pressure half-time

Pressure half-time is the duration for maximal pressure gradient to decrease by half. When velocity is used to express this quantity, it is the time that the peak stenotic velocity decreases by 30%.

Potential source of errors in calculating stenotic velocity are tachycardia, presence of severe aortic regurgitation and conditions that impact left atrial or left ventricular compliance, and/or LV relaxation. Occasionally, in mitral stenosis the early velocity descent is a ski-slope and in such cases the pressure half-time is derived by extrapolating the mid-diastolic linear descent backward, as shown in **Figure 48-17**).

The pressure half-time method has not yet been validated in calculation of tricuspid valve area.

# MURMURS

## ACC/AHA Guidelines on Echocardiography for Murmurs

A transthoracic echocardiogram with color flow and spectral Doppler is important in the evaluation of cardiac murmurs. Important information on valve structure and function,

### ACC/AHA Recommendations for Echocardiography in Patients with Murmurs

**Class I: Evidence or general agreement or both exists that the procedure is useful and beneficial**

1. Echocardiography is recommended for asymptomatic patients with diastolic murmurs, continuous murmurs, holosystolic murmurs, late systolic murmurs, murmurs associated with ejection clicks, or murmurs that radiate to the neck or back. (Level of Evidence: C)

2. Echocardiography is recommended for patients with heart murmurs and symptoms or signs of heart failure, myocardial ischemia/infarction, syncope, thromboembolism, infective endocarditis, or other clinical evidence of structural heart disease. (Level of Evidence: C)

3. Echocardiography is recommended for asymptomatic patients who have grade 3 or louder midpeaking systolic murmurs. (Level of Evidence: C)

**Class IIa: Weight of evidence/opinion in favor of usefulness/efficacy:**

1. Echocardiography can be useful for the evaluation of asymptomatic patients with murmurs associated with other abnormal cardiac physical findings or murmurs associated with an abnormal ECG or chest X-ray. (Level of Evidence: C)

2. Echocardiography can be useful for patients whose symptoms and/or signs are likely noncardiac in origin but in whom a cardiac basis cannot be excluded by standard evaluation. (Level of Evidence: C)

**Class III: Conditions for which evidence and/or general agreement exist that the procedure is not useful/effective:**

Echocardiography is not recommended for patients who have a grade 2 or softer mid-systolic murmur identified as innocent or functional by an experienced observer. (Level of Evidence: C)

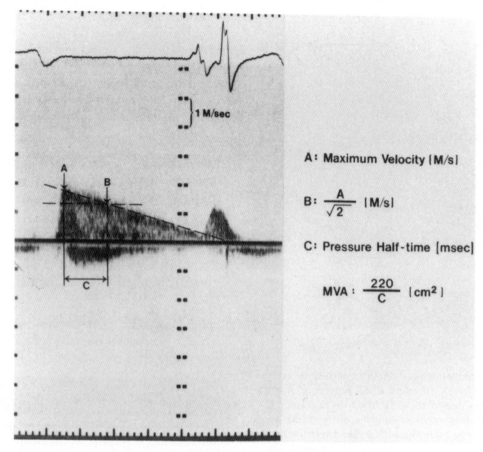

**1 M/sec**

**A:** Maximum Velocity [M/s]

**B:** $\dfrac{A}{\sqrt{2}}$ [M/s]

**C:** Pressure Half-time [msec]

**MVA :** $\dfrac{220}{C}$ [cm²]

**Figure 48-16.** Pressure half-time method for calculation of mitral valve area (MVA). (Source: From Hagan AD, DeMaria AN. Clinical Applications of Two-Dimensional Echocardiography and Cardiac Doppler. Boston: Little, Brown; 1989. With permission.)

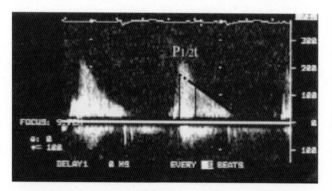

**Figure 48-17.** CW Doppler recording of transmitral velocity in a patient with mitral stenosis. Velocity pattern shows rapid early deceleration that decelerates to mid-diastole, giving rise to "ski slope" appearance. In these cases, estimating pressure half-time from the slower component of velocity descent is better, as illustrated in second cardiac cycle. (From Quinones et al. Recommendations for Quantification of Doppler Echocardiography: A Report From the Doppler Quantification Task Force of the Nomenclature and Standards Committee of the American Society of Echocardiography. *J Am Soc Echocardiogr.* 2002;15:167–84.)

chamber size, wall thickness, ventricular function, pulmonary and hepatic vein flow, and estimates of pulmonary artery pressures can be determined using transthoracic echocardiography (TTE). However, such testing may not be necessary for all patients with cardiac murmurs and usually does not add much in the evaluation of asymptomatic younger patients with short grade 1 to 2 mid-systolic murmurs and otherwise normal physical findings. On the other hand, there are patients with heart murmurs where transthoracic echocardiography may not be adequate, who instead require transesophageal echocardiography (TEE), cardiac magnetic resonance, or cardiac catheterization for better characterization of the valvular lesion.

One important point is that Doppler echocardiography is sensitive and may detect trace or mild valvular regurgitation through structurally normal tricuspid and pulmonic valves in a substantial number of young, healthy individuals and through normal left-sided valves (particularly the mitral valve) in a variable but lower percentage of patients.

# VALVULAR DISORDERS

## Mitral Stenosis

According to the ACC/AHA Guidelines, 2D and Doppler echocardiography are the diagnostic tools of choice for the assessment of mitral stenosis (MS) because the following is true of 2D-echocardiography (**Figure 48-18**):

1. It is able to identify restricted diastolic opening of the MV leaflets due to "doming" of the anterior leaflet and immobility of the posterior leaflet. Other entities that can simulate the clinical features of rheumatic MS, such as left atrial myxoma, mucopolysaccharidosis, nonrheumatic calcific MS, cor triatriatum, and a parachute MV, can be readily identified by 2D echocardiography.

2. With planimetry of the orifice area may be possible using the short-axis view.

3. It can be used to assess the morphological appearance of the MV apparatus (including leaflet mobility and flexibility, leaflet thickness, leaflet calcification, subvalvular fusion, and the appearance of commissures). These features may be important for the timing and type of intervention to be conducted. Patients with mobile noncalcified leaflets, no commissural calcification, and little subvalvular fusion may be candidates for either

balloon catheter or surgical commissurotomy/valvotomy. Wilkins score (an echocardiographic grouping based on valve flexibility, subvalvular fusion, and leaflet calcification, and the absence or presence of commissural calcium) (**Table 48-3**) is one of the methods used to assess suitability for balloon commissurotomy.

4. can be used to determine chamber size and function and other structural valvular, myocardial, or pericardial abnormalities

Doppler echocardiography can be used to:

i. determine the hemodynamic severity of the obstruction. The mean transmitral gradient can be accurately and reproducibly measured from the continuous-wave;

ii. non-invasively derive the mitral valve area using the diastolic pressure half time method (from modified Bernoulli equation) or the continuity equation. The half-time method may be inaccurate in patients with abnormalities of left atrial or LV compliance, those with associated AR, and those who have had mitral valvotomy;

iii. estimate pulmonary artery systolic pressure from the tricuspid regurgitation (TR) velocity signal; and

iv. assess severity of concomitant MR or AR;

v. determine transmitral and tricuspid velocities on exercise with formal noninvasive hemodynamic exercise testing with either a supine bicycle or upright treadmill with Doppler recordings of transmitral and tricuspid velocities. This provides measurement of both the transmitral gradient and pulmonary artery systolic pressure at rest and with exercise.

The criteria for the assessment of the severity of MS are summarized in **Table 48-4**. These criteria are applicable when heart rate is between 60 and 90 bpm.

## Mitral Regurgitation

### Acute Severe Mitral Regurgitation

In acute severe mitral regurgitation (MR), transthoracic echocardiography (TTE):

i. may demonstrate the disruption of the MV; and

ii. help provide semiquantitative information on lesion severity; however, TTE may underestimate lesion severity by inadequate imaging of the color flow jet. *Therefore, when there is hyperdynamic LV systolic function on TTE in acute heart failure, severe MR should be suspected.*

Transesophageal echocardiography (TEE) is performed in acute severe MR:

i. when the MV morphology and regurgitant severity remain in question after TTE; and

ii. to determine the anatomic etiology of acute severe MR and direct successful surgical repair.

---

**Indications for Transthoracic Echocardiography in Mitral Stenosis**

**Class I: Evidence or general agreement or both exists that the procedure is useful and beneficial**

1. Echocardiography should be performed in patients for the diagnosis of mitral stenosis (MS), assessment of hemodynamic severity (mean gradient, MV area, and pulmonary artery pressure), assessment of concomitant valvular lesions, and assessment of valve morphology (to determine suitability for percutaneous mitral balloon valvotomy). (Level of Evidence: B)

2. Echocardiography should be performed for reevaluation in patients with known MS and changing symptoms or signs. (Level of Evidence: B)

3. Echocardiography should be performed for assessment of the hemodynamic response of the mean gradient and pulmonary artery pressure by exercise Doppler echocardiography in patients with MS when there is a discrepancy between resting Doppler echocardiographic findings, clinical findings, symptoms, and signs. (Level of Evidence: C)

**Class IIa: Weight of evidence/opinion in favor of usefulness/efficacy**

Echocardiography is reasonable in the reevaluation of asymptomatic patients with MS and stable clinical findings to assess pulmonary artery pressure (for those with severe MS, every year; moderate MS, every 1 to 2 years; and mild MS, every 3 to 5 years). (Level of Evidence: C)

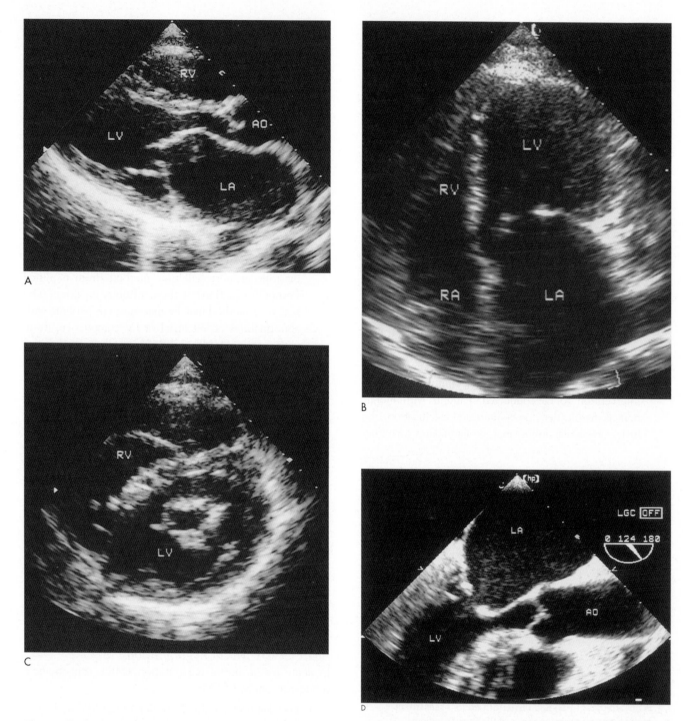

**Figure 48-18.** A. Parasternal long-axis view of MS. The LA is enlarged, mitral opening is limited, and *doming* of the anterior mitral leaflet is present. B. Apical four-chamber view in mitral stenosis. The LA is markedly dilated. C. Parasternal short-axis plane in mitral stenosis. D. Transesophageal image showing doming of the anterior mitral valve leaflet. Ao, aorta; LA, left atrium; LV, left ventricle; MS, mitral stenosis; RA, right atrium; RV, right ventricle.

### Table 48-3 • Wilkins Score

| Grade | Mobility | Subvalvular Thickening | Thickening | Calcification |
|---|---|---|---|---|
| 1 | Highly mobile value only leaflet tips restricted | Minimal thickening just below the mitral leaflets | Leaflets near normal in thickness (4 to 5 mm) | A single area of increased echo brightness |
| 2 | Leaflets mid and base portions have normal mobility | Thickening of chordal structures extending up to one third of the chordal length | Midleaflets normal, considerable thickening of margins (5 to 8 mm) | Scattered areas of brightness confined to leaflets margins |
| 3 | Value continues to move forward in diastole, mainly from the base | Thickening extending to the distal third of the chords | Thickening extending through the entire leaflets (5 to 8 mm) | Brightness extending into the midportion of the leaflets |
| 4 | No or minimal forward movement of the leaflets in diastole | Extensive thickening and shortening of all chordal structures extending down to the papillary muscles | Considerable thickening of all leaflets tissue (greater than 8 to 10 mm) | Extensive brightness throughout much of the leaflet tissue |

*Reprinted with permission from Wilkins GT, Weyman AE, Abascal VM, Block PC, Palacios IF. Percutaneous balloon dilatation of the mitral values an analysis of echocardiographic variables related to outcome and the mechanism of dilatation. Br Heart J. 1988;60:299–308(400). Adapted from Brown etal.*

### Table 48-4 • Severity of Mitral Stenosis

| | Mild | Moderate | Severe |
|---|---|---|---|
| Mean gradient (mm Hg)* | Less than 5 | 5–10 | Greater than 10 |
| Pulmonary artery systolic pressure (mm Hg) | Less than 30 | 30–50 | Greater than 50 |
| Valve area (cm²) | Greater than 1.5 | 1.0–1.5 | Less than 1.0 |

*Adapted from Bonow etal.*

## Chronic Mitral Regurgitation

An initial 2D Doppler echocardiogram is indispensable in the management of the patient with chronic MR. The echocardiogram provides:

  i. a baseline estimation of LV and left atrial size;
  ii. an estimation of LV ejection fraction; and
  iii. approximation of the severity of regurgitation quantification of the severity of MR (**Table 48-5**), as recommended by ACC/AHA Guidelines.
  v. an estimate of RVSP can be obtained from the TR peak velocity.

Changes from these baseline values are subsequently used to guide the timing of MV surgery.

The BP at the time of each study should be documented, because the afterload on the ventricle will affect the measured severity of the MR.

The initial TTE should disclose the anatomic etiology of the MR:

  i. A central color flow jet of MR with a structurally normal MV apparatus suggests the presence of functional

### Indications for Transthoracic Echocardiography in Mitral Regurgitation

**Class I: Evidence or general agreement or both exists that the procedure is useful and beneficial**

1. Transthoracic echocardiography is indicated for baseline evaluation of LV size and function, RV and left atrial size, pulmonary artery pressure, and severity of MR in any patient suspected of having MR. (Level of Evidence: C)

2. Transthoracic echocardiography is indicated for delineation of the mechanism of MR. (Level of Evidence: B)

3. Transthoracic echocardiography is indicated for annual or semiannual surveillance of LV function (estimated by ejection fraction and end-systolic dimension) in asymptomatic patients with moderate to severe MR. (Level of Evidence: C)

4. Transthoracic echocardiography is indicated in patients with MR to evaluate the MV apparatus and LV function after a change in signs or symptoms. (Level of Evidence: C)

5. Transthoracic echocardiography is indicated to evaluate LV size and function and MV hemodynamics in the initial evaluation after MV replacement or MV repair. (Level of Evidence: C)

**Class IIa: Weight of evidence/opinion in favor of usefulness/efficacy**

Exercise Doppler echocardiography is reasonable in asymptomatic patients with severe MR to assess exercise tolerance and the effects of exercise on pulmonary artery pressure and MR severity. (Level of Evidence: C)

**Class III: Conditions for which evidence and/or general agreement exist that the procedure is not useful/effective**

Transthoracic echocardiography is not indicated for routine follow-up evaluation of asymptomatic patients with mild MR and normal LV size and systolic function. (Level of Evidence: C)

### Table 48-5 • Severity of Mitral Regurgitation

| | Mitral Regurgitation | | |
| --- | --- | --- | --- |
| | **Mild** | **Moderate** | **Severe** |
| **Qualitative** | 1+ | 2+ | 3–4+ |
| Angiographic grade | | | |
| Color Doppler jet area | Small, central jet (less than 4 cm² or less than 20% LA area) | Signs of MR greater than mild present but no criteria for severe MR | Vena contracta width greater than 0.7 cm with large central MR jet (area greater than 40% of LA area) or with a wall-impinging jet of any size, swirling in LA |
| Doppler vena contracta width (cm) | Less than 0.3 | 0.3–0.69 | Greater than or equal to 0.70 |
| **Quantitative (cath or echo)** | Less than 30 | 30–50 | Greater than or equal to 60 |
| Regurgitant volume (mL per beat) | Less than 30 | 30–49 | Greater than or equal to 50 |
| Regurgitant fraction (%) | Less than 0.20 | 0.2–0.39 | Greater than or equal to 0.40 |
| Regurgitant orifice area (cm²) | | | |
| **Additional essential criteria** | | | |
| left atrial size | | | Enlarged |
| Left ventricular size | | | Enlarged |

*Adapted from Bonow et al.*

MR, which may be due to annular dilatation from LV dilatation or tethering of the posterior leaflet because of regional LV dysfunction in patients with ischemic heart disease.

ii. An eccentric color flow jet of MR with abnormalities of the MV apparatus indicates organic MR. In patients with organic MR, the echocardiogram should assess the presence of calcium in the annulus or leaflets, the redundancy of the valve leaflets, and the MV leaflet involved (anterior leaflet, posterior leaflet, or bileaflet). These factors will help determine the feasibility of valve repair if surgery is contemplated. The system proposed by Carpentier.

The anatomic and physiologic characteristics of the mitral valve help the surgeon plan the repair. Valve dysfunction is described on the basis of the motion of the free edge of the leaflet relative to the plane of the annulus (Carpentier's classification):

i. type I, normal;
ii. type II, increased, as in MVP;
iii. type IIIA, restricted during systole and diastole; and type IIIB, restricted during systole.

Multiple indicators from the Doppler examination should be used to diagnose severe MR, including the

i. color flow jet width and area;
ii. the intensity of the continuous-wave Doppler signal;
iii. the pulmonary venous flow contour;
iv. the peak early mitral inflow velocity; and
v. quantitative measures of effective orifice area and regurgitation volume (**Figure 48-19**).

In addition, there should be enlargement of the left ventricle and left atrium in chronic severe MR.

When there is discrepancy (e.g., severe MR versus ischemic MR), or if the patient has poor images on TTE, then further assessment of the severity of MR may be done using cardiac catheterization, MRI, or TEE.

## Aortic Stenosis

Echocardiography is indicated when there are symptoms that are suggestive of aortic stenosis (AS) or the presence of a systolic murmur that is grade 3/6 or greater or a single S2. Two-dimensional echocardiography (**Figure 48-20**) is valuable for evaluation of valve anatomy and function and determining the LV response to pressure overload. Doppler echocardiographic measurements of maximum jet velocity, mean transvalvular pressure gradient, and continuity equation valve area to determine the severity of aortic stenosis can be obtained in almost all patients.

Doppler evaluation of AS severity (**Table 48-6**) requires meticulous attention to technical details, with the commonest error being underestimation of disease severity due to a nonparallel intercept angle between the ultrasound beam and high-velocity jet through the narrowed valve. When measurement of LV outflow tract diameter is difficult to obtain, the ratio of outflow tract velocity to aortic jet velocity can be substituted for valve area, because this ratio is, in effect, indexed for body size. A ratio range from 0.9 to 1.0 is normal, with a ratio less than 0.25 indicating severe stenosis. Echocardiography is also used to determine LV size

valve disease. Mitral valve area can be measured accurately by the half-time method in mixed MS/MR.

- Aortic valve area would be measured inaccurately at the time of cardiac catheterization in mixed AS/AR if cardiac output were measured by either thermodilution or the Fick method. The valve area can be determined more reliably by the continuity equation from Doppler echocardiography in mixed AS/AR; however, the continuity equation calculation of valve area may not be completely independent of flow.

- Although valve area measurements by Doppler echocardiography are more accurate than those obtained at cardiac catheterization, *in general, the confusing nature of mixed valve disease makes cardiac catheterization necessary to obtain additional hemodynamic information in most patients.*

## Prosthetic Heart Valves (Figures 48-23 and 48-24)

According to ACC/AHA Guidelines, TTE is done, preferably, before TEE because great additional information can be obtained regarding cardiac function and hemodynamics by TTE that may not be otherwise available and/or may help guide the TEE.

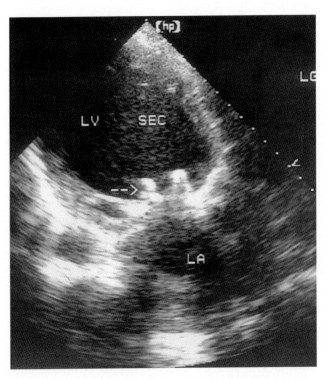

**Figure 48-24.** Apical view of a bioprosthetic valve (*arrow*) in the mitral position (two of the three prosthetic valve struts are apparent). Spontaneous echo contrast (*SEC*) is also present, secondary to systolic dysfunction and enlargement of the LV. LA, left atrium; LV, left ventricle.

Echocardiography is the preferred imaging modality for:

1. definition of abnormalities of poppet motion, annular motion;
2. the presence of thrombus or fibrin; or
3. prosthetic leaks; or
4. stenoses.

Prosthetic valve stenosis: Assessment should include Doppler technique; however, Doppler has limitations because eccentric jets may cause recording of falsely low velocities, especially in valves with central occluders. On the other hand, elevated transvalvular velocities may be seen in some small-sized prosthetic valves (especially bileaflet valves) due to pressure recovery and may not accurately represent the hemodynamic gradient. It is important to keep in mind that transvalvular gradients vary with valve type, flow, size, and heart rate, even in the normally functioning prosthesis; individual valve flow characteristics must be considered in the diagnosis of obstruction. Reevaluation is often helpful in the individual patient.

Prosthetic valve regurgitation: All prosthetic valves have some "in-built" regurgitation. Assessment of prosthetic valve regurgitation is often limited by prosthetic shadowing, particularly in the mitral position. Transthoracic Doppler and color are therefore less sensitive for detecting prosthetic valve regurgitation. TEE is particularly useful in such instances. Mechanical St. Jude's valve in the mitral position displaying

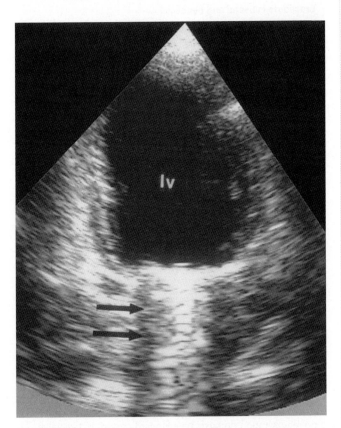

**Figure 48-23.** Apical two-chamber view of a mechanical prosthetic valve (mitral position) during systole. The LA is completely obscured by ultrasonic shadowing (*arrows*). LA, left atrium; LV, left ventricle.

a peak early velocity of >1.9 m/s without signs of obstruction is 90% sensitive and 89% specific for significant valvular regurgitation. Regurgitation of prosthetic valve in the aortic position is readily detected by transthoracic Doppler echocardiography. It is important to differentiate between the normal, central regurgitation of many mechanical prostheses and pathological paravalvular leaks. Utilization of contrast may enhance the spectral recording of both right-sided regurgitant velocities as well as the extent of the regurgitant jet.

Prosthetic valve endocarditis: Because of the reverberations, attenuation, and other image artifacts related to both mechanical valves and bioprostheses, diagnosis of prosthetic valve endocarditis by the TEE is more difficult than diagnosis of endocarditis of native valves. TTE may be helpful only when there is a large or mobile vegetation or significant regurgitation in the case of mechanical valves. Thus, TTE cannot be used to exclude the presence of small vegetations and TEE with the superior imaging quality and posterior transducer position is preferred for the assessment of prosthetic valve infective endocarditis, especially of the mitral valve and of both mitral and aortic annular areas for abscesses. Doppler techniques offer important information about the functional consequences of endocarditis of prosthetic valves, such as the existence of paravalvular leaks. It should be noted, however, that paravalvular leaks are not specific for endocarditis. Importantly, echocardiography may identify vegetations on native valves in patients with suspected prosthetic endocarditis.

# CHEST PAIN

| Indications for Echocardiography in Patients with Chest Pain |
| --- |
| **Class I: Evidence or general agreement or both exists that the procedure is useful or beneficial** |
| 1. Diagnosis of underlying cardiac disease in patients with chest pain and clinical evidence of valvular, pericardial, or primary myocardial disease |
| 2. Evaluation of chest pain in patients with suspected acute myocardial ischemia, when baseline ECG is nondiagnostic and when study can be obtained during pain or soon after its abatement |
| 3. Evaluation of chest pain in patients with suspected aortic dissection |
| 4. Chest pain in patients with severe hemodynamic instability |
| **Class III: Conditions for which evidence and/or general agreement exist that the procedure is not useful/effective** |
| 1. Evaluation of chest pain for which a noncardiac etiology is apparent Figure 48–22 |
| 2. Diagnosis of chest pain in a patient with electrocardiographic changes diagnostic of myocardial ischemia/infarction Chetlin et al. ACC/AHA Guidelines for the Clinical Application of Echocardiography. *Circulation.* 1997;95. |

# HYPERTROPHIC CARDIOMYOPATHY

**Hypertrophic cardiomyopathy** (HCM) is myocardial hypertrophy in the absence of a causative condition and is thought to be derived from genetic mutations that result in alterations in the cardiac myofilament. HCM is associated with marked genotypic, phenotypic, and clinical heterogeneity. Hypertrophy of the ventricular septum is the most common form of hypertrophy, with mid-ventricular and apical forms of hypertrophy being far less common. The pattern of ventricular septal hypertrophy is highly variable and can be divided into the morphological subtypes: reverse curvature, sigmoid, and neutral (**Figure 48-25**).

## Infective Endocarditis (Figure 48-26)

Echocardiography is useful for the detection and characterization of the hemodynamic and pathological consequences of infection. These include

- valvular vegetations;
- valvular regurgitation;

| ACC/AHA Guidelines Regarding Endocarditis in TTE |
| --- |
| **Class I: Evidence or general agreement or both exists that the procedure is useful and beneficial** |
| 1. TTE to detect valvular vegetations with or without positive blood cultures is recommended for the diagnosis of infective endocarditis. (Level of Evidence: B) |
| 2. TTE is recommended to characterize the hemodynamic severity of valvular lesions in known infective endocarditis. (Level of Evidence: B) |
| 3. TTE is recommended for assessment of complications of infective endocarditis (e.g., abscesses, perforation, and shunts). (Level of Evidence: B) |
| 4. TTE is recommended for reassessment of high risk patients (e.g., those with a virulent organism, clinical deterioration, persistent or recurrent fever, new murmur, or persistent bacteremia). (Level of Evidence: C) |
| **Class IIa: Weight of evidence/opinion in favor of usefulness/efficacy** |
| TTE is reasonable to diagnose infective endocarditis of a prosthetic valve in the presence of persistent fever without bacteremia or a new murmur. (Level of Evidence: C) |
| **Class IIb: Usefulness/efficacy is less well-established by evidence/opinion** |
| TTE may be considered for the reevaluation of prosthetic valve endocarditis during antibiotic therapy in the absence of clinical deterioration. (Level of Evidence: C) |
| **Class III: Conditions for which evidence and/or general agreement exist that the procedure is not useful/effective** |
| TTE is not indicated to reevaluate uncomplicated (including no regurgitation on baseline echocardiogram) native valve endocarditis during antibiotic treatment in the absence of clinical deterioration, new physical findings or persistent fever. (Level of Evidence: C) |

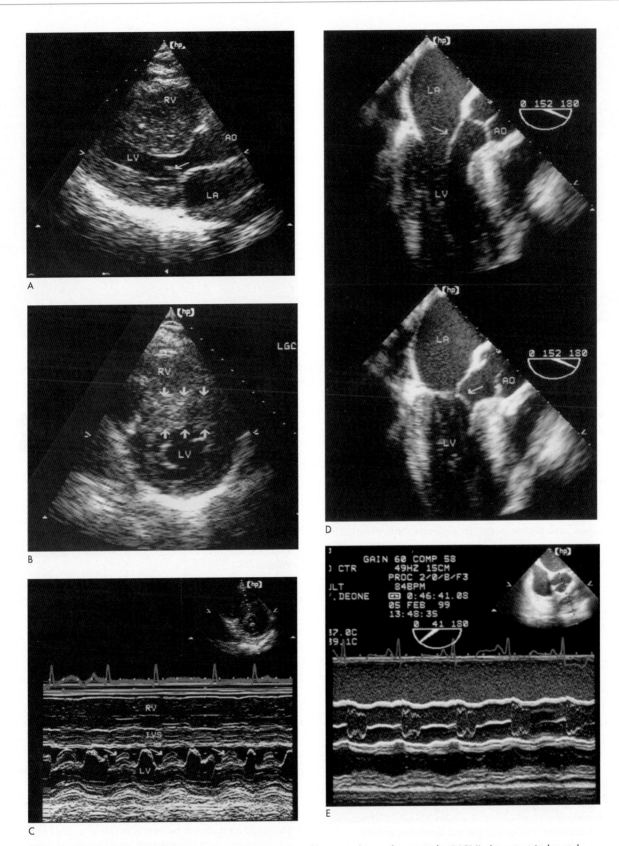

**Figure 48-25.** A. Parasternal long-axis view (during systole) of hypertrophic cardiomyopathy (HCM). Asymmetrical septal hypertrophy is present, as is systolic anterior motion of the anterior mitral valve leaflet (*arrow*). B. Parasternal short-axis view of HCM. Asymmetrical septal hypertrophy is present (*arrows*). C. Parasternal M-mode image from a patient with HCM, demonstrating systolic anterior motion of the anterior mitral valve leaflet (*arrows*). D. Transesophageal image of HCM. The aMVL appears normal during diastole (*upper panel*), but systolic anterior motion occurs during systole (*lower panel*). E. Transesophageal M-mode tracing through the AoV. Midsystolic notching and partial closure of the valve leaflets is present. aMVL, anterior mitral valve leaflet; Ao, aorta; AoV, aortic valve; IVS, interventricular septum; LA, left atrium; LV, left ventricle; RV, right ventricle.

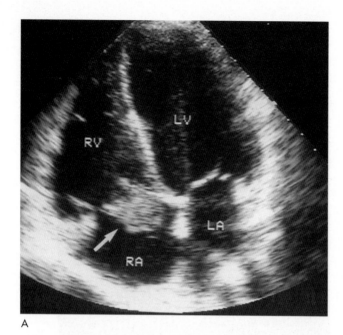

A

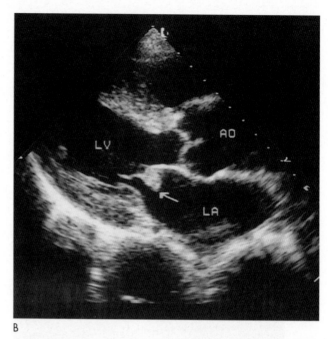

B

**Figure 48-26.** A. Apical four-chamber view demonstrating a large tricuspid valve vegetation (*arrow*). B. Parasternal long axis view demonstrating a vegetation (*arrow*) on the anterior valve leaflet; Ao, aorta; LA, left atrium; LV, left ventricle; RA, right atrium; RV, right ventricle.

- LV dysfunction; and
- associated lesions such as abscesses, shunts, and ruptured chordate.

TEE is more sensitive in detecting vegetations than TTE (especially in patients with prosthetic valves) and in determining the presence and severity of complications such as abscesses and perforations. In patients with prosthetic valves, it is reasonable to proceed directly to TEE as the first-line diagnostic test when endocarditis is suspected.

Echocardiography may be useful in the case of culture-negative endocarditis or when the source remains unclear in persistent bacteremia.

## Pericardial Disease

The pericardium typically responds to injury or disease by inflammation, which may result in an exudate (leading to pericardial effusion with or without tamponade or constriction) or thickening.

### Indications for Echocardiography in Pericardial Disease

**Class I Indications: Evidence or general agreement or both exists that the procedure is useful and beneficial**

1. Patients with suspected pericardial disease, including effusion, constriction, or effusive-constrictive process
2. Patients with suspected bleeding in the pericardial space, e.g., trauma, perforation, etc.

### Indications for Echocardiography in Pericardial Disease (continued)

3. Follow-up study to evaluate recurrence of effusion or to diagnose early constriction. Repeat studies may be goal directed to answer a specific clinical question
4. Pericardial friction rub developing in acute myocardial infarction accompanied by symptoms such as persistent pain, hypotension, and nausea

**Class IIa: Weight of evidence/opinion in favor of usefulness/efficacy**

5. Follow-up studies to detect early signs of tamponade in the presence of large or rapidly accumulating effusions. A goal-directed study may be appropriate.
6. Echocardiographic guidance and monitoring of pericardiocentesis

**Class II b**

7. Postsurgical pericardial disease, including postpericardiotomy syndrome, with potential for hemodynamic impairment
8. In the presence of a strong clinical suspicion and nondiagnostic TTE, TEE assessment of pericardial thickness to support a diagnosis of constrictive pericarditis

**Class III: Conditions for which evidence and/or general agreement exist that the procedure is not useful/effective Recommendations**

9. Routine follow-up of small pericardial effusion in clinically stable patients
10. Follow-up studies in patients with cancer or other terminal illness for whom management would not be influenced by echocardiographic findings
11. Assessment of pericardial thickness in patients without clinical evidence of constrictive pericarditis
12. Pericardial friction rub in early uncomplicated myocardial infarction or early postoperative period after cardiac surgery

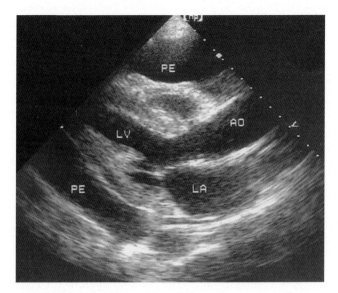

**Figure 48-27.** Large pericardial effusion (*PE*) on parasternal long-axis imaging.

## Pericardial Effusion (Figure 48-27)

Echocardiography is the procedure of choice for evaluating pericardial effusion—it provides semiquantitative assessment and qualitative information of the condition's distribution. The "echo-free" space seen around the heart in pericardial effusion can also be seen with focal epicardial fat. TTE is useful in pericardiocentesis, and TEE can be used when surface views are inadequate. Loculated effusions are often seen post-op and the classic signs of tamponade may not be apparent. In such instances elevated filling pressure and small chamber size suggests pericardial tamponade.

## Pericardial Tamponade (Figure 48-28)

As pericardial effusions increase in size they may cause tamponade. Echocardiographic signs of pericardial effusion often precede clinical signs. Signs of hemodynamic compromise in pericardial tamponade include right atrial invagination or collapse at the onset the onset of X descent and RV collapse in diastole. Although right atrial collapse is a sensitive sign of increased pressure in the pericardial space, diastolic RV collapse is more specific for hemodynamic compromise in pericardial tamponade. Doppler signs of pericardial tamponade include marked respiratory variation in transvalvular flow velocities (**Figure 48-28**), LV ejection, and LV isovolumic times. Other signs include distension of inferior vena cava that does not diminish on deep inspiration.

## Constrictive Pericarditis

There is no single echocardiographic sign diagnostic of constrictive pericarditis—a combination of echocardiographic and Doppler studies along with clinical features usually indicates the diagnosis of constrictive pericarditis. Echocardiographic signs include thickening of the pericardium, dilatation of the vena cava, flattening of LV endocardial motion in mid and late diastole, abnormalities of septal motion, mild left atrium enlargement with normal-sized left ventricle, and premature opening of the pulmonary valve. Doppler findings that support constriction include respiratory variations in flow velocities across the atrioventricular valves as well as across the LV outflow and pulmonary venous flow.

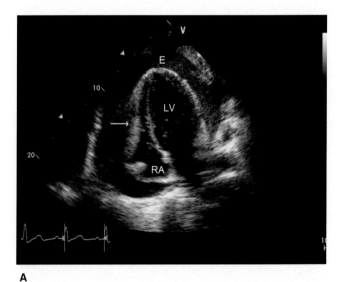

**A**

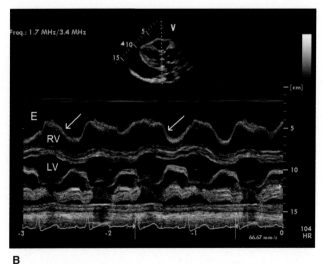

**B**

**Figure 48-28.** A. RV compression (*arrow*) in cardiac tamponade (apical 4-chamber plane). A. M-mode image of cardiac tamponade and right ventricular diastolic collapse. The *RV* free wall (*arrows*) moves posteriorly toward the interventricular septum during diastole. Ao, aorta; E, effusion; LA, left atrium; LV, left ventricle; RV, right ventricle.

# THORACIC AORTA

The entire thoracic aorta can be visualized with echocardiography in most adults. Complete aortic visualization by combined transthoracic imaging (left and right parasternal, suprasternal, supraclavicular, and subcostal windows) and TEE frequently can be achieved. High-resolution images of the aortic root, the ascending aorta, and the descending thoracic and upper abdominal aorta can be obtained by TEE. A part of the aorta that cannot be visualized with echocardiography is a small segment of the upper ascending portion adjacent to the tracheobronchial tree.

# ACKNOWLEDGEMENT

This chapter contains test verbatim from publications cited

## Suggested Readings

1. Bonow RO, Carabello BA, Chatterjee K, et al. ACC/AHA 2006 Guidelines for the Management of Patients with Valvular Heart Disease: A Report of the American College of Cardiology/American Heart Association Task Force on Practice Guidelines (Writing Committee to Revise the 1998 Guidelines for the Management of Patients with Valvular Heart Disease) developed in collaboration with the Society of Cardiovascular Anesthesiologists endorsed by the Society for Cardiovascular Angiography and Interventions and the Society of Thoracic Surgeons. *J Am Coll Cardiol.* 2006;48(3):e1–148.

2. Lang et al. Recommendations for chamber quantification: a report from the American Society of Echocardiography's Guidelines and Standards Committee and the Chamber Quantification Writing Group, developed in conjunction with the European Association of Echocardiography, a branch of the European Society of Cardiology. *J Am Soc of Echocardiogr.* 2005;18(12):1440–1463.

3. Cheitlin MD, Armstrong WF, Aurigemma GP, Beller GA, et al. ACC/AHA/ASE 2003 guideline update for the clinical application of echocardiography-summary article: a report of the American College of Cardiology/American Heart Association Task Force on Practice Guidelines (ACC/AHA/ASE Committee to Update the 1997 Guidelines for the Clinical Application of Echocardiography). *J Am Coll Cardiol.* 2003;42(5):954–970.

4. Cheitlin MD, Alpert JS, Armstrong WF, et al. ACC/AHA guidelines for the clinical application of echocardiography: executive summary. A report of the American College of Cardiology/American Heart Association Task Force on practice guidelines (Committee on Clinical Application of Echocardiography). Developed in collaboration with the American Society of Echocardiography. *J Am Coll Cardiol.* 1997;29(4):862–879.

# 49

# Transesophageal Echocardiography

Elsayed Abo-Salem and Tasneem Z. Naqvi

## ● PRACTICAL POINTS

- TEE plays an important role in the evaluation of aortic dissection, prosthetic valve diseases, infective endocarditis, cardiac source of embolization, interatrial septum and cardiac masses. Other indications are intra-operative monitoring and guiding of interventional procedures.

- TEE allows better definition of mitral valve morphology and helps to identify patients who can benefit from mitral valve repair.

- The eccentric MR jet is usually toward a leaflet with restricted mobility or away from a leaflet with excessive mobility.

- Criteria of severe MR include effective regurgitant orifice area ≥0.4 cm², MR volume ≥60 mL, regurgitation fraction ≥50%, vena contracta >0.7 cm, pulmonary vein systolic flow reversal, and mitral regurgitant color flow jet reaching the posterior wall of left atrium.

- Criteria of severe aortic regurgitation include regurgitant jet/LVOT ratio >65%, effective regurgitant orifice area ≥0.3 cm², regurgitant volume ≥60 mL, regurgitation fraction ≥50%, vena contracta of >0.6 cm, and pan diastolic flow reversal in the thoraco-abdominal aorta.

- Transthoracic echo provides limited views of the aorta, in contrast to TEE that provides high-resolution views of almost the entire length of the aorta.

- TEE findings that determine the need for surgery include size >5.5 cm for ascending aorta, >6.5 cm for descending aorta, or rapid rate of expansion (>0.5 cm in 6 months). Surgery is indicated at earlier stages in Marfan syndrome and bicuspid AV disease.

- If clinical suspicion of infective endocarditis is high (prosthetic valve, or staphylococcal bacteremia), then negative TTE will not rule out infective endocarditis and TEE should be performed.

- Atheromas at highest risk of embolization are non-calcified plaques that protrude more than 4 mm into the aortic lumen, with mobile components or ulcerated surface. The presence of aortic atheroma of 5 mm or larger increased the risk perioperative stroke rate by 6-fold.

- TEE can readily image the interatrial septum in multiple views, and is considered the primary method for the diagnosis and characterization of atrial septal defect and for monitoring of the procedure during percutaneous closure.

# INTRODUCTION

The development of transesophageal echocardiography (TEE) has rapidly progressed from M-mode to real time two-dimensional (2D) and Doppler studies and recently to three-dimensional (3D) imaging. The transducer design evolved with the development of smaller, more flexible endoscopes, and the scanning capabilities improved from monoplane to biplane to multiplane and, more recent, to 3D imaging. TEE obtains high resolution cardiac images, which has widened the diagnostic role of TEE and extended its role to the guiding and monitoring of interventional and operative procedures.

## Indications

Transthoracic echocardiography (TTE) remains the primary diagnostic technique for echocardiographic evaluation, whereas TEE is indicated for selected cases as complementary to TTE (approximately 5-10% of cases referred for echocardiography evaluation). These include the inability to obtain essential diagnostic information due to a poor transthoracic window or the inherent inability of TTE to evaluate an underlying pathology. TEE plays an important role in the evaluation of aortic dissection, prosthetic valve diseases, infective endocarditis, cardiac source of embolization, interatrial septum, and cardiac masses. Other indications are intraoperative monitoring and guiding of interventional procedures.

## Instrumentation

Preparations for TEE examination include discussion with the patient about the procedure, fasting for at least 4 hours, and removal of loose dentures. AHA/ACC guidelines for prophylaxis against infective endocarditis do not include TEE as an indication for prophylaxis. The use of conscious sedation, topical anesthetic agents, and lubricants is recommended. The transducer should be introduced gently, and the study should be initially targeted for resolving the primary issue for which TEE is being performed. Procedural risks are low in trained hands and include transient throat pain, laryngospasm, aspiration, mucosal injury, and esophageal rupture. Contraindications to TEE include esophageal stricture, diverticulum, large esophageal varices, a tumor, and recent esophageal or gastric surgery.

# NATIVE VALVULAR HEART DISEASE

TTE is the primary imaging modality for native valve disease. TEE is indicated when images of sufficient quality cannot be obtained by TTE or when detailed morphologic data are required in the diagnosis or management of the patient.

## Evaluation of Native Mitral Valve with TEE

The mitral valve apparatus is composed of the MV ring, leaflets, chordae, and papillary muscles. The proper function of the MV requires the proper function and orientation of all these elements. The mitral valve ring has a dynamic and complex saddle shaped geometry. The anterior and posterior mitral valve leaflets have several indentations dividing them into 4 segments or scallops. There are two papillary muscles, anterolateral and posteromedial, with chordae extending from each to both anterior and posterior leaflets (**Figure 49-1**).

The complete evaluation of the mitral valve leaflets can be obtained through the following views;
1. Mid esophageal 4 & 5 chamber views at 0 degrees; anteroflexion and retroflexion may be required
2. Mid esophageal 2 chamber views at 90 degrees; slight right and left turn may be required
3. Mid esophageal long axis view at 135 degrees; it cuts through the center of MV leaflets ($A_2$ & $P_2$)
4. Transgastric short axis view provides a cross-section of the mitral valve and shows all scallops of both leaflets along with the commissures

### Mitral Stenosis

TEE is routinely used before percutaneous mitral balloon valvuloplasty. It allows better definition of MV morphology with accurate scoring. TEE is also used for exclusion of significant mitral regurgitation (MR) and left atrial cavity or appendage thrombus. Evaluation and scoring of the severity of leaflet thickness, degree of leaflet mobility from margins only to the entire leaflet, leaflet calcification from margins only to the entire leaflet, and extent of involvement of subvalvular apparatus from proximal 3rd to distal 3rd allows a valve score that may then be used to determine the feasibility and success of percutaneous balloon valvuloplasty (**Figure 49-2**).

TEE is rarely required for diagnosis of mitral stenosis or assessment of severity. The underlying cause of mitral stenosis is rheumatic in 99% of cases in areas where rheumatic heart disease is rampant. Other causes include calcific mitral stenosis (which usually develops in the elderly), congenital mitral stenosis, carcinoid syndrome, systemic lupus erythematosis, and mucopolysaccharidoses. Rheumatic mitral stenosis is characterized by valve thickening and calcification (particularly of leaflet margins), commissural fusion, and chordal fibrosis and is frequently associated with MR or aortic valve disease.

Assessment of mitral stenosis severity can be done through measurement of the mitral valve area or a pressure gradient through the mitral valve as indicated in **Table 49-1**. The mitral valve area can be measured by planimetry, pressure half time (**Figure 49-3**), continuity equation, proximal

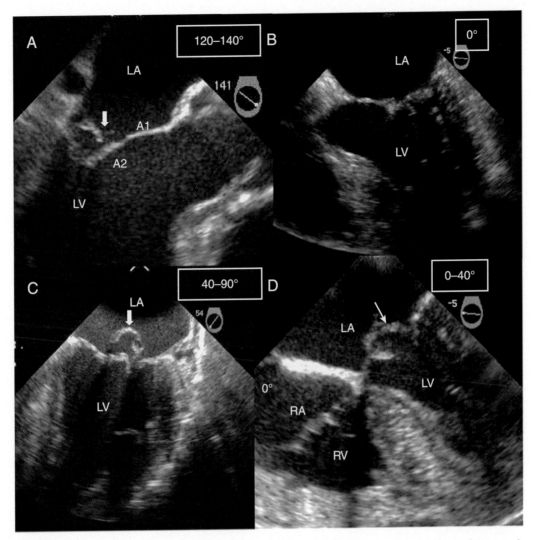

**Figure 49-1.** TEE views of mitral valve obtained in multiple angles showing various scallops of the mitral valve from 0 degrees (B and D) to 54 degrees (C) and 141 degrees (A). P2 and A2 scallops of mitral valve are shown in B, prolapsing A3 scallop (white arrow) and normal P3 scallop in D, P1, P3, and A2 scallops as well as prolapsing P2 scallop (white arrow) are shown in C, and A1 and A2 scallops and prolapsing P2 scallop (white arrow) are shown in A. The numbers on the top right of each panel indicate the range of multiple imaging TEE angles that show the representative views. LA, left atrium; RA, right atrium; RV, right ventricle; LV, left ventricle.

isovelocity surface acceleration, and 3D TEE. Planimetry is difficult in patients with previous balloon valvuloplasty or heavy calcification, and pressure half time is unreliable immediately after percutaneous balloon valvuloplasty and with rapid increase in left ventricular diastolic pressure from other causes such as aortic regurgitation or in patients with reduced LV systolic and diastolic function. A continuity equation ([TVI$_{LVOT}$ × D2$_{LVOT}$ × 0.785] / TVI$_{MV}$ TVI = time velocity integral, LVOT = left ventricular outflow tract) can be used in the absence of mitral or aortic regurgitation. The advent of 3D TEE allows precise delineation of mitral valve area by planimetry and overcomes the limitation of 2D imaging with respect to oblique cut planes.

## Mitral Regurgitation

TEE allows better definition of mitral valve morphology and helps to identify patients who can benefit from mitral valve repair. Feasibility of repair depends on the type, extent, and location of the underlying pathology (**Figure 49-1**). TEE allows better evaluation of the underlying etiology, mechanism, and severity of MR. The recent introduction of live 3D TEE has improved the utility of TEE in the evaluation of MR. Trivial MR is present in 70% of normal people (jet of a short duration not extending far from the closing mitral leaflets). The underlying cause of significant regurgitation may be due to a disease in mitral annulus, leaflets, chordae, or papillary muscles.

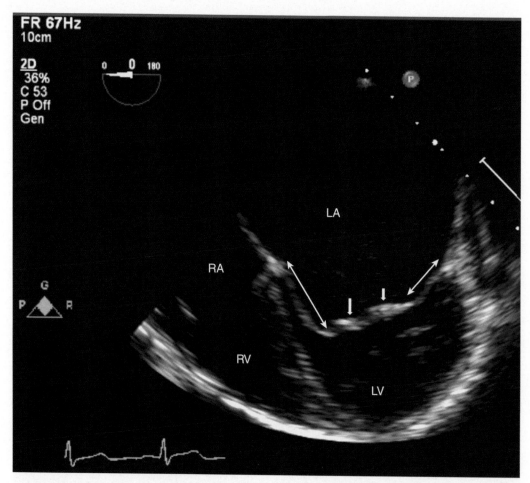

**Figure 49-2.** TEE four-chamber view showing thickening of margins of anterior and posterior mitral valve leaflets (arrowheads). The base and middle portions of the leaflets are normal (white arrows). LA, left atrium; RA, right atrium; RV, right ventricle; LV, left ventricle.

The jet of MR may be central or eccentric. The eccentric jet is usually ipsilateral to the leaflet with restricted mobility and contralateral to the leaflet with excessive mobility. Restricted leaflet motion may be organic as in rheumatic heart disease, or functional tethering of mitral valve leaflets due to displaced or ischemic papillary muscles as in dilated nonischemic or ischemic cardiomyopathy or in inferior, anterior, or lateral infarct with reverse remodeling of infarcted area that leads to displacement of papillary muscle (**Figure 49-4**). Excessive leaflet mobility may be due to mitral valve prolapse or flail MV leaflet. The flail leaflet is due to rupture chord or, occasionally, from rupture of papillary muscle due to acute myocardial infarction or trauma. This results in scallop of mitral valve leaflet or entire leaflet flowing freely in the left atrium during systole. Mitral valve prolapse results in systolic displacement of one or both mitral valve leaflets or scallops into the left atrium, beyond the plane of the mitral annulus. When prolapse occurs, most often the middle scallop of the posterior leaflet is involved (**Figure 49-1**, panel C). By allowing imaging from multiple imaging angles from 0 to 180 degrees in the long axis plane as well as by imaging in the short axis plane of the mitral valve, TEE allows precise delineation of diseased leaflet scallops and, hence, valve reparability in patients with mitral valve prolapse (**Figure 49-1**, panels A-D).

The criteria of severe MR include vena contracta (neck) of MR jet of >0.7 cm, effective regurgitant orifice area ≥0.4 cm² (<0.2 is mild), MR volume ≥60 mL (<30 mL is mild), regurgitation fraction ≥60% (<30% is mild), pulmonary vein systolic flow reversal, and mitral regurgitant color flow jet reaching the posterior wall of the left atrium. The area of regurgitant jet, relative to the size of the left atrium, is a good indicator of severity of MR. However, it is affected by gain

| Table 49-1 • Echocardiographic Criteria for Assessment of Mitral Stenosis Severity | | | |
|---|---|---|---|
| | Mild | Moderate | Severe |
| MVA (cm) | >1.5 | 1–1.5 | <1 |
| Mean gradient (mm Hg) | <5 | 5–10 | >10 |

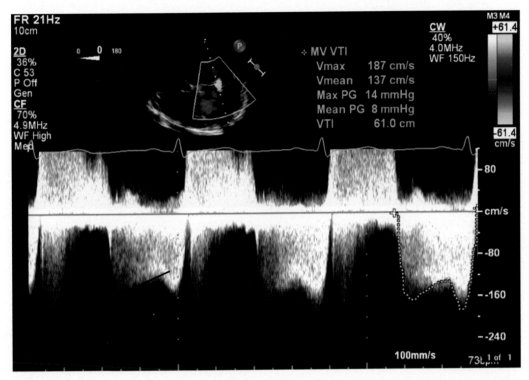

**Figure 49-3.** Echo Doppler method of assessment of mitral valve area by pressure half time (black line) and peak and mean mitral valve gradients in a patient with rheumatic mitral stenosis.

setting, pulsed repetition frequency, and direction of the jet. Effective regurgitation orifice arean can be measured through the proximal isovelocity surface area (PISA) method. Other less reliable signs of severity include dense continuous wave (CW) signal and cutoff sign of the MR signal on CW Doppler. TEE can help evaluate mechanical complications after acute myocardial infarction such as ruptured papillary muscle causing severe MR, free wall rupture and pseudo aneurysm formation when TTE evaluation often provides incomplete assessment.

## Evaluation of Native Aortic Valve with TEE

At a level 30 to 35 cm from the teeth, the aortic valve can be examined in different views. The short axis view can be obtained at 30 to 60 degrees. This shows all three leaflets simultaneously and allows planimetry of the aortic valve (**Figure 49-5**), visualization of calcification, leaflet vegetation, and central or paravalvular aortic regurgitation. Subvalvular vegetation may be missed in the short axis view.

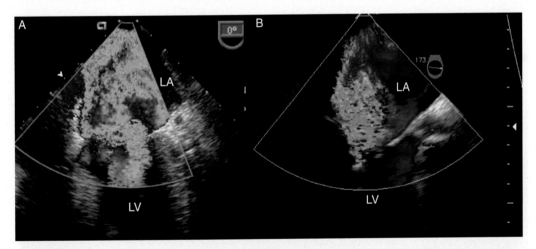

**Figure 49-4.** Eccentric mitral regurgitation jet hugging the interatrial septum and directed anteriorly due to a prolapsing P2 scallop of posterior mitral valve leaflet (white arrow). B shows central mitral regurgitation in a patient with severe aortic stenosis and coronary artery disease with prior inferior myocardial infarction. LA, left atrium; LV, left ventricle.

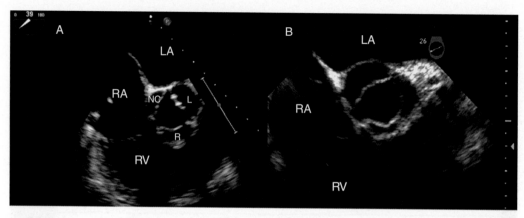

**Figure 49-5.** Short axis view of the aortic valve obtained during TEE. Noncoronary, left and right coronary cusps in a normal trileaflet aortic valve are shown in A. Note thickening of leaflet margins of left coronary cusp and restriction of cusp motion. B shows an example of bicuspid aortic valve with fish mouth appearance in systole. NC, noncoronary; L, left; R, right coronary cusps; LA, left atrium; RA, right atrium; RV, right ventricle.

Visualization of paravalvular tissue in this view allows diagnosis of a paravalvular abscess as well. The proximal portion of the main coronary artery and its division into the left circumflex and left anterior descending coronary artery can be visualized in a significant number of patients (**Figure 49-6**). Increasing the angle to 120 degrees provides a long axis view of the aortic valve and its relationship with the left atrium. Leaflet mobility, thickness, calcification, vegetation (**Figure 49-7**), and prolapse (**Figure 49-8**) can be seen. An increase in the aortic-left atrium space may indicate periaortic hematoma (**Figure 49-9**) or abscess.

Transthoracic echo provides limited views of the aorta, in contrast to TEE, which provides high-resolution views of almost the entire length of the aorta. The short axis view of the ascending aorta appears circular at 0 to 45 degrees, and the long axis view is obtained at an angle of 90 to 120 degrees. The distal ascending aorta may not be visualized

well because the left main bronchus intervening between the esophagus and aorta. The entire descending aorta can be examined by slow withdrawal of the TEE probe.

Pathologies in the proximal and ascending aorta such as aortic dissection (**Figure 49-10**), aortic aneurysm (**Figure 49-11**), aortic hematoma, aortic graft (**Figure 49-12**), and ascending aortic atheroma (**Figure 49-13**) can be seen. The use of color flow Doppler allows evaluation of the presence and location of the gradient due to obstruction, whether aortic, subaortic, or supraaortic, and calculation of the aortic valve area by a continuity equation. The presence, severity, and eccentricity of aortic insufficiency can be evaluated. Severity is assessed by vena contracta of aortic regurgitation jet, ratio of regurgitation jet width and left ventricular outflow tract diameter, effective regurgitant orifice area, aortic regurgitation jet density on CW Doppler and diastolic flow reversal in the thoraco-abdominal aorta

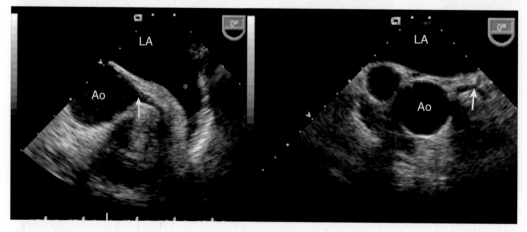

**Figure 49-6.** Short axis view of aortic root just above the level of aortic valve showing the origin of left main coronary artery (A) and division into left circumflex coronary artery and left anterior descending coronary arteries in B. Left atrial appendage cavity is indicated by white asterisk in A. Ao, aortic root.

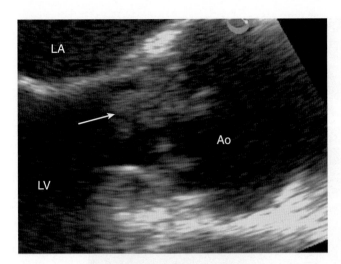

**Figure 49-7.** A close-up view showing a large mobile irregular vegetation protruding into the left ventricular outflow tract from the aortic valve (white arrow). LA, left atrium; LV, left ventricle; Ao, aortic root.

(**Figures 49-14, 49-15, 49-16** and **49-17**). Criteria of severe aortic regurgitation include, regurgitant jet/LVOT ratio >65%, effective regurgitant orifice area ≥0.3 cm$^2$ (<0.1 is mild), regurgitant volume ≥60 mL (<30 mL is mild), regurgitation fraction ≥50% (<30% is mild), vena contracta of >0.6 cm (<0.3 is mild), and pan diastolic flow reversal in the abdominal aorta.

TEE evaluation of the thoracic aortic aneurysm should include the size and morphology of the aneurysm (**Figure 49-18**) and associated aortic value diseases. The size of the aneurysm and annual expansion rate are the major TEE finding that determines the need for surgery: >5.5 cm for ascending aorta, >6.5 cm for descending aorta, or rapid rate of expansion (>0.5 cm in 6 months). Surgery is indicated at earlier stages in Marfan's syndrome and bicuspid AV disease.

TEE has a high sensitivity and specificity for diagnosis of aortic dissection. The most important diagnostic finding of aortic dissection is the presence of a mobile intimal flap (**Figure 49-19**). The entry site and, occasionally, the reentry point(s) can be seen. The differentiation between false and true lumen may be difficult. TEE can be performed quickly at bedside and allows evaluation of the potential complications such as hemopericardium, aortic regurgitation, and involvement of coronary arteries. False positive results are mostly due to reverberation arefact.

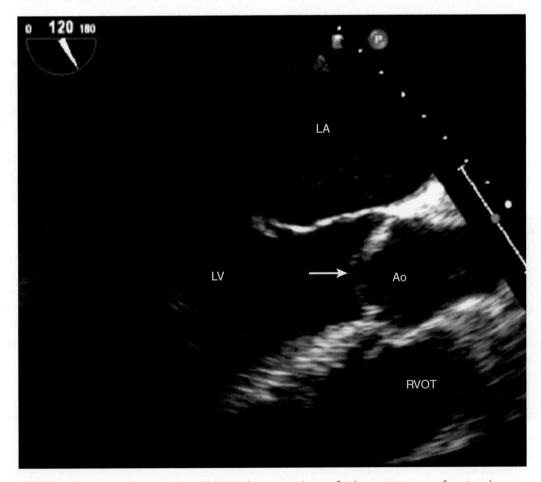

**Figure 49-8.** Long axis view obtained by TEE showing prolapse of right coronary cusp of aortic valve (white arrow). LA, left atrium; LV, left ventricle; RVOT, right ventricular outflow tract; Ao, aortic root.

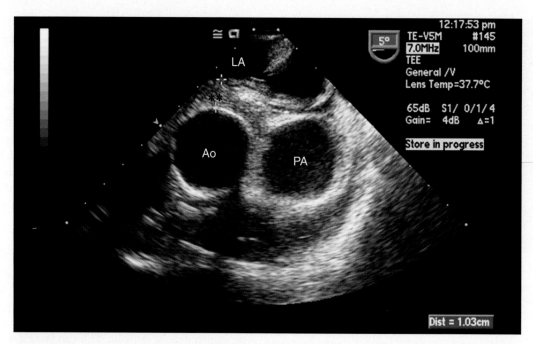

**Figure 49-9.** TEE short axis view of proximal ascending aorta and pulmonary artery. Concentric echodensity (double black asterisks) between aorta and left atrium, due to a periaortic hematoma, is shown in a patient with postaortic valve replacement. LA, left atrium; Ao, aorta; PA, pulmonary artery.

Intramural hematoma is a precursor for aortic dissection (usually in elderly patients with hypertension). It appears as an increased echodensity along the wall of the aorta corresponding to thrombus formation between the intima and adventitia without entry or exit points. Aortic penetrating ulcer is the condition in which ulceration of an aortic atherosclerotic plaque causes penetration into the media. It is important to identify this lesion because it may result in an intramural hematoma or aortic rupture. The presence of color and pulsed wave Doppler flow within a ruptured aortic plaque in patients with chest pain can be used as diagnostic criteria for a penetrating aortic ulcer and to differentiate it from an intramural hematoma or aortic dissection.

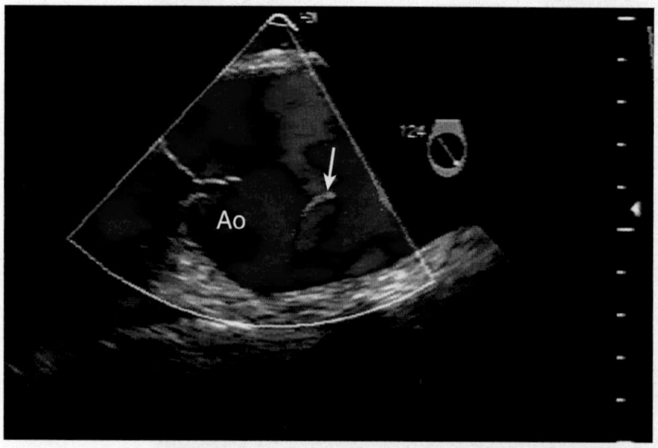

Aortic rupture is a life-threatening complication of chest trauma. TEE has the same sensitivity and specificity of aortography, computed tomography (CT), or magnetic resonance imaging (MRI). A pseudoaneurysm has a different appearance from that of a true aneurysm, with a sharply demarcated rupture site where the aorta communicates with the pseudoaneurysm.

Atherosclerotic plaques are common findings in elderly patients and were found to be an independent predictor of long-term neurologic events. Aortic plaques have irregular surfaces and shapes and may be mobile (**Figure 49-13**). Mobile and thick protruding atheromas are associated with the highest risk of stroke. A strong association has also been identified between the extent and grade of aortic atherosclerosis with coronary artery disease. Diagnosis of aortic atheroma is important before cardiac surgery, as the atheroma may be dislodged by aortic cannula or other manipulations. Manual palpation has a low sensitivity, and TEE has been proposed as an intraoperative tool for diagnosis and grading of aortic atherosclerosis plaques.

### Aortic Regurgitation

TEE allows better definition of the underlying e.g. bicuspid AV, infective endocarditis, rheumatic heart disease, Marfan's syndrome and degenerative calcification and assessment of severity of aortic regurgitation. The primary tool for assessment of aortic regurgitation severity is through measurement of the ratio of the jet width to the left ventricular outflow tract width in long axis views or the ratio of the regurgitation

**Figure 49-10.** A dilated aortic root is shown in a 36-year-old male with bicuspid aortic valve and acute back pain. Aortic dissection flap is shown within the dilated aortic root (white arrow). Ao, aortic root.

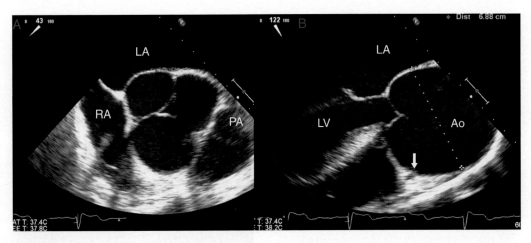

**Figure 49-11.** TEE views showing aortic root aneurysm in the short (A) and long axis (B) views. A central coaptation gap is shown in A resulting from aortic root enlargement. White arrow points at the origin of right coronary artery. LA, left atrium; LV, left ventricle; Ao, aortic root; PA, pulmonary artery; RA, right atrium; Ao, aortic root.

area at the valve orifice to the aortic orifice area in short axis views. Effective regurgitation orifice (ERO) can be calculated also by the proximal PISA profile of the aortic regurgitant jet (**Figures 49-15** and **49-16**). Measurement of regurgitation volumes and fractions can be obtained from the continuity equation using mitral inflow (if there is no significant MR).

## Aortic Stenosis

Aortic stenosis is usually associated with thickened aortic valve leaflets, systolic "doming," and decreased excursion of aortic valve leaflets (stenosis is probably severe if leaflet separation is less than 8 mm). The most common causes of aortic stenosis are bicuspid aortic valve and degenerative calcific aortic stenosis. Bicuspid aortic valve appears as fish mouth in the short axis view during systole (**Figures 49-5** and **49-20**). A "raphe" may give the appearance of three leaflets in diastole. Coarctation may be associated with bicuspid aortic valve and should be excluded. Calcific aortic stenosis involves calcification on the aortic side of the leaflets with resultant leaflet immobility. Other possible causes include

rheumatic heart disease and subvalvular or supravalvular obstruction. Rheumatic aortic stenosis is usually associated with mitral valve disease and fusion of commissures. In patients with subaortic stenosis, the membrane in the left ventricular outflow tract can be visualized more clearly by TEE.

Measurement of the aortic valve area can be done through the continuity equation using the time velocity integral of the left ventricular outflow tract and area and the time velocity integral of the aortic valve (**Figure 49-21**). An aortic valve area less than 1 cm$^2$ is considered severe. This method is not affected by aortic regurgitation severity and cardiac output but not valid in cases with dynamic or fixed subaortic obstruction. Measurement of valvular gradients will vary depending on the stroke volume.

$$LVOT_{TVI} \times LVOT_{area} = \text{stroke volume} = AVA_{TVI} \times AVA_{area}$$

TEE has an advantage over TTE in that it allows assessment of the aortic valve area by planimetry in a significant

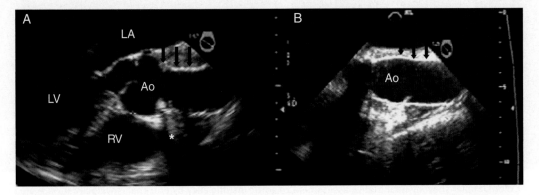

**Figure 49-12.** TEE long axis views showing normal appearances of ascending aortic graft (black arrows) in two different patients. Note the shadowing from the anterior wall of the aortic graft (white asterisk in A). LA, left atrium; LV, left ventricle; Ao, aortic root.

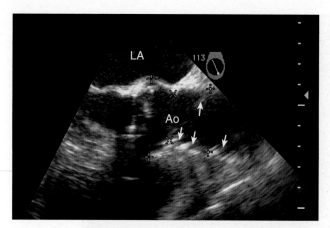

**Figure 49-13.** TEE view of ascending aorta showing marked calcification with acoustic shadowing as well as aortic atheromata (small white arrows) in an 89-year-old male undergoing aortic valve replacement and coronary artery bypass surgery for severe symptomatic aortic stenosis. Patient underwent a successful 3-vessel coronary artery bypass surgery and 23 mm Carpentier-Edwards aortic valve magna prosthesis. Postoperatively, patient remained comatose and developed left sided hemiparesis with right frontal infarct on computed tomography.

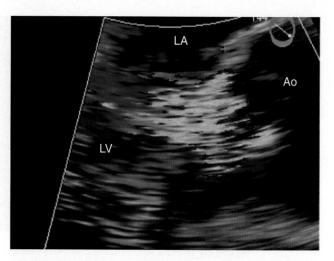

**Figure 49-14.** Color Doppler showing severe aortic insufficiency (bright blue and orange flow) in the left ventricular outflow tract in a patient with aortic valve vegetation. Note that the aortic regurgitant color Doppler jet fills the entire left ventricular outflow tract. Ao, aortic root; LA, left atrium; LV, left ventricle.

number of patients, unlike TTE. In those with severe valvular calcification, particularly those with bicuspid valve, planimetry is not feasible even with TEE.

## INFECTIVE ENDOCARDITIS

Infective endocarditis is a life-threatening disease with significant morbidity and mortality. Echocardiography plays a primary role in the diagnosis and follow-up of patients with endocarditis. The following echocardiographic findings are considered by Duke Criteria to be major criteria for diagnosis of infective endocarditis, oscillating intracardiac mass on native (**Figure 49-7**) or prosthetic valve (**Figures 49-22** and **49-23**) intracardiac periannular abscess and new partial dehiscence of prosthetic valve.

TEE has a sensitivity of 95% for vegetations more than 1 mm in size, whereas TTE has a sensitivity of 50%. If clinical suspicion of infective endocarditis is high (prosthetic valve, or staphylococcal bacteremia), then negative TTE will not rule out infective endocarditis and TEE should be

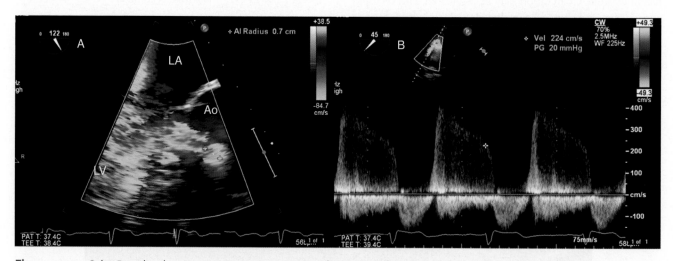

**Figure 49-15.** Color Doppler showing quantitative assessment of aortic insufficiency by proximal isovelocity surface area (PISA) method. A shows central aortic regurgitation jet by color Doppler and measurement of PISA radius (distance between white plus signs) and B shows aortic regurgitant jet by continuous wave Doppler. Peak velocity of aortic regurgitant jet is 400 cm/sec. Ao, aortic root; LA, left atrium; LV, left ventricle.

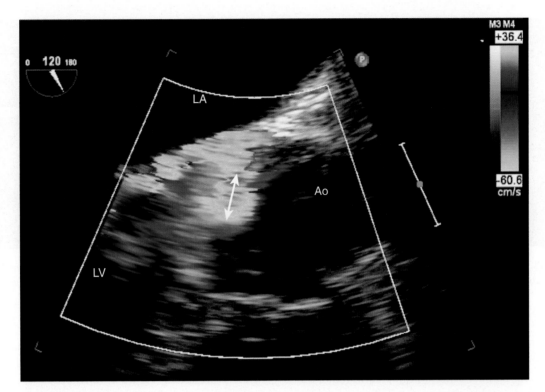

**Figure 49-16.** Color Doppler showing quantitative assessment of an eccentric aortic insufficiency jet by proximal isovelocity surface acceleration method. Note that the aortic regurgitation jet is directed toward the anterior mitral valve leaflet and running under the leaflet. Ao, aortic root; LA, left atrium; LV, left ventricle. Effective regurgitant orifice area = A = 6.28 × r2 × V/peak velocity of aortic regurgitant jet, regurgitant volume of aortic regurgitation = A × velocity time integral of aortic regurgitant jet, where *r* is the radius of PISA (shown by double headed white arrow), V = aliasing velocity (in this case = 36.4 cm/sec).

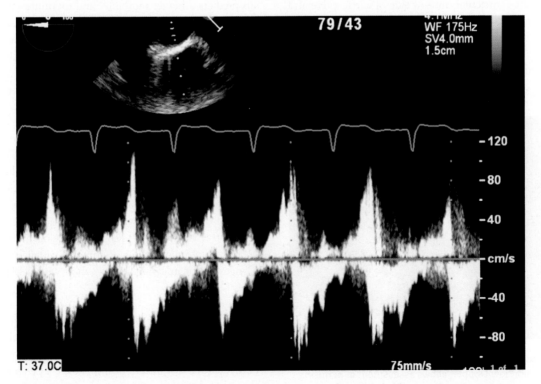

**Figure 49-17.** Diastolic flow reversal in the lower thoracic aorta of a patient with acute Type A aortic dissection and severe aortic regurgitation.

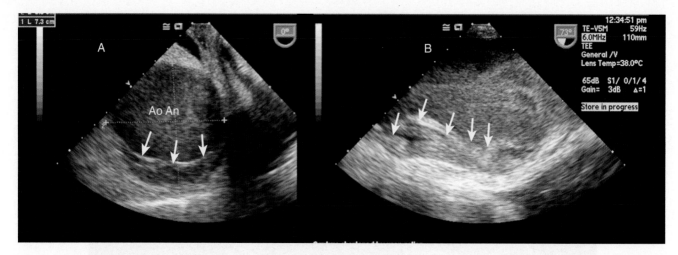

**Figure 49-18.** Descending thoracic aortic aneurysm measuring 7 × 8 cm shown in the transverse view in A and in the longitudinal view in B. Note marked stasis manifested as spontaneous contrast in A and B and thrombus lining the wall of the aorta (white arrows in A and B).

performed. In the setting of a prosthetic valve, TEE should be performed as the diagnostic method of choice. TEE is also indicated if optimal echocardiographic windows cannot be obtained (morbid obesity, etc). TEE may miss very small vegetations, paravalvular abscesses, and paravalvular fistulae, particularly when the study is performed early in the patient's illness.

Vegetations are usually found on the edge of the involved valve and are often on the low pressure side of a regurgitant valve (left ventricular outflow side of aortic valve and atrial side of mitral valve). Vegetations may also form at the site where the regurgitant jet hits the myocardial wall. Prosthetic valve vegetations usually involve the paravalvular ring (**Figures 49-22** and **49-23**) and may cause abscess

formation. Bioprosthetic valves may have evidence of infection along the valve ring but also may involve the valve leaflets themselves (**Figure 49-24**).

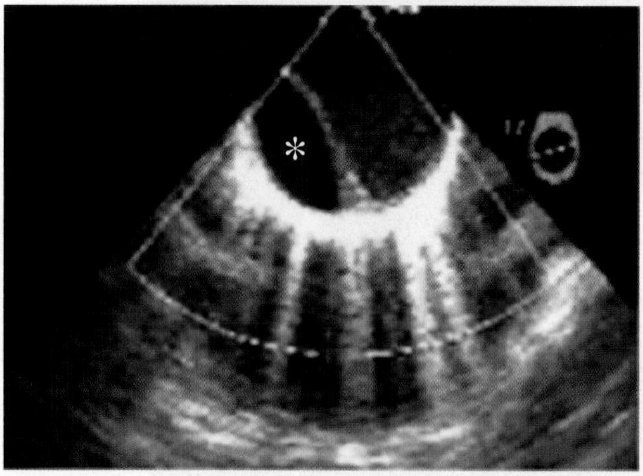

Follow-up TEE is recommended when a patient develops clinical features suggestive of complications, for example, symptoms of congestive heart failure and new atrioventricular block. An increase in vegetation size on serial echocardiography is associated with an increased risk of complications. Extension of infective endocarditis beyond the valve annulus predicts a higher morbidity and mortality rate. In native aortic valve infective endocarditis, extension occurs through the weakest portion of the annulus, which is near the membranous septum in aortic valve endocarditis. Abscesses may progress to fistulous tracts, pericarditis, and myocardial abscess. The sensitivity of TTE for detecting paravalvular abscess is low.

Acute congestive heart failure occurs more frequently in aortic valve infections (30%) than with mitral (20%) or tricuspid valve endocarditis (5%). Congestive heart failure may develop acutely from perforation of or bioprosthetic valve leaflet, rupture of infected mitral chordae, or sudden intracardiac shunts from fistulous tracts or prosthetic valve dehiscence. Congestive heart failure also may develop more insidiously as a result of progressive worsening of valvular insufficiency. Congestive heart failure is associated with a high mortality rate.

Preoperative surgical planning for patients with infective endocarditis will benefit from echocardiographic delineation of the mechanisms of valvular dysfunction or regions of myocardial disruption. Postoperative TEE should confirm the adequacy of the repair or replacement and document the successful closure of fistulous tracts.

**Figure 49-19.** Intimal dissection flap in the descending thoracic aorta. Color flow Doppler allows assessment of perfusing lumen, which in this case is for the narrower of the two lumens shown by white asterisk.

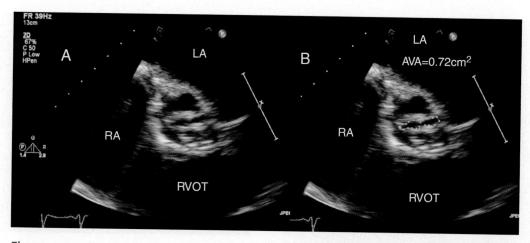

**Figure 49-20.** An example of a patient with a stenotic bicuspid aortic valve. Marked thickening of leaflet margins and restriction of cusp excursion is shown in A. Planimetry of AVA is shown in B. AVA was calculated at 0.72 cm² by planimetry (B). RA, right atrium; LA, left atrium; RVOT, right ventricular outflow tract.

## PROSTHETIC VALVE DISEASE

Imaging of prosthetic valves is usually suboptimal with TTE due to the acoustic shadowing from the mechanical prosthesis. TEE provides high resolution images of the valve and paravalvular structures. Different views for each valve are essential for evaluation of prosthetic valves and surrounding structures.

Failures of the occluder or leaflet to open or coapt properly may result from pannus overgrowth, vegetation, or thrombus formation (**Figures 49-25** and **49-26**). Dehiscence of the prosthetic valve appears as excessive motion (rocking motion) of the sewing ring. Adjacent echolucent structures may be an abscess or a fistula.

TEE provides a reliable indirect assessment of the prosthetic valve performance through peak velocity and pressure

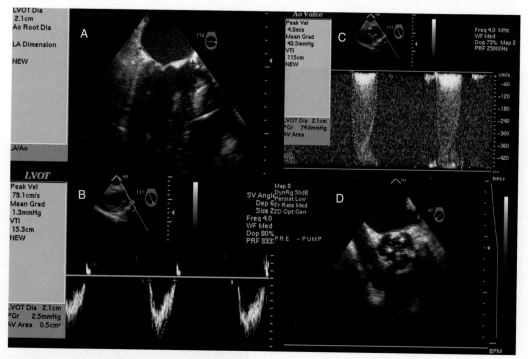

**Figure 49-21.** Case example of a 92-year-old male who underwent aortic valve replacement for severe aortic stenosis. Intraoperative measurement of aortic valve area by continuity equation is shown. Measurement of left ventricular outflow tract diameter (A), left ventricular outflow tract velocity (B), and aortic valve velocity and gradient (C) is shown. Calcified aortic valve is shown in the short axis view. Severe aortic stenosis with an aortic valve area of 0.5 cm² was calculated. Note that the presence of heavy calcification may make planimetry of aortic valve area difficult.

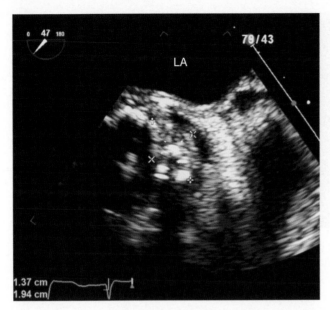

**Figure 49-22.** A moderate size vegetation measuring 14 × 19 mm is shown on a prosthetic aortic valve in short axis view. LA, left atrium.

gradients (**Figure 49-27**), effective valve orifice area, and regurgitation jets (valvular or paravalvular). The prosthetic valve velocities and pressure gradients are variable, so echocardiography should be done before hospital discharge as a baseline for follow up. The prosthetic valves are relatively stenotic with effective valve orifice less than native valve. A higher than expected gradient may be due to valve

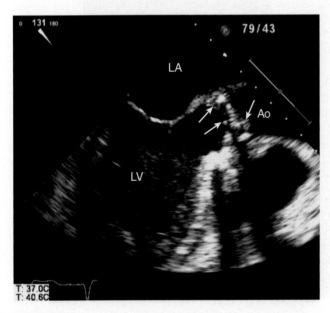

**Figure 49-23.** Three chamber view, obtained in the same patient as in Figure 49-22, showing prosthetic aortic valve with echo dense material representing vegetation (white arrows) protruding above the valve and below the valve into left ventricular outflow tract. Ao, ascending aorta; LA, left atrium; LV, left ventricle.

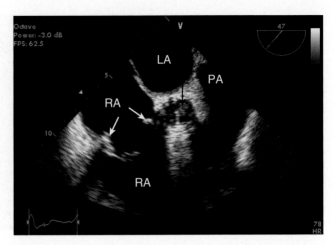

**Figure 49-24.** A bioprosthetic aortic valve is shown in short axis view. Echodense vegetations are seen within the valve ring (black arrow). Tricuspid annuloplasty ring (white arrows) is also shown. LA, left atrium; RA, right atrium; RV, right ventricle; PA, pulmonary artery.

obstruction or high cardiac output states. Assessment of effective valve orifice area and obstruction index, in such cases, will help to differentiate valve obstruction from other causes, since the effective valve orifice area is load independent.

The effective valve orifice area (EOA) can be evaluated using the continuity equation. A body surface area normalized EOA $<0.85$ cm$^2$/m$^2$ (EOA/body surface area) for an aortic valve prosthesis indicates prosthesis–patient mismatch—a term which indicates that the prosthesis chosen is too small. Many prosthetic valves have a small regurgitant flow characterized by a uniform color without aliasing. Significant regurgitation may be due to disk/ball variance, dehiscence, stuck valve, and paravalvular leaks. In general, signs indicating increased forward flow through the mitral prosthesis with

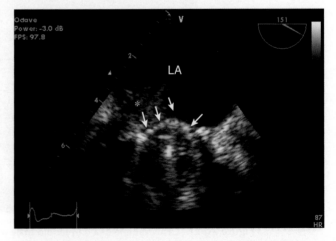

**Figure 49-25.** Vegetation protruding from prosthetic mitral valve into the left atrium during systole (white asterisk). Mitral valve disks are shown by white arrow heads. The vegetation partially blocks the mitral annulus and prevents disks from fully closing in systole. LA, left atrium.

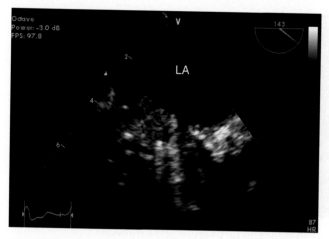

**Figure 49-26.** Vegetation on prosthetic mitral valve during diastole. The vegetation partially blocks the bileaflet disks and prevents disks from fully opening.

evidence of decreased forward cardiac output across the aortic valve point to severe MR (e.g., mitral inflow time velocity integral >40 cm with diminished aortic time velocity integral, mean mitral diastolic gradient >5–7 mm Hg, and short isovolumic relaxation time). St. Jude's valve may have three to five small back flow jets from the commissures and central portion of the valve. In general, prosthetic aortic valve jets are <1 cm$^2$ in area and project less than 1.5 cm beyond origin, whereas prosthetic mitral valve jets are less than 2 cm$^2$ in area and project less than 2.5 cm beyond origin. TEE should be performed in a patient with a mechanical or a bioprosthetic valve who develops a significant new murmur, signs of increased forward flow across the valve in the absence of a high systemic cardiac ouput state and or develops hemolysis. TEE is able to delineate presence, location and severity of paravalvular leaks. 3D TEE provides excellent surgical types views of paravalvular leaks. In addition TEE is also used for guidance during percutaneous closure of paravalvular leaks.

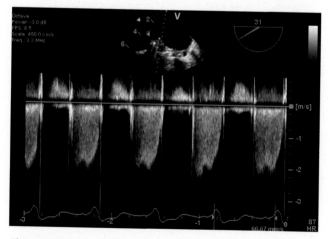

**Figure 49-27.** Markedly increased diastolic gradient across prosthetic mitral valve due to vegetation partially blocking diastolic mitral inflow.

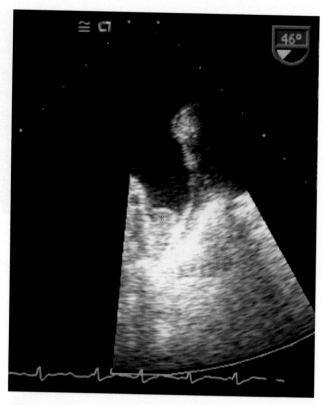

**Figure 49-28.** A triangular shaped thrombus (black asterisk) taking the shape of the left atrial appendage apex is shown in a patient with dilated cardiomyopathy and severe mitral regurgitation.

## CARDIAC SOURCE OF EMBOLI

Of the 500,000 strokes yearly in the United States, 85% are of ischemic origin. About 20% of these ischemic strokes have a cardioembolic origin and 40% are of undetermined cause (cryptogenic stroke). Cardiac embolism is the most common cause of acute limb ischemia. Evaluation of a cardiac source of embolism is a common indication for TEE study.

Cardiac sources of emboli include left atrial appendage thrombus (**Figure 49-28**), left ventricular thrombus (mostly apical), endocarditis, prosthetic valve thrombosis, atrial masses (**Figure 49-29**), fibrinous valve threads, and protruding or ulcerative aortic atheroma (**Figure 49-30**). Potential causes of cryptogenic stroke include patent foramen ovale, atrial septal aneurysm, and pulmonary arteriovenous shunt. The association of stroke with mitral annular calcification, mitral valve prolapse, and papillary fibroelastoma is not clear.

Patients with no history or clinical evidence of cardiac disease have an extremely low likelihood of positive findings on TTE. Even though TEE is superior to TTE in identifying potential sources of emboli in patients without known cardiac disease, the overall yield is increased to only 1.6%. Some authorities recommend TEE evaluation of embolic events as the initial diagnostic test for patients younger than 45 to 55 years of age.

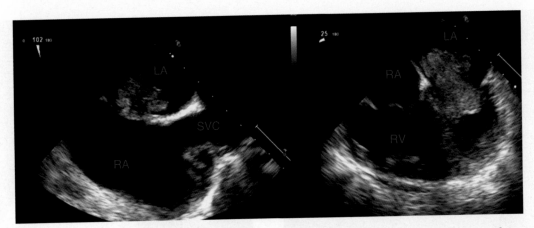

**Figure 49-29.** TEE views showing a globular mass attached to the interatrial septum at the region of fossa ovalis. The mass protrudes across the mitral valve causing turbulent color Doppler flow. LA, left atrium; RA, right atrium; RV, right ventricle; SVC, superior vena cava.

Left atrial appendage thrombus is a common source of cardiac emboli. It is usually associated with atrial flutter or fibrillation and left atrium dilation. The left atrial appendage is a complex multilobed structure with pectinate muscle, therefore, several TEE multiple imaging planes should be used (**Figure 49-31**). TEE evaluation of the left atrial appendage includes presence of thrombi and pulse wave Doppler flow patterns. Patients with normal flow patterns within the left atrial appendage (normal $46 \pm 18$ cm/s) have a low likelihood of thrombus formation.

Systemic embolization occurs in 25% of cases with infective endocarditis. Many studies have attempted to identify a high risk subset of infective endocarditis patients. The highest risk cases are those with large vegetation in anterior mitral leaflet due to staphylococci or fungi. Atrial myxoma is the most common cardiac tumor and may be associated with embolism. Polypoid and prolapsing tumors are more likely to embolize. It may also serve as a nidus for platelet and fibrin aggregation.

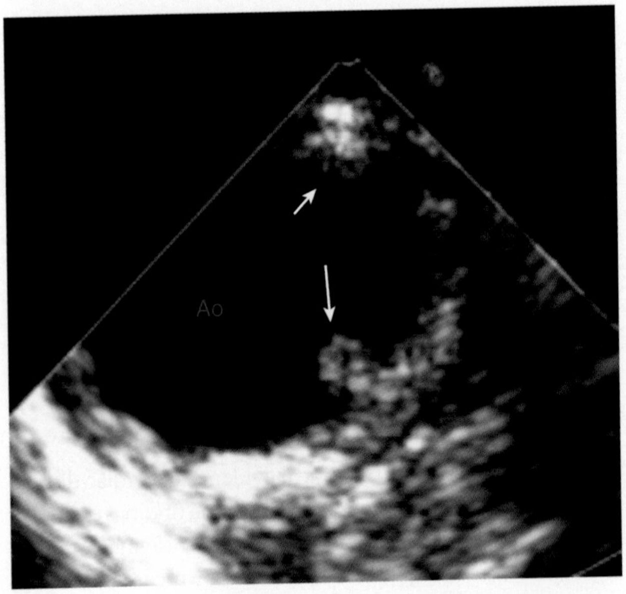

Atheromas at highest risk of embolization are noncalcified plaques that protrude more than 4 mm into the aortic lumen, with mobile components or an ulcerated surface. The presence of aortic atheroma of 5 mm or larger increased the risk perioperative stroke rate by sixfold. Patients presenting with systemic embolic events and found to have mobile aortic atheromas on TEE have a high incidence of recurrent systemic events (25%).

Patent foramen ovale (PFO) as a common cause of stroke remains somewhat controversial. There may be a higher likelihood of stroke among patients with larger size PFO, with evidence of a larger amount of shunting, or who also have an atrial septal aneurysm. Direct TEE visualization is considered the gold standard for PFO diagnosis, but peripheral injection of agitated saline with TTE has also been used to detect a right-to-left shunt. A Valsalva maneuver or repeated cough should be used to increase the diagnostic yield (**Figure 49-32**). An atrial septal aneurysm is a redundant and mobile membranous portion of the atrial septum with an excursion of more than 15 mm and a base width of 15 mm. The autopsy incidence is 1%. It is usually associated with PFO.

## TEE GUIDED CARDIOVERSION

Atrial fibrillation is the most common chronic atrial arrhythmia with a prevalence of 5% in the population older than 65 years. The annual rate of ischemic stroke is 5%, which is 5 times that of the population without atrial fibrillation. Risk factors for stroke in cases with atrial fibrillation are valvular heart disease, congestive heart failure, previous stroke, age, hypertension, and diabetes mellitus.

**Figure 49-30.** Protruding atheromata (white arrows) and thickened intimal medial layer in the aortic arch in a patient with transient ischemic attack. Ao, aorta.

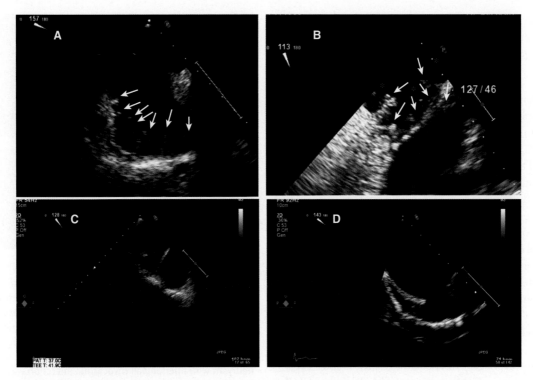

**Figure 49-31.** Left atrial appendage views in four separate patients showing variation in anatomy and size. Prominent pectinate muscles are present in A and B (white arrows). Multilobed appendage (white asterisks) in each lobe, like a cauliflower, is present in B. C and D show small appendages with no prominent pectinate muscles.

Atrial fibrillation is the most common cardiac source of emboli, and more than 90% of these emboli arise from the left atrial appendage. Twelve percent of patients with atrial fibrillation may have left atrial appendage thrombus and 2% may have left atrial cavity thrombus. The duration of atrial fibrillation and the presence of mitral stenosis are important risk factors for thrombus formation. These patients have an increased left atrium size, larger left atrial appendage with multiple lobes, and decreased appendage flow velocities. The likelihood of thrombus formation is highest in those with a spontaneous echocontrast in the left atrium. Right atrial appendage has a wide neck with a lower incidence of thrombus formation.

The left atrial appendage is a complex structure that can be readily imaged with TEE. TEE is also better than TTE for detection of thrombus within the body of the left atrium, especially the upper left atrial wall near the pulmonary veins. The right atrial appendage can be imaged with TEE. TEE can

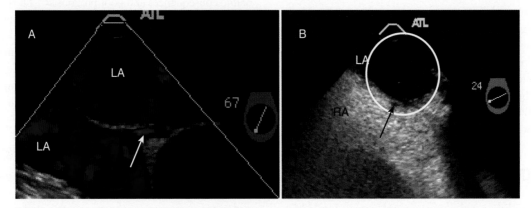

**Figure 49-32.** A TEE of the interatrial septum with color Doppler is shown in A. A small amount of flow (white arrow A) is seen in the region of foramen ovale, suggesting the possibility of patent foramen ovale. A saline contrast injection (B) shows a small amount of negative contrast in the right atrium due to L to R flow (black arrow) and a small number of bubbles (within the white circle in B) entering the left atrium from the patent foramen. LA, left atrium; RA, right atrium.

evaluate the underlying structural heart disease. Multislice computed tomography and cardiac magnetic resonance imaging appear to be less reliable than TEE for evaluation of these structures.

The risk of embolism is 3 to 7% among patients who did not receive prophylactic anticoagulation before cardioversion. The risk is higher in patients with an atrial fibrillation duration of more than 48 hours or in those with a high risk of embolism. The conventional management of these patients is empiric anticoagulation for 3 weeks before cardioversion. The other option is a TEE guided strategy to exclude the presence of left atrial thrombus before cardioversion. Drawbacks of the conventional method are longer duration of atrial fibrillation, longer duration of anticoagulation, and lack of resolution of thrombi in 20%. A subtherapeutic international normalized ratio during this period should trigger the initiation of another 3 weeks of anticoagulation. Drawbacks of the TEE guided approach are the semiinvasive approach and the rare possibility of false positive or negative results. The ACUTE (The Assessment of Cardioversion Using Transesophageal Echocardiography) and ACE (Anticoagulation in Cardioversion of Non-Valvular Atrail Fibrillation) trials proved that TEE guided cardioversion is a safe and effective alternative to the conventional method.

Patients with long-standing atrial fibrillation or valvular heart disease are not likely to remain in sinus rhythm after cardioversion and are more likely to have a left atrial stunning. Stunning of the left atrium is a delay in recovery of atrial mechanical activity with low left atrial appendage Doppler velocities despite reversion to sinus rhythm. These patients are at high risk of thromboembolism. Full anticoagulation is recommended at the time of cardioversion and continued for at least 3 weeks after cardioversion to sinus rhythm.

TEE guided ablation can be used as an alternative or supplemental to angiographic guided ablation. It can guide transseptal puncture, delineate pulmonary vein ostia, exclude left atrial thrombus, and monitor for complications such as cardiac tamponade during percutaneous intervention. Pulmonary vein stenosis is a rare but potentially life-threatening complication of catheter ablation. It may be diagnosed by TEE on the basis of dynamic evaluation of the pulmonary vein blood flow. TEE enables reliable, cost-effective, noninvasive follow-up in such patients.

## ACUTE CORONARY SYNDROME

The role of TEE in acute coronary syndromes is limited for patients with suspected aortic dissection. Additional applications of TEE in the assessment of coronary artery disease include detection of anomalous coronary arteries, detection and mapping of coronary artery fistulas, and coronary artery

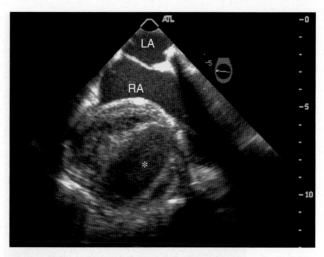

**Figure 49-33.** TEE showing a large cystic mass (white asterisk) with stasis and thrombus compressing the right atrium and basal right ventricle in a 38-year-old male with a history of St. Jude's mitral valve replacement 3 years prior to presentation following a failed repair who presented with fatigue and decreased exercise tolerance of 6 weeks duration. ECG showed new inferior q waves compared to a year ago. A right coronary psuedoaneurysm with inferior wall myocardial infarction was diagnosed on coronary angiography. LA, left atrium; RA, right atrium.

pseudoaneurysms (**Figure 49-33**). Visualization of proximal coronary vessels is possible with TEE (**Figure 49-6**). The left main coronary artery can be visualized in more than 85% of patients.

## Assessment of Mechanical Complications of Acute Myocardial Infarction

Mechanical complications of myocardial infarction include left ventricular free wall rupture (**Figure 49-34**), formation of a ventricular septal defect, and development of significant MR. These complications often occur in the early days after myocardial infarction and usually result in adverse hemodynamic consequences and poor prognosis. TTE is the primary tool for evaluation of these patients with suspected acute complications. TEE is indicated whenever the data obtained from TTE are not sufficient, due to poor image quality, or further diagnostic detail on the underlying pathology is needed. TEE monitoring during surgical repair of complication of myocardial infarction listed above is also helpful.

## Intraoperative Echocardiography During Coronary Artery Bypass Surgery

The use of TEE during coronary artery bypass surgery is associated with improved outcome among high risk patients undergoing emergency surgery or associated with hemodynamic disturbances. TEE may be particularly useful during off pump coronary artery bypass surgery, where hemodynamic instability and coronary ischemia are possible during positioning of the heart for distal coronary anastomosis.

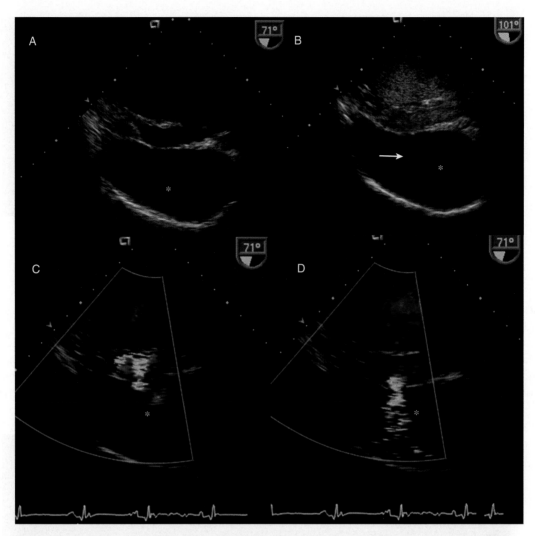

**Figure 49-34.** Left ventricular pseudoaneurysm in a patient post lateral wall myocardial infarction. Thin anterolateral wall communicating with a pseudoaneurysm space (white asterisk) is shown in A to D. Injection of Optison contrast agent that traverses the pulmonary circulation to appear into LV cavity shows contrast appearing in the pseudoaneurysm (white arrow) due to communication with the left ventricular cavity (B). C shows color Doppler flow from the pseudoaneurysm into the LV cavity and D shows color flow entering into the pseudoaneurysm from LV cavity in systole. To and fro flow into pseudoaneurysm is therefore present in systole and diastole.

TEE can assist at each stage of coronary artery bypass surgery. It supplements an incomplete cardiac workup and assists in the conduct of circulatory management and vascular cannulation including correct placement of coronary sinus catheters (**Figure 49-35**), an endoaortic clamp, and an intraaortic balloon pump. The presence of atheromatous plaques in the ascending aorta is associated with increased risk of postoperative stroke **Figure 49-13**, and modification of the surgical technique is required to avoid disruption of the plaque.

Monitoring of ventricular function and ischemia is essential during coronary artery bypass surgery. Patients who exhibit new wall motion abnormality during bypass surgery are at increased risk of morbidity and mortality. Other possible causes of new wall motion abnormalities are cardiac pacing, bundle branch block, and distortion of the heart.

## CONGENITAL HEART DISEASE

Congenital heart disease comprise of cardiac birth defect and occurs in about 1% of live births. TTE provides adequate information in the majority of patients. TEE plays an important role in selected cases with congenital heart disease (**Figure 49-36**). It allows better definition of interatrial septum, pulmonary veins, patent ductus arteriosus, and chordal attachment and has been used during such interventions as closure of an atrial septal defect, patent ductus arteriosus,

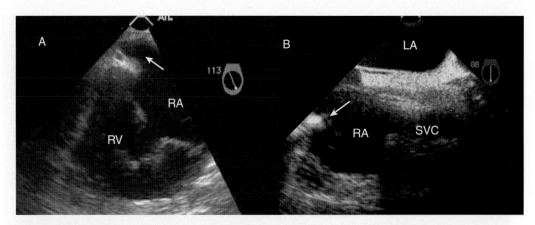

**Figure 49-35.** A shows tricuspid inflow view by TEE during coronary sinus cannulation. White arrow in A points to the coronary sinus. B shows coronary sinus cannula (white arrow) placed in the coronary sinus. RA, right atrium; RV, right ventricle; LA, left atrium; SVC, superior vena cava.

and aortic and pulmonic balloon valvuloplasty. TTE is often superior to TEE in the evaluation of a ventricular septal defect. The use of TEE in children is restricted to carefully selected cases, because the TTE usually provides excellent images and TEE is requires general anesthesia. Cyanotic patients must be monitored with particular care during TEE.

An atrial septal defect makes up approximately 10% of congenital heart disease. Types of atrial septal defect include secundum type, premium type, sinus venosus type, and coronary sinus defect. TTE is associated with a significant percentage of false positive and negative results. TEE can readily image the interatrial septum in multiple views and

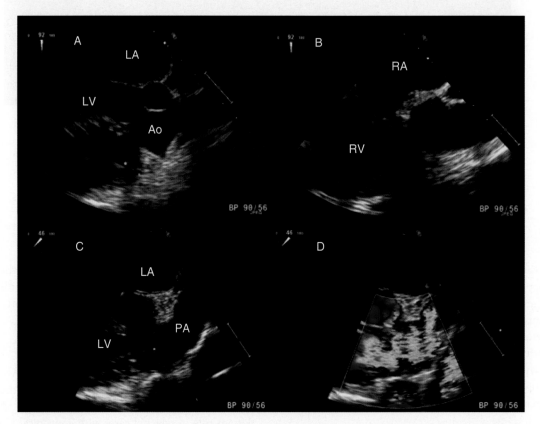

**Figure 49-36.** Tetralogy of Fallot in a 24-year-old Hispanic female. TEE views show overriding aorta (A), right ventricular dilation and hypertrophy (B), ventricular septal defect (C), and markedly turbulent flow across right ventricular outflow tract due to subpulmonic stenosis (D). Left to right flow across VSD is also shown (D). LA, left atrium; RA, right atrium; RV, right ventricle; LV, left ventricle; PA, pulmonary artery; Ao, aortic root.

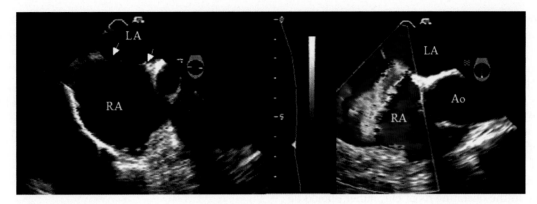

**Figure 49-37.** A secundum atrial septal defect with anterior and posterior margins (white arrows) is shown in A. Left to right flow across the atrial septal defect and measurement of atrial septal defect size in the anteroposterior plane is shown in B.

is considered the primary method for diagnosis of an atrial septal defect. TEE is recommended in any patient with an unexplained dilation of the right side of the heart. The following views can be used for evaluation of the interatrial septum: four chamber view, short axis view of the aortic valve, and bicaval view (**Figure 49-37**).

Diagnosis of an atrial septal defect should include the following anatomical data—site, size, associated anomalies, and feasibility of percutaneous closure—and the following hemodynamic data—the degree of shunt and pulmonary artery pressure. A premium atrial septal defect is a part of a partial or complete endocardial cushion defect. A sinus venosus defect is frequently associated with anomalous pulmonary venous drainage. A coronary sinus defect may be associated with persistent left-sided superior vena cava, secundum atrial septal defect, and rarely, unroofed coronary sinus.

TEE plays an important role in patient selection for percutaneous closure of an atrial septal defect and monitoring of the procedure. A margin of at least 5 mm is required for successful closure. The size of the defect will determine the size of the occlusive device. The defect may be oval, and the largest diameter should be used. Before the device is released, one should exclude the residual shunt and obstruction of the mitral valve, coronary sinus, and right upper pulmonary vein orifice.

## CRITICAL ILLNESS

TTE is recommended for critically ill patients with unexplained hemodynamics or hypoxemia and cases with a clinical suspicion of serious underlying heart pathology. The yield of TTE is lower in critically ill cases, particularly in the mechanically ventilated cases. TEE is indicated in cases with poor acoustic window or cases with a suspicion of endocarditis, prosthetic valve malfunction, or aortic dissection.

TEE can provide important hemodynamic data, for example, right atrial and pulmonary artery pressures, hepatic veins, inferior vena cava, left ventricular systolic function, and ventricular preload. With positive pressure ventilation, the jugular venous pressure may be increased and left ventricular preload decreased. In post cardiac surgical patients, TEE can detect focal cardiac tamponade that is very difficult to evaluate by TTE due to poor images from chest wall bandages, chest tubes, and a poor acoustic window due to pericardial hematoma. TEE can detect a dynamic left ventricular outflow gradient that develops particularly in patients post mitral valve repair and post aortic valve replacement for aortic stenosis. Management in these patients, who are often hypotensive with decreased cardiac output, is volume repletion, beta-blockade, and calcium channel blockade rather than diuretics and inotropes. TEE plays an important role in the case of left ventricular assist device implantation. It is essential for case selection, guiding the procedure, optimizing device performance, and evaluating device dysfunction.

The main pulmonary artery, right pulmonary artery, and proximal part of the left pulmonary artery can be evaluated with TEE. Thrombi within these segments can be readily imaged with TEE. These thrombi can be occasionally seen as a thrombus in transit within the right atrium. Blunt chest injury may commonly result in myocardial contusion, traumatic ventricular septal defect, tricuspid/mitral valve trauma, and hematoma or dissection of the aorta. Deceleration may result in an injured thoracic artery despite lack of external evidence of chest trauma.

### Intraoperative TEE

Echocardiography was introduced into the cardiac operating room in the early 1980s with epicardial scanning. Recently, TEE has been widely used by anesthesiologists during cardiac surgery and in the early postoperative period. After the patient is anesthetized, the TEE probe is inserted to obtain baseline data about the underlying pathology and associated pathologies. TEE offers the advantage of not interfering with the surgical procedure, and it also allows continuous monitoring during surgery.

Intraoperative TEE after induction of anesthesia may not be the best method to reliably identify severity of mitral, aortic, or tricuspid regurgitation due to the afterload reducing effect of cardiac anesthesia. Hence, a decision on the severity of valvular regurgitation should not be made for the first time in the operating room but, rather, should be identified prior to surgery. On the other hand, severity of stenotic lesions can be reliably identified during prebypass TEE findings, which can help in decision making about the surgical procedure. New findings are likely to alter surgery or management in 4% of cases. It is of particular importance in cases undergoing reconstructive cardiac surgery. These surgeries are individualized procedures and the outcome is less predictable than that of valve replacement. TEE has also been recommended to help determine the extent of ventricular myomectomy to be performed in patients with hypertrophic obstructive cardiomyopathy. The presence of atheromatous plaques in the ascending aorta is associated with increased risk of postoperative stroke, and modification of the surgical technique is required to avoid disruption of the plaque.

Continuous monitoring of the left ventricular function can be done with TEE without interfering with the surgical field. Several authors have documented the value of TEE in the early detection of myocardial ischemia. In the growing area of "off-pump" bypass surgery, TEE is an indispensable tool for the monitoring of surgical procedures. TEE is very helpful in guiding correct positioning of the balloon tip in the descending aorta during insertion.

After the patient comes off the bypass pump, TEE is repeated to assess the results of the operation. TTE is often unsatisfactory after open chest surgery for various reasons including the presence of air and tubes in the operative field. It prompts immediate revision of significant residual defects and helps in weaning patients from cardiopulmonary bypass or ventricular assist devices. It is especially useful for the detection of air in the left side of the heart before removal of aortic cannula, evaluation of global and regional function, assessment of the filling status of the left ventricle, and detection of pericardial effusion or hematoma within the pericardial space after an operation.

## Other Indications

TEE is superior to TTE in delineating cardiac masses and masses adjacent to the heart, such as in the pulmonary arteries and mediastinum (**Figure 49-38**). It is particularly useful for differentiating structural features, such as the site of attachment, consistency in cystic versus solid, and infiltration into surrounding structures, that are useful for differentiating thrombi and benign from malignant neoplasms. TEE is also useful in the detection of thrombi lying in the proximal portion of the pulmonary arteries. TEE affords a clear view into the superior vena cava and thrombi attached to pacemaker wires or intravenous lines.

## Three-dimensional TEE

Recently, live TEE technology has been introduced. The utility of this method is being evaluated, however, the technique appears to be beneficial compared to 2D TEE in the evaluation of mitral valve and paravalvular structures. Delineation of mitral valve scallop/scallops involved helps in planning and determining feasibility of surgical repair. Location and extent of paravalvular leaks in patients with bioprosthetic and prosthetic valves (**Figures 49-39** and **49-40**) seem to be significantly enhanced by 3D TEE compared to 2D TEE, thus allowing determination of feasibility of percutaneous repair as well as allowing guidance during the procedure. TEE allows assessment of the size and shape of an atrial septal defect, thus assisting with planning an appropriate procedure and placement of an interatrial septal device of correct size.

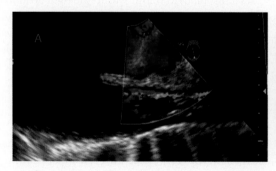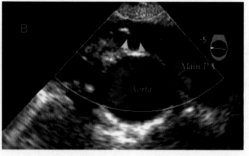

**Figure 49-38.** Tumor in a 27-year-old Asian female infiltrating superior vena cava causing turbulent color Doppler flow (A). Location of primary tumor is shown in right pulmonary artery in B (colored arrowheads).

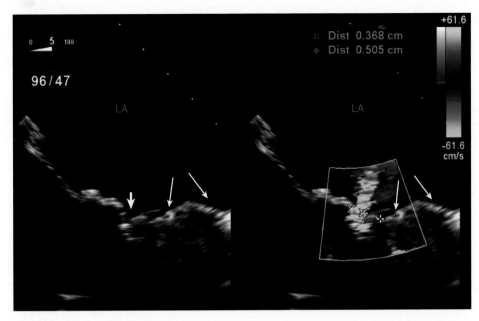

**Figure 49-39.** Bileaflet St. Jude's valve is shown in the mitral position in a 35-year-old female with history of rheumatic valve disease and prosthetic mitral and aortic valves. Prosthetic mitral valve disks are shown in systole in a closed position (white arrows). A gap (white arrowhead) in the paravalvular tissue with paravalvular systolic flow is seen located in the medial position between mitral valve and aortic valve. LA, left atrium.

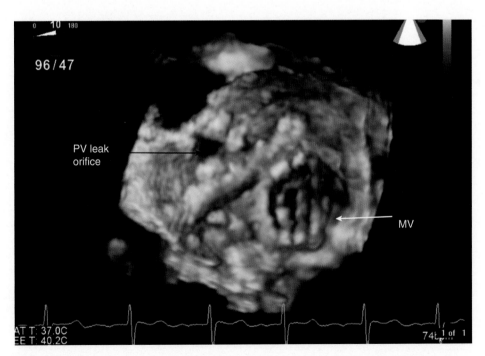

**Figure 49-40.** Three-dimensional TEE showing a bileaflet valve in the mitral position. Location and extent of paravalvular leak is clearly visualized. The leak is present between prosthetic aortic and mitral valves and is closer to aortic than the mitral valve.

## Suggested Readings

1. Peterson G, Brickner M and Reimold S. Transesophageal Echocardiography: Clinical Indications and Applications. *Circulation*. 2003;107;2398–2402.

2. Van den Brink. Evaluation of Prosthetic Heart Valves by Transesophageal Echocardiography: Problems, Pitfalls, and Timing of Echocardiography. Seminars in Cardiothoracic and Vascular Anesthesia, Vol 10, No 1 (March), 2006:89–100.

3. Evangelista A and Gonzalez-Alujas T. Echocardiography in infective endocarditis. *Heart*. 2004;90;614–617.

4. Eltzschig H, Rosenberger P, Löffler M, Fox J, Aranki S, and Shernan S. Impact of Intraoperative Transesophageal Echocardiography on Surgical Decisions in 12,566 Patients Undergoing Cardiac Surgery. *Ann Thorac Surg*. 2008;85: 845–852.

5. Poelaert J, Trouerbach J, Buyzere M, Everaert J and Colardyn F. Evaluation of Transesophageal Echocardiography as a Diagnostic and Therapeutic Aid in a Critical Care Setting. *Chest*. 1995;107:774–779.

# 50

# Stress Echocardiography

STEPHEN G. SAWADA AND ATHANASIOS THOMAIDES

## ● PRACTICAL POINTS

- Bicycle stress echocardiography enables imaging during peak exercise which may improve the sensitivity for detection of singie vessel disease.

- Contrast agents may improve endocardial border visualization and are recommended when 2 or more segments in a particular echocardiographic view are not adequately visualized.

- Stress –induced wall motion abnormalities may occur because of ischemia in the absence of obstruction of major coronary vessels.

- Appropriateness criteria for stress echocardiography have been published which provide a resource for determining appropriate indications for performance of stress echocardiography.

- The "biphasic" wall motion response to dobutamine has a high positive predictive value for detection of myocardium that will improve in function with revascularization.

- The utility of stress echocardiography for risk stratification of patients with known or suspected coronary disease has been documented in numerous studies.

## INTRODUCTION

Stress echocardiography is a universally employed modality in the noninvasive diagnosis and risk stratification of patients with suspected or known coronary artery disease. New applications continue to be established for this technique more than 20 years after the initial studies that introduced stress echocardiography as a versatile, safe, and accurate technique for the diagnosis of coronary artery disease (CAD).

In the setting of a fixed coronary obstruction, an increase in myocardial oxygen demand produced by exercise or catecholamine stress results in myocardial oxygen supply-demand imbalance and ischemia. Reduction in myocardial thickening and wall motion is a relatively early manifestation of ischemia, usually preceding the development of electrocardiographic abnormalities and symptoms. Myocardial oxygen supply-demand imbalance is greatest in the subendocardium, the inner myocardial layer that contributes the most to myocardial wall thickening. Regional reductions in myocardial thickening and wall motion are readily detected by two-dimensional echocardiography, which utilizes multiple tomographic imaging planes to assess function in all coronary artery distributions. Digital image acquisition and storage permits easy and direct visual comparison of cine loops obtained at baseline and with stress to determine the presence or absence of abnormalities in wall thickening or wall motion. Regional function is graded using a system that assigns a higher score with increasing severity of wall motion abnormality (1 = normal, 2 = hypokinetic, 3 = akinetic) and a 16- or 17-segment representation of the left ventricle (**Figure 50-1**). Myocardial segments can be grouped according to their coronary supply (left anterior descending [LAD], right coronary [RCA], and left circumflex [LCX]) with the recognition that there is variability in coronary supply of various segments including the apical lateral (LAD or LCX territory) and apical inferior (LAD or RCA territory) segments. Visual assessment of wall thickening and wall motion is a challenging exercise even for those with Level 2 or 3 training in echocardiography. Interpretation of at least 100 stress echocardiograms under the supervision of an expert is considered the minimum experience necessary before independent interpretation of studies. Considerably more experience is desirable as the accuracy of wall motion analysis has been shown to be greatest in those who have extensive experience in the technique.

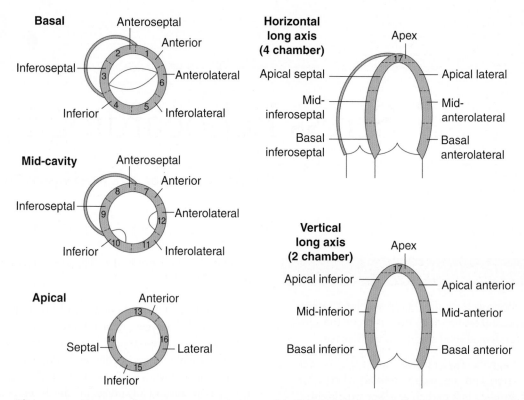

**Figure 50-1.** Diagram of 17-segment representation of the left ventricle with basal, mid, and apical short axis planes and 4 chamber and 2 chamber planes. (Adapted from Cerqueira MD et al, 2001.)

## STRESS METHODS

Various means of producing myocardial stress can be used with echocardiography. As a general rule, exercise is preferred over nonexercise methods if the patient can perform adequate dynamic exercise. Knowledge of the patient's exercise capacity contributes significant prognostic information. **Table 50-1** lists the major modalities of stress and their relative utility, advantages, and disadvantages.

Initial exercise echocardiography studies were conducted with treadmill exercise, which has the advantage of being the most familiar form of exercise in this country. The disadvantage of treadmill exercise is that imaging is limited to the postexercise period where rapid image acquisition is required by an expert sonographer. The success of treadmill exercise echocardiography hinges on the fact that wall motion abnormalities produced by demand ischemia persist for at least a short time after exercise is completed. The persistence of wall motion abnormalities poststress is in part due to myocardial stunning, which depends on the severity and extent of obstructive CAD.

The use of bicycle exercise permits imaging during exercise that, theoretically, might provide a higher sensitivity than treadmill exercise. Peak heart rate–systolic blood pressure product is often comparable between the two forms of exercise with the achieved heart rate higher with treadmill

exercise and systolic blood pressure higher with bicycle exercise, owing to an element of isometric stress with the latter method. There are few head-to-head comparisons of the sensitivity of peak bicycle exercise imaging and post-treadmill exercise imaging. Peak bicycle exercise imaging may yield more extensive wall motion abnormalities in those with coronary disease and have enhanced sensitivity for detection of single vessel disease compared with treadmill exercise. Bicycle exercise also has the advantage of permitting Doppler interrogation during exercise, enabling evaluation of left ventricular diastolic function and valvular function.

Pharmacologic stress echocardiography is primarily utilized in patients who cannot perform dynamic exercise. In this country, dobutamine is the most widely used agent. In the most commonly employed dosing regimen, dobutamine is first given at a low dose (5 µg/kg/min) and then increased to 10 µg/kg/min after 2 to 3 minutes. The dose is increased by 10 µg/kg/min increments every 2 to 3 minutes thereafter to a peak dose of 40 or 50 µg/kg/min. This dosing protocol, although never achieving a steady state drug level, provides a progressive increase in heart rate that simulates the increase in heart rate with exercise. In approximately 30% of patients, supplemental atropine, in divided doses up to a total of 2.0 mg, is needed to block vagal suppression of the heart rate response to dobutamine. Dobutamine stress has the advantage of being physiologically similar to exercise

| Table 50-1 • Stress Echo Modalities | | | | | |
|---|---|---|---|---|---|
| **Method** | **Procedure** | **Advantages** | **Disadvantages** | **Sensitivity** | **Specificity** |
| Treadmill | rest, immediate postexercise imaging | most familiar type of stress | imaging after exercise requires sonographer expertise for rapid image acquisition | high | high |
| Supine or upright bicycle | rest, early stage, peak and post imaging | permits peak exercise imaging, valve function can be assessed | lower peak heart rates than treadmill, supine exercise difficult in lung disease patients | high; may be higher than with treadmill, more extensive ischemia than with treadmill | high |
| Dobutamine | doses to 40 or 50 µg/kg/min; atropine often needed; rest, low, peak dose imaging | similar BP, HR changes to exercise, high quality images, valve function can be assessed | requires IV access, higher rate of side effects than exercise | moderate to high; reduced in patients with concentric remodeling | high |
| Vasodilator, adenosine, dipyridamole | 0.84 mg/kg dip dose; atropine needed; rest, early stage, late stage imaging | shorter infusion times compared to dobutamine, coronary flow, myocardial perfusion can be assessed | requires IV access, less physiologic than dobutamine stress | moderate to high | high |
| Transesophageal pacing | pacing catheter required; pacing up to 100% of age-predicted max HR; imaging at rest, 85% of max HR, max HR | short duration of stress | requires swallowing of pacing catheter, atropine may be needed for AV block | very high | high |

and is similar to the hemodynamic stress experienced by patients undergoing noncardiac surgery.

Dobutamine stress requires placement of intravenous access and is more labor and time intensive than exercise stress. Studies have shown that dobutamine stress may have decreased sensitivity in patients with concentric remodeling where LV cavity size is small and relative wall thickness is increased. In this setting, vasodilation caused by dobutamine may decrease wall stress and reduce the frequency of ischemia in patients with limited disease. Accelerated dobutamine and atropine infusion protocols have been shown to safely allow reduction in the duration of stress. Reversal of the effects of dobutamine using intravenous metoprolol or esmolol is routinely employed in many laboratories. This limits the duration of side effects experienced by the patient, effectively treats symptomatic ischemia, and reduces the time required for postinfusion monitoring. Studies have also shown that ischemic wall motion abnormalities may be unmasked by beta-blocker administration and imaging shortly after giving beta-blockers may enhance the sensitivity of the test. The safety of dobutamine stress echocardiography has been investigated in a number of large-scale studies. Life-threatening complications occur in 1 of every 2,000 studies.

The contraindications to dobutamine stress are similar to those for exercise stress. Laboratories should be prepared to rapidly reverse dobutamine stress in individuals with a history of symptomatic ischemia or severe coronary disease.

Vasodilator stress echocardiography utilizing high dose dipyridamole (0.84 mg/kg over 10 min) infusion with supplemental atropine is an alternative to dobutamine stress in patients who cannot exercise. The method is less commonly employed in the United States compared to Europe in part because of the low cost of dobutamine in this country, the requirement for high dose dipyridamole, and unfamiliarity with the vasodilator method. There are few comparative studies that have investigated the accuracy of dobutamine versus vasodilator stress in the same patient population. The available data suggest that adenosine stress has lower sensitivity than dobutamine stress. The safety of vasodilator stress is well validated and it has the advantage of permitting easier assessment of myocardial perfusion using echocardiographic contrast agents compared to dobutamine stress. Currently, no contrast agents have been approved for use in this country for assessment of myocardial perfusion, but a wealth of studies have demonstrated the utility of vasodilator stress with contrast perfusion imaging for detection of coronary disease.

Vasodilator stress also enables assessment of coronary flow velocity using transthoracic Doppler recordings of the left anterior descending coronary artery. This technique is underutilized in the United States but has been shown to be a useful adjunct to wall motion analysis for detection of coronary disease.

Transesophageal atrial pacing stress echocardiography is an alternative method to pharmacologic stress in patients who cannot exercise. The feasibility, safety, and accuracy of this method has been well validated in studies primarily from the Mayo Clinic. A specially designed catheter is placed orally or intranasally into the midesophagus after topical anesthesia. Pacing thresholds in the range of 10 mA are usually required and are generally well tolerated. Very high sensitivity for coronary disease can be obtained by echocardiographic imaging at paced rates of 85% and 100% of the patient's age predicted maximal heart rate. Pacing stress echocardiography requires a shorter duration of stress compared with pharmacologic stress, and higher quality images may be obtained in the absence of respiratory artifact and cardiac motion that may result from vasodilator or dobutamine stress, respectively. Pacing stress echocardiography has the disadvantage of being invasive and atropine may be required in some individuals because of AV nodal block. Studies have also shown that effective stress can be achieved in patients with permanent pacing devices and an atrial lead.

Pacing stress echocardiography using a ventricular lead can provide desired levels of stress but necessitates assessment of wall motion in the setting of dysynchronous septal contraction, as would be encountered in a patient with left bundle branch block. Assessment of ischemic wall motion abnormalities is more difficult in the setting of abnormal septal motion and requires evaluation of septal thickening and apical wall motion to distinguish between septal dysynchrony and LAD ischemia.

Additional forms of stress have been combined with echocardiography including arm ergometry, handrip, cold pressor, mental stress, squatting, and ergonovine stimulation. The use of handgrip at peak exercise has been shown to be a useful adjunct to pharmacologic stress by increasing wall stress. The safety and utility of ergonovine stress echocardiography have been demonstrated for detection of patients with coronary vasospasm.

# ECHOCARDIOGRAPHIC DETECTION OF CORONARY ARTERY DISEASE

We have briefly described the process of assessment of regional function with echocardiography in the introduction. A detailed description of analysis of regional function is

beyond the scope of this review. However, a basic knowledge of factors that influence both global and regional left ventricular function is important for both those who refer patients for stress echocardiography and those who are engaged in interpretation of these studies. Studies utilizing quantitative techniques have shown that there is regional heterogeneity in the timing and magnitude of wall motion and thickening between different regions of the myocardium in normal individuals without coronary disease. Myocardial segments that are in close proximity to the mitral or aortic annulus may appear to contract less in radial or transverse planes than segments that are not tethered to fibrous structures. Motion of the entire heart (cardiac translation) can occur with marked increases in global left ventricular contractility that occur with dobutamine stress, making detection of ischemic wall motion abnormalities more difficult.

Knowledge of the normal ventricular volume responses to the various modalities of stress can aid in identification of patients with cardiovascular disease. Normal subjects undergoing treadmill exercise typically have smaller end systolic volumes and increased ejection fraction postexercise compared to baseline. An increase in end-systolic volume or lack of improvement in global function may indicate the presence of extensive ischemia or an underlying cardiomyopathy. **Figure 50-2** is an example of a patient with LAD ischemia who has apical cavity dilation with stress. Bicycle exercise produces variable changes in cardiac volumes. A reduction in end-systolic volume and a prominent increase in ejection fraction are less likely to occur in normal individuals with bicycle exercise compared with treadmill stress. Dobutamine stress produces greater increases in global contractility than either treadmill or bicycle stress and reduction in cavity volume is the rule in normal individuals. Cavity dilation is infrequent with dobutamine stress even in the setting of left main disease. Modest declines in systolic blood pressure are common with dobutamine and vasodilator stress and are not specific markers of ischemia.

## Accuracy of Stress Echocardiography

Data pooled from numerous stress echocardiography studies employing coronary angiography as the reference standard

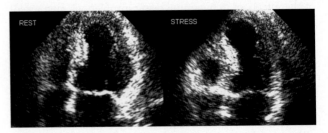

**Figure 50-2.** Rest and posttreadmill stress 4-chamber images at end systole in a patient with ischemia in the LAD distribution. The apex is dilated and severely hypokinetic with stress.

Patients with good exercise capacity and a normal exercise echocardiogram (no baseline or stress-induced wall motion abnormalities) are at very low risk with a less than 1% annual rate of myocardial infarction or cardiac death. These subjects remain at low risk for at least several years following their stress study. The risk of patients with normal exercise echocardiograms who have diabetes, advanced chronic kidney disease, or poor exercise capacity may increase after 2 to 3 years following their stress study.

Provided that adequate stress is achieved, a normal pharmacologic stress echocardiogram also identifies patients at low risk. However, because of a higher pretest prevalence of CAD, individuals who cannot exercise, such as those with peripheral vascular disease, remain at slightly higher risk compared to those who have normal exercise echocardiograms.

Poor exercise capacity, a history of infarction, and the presence of resting and/or stress-induced wall motion abnormalities identify patients at increased risk. Risk progressively increases with an increasing amount of myocardium with resting and/or stress-induced wall motion abnormalities. A reduction in global function at rest or with stress, evidence for multivessel disease with baseline or stress-induced wall motion abnormalities in more than one coronary territory, and cavity dilation with stress are markers of high risk. Echocardiographic assessment of left ventricular wall thickness, left atrial volume, and diastolic function provide additional risk stratification information.

## RESEARCH ADVANCES

Recent advances in three-dimensional (3D) echocardiography include real-time image acquisition that has extended the application of 3D imaging to stress echocardiography. An advantage of 3D full-volume imaging is that more regions of the left ventricle can be assessed than are possible using two-dimensional (2D) imaging. In addition, more accurate chamber volumes can be obtained. Disadvantages of the 3D technique include lower frame rates and the need for high quality images.

The reliance on qualitative visual assessment of regional wall thickening and motion has been viewed as a limitation of stress echocardiography. The accuracy and reproducibility of visual assessment of regional function are decreased in the hands of nonexperts. A potential solution to this problem is the development of quantitative analysis techniques, which are an increasing focus of research. Automated border detection, tissue Doppler imaging, and most recent, strain and strain rate imaging are advanced methods of assessing regional function that are now available on most ultrasound manufacturers' systems. Strain and strain rate imaging enable assessment of the magnitude of regional shortening or thickening and the velocity of regional shortening in localized areas of the myocardium. Strain and strain rate imaging are not affected by tethering and translational cardiac motion, which complicates visual assessment of regional function. These newer, quantitative methods have shown promise as adjuncts to visual assessment of regional function in an increasing number of published investigations.

## Suggested Readings

1. Douglas PS, Khandheria B, Stainback RF, et al. ACCF/ASE/ACEP/AHA/ASNC/SCAI/SCCT/SCMR 2008 appropriateness criteria for stress echocardiography: A report of the American College of Cardiology Foundation Appropriateness Criteria Task Force, American Society of Echocardiography, American College of Emergency Physicians, American Heart Association, American Society of Nuclear Cardiology, Society for Cardiovascular Angiography and Interventions, Society of Cardiovascular Computed Tomography, and Society for Cardiovascular Magnetic Resonance. *J Am Coll Cardiol.* 2008;51:1127–1147.

2. Pellikka PA, Nagueh SF, Elhendy AA, Kuehl CA, Sawada SG. Stress echocardiography: Recommendations for performance, interpretation and application. *J Am Soc Echocardiogr.* 2007;20:1021–1034.

3. Armstrong WF, Ryan T. Stress echocardiography from 1979 to present. *J Am Soc Echocardiogr.* 2008;21:22–28.

4. Armstong WF, Zoghbi W. Stress echocardiography: Current methodology and clinical applications. *J Am Coll Cardiol.* 2005;45:1739–1747.

5. Cerqueira MD, Weissman NJ, Dilsizian V, et al. Standardized myocardial segmentation and nomenclature for tomographic imaging of the heart: A statement of healthcare professionals from the Cardiac Imaging Committee of the Council on Clinical Cardiology of the American Heart Association. *Circulation.* 2001;105:539–542.

# 51

# Positron Emission Tomography

SHARMILA DORBALA AND MARCELO F. DI CARLI

## ● PRACTICAL POINTS

- Cardiac PET is increasingly being used in clinical practice.

- O-15 labeled water is an ideal radiotracer with linear uptake in relation to myocardial blood flow.

- Myocardial perfusion imaging with N-13 ammonia and rubidium-82 PET is highly sensitive and specific for identification of obstructive CAD.

- The overall diagnostic accuracy of PET MPI is higher compared to nonattenuation corrected SPECT (from higher specificity).

- The prognostic value of MPI with PET is excellent and comparable to that described with SPECT.

- Cardiac PET imaging with FDG is the most accurate test for diagnosis of myocardial viability.

- Assessment of inotropic contractile reserve with low dose dobutamine improves the specificity of identification of viable myocardium.

- There are no published randomized clinical studies demonstrating the utility of viability assessment in predicting recovery of function and outcomes following revascularization. However, extensive literature supports the role of viability assessment with FDG PET in predicting improvement in left ventricular ejection fraction, heart failure symptoms, and natural history following revascularization.

- The prognostic value of FDG imaging depends not only on the magnitude of viable myocardium, but also on several other factors, such as the baseline left ventricular ejection fraction, degree of remodeling of the left ventricle, and time to revascularization.

## INTRODUCTION

Cardiac positron emission tomography (PET) is a well-validated technique to evaluate myocardial perfusion and metabolism. Although long viewed as a research technique, the clinical use of cardiac PET imaging has increased significantly over the past five years. This is being driven primarily by increasing availability of PET scanners driven by oncology applications. Also, rubidium-82, a generator-produced perfusion radiotracer, as well as F-18-labeled fluoro-deoxyglucose (FDG) enables the use of PET in institutions without a cyclotron. PET images have higher spatial and temporal resolution and depth-independent attenuation correction. Each of these factors has contributed to the growing interest and clinical use of cardiac PET.

Positron emission tomography is a radionuclide technique wherein a radioactive tracer emitting positrons (511-kEV gamma rays) is used to study myocardial blood flow or physiology. The positrons travel a few millimeters in the tissue, collide with neighboring electrons, and release two 511-kEV photons. These pairs of photons are imaged in a coincidence detection mode using a PET scanner. PET scanners are available in two different configurations: a dedicated PET scanner or a hybrid PET/CT scanner. Dedicated PET scanners use a rotating line source or a germanium (Ge) rod source for transmission imaging, whereas PET/CT scanners use a low-dose CT scan of the chest for transmission imaging and attenuation correction. The majority of new PET scanner installations are hybrid PET/CT scanners. Cardiac PET scans have a spatial resolution on the order of 4–8 mm.

# PET RADIOTRACERS

There are several radiotracers available for cardiac PET imaging. Of these the FDA approved radiotracers for clinical use include N-13 ammonia and rubidium-82 (myocardial perfusion tracers) and FDG (myocardial glucose metabolism tracer) (**Table 51-1**).

## N-13 Ammonia

This is a cyclotron-producing radiotracer with a half-life of 9.96 minutes. The exact mechanism of N-13 ammonia transport into the myocytes is not known. It has been suggested that N-13 ammonia undergoes passive diffusion across the cell membrane or active transport via the sodium potassium ATPase pump. It is an excellent radiotracer with a very high extraction fraction and linear uptake in relation to myocardial blood across a wide range of blood flow values. Myocardial blood flow can be well-assessed semiquantitatively (visually), and it also can be quantified using tracer kinetic modeling (myocardial blood flow in mL/gm/min). N-13 ammonia's relatively long half-life enables its use with in either exercise or pharmacological stress testing.

## Rubidium-82

This is a generator-produced radiotracer with a half-life of 76 seconds. It is supplied by a strontium generator, which is replaced every 4 weeks (due to the long half-life of the parent compound strontium, 28 days). Rubidum-82 has thallium-like kinetics and enters the myocyte via the myocardial K-channels. Rb-82 is a good radiotracer with an adequate extraction fraction and plateau peak radiotracer concentration at high blood flow values. The short half-life makes it ideal for use with pharmacological stress testing, but less amenable to use in exercise stress imaging.

## O-15 Water

This is a cyclotron-produced radiotracer with a half-life of 2.15 minutes. This is an ideal radiotracer for imaging myocardial blood flow, because of its linear uptake in relation to myocardial blood flow even at high flow rates induced by vasodilator stress. This radiotracer is freely diffusible and makes semiquantitative interpretation of images difficult (due to the need for subtraction of background blood pool activity). However, myocardial blood flow can be well quantified using tracer kinetic modeling. O-15 water is therefore widely used in research studies for quantitative estimation of myocardial blood flow.

## F-18 Fluoro-deoxy Glucose (FDG)

This is the primary radiotracer used clinically for myocardial viability assessment with PET. FDG is a cyclotron-produced radiotracer with a half-life of 109 minutes, permitting transportation of unit doses to sites without an on-site cyclotron. FDG competes with glucose and is transported into the myocyte by facilitated transport via glucose transporters, and then it becomes trapped in the myocyte following phosphorylation by hexokinase. The magnitude of FDG uptake is indicative of myocardial glucose uptake and metabolism and is used clinically to study myocardial viability. Patients are typically studied in a glucose-loaded state. Appropriate preparation of patients with insulin and glucose is critical to ensure adequate image quality. Details of the preparation of a patient for the FDG PET study are beyond the scope of this chapter; readers

| Table 51-1 • Commonly Used PET Radiotracers | | | | |
|---|---|---|---|---|
| **Radiotracer** | **Half-Life** | **Type of Stress** | **Uptake Mechanism** | **Imaging Process** |
| **Perfusion tracers** | | | | |
| N-13 ammonia* | 10 min | Exercise or Pharmacological | Passive diffusion | Perfusion |
| O-15 water | 2 min | Pharmacological | Passive diffusion | Blood flow, perfusible tissue |
| Rubidium-82* | 75 sec | Pharmacological | Active uptake K+ like | Perfusion, viability |
| **Metabolic tracers** | | | | |
| F-18 fluorodeoxy glucose* | 110 min | | Passive | Glucose transport, hexokinase |
| C-11 palmitate | 20 min | | | Oxidative metabolism (TCA cycle turnover) |
| C-11 acetate | 20 min | | | Fatty acid metabolism |
| C-11 glucose | 20 min | | | Glucose metabolism |

*FDA approved radiotracers for clinical use.*

21. Allman KC, Shaw LJ, Hachamovitch R, Udelson JE. Myocardial viability testing and impact of revascularization on prognosis in patients with coronary artery disease and left ventricular dysfunction: a meta-analysis. *J Am Coll Cardiol.* 2002;39:1151–1158.

22. Di Carli MF, Davidson M, Little R, et al. Value of metabolic imaging with positron emission tomography for evaluating prognosis in patients with coronary artery disease and left ventricular dysfunction. *J Am J Cardiol.* 1994;73:527–533.

23. Eitzman D, al-Aouar Z, Kanter HL, et al. Clinical outcome of patients with advanced coronary artery disease after viability studies with positron emission tomography. *J Am Coll Cardiol.* 1992;20:559–565.

24. Lee KS, Marwick TH, Cook SA, et al. Prognosis of patients with left ventricular dysfunction, with and without viable myocardium after myocardial infarction. Relative efficacy of medical therapy and revascularization. *Circulation.* 1994;90:2687–2694.

25. Di Carli MF, Hachamovitch R, Berman DS. The art and science of predicting post revascularization improvement in left ventricular (LV) function in patients with severely depressed LV function. *J Am Coll Cardiol.* 2002;40:1744–1747.

26. Beanlands RS, Ruddy TD, deKemp RA, et al. Positron emission tomography and recovery following revascularization (PARR-1): the importance of scar and the development of a prediction rule for the degree of recovery of left ventricular function. *J Am Coll Cardiol.* 2002;40:1735–1743.

27. Yamaguchi A, Ino T, Adachi H, et al. Left ventricular volume predicts postoperative course in patients with ischemic cardiomyopathy. *Ann Thorac Surg.* 1998;65:434–438.

28. Tarakji KG, Brunken R, McCarthy PM, et al. Myocardial viability testing and the effect of early intervention in patients with advanced left ventricular systolic dysfunction. *Circulation.* 2006;113:230–237.

29. Shan K, Constantine G, Sivananthan M, Flamm SD. Role of cardiac magnetic resonance imaging in the assessment of myocardial viability. *Circulation.* 2004;109:1328–1334.

# Nuclear Cardiac Imaging: A Primer

Rami Kahwash

## INTRODUCTION

Over the past decade, the number of nuclear cardiac imaging procedures in the United States has exceeded the number of noncardiac ones by a significant margin. Myocardial nuclear imaging is a noninvasive technique that uses the properties of radioactive tracers in providing valuable cardiac diagnostic and prognostic data related to myocardial perfusion and ventricular function. Recently, positron emission tomographic (PET) cardiac imaging has become a favored technique implemented in modern clinical practice to assess myocardial viability prior to surgical and percutaneous coronary revascularization. This chapter will review the basics of cardiac nuclear imaging and its role in clinical cardiology.

## PERFORMANCE OF CARDIAC NUCLEAR IMAGING

### Radioactive Nuclear Tracers

Several radioactive nuclear tracers have been implemented in nuclear cardiac imaging and vary substantially in their properties. After administration to the body, nuclear tracers get extracted from the blood stream by the heart in an amount that is proportionate to myocardial blood perfusion. Due to their instability, once inside the cells, they undergo spontaneous decay. This fundamental property of the radioactive agents generates electromagnetic energy (photons) that exits the body in the form of X-rays and gamma rays. When these high energy electromagnetic rays are captured by highly specialized detectors, they can be converted to produce nuclear images. The ideal tracer should be nontoxic, readily available, and able to emit high energy photons without exposing the patient to significant radiation risk.

### Gamma Camera (Illustration 52-1)

The gamma camera is used to capture photons and convert their energy into actual images. A standard gamma camera consists of three major components: a lead collimator, sodium iodide crystals, and photomultiplier tubes. The metal

**Gamma camera**

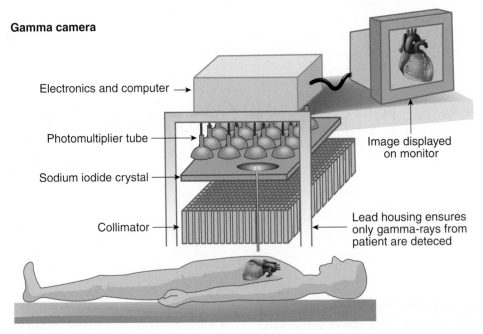

**Illustration 52-1.** Major components of Gamma camera

honeycomb-shaped collimator has holes that help filter low energy, scattered photons produced by tissue attenuation. This allows the focus of the high energy emitted photons originated from the myocardial cell to reach the iodide crystals. Spatial resolution of the images increases when the ratio of the hole's diameter to length decreases. This of course happens at the expense of count sensitivity (number of photons striking the crystal per unit of time). When photons exit the collimator, they strike the sodium iodide crystals and generate light proportionate to the quantity and energy of the photons. The function of the photomultiplier tubes is to convert light produced by the iodide crystal into energy after amplifying it thousands of times. Special circuits and software convert the energy produced into actual images that reflect the nuclear activities in the myocardium. Only signals from a predetermined energy range finally get processed into actual images in order to eliminate the "fuzzy" effect of scattered photons, which tend to have a lower energy level.

## MYOCARDIAL SPECT IMAGING

SPECT images are planar images obtained from multiple fixed cameral projections in relation to the body (anterior, left anterior oblique, and left lateral). Myocardial nuclear images then get processed in short axis, vertical long axis, and horizontal long axis. Using this method, the left ventricle is divided into the standard 17 segments (**Figures 52-1** and **52-2**). Each segment is given a score from zero to four depending on its uptake of the nuclear tracer. A score of zero is given to segments with normal nuclear uptake and a score of four is given to complete absence of nuclear uptake. Scores

of one, two, and three are given to mild, moderate, and severe decreases in nuclear uptake, respectively. Rest and stress images are analyzed carefully and a summed score is given. Reversible defects are the hallmark of ischemia and imply defects present at stress and absent at rest. On the contrary, fixed defects are the ones present at both rest and exercise and imply scar tissue. Partial reversibility is seen in nontransmural scars. Reverse redistribution, where the defect seen at rest disappears at stress, is seen in acute myocardial infarction and with artifact (**Table 52-1**). The severity of the defect

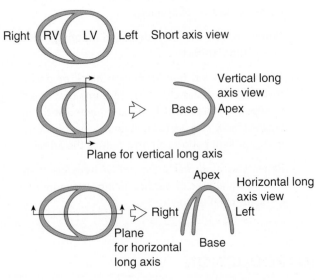

**Figure 52-1.** Cardiac plane definition and display for tomographic imaging modalities. Source: American Heart Association scientific statement, *Circulation.* 2002;105:539. (From AHA, there is fee required, appreciate your help/advise)

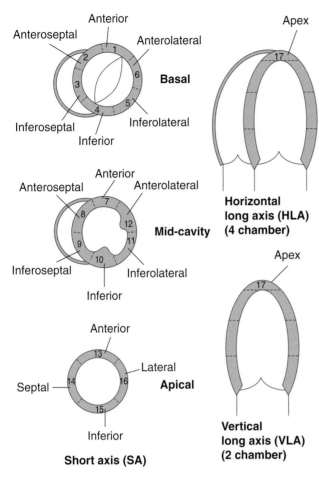

**Figure 52-2.** Diagram of vertical long-axis (VLA, approximating the two-chamber view), horizontal long-axis (HLA, approximating the four-chamber view), and short-axis (SA) planes showing the name, location, and anatomic landmarks for the selection of the basal (tips of the mitral valve leaflets), mid-cavity (papillary muscles), and apical (beyond papillary muscles, but before cavity ends) short-axis slices for the recommended 17-segment system. (Source: American Heart Association scientific statement, *Circulation.* 2002;105:539. From AHA, fee applied)

reversibility is further classified based on the difference in the summed scores between rest and stress images: low, if the summed scores difference between rest and stress images is less than three; moderate, when between three and seven; and severe, when more than seven.

| Table 52-1 • Simplistic Approach in Interpreting Stress SPECT Study | | |
|---|---|---|
| **Rest SPECT** | **Stress SPECT** | **Conclusion** |
| Normal | Normal | Normal |
| Normal | Abnormal | Reversible defect (ischemia) |
| Abnormal | Abnormal | Fixed defect (scar) |
| Abnormal | Normal | Seen in acute myocardial infraction consider artifact |

# MYOCARDIAL PET IMAGING

Positron emission tomographic cardiac imaging has been increasingly implemented in clinical practice in recent years. It is the preferred noninvasive technique to assess left ventricular myocardial viability prior to coronary revascularizations. In contrary to SPECT, nuclear tracers in PET eject a positron (positive particle) that interacts with a nearby electron (negative particle), causing annihilation of the two original particles and the production of paired high energy (511 KeV) photons. These coupled photons split, exiting the body in opposite directions, exactly 180°s apart. PET cameras consist of multiple circular formations of gamma ray detectors capable of distinguishing coupled photons produced by the same annihilation event from other uncoupled photons produced by tissue attenuations (**Illustration 52-2**). In addition to its role in the assessment of myocardial perfusion, PET has an advantage over SPECT of evaluating myocardial metabolic activity through the uptake of 2-fluoro-2-deoxyglucose (FDG) by the viable cells. Perfusion-metabolic mismatch is the hallmark of viable myocardium (presence of perfusion defect and preserved uptake of FDG) (**Table 52-2**). This property has become increasingly important in guiding revascularization and restoring blood flow to areas of viable myocardium, which subsequently improves left ventricular function. The PET technique is superior to SPECT in achieving a spatial and temporal resolution of myocardial perfusion imaging due to the ability of identification and correction of attenuation artifacts.

# ECG-GATED IMAGING PROCESSING TECHNIQUE

ECG-gated images are obtained with an electrocardiogram gating technique that allows the integrating of the cardiac cycle into image acquisition and processing. The R-R intervals of the patient's actual ECG are divided into 8 or 16 frames. Images of each frame from each cardiac cycle are added up, averaged, and reconstructed over a predefined period of time. By doing that, the gated technique provides us with a dynamic assessment of the wall motion and global ejection fraction of the ventricle. This technique can be used in both SPECT and PET images. Technetium-99m Sestamibi is the preferred nuclear tracer in gated SPECT studies due to its high count rate, whereas Nitrogen-13 Ammonia is the preferred tracer for gated PET imaging due to its long tissue retention.

# RADIONUCLIDE VENTRICULOGRAPHY

Nuclear cardiac images are helpful in the assessment of ventricular function, wall motion, and chamber sizes. Two techniques are commonly used: first-pass imaging and gated radionuclide ventriculography (multiple-gated acquisition

**Basic physics of positron emission tomography**

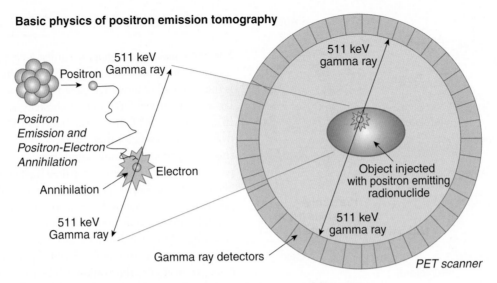

**Illustration 52-2.** Basic physics of positron emission tomography (PET).

[MUGA]). In the first-pass imaging technique, a bolus of the radioactive tracer is given intravenously, and then a series of nuclear images is acquired by a high count camera while the nuclear tracer bolus passes through the cardiac chambers. The measurement of the heart chamber's size is averaged over 5 to 15 beats and calculated. The left ventricular ejection fraction can be calculated from the following formula:

LVEF = (end diastolic counts – end systolic counts / end diastolic counts).

First-pass studies can also be used to assess myocardial ischemia by comparing regional wall motion in response to exercise.

In MUGA, red blood cells are labeled with the nuclear tracer and injected into the patient through an intravenous route. Using the patient's own ECG, dynamic images are obtained over hundreds of cardiac cycles and then averaged together. This will allow the images to be played in a ciné loop that provides time-averaged calculations of the ejection fraction using the same formula as in the first-pass imaging technique. Similar to the first-pass technique, stress MUGA images can be used to assess ischemia by analyzing regional wall motion in response to stress compared to rest.

## Table 52-2 • Simplistic Approach in Interpreting Viability PET Study

| Perfusion | Metabolism | Conclusion |
|-----------|-----------|-----------|
| Normal | Normal | Normal |
| Abnormal | Normal | Viable |
| Abnormal | Abnormal | Scar |

# RADIOACTIVE TRACERS

## SPECT Radioactive Tracers

### Thallium-201
Property similar to Potassium
Requires cyclotron for production
Long half life (73 hours)
Low energy produced (80 KeV) makes it susceptible to scatter and attenuation artifacts
Long half life prohibits the use of high doses
Redistribution property allows its use in the assessment of viability

### Technetium-99m Labeled Agents
Does not require cyclotron for production
Higher energy (140KeV) makes it less susceptible to attenuation artifacts than Thallium-201
Shorter half life allows administration of higher doses than Thallium-201
High count rate allows its use in acquiring ECG-gated studies
Minimum retribution, not commonly used in viability assessment

# PET RADIOACTIVE TRACERS FOR PERFUSION ASSESSMENT

## Rubidium-82

Metabolized similar to potassium
Does not require cyclotron for production
Very short half life (76 seconds), on site production needed

## Nitrogen-13 Ammonia

Requires cyclotron for production
Short half life (10 minutes), on site production needed
Long tissue retention allows its use in ECG-gated studies

## Oxygen-15 water

Requires cyclotron for production
Short half life (2.1 minutes), on site production needed
Uptake by tissue is linear to blood flow

# PET RADIOACTIVE TRACERS FOR METABOLISM ASSESSMENT

## 2-fluoro-2-deoxyglucose (FDG)

Metabolized similar to glucose
Trapped inside the viable cells after phosphorylation to FDG-6-phosphate
Uptake indicates viability in areas of compromised perfusion

# ASSESSMENT OF VIABILTY WITH THALLIUM-201

A unique property of Thallium-201 is the delayed redistribution. After the initial increase in blood concentration following its injection, Thallium-201 leaves the blood stream and enters the cells. Thallium-201 then leaves the cell and returns to the blood stream when its blood concentration decreases. The area of the myocardium with an impaired flow slows down Thallium-201's ability to move in and out of the cells. As a result of this phenomenon, areas that first had a perfusion defect might get better nuclear uptake on delayed images. This implies a viable tissue and suggests further benefits from revascularizations.

# IMAGING PROTOCOLS

Several imaging protocols are used in clinical practice. These include a same-day rest and stress with single isotope, a 2-day protocol with the same isotope, or a dual isotope study where different isotopes are used for stress and rest. During acquisitions, a total of 60 to 64 projections is acquired over a 180° arc while the patient is in a supine position. Prone images are sometimes performed to decrease the chance of diaphragmatic attenuation artifact. Several types of artifact can potentially occur during acquisitions of images. These can be related to the patient or to the equipment. Attenuations from breast tissue, the chest wall, the diaphragm, and the patient's motion are common causes of artifact. The dyssynchronous septum in patients with a left bundle branch block or a paced rhythm can cause a septal artifact, which can be augmented by increasing the heart rate; therefore, stressing with vasodilators (adenosine or dipyridamole) can reduce the problem of septal artifact.

# CLINICAL APPLICATION OF NUCLEAR CARDIAC IMAGING

## Diagnostic Assessment

Stress SPECT is most useful in diagnosing coronary artery disease in patients who belong to the intermediate risk category. The sensitivity and specificity of myocardial perfusion SPECT in detecting coronary artery disease is 87% and 73% for exercise SPECT and 89% and 75% in vasodilator SPECT, respectively. Stress SPECT has an advantage over stress echo in patients with poor echo windows due to obesity and chronic pulmonary disease or in patients with a paced rhythm or left bundle branch block.

## Prognostic Assessment

Stress SPECT prognostic values have been studied and validated extensively in the past. It is already proven that patients with normal stress SPECT have less than a 1% annual risk of cardiac death and nonfatal myocardial infarction. This does not hold true, however, in patients with diabetes and those with abnormal ECG responses to stress with vasodilators. Both the size and severity of the perfusion defects are major factors in determining the prognosis of patients with known coronary artery disease. Prognostic values of stress SPECT are well validated in the elderly, women, and diabetic patients as well as those undergoing noncardiac surgeries.

# FUTURE DIRECTIONS

Incorporations of nuclear cardiac imaging techniques into new diagnostic modalities, such as CT technology, offer the promise of comprehensive diagnostic and prognostic cardiac assessments of patients with known or suspected heart disease. The expanding of PET technology will allow us to further evaluate patients with microvascular dysfunction.

# LIMITATIONS

Despite the vast improvement in cardiac imaging techniques, it still requires skills in patient selection, preparation, image acquisition, and interpretation of data. The need of an on-site cyclotron in addition to the short half life of some tracers limits its use to large medical facilities. Radiation exposure, increased time consumption, and the high costs of material and equipment used in performing nuclear studies make it less appealing when compared to other imaging modalities such as echocardiography and MR.

## Suggested Readings

1. American Heart Association, American College of Cardiology, and Society of Nuclear Medicine. Standardization of cardiac tomographic imaging. *Circulation*. 1992;86: 338–339.

2. American Society of Nuclear Cardiology. Imaging guidelines for nuclear cardiology procedures, Part 2. *J Nucl Cardiol*. 1999;6:G47–G84.

3. Standardized myocardial segmentation and nomenclature for tomographic imaging of the heart: A statement for healthcare professionals from the Cardiac Imaging Committee of the Council on Clinical Cardiology of the American Heart Association. *Circulation*. 2002 Jan 29;105(4):539–542.

# Cardiovascular Nuclear Stress Testing

Aman M. Amanullah, Daniel S. Berman,
Rory Hachamovitch, and Guido Germano

## ● PRACTICAL POINTS

- Exercise is the preferred form of stress for SPECT-MPI; however, vasodilators are preferred in patients with LBBB and paced ventricular rhythm, due to the possibility of perfusion defects with higher heart rates.

- The average sensitivity is 87% and specificity 73% for exercise SPECT and similar for vasodilators SPECT.

- A normal scan is generally associated with a less than 1% annual risk of cardiac death or MI, depending on the clinical state.

- In occasional patients, the possibility of extensive CAD can be "missed" due to balanced reduction of flow. Some of these patients have other high risk markers, such as LV transient ischemic dilation, a rest to poststress fall in LVEF, or increased lung uptake tracer.

- Mildly abnormal scans have been reported to be associated with an intermediate risk for MI but a low risk for subsequent mortality.

- Survival benefit was present for patients undergoing medical therapy versus revascularization in the setting of no or mild ischemia, whereas patients undergoing revascularization had an increased benefit over medical therapy in patients with moderate to severe ischemia.

- The risk of cardiac events in diabetics with abnormal SPECT-MPI is higher than in nondiabetics throughout the range of perfusion abnormalities.

- When the coronary artery calcium score is less than 400, the rate of SPECT-MPI abnormalities is low; however, when the score exceeds 400, the rate of an ischemic SPECT-MPI is elevated.

- In patients presenting to the ED with chest pain with a low-intermediate likelihood of an ACS, a normal SPECT-MPI study has a 99% negative predictive value.

- SPECT-MPI can be used to distinguish viable but nonfunctioning myocardium that can improve with revascularization from nonviable myocardium.

The major applications of cardiovascular stress testing with single-photon emission computed tomography (SPECT) or positron emission tomography (PET) myocardial perfusion imaging (MPI) include the detection of significant coronary artery disease (CAD) as well as the assessment of short- and long-term prognosis, that is, to separate patients at high risk from those at low risk for future events in order to guide patient management decisions. Since its beginnings in the early 1970s, clinical nuclear cardiology has evolved

substantially, gaining both technical sophistication and enhanced imaging capabilities. It is important that in parallel to these developments, an extensive literature supporting the clinical and cost-effectiveness of this modality has developed. Today, state-of-the-art nuclear cardiology allows for the objective measurement of both myocardial function and relative regional myocardial perfusion at rest and stress, providing accurate risk assessment in a wider variety of patient subsets. The most commonly performed imaging procedure for cardiovascular nuclear perfusion is SPECT, but increasingly PET is also being used for this purpose. This chapter will primarily deal with SPECT-MPI; however, almost all comments apply equally to PET-MPI.

The SPECT or PET cameras capture the timing and location of the photon/crystal interaction, convert the information into digital data, and reconstruct the data into a three-dimensional volume set that is most commonly displayed as a series of slices (tomograms). The final SPECT or PET displays represent the distribution of perfusion in the myocardium. The use of ECG-gating during acquisition ("gated SPECT" or "gated PET") allows assessment of ventricular function as well as perfusion. PET-MPI is usually combined with computed tomography (CT) (PET/CT), and SPECT/CT is becoming more common. The addition of the CT is usually for attenuation correction (reducing artifact caused by nonuniform soft tissue attenuation) as well as for assessing coronary artery calcium.

# EXERCISE AND PHARMACOLOGIC STRESS TO INDUCE CORONARY HYPEREMIA

The basic physiologic concept underpinning of the use of rest and stress MPI for assessment of myocardial perfusion is that coronary arteries with significant stenosis cannot increase blood flow maximally during stress, thus causing a relative perfusion deficit when compared with regions supplied by nonstenosed vessels. Typically, coronary stenosis has been defined using a 50% diameter narrowing, but it is increasingly being recognized that a 70% stenosis criterion more accurately defines a threshold for inducible ischemia. SPECT- and PET-MPI generally do not detect subclinical coronary atherosclerosis without stenosis, with the possible exception of regions supplied by a rupture-prone plaque, in which vasoconstriction rather than vasodilation might be seen with stress.

Exercise is the preferred form of stress for SPECT-MPI, as it provides information on functional capacity, exercise-induced ECG changes, arrhythmias, blood pressure and heart rate response, as well as heart rate recovery, all of which have important diagnostic and prognostic implications. In patients with exertional symptoms, it also provides an opportunity to provoke and reproduce ischemic symptoms during maximal physical effort and correlate these with the presence, location, and extent of perfusion abnormalities on SPECT. A list of high risk ECG stress test variables is shown in **Table 53-1**.

Pharmacologic stress agents are broadly divided into two types: vasodilator agents, which include dipyridamole, adenosine, and regadenoson; and adrenergic agents such as dobutamine. With rubidium-82 PET, only pharmacologic stress is available due to the very short half-life of the tracer. Although exercise is the preferred modality for inducing coronary hyperemia with SPECT-MPI, a substantial number of patients

| Table 53-1 • High Risk Exercise Stress ECG Variables |
| --- |
| 1. Achievement of <4 METS |
| 2. ST-segment depressions appearing in greater than 5 leads |
| 3. ≥2.0-mm ST-segment depression |
| 4. ≥1.0-mm ST-segment depression in stage 1 of Bruce Protocol |
| 5. ST-segment depression lasting longer than 5 minutes in the recovery period |
| 6. An abnormal exercise blood pressure response to increasing levels of work load |
| 7. Exercise-induced ventricular arrhythmias |
| 8. Poor heart rate recovery when exercise ceases |

have exercise limitations or cannot achieve more than 85% of the maximum predicted heart rate for age, lowering the workload achieved and, thus, the sensitivity of SPECT-MPI. When normal, submaximal-stress SPECT-MPI studies must be considered nondiagnostic due to the possibility that potential ischemia was not provoked. The ACC/AHA/ASNC guidelines for the clinical use of cardiac radionuclide imaging consider inability to exercise in a patient with intermediate-to-high likelihood of CAD as a Class 1 indication for the use of pharmacologic stress. Other Class I indications for vasodilator (adenosine, regadenoson, or dipyridamole) stress SPECT-MPI include patients with left bundle branch block (LBBB) or paced ventricular rhythm, as these patients may have heart-rate related perfusion defects on exercise or dobutamine SPECT-MPI without having CAD.

Adenosine is a potent coronary vasodilator. Its vasodilatory effect is predominantly mediated by stimulation of $A_{2a}$ receptors. It has a short half-life of less than 10 seconds and a rapid onset of action. Regadenoson is a selective $A_{2a}$ adenosine receptor agonist that has recently been approved by FDA for vasodilator stress SPECT-MPI. It is administered as a single rapid intravenous injection followed by tracer injection, and the protocol is completed in less than 1 minute. Recent studies have demonstrated that the image quality and diagnostic accuracy of regadenoson and adenosine SPECT-MPI are similar. Dipyridamole acts indirectly by blocking the intracellular transport of adenosine and inhibiting adenosine deaminase, responsible for intracellular breakdown of adenosine.

When possible, low level exercise is generally combined with vasodilator stress testing. Although no definite advantage in the diagnostic yield has been demonstrated, this addition is associated with fewer side effects and less extracardiac tracer uptake, improving image quality and the ability to image earlier after stress.

Intravenous graded dobutamine infusion is used in patients in whom vasodilator pharmacologic stress is contraindicated because of bronchospastic airways disease or being under the influence of methyxanthines, which may block the action of the vasodilators. Dobutamine has a relatively rapid onset of

## Table 53-2 • Contraindications to Pharmacologic Stress Testing

### Contraindications to dipyridamole or adenosine

Severe obstructive lung disease

Second- or third-degree AV block without a functioning pacemaker

Acute MI or unstable coronary syndrome (<24 hr)

Systolic blood pressure < 90 mm Hg

Hypersensitivity to adenosine or dipyridamole

Intake of xanthine-containing compounds within the previous 12 hr

### Contraindications to dobutamine

Acute coronary syndrome (<4 d)

Severe aortic stenosis or hypertrophic obstructive cardiomyopathy

Uncontrolled hypertension

Uncontrolled atrial arrhythmias

Uncontrolled heart failure

Severe ventricular arrhythmias

Large aortic aneurysms

Narrow-angle glaucoma, myasthenia gravis, obstructive uropathy, or obstructive gastrointestinal disorders

*Source: Elhendy A et al, J Nucl Med. 2002;43:1634–1646.*

action with a half-life of approximately 2 minutes and is used in a stepwise fashion to a maximum of 40 mcg/kg/min. At low dose of dobutamine infusion (5-10 mcg/kg/min), there is an increase in myocardial contractility, thus allowing viability assessment. At higher dose (beyond 10 mcg/kg/min), there is a progressive increase in heart rate and contractility, leading to an increase in oxygen demand and myocardial blood flow.

The standard contraindications to pharmacologic stress are listed in **Table 53-2**. Vasodilator stress protocols are shown in **Table 53-3**.

## SPECT/PET IMAGE ANALYSIS AND INTERPRETATION

SPECT/PET-MPI images are generally interpreted by visual analysis, with semiquantitative visual analysis being

## Table 53-3 • Vasodilator Stress Protocol

| Stressor | Dose | Duration | Isotope Injection |
|---|---|---|---|
| Dipyridamole | 142 mcg/kg/min | 4 min by hand infusion or pump | 3 min after completion of infusion |
| Adenosine | 140 mcg/kg/min | 5 or 6 min infusion by pump | at 3 min into infusion |
| Regadenoson | 0.4 mg | i.v. bolus in 10 sec followed by saline flush | 30 sec after saline flush |

recommended. Increasingly, quantitative computer analysis is used in conjunction with visual interpretation, providing automatic objective interpretation and minimizing the subjectivity in image interpretation. For visual analysis, the important elements include the presence, size, location, and severity of the perfusion defect and whether the defect is reversible (present only at stress images implying stress-induced myocardial ischemia), or fixed (non-reversible present both at stress and rest images, often implying infarcted or scarred myocardium). For semiquantitative visual analysis, the left ventricle is divided into a 17-segment model (**Figure 53-1**); each segment is assigned a perfusion score. A commonly used scoring system is as follows: 0 = normal perfusion, 1 = mildly reduced perfusion, 2 = moderately reduced perfusion, 3 = severely reduced perfusion, and 4 = absence of tracer uptake. Scores of all 17 segments are added to both stress and rest images to create a summed stress score (SSS) and a summed rest score (SRS). SSS represents the extent and severity of stress perfusion defect while SRS represents the extent of resting hypoperfusion or infarction. The summed difference score (SDS) derived by subtracting SRS from SSS represents the extent and severity of stress-induced myocardial ischemia (**Figure 53-2**). Quantitative analysis of SPECT-MPI or PET-MPI is generally displayed by creating a polar-map display of myocardial perfusion at rest and stress. The quantitative perfusion study can show the extent and severity of a global perfusion abnormality, an abnormality within vascular territories, as well as the extent of a reversible and fixed defect (**Figure 53-3**). With either quantitative or visual perfusion defect assessments, the percentage myocardium abnormal stress and rest and the percentage myocardium ischemia can be expressed, allowing a more intuitive understanding of the magnitude of perfusion defect that was provided by the SSS, SRS, and SDS.

ECG gating of SPECT- or PET-MPI is now routinely used to complement the perfusion information by providing assessment of both global and regional systolic function including left ventricular ejection fraction (LVEF), end-diastolic volume, and end-systolic volume (ESV). Diastolic function parameters such as peak filling rate (PFR), time to PFR, peak ejection rate (PER), time to PER, and so on can also be assessed but are less commonly used.

## SENSITIVITY AND SPECIFICITY OF EXERCISE AND PHARMACOLOGIC SPECT-MPI AND PET-MPI FOR DETECTION OF CAD

A pooled analysis from the 2003 ACC/AHA/ASNC radionuclide imaging guidelines involving 4,480 patients from 33 studies undergoing exercise SPECT-MPI demonstrated a sensitivity of 87% (range from 71 to 97%) and specificity of 73% (range from 36 to 100%) for detecting CAD defined

## Myocardial perfusion SPECT 17-segment scoring

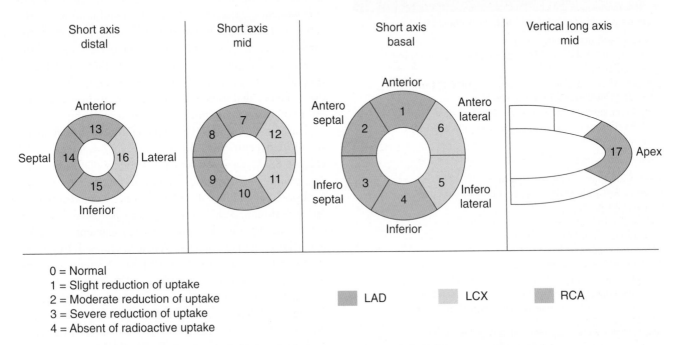

0 = Normal
1 = Slight reduction of uptake
2 = Moderate reduction of uptake
3 = Severe reduction of uptake
4 = Absent of radioactive uptake

LAD          LCX          RCA

**Figure 53-1.** Standard segmental myocardial display for semiquantitative visual analysis in a 17-segment model.

by greater than 50% stenosis. The relatively low specificity of SPECT-MPI may be related to artifacts and motion during image acquisitions but in most studies is related to post-test-referral bias (verification bias) in which patients with positive studies are much more likely to undergo coronary angiography. Verification bias also has the effect of raising the apparent test sensitivity. Methods for correcting for verification bias have been described but, to date, have not been employed in most literature reports. To assess the specificity of stress SPECT/PET-MPI, the "normalcy rate" is commonly employed, which is defined by the frequency of the test being

normal in subjects with a very low pretest likelihood of CAD (<5%). The normalcy rate of SPECT-MPI and PET-MPI has consistently been above 90%. Attenuation correction with PET or SPECT and the use of ECG gating can improve the accuracy of SPECT/PET-MPI. For SPECT-MPI, prone imaging, as a complement to supine imaging, also improves test specificity by shifting soft-tissue attenuation.

The sensitivity and specificity of vasodilator pharmacologic stress SPECT-MPI are similar to those reported with exercise

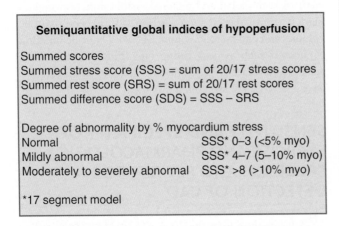

**Semiquantitative global indices of hypoperfusion**

Summed scores
Summed stress score (SSS) = sum of 20/17 stress scores
Summed rest score (SRS) = sum of 20/17 rest scores
Summed difference score (SDS) = SSS − SRS

Degree of abnormality by % myocardium stress
Normal                              SSS* 0–3 (<5% myo)
Mildly abnormal                     SSS* 4–7 (5–10% myo)
Moderately to severely abnormal     SSS* >8 (>10% myo)

*17 segment model

**Figure 53-2.** Scoring perfusion defects in each individual segment for deriving summed perfusion parameters, which incorporate the global extent and severity of perfusion abnormality. (Adapted from Berman DS et al, 2004.)

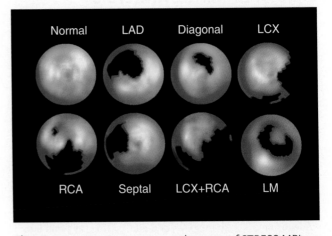

**Figure 53-3.** Quantitative stress polar maps of STRESS MPI showing typical vascular perfusion patterns. Black represents regions of quantitative perfusion defect when compared to normal limit files.

SPECT-MPI. The 2003 ACC/AHA/ASNC radionuclide imaging guidelines summarize sensitivity and specificity from 17 studies involving 2,465 catheterized patients. The average sensitivity was 89% and specificity was 75%, results similar to exercise SPECT-MPI studies, uncorrected for verification bias. The diagnostic accuracy of dobutamine SPECT-MPI studies are similar to exercise and vasodilator stress SPECT-MPI. PET-MRI appears to have slightly higher sensitivity and specificify than SPECT-MPI.

## RISK STRATIFICATION

### Principles

A risk-based approach is a newer, widely used paradigm in the management of patients with suspected CAD in whom symptoms are nonlimiting. As a general guideline, risk categories, as defined by ACC/AAHA stable angina guidelines, are based on annual cardiac mortality: (1) low risk (less than 1% per year), (2) intermediate risk (1-3% per year), and (3) high risk (greater than 3% per year). With respect to appropriate selection of patients for risk stratification, the basic concept underlying the use of nuclear stress testing is that only those patients who can be successfully stratified in terms of survival benefit would be appropriate for stress SPECT-MPI. Since the mortality risk for patients undergoing revascularization is at least 1%, symptomatic patients with a less than 1% annual mortality rate would not appear to accrue a survival benefit with revascularization. A greater than 3% annual mortality rate is a threshold to identify patients with symptoms whose mortality rate might be improved by revascularization. Thus, SPECT-MPI is most appropriate in patients with less than 1% annual mortality and intermediate or high likelihood of CAD. Depending on the underlying clinical risk of the patients being tested, the exact level of these risk thresholds would vary. Many of the major determinants of prognosis in CAD are assessed by measurements of stress-induced perfusion and function, including extent of infarcted myocardium and of jeopardized ("ischemic") myocardium (supplied by vessels with hemodynamically significant stenosis) and the degree of jeopardy (severity of the individual coronary stenosis). As suggested above, the stability (or instability) of the CAD process is an additional factor influencing the ability of a coronary vessel to increase flow during stress. It has been observed that most myocardial infarctions occur in regions supplied by vessels with less than 50% diameter narrowing before the acute event and thus might not be expected to produce a perfusion defect; in general, MPI is insensitive for detecting less than 50% stenoses. Nonetheless, a normal SPECT-MPI is associated with a low risk of either cardiac death or nonfatal myocardial infarction (MI). A vasoconstrictive response to stress due to endothelial dysfunction in unstable plaques may explain the ability of a normal SPECT to be associated with low cardiac death rate. Additional factors include that patients with severe CAD may have more numerous mild plaques subject to rupture than patients without severe stenosis.

## RISK STRATIFICATION IN PATIENTS WITH SUSPECTED OR KNOWN CAD

Stress SPECT-MPI is an integral part of the evaluation of symptomatic patients for CAD and is commonly used in patients at intermediate postexercise treadmill testing (ETT) risk or with resting ECG abnormalities. As with diagnostic testing, if the patient's rest ECG is uninterpretable for purposes of stress testing, direct referral to SPECT-MPI is effective in prognostic stratification.

### Incremental Prognostic Value of SPECT-MPI

The clinical value of SPECT-MPI for prognostic assessment of CAD results from the incremental or added prognostic information yielded by this modality over all pretest data (clinical, historical, and stress data). Stress SPECT-MPI variables have been shown to have incremental prognostic value when added to prognostic stress ECG variables such as Duke Treadmill Score, a well-established and validated instrument that integrates the presence and magnitude of exercise-induced ST segment depression, exercise duration, and the presence of limiting angina. In a group of 2,200 patients with suspected CAD referred for exercise nuclear testing, information from SPECT-MPI added incremental prognostic information to each of the Duke Treadmill Score risk categories (low, intermediate, and high) (**Figure 53-4**). Studies have also demonstrated the incremental prognostic value of SPECT-MPI over clinical, stress, and even angiographic data.

### Prognostic Value of Normal SPECT-MPI

A synthesis of available data reveals that a normal scan is generally associated with a less than 1% annual risk of cardiac death or MI. A metanalysis of the prognostic value of a normal stress perfusion scan ($N = 29,788$) reveals that the annual risk of MI or cardiac death after a normal perfusion scan is 0.5% (95% CI 0.3-0.7%). This low event rate associated with a normal scan is critical in applying nuclear test information to risk stratification, since in the absence of limiting symptoms, patients with normal perfusion scans can often be managed conservatively.

Despite the low risk associated with normal SPECT studies, a limited number of studies have reported somewhat higher levels of risk. A study examining predictors of risk and its temporal characteristics in a series of 7,376 patients

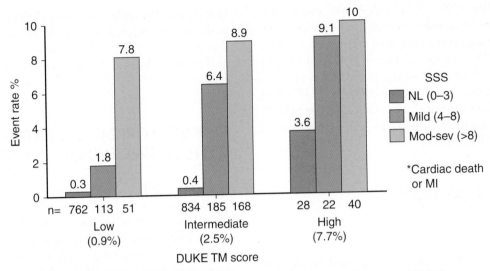

**Figure 53-4.** Rates of cardiac events as a function of the results of exercise stress SPECT in patients with low, intermediate, and high Duke Treadmill Scores. (Adapted from Hachamovitch R. et al, *Circulation*. 1996;905–914.)

with normal stress SPECT-MPI identified the use of pharmacologic stress and the presence of known CAD (**Figure 53-5A**), diabetes mellitus (in particular, female diabetics), and advanced age as markers of increased risk and shortened time to a hard event (e.g., risk in the 1st year of follow-up was less than in the 2nd year). Hence, a dynamic temporal component of risk was present and the existence of a "warranty" period for specific patient groups was defined (**Figure 53-5B**). This increased risk after normal SPECT in subsets of patients is due to the presence of comorbidities that increase baseline risk of all patients (diabetes mellitus, age, inability to exercise, prior CAD, and dyspnea as the presenting symptom). In occasional patients, extensive CAD is "missed" due to balanced reduction of flow. The latter would lead to a severe underestimation of the extent of ischemia by SPECT-MPI. Although many of these patients can be detected by ancillary markers, such as LV transient ischemic dilation, a rest to poststress fall in LVEF, or increased lung tracer uptake, in some patients with high-risk anatomic lesions, SPECT-MPI will appear normal. In an observational registry of SPECT-MPI, 13% of patients with left main coronary artery disease were not identified as being at high risk by SPECT-MPI.

## Extent of Perfusion Defect and Outcome

### Mildly Abnormal SPECT-MPI

Mildly abnormal scans have been reported to be associated with an intermediate risk for MI but a low risk for subsequent mortality; however, risk assessment in an individual patient is improved by taking into account findings other than those of the scan alone. The presence of high risk

clinical or historical markers identifies a subset of patients at greater risk for any level of scan abnormality, that is, prescan data yield incremental prognostic information over SPECT-MPI results (**Figure 53-6**). Hence, although patients with mildly abnormal SPECT-MPI results generally are at low risk of cardiac death, the risk has been shown to be higher in a variety of subgroups with significant comorbidities and presentations (e.g., advanced age, diabetes mellitus, atrial fibrillation, pharmacologic stress, reduced LV function, and dyspnea).

### Moderately to Severely Abnormal SPECT-MPI

This category of scan abnormality is associated with the highest levels of risk. Anticipated patient risk is greatest in patients with high risk cardiovascular comorbidities, increased left ventricular size, reduced LV function, extensive scar, and so on. As discussed below, patients with extensive ischemia appear to be those most likely to benefit from revascularization as opposed to conservative management.

## USING SPECT-MPI FOR MEDICAL DECISION MAKING: IDENTIFICATION OF TREATMENT BENEFIT

A major step forward is the recently evolved paradigm indicating that rather than identify patient risk, the role of SPECT-MPI in a testing strategy is the identification of patients who may accrue a survival benefit from revascularization as opposed to those who lack a survival benefit from this procedure and, conversely, which patients will have a superior survival with medical therapy alone. In a study examining 10,627 patients without prior MI or

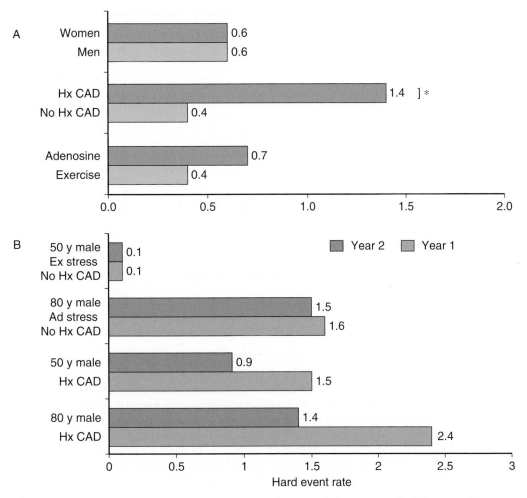

**Figure 53-5.** Annual rates of hard events in patients after normal SPECT-MPI. The following subgroups are shown: women versus men, patients with and without history (Hx) of CAD, and patients undergoing adenosine versus exercise stress. A significant risk is noted in the patients with Hx CAD. *p < 0.001. A. Rates of hard events in 1st and 2nd years of follow-up after normal SPECT-MPI. Four examples are given: a 50-year-old male undergoing exercise stress with no history of CAD, an 80-year-old male undergoing adenosine stress with no history of CAD, a 50-year-old male with a history of CAD, and an 80-year-old male with a history of CAD. In patients with no history of CAD, the event rates in the 1st and 2nd years after SPECT-MPI are not different; however, the event rate for normal SPECT-MPI goes up significantly with increased patient risk. In patients with previous CAD, the event rates in the 2nd year after SPECT-MPI were greater than in the 1st year and there is additional increase in the event rate with clinical risk. B. (Adapted from Hachamovitch R. et al, *J Am Coll Cardiol.* 2003;41:1329–1340.)

revascularization who underwent stress SPECT-MPI, a survival benefit was present for patients undergoing medical therapy versus revascularization, in the setting of no or mild ischemia, whereas patients undergoing revascularization had an increasing survival benefit over patients undergoing medical therapy, when moderate to severe ischemia was present (>10% of the total myocardium ischemia) (**Figure 53-7**). This survival benefit was particularly striking in higher risk patients. These results have been extended to incorporate gated SPECT-MPI EF information. In assessing treatment options in an individual patient, cardiac risk factors, comorbidities, and EF all have to be considered along with ischemia in order

to determine the potential advantages of a specific therapeutic strategy.

## Use of SPECT-MPI in Guiding Decisions for Catheterization

SPECT-MPI results considerably influence post–SPECT-MPI clinical decision making. In patients undergoing SPECT-MPI, the extent and severity of reversible defects are the principal factors driving subsequent resource utilization, with statistical analysis suggesting that more than 80% of the information governing the decision for catheterization comes from the amount of ischemia observed.

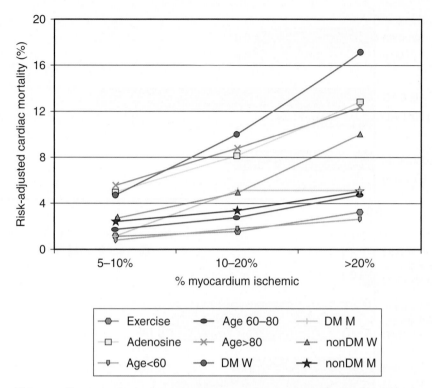

**Figure 53-6.** Rates of risk-adjusted cardiac mortality as a function of percentage myocardium ischemia (5-10%, 10-20%, and >20%) in medically treated patients (exercise vs. adenosine stress; patients aged <60 years, 60-80 years, and >80 years; diabetic men vs. women and nondiabetic men and women). Although predicted cardiac mortality increases with increasing percentage myocardium ischemia, the rates at any level of ischemia vary widely as a function of clinical information. (Based on data from Hachamovitch et al, *Circulation.* 2003;107:2900–2907.)

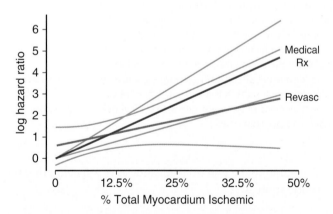

**Figure 53-7.** Relationship between percentage myocardium ischemia and log of the hazard ratio in 10,647 patients treated either with medical therapy (dashed line) or early revascularization (<60 days post–SPECT-MPI) (solid line), based on multivariable modeling. In the setting of little or no ischemia, medical therapy is associated with superior survival; with increasing amounts of ischemia, a progressive survival benefit with revascularization over medical therapy is present. 95% confidence intervals are shown (closely dotted lines) based on (data from Hachamovitch et al, *Circulation.* 2003;107:2900–2907.)

Among patients with normal scans, only a small proportion undergo early post–SPECT-MPI cardiac catheterization, usually as a result of clinical symptomatology. Regarding the cost-effectiveness of this approach, Shaw et al, in a multicenter study of 11,249 patients, showed that strategies of direct referral to catheterization and referral to SPECT-MPI with selective subsequent catheterization produced a substantial reduction (31-50%) in costs for all levels of pretest clinical risk in favor of the noninvasive approach (**Figure 53-8**), with essentially identical outcomes as assessed by cardiac death and MI rates.

A recent landmark study addressed how SPECT testing may shape clinical outcomes in the nonrandomized nuclear substudy of the Clinical Outcomes Utilizing Revascularization and Aggressive Drug Evaluation (COURAGE) trial. In the nuclear substudy, there were suggestive data that in the patients with moderate-to-severe ischemia by SPECT-MPI (>10% using a computer-based quantitative measure of ischemia), there may be a benefit in event-free survival, when a strategy of early percutaneous coronary intervention (PCI) plus optimal medical therapy is used.

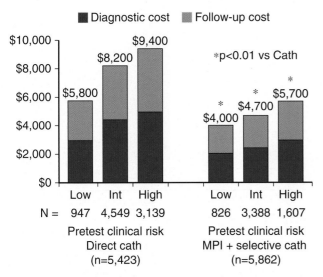

**Figure 53-8.** Comparative cost between screening strategies employing direct catheterization (Cath) and myocardial perfusion imaging (MPI) with selective Cath. Low, Int, and High represent low risk, intermediate risk, and high risk subsets of the patients with stable angina. Shown are the initial diagnostic costs (solid bars) and follow-up costs including costs of revascularization (gray bars). A 30 to 41% reduction in costs was noted in each category. Hard event rates were similar to the two strategies, but the revascularization rate was twice as high in the direct cath group. (Reproduced with permission from Shaw LJ et al, *J Am Coll Cardiol.* 1999;33:661–669.)

Given the absence of information to date indicating that PCI is superior to medical therapy in stable CAD, this interesting information may form the basis for a new randomized clinical trial.

## Potential Underestimation of the Risk Stratification by SPECT-MPI

Although there is strong evidence that SPECT-MPI is effective in the prognostic stratification, the current data on risk stratification by SPECT-MPI may actually underestimate the strength of this modality due to a prognostic counterpart to the diagnostic verification bias described above. The current prognostic data are entirely composed of patients undergoing medical therapy after testing, since prognostic assessment of noninvasive testing using observational data series dictate that patients undergoing early revascularization after testing be removed or censored from prognostic analyses due to the relationship between the referral to revascularization and the test results. Thus, with increasing physician acceptance and the strong dependence of post–SPECT-MPI referral to revascularization on the SPECT-MPI results, a posttest referral bias may develop that results in an underestimation of the prognostic value of this test due to the revascularization (and censoring) of the highest risk patients.

## Added Value of Gated SPECT-MPI: Integrated Clinical Algorithms

Gated MPI has now become routine with SPECT and PET. Studies have shown that poststress LVEF and LV ESV, as measured by gated SPECT, provide incremental information over the perfusion defect assessment in the prediction of cardiac death. In a report of 6,713 patients, using separate criteria for EF and ESV for men and women, Sharir et al reported that perfusion (percentage myocardium ischemia) and function (LVEF or ESV) provided incremental prognostic information regarding cardiac death and hard events (**Figure 53-9**), with particularly high event rates noted in women with reduced function and greater than 10% myocardium ischemia.

### High Risk SPECT Variables

A list of high risk SPECT variables is shown in **Table 53-4**. The assessment of poststress wall motion abnormalities on gated SPECT MPI is a sign of exercise-induced stunning and a marker of severe CAD. One of the most powerful predictors of high risk CAD on exercise SPECT-MPI is transient ischemic dilation of the LV cavity. This reversible LV cavity dilation is thought to represent diffuse subendocardial ischemia (relatively less tracer uptake in the subendocardium during stress creating the appearance of an enlarged cavity) or true poststress LV dilation. This finding is associated with higher incidence of severe and extensive CAD and a worse outcome than in patients without this finding.

Pulmonary uptake of radioactivity, as determined by the measurement of lung/heart ratios of radioactivity, has been shown to be of prognostic importance.

## USE OF SPECT-MPI IN SPECIFIC PATIENT POPULATIONS

Large databases have been accumulated in nuclear cardiology, resulting in evidence documenting the effectiveness of SPECT-MPI for risk stratification of appropriately selected patients. This evidence has resulted in many Class I indications for the use of stress SPECT-MPI. Several specific lines of evidence are described below.

## Evidence Supporting Nuclear Imaging for Patients with an Intermediate Risk or Indeterminate Treadmill Test

Several reports support nuclear testing in patients with uninterpretable or intermediate exercise ECG response. As described earlier, patients with an intermediate Duke Treadmill Score and an intermediate risk of hard events, but a normal SPECT MPI scan, had very low event rates

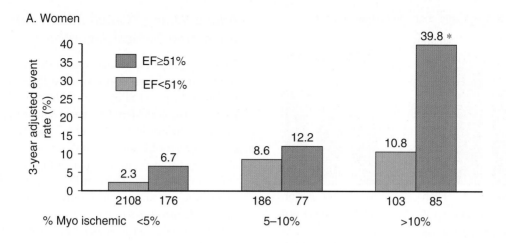

A. Women

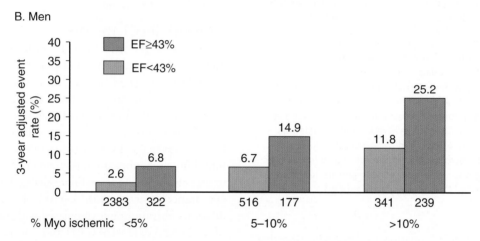

B. Men

**Figure 53-9.** Three-year adjusted cardiac hard event rates in women (A) and men (B) as a function of the amount of ischemia (percentage myocardium ischemia) and gender specific normal/abnormal ejection fraction (EF). (Reproduced with permission from Sharir T et al, *J Nucl Cardiol.* 2006;13:495–506.)

| Table 53-4 • High Risk SPECT Imaging Variables |
|---|
| 1. Multiple perfusion defects >1 coronary supply region (multivessel CAD scan pattern) |
| 2. An extensive area of stress-induced hypoperfusion, even if confined to the territory of a single coronary artery (e.g., proximal left anterior descending coronary artery scan pattern) |
| 3. A high ischemic burden reflected by multiple reversible defects |
| 4. Transient ischemic left ventricular cavity dilation |
| 5. Multiple abnormal regional wall motion or thickening abnormalities, even if not associated with perfusion defects |
| 6. A gated SPECT ejection fraction of <40% |
| 7. Increased end-systolic volumes on quantitative SPECT |
| 8. Increased lung heart ratio of thallium uptake when thallium-201 is used for exercise imaging |
| 9. Extensive ischemia as defined by >10% myocardium by visual or quantitative methods |

*Source: Modified by Beller GA, 2005.*

and were infrequently catheterized. Those with moderately abnormal scans had intermediate rates of events and catheterization, and those with moderately to severely abnormal scans had higher rates of events and catheterization.

## Evidence Supporting Nuclear Imaging for Patients with Normal Resting ECG Unable to Exercise

In patients unable to exercise, there is a clear consensus in support of pharmacologic stress imaging as the initial test in symptomatic male and female patients with intermediate or high pretest likelihood of CAD unable to achieve maximal exercise levels. As reported by the recent AHA consensus statement on cardiac imaging in women, functionally impaired patients (e.g., <5 metabolic equivalent (METs) of exercise) have at least a 2% per year risk of cardiac death or MI, ranking them as having event rates equivalent to patients with established coronary heart disease. The higher event rates than in exercising patients are driven by excessive comorbidity and risk factor burden. Vasodilator stress SPECT-MPI has been shown to be effective for both CAD diagnosis and risk stratification for patients who have a normal resting ECG and an intermediate to high likelihood of CAD but are unable to exercise.

## Evidence Supporting Nuclear Imaging for Patients with Diabetes Mellitus

SPECT-MPI has been reported to be particularly effective in risk stratification of patients with diabetes. The risk of cardiac events in diabetics with abnormal SPECT-MPI is higher than in nondiabetics throughout the range of perfusion abnormalities. However, even when diabetic patients have normal SPECT-MPI studies, the event rate is higher and events occur sooner in diabetic compared to nondiabetic patients. Routine screening of asymptomatic diabetic patients is not recommended by current appropriate use criteria; as noted below, however, if coronary artery calcium by CT is performed, diabetics have a higher frequency of a coronary calcium score of more than 400-a score that by appropriateness criteria merits further evaluation by SPECT-MPI.

## Evidence Supporting Nuclear Imaging for Patients with Left Bundle Branch Block

Current guidelines support cardiac imaging in symptomatic patients with LBBB. The sensitivity for left anterior descending stenosis was similar (on average 89%) with exercise and vasodilator SPECT-MPI, but a higher specificity was found for vasodilator stress (81%) as compared to exercise (36%) SPECT-MPI. Vasodilator stress is recommended over exercise for SPECT-MPI and has been shown to be a predictor of cardiac events in LBBB patients. Patients with LBBB and normal SPECT-MPI have demonstrated very low event rates over time. In contrast, patients with LBBB and "high risk" perfusion findings on SPECT-MPI have high event rates. Although there are fewer reported studies regarding patients with ventricular pacemakers, expert consensus is that these patients should have vasodilator stress when undergoing SPECT-MPI, similar to patients with LBBB.

## Evidence Supporting Nuclear Imaging for Patients with LVH, Atrial Fibrillation, and those with Shortness of Breath

In patients with left ventricular hypertrophy (LVH), exertional ST-segment depression is frequently associated without significant epicardial CAD. SPECT-MPI has been shown to be similarly effective in patients with and without LVH for identifying obstructive disease and for risk stratification.

In asymptomatic patients with new onset atrial fibrillation, the use of stress SPECT-MPI in patients with a high pretest risk is considered appropriate in view of a higher baseline clinical risk resulting in higher expected cardiac events. A recent observational report in 16,048 patients on the prognostic value of SPECT-MPI in patients with atrial fibrillation showed that an annual rate of cardiac death in patients with normal SPECT-MPI was 1.6% per year for those with atrial fibrillation and 0.4% for the remaining cohort of nonatrial fibrillation patients ($p < 0.001$).

Patients presenting with unexplained shortness of breath have been shown to have as high a cardiac death event rate as patients with typical angina and have a greater frequency of cardiac death as a function of SPECT-MPI ischemia than patients presenting with atypical chest pain syndromes.

## Evidence Supporting Nuclear Imaging for Elderly Patients

With the increasing age of the population and the increasing prevalence of CAD as a function of age, large numbers of elderly patients are requiring diagnostic and/or prognostic assessment for CAD. The Duke Treadmill Score, useful in many patient subsets, has been reported to be less effective in risk stratification of elderly patients. The Mayo Clinic and Cedars-Sinai groups have reported that SPECT-MPI provides effective risk stratification in elderly men and elderly women. Pharmacologic stress testing is increasingly being applied in the elderly, who frequently are unable to exercise adequately, and the elderly make up a high proportion of patients undergoing pharmacologic stress imaging. Consistent with data on other functionally impaired patients, the prognostic value of SPECT-MPI in the elderly is associated with higher cardiac event rates for normal to severely abnormal test results. These results have been extended to dobutamine stress. Of note, patients requiring dobutamine stress SPECT-MPI appear to have an even greater rate of cardiac events, as a function of the amount of ischemia, than do patients undergoing vasodilator stress, likely due to greater comorbidities. Therapeutic benefit for mortality in very elderly patients with extension ischemia on SPECT-MET has recently been shown.

## Evidence Supporting Nuclear Imaging after Coronary Calcium Screening or CT coronary angiography

In patients with high risk coronary calcium scores (CCS), referral to SPECT-MPI has been evaluated in numerous studies. Data from the published studies are consistent in that when the CCS is less than 400, the rate of SPECT-MPI abnormalities is low. When the CCS exceeds 400, the rate of an ischemic SPECT-MPI is elevated and has been reported to be as high as 47% in some populations. Recent consensus documents and the recent ACC appropriateness criteria support the use of SPECT-MPI in patients with a high risk CCS greater than or equal to 400.

## Evidence Supporting Nuclear Testing for Patients after PCI and after CABS

In patients with PCI, exercise or vasodilator SPECT/PET-MPI can be helpful in detecting the presence and location of restenosis. Stress SPECT/PET-MPI is currently recommended by ACC/AHA for assessment of restenosis in newly symptomatic post-PCI patients. Although routine performance of SPECT/PET-MPI is not recommended in asymptomatic post-PCI patients, important information may be obtained in symptomatic patients for guiding clinical decisions regarding subsequent catheterization and reinterventions.

In post-CABS patients with new symptoms, SPECT-MPI can identify the presence and extent of ischemia and can accurately detect the presence and location of the graft stenosis. In such patients, SPECT-MPI can guide the need for cardiac catheterization.

Whereas SPECT-MPI has been shown to be capable of risk-stratifying post-CABS patients, routine assessment with stress SPECT-MPI in asymptomatic patients after CABS is not recommended by current ACC/AHA guidelines. Although some studies suggest that SPECT-MPI should be considered 5 or more years after CABS in asymptomatic patients. Moderate to severe ischemia in these patients is useful in determining the need for repeat catheterization.

## Evidence Supporting Nuclear Imaging for Preoperative Risk Assessment in Noncardiac Surgery Patients

A large body of literature exists documenting the effectiveness of nuclear stress testing in patients undergoing peripheral vascular surgery. Previous guidelines suggested that nuclear testing is best reserved for patients with an intermediate risk of a cardiac event undergoing an intermediate risk to high risk procedure and who have limited exercise capacity. The guidelines were rewritten in 2007. Consideration of noninvasive stress testing is recommended in patients with three or more clinical risk factors and poor functional capacity (less than 4 METs) undergoing vascular surgery if it will change management (Class IIa) and patients with 1-2 clinical risk factors and poor functional capacity who require intermediate-risk or vascular surgery if it will change management (Class IIb). These specific risk factors include: history of ischemic heart disease, heart failure, cerebrovascular disease, diabetes mellitus, and renal insufficiency.

## High Pretest Likelihood of CAD

The ACC appropriateness criteria support SPECT-MPI for high likelihood patients who have an interpretable or uninterpretable ECG as well as for those able or unable to exercise. Evidence on risk assessment of this group with SPECT-MPI has been published and a strategy incorporating initial testing with SPECT-MPI in these patients has been shown to be cost-effective when used to guide the decision for catheterization.

Other high likelihood patients include those asymptomatic individuals with a high Framingham risk score or those classified as CHD risk equivalents, including diabetics and those with peripheral arterial disease. The ACC appropriateness criteria support the use of SPECT-MPI in patients with a high Framingham risk score or a coronary artery calcium (CAC) score ≥400, indicating a high atherosclerotic plaque burden. In addition, evidence supports SPECT-MPI as a highly useful test for diagnosis and prognosis in obese patients, preferably using Tc-99m agents with attenuation correction or prone and supine imaging, combined with quantitation and ECG gating. There is also enough evidence supporting nuclear imaging for prognostic stratification of African American and Hispanic patients who generally have higher risk burden than the Caucasian population.

## EVALUATION OF ACUTE CHEST PAIN

For patients with normal or nondiagnostic initial ECGs on presentation to the emergency department (ED), an important clinical problem is to distinguish those with acute coronary syndromes requiring hospital admission from those who may be safely discharged. [99m]Tc-sestamibi or tetrofosmin SPECT-MPI with injection during chest pain provides an excellent opportunity to reduce clinical indecision in the acute evaluation of chest pain (**Figure 53-10**). In patients presenting to the ED with chest pain but a low-intermediate likelihood of an acute coronary syndrome, a normal rest [99m]Tc-sestamibi or tetrofosmin SPECT-MPI study has a 99%

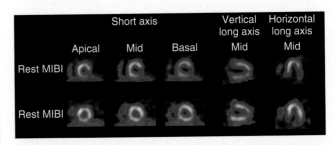

**Figure 53-10.** Resting sestamibi (MB) injected during chest pain in emergency department (top) and 3 days post-PCI of the left circumflex coronary artery (LCX) (bottom) in a patient with no EGG or enzyme abnormalities. Clear evidence of extensive myocardial salvage in LCX territory is shown.

## Table 54-1 • Appropriateness Criteria for Cardiac MRI

| Indication | | Appropriateness Criteria (Median Score) |
|---|---|---|
| | **Detection of CAD: symptomatic—evaluation of chest pain syndrome (use of vasodilator perfusion CMR or debutamine stress funtion CMR)** | |
| 3. | • Intermediate pre-test probability of CAD<br>• ECG uninterpretable OR unable to exercise | A (7) |
| | **Detection of CAD: symptomatic—evaluation of intra-cardiac structures (use of MR coronary angiography)** | |
| 8. | • Evaluation of suspected coronary anomalies | A (8) |
| | **Risk assessment with prior test results (use of vasodilator perfusion CMR or dobutamine stress function CMR)** | |
| 13. | • Coronary angiography (catheterization of CT)<br>• Stenosis of unclear significance | A (7) |
| | **Structure and fuction—evaluation of ventricular and valvular function procedures may include LV/RV mass and volumes, MR angiography, quantification of valvular disease, and delayed contrast enhancement** | |
| 18. | • Assessment of complex congenital heart disease including anolalies of coronary circulation great vessels, and cardiac chambers and valves<br>• Procedures may include LV/RV mass and volumes, MR angiography, quantification of valvular disease, and contrast enhancement | A (9) |
| 20. | • Evaluation of LV function following myocardial infarction OR in heart failure patients<br>• Patients with technically limited images from echocardiogram | A (8) |
| 21. | • Quantification of LV function<br>• Discordant information that is clinically significant from prior tests | A (8) |
| 22. | • Evaluation of specific cardiomyopathies (infiltrative [anoyloid sarcoid], HCM, or due to cardiotoxic therapies)<br>• Use of delayed enhancement | A (8) |
| 23. | • Characterization of native and prosthetic cardiac valves—including planimetry of stenotic disease and quantification of regurgitant disease<br>• Patients with technically limited images from echocardiogram of TEE | A (8) |
| 24. | • Evaluation for arrythmogenic right ventricular cardiomyopathy (AEVC)<br>• Patients presenting with syncope or ventricular arrhythmia | A (9) |
| 25. | • Evaluation of myocarditis or myocardial infarction with normal coronary arteries<br>• Positive cardiac enzymes without obstructive atherosclerosis on angiography | A (8) |
| | **Structure and fuction—evaluation of intra- and extra-cardiac structures** | |
| 26. | • Evaluation of cardiac mass (suspected tumor or thrombus)<br>• Use of contrast for perfusion and enhancement | A (9) |
| 27. | • Evaluation of pericardial conditions (pericardial mass, constrictive pericarditis) | A (8) |
| 28. | • Evaluation for aortic dissection | A (8) |
| 29. | • Evaluation of pulmonary veins prior to radiofrequency ablation for atrial fibrillation<br>• Left atrial and pulmonary venous anatomy including dimensions of veins for mapping purposes | A (8) |
| | **Detection of myocardial scar and viability—evaluation of myocardial scar (use of late gadolinium enhancement)** | |
| 30. | • To determine the location, and extent of myocardial necrosis including 'no reflow' regions<br>• Post acute myocardial infarction | A (7) |
| 32. | • To determine viability prior to revascularization<br>• Establish likelihood of recovery of function with revascularization (PCI or CABG) or medical therapy | A (9) |
| 33. | • To determine viability prior to revascularization<br>• Viability assessment by SPECT or dobutamine echo has provided "equivocal or indeterminate" results | A (9) |

*From Hendel RC, et al. Appropriateness Criteria for CCT/CMR, JACC. 2006:1488.*

thickening with systole of less than 1 mm is most likely a myocardial scar. Cine MRI can also detect complications of myocardial infarction, such as ventricular septal defect, mitral regurgitation, flail mitral leaflet, ventricular thrombus, right ventricular dysfunction, and pericardial effusions.

Microvascular obstruction is indicative of inadequate myocardial tissue perfusion even after restoration of epicardial blood flow in the infarct territory. Microvascular obstruction is identified on CMR as a hypoenhanced subendocardial area of the myocardium on the first pass perfusion images. Microvascular obstruction on CMR has been shown to be a poor prognostic indicator for subsequent cardiovascular events in acute myocardial infarction patients (**Figure 54-1**).

Infarct location and extent can be readily assessed on delayed hyperenhancement images (**Figure 54-2**). CMR is more sensitive in detecting infarct compared to SPECT nuclear imaging at 7 days in acute myocardial infarction patients treated with percutaneous coronary intervention. In the acute and chronic myocardial infarction patient, late gadolinium hyperenhancement of the subendocardium reflects irreversibly damaged tissue, and in areas of akinesis, the transmural extent of infarcted tissue can also be characterized (**Figure 54-3**). Infarct sizing is accurate and reproducible with CMR. The transmural extent of hyperenhancement can predict global and segmental functional recovery, as the transmural extent of hyperenhancement increases and the likelihood of functional recovery is lessened (**Figure 54-4**).

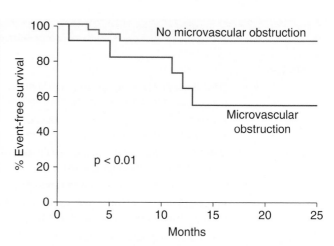

**Figure 54-1.** Microvascular obstruction provides prognostic information in acute myocardial infarction patients. Event free survival was significantly lower in patients with evidence of microvascular obstruction compared to those without microvascular obstruction. (From Wu et al. Prognostic Significance of Microvascular Obstruction by Magnetic Resonance Imaging in Patients With Acute Myocardial Infarction. *Circulation.* 1998;97:765–772.)

Transmural delayed hyperenhancement indicates no functional recovery even after revascularization with stents or bypass. Myocardial segments with scar formation and wall motion abnormalities are indicative of nonviable tissue. In myocardial areas with segmental dysfunction and no delayed hyperenhancement, there is no myocardial scar or fibrosis;

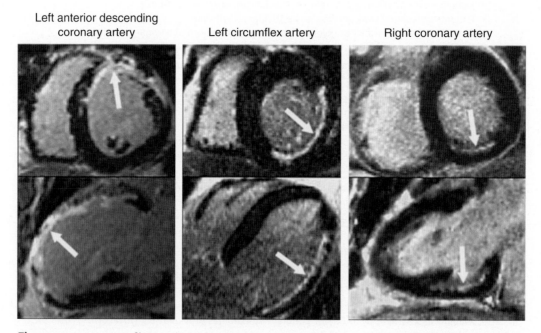

**Figure 54-2.** Location of hyperenhancement in relation to coronary artery territory. Infarcted tissue can be seen on delayed hyperenhancement short-axis and long-axis images. The pattern of hyperenhancement correlates with the three different coronary perfusion territories. (Adapted from Kim RJ et al, The use of contrast-enhanced magnetic resonance imaging to identify reversible myocardial dysfunction. *N Engl J Med.* 2000;343: 1445–1453.)

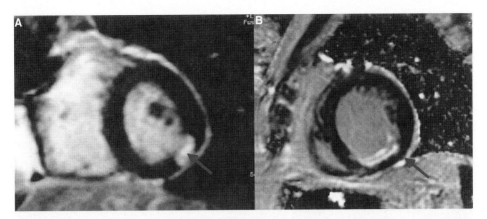

**Figure 54-3.** Transmural extent of infarcted tissue. Short-axis delayed contrast images demonstrating transmural scar of the inferolateral (A) and subendocardial scar of the inferior wall (B). (Adapted from Poon M, Dinh H, Fuster V: Magnetic Resonance imaging of the heart. In Fuster V, et al, eds. *The Heart,* 11th New York: McGraw-Hill; 2004:629–645.)

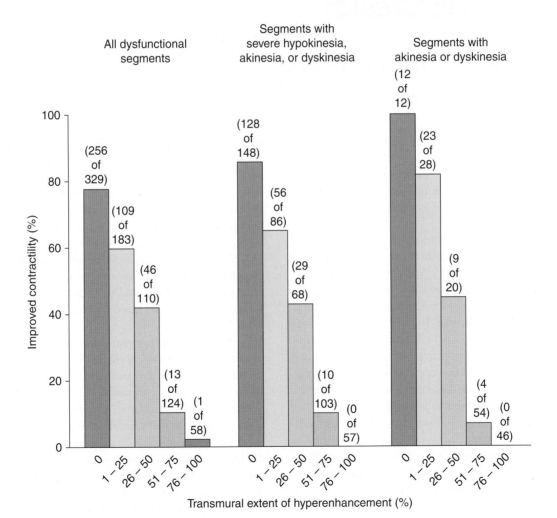

**Figure 54-4.** Relationship of myocardial scar versus likelihood of improved contractility. As the transmural extent of myocardial scars increases, improvement in contractility decreases. Segments with no or mild subendocardial scars are more likely to have improved contractility. (Adapted from Kim RJ et al,. The use of contrast enhanced magnetic resonance imaging to identify reversible myocardial dysfunction. *N Engl J Med.* 2000;343:1445–1453.)

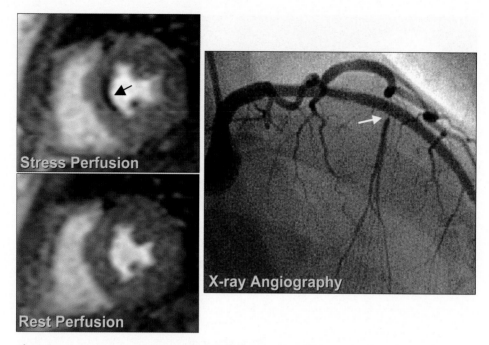

**Figure 54-5.** Inducible perfusion defect involving subendocardial septal wall on stress perfusion image (black arrow), which normalizes on rest perfusion image. Angiography demonstrates significant ostial disease in the septal branch of the left anterior descending artery (white arrow). (Source: Fuster V, O'Rourke RA, Walsh RA, Pool-Wilson P: *Hurst's The Heart*, 12th ed. http://www.accessmedicine.com)

therefore, these areas are considered viable. In dysfunctional myocardium with hyperenhancement patterns that are less than 50%, the transmural extent may have functional recovery after revascularization. Newer imaging protocols with T2 weighted images can also identify myocardial edema.

Stress CMR can also be performed to diagnose myocardial ischemia from epicardial and microvascular disease as part of the evaluation of chest pain. Stress agents include dobutamine, dipyridamole, and adenosine; in addition, recent stress exams have been performed on a MRI compatible treadmill. Assessment for wall motion abnormalities on cine MRI is performed prior to and during dobutamine infusion. Improvement in left ventricular regional thickening with low dose dobutamine has been shown to predict segmental functional recovery (viability) with revascularization. The sensitivity of dobutamine stress CMR increases with myocardial tagging techniques. Dipyridamole and adenosine both evaluate the myocardial perfusion reserve index (perfusion defects) to identify ischemic segments (**Figure 54-5**); in addition, wall motion abnormalities can sometimes be seen with adenosine infusion.

## Nonischemic Cardiomyopathy

Assessment and differentiation of ischemic versus nonischemic cardiomyopathy can be performed. The CMR exam for the assessment of nonischemic cardiomyopathy includes regional and global wall motion analysis with cine MRI, tissue characterization with various imaging protocols (T1 and T2 weighted images, fat suppression, T2 star), and characterization of myocardial hyperenhancement on delayed contrast images. Ischemic cardiomyopathy has the typical pattern of subendocardial or transmural hyperenhancement. Epicardial or mid-myocardial hyperenhancement is indicative of nonischemic cardiomyopathy (**Figure 54-6**). Hyperenhancement can be seen in myocarditis, hypertrophic cardiomyopathy, and infiltrative cardiomyopathies such as amloydosis and hemochromatosis.

Hypertrophic cardiomyopathy has a similar distinctive pattern as seen in echocardiography. There is asymmetrical, septal, or global left ventricular hypertrophy. Patients with hypertrophic obstructive cardiomyopathy have a dynamic obstruction of the left ventricular outflow tract (**Figure 54-7**). In this scenario, systolic anterior motion of the mitral valve, mitral regurgitation, and turbulence across the left ventricular outflow tract can be seen. Delayed contrast images may demonstrate patchy hyperenhancement in areas of collagen deposition and are associated with myocardial disarray. Prognostic information regarding this pattern of hyperenhancement is unknown, but it has been shown to be associated with sudden cardiac death and progressive left ventricular dilation. Those patients who have undergone alcohol septal ablation will have localized hyperenhancement of the basal septum in the territory that was ablated.

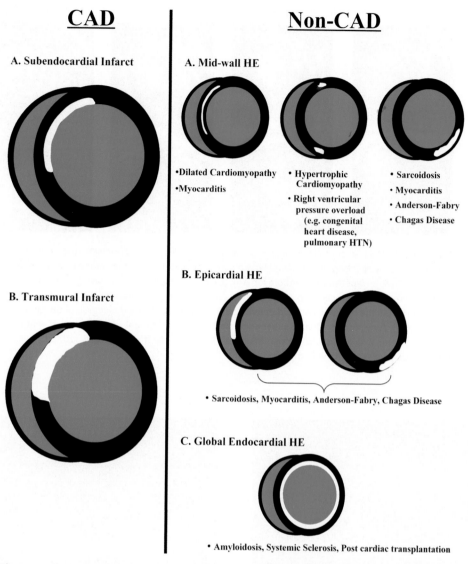

**Figure 54-6.** Pattern of hyperenhancement in CAD versus non-CAD patients. (Shah DJ, Kim RJ; magnetic resonace of myocardial viability. In Edelman RR ed. clinical magnetic imaging, 3rd ed. New York; Elsevier.)

Amyloidosis is seen as diffuse ventricular hypertrophy and dilated atria. Diffuse subendocardial or transmural hyperenhancement is seen on delayed contrast images.

Cardiac sarcoidosis has areas of myocardial edema, which is seen as increased signal intensity on T2 weighted images, and hypertrophy of the left ventricular walls. Patchy hyperenhancement in a noncoronary territory pattern can be seen and also has been shown to regress after steroid treatment (**Figure 54-8**). Myocardial iron overload is demonstrated by reduced myocardial T2 star images secondary to iron deposition resulting in increased myocardial inhomongenities. Myocarditis can be seen as mid-myocardial hyperenhancement (typically the lateral wall) on delayed images with a corresponding wall motion abnormality.

Arrhythmogenic right ventricular dysplasia (ARVD) is frequently diagnosed using the McKenna criteria. MRI findings in ARVD include abnormal RV morphology (dilated RV, focal RV aneurysms), abnormal RV function, abnormal signal intensity, and enhancement of the RV wall secondary to fibro fatty replacement of the muscular myocardium.

## Valvular Heart Disease

CMR can detect valvular stenosis and regurgitation as well as determine chamber sizes and ejection fraction. Similar to regurgitant lesions in echocardiography, proximal isovelocity surface area (PISA) can be seen in CMR and is directly related to the amount of regurgitation. Regurgitant flow is often seen as a signal void area due to the high velocity of the regurgitant jet (**Figure 54-9**).

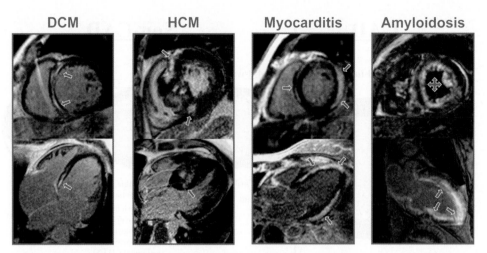

**Figure 54-7.** Delayed contrast enhancement patterns in patients with nonischemic cardiomyopathy. Dilated cardiomyopathy (DCM): Hyperenhancement of the mid-wall of the interventricular septum (arrows). Hypertrophic cardiomyopathy (HCM): Multiple patchy areas of hyperenhancement within the mid-myocardium of the septum (arrows) but not lateral wall. Myocarditis: Hyperenhancement in the mid-wall of the interventricular septum and epicardial region of the lateral LV wall (arrows). Amyloidosis: Diffuse subendocardial hyperenhancement of the entire left ventricle. (Source: Fuster V, O'Rourke RA, Walsh RA, Pool-Wilson P: *Hurst's The Heart*, 12th ed. http://www.accessmedicine.com)

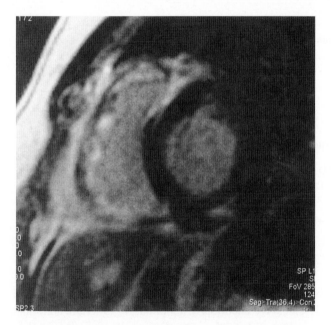

**Figure 54-8.** Sarcoidosis. Delayed contrast imaging reveals patchy hyperenhancement of the RV free wall secondary to scarring or fibrosis from cardiac sarcoidosis. (Adapted from Poon M, Dinh H, Fuster V: Magnetic Resonance Imaging of the heart. In: Fuster V, et al., eds. *The Heart*, 11th ed. New York: McGraw-Hill; 2004:629–645.)

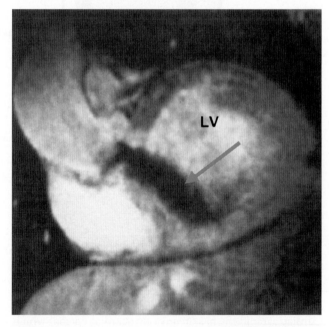

**Figure 54-9.** Severe aortic regurgitation. High velocity turbulent regurgitant jets into the left ventricle from severe aortic regurgitation can be seen as a signal void area on cine images. (Adapted from Poon M, Dinh H, Fuster V: Magnetic Resonance Imaging of the heart. In Fuster V, et al., eds. *The Heart*, 11th ed. New York, McGraw-Hill; 2004:629–645.)

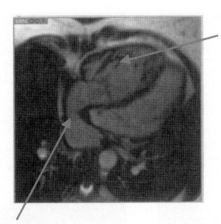

**Systemic ventricle**

**Mustard's Baffle**

**Figure 54-10.** Congenital heart disease. Post Mustard repair for transposition of the great vessels, demonstrating a baffle shunting pulmonary venous blood to the systemic ventricle. (Adapted from Poon M, Dinh H, Fuster V: Magnetic Resonance Imaging of the heart. In: Fuster V, et al., *The Heart,* 11th eds. New York: Mc Graw-Hill 2004;629–645.)

Phase velocity mapping with CMR is similar to Doppler echocardiography and provides quantitative information regarding the amount of regurgitation or degree of stenosis. Planimetry of the valves can also be performed to assess degree of valvular stenosis.

## Congenital Heart Disease

CMR is a great investigative tool for congenital heart disease, especially the complex or postsurgical cases (**Figure 54-10**). Chamber dimensions and functions can be calculated. Assessment for an intracardiac shunt is performed by measuring pulmonary and systemic blood flows with phase velocity mapping techniques and then calculating the ratio. In addition, the origins of the coronary arteries as well as morphology of the aortic and pulmonic vessels can be studied.

## Masses

Myxoma is the most common primary benign tumor of the heart. Myxomas typically have an interatrial septal attachment, with a 4:1 predilection for the left atrium compared to the right atrium (**Figure 54-11**). These tumors are isointense (similar intensity as myocardium) on T1 images and hyperintense (high signal or intensity compared to myocardium) on T2 images. Cine MRI images allow visualization of the tumor throughout the cardiac cycle, including the extent of invasion into the atrial cavity as well as prolapse of the mass into the respective ventricle. Lipomatous atrial septal hypertrophy is often diagnosed as an echogenic mass on echocardiogram and has a low association with obesity and cardiac arrhythmias. The interatrial septum often has a "bar bell" appearance.

The lipomatous septum is bright (hyperintense) on T1 images and the signal is suppressed on T1 fat saturation images. Atrial lipomas are located in the atrial wall, are hyperintense on T1 images, and are suppressed on T1 fat saturation images with similar tissue characterizations to the lipomatous septal hypertrophy (**Figure 54-12**). The christa terminalis, chiari network, and eustachian valve are frequent echo findings that prompt CMR evaluation for tumor.

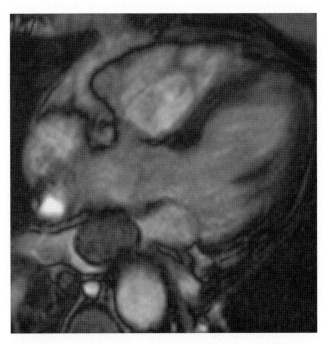

**Figure 54-11.** Myxoma. Cine MRI sequence demonstrating left atrial myxoma, which is attached to the interatrial septum.

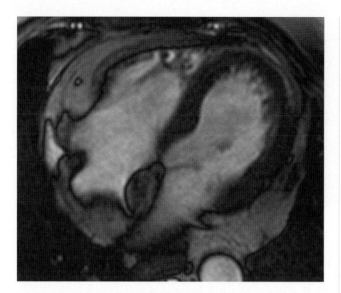

**Figure 54-12.** Lipomatous hypertrophy seen within the interatrial septum and right atrial free wall.

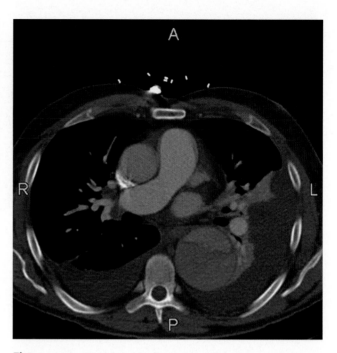

**Figure 54-13.** Type B aortic dissection. Dilated descending thoracic aorta with a dissection flap, small true lumen, and large false lumen. Normal caliber ascending aorta.

Primary malignant tumors of the heart include angiosarcomas, rhabdomyosarcoma, other sarcomas, mesothelioma, and primary lymphoma. Thrombus is frequently mistaken as a mass or difficult to definitively diagnosis on echo, but cardiac MRI has a high sensitivity for left ventricular and atrial thrombi.

## Pericardium

Normal pericardial thickness is less than 3 mm and it has low signal intensity. Pericardial effusions can be easily seen and differentiated from the pericardium, since the effusions typically have a bright signal on cine MRI images, whereas the pericardium is dark. Postgadolinium enhancement of the pericardium is indicative of a possible inflammatory process involving the pericardium. CMR helps in the diagnosis of loculated pericardial effusions, constrictive pericarditis, congenital absence of the pericardium, and tumor invasion of the pericardium. Real time imaging in patients with constrictive pericarditis can demonstrate the interrelationship of ventricular filling and septal wall motion with the respiratory cycle, similar to the pattern seen on echocardiography.

## Aortic Disease

CMR can be utilized to evaluate aortic dissections (**Figure 54-13**), including assessment of dissection flaps, true and false lumens, and extent of the dissection. In addition, aortic imaging is useful in the assessment of congenital heart disease, allowing assessment of not only the aorta for coarctation and patent ductus arterious (PDA) but also aortic arch anomalies and origins of the coronary arteries. Thoracic and abdominal aortic aneurysms can be imaged and followed over time for changes. The aortic images can be reconstructed into a 3D display. CMR is not recommended in hemodynamically unstable patients due to difficulties in adequately monitoring the patient during the test as well as prolonged imaging time compared to CT or transesophageal echocardiogram (TEE).

## CARDIAC CT

Cardiac CT is a rapidly developing technology, with newer generation scanners being developed rapidly. It requires an X-ray beam to pass through the patient, which is then attenuated prior to striking the scintillation crystals of the detector array. The X-rays are converted to light, which is then converted to an electrical charge by photodiodes. This is translated into a digital signal by electronics. CT scanners have undergone significant advancement over recent years, moving from a pencil beam X-ray with a single detector element to a wide beam fan X-ray with an arc of detector elements. There are two types of scanners: electron beam computed tomography (EBCT) and multidetector computed tomography (MDCT). EBCT involves a large stationary anode and has a lower spatial resolution. First-generation scanners had a single detector element so there was a pencil beam of X-ray. The scan time was very slow. Second-generation scanners had multiple detector elements and a narrow fan beam of X-ray with a slow scan speed. First- and second-generation scanners required translation of the tube and detector to scan, which alternated with rotation of the scan, thus creating long scan times. Third-generation scanners' detector elements are in an arc, so there is a wide fan beam of X-ray. Only rotation without translation is required; therefore, the scan speed is faster.

It is a test that can be performed within a few minutes. The data obtained are three-dimensional, allowing the viewer to manipulate the images into different planes. CT has a higher spatial resolution and lower temporal resolution compared to MRI. Depending on the type of scanner, type of scan, and patient factors, the radiation dose can vary and, in some cases, may even be more than conventional coronary angiography. Iodine contrast is administered, therefore, patients must be screened for this allergy.

A variety of postprocessing techniques is available. Maximal intensity projection (MIP) is utilized with a stack of images, depending on the chosen slice thickness. CT values are assigned to each pixel and the image is determined from the maximum value of all the pixels in the stack at that particular location. Curved multiplanar reformat (MPR) images follow the course of the vessel; the image has no plane name, but the entire vessel is depicted in one image. The vessel needs to be reviewed in multiple planes with the curved MPR technique. Volume rendered images are beautiful three-dimensional images that are visually appealing but nondiagnostic for assessment of atherosclerosis (**Figure 54-14**).

CT is not without risk, and one of the most concerning risks is the amount of radiation exposure to the patient. On average, the background radiation of the general public is 3 mSv a year; in comparison, a chest X-ray is 0.1 mSv. The average effective radiation dose is 0.7 to 2.0 mSV for calcium scoring and 18 to 20 mSv for CT angiography. Women are at a greater risk for cancer from radiation exposure secondary to the breast tissue being radiosensitive. Any lowering of radiation will decrease risk of cancer. ECG-triggered dose modulation (pulse modulation) limits image quality and decreases radiation during certain preset phases of the cardiac cycle by reducing tube current in phases of the cardiac cycle, which are more likely to have suboptimal coronary artery images.

## Calcium Scoring

Calcium scoring is a simple and reproducible test that identifies calcium within the coronary artery tree (**Figure 54-15**). Presence of calcium within the coronary arteries is indicative of atherosclerosis, as it is the only known process to result in deposition of calcium within

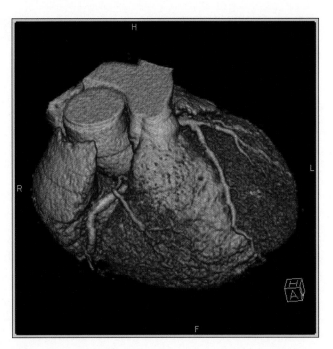

**Figure 54-14.** Volume rendered images. Visually appealing images, which provide limited assessment for quantification of coronary stenosis.

the intima, and it begins many years prior to the development of symptoms or hemodynamically significant lesions. Therefore, coronary artery disease is identified on CT much earlier than it would be identified on stress tests. Intimal calcification is present in both obstructive and nonobstructive lesions, therefore, coronary artery calcification is specific for detection of atheromatous plaque, but it is not specific for detection of an obstructive lesion. The most widely used method for quantifying coronary calcification is the Agatston score. Calcium scoring of the coronary arteries provides a quantitative measure of the atherosclerotic burden, but it does not provide

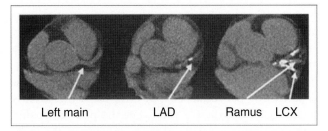

Left main      LAD      Ramus LCX

**Figure 54-15.** Coronary calcification. Electron beam CT of the left coronary system in three different patients. There is no coronary artery calcium on the left image. There is mild to moderate coronary calcium on the center image and severe extensive coronary artery calcium on the right image. (From Rumberger JA et al., Electron beam CT colonary calcium scanning: *a review Mayo clin Proc.* 1999;74:243–252.)

**Table 54-2 • Coronary Artery Calcium Score and Extent of Plaque Burden[*†]**

| EBCT Calcium Score | Plaque Burden | Probability of Significant CAD | Implications for CV Risk | Recommendations |
|---|---|---|---|---|
| 0 | No identifiable plaque | Very low, generally <5% | Very low | Reassure patient while discussing general public health guidelines for primary prevention of CV diseases |
| 1–10 | Minimal identifiable plaque burden | Very unlikely, <10% | Low | Discuss general public health guidelines for primary prevention of CV diseases |
| 11–100 | Definite, at least mild atherosclerotic plaque burden | Mild or minimal coronary stenoses likely | Moderate | Counsel about risk factor modification, strict adherence with NCEP ATP II primary prevention cholesterol guidelines, daily ASA† |
| 101–400 | Definite, at least moderate atherosclerotic plaque burden | Nonobstructive CAD highly likely, although obstructive disease possible | Moderately high | Institute risk factor modification and secondary prevention NCEP ATP II guidelines. Consider exercise testing for further risk stratification |
| >400 | Extensive atherosclerotic plaque burden | High likelihood (≥90%) of at least 1 "significant" coronary stenosis. | High | Institute very aggressive risk factor modification. Consider exercise or pharmacologic stress imaging to evaluate for inducible ischemia |

*See text for more details.
†ASA = acetaminophen; CAD = coronary artery disease; CV = cardiovascular; EBCT = electron beam computed tomography; NCEP ATP II = National Cholesterol Education Program (Adult Treatment Panel II).
From Rumberger JA et al., Electron beam CT colonary calcium scanning: a review Mayo clin Proc. 1999;74:243–252.

information on severity of epicardial luminal narrowing (**Table 54-2**). Assessment for progression of atherosclerosis can be serially monitored and helps determine the significance of treatment.

## CT Angiography

CT angiography (CTA) of the coronary arteries has become increasingly available and is a relatively new technology. Assessment of the coronary arteries not only has the inherent limitations of standard CT but also is affected by the movement of the heart throughout the cardiac cycle.

Numerous studies have examined the diagnostic accuracy of CTA compared to conventional invasive coronary angiography. The sensitivity of CTA is greater than 85% and the specificity is greater than 90% with 64-slice scanners. There is higher accuracy on a per-patient basis as opposed to a per-segment basis. CTA has a consistently high negative predictive value, but the positive predictive value is lower, owing to the experience of the technologist (both with performing the scan and preparing the patient) and the experience of the interpreting physician. CTA can quantify stenoses, but there can be wide limits of agreement between CTA and quantitative coronary angiography (**Figure 54-16**). For example, CTA can

overestimate the degree of stenosis in less significant lesions and underestimate the degree of stenosis in significantly obstructive lesions.

CTA does not have the ability to reliably differentiate between high grade stenosis and coronary artery occlusion because of the decreased spatial resolution to see the small lumen, and in either case, the vessel lumen appears interrupted. Long interruptions of the coronary vessel are typically secondary to total occlusion (**Figure 54-17**). It is difficult to assess collateral flow. CTA can be used to predict percutaneous recanalization success; the two key predictors are the length of the lesion and the extent of calcification. Recanalization success occurs more often in lesions that are shorter and have less calcification. There are a few studies that have shown that acute coronary syndrome plaques tend to have more positive remodeling, less frequent calcification, and lower density compared to stable plaques. Stable plaque is often calcified and has a higher density, whereas lipid rich plaque has a lower density.

## Evaluation of the Symptomatic Patient

Exclusion of significant coronary artery disease can be performed with CTA in symptomatic patients with an

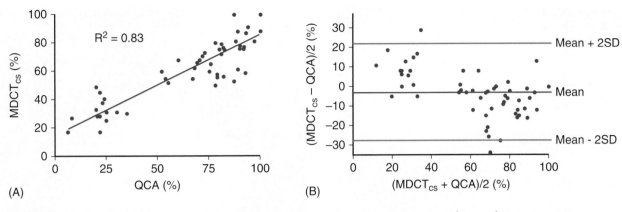

**Figure 54-16.** Correlation of CTA stenosis to cath QCA. Coronary artery stenosis on CT correlates with quantitative coronary angiography (cardiac cath), but there can be wide limits of agreement between the two. (Adapted from Curry Rc, et al,. Accuracy of 16-slice multidetector CT to quantify the degree of coronary artery stenosis: Assessment of cross-sectional and longitudinal vessel reconstructions. *European Journal of Radiology.* 2006 March; 57(3):345–350.)

intermediate risk of CAD or in those with atypical chest pain. CTA is useful in symptomatic patients with equivocal stress test results, such as when there is a discrepancy between ECG findings and imaging findings (perfusion or wall motion abnormalities). CTA is not routinely recommended for the assessment of symptomatic patients with known CAD. Many coronary stents are not evaluable by CTA and higher temporal resolution is needed, but it is possible with larger stents (>3 mm) and in thinner patients. In post-CABG patients, CTA can be used for assessment of symptoms in those who are felt to be at a high risk for undergoing cardiac catheterization and provides information regarding graft patency (**Figure 54-18**). CTA is an important diagnostic tool in patients undergoing redo open heart surgery,

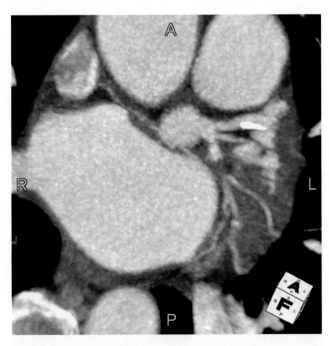

**Figure 54-17.** Chronic total occlusion. Interruption of the proximal circumflex artery is seen due to a total occlusion of the vessel. The distal vessel opacifies with contrast, which is highly indicative of the vessel filling by collateral flow.

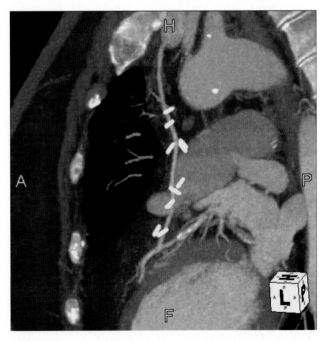

**Figure 54-18.** Post-CABG patients. CTA helped identify patency of this LIMA graft to the mid LAD. The bright structures along the graft are surgical clips that can sometimes hinder the visualization of the graft lumen. For patients undergoing repeat surgery, CTA can also demonstrate the distance between the bypass graft and the chest wall.

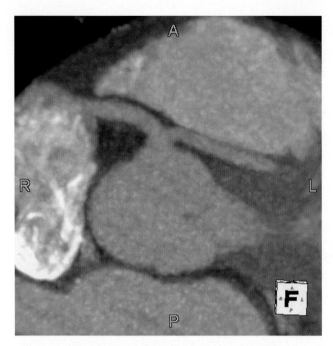

**Figure 54-19.** Coronary anomalies. The left anterior descending artery arises from the right coronary artery and then traverses between the aorta and pulmonary artery to the left ventricle.

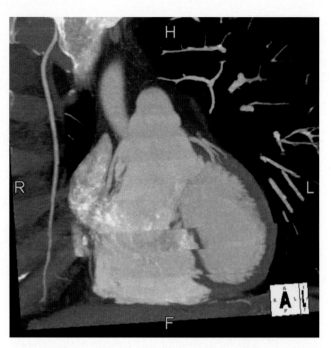

**Figure 54-20.** Artifacts. Stair step artifact secondary to extrasystolic beats or heart rate variability can be seen on sagittal or coronal views as misalignment of the imaging slabs.

because the relationship of the bypass vessels to the thorax can be determined, which helps determine the surgical approach. CTA can aid the diagnosis of coronary anomalies that may contribute to symptoms or sudden cardiac arrest (**Figure 54-19**).

## Artifacts

Calcium within the vessel results in a blooming appearance of the calcium due to partial volume effects, thus, calcified plaques appear larger than their size. Partial volume effects can be reduced with higher spatial resolution. Streak artifacts are produced by metal from ECG clips, prosthetic valves, pacemaker wires, sternal wires, and stents. Beam hardening artifact is seen as a dark area adjacent to calcium and occurs due to the filtering of X-ray by high density objects. Motion artifacts result in blurring of the image and can occur with faster heart rates or breathing during image acquisition. Motion artifacts can be reduced with multisegment reconstruction and decreased heart rates. Misalignment or step artifacts occur when there is an irregular heart rate or breathing during image acquisition (**Figure 54-20**).

An absolute contraindication to CTA is the inability of the patient to hold his or her breath or cooperate; relative contraindications include very heavily calcified vessels (**Figure 54-21**), frequent ectopy, atrial fibrillation, elevated

heart rate despite beta-blockade, and severe contrast allergy. The appropriateness criteria for cardiac CTA are located in **Table 54-3**. There are many noncoronary CT findings that need to be identified as well; these findings may include chamber enlargement, intra/extracardiac masses, valvular function, pulmonary embolus, aortic dissection, lung nodules, and tumors.

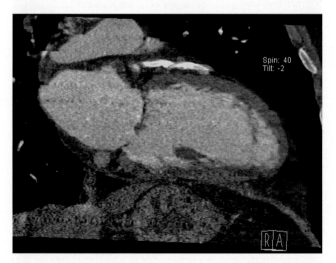

**Figure 54-21.** Coronary calcification. Severe calcification within the LAD that precludes diagnostic assessment of the vessel.

## Table 54-3 • Appropriateness Criteria for Cardiac CT

| Indication | | Appropriateness Criteria (Median Score) |
|---|---|---|
| | **Detection of CAD: symptomatic—evaluation of chest pain syndrome (use of CT angiogram)** | |
| 2. | • Intermediate pre-test probability of CAD<br>• ECG uninterpretable OR unable to exercise | A (7) |
| | **Detection of CAD: symptomatic—evaluation of intra-cardiac structures (use of CT angiogram)** | |
| 4. | • Evaluation of suspected coronary anomalies | A (9) |
| | **Detection of CAD: symptomatic—acute chest pain (use of CT angiogram)** | |
| 6. | • Intermediate pre-test probability of CAD<br>• No ECG change and serial anaymes negative | A (7) |
| | **Detection of CAD with prior test Results—Evaluation of chest pain syndrome (use of CT angiogram)** | |
| 16. | • Uninterpretable or equivocal stress test (exercise, perfusion, or stress echo) | A (8) |
| | **Structure and function—morphology (use of CT angiogram)** | |
| 28. | • Assessment of complex congenital heart disease including anomalies of coronary circulation, great vessels, and cardiac chambers and valves | A (7) |
| 29. | • Evaluation of coronary arteries in patients with new coset heart failure to assess etiology | A (7) |
| | **Structure and function—evaluation of intra- and extra-cardiac structures (use of CT cardiac)** | |
| 33. | • Evaluation of cardiac mass (suspected tumor or thrombus)<br>• Patients with technically limited images from echocardiogram, MRI, or TEE | A (8) |
| 34. | • Evaluation of pericardial conditions (pericardial mass, constrictive pericarditis, or complications of cardiac surgery)<br>• Patients with technically limited images from echocardiogram, MRI, or TEE | A (8) |
| 35. | • Evaluation of pulmonary vein anatomy prior to invasive radiofrequency ablation for atrial fibrillition | A (8) |
| 36. | • Noninvasive coronary vein mapping prior to placement of biventricular pacemaker | A (8) |
| 37. | • Noninvasive coronary arterial mapping, including internal mammary artery price to repeat cardiac surgical revascularization | A (8) |
| | **Structure and function—evaluation of aortic and pulmonary disease (use of CT angiogram\*)** | |
| 38. | • Evaluation of suspected aortic dissection or thoracic aortic aneurysm | A (9) |
| 39. | • Evaluation of suspected pulmonary embolism | A (9) |

*Non-gated, CT angiogram which has a sufficiently large field of view for these specific indications
Adapted from Hendel RC et al, Appropriateness Criteria for CCT/CMR. JACC 2006:1483.

## Suggested Readings

1. Hendel RC, Patel MR, Kramer CM, Poon M, et al. Appropriateness criteria for CCT/CMR. JACC. 2006;48(7);1475–1497.

2. Kim RJ, Wu E, Rafael A, Chen EL, et al. The use of contrast-enhanced magnetic resonance imaging to identify reversible myocardial dysfunction. N Engl J Med. 2000 Nov 16;343(20):1445–1453.

3. Mahmarian JJ. Computed tomography of the heart. In: Fuster V, Alexander RW, O'Rourke RA, eds. Hurst's The Heart. New York: McGraw Hill; 2004;599–628.

4. Poon M, Dinh HV, Fuster V. Magnetic resonance imaging of the heart. In: Fuster V, Alexander RW, O'Rourke RA, eds. Hurst's The Heart. New York: McGraw Hill; 2004;629–646.

5. Rumberger JA, Brundage BH, Rader DJ, et al. Electron beam computed tomographic coronary calcium scanning: A review and guidelines for use in asymptomatic persons. Mayo Clin Proc. 1999;74:243–252.

6. Wu et al. Prognostic significance of microvascular obstruction by magnetic resonance imaging in patients with acute myocardial infarction. Circulation. 1998;97:765–772.

# 55

# Selection of Stress Testing

KELLEY R. BRANCH AND PETER J. CAWLEY

## ● PRACTICAL POINTS

**Stress modality**

Exercise/treadmill stress

- Indications
  - Preferred method for any stress testing
  - Possible myocardial ischemia
  - Asymptomatic with moderate to high Framingham risk and high-risk occupation
  - Asymptomatic with high Framingham risk

- Cautions
  - Absolute
    - Acute myocardial infarction (within 2d)
    - High-risk unstable angina
    - Uncontrolled cardiac arrhythmias causing symptoms or hemodynamic compromise
    - Symptomatic severe aortic stenosis
    - Uncontrolled symptomatic heart failure
    - Acute pulmonary embolus or pulmonary infarction
    - Acute myocarditis or pericarditis
    - Acute aortic dissection
  - Relative
    - Left main coronary stenosis
    - Electrolyte abnormalities
    - Severe arterial hypertension—systolic BP >200, diastolic BP >110 mm Hg
    - Tachyarrhythmias or bradyarrhythmias

    - Hypertrophic cardiomyopathy and other forms of outflow tract obstruction
    - Inability to exercise adequately
    - High-degree atrioventricular block
    - Severe aortic stenosis
    - Left bundle branch block (LBBB)

Dobutamine

- Indications
  - Inability to exercise to goal
  - Reactive airway disease, if pharmacologic stress is needed
  - Possible low-output, low-gradient valvular disease

- Cautions
  - History of inducible ventricular arrhythmia
  - Baseline hypertension SBP >200, DBP >110 mm Hg
  - Cannot discontinue beta-blocker
  - LBBB, if SPECT is used

Vasodilator (dipyridamole or adenosine)

- Indications
  - Inability to exercise to goal
  - LBBB, when coupled with SPECT

- Cautions
  - Reactive airway disease
  - High grade AV nodal block or inducible heart block
  - Baseline hypotension

(continued)

## ● PRACTICAL POINTS (continued)

**Imaging modality coupled with a stress test above**

ECG alone (no imaging)

- Indications
  - ○ Able to exercise
  - ○ ECG interpretable
  - ○ Intermediate pretest probability
- Cautions
  - ○ Paced or LBBB rhythm
  - ○ ST depressions ≥ 1 mm
  - ○ Preexcitation
  - ○ Established CAD diagnosis without need for risk or ischemic assessment

Stress SPECT

- Indications
  - ○ Intermediate pretest probability for CAD
    - – Includes acute and chronic chest pain, chest pain, and new heart failure
  - ○ High pretest probability for CAD
    - – Nonevaluable ECG –OR- cannot exercise
  - ○ Moderate Framingham risk and heart failure without chest pain
  - ○ Moderate to high Framingham risk
    - – High-risk occupation
  - ○ Agatston calcium score ≥ 400
  - ○ Idiopathic ventricular tachycardia
  - ○ Preoperative evaluation, intermediate to high-risk surgery
- Cautions
  - ○ Obesity or high likelihood of soft tissue attenuation
  - ○ Irregular heart rates, if gating is required
  - ○ Asymptomatic at low Framingham risk or with stable symptoms, < 1 year from last test

Stress echocardiography

- Indications
  - ○ Low pretest probability, uninterpretable ECG, and cannot exercise—symptomatic
  - ○ Intermediate or high pretest probability
    - – Includes new LV dysfunction, atrial fibrillation
  - ○ Equivocal prior stress test
  - ○ Evaluation of medically managed CAD patients with worsening symptoms
  - ○ Agatston calcium score ≥ 400
  - ○ Viability
  - ○ Equivocal aortic stenosis with low cardiac output (dobutamine)
  - ○ Asymptomatic severe MR or AI
  - ○ Preoperative evaluation, intermediate to high-risk surgery
- Cautions
  - ○ Suboptimal windows
    - – Obesity and lung disease (contrast may help)
  - ○ Asymptomatic at low Framingham risk or with stable symptoms, < 1 year from last test

Stress MRI (dipyridamole or dobutamine)

- Indications
  - ○ Not well defined, but likely similar to SPECT and echo
- Cautions
  - ○ Low pretest probability
  - ○ Cannot hold breath for imaging
  - ○ Ferromagnetic metal (pacemakers, ICD, etc.)
  - ○ Arrhythmias that impair reconstruction
  - ○ Reactive airway disease
  - ○ Severe claustrophobia

---

Selection of appropriate stress testing is determined by multiple patient- and technique-specific factors. Obviously, none of these noninvasive tests are perfect and each test has certain strengths and limitations. In many cases, complementary tests are used for diagnosis and decisions for treatment. In clinical practice, test selection and interpretation are individualized for each patient, and for this reason, the cardiology boards commonly use these appropriateness questions throughout the examination either as the question itself ("What test would be the best?") or as a springboard to test other knowledge ("Of the possible agents for the stress test, what would be contraindicated given the patient's medical history?").

This chapter will serve to incorporate the knowledge reviewed in the previous chapters into instructive cases that will mimic the board format as well as your patients in clinical practice. This chapter should be used to solidify your knowledge of noninvasive testing or point out certain weaknesses that should be reviewed further. This chapter will not

# Heart Failure

# 56

# Molecular Mechanisms of Heart Failure

ANGELA G. BRITTSAN AND DOUGLAS B. SAWYER

## ● PRACTICAL POINTS

- There does not appear to be one common pathway that can be targeted to reverse the pathological remodeling of the heart, but several complex signaling cascades contribute.

- The two basic patterns of cardiac hypertrophy are concentric (where sarcomeres are added in parallel fashion due to systolic wall stress) and eccentric (where sarcomeres are added in series due to diastolic wall stress).

- $\beta$-adrenergic receptor ($\beta$-AR) signaling regulates dynamic changes in myocardial function, with $\beta_1$-AR isoform predominant over $\beta_2$-AR.

- Calcium ($Ca^{2+}$) is the central second messenger involved in the translation of electrical signals into mechanical activity in the heart, with alterations in $Ca^{2+}$ homeostasis resulting in contractile dysfunction and malignant arrhythmias.

- The $Ca^{2+}$-cycling defects identified in failing hearts are (a) reduced $Ca^{2+}$ transients, (b) impaired sarcoplasmic

reticulum (SR) $Ca^{2+}$-release that is associated with a diastolic $Ca^{2+}$ leak, and (c) reduced SR $Ca^{2+}$-uptake.

- Degradation of the extracellular matrix, primarily composed of Type I collagen, has been noted in dilated cardiomyopathy due to an imbalance of matrix metalloproteinases and inhibitors.

- In the failing heart, studies have shown there is a progressive loss of myocytes through apoptotic, necrotic, or autophagic cell death pathways.

- The neurohormonal cascade contributes to progressive myocardial remodeling, from prolonged activation of both the sympathetic (beta-adrenergic receptors) and renin-angiotensin-aldosterone systems.

- Inflammation, with increased levels of cytokines (TNFα and IL-1), has also been shown to play a significant role in the pathogenesis of heart failure and cardiac remodeling.

Heart failure is a clinical syndrome that develops when the heart is unable to pump the amount of blood needed to meet the body's metabolic demands at rest and/or with exertion at normal filling pressures. Symptoms of fatigue, dyspnea, fluid retention, and exercise intolerance manifest from this imbalance of supply and demand and supraphysiologic end-diastolic pressures. Over the past several decades, there have been intense research efforts aimed at elucidating the mechanisms of heart failure and understanding the pathophysiology of the failing ventricle.

Despite the medical advances made in understanding this disease, the prevalence of heart failure continues to increase with associated high rates of morbidity and mortality that affect our society with extraordinary social and economic costs.[1] Thus, there continues to be great interest and dedication invested in better understanding the pathophysiology of heart failure, elucidating the molecular mechanisms involved in the progression of heart failure and targeting novel therapeutic strategies to prevent further deterioration of left ventricular function, as well as decreasing the prevalence, morbidity, and mortality associated with this disease.

The cardiovascular system responds with compensatory measures to preserve cardiovascular homeostasis in the setting of left ventricular dysfunction including the activation of the sympathetic nervous system and the renin-angiotensin-aldosterone system. In the short term, this adaptation increases cardiac output and maintains adequate blood flow to vital organs; however, over a long period of time, sustained sympathetic and neurohormonal activation as well as enhanced release of endothelin, cytokines, and growth factors trigger intracellular signal transduction cascades that are maladaptive for the heart and alter cellular and organ morphology and function. This results in adverse effects on cardiac structure through the process known as ventricular remodeling. Different types of stress stimuli couple with different signal pathways, as demonstrated in **Figure 56-1**. For example, protein kinase A (PKA), protein kinase C (PKC), mitogen-activated protein kinase (MAPK), calcineurin, and $Ca^{2+}$/calmodulin-dependent kinase II (CaMKII) are some of the kinases and phosphatases activated and involved in the intracellular signaling pathways that regulate and modulate gene transcription in the heart. Although it is not the focus of this chapter to review each individual signal transduction cascade identified in heart failure, it is important to point out that there does not appear to be one common pathway that can be targeted to reverse the pathological remodeling of the heart; rather, several complex signaling cascades contribute in parallel to alter the phenotype of the cardiomyocyte and molecular regulation of the heart.

In this chapter, we focus on the molecular mechanisms of heart failure, specifically the patterns of left ventricular hypertrophy and alterations observed in β-adrenergic receptor signal transduction, excitation-contraction (EC) coupling[2] and $Ca^{2+}$-handling, myofilament and cytoskeletal proteins, the extracellular matrix, and cell death.

## PATTERNS OF HYPERTROPHY

Two basic patterns of cardiac hypertrophy occur in response to hemodynamic overload. When the ventricle is subjected to sustained systolic wall stress (or pressure overload as occurs in systemic hypertension and aortic stenosis), the cardiomyocyte increases its cross-sectional area and adds sarcomeres in a parallel fashion.[2,3] This results in a pattern of hypertrophy characterized by increased ventricular wall thickness and is referred to as concentric hypertrophy (**Figure 56-2**). In addition, there is an accumulation of collagen between myocytes in concentric hypertrophy that is associated with ventricular stiffening and contributes to impaired diastolic dysfunction. In contrast, when there is increased ventricular diastolic wall stress (or volume overload as occurs in mitral and aortic insufficiency), the cardiomyocyte increases its length by

adding sarcomeres in a series.[2,3] This results in a pattern of hypertrophy characterized by increased internal ventricular dimension referred to as eccentric hypertrophy (**Figure 56-2**). Eccentric hypertrophy is associated with increased turnover of collagen, contributing to the increased chamber diameter. In each of these patterns of hypertrophy, the cardiomyocyte's response to a specific type of biomechanical stress is mediated by the release of various neurohormones, growth factors, cytokines, or reactive oxygen species, which subsequently activate different signal transduction cascades that alter the expression levels of a number of genes.[4]

In hypertrophy, the growth of myocytes is activated by small molecules such as adrenergic agonists and prostaglandins, as well as the release of peptides (e.g., endothelin-1 and angiotensin II), growth factors (e.g., IGF-1, neuregulin-1), and cytokines (e.g., IL-6/cardiotropin 1). Some of these signals are known to play a role in the physiologic growth of the heart (IGF-1 and cardiotrophin 1) and conceptually may be triggers for adaptive hypertrophy. Others are primarily considered stimuli for maladaptive hypertrophy (endothelin-1 and angiotensin II). There are many signaling molecules that have been associated with hypertrophy, including (a) receptor tyrosine kinases, cytokine, and G-protein coupled receptors; (b) serine/threonine kinases (such as Akt, MAPK, and CaMKII); (c) transcription factors (including STAT3, MEF2, and NFAT); and (d) protein phosphatases (such as calcineurin). Each of these has been implicated in both adaptive, physiological hypertrophy as well as pathological hypertrophy. A key determinant appears to be the duration and magnitude of activation of a given pathway, with prolonged and greater degrees of activation, in general, being associated with the promotion of pathological remodeling.

## ALTERATIONS IN SIGNALING PATHWAYS

### Alterations in β-Adrenergic Receptor Signal Transduction

β-adrenergic receptor (β-AR) signaling is known to critically regulate dynamic changes in myocardial function.[5] β-ARs are part of a superfamily of G-protein-coupled receptors (GPCRs). There are two main isoforms of β-ARs expressed in the heart, $β_1$-AR and $β_2$-AR. $β_1$-AR is the predominant isoform expressed. In the nonfailing heart, studies have shown the $β_1$-AR:$β_2$-AR ratio to be 70:30.[6] Both $β_1$- and $β_2$-ARs activate $G_s$ and couple to adenylyl cyclase, generating increased levels of cAMP that activates PKA. PKA is involved in the phosphorylation of several downstream targets, such as the L-type $Ca^{2+}$ channel, ryanodine receptor, phospholamban, troponin I, myosin binding protein-C, and titin, which results in enhanced cardiac inotropy and lusitropy. Increased chronotropy results from cAMP directly

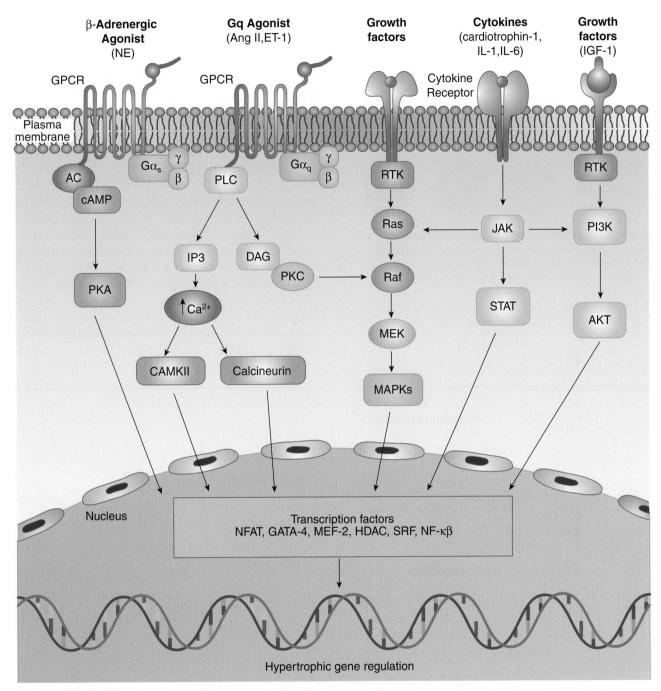

**Figure 56-1.** Signal transduction cascades involved in left ventricular remodeling. A schematic illustration of common signaling pathways involved in altering cardiomyocyte function and growth. Stress stimuli (catecholamines, neurohormones, cytokines, and growth factors) bind to cell surface receptors, activating intracellular signaling pathways that influence and regulate the expression of cardiac hypertrophic genes. β-AR, β-adrenergic receptor; GPCR, G-protein coupled receptor; RTK, receptor tyrosine kinase; NE, norepinephrine; ET-1, endothelin-1; AngII, angiotensin II peptide; TNF-α, tumor necrosis factor-α; NRG, neuregulin; IL-1, interleukin-1; IGF-1, insulin growth factor-1; AC, adenylyl cyclase; cAMP, cyclic adenosine monophosphate; PKA, cyclic AMP protein kinase; PLC, phospholipase C; JAK, Janus kinase; STAT, signal transducer and activator of transcription; PI3K, phosphatidylinositol 3-kinase; PKC, protein kinase C; DAG, diacylglycerol; MAPK, mitogen-activated protein kinase; IP3, inositol (1,4,5)-triphosphate; CAMKII, calcium/calmodulin- dependent protein kinase II; MEK, mitogen-activated protein kinase kinase; NFAT, nuclear factor of activated T cells; GATA4, GATA binding protein 4; MEF2, myocyte enhancer factor 2; HDAC, histone deacetylase; SRF, serum response factor; NF-κB, nuclear factor κB.

LV remodeling in heart failure

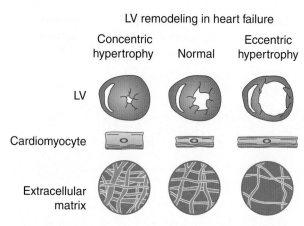

**Figure 56-2.** Left ventricular remodeling. In response to the different types of hemodynamic overload, phenotypically distinct changes occur in the morphology of myocytes and in the extracellular matrix resulting in different patterns of cardiac hypertrophy.

stimulating the hyperpolarization-activated cyclic nucleotide-gated cation channel. In addition to coupling with $G_s$, the $\beta_2$-ARs also have the ability to couple with $G_i$, which has been shown to decrease cAMP levels, mediate antiapoptotic effects (via activation of Akt/protein kinase B and phosphatidylinositol 3-kinase kinases)[7], and regulate cardiac hypertrophy (via activation of MAPK pathways)[8].

The cardiomyocyte also has the ability to modulate β-adrenergic signaling when sustained β-AR stimulation occurs through a process called desensitization.[9] Desensitization occurs via two pathways: phosphorylation of the β-AR's cytoplasmic tail by PKA or by a G-protein-coupled receptor kinase called β-agonist receptor kinase (βARK). It is interesting that desensitization of the β-AR by βARK also involves another protein called β-arrestin, which is a scaffolding protein. Phosphorylation of the β-AR by βARK increases the binding affinity of β-arrestin for the receptor's cytoplasmic loop that results in impaired G-protein binding and reduced receptor responsiveness, as well as internalization of the ligand bound receptor to clathrin coated pits (**Figure 56-3**).[9]

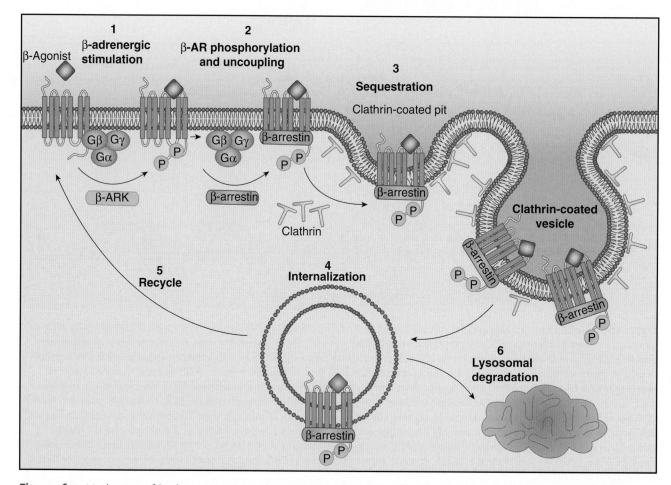

**Figure 56-3.** Mechanism of β-adrenergic receptor desensitization. Activation of β-adrenergic receptors results in the stimulation of β-adrenergic receptor kinase (β-ARK), phosphorylation, and the uncoupling of the β-adrenergic receptor. This subsequently is followed with the recruitment and binding of β-arrestin and the internalization of the ligand-receptor complex. β-AR, β-adrenergic receptor; β-ARK, β-adrenergic receptor kinase.

In the setting of heart failure, there is pronounced activation of the sympathetic nervous system that has been shown to be inversely correlated with survival.[10] A reproducible collection of biochemical defects has been observed in the β-AR signaling pathway of failing hearts. There is a marked selective downregulation of $\beta_1$-ARs (~50%) with no change in $\beta_2$-AR levels.[11,13] In addition, the functional coupling of the remaining receptors to the $G_s$-adenylyl cyclase system is reduced.[14] Furthermore, in failing hearts, the βARK activity and mRNA levels are increased, and this appears to contribute to β-AR desensitization.[15] Thus, although ventricular systolic function is decreased in the setting of heart failure, reduced sensitivity of myocardium via receptor downregulation and desensitization prevents sustained inotropic response.

Whether or not adrenergic desensitization is an adaptive mechanism to reduce the cytotoxicity associated with sustained adrenergic signaling (see below), it is very clear that pharmacologic desensitization of adrenergic signaling in systolic heart failure with β-AR blockers is beneficial and prevents adverse myocardial remodeling as well as arrhythmias. However, research elucidating the role of βARK in various animal models of heart failure suggests that βARK mediated activity in the setting of heart failure is adaptive. Different transgenic mouse models of heart failure demonstrate improved β-adrenergic signaling and hemodynamics, reduced hypertrophy, and increased survival with overexpression of a C-terminal βARK peptide, which functions as a βARK inhibitor.[12,16,17,18,19] Similar findings were demonstrated in failing human cardiomyocytes after adenoviral-mediated gene transfer of the βARK inhibitory peptide.[20] Thus, these findings suggest that increased βARK activity contributes to the progression of heart failure. How these findings integrate with the known therapeutic effects of β-AR blockers remains to be fully elucidated.

## Alterations in Excitation-contraction Coupling and Ca²⁺- Handling

Excitation-contraction coupling is a highly coordinated and regulated process in the cardiomyocyte. Calcium ($Ca^{2+}$) is the central second messenger involved in the translation of electrical signals into mechanical activity in the heart. Alterations in $Ca^{2+}$ homeostasis result in contractile dysfunction and malignant arrhythmias, as seen in failing hearts. During an action potential, $Ca^{2+}$ enters the myocyte via voltage-activated L-type $Ca^{2+}$ channels as illustrated in **Figure 56-4**. This small influx of $Ca^{2+}$ is called trigger $Ca^{2+}$, which induces a much larger release of $Ca^{2+}$ from the sarcoplasmic reticulum (SR) via the SR $Ca^{2+}$ release channel known as the ryanodine receptor (RyR2). This process is called $Ca^{2+}$-induced $Ca^{2+}$-release.[21] Increased cytosolic concentrations of $Ca^{2+}$ activate the myofilaments via the binding of $Ca^{2+}$ to troponin C, resulting in the displacement

of tropomyosin and allowing actin-myosin cross-bridge formation to take place. For relaxation to occur, the cytosolic concentration of $Ca^{2+}$ must decrease in order to allow $Ca^{2+}$ to dissociate from troponin. $Ca^{2+}$ returns to diastolic levels primarily via two pathways. A large proportion of the cytosolic $Ca^{2+}$ (70%) is sequestered into the SR via the SR $Ca^{2+}$-ATPase (SERCA2a) and a smaller amount (28%) is removed toward the extracellular space via the Na+/ $Ca^{2+}$ exchanger (NCX) located in the sarcolemma.[21] The remaining $Ca^{2+}$ in the cytosol is removed by the sarcolemma $Ca^{2+}$-ATPase and the mitochondrial $Ca^{2+}$ uniporter (**Figure 56-4**). Sequestration of $Ca^{2+}$ into the SR by SERCA2a is regulated by the phosphoprotein phospholamban (PLB). In its dephosphorylated state, PLB inhibits SERCA2a activity. PLB can be phosphorylated by PKA or CaMKII, thereby releasing its inhibition on SERCA2a and consequently increasing SR $Ca^{2+}$-uptake activity.[22] Thus, for the myocyte to be in a steady state with respect to $Ca^{2+}$ balance, the amount of $Ca^{2+}$ removed from the cell during relaxation must equal the amount of $Ca^{2+}$ entering the cell on a beat to beat basis. Furthermore, the amount of $Ca^{2+}$ released from the SR by the RYR2 must equal the amount of $Ca^{2+}$ resequestered into the SR by SERCA2a. When abnormalities in $Ca^{2+}$-handling manifest, the heart develops problems with electrical and mechanical coupling, resulting in arrhythmias as well as problems with contraction and relaxation.[23,24,25,26,27] The $Ca^{2+}$-cycling defects identified in failing hearts are (a) reduced $Ca^{2+}$ transients, (b) impaired SR $Ca^{2+}$-release that is associated with a diastolic $Ca^{2+}$ leak, and (c) reduced SR $Ca^{2+}$-uptake.

### SR Ca²⁺-Uptake

In failing hearts, SR $Ca^{2+}$-uptake has been shown to be markedly impaired and this is associated with decreased levels of SERCA2a protein expression and activity.[24,25,27] It is interesting that in animal models of heart failure, overexpression of SERCA2a in diseased hearts has been shown to result in the recovery of cardiac contractility.[28] Thus, SERCA2a appears to play a critical role in $Ca^{2+}$ regulation and is being pursued as a target for the treatment of heart failure. In fact, clinical trials are currently under way assessing a strategy of virally mediated overexpression of SERCA2a in humans.

In addition to reduced levels of SERCA2a expression, the phosphorylation status of PLB is decreased in heart failure, which should further reduce SERCA2a activity. As discussed, the stimulatory effects of β-adrenergic stimulation on cardiomyocyte contractility are mediated by the phosphorylation of several key phosphoproteins in the heart by PKA, including PLB. In order to maintain a balance of the status of phosphorylation/dephosphorylation in these regulatory phosphoproteins, protein phosphatases must oppose the actions of kinases to attain biochemical and functional phosphorylation homeostasis. Protein phosphatase-1 (PP1) is a major phosphatase in the heart

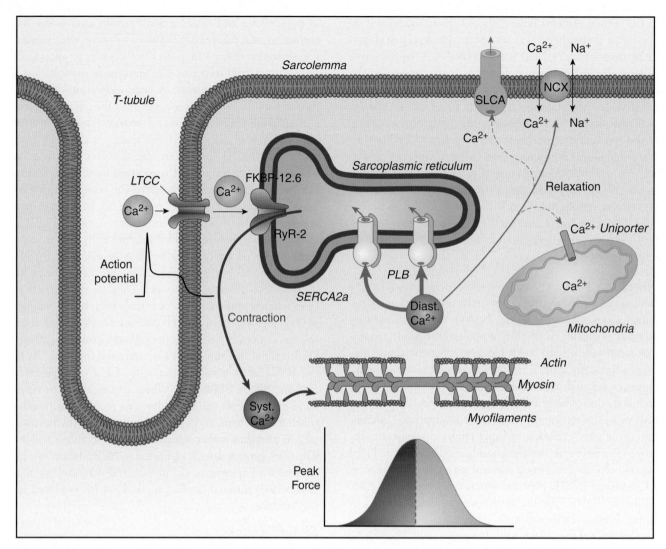

**Figure 56-4.** Calcium handling in the cardiomyocyte. Calcium handling is the central coordinator of cardiac contraction and relaxation. Sarcomere contraction is initiated by $Ca^{2+}$-induced $Ca^{2+}$ release. For relaxation to occur, $Ca^{2+}$ is sequestered predominantly by the sarcoplasmic reticulum (70%) via the SR $Ca^{2+}$-ATPase and the $Na^+/Ca^{2+}$ exchanger (28%). SERCA2a, sarcoplasmic/endoplasmic reticulum; $Ca^{2+}$, calcium; $Ca^{2+}$-ATPase 2a; PLB, phospholamban; NCX, $Na^+/Ca^{2+}$ exchanger; RYR-2, ryanodine receptor-2; Syst. $Ca^{2+}$, systolic calcium; Dias. $Ca^{2+}$, diastolic calcium.

that has been shown to dephosphorylate PLB, among many other phosphoproteins. Furthermore, in heart failure, PP1 activity has been shown to be increased and this has been linked to depressed SR $Ca^{2+}$-uptake as well as depressed levels of PLB phosphorylation. A transgenic mouse model, overexpressing PP1 in the heart, developed dilated cardiomyopathy and exhibited impaired relaxation. These results suggest that PP1 may also play a role in the progression of heart failure.[29]

PP1 is also regulated by an endogenous inhibitor called inhibitor-1 (INH-1). INH-1 regulation of PP1 is an additional layer of complexity to the PKA and PP1 regulation of PLB's phosphorylation status. PKA phosphorylates INH-1 and this posttranslational modification result in a potent inhibition of PP1 activity by INH-1.[30] As a result,

PKA phosphorylation of INH-1 and PLB facilitates an increase in cardiac contractility in an unopposed manner. In addition, overexpression of INH-1 or of a constitutively active form of INH-1 has been shown to augment cardiac contraction and relaxation, both in vitro and in vivo.[30,31] In contrast, decreased activity and/or reduced expression levels of INH-1 have been shown to be associated with cardiac dysfunction in animal models and in humans with heart failure.[29,32] Furthermore, when INH-1 is phosphorylated by PKCα (which is activated by the binding of either angiotensin II or endothelin to $G_q$-coupled receptors), it no longer inhibits PP1 but actually activates PP1 and facilitates the dephosphorylation of PLB.[33,34] Thus, aberrant neurohormonal signaling and depressed $Ca^{2+}$ cycling are associated with an imbalance of kinase and phosphatase activities that confer a heart failure phenotype.

future we may obtain microRNA profiles from patients that will be used to dictate their personalized treatment regimen for their heart failure. Increasing evidence also suggests that the heart has regenerative potential in the form of undifferentiated cells residing in both the bone marrow and heart that can differentiate to myocytes, replacing and repairing injured myocardium. Ongoing studies will help to elucidate the degree that these cells can be manipulated to affect repair after the development of heart failure. These areas of research may revolutionize our understanding of heart failure and affect our success in treating this chronic disease.

## ACKNOWLEDGMENTS

We thank Mr. Dennis E. Mathias for the artistic contribution provided in generating the figures published in this chapter.

## References

1. Lloyd-Jones D, et al. Heart disease and stroke statistics–2009 update: A report from the American Heart Association Statistics Committee and Stroke Statistics Subcommittee. *Circulation*. 2009;119(3):e21–181.

2. Opie LH, et al. Controversies in ventricular remodelling. *Lancet*. 2006;367(9507):356–367.

3. Katz AM. Maladaptive growth in the failing heart: The cardiomyopathy of overload. *Cardiovasc Drugs Ther*. 2002;16(3): 245–249.

4. Hunter JJ, Chien KR. Signaling pathways for cardiac hypertrophy and failure. *N Engl J Med*. 1999;341(17):1276–1283.

5. Rockman HA, Koch WJ, Lefkowitz RJ. Seven-transmembrane-spanning receptors and heart function. *Nature*. 2002;415(6868):206–212.

6. Brodde OE, Michel MC. Adrenergic and muscarinic receptors in the human heart. *Pharmacol Rev*. 1999;51(4):651–690.

7. Communal C, et al. Opposing effects of beta(1)- and beta(2)-adrenergic receptors on cardiac myocyte apoptosis: Role of a pertussis toxin-sensitive G protein. *Circulation*. 1999;100(22):2210–2212.

8. Molkentin JD, Dorn GW II. Cytoplasmic signaling pathways that regulate cardiac hypertrophy. *Annu Rev Physiol*. 2001;63:391–426.

9. Lefkowitz RJ. G protein-coupled receptors. III. New roles for receptor kinases and beta-arrestins in receptor signaling and desensitization. *J Biol Chem*. 1998;273(30):18677–18680.

10. Ungerer M, et al. Expression of beta-arrestins and beta-adrenergic receptor kinases in the failing human heart. *Circ Res*. 1994;74(2):206–213.

11. Lohse MJ, Engelhardt S, Eschenhagen T. What is the role of beta-adrenergic signaling in heart failure? *Circ Res*. 2003;93(10):896–906.

12. Tevaearai HT, Koch WJ. Molecular restoration of beta-adrenergic receptor signaling improves contractile function of failing hearts. *Trends Cardiovasc Med*. 2004;14(6):252–256.

13. Bristow MR, et al. Beta 1- and beta 2-adrenergic-receptor subpopulations in nonfailing and failing human ventricular myocardium: Coupling of both receptor subtypes to muscle contraction and selective beta 1-receptor down-regulation in heart failure. *Circ Res*. 1986;59(3):297–309.

14. Colucci WS. The effects of norepinephrine on myocardial biology: Implications for the therapy of heart failure. *Clin Cardiol*. 1998;21(12 Suppl 1):I20–I24.

15. Leineweber K, et al. Ventricular hypertrophy plus neurohumoral activation is necessary to alter the cardiac beta-adrenoceptor system in experimental heart failure. *Circ Res*. 2002;91(11):1056–1062.

16. Rockman HA, et al. Expression of a beta-adrenergic receptor kinase 1 inhibitor prevents the development of myocardial failure in gene-targeted mice. *Proc Natl Acad Sci USA*. 1998;95(12):7000–7005.

17. Harding VB, et al. Cardiac beta ARK1 inhibition prolongs survival and augments beta blocker therapy in a mouse model of severe heart failure. *Proc Natl Acad Sci USA*. 2001;98(10):5809–5814.

18. Freeman K, et al. Alterations in cardiac adrenergic signaling and calcium cycling differentially affect the progression of cardiomyopathy. *J Clin Invest*. 2001;107(8):967–974.

19. Hansen JL, et al. Role of G-protein-coupled receptor kinase 2 in the heart–do regulatory mechanisms open novel therapeutic perspectives? *Trends Cardiovasc Med*. 2006;16(5):169–177.

20. Williams ML, et al. Targeted beta-adrenergic receptor kinase (betaARK1) inhibition by gene transfer in failing human hearts. *Circulation*, 2004;109(13):1590–1593.

21. Bers DM. Cardiac excitation-contraction coupling. *Nature*. 2002;415(6868):198–205.

22. Waggoner JR, Kranias EG. Role of phospholamban in the pathogenesis of heart failure. *Heart Fail Clin*. 2005;1(2): 207–218.

23. Yano M. Ryanodine receptor as a new therapeutic target of heart failure and lethal arrhythmia. *Circ J*. 2008;72(4): 509–514.

24. Kranias EG, Bers DM. Calcium and cardiomyopathies. *Subcell Biochem*. 2007;45:523–537.

25. Ikeda Y, Hoshijima M, Chien KR. Toward biologically targeted therapy of calcium cycling defects in heart failure. *Physiology (Bethesda)*. 2008;23:6–16.

26. Chelu MG, Wehrens XH. Sarcoplasmic reticulum calcium leak and cardiac arrhythmias. *Biochem Soc Trans*. 2007;35 (Pt 5):952–956.

27. Bers DM. Altered cardiac myocyte Ca regulation in heart failure. *Physiology (Bethesda)*. 2006;21:380–387.

28. Kawase Y, Hajjar RJ. The cardiac sarcoplasmic/endoplasmic reticulum calcium ATPase: A potent target for cardiovas-

cular diseases. *Nat Clin Pract Cardiovasc Med.* 2008;5(9): 554–565.

29. Carr AN, et al. Type 1 phosphatase, a negative regulator of cardiac function. *Mol Cell Biol.* 2002;22(12):4124–4135.

30. El-Armouche A, et al. Evidence for protein phosphatase inhibitor-1 playing an amplifier role in beta-adrenergic signaling in cardiac myocytes. *FASEB J.* 2003;17(3):437–439.

31. Pathak A, et al. Enhancement of cardiac function and suppression of heart failure progression by inhibition of protein phosphatase 1. *Circ Res.* 2005;96(7):756–766.

32. El-Armouche A, et al. Decreased protein and phosphorylation level of the protein phosphatase inhibitor-1 in failing human hearts. *Cardiovasc Res.* 2004;61(1):87–93.

33. Rodriguez P, et al. Identification of a novel phosphorylation site in protein phosphatase inhibitor-1 as a negative regulator of cardiac function. *J Biol Chem.* 2006;281(50): 38599–38608.

34. Braz JC, et al. PKC-alpha regulates cardiac contractility and propensity toward heart failure. *Nat Med.* 2004;10(3): 248–254.

35. Marks AR. Ryanodine receptors/calcium release channels in heart failure and sudden cardiac death. *J Mol Cell Cardiol.* 2001;33(4):615–624.

36. Morita H, Seidman J, Seidman CE. Genetic causes of human heart failure. *J Clin Invest.* 2005;115(3):518–526.

37. Westermann D, et al. Diltiazem treatment prevents diastolic heart failure in mice with familial hypertrophic cardiomyopathy. *Eur J Heart Fail.* 2006;8(2):115–121.

38. Badorff C, et al. Enteroviral protease 2A cleaves dystrophin: Evidence of cytoskeletal disruption in an acquired cardiomyopathy. *Nat Med,* 1999;5(3):320–326.

39. Zheng QS, et al. Dystrophin: From non-ischemic cardiomyopathy to ischemic cardiomyopathy. *Med Hypotheses.* 2008;71(3):434–438.

40. Granzier H, et al. Titin: Physiological function and role in cardiomyopathy and failure. *Heart Fail Rev.* 2005;10(3): 211–223.

41. Lim CC, Sawyer DB. Modulation of cardiac function: Titin springs into action. *J Gen Physiol.* 2005;125(3):249–252.

42. D'Armiento J. Matrix metalloproteinase disruption of the extracellular matrix and cardiac dysfunction. *Trends Cardiovasc Med.* 2002;12(3):97–101.

43. Kim TH, et al. Expression and activation of pro-MMP-2 and pro-MMP-9 during rat liver regeneration. *Hepatology.* 2000;31(1):75–82.

44. Thomas CV, et al. Increased matrix metalloproteinase activity and selective upregulation in LV myocardium from patients with end-stage dilated cardiomyopathy. *Circulation.* 1998;97(17):1708–1715.

45. Li YY, et al. Differential expression of tissue inhibitors of metalloproteinases in the failing human heart. *Circulation.* 1998;98(17):1728–1734.

46. Kang PM, Izumo S. Apoptosis in heart: Basic mechanisms and implications in cardiovascular diseases. *Trends Mol Med.* 2003;9(4):177–182.

47. Diwan A, Dorn GW II. Decompensation of cardiac hypertrophy: Cellular mechanisms and novel therapeutic targets. *Physiology (Bethesda).* 2007;22:56–64.

48. Mann D. Pathophysiology of heart failure. In: Braunwald E, ed. *Braunwald's Heart Disease: A Textbook of Cardiovascular Medicine.* Philadelphia: Saunders; 2008:541–560.

49. van Rooij E, Marshall WS, Olson EN. Toward microRNA-based therapeutics for heart disease: The sense in antisense. *Circ Res.* 2008;103(9):919–928.

50. Divakaran V, Mann DL. The emerging role of microRNAs in cardiac remodeling and heart failure. *Circ Res.* 2008;103(10):1072–1083.

# 57

# Pathophysiology of Heart Failure

STUART D. KATZ

## ● PRACTICAL POINTS

- Heart failure is a pathophysiological condition in which a primary abnormality in cardiac structure and/or function compromises the heart's ability to pump blood commensurate with the body's metabolic requirements at normal cardiac filling pressures.

- The clinical manifestations of heart failure can best be explained by considering the complex interaction of cardiac, vascular, and other neural and endocrine factors that regulate distribution of blood in regional organ circulations.

- The initial event that triggers the development of heart failure may be an acute or subacute injury with segmental or diffuse loss of myocytes, chronic injury related to long-term changes in loading conditions of the heart, intrinsic defects in myocyte function, or infiltrative diseases that compromise myocyte function.

- The process of ventricular remodeling is critically important to the current understanding of the pathophysiology of heart failure, as the characteristic changes in ventricular size and function in response to injury are closely linked to disease progression and survival.

- The nature of the changing loading conditions (as the primary determinant of myocyte hypertrophy)

- and other autocrine, paracrine, endocrine, and autonomic factors (as modifiers of the hypertrophic response to changing load) dictate the form of ventricular remodeling (concentric vs. eccentric).

- The remodeling process induced by altered loading conditions and neurohormonal activation leads to progressive dilation and hypertrophy of the ventricle.

- Resting ejection fraction or other parameters of resting left ventricular hemodynamic performance are not closely correlated to the degree of exercise intolerance.

- Attenuated vasodilatory capacity of resistance arterioles contributes to reduced aerobic capacity by limiting exercise-induced skeletal muscle hyperemia and may contribute to disease progression by increasing afterload on the injured ventricle, and by reducing myocardial flow reserve.

- Abnormalities in skeletal muscle metabolism contribute to impaired exercise endurance at submaximal work rates in heart failure.

- The diastolic heart failure syndrome is likely attributable to a combination of ventricular factors that alter diastolic filling properties and vascular factors that alter cardiac preload and afterload.

Heart failure is a pathophysiological condition in which a primary abnormality in cardiac structure and/or function compromises the heart's ability to pump blood commensurate with the body's metabolic requirements at normal cardiac filling pressures. For the purposes of the scope of this chapter, this definition of heart failure intentionally excludes related entities in which a heart failure syndrome may be induced by the effects of extraordinary loading conditions on a structurally and functionally normal heart (high output heart failure related to severe anemia or arteriovenous fistulae, severe sodium and water overload related to primary kidney disease, or hypertensive crisis). However, this definition does not exclude the role of extracardiac factors as important determinants of the progression and clinical manifestations of disease. Indeed, although the majority of clinical heart failure syndromes can be traced back to an index myocardial injury event, the clinical manifestations of heart failure can best be explained by considering the complex interaction of cardiac,

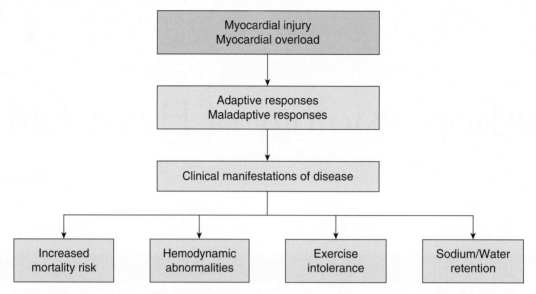

**Figure 57-1.** Overview of the pathophysiology of heart failure. Successive models of disease pathophysiology have been developed based on cumulative clinical observations and technological advancements. Common themes to the current understanding of heart failure is that an initiating event of myocardial injury and/or overload leads to adaptive and maladaptive responses which are ultimately linked to the clinical manifestations of disease. Other models presented in the chapter link the initial injury to a distinct aspect of disease progression and/or manifestations.

vascular, and other neural and endocrine factors that regulate distribution of blood in regional organ circulations.

Heart failure pathophysiology can best be understood from a historical perspective of successive models developed over time, as advances in technology have provided additional insight into the underlying molecular, structural, and hemodynamic factors associated with the clinical manifestations of disease. There are some caveats to consider for interpretation of the models presented in this chapter. Many of the more recent investigations of molecular and cellular changes in response to myocardial injury are derived from experimental observations in rodents, with some supporting data available from larger mammals or humans. Although the relatively scant human data are generally consistent with experimental observations, there are well-recognized interspecies differences in cardiovascular physiology and dissimilarities between the nature and time course of experimental versus clinical myocardial injury that may limit extrapolation of animal model findings to human disease states. It is also important to note that in many instances, it is not possible to definitively discern which abnormalities are critical to disease progression or merely markers of the disease process (epiphenomena). Several currently accepted models of the pathophysiology of heart failure are presented in this chapter. A schematic view of the interrelated themes of these models is provided in **Figure 57-1**.

## CAUSES OF HEART FAILURE

The initial event that triggers the development of heart failure may be an acute or subacute injury with segmental or diffuse loss of myocytes, chronic injury related to long-term

changes in loading conditions of the heart, intrinsic defects in myocyte function, or infiltrative diseases that compromise myocyte function (**Table 57-1**). In the United States, myocardial infarction is the most common cause of heart failure. Hypertension is a common risk factor for heart failure, but a causative role has not been definitively determined. In many patients, no specific etiology can be identified from clinical history and diagnostic testing. Endomyocardial biopsy is not routinely recommended for diagnosis of the cause of heart failure but may be considered if the clinical setting suggests an etiologic factor with known specific treatment options. The myocyte is a highly differentiated cell type with a limited repertoire of responses to injury. Accordingly, many features of the pathophysiology of heart failure remain consistent regardless of the type of initial injury to the heart.

## ADAPTIVE AND MALADAPTIVE RESPONSES TO VENTRICULAR INJURY

### Adaptive Responses to Myocardial Injury

The heart is a volume driven pump, responding on a beat-by-beat basis to changes in preload delivered to the ventricles during the diastolic phase of the previous cardiac cycle. The Frank-Starling mechanism relating myocardial stretch (end-diastolic volume or preload) to the force of contraction is the underlying basis for these physiological adaptations to short-term changes in preload (**Figure 57-1**). In normal physiological settings, increased contractility related to the Frank-Starling mechanism occurs over a relatively small range of increased preload corresponding to left ventricular end-diastolic

| Table 57-1 • Causes of Heart Failure |
| --- |
| **1. Myocardial injury** |
| Myocardial infarction |
| Myocarditis (all causes, including peripartum cardiomyopathy) |
| Cardiac toxins (alcohol, cocaine, cobalt) |
| Anthracyclines and other chemotherapeutic agents |
| Sarcoidosis |
| Collagen vascular diseases |
| Infectious diseases (viral-associated, tick-borne disease, and Chagas disease) |
| Irradiation injury |
| Pheochromocytoma and carcinoid syndrome |
| **2. Myocardial overload** |
| Aortic stenosis |
| Aortic regurgitation |
| Mitral regurgitation |
| Pulmonary artery hypertension (primary and secondary) |
| Congenital heart disease |
| Acquired shunts (ventricular septal defect, coronary fistula) |
| **3. Intrinsic defects of the myocyte** |
| Nutritional deficiencies (thiamine, selenium) |
| Thyroid deficiency |
| Right ventricular dysplasia |
| Genetic diseases |
|     Primary cardiomyopathy phenotype (hypertrophic and dilated cardiomyopathy) |
|     Muscular dystrophies |
|     Glycogen storage diseases |
|     Hemachromatosis |
|     Carnitine deficiency |
|     Kearns-Sayres syndrome |
| **4. Infiltrative diseases of the myocardium** |
| Amyloidosis |
| Endomyocardial fibrosis |
| Hypereosinophilic syndromes |
| Invasive tumors |

## Subacute Response to Myocardial Injury

Within the first hours to days after myocardial infarction, there are structural changes in the left ventricle characterized by expansion of the infarct zone (a passive process likely related to changes in connective tissue matrix after ischemic injury) and a complex rearrangement of myocytes within the ventricular wall in noninfarcted areas (myocyte slippage and ventricular wall thinning). These two short-term processes, distinct from the normal physiology of the Frank-Starling relationship (preload dependent changes in sarcomere length), and the longer-term pathophysiological ventricular remodeling processes (which are characterized by myocyte hypertrophy as described below) increase the end-diastolic volume of the injured ventricle (**Figure 57-2**). Increased ventricular dimension increases cardiac wall tension linearly by a factor proportional to the radius raised to the first power (per the Laplace equation; see below) but increases the ventricular diastolic volume by a factor proportional to the third power of the radius (according to volumetric formulae).

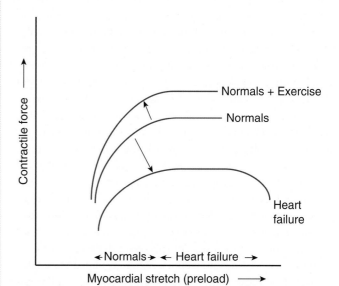

**Figure 57-2.** The Frank-Starling relationship. This graph represents the idealized conceptual physiological relationship between cardiac muscle stretch and muscle contractile performance in normal subjects at rest, normal subjects during exercise, and heart failure subjects. In normal physiology, increased preload within the physiological range (corresponding to left ventricular end-diastolic pressures <10 mm Hg) is associated with increased contractile performance. Exercise-induced adrenergic stimulation increases contractile performance in normal subjects without further increase in preload. In heart failure, the relationship between preload and contractile performance is shifted downward. Most heart failure subjects have preload above the normal range (end-diastolic pressure >10 mm Hg), corresponding to a flat portion of the curve in which further increases in preload are not associated with increased contractile performance. The response to adrenergic stimulation is also blunted in failing myocardium. There is no true descending limb of the Starling curve (preload dependent decrement in contractile performance), but forward stroke volume may decrease at high preload due to functional mitral regurgitation.

pressure of <10 mm Hg. The maximum augmentation in contractile force in response to additional preload occurs at a sarcomere length of 2.2 $\mu$M. In response to physiological stress such as exercise, increased adrenergic stimulation and a positive force-frequency relationship further enhance cardiac contractile performance without further increase in preload. In pathophysiological settings, the acute response to myocardial injury is mediated by the same adaptive mechanisms. However, the increase in stroke volume is typically reduced due to loss of functioning myocardium, decreased contractile state of the myocardium, and/or severely abnormal loading conditions that limit the effectiveness of these mechanisms. The result is a shift of the Frank-Starling curve downward and to the right with reduction in the stroke volume reserve despite higher ventricular preload. There is no evidence of a true descending limb of the Frank-Starling mechanism in human heart failure, but forward stroke volume may decrease at high preload due to functional mitral valve regurgitation.

In the setting of myocardial injury with decreased ejection fraction, the increase in diastolic dimension serves to augment stroke volume with only a modest increase in myocardial energy requirements. However, increased wall stress associated with ventricular enlargement and the fact that the relatively small changes in diastolic volumes are insufficient to normalize stroke volume ultimately contribute to maladaptive ventricular remodeling and progressive decline in the contractile performance of the injured ventricle.

## Ventricular Remodeling

The term "remodeling" was first utilized to describe the process of progressive ventricular dilation and contractile dysfunction observed after myocardial infarction but is now used more broadly to describe structural and functional changes in the myocardium in response to any injury or change in loading conditions. The process of ventricular remodeling is critically important to the current understanding of the pathophysiology of heart failure, as the characteristic changes in ventricular size and function in response to injury are closely linked to disease progression and survival. Current understanding of the pathophysiology of ventricular remodeling is based on the concept that short-term adaptations to acute injury that serve to augment contractility lead to long-term maladaptive changes in myocyte structure and function. Myocytes sense systolic and diastolic wall stress within the ventricular wall and adapt to changing loading conditions by changing their size and shape in order to restore these physical forces towards the physiological range. The Laplace equation provides a simplified mathematical formula (based on a perfect cylinder) that is useful for estimating directional changes in wall stress in the more complex geometry of the left ventricle (**Figure 57-3**). Increased mechanical stretch of myocytes is associated with rapid activation of signaling cascades (phosphotidylinositol, protein kinase C, raf-1, and extracellular signal–regulated protein kinase) that trigger gene transcription programs for increased synthesis of proteins associated with myocyte hypertrophy (atrial natriuretic peptide, skeletal alpha-actin, and beta myosin heavy chain). There is a transcriptional shift towards expression of the fetal isozymes of many contractile proteins, with similar function but distinct kinetics from that of the adult forms. Increased end-systolic wall stress (e.g., aortic stenosis) induces hypertrophy with production of additional sarcomeres in parallel (concentric remodeling). Increased end-diastolic wall stress (e.g., aortic insufficiency) induces hypertrophy with production of additional sarcomeres in series (eccentric remodeling). The nature of the changing loading conditions (as the primary determinant of myocyte hypertrophy) and other autocrine, paracrine, endocrine, and autonomic factors (as modifiers of the hypertrophic response to changing load as described below) dictate the form of ventricular remodeling (**Figure 57-3**). In most instances, since changes in end-systolic and end-diastolic wall stress after injury are interdependent, there is a combination of eccentric and concentric remodeling that leads to development of a dilated hypertrophied ventricular chamber with transformation from the normal ellipsoid shape towards a more spherical shape. The hypertrophic changes in the heart can be considered adaptive or compensatory, as they serve to reduce wall stress and preserve stroke volume in the setting of cardiac injury. The hypertrophic response is often associated with prolonged periods of time (years, even decades) of clinically silent, "compensated" left ventricular systolic dysfunction. While patients in this stage of the disease may appear "compensated," the contractile function of the remodeled ventricle remains impaired, in part because the increases in wall thickness do not fully normalize myocardial wall stress, and in part due to fundamental changes in myocyte excitation contraction coupling and ventricular interstitium that occur in the setting of pathological hypertrophy. Ultimately, the clinically compensated state of left ventricular systolic dysfunction progresses towards greater dilation and hypertrophy and, eventually, development of symptomatic disease.

# MYOCARDIAL CHANGES ASSOCIATED WITH PATHOLOGICAL HYPERTROPHY

## Changes in Excitation Contraction Coupling

Failing myocardium is characterized by decreased isometric force generation at a given preload, decreased isotonic velocity of contraction at a given afterload, delayed relaxation postcontraction, loss of contractile reserve in response to catecholamine stimulation, and development of a negative force-frequency relationship. Impaired contractile performance is associated with changes in excitation contraction coupling in the myocyte. Altered expression of contractile proteins, characterized by reduction in myofibrillar ATPase activity and reversion from expression of the adult alpha myosin heavy chain isoform to the fetal beta myosin heavy chain isoform is associated with decreased velocity of contraction and relaxation. Changes in expression of other regulatory proteins including myosin light chain, tropomyosin, troponin, and altered cytoskeletal proteins may also impact contractile function. Calcium cycling within the failing myocyte is also known to be markedly abnormal with altered expression and regulation of key calcium cycling proteins including the ryanodine receptors, calcium adenosine triphosphatase of the sarco(endo)plasmic reticulum (SERCA2), phospholamban, and the sodium-calcium exchanger. The net result of these abnormalities is a decrease and delay in the calcium transient triggered by the action potential, decreased and delayed calcium re-uptake into the sarcoplasmic reticulum, and increased diastolic sarcolemmal calcium levels. These changes in calcium handling not only negatively impact the force

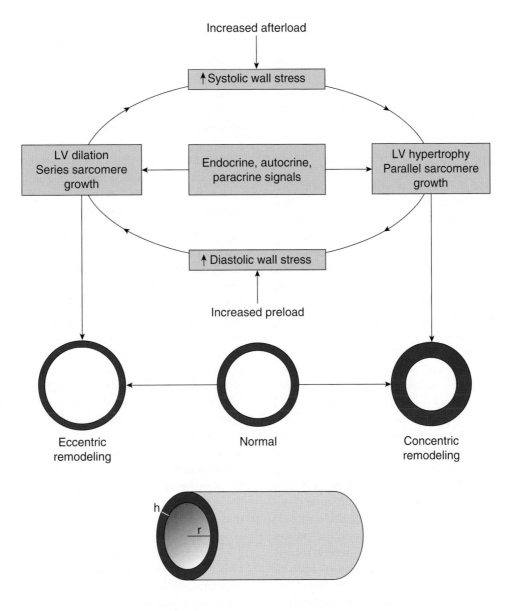

Laplace equation: Wall stress = $\dfrac{\text{Pressure} \times \text{Radius (r)}}{2 \times \text{Thickness (h)}}$

**Figure 57-3.** Determinants of ventricular remodeling. Ventricular dilation and hypertrophy after myocardial injury is thought to be a critical determinant of heart failure progression. Myocytes sense physical forces in the ventricular wall and adjust their size and shape in order to restore systolic and diastolic wall stress to the physiological range. The Laplace equation, which describes determinants for wall stress in a perfect cylinder, can be used to estimate directional changes in the more complex geometry of the left ventricle. The Laplace equation predicts that increased wall tension associated with increased pressure or chamber radius can be offset by a compensatory increase in wall thickness. Increased afterload (pressure) primarily increases end-systolic wall stress and leads to increased sarcomere replication in parallel with concentric remodeling of the ventricle. Increased preload (chamber radius) primarily increases end-diastolic wall stress and leads to increased sarcomere replication in series with eccentric remodeling of the ventricle. Neurohormonal responses to altered loading conditions also modify the remodeling process. In most clinical settings, interdependent increases in systolic and diastolic wall stress and altered neurohormonal milieu leads to a structurally remodeled ventricle characterized by dilation and hypertrophy.

and velocity of contraction but also alter diastolic function, increase risk of ventricular arrhythmias, and activate hypertrophic signaling transcription factors. Since there are no currently available clinical interventions to directly impact contractile protein and/or calcium handling, it is uncertain whether these changes are causally associated with disease progression.

## Myocardial Energetics

Myocardial substrate utilization in advanced experimental and clinical heart failure is characterized by decreased fatty acid oxidation and increased glucose oxidation. Enzymes for fatty acid utilization are down-regulated and translocation of the myocardial glucose transporter GLUT-4 is increased in the failing heart. Alterations in the expression and activity of the peroxisome proliferator-activated nuclear receptors are thought to play an important role in the altered substrate utilization in hypertrophied and failing myocardium. Experimental studies on the potential role of mitochondrial dysfunction have yielded conflicting data, but it is possible that alterations in mitochondrial structure and/or function may decrease efficiency of ATP generation and increase reactive oxygen species generation in the myocardium. Increased mitochondrial production of reactive oxygen species may contribute to the progression of ventricular remodeling by stimulating hypertrophic signaling pathways. The net effect of the changes in substrate utilization and mitochondrial function is a decrease in myocardial energy reserves, characterized by decreased creatinine kinase activity, decreased concentrations of phosphocreatine, reductions in the phosphocreatine/ATP ratio, and decreased availability of ATP for myocyte contraction and calcium cycling. Although experimental genetic models and human genetic diseases associated with inborn errors of energy metabolism may manifest hypertrophic or dilated cardiomyopathy phenotypes, it is uncertain whether the observed changes in myocardial energy stores contribute to progression of disease in other acquired forms of human heart failure.

## Ventricular Wall Interstitium

Ventricular remodeling is characterized by accumulation of increased fibrillar type I and type III collagens in the myocardial interstitium and a complex re-arrangement of myocytes and connective tissue within the ventricular wall with resultant dramatic changes in ventricular size and shape. These changes in the interstitium are mediated by increased cardiac fibroblast collagen production (stimulated by angiotensin II, aldosterone, and other neurohormonal signaling molecules) and altered regulation of the collagen matrix structure by matrix metalloproteinases and endogenous tissue inhibitors of metalloproteinases. In animal models, postinfarction ventricular enlargement is associated with increased activity of matrix metalloproteinases and can be attenuated with pharmacological inhibition of

matrix metalloproteinase activity. In human heart failure, the importance of matrix metalloproteinase activation in ventricular remodeling is uncertain, as there are currently no clinical tools for directly assessing enzyme activity in the intact heart. Increased serum markers of collagen turnover after myocardial infarction are associated with increased risk of mortality. However, a randomized clinical trial of pharmacological matrix metalloproteinase inhibition in post myocardial infarction patients did not demonstrate evidence of decreased left ventricular remodeling at 90 days.

## Apoptosis and Progression of Disease

Apoptosis is a biological process of regulated cell death that has been implicated in the pathophysiology of disease progression in heart failure. Both necrosis and apoptosis contribute to the loss of myocytes after myocardial infarction. Many of the factors associated with hypertrophic signaling in the postinjury ventricular remodeling process (adrenergic signaling, angiotensin II, proinflammatory cytokines, reactive oxygen species) are also known to be associated with caspase activation and proapototic signaling in myocytes in experimental settings. In animal models, very low rates of experimentally controlled apoptosis induce dilated cardiomyopathy and heart failure. In participants, the data on the rates of apoptosis as a mechanism of disease progression are inconsistent, but most studies indicate that myocyte apoptosis does occur at very low rates in the human heart, with greater rates of apoptosis in failing hearts when compared with that in normal hearts. Since even very low rates of apoptosis would eventually lead to complete loss of myocytes over decades, the presence of apoptosis in the heart strongly suggests the existence of a homeostatic mechanism for creation of new functional myocytes to replace those lost to the apoptotic process. Myocytes are a terminally differentiated cell type that does not undergo cell division. Recent findings provide evidence for the presence of a population of regenerative progenitor cells within the myocardium. These data suggest that progression of heart failure may be attributable to an imbalance between the rates of myocyte apoptosis and regeneration that leads to a cumulative loss of functioning myocytes. This model of the disease suggests that augmentation of the cardiac regeneration process with stem cells or specific transcription factors may have therapeutic potential in heart failure. Further work is needed to determine if apoptotic cell loss is a direct determinant of disease progression in heart failure.

## Reverse Remodeling

Extremely low wall tension conditions during prolonged mechanical circulatory support with a left ventricular assist device are associated with dramatic reduction in ventricular size. Limited data in human subjects indicate that reverse chamber remodeling after mechanical support is associated with regression of myocyte hypertrophy and improvements in myocyte

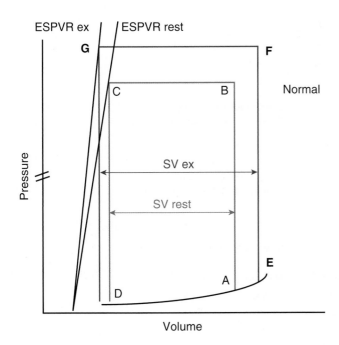

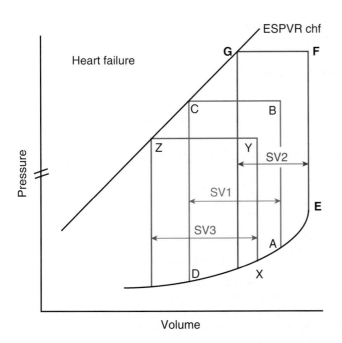

**Figure 57-6.** Hemodynamic model of heart failure. Idealized pressure volume loops representing the systolic and diastolic phases of the cardiac cycle for normal and failing hearts. The end-diastolic pressure volume relationship and slope of the end-systolic pressure volume relationship (ESPVR, an index of myocardial contractile function) provide a conceptual framework for characterizing intrinsic pump function of the ventricle. In normal physiology (top panel cycle ABCD), the ventricle fills during diastole over a flat portion of the diastolic pressure volume curve (points D to A) with little change in diastolic pressure. The slope of the end-systolic pressure volume relationship is steep. In response to exercise (cycle EFG), there is a modest increase in preload (still on the flat portion of the curve, with little increase in end-diastolic pressure) and a shift in the slope of the ESPVR upward and to the left (greater contractile state mediated by the Frank-Starling mechanism and adrenergic stimulation). The net result is increased stroke volume (SV ex) with little change in preload. In the resting failing heart (bottom panel, cycle ABCD), the diastolic pressure volume relationship is shifted substantially to the right, characterized by large increases in diastolic volume and moderate increases in diastolic pressures, and normal stroke volume (SV1). The slope of the ESPVR is shifted downward and to the right (decreased contractile state). In response to exercise (cycle EFG), the increased preload is associated with large increases in diastolic filling pressure. The myocardial response to adrenergic stimulation is blunted and there is little or no shift in the ESPVR slope, with resultant decrease in stroke volume (SV2). Conversely, administration of an arterial vasodilator drug (cycle XYZ) is associated with reduction in end-diastolic volume to a flatter portion of the curve. The reduced slope of the ESPVR results in an exaggerated augmentation of stroke volume in response to afterload reduction (SV3).

muscle blood flow, and skeletal muscle oxygen utilization) also play an important role in the pathophysiology of exercise intolerance in patients with CHF (**Figure 57-7**). In normal physiology, exercise-induced increases in cardiac output are distributed to the active skeletal muscle mass due to metabolic vasodilation in this regional circulation. In patients with severe heart failure, chronically reduced peripheral blood flow (altered shear stress signal), vascular wall edema, activation of cytokines and local tissue growth factors, and vascular endothelial dysfunction decrease maximal vasodilatory capacity in the skeletal muscle circulation. Vascular endothelium dysfunction in

heart failure is characterized by reduced bioavailability of nitric oxide and increased release of endothelin-1, vasoconstricting prostaglandins, and superoxide anion. In a manner analogous to the ventricular remodeling process, the combination of chronic reduction in shear stress, altered hormonal milieu, and endothelial dysfunction are associated with a vascular structural remodeling process that increases systemic vascular resistance. Attenuated vasodilatory capacity of resistance arterioles contributes to reduced aerobic capacity by limiting exercise-induced skeletal muscle hyperemia and may contribute to disease progression by increasing afterload on the injured

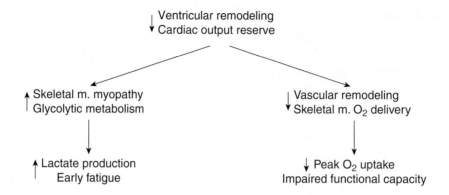

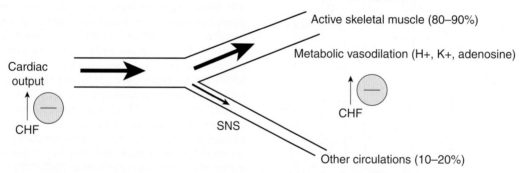

**Figure 57-7.** Pathophysiology of exercise intolerance in heart failure. Functional capacity in heart failure is determined by a complex interaction between myocardial contractile performance during exercise, vascular distribution of cardiac output during exercise, and skeletal muscle oxygen utilization during exercise. Skeletal muscle metabolic changes are associated with increased fatigue at submaximal exercise levels. Vascular changes are associated with reduced peak oxygen uptake at maximal exercise. As shown in the table, a compensated heart failure patient with ejection fraction (EF) of 0.30 and increased left ventricular end-diastolic volume (LVEDV) and left ventricular end-systolic volume (LVESV) may have normal stroke volume (SV) and cardiac output (CO) at rest. However, in response to exercise, limited ability to increase preload, contractility and heart rate are associated with a 50% decrease in maximal cardiac output reserve. As shown in the bottom figure, normal distribution of blood during exercise is regulated by generalized vasoconstriction mediated by activation of the sympathetic nervous system (SNS) and metabolic vasodilation in the active skeletal muscle. The regional vasodilation delivers close to 90% of available cardiac output to the active skeletal muscle in normal subjects. In heart failure, reduced cardiac output reserve and attenuated skeletal muscle vasodilation during exercise reduces the total and proportional regional blood flow available to the active skeletal muscle.

ventricle and by reducing myocardial flow reserve. The severity of vascular endothelial dysfunction is an independent risk factor for increased mortality in heart failure patients. Abnormalities in skeletal muscle metabolism

also contribute to impaired exercise endurance at submaximal work rates in heart failure. Deconditioning and chronic activation of neurohormonal and inflammatory cytokine systems are associated with changes in skeletal muscle mass, fiber composition, aerobic enzyme content, mitochondrial structure and function, and microcirculatory structure and function. These changes are associated with increased skeletal muscle anaerobic metabolism and early fatigue at low work rates independent of the nutritive blood flow. Although these changes in vascular and skeletal muscle occur secondary to the progressive ventricular remodeling process, the severity of aerobic impairment is strongly associated with increased mortality risk. Therapies directed at reversal of these peripheral abnormalities are associated with improved exercise capacity and quality of life in heart failure.

## Edema Formation

Early models of the pathophysiology of heart failure were developed to address the process of edema formation, since the most prominent signs and symptoms of decompensated heart failure are related to pulmonary, sphlachnic, and lower extremity edema formation. The cardiorenal model of heart failure (**Figure 57-8**) is generally accepted to best represent the underlying mechanisms of edema formation in most patients with heart failure. Myocardial injury leads to reduced contractile function and underfilling of the arterial vascular space (hypotension). Activation of the sympathetic nervous system, the renin-angiotensin-aldosterone system, and non-osmotic secretion of vasopressin promote

renal sodium retention by increasing filtration fraction in the glomerulus secondary to vasoactive effects on the afferent and efferent arterioles, and direct signaling effects on renal proximal and distal tubules and collecting ducts. Intrinsic changes in glomerular and tubular function (glomerulo-tubular feedback via adenosine receptor type 1 signaling, distal tubular cell hypertrophy, increased neutral endopeptidase, and phosphodiesterase type 5 activity) attenuate the counter-regulatory renal effects of natriuretic peptides and also play an important role in the pathogenesis of diuretic resistance. In normal physiology, sodium and water retention would homeostatically increase ventricular preload and cardiac output. In contrast, the response to increased preload is severely attenuated in failing myocardium, so cardiac output remains decreased and leads to an unregulated sodium and water retention, overfilling of the vascular space, and elevated pressures in the pulmonary and systemic venous circulations. The increased hydrostatic forces in the capillaries induced by elevated venous pressures lead to pulmonary, lower extremity, and sphlachnic edema formation.

## Diastolic Heart Failure

Approximately 50% of heart failure cases are associated with normal ejection fraction. This clinical entity has been called "heart failure with preserved ejection fraction" or "diastolic heart failure." This clinical entity is distinct from genetic forms of hypertrophic cardiomyopathy and is commonly associated with female gender, advanced age, and a history of hypertension. The pathophysiology of this entity appears to be distinct from that discussed above after myocardial injury (**Figure 57-9**). Some investigators have identified abnormalities in the diastolic phase of the cardiac cycle as the primary cause of this disorder. The factors contributing to abnormal diastolic function are not well characterized but may be related to changes in myocyte diastolic calcium handling, changes in the passive properties of the ventricular wall as determined by its connective tissue composition. The net effect is a shift of the diastolic pressure volume curve upward and to the left. Other investigators have suggested that the alterations in cardiac filling pressures observed in this condition are not due to intrinsic changes in cardiac diastolic function but, rather, are related to chronic changes in arterial and venous tone that alter ventricular loading conditions. Increased aortic stiffness is associated with increased velocity of pressure wave reflections that increase the forces that oppose ejection of blood into the aorta (input impedance). Decreased venous capacitance in the sphlachnic and skeletal muscle circulations may displace blood into the thoracic veins and increase pulmonary venous pressures. In many patients, the diastolic heart failure syndrome is likely attributable to a combination of both ventricular and vascular factors. Chronic kidney disease is common in this population and

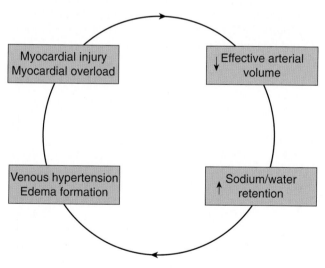

**Figure 57-8.** Cardiorenal model of disease. Decreased contractile performance in response to myoacardial injury or overload reduces cardiac output and the effective arterial volume. The reduction in arterial filling is associated with increased sodium and water retention mediated by neurohormonal activation and intrinsic renal mechanisms. Sodium and water retention increases venous pressures and in normal physiology increases cardiac output. In failing myocardium, the attenuated response to increased preload fails to increase cardiac output and leads to excessive sodium and water retention, systemic and pulmonary venous hypertension, and formation of interstitial edema due to increased hydrostatic forces.

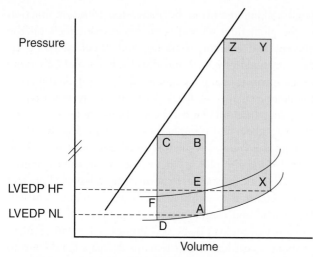

**Figure 57-9.** Pathophysiology of diastolic heart failure. Idealized pressure volume loops representing changes in myocardial function and/or loading conditions may contribute to the pathophysiology of diastolic heart failure. Normal cardiac function is represented by cycle ABCD. An alteration in the diastolic calcium re-uptake or changes in the physical properties of the ventricular wall can shift the diastolic pressure volume relationship upward, leading to elevated diastolic filling pressures with normal ventricular volumes (cycle EBCF). Alternatively, large increases in afterload (induced by increased stiffness of conduit arteries, increased pulse wave velocity, and reflected pressure waves returning to the proximal aorta during early systole) in combination with reduced venous capacitance and displacement of venous blood into the thoracic space shift the diastolic filling rightward along a normal curve to high diastolic filling pressures (cycle XYZ). In both cases, the left ventricular end-diastolic pressures (LVEDP) are elevated to a similar degree (dashed lines). For clarity, these two explanations for diastolic heart failure are illustrated as distinct entities, but in many patients a combination of altered diastolic filling properties and altered loading conditions likely contribute to the hemodynamic abnormalities associated with heart failure.

may also contribute to overfilling of the venous vascular space due to excess sodium and water retention. The net result is increased cardiac filling pressures and decreased stroke volume reserve comparable to that observed in patients' systolic dysfunction. The effects of reduced cardiac output reserve on exercise intolerance and renal sodium and water retention are also comparable in the two groups. There are few clinical trial data to identify important causal pathways in the pathophysiology of disease progression in this entity. In contrast to patients with myocardial injury and systolic dysfunction, pharmacological inhibition of the renin-angiotensin system has not been associated with decreased mortality risk when compared with placebo in clinical trials of patients with preserved ejection fraction.

## Suggested Readings

1. Francis GS. Pathophysiology of chronic heart failure. *Am J Med.* 2001;110 Suppl 7A:37S–46S.

2. Mann DL, Bristow MR. Mechanisms and models in heart failure: The biomechanical model and beyond. *Circulation.* 2005;111:2837–2849.

3. Katz AM. Pathophysiology of heart failure: Identifying targets for pharmacotherapy. *Med Clin North Am.* 2003;87: 303–316.

4. Colucci WS, Braunwald E. Pathopysiology of heart failure. In: Braunwald E, Zipes DP, Libby P, eds. *Heart Disease,* 6th ed. Philadelphia, PA: W.B. Saunders Company; 2001.

5. Francis GS, Tang HW, Sonnenblick EH. Pathophysiology of heart failure. In: Fuster V, Alexander RW, O'Rourke RA, eds. *Hurst's The Heart, 11th ed.* New York, NY: McGraw-Hill Medical Publishing Division; 2004.

# · 58

# Diastolic Heart Failure

MUHAMED SARIC AND ITZHAK KRONZON

## ● PRACTICAL POINTS

- Diastole starts with the closure of the aortic valve and ends with the closure of the mitral valve.

- It consists of four phases: isovolumic relaxation time (IVRT), early or rapid ventricular filling, diastasis, and late filling or atrial contraction phase.

- During IVRT, there is no blood flow or filling from the atria to the ventricles; it represents the time period between the aortic valve closure and the mitral valve opening.

- Diastolic dysfunction is characterized by abnormal active and passive relaxation properties of the left ventricle (LV), a rise in the LV diastolic pressures, and a rise in the left atrial (LA) pressures aimed at maintaining an LA to LV pressure gradient that is necessary for LV filling.

- Pseudonormal and restrictive patterns arise because the elevation in the LA to LV pressure gradient leads to an increase in the mitral E wave peak velocity, an increase in the mitral E/A ratio, and a shortening of both IVRT and DT.

- An abnormal relaxation pattern (Grade I or mild LV diastolic dysfunction) is characterized by IVRT

prolongation, a mitral A wave taller than the E wave (E < A), a prolonged deceleration time (DT) of the mitral E wave, and a taller S wave than D wave on pulmonary venous flow velocity.

- A pseudonormal relaxation pattern (Grade II or moderate LV diastolic dysfunction) is characterized by an E/A ratio between 1 and 2.

- A restrictive filling pattern (Grade III or severe LV diastolic dysfunction) occurs when the E/A becomes >2 and the DT of the mitral E wave shortens to below 150 msec.

- True diastolic heart failure is a result of an upward and leftward shift in the EDPVR curve as a result of the combined effects of impaired LV relaxation and increased LV stiffness, which leads to LV end-diastolic pressure elevation even at normal or low LV filling volumes.

- About 50% of patients presenting with signs and symptoms of heart failure have a normal or near-normal ejection fraction (HFNEF) without another explanation; risk factors for HFNEF include age, female gender, systemic hypertension, LV hypertrophy, and diabetes mellitus.

## INTRODUCTION

Ventricular diastole (from the Greek derivation for διαστολη diastolê—"dilation") is the filling portion of the cardiac cycle, which has traditionally been defined by events heard during cardiac auscultation. It starts with the closure of the aortic valve and ends with the closure of the mitral valve. Electrocardiographically, mechanical diastole lasts from the peak of the T wave to the peak of the R wave.

## NORMAL AND ABNORMAL LV VENTRICULAR DIASTOLIC FUNCTION

The diastolic period during sinus rhythm is divided into four phases: (1) isovolumic relaxation time (IVRT) between the aortic valve closure and the mitral valve opening devoid of blood flow from the atria into the ventricles; (2) early or rapid ventricular filling (RVF); (3) diastasis, an intermezzo period with usually little or no appreciable ventricular filling;

677

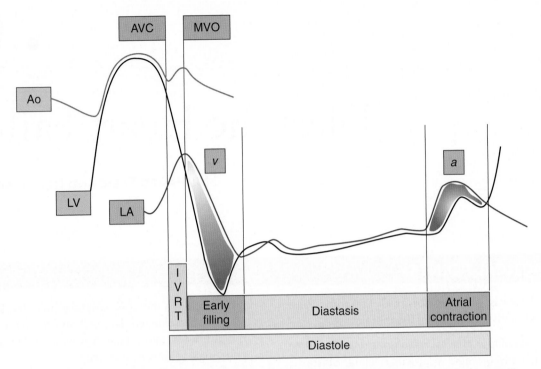

**Figure 58-1.** Phases of diastole based on the intracardiac pressure measurement of the left atrium (LA), left ventricle (LV), and the aorta (Ao): [1] IVRT, isovolumic relaxation time; [2] E, early or passive filling phase; [3] diastasis; [4] A, atrial kick. AVC, aortic valve closure. MVO, mitral valve opening. v, ventricular wave; **a**, atrial wave of LA pressure curve.

and (4) late filling or atrial contraction phase (**Figure 58-1**). The atrial contraction phase is either abolished or becomes asynchronous with other ventricular events during atrial arrhythmias and atrioventricular block.

These four phases occur simultaneously in the right and left ventricles. In this chapter, we will concentrate on the events in the left ventricle.

## Echocardiographic Correlates of Diastolic Phases

After placing a pulsed spectral Doppler sample volume at the mitral leaflet tips, one obtains a flow velocity recording (depicted in **Figure 58-2**), a horizontal axis representing time, and a vertical axis representing blood velocity.

During each of the two filling phases, a distinct antegrade (above the baseline) wave is inscribed: E wave during rapid ventricular filling, and A wave during atrial contraction. As seen in **Figure 58-1**, the flow of blood from the left atrium into the left ventricle is the result of the left atrial pressure exceeding the left ventricular pressure in those two phases of diastole.

The time interval between the peak of the E wave and the end of the E wave is referred to as deceleration time (DT)

and is inversely related to the rate of left ventricular relaxation and the magnitude of the pressure gradient between the left atrium and the left ventricle.

Because no ventricular filling occurs during IVRT, a flat line is inscribed on the echocardiographic flow velocity tracings. The length of this line segment represents the duration of IVRT. Like DT, IVRT is inversely related to the rate of left ventricular relaxation and the magnitude of the pressure gradient between the left atrium and the left ventricle. Normal E, A, DT, and IVRT values are given in **Table 58-1**.

Because no appreciable filling occurs during diastasis in normal individuals, a flat line is usually inscribed between the E and A waves. The length of this line segment is inversely related to heart rate. Given the absence of significant flow during diastasis, tachycardia (unless extreme) is not detrimental to left ventricle filling in a normal individual.

When left ventricular relaxation is delayed, early left ventricular filling may continue past the E wave into the diastasis. The presence of an antegrade wave (sometimes referred to as L wave) in diastasis with a peak velocity ≥20 cm/sec is indicative of left ventricular diastolic dysfunction (**Figure 58-3**).

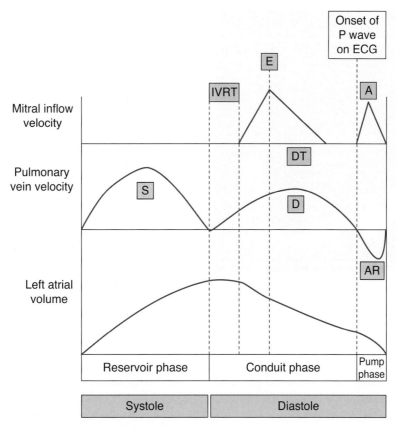

**Figure 58-2.** Schematic representation of mitral and pulmonary venous flow velocity patterns, and left atrial volume. Mitral inflow: IVRT, isovolumic relaxation time; E, early filling; DT, deceleration time; A, atrial contraction. Pulmonary vein: S, systolic; D, diastolic wave; AR, atrial reversal wave.

## Filling in Early Versus Late Diastole in a Normal Ventricle

Ventricular filling is driven primarily by a pressure gradient between the left atrium and the left ventricle. However, the pressure difference during rapid ventricular filling arises from a fundamentally different reason compared to the atrial contraction phase.

| Table 58-1 • Normal Values of Mitral Inflow Parameters | | | |
|---|---|---|---|
| **Mitral Value Parameter** | **AGE (years)** | | **Change with Age** |
| | **<50** | **>50** | |
| IVRT (msec) | 65–89 | 73–107 | ↑ |
| $E_{max}$ (cm/s) | 58–86 | 48–76 | ↓ |
| DT (msec) | 159–199 | 174–246 | ↑ |
| $A_{max}$ (cm/s) | 30–50 | 45–73 | ↑ |
| $E_{max}/A_{max}$ | 1.3–2.5 | 0.8–1.4 | ↓ |

*IVRT, isovolumic relaxation time; DT, deceleration time; E, early or passive filling phase; A, atrial kick.*

During rapid ventricular filling in a normal individual, the left ventricular pressure falls below the left atrial pressure through active and passive relaxation of the left ventricle. In contrast, during the atrial contraction phase, the left ventricular filling occurs because the left atrial pressure rises above the left ventricular pressure. In other words, the rapid ventricular filling phase is primarily driven by active relaxation of the left ventricle, whereas the atrial contraction phase is driven by the systolic properties of the left atrium. In a normal individual, the rapid filling phase flow accounts for about three quarters of the total diastolic flow volume, and the atrial contraction phase for the remaining one quarter of the total.

## Mechanical Performance of Left Ventricle During Diastole

Left ventricular dilation during diastole involves both active and passive forces.

### Active Relaxation

Left ventricular relaxation in early diastole is a load-dependent and energy consuming process. The energy in the form of adenosine triphosphate (ATP) is used

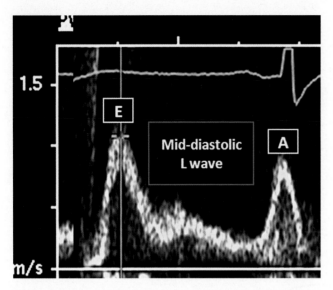

**Figure 58-3.** Mid-diastolic wave. Spectral Doppler recordings of the mitral blood inflow reveal abnormal mid-diastolic L wave of an A peak velocity ≥20 cm/sec, indicative of left ventricular myocardial dysfunction.

to uncouple actin-myosin bridges and to remove cytosolic calcium ions into the sarcoplasmic reticulum via SERCA (sarco/endoplasmic reticulum $Ca^{2+}$ ATP-ase).

At the end of the preceding ventricular systole, the left ventricle completes its torsional deformation and assumes a shape similar to that of a wrung towel. The untwisting of the left ventricular apex in the counterclockwise direction and the ventricular base in the clockwise fashion is the first mechanical event of diastole. As a result, the left ventricle undergoes lengthening in its long and short axes (longitudinal and circumferential strains become positive), and its wall decreases in thickness (radial strain becomes negative).

These mechanical events of active myocardial relaxation of the ventricle start with the onset of IVRT and are essentially completed by the end of the rapid filling phase but occasionally may extend into diastasis. The gold standard for the assessment of active myocardial relaxation is the time constant $\tau$ (tau), calculated from the left ventricular pressure curve obtained invasively by high-fidelity pressure transducers during cardiac catheterization. The value of $\tau$ represents the time constant of the exponential decay of the left ventricular pressure during IVRT. A $\tau$ value that is longer than 48 milliseconds indicates abnormal LV relaxation.

Echocardiographically, active relaxation properties are assessed either indirectly from the mitral blood flow velocity tracings or directly by tissue Doppler recordings from the mitral annulus.

Abnormal left ventricular relaxation (unless masked by concomitant left atrial pressure elevation) is characterized by prolongation of both IVRT and DT; these two parameters shorten with the rise of left atrial pressure.

By combining the color Doppler and M mode imaging over the left ventricle during diastole, one can determine the rate at which the E wave propagates from the mitral leaflet tips to the left ventricular apex; this rate is referred to as flow propagation velocity or Vp. The more impaired the left ventricular relaxations are, the lower the value of Vp (**Figure 58-4**).

Using the tissue Doppler technique after placing the sample volume at the level of either medial or lateral mitral annulus, one can record the velocities of left ventricular lengthening in the longitudinal direction during diastole (as well as shortening during ventricular systole). During diastole, tissue Doppler recordings reveal two negative (below the baseline) waves that are simultaneous with the blood velocity E and A waves; they are referred to as E′ and A′ waves. The more impaired the left ventricular relaxations are, the lower the peak E′ velocity (**Figure 58-4**). The amplitude of the E′ wave continues to decline with the worsening of left ventricular diastolic dysfunction and, in principle, is not affected by left atrial pressure (preload). In other words, E′ may be considered as a surrogate of tau.

### Passive Recoil

Active ventricular relaxation is augmented by the passive recoil of the ventricular myocardium, pericardium, and the surrounding thoracic tissue. The passive diastolic property of the ventricle is expressed as either the ventricular stiffness (dP/dV) or its inverse, the LV compliance (dV/dP), where P is the LV pressure and V is the LV volume.

This relationship between LV volume and pressure has traditionally been studied at end-diastole using the end-diastolic volume-pressure relationship (EDVPR) curve. This curve represents the lower boundary of a series of LV volume-pressure curves obtained at various preloads (see chapter on cardiac catheterization).

Because EDPRV is not linear, the stiffness varies along the EDVPR curve; the LV becomes stiffer as the end-diastolic volume increases. In addition, when the LV myocardium hypertrophies (as in hypertrophic cardiomyopathy) or accumulates inelastic extracellular matrix substances (as in myocardial fibrosis or amyloidosis), the EDVRP curve shifts upward and leftward. This shift indicates that LV end-diastolic pressure has risen above normal levels, even at normal LV filling volumes. Conversely, when the LV remodeling leads to an increase in end-diastolic volume (as in systolic LV dysfunction), the EDVPR curve shifts downward and rightward (**Figure 58-5**).

**(2) PSEUDONORMAL FILLING PATTERN** (Grade II or moderate LV diastolic dysfunction) is characterized by an E/A ratio between 1 and 2.

**(3) RESTRICTIVE FILLING** (Grade III or severe LV diastolic dysfunction) occurs when the E/A becomes greater than 2 and the deceleration time of the mitral E wave shortens to below 150 msec.

It is important to emphasize that E/A and D/S ratios reflect, primarily, the magnitude of the pressure gradients between respective cardiac chambers (LA to LV pressure gradient in the case of E/A ratio, and pulmonary vein to LA pressure gradient in the case of D/S ratio). Thus, these ratios by themselves cannot tell us whether the left ventricular diastolic function is normal or abnormal.

For instance, the same 3-mm Hg pressure gradient between the left atrium and the left ventricle (and thus the same E/A and D/S ratios) may occur with normal filling pressures (as in a young individual whose mean LA may be 5 and the LV pressures may be 2 mm Hg during the rapid filling phase), as well as in someone with left ventricular dysfunction whose mean LA and LV pressures are 17 and 14 mm Hg, respectively.

Because pseudonormal and restrictive patterns reflect both abnormal LV relaxing properties and elevated filling pressures, maneuvers that diminish LA pressure (such as Valsalva maneuver or diuresis) will lead to a decrease in the E/A and D/S ratios. Thus, a restrictive pattern may turn into a pseudonormal pattern, and the pseudonormal pattern may revert to an abnormal relaxation pattern after such maneuvers. A decrease of ≥50% in the E/A ratio is highly specific for elevated LV filling pressures and is an important discriminator between normal and abnormal filling patterns. One should also use the left atrial volume to differentiate normal from abnormal filling patterns. In the absence of left atrial enlargement, abnormal (pseudonarmal and restrictive) filling patterns are unlikely.

**(4) IRREVERSIBLE RESTRICTIVE PATTERN** (Grade IV diastolic dysfunction). Individuals with a restrictive filling pattern, in whom the E/A ratio does not change significantly after preload-lowering maneuvers, have an extremely severe form of diastolic dysfunction (Grade IV). They have an extremely poor prognosis with a survival rate of less than 50% at 2 years.

## Echocardiographic Estimation of LV Filling Pressures

In general, estimation of instantaneous filling pressures by echocardiography is based on a ratio of a peak blood velocity during rapid ventricular filling (the height of the mitral E wave is directly proportional to the LA to LV pressure gradient)

| Table 58-4 • Left Atrial (LA) Pressure Estimation by E/E' Ratio | |
|---|---|
| **E/E'** | **LA Pressure** |
| <8 | Normal |
| 8–15 | Can't Tell |
| >15 | High |

and the corresponding marker of LV relaxation (either the E' velocity of the mitral annular tissue Doppler, or the Vp). Left atrial pressure estimation by E/E' ratio is given in **Table 58-4**.

Mean pulmonary artery wedge pressure (PAWP) can be estimated from the following two equations:

[Equation 1]     $PAWP = 1.9 + 1.24 \times E/E'$

[Equation 2]     $PAWP = 4.6 + 5.27 \times \dfrac{E}{Vp}$

Elevation of LV filling pressures occurs in symptomatic heart failure and the degree of pressure elevation correlates well with the magnitude of the patient's symptoms. It is important to emphasize that the filling pressure elevation in systolic heart failure occurs with increased LV volumes (a rightward and downward shift in the diastolic pressure-volume relationship compared to normal), whereas the pressure elevation in diastolic heart failure occurs at normal or small LV volumes (a leftward and upward shift in the diastolic pressure-volume relationship compared to normal). These changes are depicted in **Figure 58-5**. Normal LV end-diastolic volume index is ≤75 mL/m², whereas the normal end-systolic volume index is ≤30 mL/m².

## Left Atrial Volume as an Indicator of LV Diastolic Dysfunction

The E/E' and E/Vp ratios mentioned above give only a point estimate of the filling pressures at a particular moment in time. Left ventricular dysfunction is characterized by chronically elevated LA pressures resulting in left atrial enlargement. Thus, an increase in LA size is an indicator of chronically elevated filling pressures. The higher the grade of LV diastolic dysfunction, the larger the LA size is. The LA size should be expressed as LA volume indexed for body surface area; LA anteroposterior diameter should not be used for such a purpose, as it poorly correlates with the actual LA volume.

Although chronic LV diastolic dysfunction invariably leads to LA enlargement, not all LA enlargements are due to LV diastolic dysfunction. LA enlargement due to chronic volume overload (such as with mitral regurgitation or in marathon runners) or pressure overload due to valvular disease (such as mitral stenosis) should be excluded before attributing LA enlargement to LV diastolic dysfunction.

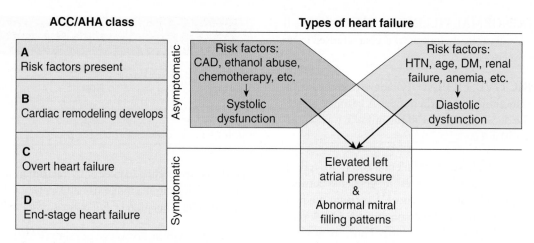

**Figure 58-9.** Types and stages of heart failure. Stages A, B, C, & D refer to the American College of Cardiology (ACC) and American Heart Association classification of heart failure. CAD, coronary artery disease; HTN, systemic hypertension; DM, diabetes mellitus.

## DIASTOLIC HEART FAILURE

Heart failure, whether systolic or diastolic, has classically been recognized as a clinical triad of breathlessness, fatigue, and fluid overload. Breathlessness is caused by elevated left atrial pressure, which leads to alteration of diastolic filling patterns as visualized echocardiographically by mitral and pulmonary venous Doppler flow velocity indices. The LA pressure is either normal or mildly elevated in individuals with the abnormal relaxation pattern. It is moderately elevated in individuals with the pseudonormal pattern and severely elevated in those with the restrictive pattern. In other words, mitral and pulmonary venous Doppler flow indications are well correlated with the severity of the patient's heart failure symptoms. However, it is important to emphasize that the mitral and pulmonary venous Doppler flow indices alone cannot differentiate between diastolic and systolic heart failure. By observing Doppler filling indices, one can conclude whether the LA pressure during diastole is normal or abnormal but not infer whether the LV diastolic function is normal or abnormal.

True diastolic heart failure is a result of an upward and leftward shift in the EDPVR curve as a result of the combined effects of impaired LV relaxation and increased LV stiffness, which leads to LV end-diastolic pressure elevation even at normal or low LV filling volumes. In contrast, systolic heart failure is characterized by LA pressure elevation only at high filling volumes due to a rightward and downward shift in the EDRPV curve. As seen in **Figure 58-5**, the same LA pressure elevation (and consequently the same LV Doppler filling indices) can be observed in patients with either diastolic or systolic heart failure.

It is now recognized that this symptomatic phase (ACC/AHA Stages C and D; **Figure 58-9**) is a late manifestation of a disease process that might have started years or even decades earlier. In AHA/ACC Stage A, diastolic heart failure is initiated by disease-specific risk factors (such as age and hypertension). In Stage B, LV remodeling occurs, characterized by an increase in left ventricular wall thickness (concentric LV hypertrophy) and progressive left atrial enlargement.

Once patients reach Stage C, they can be in any of the four New York Heart Association symptom classes (Class I: symptoms only at levels of exertion that would limit normal individuals; Class II: symptoms on ordinary exertion; Class III: symptoms at less-than-ordinary exertion; or Class IV: symptoms at rest). Stage D is characterized by Class IV symptoms.

## TYPES OF DIASTOLIC HEART FAILURE

There is no universally agreed upon definition of diastolic heart failure (DHF). It may occur in conjunction with either normal or abnormal LV systolic function.

Conceptually, isolated DHF could be defined as a combination of signs and symptoms of heart failure and LV diastolic dysfunction. The clinical impression of heart failure can be corroborated by objective signs of pulmonary vascular congestion on a chest radiograph, increased brain natriuretic peptide (BNP) serum levels, and the demonstration of elevated left atrial pressures either invasively or echocardiographically.

A direct demonstration of LV diastolic dysfunction would require a determination of abnormal values of tau and LV stiffness modulus, as well as the demonstration of a pathologic substrate through an endomyocardial biopsy. However, such measurements are complex and, as pointed earlier, not routinely used in clinical practice. As a consequence, there are only very few conditions with well-characterized LV diastolic dysfunctions that lead to DHF. These include hypertrophic cardiomyopathy (discussed elsewhere) and infiltrative cardiomyopathies, which are discussed below.

Instead, the presence of LV diastolic dysfunction in most patients with presumed DHF is inferred. In such individuals, LV diastolic dysfunction is suspected because they present with heart failure in the setting of normal or near-normal LV systolic function (LV ejection fraction ≥50%), normal or small LV diastolic volumes, and no significant valvular heart disease. Because the stiffness is defined as dP/dV, the presence of elevated filling pressures in the setting of normal LV volume is indicative of increased LV stiffness and, by extension, true LV diastolic dysfunction.

According to an American Heart Association position paper from 2000, DHF can be defined as either probable or definitive. *Probable* DHF is simply defined as the presence of clinical signs and symptoms of heart failure within 72 hours of detecting normal or near-normal LV systolic function and no significant valvular disease. The diagnosis of *definitive* DHF also requires detection of abnormal LV diastolic function by Doppler echocardiography.

Because a definitive diagnosis of DHF requires extensive expertise in echocardiographic assessment of LV diastolic function, epidemiologic studies routinely define DHF along the probable DHF criteria. Because LV diastolic dysfunction is infrequently measured directly in such studies, some prefer the term *heart failure with normal LV ejection fraction* (HFNEF) to that of DHF, when applied to patients in these studies.

In 2007, the European Society of Cardiology made the DHF diagnostic criteria even more stringent; it defined isolated DHF as a condition with clinical signs and symptoms of heart failure, normal LV systolic function, abnormal Doppler filling patterns, and the presence of elevated LV filling pressures (defined as one or more of the following: LV end-diastolic pressure >16 mm Hg; mean pulmonary artery wedge pressure >12 mm Hg; and an E/E' >15) in the setting of normal LV end-diastolic volume index (≤75 mL/m$^2$).

## DIASTOLIC HEART FAILURE DUE TO INFILTRATIVE DISORDERS

Infiltrative myocardial disorders (restrictive cardiomyopathies) are rare causes of DHF. Although such cardiomyopathies are infrequent, the presence of DHF in affected individuals is the norm. LV distensibility in these patients decreases due to deposition of various substances either in the extracellular matrix of the heart muscle (such as proteins in amyloidosis and myocardial fibrosis; and small molecules in hyperoxaluria) or in the cardiac lysosomes.

| Table 58-5 • Characteristics of the three most Common forms of Amyloidosis | | | |
|---|---|---|---|
| Amyloidosis Type | Amyloid Deposit | Underlying Disease | Risk of Cardiac Involvement |
| AL | Monoclonal IG Light Chains | Multiple Myeloma | 50% |
| AA | Serum Amyloid Protein | Chronic Inflammation | 10% |
| Familial | Transthyretin (Prealbumin) | Gene Mutation | 5% |

AMYLOIDOSIS is a systemic multiorgan disorder caused by extracellular deposition of normally soluble amyloidogenic proteins in various organs including the heart. Amyloid fibrils are formed by a variety of genetically unrelated proteins that share the same folding pattern (β-pleated sheets). The characteristics of the three most common forms of amyloidosis are given in **Table 58-5**. Although amyloidosis is the most common form of restrictive cardiomyopathy, its prevalence in the general population is very low (acquired systemic amyloidosis occurs in 1 in 100,000 US person-years).

MYOCARDIAL FIBROSIS occurs due to excessive deposition of collagen fibers in the extracellular matrix. It is often seen in patients with left ventricular hypertrophy due to systemic hypertension and, thus, may be the contributing factor to at least some forms of heart failure with the normal LVEF. It also occurs following chest radiation and in late stages of *Trypanosoma cruzi* infection. Frequently, myocardial fibrosis has no apparent cause and is then referred to as being idiopathic.

HYPEROXALURIA is characterized by calcium oxalate deposits in various organs including the myocardium, the kidneys, and the liver.

LYSOSOMAL STORAGE DISORDERS are due to lysosomal enzyme deficiencies that lead to the inability to break down normal cellular constituents. Lysosomal deposits include lipids (as in Gaucher's and Nieman-Picks disease), mucopolysaccharides (as in Hurler's disease), and gangliosides (as in Tay-Sachs disorder). Gaucher's disease is the most common lysosomal storage disease and is characterized by a marked increase in LV wall thickness and stiffness.

## HEART FAILURE WITH NORMAL LV EJECTION FRACTION (HFNEF)

Epidemiologic surveys and case-control studies, in both inpatient and outpatient settings, have demonstrated that, currently, about 50% of patients presenting with signs and symptoms of heart failure have a normal or near-normal ejection fraction, no significant valvular disease, and no evidence for hypertrophic or restrictive cardiomyopathy.

Age is the major risk factor for HFNEF; the older the studied population, the higher the prevalence of HFNEF compared to systolic heart failure. With the rapidly aging population, HFNEF is expected to become the dominant form of heart failure in the near future. Other risk factors include female gender, systemic hypertension, LV hypertrophy (LV mass index $>95$ g/m$^2$ in women and $>115$ g/m$^2$ in men), and diabetes mellitus.

Because these individuals present with clinical signs and symptoms of heart failure in the setting of normal or near-normal LV systolic function (LV ejection fraction $\geq 50\%$), normal or small LV diastolic volumes, and no significant valvular heart disease, they are presumed to have diastolic heart failure. However, there is a paucity of data in these individuals on the presence of true LV diastolic dysfunction as defined by abnormal tau and LV stiffness modulus values. Because true LV diastolic dysfunction has not been demonstrated directly in large groups of such patients, some researchers believe that the term *diastolic heart failure* should not be applied to these patients; instead, they propose *heart failure with normal LV ejection fraction* as a more neutral term for this disorder.

Indeed, HFNEF is a syndrome in which the LV filling pressure elevation is only partly explained by an intrinsic LV diastolic dysfunction, because there is often a contribution from an increase in afterload (elevated systemic blood pressure; stiff aortic wall) and/or preload (anemia; renal failure). In one study, the mortality and morbidity of HFNEF was shown to be lower than that of systolic heart failure.

## DIAGNOSIS OF DHF

Symptoms and signs of DHF are similar to those of systolic heart failure. Symptoms include fatigue and breathlessness including dyspnea on exertion, orthopnea, and paroxysmal nocturnal dyspnea. On physical exam, one finds pulmonary râles and peripheral edema. Cardiac auscultation may reveal either an S4 gallop (in Grade I LV diastolic dysfunction) or an S3 gallop (in Grades II-IV).

A chest radiograph reveals left atrial enlargement and pulmonary vascular congestion. Electrocardiographic (ECG) findings in HFNEF often include signs of left atrial enlargement and left ventricular hypertrophy. In contrast, an ECG in patients with cardiac amyloidosis usually has diminished voltage, as the wall thickening in

these cardiomyopathies is due to deposits of electrically inert substances. In fact, the discrepancy between the low QRS voltage on the ECG and the apparent LV hypertrophy (or more precisely, LV wall thickening) on echocardiography is frequently the first diagnostic clue that the patient might have restrictive cardiomyopathy, such as amyloidosis.

Just as in systolic heart failure, a laboratory test for DHF often reveals an elevation of plasma brain natriuretic peptide (BNP). In HFNEF, lab tests frequently reveal anemia and some degree of renal insufficiency.

Echocardiography plays the central role in the diagnosis of DHF; it provides information in the following four areas:

1. ESTIMATION OF THE FILLING PRESSURES (e.g., LA pressures by E/E' ratio, pulmonary wedge pressure by E/Vp, and LV pre-A diastolic pressure by the pulmonary vein AR duration of more than 30 msec compared to mitral A wave). The finding of elevated pressure within 72 hours of presentation helps differentiate DHF from other causes of breathlessness. A serial filling pressure estimation may also be helpful in monitoring therapy in acute setting.

2. DETERMINATION OF LV EJECTION FRACTION. Normal LV ejection fraction excludes systolic dysfunction.

3. DETERMINATION OF MITRAL AND PULMONARY VENOUS FLOW PATTERNS (normal, abnormal relaxation, pseudonormalization, and restrictive filling). A pseudonormal pattern in middle-age and elderly patients may be distinguished from the normal pattern by the presence of $S < D$ in pulmonary vein tracings, diminished E' velocity or Vp, and an AR – A wave duration of $>30$ msec. The filling pattern and the grade of LV diastolic dysfunction may change over time in the same patient; they may worsen as the disease progresses (as has been clearly shown in amyloidosis) or may improve (if it occurs following diuretic therapy and the decrease in filling pressures.

4. CALCULATION OF LA VOLUME. The presence of an increased LA volume in the absence of a chronic volume overload or mitral valve disease is indicative of chronically elevated LA pressures and thus supports the diagnosis of DHF. Conversely, if one is contemplating the diagnosis of a pseudonormal filling pattern (Grade II LV diastolic dysfunction) but finds a normal LA volume, a diagnosis different from DHF should be considered.

5. CALCULATION OF LV VOLUME AND MASS. In both HFNEF and restrictive cardiomyopathies, the LV wall thickness is increased and, thus, the calculated LV mass is increased (LV mass index $>95$ g/m$^2$

## Table 59-1 • Commonly Used Diuretics in Heart Failure

| Drug | Initial Dose to Maximum Daily Dose (Oral) or to Maximal Single Dose (Intravenous) | Mechanism of Action |
|---|---|---|
| **Loop diuretics** | | |
| Furosemide oral | 20-40 mg once or twice daily to 600 mg | Inhibit $Na^+$ and $Cl^-$ reabsorption by blocking the $Na^+-K^+-2Cl^-$ cotransporter in thick ascending limb of loop of Henle leading to free water excretion. |
| Intravenous | 40-160-200 mg | |
| Infusion | 40 mg IV load, then 10-40 mg/hr | |
| Bumetanide oral | 0.5-1.0 mg once or twice daily to 10 mg | |
| Intravenous | 1.0 mg to 4-8 mg | |
| Infusion | 1 mg IV load, then 0.5-2 mg/hr | |
| Torsemide oral | 10-20 mg once daily to 200 mg | |
| Intravenous | 10 mg to 100-200 mg | |
| Infusion | 20 mg IV load, then 5-20 mg/hr | |
| **Thiazide diuretics** | | |
| Chlorothiazide* (intravenous) | 250-500 mg once or twice to 1000 mg | Block the $Na^+Cl^-$ cotransporter in distal convoluted tubules thereby inhibiting $Na^+/Cl^-$ reabsorption. |
| Metolazone* | 2.5 mg once to 20 mg | |
| Hydrochlorothiazide | 25 mg once or twice to 200 mg | |

*Thiazides with more potent diuretic effects.*
*Ethacrynic acid is the only loop diuretic without a sulfa moiety and may be used in sulfa-allergic patients. It is not commonly available in the United States.*

*Thiazide diuretics:* hypokalemia, increased serum cholesterol and triglycerides, impaired glucose tolerance, diabetes mellitus. Metolazone can cause profound hyponatremia, hypokalemia, and volume depletion.

## Diuretic Resistance

*Definition:* Unresponsiveness to higher doses of loop diuretics.

*Potential causes:* Potential causes are increased dietary sodium intake, concomitant use of agents that can block the effects of diuretics (e.g., NSAIDs, COX-2 inhibitors), significant impairment of renal function or perfusion, worsening HF resulting in bowel edema and intestinal hypoperfusion with poor absorption of the diuretic when given orally.

*Treatment:* Restrict sodium intake, intravenous diuretics, use of two or more diuretic classes in combination, use of diuretics together with drugs that increase renal blood flow (e.g., positive inotropes).

## DIGITALIS

The positive inotropic effects of digitalis have not translated into robust clinical benefit in clinical trials. Thus, the use of digitalis in HF has acquired a more secondary role.

## Mechanism of Action

Digitalis inhibits the $Na^+/K^+$ ATPase, ultimately resulting in increased intracellular calcium. This results in (a) increased inotropy and (b) decreased conduction through the SA and AV nodes.

## Clinical Outcomes

The main DIG trial randomized 6800 patients with HF, LVEF <45%, and sinus rhythm to digoxin or placebo. At 3 years follow-up, digoxin had a neutral effect on mortality but resulted in 28% reduction in HF hospitalization. The PROVED and RADIANCE trials demonstrated that discontinuation of digoxin resulted in higher frequency of worsening HF.

## Indications

Digoxin can be used in:

1. Patients with persistent symptoms of HF despite treatment with diuretics, ACE-I, and beta-blockers (Stage C and D, NYHA II-IV) (ACC/AHA Class IIa recommendation, Level of evidence: B).
2. LV systolic dysfunction and atrial fibrillation (for rate control), often in addition to beta-blockers, which are more effective in controlling ventricular response especially during exercise.

Of note, a retrospective analysis of the DIG trial demonstrated increased risk of death in women randomized to digoxin. With the relatively small benefit with digoxin (compared to other HF medications) and the potentially worse outcome in women, some physicians do not use digoxin in women with HF. (This is not a guideline recommendation and is left up to the discretion of the physician.)

Furthermore, caution is recommended when withdrawing digoxin in patients who are tolerating it well.

## Recommended Dosing

0.125-0.25 mg daily is recommended. Since there is no clear serum level–response relationship, in HF patients, 0.125 mg daily is typically used to prevent digitalis toxicity, especially in more advanced HF patients who have renal insufficiency or rapidly changing renal function (with diuresis, worsening cardiac function, addition of ACE-I or ARB, etc.). Loading doses are not indicated when digoxin is initiated for HF treatment.

Serum concentration is rarely checked to assess for therapeutic target but is usually checked to assess for toxicity. The recommended serum concentration to avoid toxicity is 0.5-1.0 ng/mL. Post-hoc analyses have demonstrated increasing mortality as levels exceed 1 ng/mL.

## Adverse Effects

Overt digitalis toxicity is commonly associated with serum digoxin levels >2 ng/mL. However, toxicity may occur with lower digoxin levels, especially if hypokalemia, hypomagnesemia, hypothyroidism, renal insufficiency, or lower body mass coexist.

Symptoms of digitalis toxicity include fatigue, gastrointestinal symptoms (e.g., anorexia, nausea, vomiting, diarrhea, abdominal pain), neurological complaints (e.g., headache, dizziness, visual disturbances such as yellow-green halos, disorientation, and confusion), and cardiac arrhythmias such as bradycardia, ventricular ectopy, atrial arrhythmias (may be seen together with high degree AV block, e.g., atrial flutter with >4:1 block or atrial fibrillation with heart block resulting in a slow, regular ventricular response), and ventricular arrhythmias. Accelerated junctional rhythm and bidirectional ventricular tachycardia are more specific for digitalis toxicity.

Medications that can increase digitalis levels and cause toxicity: amiodarone, clarithromycin, erythromycin, tetracycline, itraconazole, cyclosporine, verapamil, diltiazem, or quinidine. Rifampin enhances digoxin metabolism and lowers its levels. Thus, stopping rifampin can lead to digoxin accumulation and toxicity.

## Treatment of Digitalis Toxicity

- Charcoal for drug adsorption in GI tract (within 6-8 hours of ingestion)
- Correct hypokalemia and hypomagnesemia
- Digoxin-specific Fab fragments are indicated in patients with symptomatic arrhythmias, hemodynamic instability, hyperkalemia (K > 5.0 mEq/L), digoxin level >10 ng/mL.

- Hemodialysis or hemofiltration are not effective in removing digoxin.

# RENIN ANGIOTENSIN ALDOSTERONE ANTAGONISTS

Activation of the renin-angiotensin-aldosterone system (RAAS) plays a crucial role in the development and progression of HF. Deleterious effects of the RAAS in HF are mediated primarily through increased levels of angiotensin II. Angiotensin II is an extremely potent vasoconstrictor and produces sodium retention (via aldosterone and renal vasoconstriction) and fluid retention (via antidiuretic hormone), thereby promoting the HF state. At the cellular level, angiotensin II promotes hypertrophy, contributing to remodeling of the left ventricle and alterations in the vasculature. Blocking the RAAS cascade at different levels has been shown to reduce the progression of HF and improve long-term outcome.

# ANGIOTENSIN CONVERTING ENZYME INHIBITORS (ACE-I)

## Mechanism of Action

ACE-I inhibit the angiotensin converting enzyme (ACE) that converts angiotensin I to angiotensin II. By decreasing the production of angiotensin II, ACE-I decrease the deleterious effects of angiotensin II. Furthermore, ACE is involved in the degradation of bradykinin (which acts as a vasodilator through the release of nitric oxide) and prostaglandin, along with having antimitotic, antithrombotic, and natriuretic actions. Some beneficial effects of ACE-I may be due to inhibition of ACE-mediated bradykinin degradation. Acutely, the beneficial clinical effects of ACE-I are attributed to their vasodilatory properties (resulting in decreased afterload). Chronically, their neurohormonal effects appear more important.

## Clinical Outcomes

Numerous trials have demonstrated that ACE-I improve HF symptoms, reduce HF hospitalizations, and improve survival in patients with LV systolic dysfunction (**Tables 59-2** and **59-3**).

## Indications

ACE-I are indicated in all patients with LV systolic dysfunction, with or without HF (i.e., Stages B-D and NYHA Class I-IV), irrespective of etiology of HF.

The starting and target doses of ACE-I recommended for HF are displayed in **Table 59-4**.

| Table 59-2 • Clinical Trials of ACE-I in Post Myocardial Infarction HF/LV Systolic Dysfunction | | | |
|---|---|---|---|
| **Trial** | **Study Population** | **Study Drug Target Dose** | **Outcome with Drug vs. Placebo** |
| AIRE (n = 1986) | post-MI HF | ramipril, 5 mg twice daily | 27% ↓ mortality |
| SAVE (n = 2231) | post-MI LVEF <40% without HF | captopril, 50 mg three times daily | 19% ↓ mortality, 37% ↓ severe HF, 25% ↓ recurrent MI |
| TRACE (N = 2606) | post-MI LVEF ≤35% | trandolapril, 4 mg once daily | 22% ↓ mortality, 29% ↓ severe HF |

*HF, heart failure; LV, left ventricular; MI, myocardial infarction; LVEF, left ventricular ejection fraction.*

## Adverse Effects

- Hypotension, worsening renal function, hyperkalemia, cough (5-10%, up to 50% in Chinese), angioedema (rare, with an incidence of <1%; more frequent in African Americans).
- A dry, nonproductive cough may occur, presumed secondary to increased bradykinin levels; alternative causes of cough should be excluded before the ACE-I are stopped. Cough and angioedema usually occur within a few weeks of initiation but have been noted months to years after starting ACE-I.

## Contraindications

Angioedema or anuric renal failure during prior exposure to ACE-I; hyperkalemia, pregnancy, bilateral renal artery stenosis.

## Caveats When Using ACE-I

Caution in initiation or uptitration of ACE-I is advised if:

- Systolic BP <80-90 mm Hg
- Creatinine >3 mg/dL
- Potassium >5.5 mmol/L

ACE-I should be started at low doses and gradually increased to target doses used in clinical trials. If target doses cannot be reached (e.g., because of hypotension, hyperkalemia, renal insufficiency), the highest tolerated dose should be used. The ATLAS trial (Assessment of Treatment with Lisinopril and Survival) demonstrated that HF patients taking higher doses of lisinopril had a trend toward lower cardiovascular mortality and had significantly fewer hospitalizations for any cause and for HF, as compared to patients on low dose lisinopril.

A beta-blocker can be initiated soon after ACE-I initiation (if patient is euvolemic) and does not have to be delayed until target ACE-I dose has been reached. Both should gradually be uptitrated, as tolerated.

# ANGIOTENSIN RECEPTOR BLOCKERS (ARBS)

## Mechanism of Action

Angiotensin receptor blockers (ARBs) selectively block the binding of angiotensin II to the angiotensin II receptor, Type 1 ($AT_1$). This results in a decrease in arterial vasoconstriction, decrease in sympathetic tone, and attenuation of myocardial hypertrophy. Because angiotensin II stimulates aldosterone production, aldosterone levels are also reduced, resulting in a decrease in $Na^+/Cl^-$ absorption, $K^+$ excretion, and water retention.

The premise for the introduction of ARBs is that ACE-I do not completely suppress angiotensin II levels in patients with HF. In fact, angiotensin II levels appear to gradually increase on chronic ACE-I therapy, likely due to various

| Table 59-3 • Clinical Trials of ACE-I in Chronic Heart Failure | | | |
|---|---|---|---|
| **Trial** | **Study Population** | **Study Drug Target Dose** | **Outcome with Drug vs. Placebo** |
| SOLVD prevention (n = 4228) | LVEF < 35%, on no treatment for HF | Enalapril, 10 mg twice daily | no difference in mortality, 29% ↓ death or HF development |
| SOLVD treatment (n = 2569) | Chronic HF (Class II-III) and LVEF < 35% | Enalapril, 10 mg twice daily | 16% ↓ mortality, 26% ↓ death or HF hospitalization |
| CONSENSUS I (n = 253) | NYHA Class IV HF | Enalapril, 20 mg twice daily | 40% ↓ 6-month, 27% ↓ overall mortality, NYHA class improved |

*HF, heart failure; LVEF, left ventricular ejection fraction.*

**Table 59-4 • ACE-I Recommended in Heart Failure**

| ACE-I | Initial Daily Dose | Maximum Daily Dose |
|---|---|---|
| Captopril | 6.25 mg 3 times | 50 mg 3 times |
| Enalapril | 2.5 mg twice | 10 to 20 mg twice |
| Lisinopril | 2.5 to 5 mg once | 20 to 40 mg once |
| Fosinopril | 5 to 10 mg once | 40 mg once |
| Perindopril | 2 mg once | 8 to 16 mg once |
| Quinapril | 5 mg twice | 20 mg twice |
| Ramipril | 1.25 to 2.5 mg once | 10 mg once |
| Trandolapril | 1 mg once | 4 mg once |

alternative non-ACE pathways that convert angiotensin I to angiotensin II. ARBs were therefore developed for more complete inhibition of angiotensin II by directly blocking the angiotensin receptor.

## Clinical Outcomes (Tables 59-5 and 59-6)

Trials comparing ARBs to ACE-I in chronic HF have demonstrated that ARBs are equivalent to ACE-I with respect to morbidity and mortality outcomes (trials using valsartan and candesartan); however, a trend toward improved outcomes was noted with ACE-I in a trial comparing captopril to losartan. In light of the greater amount of data and experience with ACE-I compared to ARBs, ACE-I continue to be the recommended first-line agents for patients with HF and depressed LVEF. ARBs are recommended in patients with HF who are intolerant of ACE-I. The Val-HeFT and the CHARM-Added trials assessed the addition of ARBs to ACE-I on morbidity and mortality in patients with HF and LV systolic dysfunction. Both trials demonstrated a reduction in HF hospitalizations when an ARB was added to an ACE-I with modest reduction in cardiovascular mortality only in CHARM-Added.

## Indications

ARBs are indicated in patients with LV systolic dysfunction in the following scenarios:

- Patients who are intolerant of ACE-I because of intractable cough or angioedema (Stages A-D, NYHA Class I-IV).
- ARBs can be added to ACE-I if patients continue to have HF symptoms or uncontrolled hypertension despite target doses of ACE-I and beta-blockers.
- If patients are on ACE-I but are unable to tolerate beta-blockers and have persistent symptoms (Heart Failure Society of America recommendation).

The ARBs recommended in HF with LV systolic dysfunction and their dosing are presented in **Table 59-7**.

## Adverse Effects

ARBs are as likely as ACE-I to produce hypotension, worsening renal function, and hyperkalemia. Otherwise, ARBs are better tolerated than ACE-I. The incidence of cough is much lower in ARBs (~1%) compared to ACE-I (5-10%), and the incidence of angioedema with ARB is extremely rare. Guidelines recommend that ARBs may be considered in patients who have had angioedema while taking ACE-I, however, extreme caution is advised.

## ALDOSTERONE ANTAGONISTS

Aldosterone antagonists were investigated in the treatment of HF, because treatment with ACE-I and ARBs suppresses aldosterone levels incompletely, owing to non-angiotensin-mediated stimulation of aldosterone. In addition to fluid retention, aldosterone has adverse effects on cardiac structure

**Table 59-5 • Clinical Trials of ARBs in Post Myocardial Infarction Heart Failure**

| Trial; Number of Patients | Study Population | Study Drug Target Dose | Comparator | Outcome |
|---|---|---|---|---|
| OPTIMAAL (n = 5477) | post-MI, HF LVEF <35% or LVEDD >65 mm | losartan, 50 mg daily | captopril, 50 mg three times daily | trend toward 13% ↑ mortality with losartan; trend toward 16% ↑ HF hospitalization |
| VALIANT (n = 14,500) | post-MI, with HF or LVEF <35% | valsartan, 160 mg twice daily | captopril, 50 mg three times daily OR combination of valsartan, 80 mg twice daily, and captopril, 50 mg three times daily | similar mortality in all 3 groups |

*HF, heart failure; MI, myocardial infarction; LVEF, left ventricular ejection fraction; LVEDD, left ventricular end-diastolic diameter.*

*Indications.* ADHF, especially in the presence of:
- increased afterload (e.g., hypertensive ADHF).
- significant mitral regurgitation.

*Dosage.* Start at 10 mcg/min (0.3-0.5 mcg/kg/min) and uptitrate every 5-15 minutes as tolerated to achieve a mean arterial pressure of 65-70 mm Hg or systolic blood pressure of 90-100 mm Hg. Maximum recommended dose is 400 mcg/min (<4-5 mcg/kg/min).

Adverse Effects. Adverse effects may include hypotension, coronary steal phenomenon (thus, not indicated in patients with acute coronary syndromes), nausea/vomiting, abdominal discomfort, cyanide toxicity, and methemoglobinemia.

Rebound hypertension is possible if SNP is stopped abruptly, thus, gradual tapering is recommended.

Thiocyanate toxicity is rare, however, it occurs more often with hepatic dysfunction, renal insufficiency, and exposure to higher doses (>250 mcg/min) for >48 hours.

## Nesiritide

*Mechanism of Action.* Nesiritide is recombinant B-type natriuretic peptide (BNP) that, through the cGMP pathway, leads to vasodilation, natriuresis, and diuresis.

*Clinical Outcome.* Trials have shown an improvement in filling pressures and symptoms of volume overload with nesiritide in ADHF, but no trial has demonstrated long-term morbidity or mortality benefit. Although approved for the treatment of ADHF, its benefit over other vasodilators is not clear. Recent retrospective analyses have raised concern for possible adverse effects on renal function and survival, based on which a large prospective trial is ongoing.

*Dosage.* 2 mcg/kg (bolus), followed by continuous infusion at 0.01 mcg/kg/min.

*Adverse Effects. Adverse effects may include* hypotension, headaches, and worsening renal function.

## INOTROPES

Inotropes are mainly initiated in Stage D or in NYHA Class IV HF patients. Two main groups of inotropes are used: phosphodiesterase inhibitors and beta-agonists.

The mechanisms of action, dosing, and adverse effects of the commonly used agents in ADHF are detailed in **Table 59-13**. Of note, milrinone may be preferred over dobutamine in patients already taking beta-blockers and may be more effective in the presence of significant secondary pulmonary hypertension. However, due to greater vasodilation, milrinone causes more hypotension than dobutamine. In addition, milrinone has a more prolonged duration of action, especially with renal dysfunction. Furthermore, if hypotension is an issue, dopamine, which has greater alpha-blocking vasoconstrictor activity in addition to its beta-agonist effects at medium to high doses (5-25 mcg/kg/min), may be required. More potent vasoconstrictors such as epinephrine and norepinephrine may be needed for severe hypotension.

## Clinical Outcomes

Inotropes have been shown to improve hemodynamics (increase cardiac output, decrease filling pressures, promote

| Table 59-13 • Inotropes in Heart Failure | | | | |
|---|---|---|---|---|
| Inotrope | Mechanism of Action | Hemodynamic Effect | Dosing | Adverse Effects |
| **Milrinone** | phosphodiesterase III inhibitor | positive inotropy and vasodilation | 0.25-0.75 mcg/kg/min | hypotension, arrhythmias (atrial and ventricular), rare thrombocytopenia |
| **Dobutamine** | predominant β-1 agonist (weak β-2 and α-1 agonist) | positive inotropy and positive chronotropy | 2.5-20 mcg/kg/min | sinus tachycardia, arrhythmias (atrial and ventricular), development of tolerance, eosinophilic myocarditis with peripheral eosinophilia (rare) |
| **Dopamine** | <5 mcg/kg/min: mesenteric and dopaminergic receptors; 5-10 mcg/kg/min: β-1 and dopaminergic receptors; >10 mcg/kg/min: β-1 and α-receptors | low dose: mesenteric vasodilation, some inotropy; medium dose: positive inotropy and chronotropy; high doses: positive inotropy, chronotropy, and peripheral vasoconstriction | 1-20 mcg/kg/min | arrhythmias similar to dobutamine |

diuresis) and HF symptoms (symptoms of volume overload and low output). However, no inotrope has been shown to improve survival. On the contrary, the majority of prospective trials demonstrated increased mortality in HF patients routinely treated with inotropes.

## Indications

Because of worse outcomes with inotropic therapy, guidelines recommend chronic intravenous intropic therapy only if standard HF therapy and attempts at weaning the inotropes repeatedly fail. In the acute setting, they should be used only in patients with ADHF who do not respond to or are unable to tolerate intravenous vasodilator therapy.

Thus, inotropic therapy can be considered for:

- temporary in-hospital use for ADHF with markedly reduced cardiac output and end-organ hypoperfusion.
- as a bridge to heart transplantation in hospitalized patients or in a subgroup of patients awaiting transplantation at home who have an implanted defibrillator to reduce the risk of sudden death.
- as palliation to allow patients to die with comfort (Class IIb indication, Level of evidence: C).
- routine intermittent infusions of positive inotropic agents are not recommended for patients with refractory end-stage HF (Class III indication, Level of evidence: B).

## NEWER MEDICATIONS

### Vasopressin Antagonists

Vasopressin or ADH is an endogenous peptide hormone that is released from the posterior pituitary and increases free water absorption in the distal convoluted tubules and collecting tubules of the kidney. Vasopressin receptor antagonists have been investigated in several prospective HF trials. Tolvaptan (a selective V2 antagonist) has been the most extensively studied vaptan in HF and is now FDA approved for the treatment of hyponatremia in the setting of HF. Treatment with tolvaptan has been shown to decrease body weight, reduce edema, and normalize serum sodium in patients with hyponatremia. However, no significant impact on morbidity and mortality has been demonstrated.

### Calcium Sensitizers

The proarrhythmic properties of inotropes have been attributed to calcium influx into the myocyte and intracellular calcium overloading. Calcium sensitizers increase the sensitivity of the myocardial contractile apparatus to calcium without increasing intracellular calcium concentration, theoretically allowing for positive inotropic action without proarrhythmic effects. Levosimendan, the most widely studied calcium sensitizer, has been demonstrated to reduce PCWP, right atrial, and pulmonary artery pressures and increase stroke volume and cardiac index in patients with ADHF. Clinically, improvement in dyspnea and fatigue was demonstrated. In the REVIVE II trial, levosimendan compared to placebo resulted in clinical improvement in HF symptoms and a shorter hospital stay. Mortality at 90 days did not differ significantly between groups, although there were more deaths in the levosimendan group. The SURVIVE trial compared levosimendan to dobutamine in ADHF. The primary end-point of mortality at 180 days was not significantly different between levosimendan and dobutamine. However, there was a trend toward lower mortality in the levosimendan arm. Calcium sensitizers are not approved for HF in the United States.

### Statins

Several retrospective analyses and smaller prospective trials have indicated beneficial effects of HMG coenzyme A reductase inhibitors (statins) in patients with HF, potentially as a result of the statins' pleiotropic effects. Two prospective randomized trial, the CORONA trial, and Gissi-HF trial, compared rosuvastatin to placebo in patients with ischemic and non-ischemic cardiomyopathy. Treatment with rosuvastatin did not confer significant clinical benefit. Therefore, currently, statins are not indicated in all HF patients but should be used in patients with known coronary artery disease and elevated levels of low-density lipoprotein cholesterol, as recommended by the lipid guidelines.

### Suggested Readings

1. Hunt, SA, et al. ACC/AHA 2005 guideline update for the diagnosis and management of chronic heart failure in the adult. *Circulation.* 2005;112:e154-e235.

2. Heart Failure Society of America. 2006 comprehensive heart failure practice guideline. *Journal of Cardiac Failure.* 2006;12:e1-e122.

3. Mann, DL. Management of heart failure patients with reduced ejection fraction. In: Libby P, Bonow RO, Mann DL, Zipes DP, eds. *Braunwald's Heart Disease: A Textbook of Cardiovascular Medicine.* Philadelphia, PA: Saunders, An Imprint of Elsevier; 2007:611–640.

# .60

# Restrictive Cardiomyopathy

Dhaval Shah and Mandeep R. Mehra

## ● PRACTICAL POINTS

- A clinically oriented classification system for cardiomyopathies based on ventricular morphology and function divides the disorders into the following phenotypes: hypertrophic, dilated, restrictive, arrhythmogenic right ventricular cardiomyopathy, and unclassified.

- Restrictive left ventricular physiology is defined as increased stiffness of the myocardium, which causes the ventricular pressure to rise disproportionately higher than the increase in ventricular volume.

- In restrictive cardiomyopathies (RCM), there is a normal or increased ventricular wall thickness with normal or reduced ventricular volumes.

- In RCM, elevated filling pressures are needed to maintain cardiac output, but result in volume overload and right-sided or left-sided congestion, leading to diastolic heart failure.

- The diagnostic approach to RCM first involves ruling out constrictive pericarditis, due to similar symptoms, and excluding a secondary cause of restrictive cardiomyopathy.

- Both constrictive and restrictive disease present with a "dip and plateau" pattern on cardiac catheterization hemodynamics, but RCM is associated with LVEDP often >5 mm Hg greater than RVEDP, RV systolic pressure >50 mm Hg, RVEDP < one-third of RV systolic pressure, and concordant changes in RV and LV pressure with inspiration/expiration.

- Treatment of RCM involves diuretics for symptoms of heart failure, treatment of arrhythmias, and trying to maintain sinus rhythm to maintain atrial contraction for ventricular filling.

- Types of amyloidosis included primary (AL), familial (transthyretin), senile (transthyretin), and secondary (AA); treatment is supportive, but chemotherapy is used in primary amyloidosis.

- Sarcoidosis leads to RCM, varying from subclinical diastolic dysfunction, to systolic dysfunction, to acute presentation with sudden death or high-degree heart block.

- Endomyocardial fibrosis is primarily a disease of the tropics with insidious onset and poor prognosis.

Cardiomyopathies are grouped into specific morphological and functional phenotypes. A clinically oriented classification system for cardiomyopathies based on ventricular morphology and function remains the most useful method for diagnosing and treating patients with heart muscle disease. Accordingly, cardiomyopathies are now divided into the following phenotypes: hypertrophic, dilated, restrictive, arrhythmogenic right ventricular cardiomyopathy, and unclassified, with each phenotype subclassified into familial and nonfamilial forms.

Restrictive left ventricular physiology is defined as increased stiffness of the myocardium, which causes the ventricular pressure to rise disproportionately higher than the increase in ventricular volume. In restrictive cardiomyopathies, there is a restrictive ventricular physiology in the presence of normal or increased ventricular wall thickness. The diastolic and systolic ventricular volumes are either normal or reduced. Restrictive cardiomyopathy (RCM) occurs in a wide range of different pathologies. Nonfamilial cardiomyopathy may be idiopathic or result from various systemic disorders,

**Table 60-1 • Etiology of Restrictive Cardiomyopathy (RCM)**

| Familial Causes | Nonfamilial Causes |
|---|---|
| 1. Familial, unknown gene | idiopathic |
| 2. Sarcomeric protein mutations:Troponin I (RCM +/− HCM) Essential light chain of myosin | amyloid (AL/prealbumin) |
| 3. Familial amyloidosis: Transthyretin (RCM + neuropathy) Apolipoprotein (RCM + nephropathy) | scleroderma |
| 4. Desminopathy | endomyocardial fibrosis: a. hypereosinophilic syndrome b. idiopathic c. chromosomal cause d. drug (serotonin, methysergide, ergotamine, mercurial agents, busulfan) |
| 5. Pseuxanthoma elasticum | carcinoid heart disease |
| 6. Anderson–Fabry disease | metastatic cancers |
| 7. Haemochromatosis | radiation |
| 8. Glycogen storage disease | drugs (anthracyclines) |

*Reprinted with permission from Elliott P, Andersson B, Arbustini E, et al. Classification of the cardiomyopathies: A position statement from the European Society of Cardiology working group on myocardial and pericardial diseases. European Heart Journal. 2008;29:270–276. doi:10.1093/eurheartj/ehm342.*

**Table 60-2 • Clinical History and Potential Causes of Restrictive Cardiomyopathy**

| History | Potential Causes of Restrictive Cardiomyopathy |
|---|---|
| Previous malignancy | radiation, anthracycline, doxorubicin |
| Drug intake | L-tryptophan, chloroquine |
| Weight loss | amyloidosis |
| Renal impairment | cystinosis, scleroderma, mitochondrial myopathy, amyloidosis, Fabry's disease |
| Gastrointestinal problems | scleroderma, mitochondrial myopathy, carcinoid, amyloidosis |
| Pulmonary problems | scleroderma, carcinoid, Churg-Strauss syndrome |
| Flushing | carcinoid |
| Allergic rhinitis | Churg-Strauss syndrome |
| Nasal polyps | Churg-Strauss syndrome |
| Diabetes mellitus | hemochromatosis, mitochondrial myopathy |
| Hepatic problems | hemochromatosis, amyloidosis |
| Acroparesthesias | Fabry's disease |
| Bone pain | multiple myeloma |
| Fever | reactive arthritis |
| Arthralgia | reactive arthritis |
| Muscle weakness and wasting | neuromuscular disorders like desminopathy, mitochondrial myopathy, polymyositis, dermatomyositis, chloroquine myopathy |

*Reprinted with permission from Stöllberger C, Finsterer J. Extracardiac medical and neuromuscular implications in restrictive cardiomyopathy. Clin. Cardiol. 2007;30:375–380.*

like amyloidosis, sarcoidosis, carcinoid heart disease, and scleroderma. Similarly, it is also suggested that cardiac amyloidosis should be listed in the differential diagnosis of both hypertrophic (HCM) and restrictive cardiomyopathy. Thus, cardiac amyloidosis has been considered as a separate entity (see **Table 60-1**).

# CLINICAL FEATURES

Clinical characteristics of restrictive cardiomyopathy can be divided into cardiac and noncardiac features.

## Cardiac Features

Restrictive cardiomyopathy leads to diastolic dysfunction, which means that elevated filling pressures are needed to maintain cardiac output. Elevated filling pressures result in volume overload and right-sided or left-sided congestion, leading to diastolic heart failure. Thus, the most common symptoms are dyspnea (71%), edema (46%), palpitations (33%), fatigue (32%), orthopnea (22%), and chest pain (22%). Most common clinical signs are jugular venous distension (52%), systolic murmur (46%), third heart

sound (27%), pulmonary rales (18%), ascites (15%), and edema (15%).

## Extracardiac Clinical Features

In a patient with suspected restrictive cardiomyopathy, an underlying systemic disorder should always be sought before labeling it as idiopathic. The following tables summarize the symptoms and signs seen in various systemic diseases that can cause restrictive cardiomyopathy (see **Table 60-2** and **60-3**).

# DIAGNOSTIC APPROACH TO RESTRICTIVE CARDIOMYOPATHY

There are two very important steps in the diagnostic approach to a patient with suspected restrictive cardiomyopathy. First, we must rule out constrictive

| Table 60-3 • Clinical Examination and Potential Causes of Restrictive Cardiomyopathy ||
|---|---|
| **Abnormality** | **Potentially Indicates** |
| Skin fibrosis | scleroderma |
| Raynaud's phenomenon | scleroderma |
| Nail dystrophy | amyloidosis |
| Hyperpigmentation | hemochromatosis, POEMS syndrome* |
| Angiokeratoma | Fabry's disease |
| Purpura | multiple myeloma |
| Porokeratosis of Mibelli | primary cardiac amyloidosis |
| Skin infiltrates | multiple myeloma, amyloidosis |
| Yellowish reticulated skin lesions | pseudoxanthoma elasticum |
| Skeletal abnormalities | Gaucher's disease |
| Joint abnormalities | Gaucher's disease, amyloidosis, reactive arthritis |
| Arthritis | hemochromatosis |
| Bronchospasm | Churg-Strauss syndrome, carcinoid |
| Hepatomegaly | amyloidosis, Gaucher's disease |
| Splenomegaly | amyloidosis, Gaucher's disease, POEMS syndrome,* cystinosis |
| Macroglossia | amyloidosis |
| Muscle weakness and wasting | neuromuscular disorders as listed in Table 60-2 |

*POEMS syndrome: polyneuropathy, organomegaly, endocrinopathy, M-protein, skin changes. Reprinted with permission from Stöllberger C, Finsterer J. Extracardiac medical and neuromuscular implications in restrictive cardiomyopathy. Clin. Cardiol. 2007;30:375–380.

pericarditis, since constrictive pericarditis presents with similar symptoms and can be potentially cured by surgery. Second, we must exclude a secondary cause of restrictive cardiomyopathy.

## DIFFERENCES BETWEEN RESTRICTIVE CARDIOMYOPATHY AND CONSTRICTIVE PERICARDITIS

### Clinical Examination

One sign that is classical to constrictive pericarditis is pericardial knock, which occurs before S3 but after an opening snap during the cardiac cycle. In restrictive cardiomyopathy, S4 (early stage) or S3 (late stage) may be present and regurgitant murmurs are more common. However, since most other clinical signs are similar, clinicians have to rely on other diagnostic tests to differentiate between the two conditions.

### Role of Brain Natriuretic Peptide (BNP)

Brain natriuretic peptide is released by ventricular muscle in response to ventricular muscle stretch. Therefore, levels are elevated in most patients with heart failure. In patients with idiopathic constrictive pericarditis, there is external constriction of the heart, rather than a primary abnormality of the myocardium. Therefore, BNP levels are lower in patients with idiopathic constrictive pericarditis compared to patients with restrictive cardiomyopathy. However, BNP levels cannot be used to differentiate secondary constrictive pericarditis and restrictive cardiomyopathy since both the heart and pericardium are diseased in secondary pericarditis. Similarly, utility of BNP levels is limited in patients with coexisting constrictive pericarditis and renal failure.

### Chest X-ray

Calcifications may sometimes be seen in patients with constrictive pericarditis. Since it does not give any information about the pathophysiological abnormality, it is of limited use to the clinician in differentiating these two diseases in the modern era.

### Electrocardiography

In restrictive cardiomyopathy low voltage tracing (amyloidosis), atrial fibrillation or conduction disturbances are common.

### Echocardiography

Echocardiography is the main diagnostic procedure used to differentiate between restrictive cardiomyopathy and constrictive pericarditis since it is noninvasive and less time consuming. Also, various stages of diastolic dysfunction can be characterized. Understanding the pathophysiology of these two diseases is important to interpret the results of echocardiography.

### Pathophysiology

In constrictive pericarditis, due to external constriction of the heart, there is dissociation of pressures within the heart and thoracic cavity during the respiratory cycle. This causes decreased pulmonary diastolic blood flow and decreased left ventricular filling during inspiration, but the total volume of blood entering the heart during the respiratory cycle is unchanged. Therefore, right ventricular filling increases during inspiration and causes the interventricular septum to move to the left. Opposite changes are seen during expiration. In restrictive cardiomyopathy, both ventricular relaxation and compliance are affected and there is no change in ventricular filling during the respiratory cycle.

These physiologic abnormalities can be evaluated by two-dimensional, M-mode, Doppler, and myocardial (tissue Doppler) imaging. The various parameters measured are isovolumic relaxation time (IVRT), mitral inflow and pulmonary venous Doppler flow velocities, tissue Doppler mitral annular velocities, and color M-mode measured mitral inflow propagation velocity (Vp).

## Two-dimensional Echocardiography

The classic feature in restrictive cardiomyopathy is small ventricular cavities and large atria. In amyloidosis, the ventricular walls may be thickened and a "granular sparkling" myocardial texture may be seen. In constrictive pericarditis, the classic findings include pericardial calcification and adhesion, and septal bounce in early diastole. The inferior vena cava is plethoric in both the conditions.

## Color M-mode and Doppler Echocardiography

Flow propagation velocity (Vp) is inversely proportional to time constant of relaxation. Since relaxation is affected in myocardial restriction, Vp is decreased in restrictive cardiomyopathy.

In constrictive pericarditis, there is rapid filling of the ventricles (75%) in the first 25% of diastole. Due to reduced compliance of the heart, there is an abrupt decline in ventricular filling during mid-diastole. Therefore Vp is rapid in constrictive pericarditis during early diastole and a slope of >100 cm/s for the first aliasing contour has a 74% sensitivity and 91% specificity to diagnose constriction and thus differentiate these two conditions.

A >10% variation in early mitral inflow peak velocity during the respiratory cycle has 84% sensitivity and 91% specificity to diagnose constrictive pericarditis. Some patients might not show this variation because of increased left atrial pressure, and various maneuvers that decrease the preload can be used to unmask this variation and help to classify their disease. Also, in restriction, mitral and tricuspid flow velocity decrease during atrial contraction.

Isovolumic relaxation time shows greater than 25% variation with respiration in constriction. Both conditions lead to shortening of mitral and tricuspid deceleration times but there is further shortening with inspiration in patients with restriction. Diastolic mitral and tricuspid regurgitation is also more common in patients with restriction.

A >18% variation in pulmonary venous diastolic flow also diagnoses constriction with a sensitivity of 79% and specificity of 91%. Rapid volume expansion increases this variation more and can further help to differentiate constrictive pericarditis from restrictive cardiomyopathy. Additionally, in restrictive cardiomyopathy there is a decreased pulmonary venous systolic to diastolic blood flow ratio (<0.5).

## Myocardial (Tissue Doppler Imaging)

Mitral annular velocity (E') of >8 cm/s is seen in constrictive pericarditis and it is markedly reduced in restriction. This cut-off value has a sensitivity of 95% and specificity of 96%. It has been shown that combining E' with systolic mitral annular velocity (S') and the time difference between the onset of mitral inflow and onset of E' has higher sensitivity. In patients with no respiratory variation in transmitral velocities, E' can be used to differentiate between these two diseases (see **Figure 60-1** and **60-2**).

## Cardiac Catheterization

If Doppler echocardiography is unable to differentiate, then measuring of intracardiac hemodynamics becomes important. Both the conditions show a characteristic rapid decline and rapid rise of ventricular pressure to a plateau in early diastole (dip and plateau or square-root sign). Left ventricular end diastolic pressure (LVEDP) is often 5 mm Hg greater than right ventricular end diastolic pressure (RVEDP) in restriction. In constriction, RV systolic pressure is <50 mm Hg and RVEDP is greater than one-third of RV systolic pressure. The characteristic respiratory variation in ventricular pressures can also be seen in constrictive pericarditis. Recently, it has been shown that the ratio of right ventricular to left ventricular systolic area during the respiratory cycle accurately differentiates these two diseases.

## CT Scan/MRI (Magnetic Resonance Imaging)

Pericardial thickening of >4 mm in constrictive pericarditis helps to differentiate it from restrictive cardiomyopathy. Real-time cine MRI shows increased ventricular coupling in patients with constriction and thus is helpful in patients with normal thickness of pericardium.

## Endomyocardial Biopsy

In cases where the diagnosis remains unclear, endomyocardial biopsy can be done and it may reveal a specific disease causing restriction. Normal appearing myocytes support the diagnosis of constrictive pericarditis.

## INVESTIGATIONS TO RULE OUT SECONDARY CAUSES OF RESTRICTIVE CARDIOMYOPATHY

Depending on the clinical history and examination, the following investigations can be done to rule out secondary nonfamilial causes of restriction (see **Table 60-4** and **60-5**).

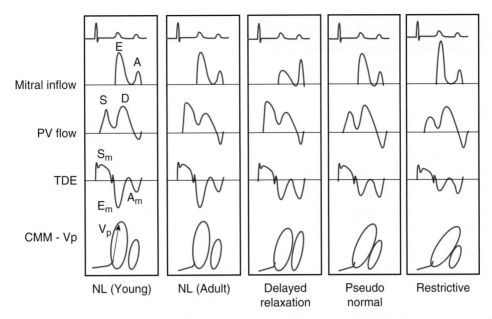

**Figure 60-1.** Stages of diastolic function as assessed by Doppler echocardiography mitral inflow, pulmonary venous flow, tissue Doppler, and color M-mode. Using an integrated approach with these four modalities, the stages of diastolic dysfunction can be determined. A, mitral A-wave velocity; Am, tissue Doppler atrial contraction wave; CMM-vp, color M-mode flow propagation velocity; D, pulmonary venous diastolic wave; E, mitral E-wave velocity; Em, tissue Doppler early filling wave; PV, pulmonary vein; S, pulmonary venous systolic wave; Sm, tissue Doppler systolic wave; TDE, tissue Doppler echocardiography; Vp, color M-mode flow propagation velocity. (Reprinted with permission from Asher CR, Klein AL. Diastolic heart failure: Restrictive cardiomyopathy, constrictive pericarditis, and cardiac tamponade: Clinical and echocardiographic evaluation. *Cardiology in Review*. 2002;10(4):218–229.)

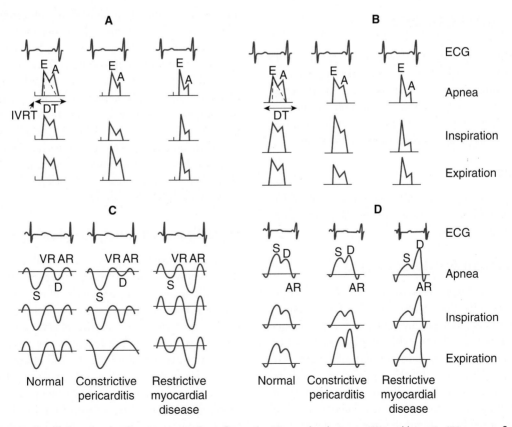

**Figure 60-2.** Diagram of left (A) and right (B) ventricular inflow velocities and pulmonary (C) and hepatic (D) venous flows during different phases of respiration differentiating constrictive pericarditis and restrictive cardiomyopathy as assessed by echocardiography. (Reprinted with permission from Asher CR, Klein AL. Diastolic heart failure: Restrictive cardiomyopathy, constrictive pericarditis, and cardiac tamponade: Clinical and echocardiographic evaluation. *Cardiology in Review*. 2002;10(4):218–229.)

| **Table 60-4 • Investigations in Restrictive Cardiomyopathy** | |
|---|---|
| **Investigation** | **Disease Diagnosed** |
| Transferrin saturation, serum ferritin | hemochromatosis |
| Alpha-galactosidase A levels | Fabry's disease |
| Glucocerebrosidase levels | Gaucher's disease |
| Endomyocardial biopsy | Churg-Strauss syndrome, lymphoma, multiple myeloma, endomyocardial fibrosis, pseudoxanthoma elasticum |
| Biopsy of affected organs | scleroderma, amyloidosis |
| Cystine levels, corneal slit lamp examination | cystinosis |
| Cardiac MRI, nuclear medicine | sarcoidosis |
| Peripheral blood eosinophilia | hypereosinophilic syndrome |
| Urinary 5-HIAA | carcinoid syndrome |

Abbreviations: MRI, magnetic resonance imaging. Reprinted with permission from Stöllberger C, Finsterer J. Extracardiac medical and neuromuscular implications in restrictive cardiomyopathy. Clin. Cardiol. 2007;30:375–380.

# CARDIAC AMYLOIDOSIS

Amyloid is defined as extracellular tissue deposition of insoluble fibrillar proteins, which have a characteristic appearance in an electron microscope, show apple green birefringence under polarizing light microscopy, and have an affinity for Congo red. Multiple organs can be involved in amyloidosis, but involvement of the heart confers a worst prognosis.

## Classification

Cardiac amyloidosis is classified into immunoglobulin (AL), secondary (reactive), hereditary, age related, and hemodialysis-associated amyloidosis.

## Immunoglobulin Amyloidosis (AL)

In immunoglobulin amyloidosis, there is excess production of immunoglobulin light chain protein (AL). This is seen in primary amyloidosis, multiple myeloma, and other plasma cell disorders. It is a rare disease with an incidence of 5.1 to 12.8 per million person-years and accounts for 85% of newly diagnosed amyloidosis cases. In primary amyloidosis, there is clonal proliferation of plasma cells and up to 5 to 10% of plasma cells produce a light chain isotype. Laboratory studies show monoclonal light chains in urine or serum protein electrophoresis with a lambda to kappa ratio of 2:1. Bone marrow biopsy may reveal plasma cell proliferation with excessive light chain staining.

Multiple organ systems are affected in immunoglobulin amyloidosis. The heart is most commonly involved in about 70% of patients. There may be asymptomatic ECG abnormalities before onset of heart failure. Heart failure confers worst prognosis with median survival of 0.75 years. Heart failure symptoms are predominantly of the right side. The most common ECG abnormalities seen are low limb voltage or pseudo infarction pattern. Involvement of the His-Purkinje system is common, leading to prolongation of the infra-His (HV) conduction, which is associated with a high prevalence of sudden death in these patients.

Extracardiac involvement is also common. Fatigue and weakness are the most common symptoms and patients are frequently misdiagnosed with flu when these are presenting symptoms. Carpal tunnel syndrome may be present for years before amyloidosis is diagnosed. Gastrointestinal involvement is common, leading to weight loss and hepatomegaly. Nephrotic syndrome results from involvement of the kidney and macroglossia sufficient to cause problems with breathing, speech, mastication, and deglutition may also be seen.

## Secondary (AA) Amyloidosis

This type results from deposition of serum amyloid A (SAA) protein, an acute phase reactant in response to inflammation. However, due to decreased incidence of chronic infections such as tuberculosis, osteomyelitis, and bronchiectasis, this form is less commonly seen in Western countries. It can still be seen in patients with chronic inflammatory diseases such as rheumatoid arthritis, inflammatory bowel disease, and familial Mediterranean fever. Secondary amyloidosis mostly causes renal disease, with hepatomegaly and/or splenomegaly seen in 10% of patients. Heart involvement is rare and does not lead to any clinically significant heart failure.

## Hereditary (Familial) Amyloidosis

Familial amyloidosis is an autosomal dominant disease that is caused by mutation in either transthyretin (TTR) or apolipoprotein. Transthyretin mutation is much more common than apolipoprotein. Transthyretin is a thyroid binding protein found in the plasma and cerebrospinal fluid. It is primarily produced in the liver and in small amounts in the choroid plexus and retina. The gene for TTR is located on chromosome 18 and to date more than 100 TTR gene mutations have been identified. Out of these, more than 80 have been found to have amyloidogenic properties. The most common mutation causing cardiac disease is methionine-for-valine substitution at position 30 (Val30Met). Other mutations causing significant heart disease include serine-for-isoleucine substitution at

## Table 60-5 • Differences Between Restrictive Cardiomyopathy and Constrictive Pericarditis

| Evaluation Type | Restrictive Cardiomyopathy | Constrictive Pericarditis |
|---|---|---|
| Physical examination | S4 (early disease), S3 (advanced disease), apical impulse may be prominent, regurgitant murmurs common | pericardial knock may be present, apical impulse usually not palpable, regurgitant murmurs uncommon |
| BNP levels | increased | low in primary constrictive pericarditis |
| Chest X-ray | no calcifications | calcification sometimes seen |
| Electrocardiography | low voltage (especially in amyloidosis), pseudoinfarction, left-axis deviation, atrial fibrillation, conduction disturbances common | low voltage (<50%) |
| Two-dimensional echocardiography | small LV cavity with large atria, increased wall thickness sometimes seen (especially thickened interatrial septum in amyloidosis), thickened cardiac valves and granular sparkling texture in amyloidosis | normal wall thickness, pericardial thickening seen, prominent early diastolic filling with abrupt displacement of interventricular septum |
| Mitral inflow | no respiratory variation of mitral inflow, E/A ratio >2 | inspiration decreases mitral inflow and expiration shows opposite changes |
| Pulmonary vein | blunted S/D ratio (0.5), prominent and prolonged AR, no respiratory variation in D wave | S/D ratio = 1, inspiration decreases PV, S and D waves and expiration shows opposite changes |
| Tricuspid inflow | mild respiration variation of tricuspid inflow E wave, E/A ratio >2, TR peak velocity no significant change with respiration | inspiration increases tricuspid inflow E waves and TR peak velocity and expiration shows opposite changes |
| Hepatic vein | blunted S/D ratio, inspiration increases reversal | inspiration = minimal increase in HV, S and D flows, and expiration decreases diastolic flow and increases reversal |
| Color M-mode | slow flow propagation | rapid flow propagation (≥100 cm/s) |
| Mitral annular motion | low velocity early filling (<8 cm/s) | high velocity early filling (≥8 cm/s) |
| Cardiac catheterization | "dip and plateau," LVEDP often >5 mm Hg greater than RVEDP, RV systolic pressure >50 mm Hg, RVEDP < one-third of RV systolic pressure | "dip and plateau," RVEDP and LVEDP usually equal, inspiration increases RV systolic pressure and decreases LV systolic pressure, expiration causes opposite changes |
| Endomyocardial biopsy | may reveal the specific cause | normal or shows nonspecific myocardial fibrosis or hypertrophy |
| CT/MRI | normal pericardium | thickened pericardium |

*Abbreviations: BNP, brain natriuretic peptide; LV, left ventricular; E/A mitral E to A wave ratio; S/D systolic to diastolic flow ratio; A R aortic regurgitation; PV, pulmonary vein; TR tricuspid regurgitation; LVEDP, left ventricular end diastolic pressure; RVEDP, right ventricular end diastolic pressure; CT, computerized axial tomography scan; MRI, magnetic resonance imaging. Reprinted with permission from Asher CR, Klein AL. Diastolic heart failure: Restrictive cardiomyopathy, constrictive pericarditis, and cardiac tamponade: Clinical and echocardiographic evaluation. Cardiology in Review. 2002;10(4):218–229.*

position 84 and alanine-for-threonine substitution at position 60.

Familial amyloidosis with Val30Met mutation was considered to be endemic to certain parts of the world, like Oporto in Portugal, the northern part of Sweden, and Arao and Ogawa in Japan. However, in the past 20 years, this disease has been found in many nonendemic areas with different genetic mutations and phenotypic presentations. Patients with Val30Met mutations from endemic areas tend to be younger at onset of disease and have various conduction abnormalities without significant heart failure. In contrast, patients with Val30Met mutation from nonendemic areas

and with non-Val30Met mutations tend to have the disease at an older age with an increased frequency of heart failure.

Transthyretin familial amyloidosis primarily leads to progressive peripheral and autonomic neuropathy. Patients develop ascending sensory and motor neuropathy and often become wheelchair dependent. Autonomic neuropathy causes impotence, incontinence, orthostatic hypotension, and constipation. In elderly black persons, a unique form is seen without neurologic symptoms. These patients have isoleucine 122 gene mutation of the TTR DNA. However, its phenotypic presentation is variable and the penetration of the disease is not clear.

## Age-related Amyloidosis

Age-related amyloidosis can be divided into senile systemic and isolated atrial amyloidosis.

Senile systemic amyloidosis results from deposition of wild type transthyretin, primarily affecting the heart. It is primarily seen in elderly men and affects almost a quarter of people over the age of 85 years. History of myocardial infarction and variations in the alpha-2-M and tau genes are also associated with this disorder. Heart failure is not as severe and disease course is less progressive than primary amyloidosis. However, the failure to recognize the disease early in the course can lead to clinically significant heart failure.

Isolated atrial amyloidosis in contrast is seen more commonly in elderly females. It occurs due to deposition of atrial natriuretic peptide, released by atria as a result of increased wall stretch. Therefore, it can also be seen in patients with valvular heart disease and atrial fibrillation.

However, it does not lead to any clinically significant heart disease.

## Hemodialysis-related Amyloidosis

B-2 microglobulin accumulates in chronic renal failure patients when dialysis cannot effectively clear it. The deposits are primarily in the joint with minimal involvement of the heart. Renal transplantation helps decrease the deposits, thus improving the joint pain (See **Table 60-6**).

## Pathophysiology and Clinical Manifestations

Of the different subtypes of amyloidosis mentioned above, only primary, hereditary, and senile amyloidosis cause significant cardiac involvement and, thus, heart failure. Thus, the clinical findings in amyloidosis include dilated or restrictive cardiomyopathy, congestive heart failure, coronary insufficiency, valvular dysfunction, pericardial tamponade,

### Table 60-6 • Classification of Cardiac Amyloidosis

| | Amyloidosis Type | | | | | |
| | Primary | Hereditary (ATTR) | Senile Systemic (ATTR) | Isolated Atrial Amyloidosis | Reactive (AA) | Dialysis-related (B-2 Microglobulin) |
|---|---|---|---|---|---|---|
| Protein | Light chain | Mutant TTR | TTR | Atrial natriuretic factor | Amyloid A | B-2 microglobulin |
| Cardiac Involvement | 22–34% | Variable | Common | Limited to heart | < 10% | Unknown, asymptomatic |
| Median Survival, mo. | 13 (4 mo if heart failure present at diagnosis) | 70 | 75 | — | 24.5% | — |
| Extracardiac Manifestations | Renal failure, proteinuria, autonomic dysfunction, macroglossia, purpura, neuropathy, carpal tunnel syndrome | Severe neuropathy, autonomic dysfunction, renal failure, blindness | Diffuse organ involvement | None | Renal failure, proteinuria, hepatomegaly associated with chronic inflammatory conditions | Arthralgias, carpal tunnel syndrome, arthropathies, bone cyst, pathologic fractures |
| Diagnostic Testing | SPEP, UPEP, bone marrow biopsy tissue analysis revealing plasma cell dyscrasia, kappa and lambda chain antiserum staining | ATTR antiserum staining, serum TTR isoelectric focusing, restriction fragment length polymorphism analysis | TTR and serum staining | Atrial natriuretic factor antiserum staining | Target organ biopsy specimen analysis, AA antiserum staining | Synovial and bone specimen analysis, B-2 microglobulin antiserum, serum B-2 microglobulin concentration |

*SPEP, serum protein electrophoresis; TTR, transthyretin; UPEP, urine protein electrophoresis.*

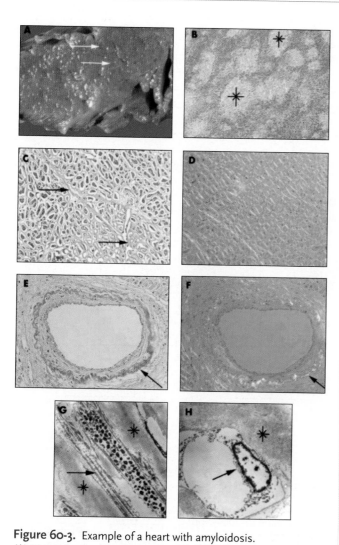

**Figure 60-3.** Example of a heart with amyloidosis.
(A) Macroscopic view showing nodules with amyloid (arrows).
(B) Microscopic view showing eosinophilic areas containing amyloid (asterisks); original magnification, × 100. (C) Microscopic view showing eosinophilic bands, containing amyloid, around individual cardiomyocytes (arrows); original magnification, × 100.
(D) Microscopic view (same figure as C) showing apple green birefringence under polarized light; original magnification, × 100.
(E) An intramyocardial artery showing Congo red stained amyloid (arrow); original magnification, × 400. (F) An intramyocardial artery (same figure as E) showing apple green birefringence under polarized light; original magnification, × 400. (G) Amyloidosis is characterized by the deposition of fine fibrillar material (asterisk) in and around cardiomyocytes (arrow); original magnification, × 10,000. (H) Amyloidosis is characterized by the deposition of fine fibrillar material (asterisk) around small vessels; arrow, endothelial cell; original magnification, × 15,000. (Reprinted with permission from Kholová I, Niessen HWM. Amyloid in the cardiovascular system: A review. *J Clin Pathol.* 2005;58:125–133. doi:10.1136/jcp.2004.017293)

increased sensitivity to digitalis, and atrial thrombosis and embolization (see **Figure 60-3**).

Diagnosis and management of cardiac amyloidosis can be summarized as follows (see **Figure 60-4**):

# ENDOMYOCARDIAL FIBROSIS (EMF)

Endomyocardial fibrosis is primarily a disease of the tropics, although cases have been reported out of these regions. However, it is still mostly found in sub-Saharan Africa. Uganda particularly has a high prevalence of this disease, where it shows a bimodal peak at age 10 and 30 with adult EMF affecting women twice as much as men. EMF has been frequently compared to Loeffler's endocarditis, which is seen primarily in the temperate regions.

Various theories have been proposed for the pathophysiology of endomyocardial fibrosis. The most prominent one is the eosinophil hypothesis. It has been suggested that parasitic infections in these regions cause eosinophilia and subsequent cardiac damage occurs due to various toxins released by the eosinophils. However, the similarities between the fibrotic stage of Loeffler's endocarditis and EMF as well as the mismatch between the geography of EMF and the prevalence of parasite-induced eosinophilia have raised questions for this hypothesis.

The main pathology in EMF is fibrosis of the endocardium and, to a lesser extent, of the inflow tract and apex of ventricular myocardium in one or both of the ventricles. This results in endocardial rigidity, atrial regurgitation, and restriction to diastolic filling of the ventricles. There is characteristic enlargement of the atria with normal sized ventricles. The characteristic echocardiographic appearance is obliteration of the apex of the involved ventricle and grossly dilated atria. There is also thickening of the posterior left ventricular wall in patients with left heart involvement and thickening of the anterior interventricular septum in patients with right sided involvement. Ventriculography also shows the obliteration of the apical region and, along with echocardiography, helps in establishing the diagnosis. Therefore, endomyocardial biopsy is not essential for diagnosis.

Prognosis for EMF is poor and most patients die within 2 years of diagnosis. Patients typically have an insidious onset of the disease, which gradually progresses to heart failure. Atrial fibrillation can be seen in patients with right ventricular disease. Other ECG findings include low QRS voltage, first-degree heart block, and atrial enlargement.

# OTHER INFILTRATIVE DISORDERS

Fabry's disease is an X-linked disease that causes deficiency of the enzyme ceramide trihexosidase in the lysosomes. As a result, there is deposition of a glycolipid in many different tissues throughout the body, including the heart. The disease has complete phenotypic presentation in males and incomplete phenotypic appearance in females.

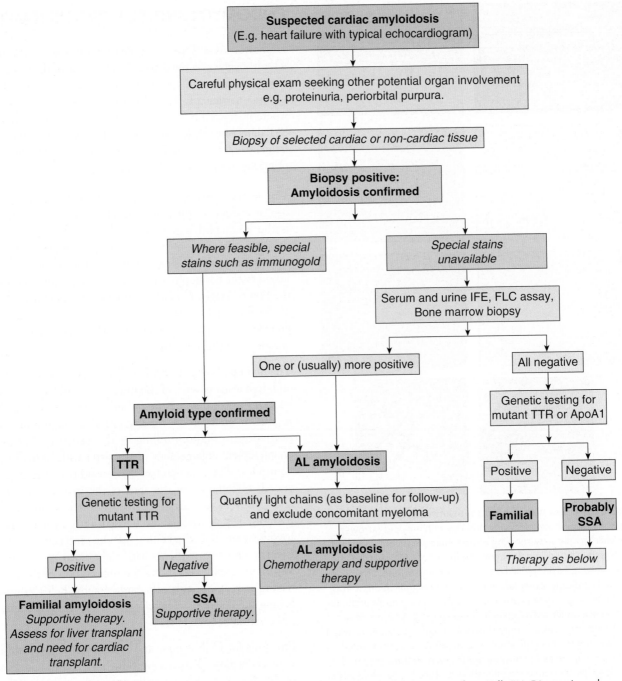

**Figure 60-4.** Diagnosis and management of cardiac amyloidosis. (Reprinted with permission from Falk RH. Diagnosis and management of the cardiac amyloidoses. *Circulation.* 2005;112:2047–2060.)

Sarcoidosis can also affect the heart, primarily causing interstitial inflammation. This leads to diastolic dysfunction and restrictive cardiomyopathy. With progression of the disease, there is fibrosis of the myocardium causing systolic dysfunction. The course of the disease is variable with many patients having subclinical diastolic dysfunction, while rarely some patients might show an acute presentation with sudden death or high-degree heart block. Myocardial imaging (thallium-201 or gallium-67) may show areas of myocardial involvement. Endomyocardial biopsy is also useful in the diagnosis of sarcoidosis, however, a negative biopsy doesn't necessarily rule out the diagnosis.

In carcinoid syndrome, high circulating levels of 5-hydroxyindoleacetic acid lead to proliferation of fibroblasts and formation of fibrous plaques. These plaques are found mainly over the tricuspid and pulmonary valves and the right ventricular endocardium. This can lead to tricuspid regurgitation, which is the predominant finding in carcinoid heart disease.

# TREATMENT OF RESTRICTIVE CARDIOMYOPATHY

## Symptomatic Therapy

Diuretics are the mainstay of treatment to relieve the symptoms of heart failure. However, excessive diuresis can cause hypotension and should be avoided. Any associated arrhythmia should be promptly and adequately treated as atrial contraction is important for ventricular filling. Therefore, sinus rhythm should be maintained. Amiodarone can be used, or in advanced conduction system disease, a pacemaker can be implanted. When a patient with cardiac sarcoidosis presents with life-threatening ventricular arrhythmia, an automatic implantable defibrillator can be used. Patients with restrictive cardiomyopathy, especially those having atrial fibrillation, valvular regurgitation, or low cardiac output, are at increased risk of atrial thrombus formation and embolization. These patients should receive anticoagulation with warfarin. In severe cardiac amyloidosis, there might be thrombus formation even in the presence of normal sinus rhythm and it is prudent to anticoagulate in such patients.

## Specific Therapy

### Amyloidosis

For symptomatic therapy, digoxin should be avoided as it binds to amyloid fibrils and leads to toxic side effects. Similarly, negative inotropic agents like calcium channel blockers and ACE inhibitors should be avoided as these patients often have autonomic dysfunction and orthostatic hypotension.

Definitive treatment for AL amyloidosis is oral chemotherapy with melphalan to stop plasma cell production of the amyloid paraproteins. However, treatment benefit is limited as most patients have extensive involvement of the heart at the time of diagnosis. This increases the peritreatment mortality rates. Patients with normal ejection fraction, absence of heart failure, and minimal involvement of other organ systems benefit the most from treatment. In such patients, combined treatment with high dose melphalan and bone marrow transplantation has shown to improve survival and quality of life. A limited number of patients with no significant extracardiac disease have been successfully treated with a combination of melphalan, bone marrow transplant, and heart transplant.

Hereditary amyloidosis can be treated by liver transplantation as the mutant TTR protein is produced by the liver. Liver transplantation in these patients has a good success rate with 5-year survival rates reported to be 60-77%. However, these benefits are limited in patients with minimal involvement of the heart. In selected cases with extensive myocardial involvement, combined heart and liver transplantation has been found to be successful. Senile systemic amyloidosis has a very good prognosis and responds well to symptomatic management of heart failure.

### Endomyocardial Fibrosis

This disease can be successfully treated with cardiac surgery. Surgical therapy consists of excision of the fibrotic endocardium with or without replacement of the mitral and/or tricuspid valves. A 10-year survival rate with this treatment has been found to be approximately 70%.

Treatment of other disorders causing restrictive cardiomyopathy can be summarized as follows:

## Suggested Readings

1. Kushwaha SS, Fallon JT, Fuster V. Restrictive cardiomyopathy. *N Engl J Med.* 1997;336:267–276.

2. Ha J-W, Ommen SR, Tajik AJ, et al. Differentiation of constrictive pericarditis from restrictive cardiomyopathy using mitral annular velocity by tissue Doppler echocardiography. *Am J Cardiol.* 2004;94:316–319.

3. Francone M, Dymarkowski S, Kalantzi M, Rademakers FE, Bogaert J. Assessment of ventricular coupling with real-time cine MRI and its value to differentiate constrictive pericarditis from restrictive cardiomyopathy. *Eur Radiol.* 2006;16:944–951.

4. Shah KB, Inoue Y, Mehra MR. Amyloidosis and the heart: A comprehensive review. *Arch Intern Med.* 2006;166:1805–1813.

5. Falk RH. Diagnosis and management of the cardiac amyloidoses. *Circulation.* 2005;112:2047–2060.

# 61

# Devices for Heart Failure

AYESHA HASAN

## ● PRACTICAL POINTS

- Improved survival has been shown with both implantable cardioverter defibrillator (ICD) and cardiac resynchronization therapy (CRT), alone or in combination, in symptomatic heart failure patients.

- The MADIT trials established the mortality benefit of prophylactic ICD therapy in ischemic heart failure with risk stratification based on the presence of coronary artery disease and ejection fraction.

- SCD-HeFT is a landmark clinical trial demonstrating that ICD prophylaxis was effective in the primary prevention of mortality, regardless of ischemic or nonischemic etiology of heart failure.

- Concerning medical therapy for suppression of ventricular arrhythmias, SCD-HeFT also confirmed that the use of amiodarone does not improve survival when used for suppression of ventricular arrhythmias in this patient population.

- The current ACC/AHA/HRS 2008 recommendations for primary prevention ICD include an ejection fraction less than or equal to 35% for patients with symptomatic heart failure (NYHA Class II and III) and either ischemic (greater than 40 days out from a myocardial infarction) or nonischemic disease.

- Current recommendations also include NYHA Class I patients with ischemic disease with an ejection fraction less than or equal to 30% (based on MADIT II inclusion criteria).

- Current CRT indications are based on QRS duration from the landmark CRT trials; use of dyssynchrony studies in narrow QRS patients is not part of guidelines at this time.

## INTRODUCTION

Device therapy has been well established as the standard of care in appropriate patients in the chronic heart failure population. In fact, device therapy, in addition to pharmacologic therapy, is now considered evidence-based treatment in these patients, supported by numerous clinical trials. Improved survival has been shown with both implantable cardioverter-defibrillator (ICD) and cardiac resynchronization therapy (CRT), alone or in combination, in symptomatic heart failure patients. Although almost half of heart failure mortality is associated with ventricular tachyarrhythmias, mortality in advanced clinical disease (New York Heart Association, NYHA Class III and IV) results more often from worsening heart failure. The survival benefit

associated with CRT alone is attributed partly to synchronization of ventricular dyssynchrony through simultaneous pacing of the right and left ventricles, thereby improving the pump function of the heart. CRT also improves symptoms [in terms of functional class, 6-minute hall walk (6MW), and quality of life (QOL)] in refractory heart failure, all of which have been primary endpoints of early CRT trials.

The use of these strategies is now driven by guideline statements, issued by the American College of Cardiology (ACC), American Heart Association (AHA), Heart Failure Society of America (HFSA), European Society of Cardiology (ESC), and the Heart Rhythm Society (HRS, formerly the North American Society for Pacing and Electrophysiology). With increasing studies and available literature, ICD and

CRT indications have changed and will inevitably continue to expand as the field advances. Updated guidelines from major societies regarding appropriate use of such devices in heart failure management will be reviewed in this chapter with an emphasis on the recent ACC/AHA/HRS 2008 joint statement, along with highlights from the landmark clinical trials. Focus will be on Class I and Class III indications, along with reviewing randomized trial data, as this represents material that will be tested on the cardiovascular board examination.

# DEFIBRILLATORS IN CHRONIC HEART FAILURE

As we gain experience with device therapy in chronic heart failure, we are improving the process of risk stratifying appropriate candidates for "primary" implantable defibrillator therapy or those who are at risk of ventricular arrhythmias. Therefore, ICDs in these patients are considered primary prevention devices, compared to "secondary" prevention, when ICDs are implanted in those who have survived a cardiac arrest or had documented sustained ventricular tachycardia or syncope of unknown etiology in the setting of systolic dysfunction. The term *sudden cardiac death* (SCD) refers to a cardiac cause that results in death soon after the onset of symptoms. Despite advances in the prevention of SCD, it remains a major cause of mortality, which is especially the case in chronic heart failure. Guidelines have been endorsed by the major international societies, such as the American College of Cardiology, American Heart Association, European Society of Cardiology, and the Heart Rhythm Society; as new data surface, a joint statement was issued from the ACC, AHA, and HRS in 2008 reviewing the available trial data and ongoing issues regarding management of ventricular arrhythmias and preventing sudden cardiac death in this patient population. For practical purposes, this chapter will focus on this recent guideline statement, rather than comparing it to the earlier 2005 ACC/AHA and 2006 HFSA Practice Guideline statements.

The first successful ICD implant was in the 1970s, and the technology continues to advance. Current devices are capable of improved arrhythmia discrimination, "painless" therapy with antitachycardia pacing for ventricular arrhythmias, low energy cardioversion, high energy defibrillation, and bradycardia pacing. The majority of devices are implanted in the pectoral area, in a subcutaneous or submuscular position, with venous access obtained through the subclavian or axillary veins (**Figure 61-1**).

## Review of Clinical Trials

Early ICD mortality trials compared device therapy to antiarrhythmic drug therapy with amiodarone or sotalol in a

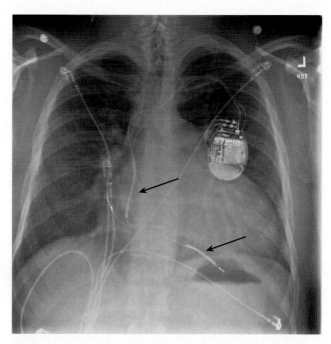

**Figure 61-1.** Chest radiograph of a dual chamber defibrillator system implanted for primary prevention in a patient with dilated cardiomyopathy. Right ventricular lead is a dual coil lead placed in the apex. Arrows mark the proximal (or superior vena cava coil) and distal coils. (*Chest radiograph obtained from the Ohio State University Medical Center.*)

high risk patient population, patients who either had documented ventricular arrhythmias or cardiac arrest or were post-myocardial infarction without advanced heart failure. Subsequent trials focused on primary prevention in the heart failure population, initially in those with documented ventricular arrhythmias and later based on ejection fraction as risk stratification. Details of the individual clinical trials can be found in **Table 61-1**, which summarizes the inclusion criteria, primary endpoint, and results.

### MADIT Clinical Trials: MADIT I and II

The Multicenter Automatic Defibrillator Trials (MADIT) evaluated prophylactic use of an ICD as primary prevention in high risk patients with coronary artery disease. The first study, MADIT I, enrolled patients who had documented ventricular arrhythmias, a history of asymptomatic nonsustained ventricular tachycardia (from 3 to 30 beats), and inducible, nonsuppressible sustained ventricular tachycardia on electrophysiology (EP) study. Patients had NYHA Class I-III heart failure, had an ejection fraction less than or equal to 35%, and were greater than 3 weeks post-myocardial infarction. Patients were treated with conventional medical therapy, which included antiarrhythmics at the physician's discretion (usually amiodarone), or were assigned to an ICD in addition to conventional medical therapy. The study was small with 196 patients; a large survival benefit was noted in the ICD group of 54% (HR 0.46, 95% CI

## Table 61-1 • Summary of Clinical Trials of ICD Therapy in Chronic Heart Failure

| Clinical Trial | N | Inclusion | Control/ Treatment Group | Primary Endpoint | Results |
|---|---|---|---|---|---|
| MADIT I | 196 | NYHA Class I-III, remote MI, EF ≤35%, history of documented VT[†] | medical therapy/ ICD | all-cause mortality | 54% relative reduction with ICD* |
| MADIT II | 1232 | NYHA Class I-III, remote MI, EF ≤30% | medical therapy/ ICD | all-cause mortality | 31% relative reduction with ICD* |
| DEFINITE | 488 | NYHA Class I-III, dilated cardiomyopathy, EF ≤35%, history of documented VT[§] | medical therapy/ ICD | all-cause mortality | 35% relative reduction with ICD (NS) |
| SCD-HeFT | 2520 | NYHA Class II-III, history of CAD or dilated cardiomyopathy, EF ≤35% | medical therapy/ ICD | all-cause mortality | 23% relative reduction with ICD* |

*Significant p value <0.05.
[†]NSVT and nonsuppressible inducible VT on EPS.
[§]NSVT or ≥10 PVCs/hr.
*Abbreviations:* NYHA, New York Heart Association; MI, myocardial infarction; EF, ejection fraction; VT, ventricular tachycardia; ICD, implantable cardioverter defibrillator; NS, nonsignificant; CAD, coronary artery disease; NSVT, nonsustained ventricular tachycardia; PVC, premature ventricular contraction.

0.26-0.82, $p = 0.009$). Subgroup analysis revealed that ICD prophylaxis in higher risk heart failure patients (defined as an ejection fraction <26%, heart failure requiring therapy, and QRS ≥120 ms) independently predicted improved survival, with survival benefit proportional to the number of risk factors. A concern regarding this trial involves the inclusion criteria of sustained ventricular tachycardia during EP study that was not suppressible by procainamide, questioning whether patients in the drug therapy arm were likely to respond to pharmacologic therapy. This limitation was addressed in MADIT II with enrollment of a lower risk heart failure population.

MADIT II was a much larger trial, enrolling 1,232 patients, and did not require a history of documented ventricular tachyarrhythmias or EP study. Risk stratification was based on a more stringent ejection fraction criteria of 30% or less (compared to 35% in MADIT I) and the presence of coronary artery disease with patients at least 40 days post-myocardial infarction. The ICD group was compared to a control group of conventional medical therapy, with similar percentages of patients taking standard medical therapy in both groups, at the last follow-up visit. A large benefit from ICD therapy was found and resulted in early termination of the study. A 31% reduction in all-cause mortality was noted in the ICD group ($p = 0.016$), attributed to a reduction in sudden cardiac death. Sudden cardiac death occurred in 10% of the conventional medical therapy group compared to 3.8% of the ICD group ($p < 0.01$).

Post-hoc analysis of MADIT II results evaluated the influence of the length of time from myocardial infarction to device implant on the observed survival benefit. The mortality benefit after ICD prophylaxis was not seen until 9 *months* post-device implantation, suggesting that ICD therapy

might not be effective early after a myocardial infarction. There was also a trend toward an increased incidence of heart failure hospitalization in the ICD group, possibly related to detrimental effects of right ventricular pacing or ICD shocks on the myocardium. The MADIT trials established the mortality benefit of prophylactic ICD therapy in ischemic heart failure with risk stratification based on the presence of coronary artery disease and ejection fraction.

### Definite

The Defibrillators in Nonischemic Cardiomyopathy Treatment Evaluation (DEFINITE) was designed to investigate the role of primary prevention ICD in patients with a nonischemic etiology of heart failure. The ejection fraction cut-off for this trial was slightly higher than in MADIT II at less than or equal to 35%, and patients were required to have ambient arrhythmias (frequent premature ventricular contractions or nonsustained ventricular tachycardia). Although ICD prophylaxis resulted in significantly reduced arrhythmic death and a trend toward reduction in the primary endpoint of all-cause mortality, the study was underpowered with a lower than expected mortality rate of 14.1% in the control arm of conventional medical therapy. The inclusion of Class I patients, constituting 22% of total enrolled patients, might also have contributed to the lower than expected mortality rate.

### SCD-HeFT

The Sudden Cardiac Death Heart Failure Trial enrolled both ischemic and nonischemic heart failure patients, NYHA Class II or III, with an ejection fraction less than or equal to 35%. This was a large trial enrolling 2,520 patients, randomized to one of three groups: conventional medical therapy in all groups plus placebo, amiodarone, or an ICD. It was designed to address not only the role of ICD therapy but also the effect of amiodarone on heart failure mortality. By enrolling 52% ischemic and 48% nonischemic patients, the study also expanded on questions remaining from the DEFINITE trial, regarding the use of ICD as primary prevention in nonischemic patients. During 60 months of follow-up, there was no difference in the primary endpoint of all-cause mortality with the addition of amiodarone to standard medical therapy. However, implant of an ICD produced a significant 23% relative risk reduction and 7.2% absolute risk reduction in all-cause mortality at 5 years, compared to the control of optimal medical therapy. The study is a landmark clinical trial as it demonstrated that ICD prophylaxis was effective in the primary prevention of mortality, regardless of ischemic or nonischemic etiology of heart failure. It also confirmed that the use of amiodarone to suppress ventricular arrhythmias does not improve survival in this patient population.

## CABG-Patch Trial and DINAMIT

The previously discussed trials excluded patients who had recent coronary artery bypass surgery or recent myocardial infarction (MI). The CABG-Patch Trial and DINAMIT studies enrolled such patients in order to study the effect of timing on ICD benefit. The Coronary Artery Bypass Graft Patch (CABG-Patch) Trial compared prophylactic ICD at the time of coronary artery bypass surgery to standard medical therapy in patients with an ejection less than 35%. No significant reduction in mortality was observed with ICD therapy. Similarly, no survival benefit was noted in The Defibrillators in Acute Myocardial Infarction Trial (DINAMIT) when prophylactic ICD was implanted in patients who had a recent myocardial infarction (<40 days post-MI). Although negative studies, these trials are important as they have contributed to our current guideline criteria, where we exclude patients as primary prevention candidates until they are 40 days status post-myocardial

infarction and have had time to document an improvement in systolic function after revascularization procedures.

## Indications for Primary Prevention Devices

Previous guidelines for ICD therapy in heart failure were based on ACC/AHA recommendations from 2005. Several studies have been published since the latest statement; therefore, updated joint recommendations were published in 2008, ACC/AHA/HRS Guidelines for Device-Based Therapy: Executive Summary. Standard ACC/AHA definitions of the level of evidence and categorization of that evidence are listed in **Table 61-2**.

ACC/AHA 2005 guidelines acknowledge the risk of SCD in heart failure and recommend an ICD as primary prevention in symptomatic patients with an ejection fraction of less than or equal to 30% and either ischemic or nonischemic causes of systolic dysfunction. However, controversy developed regarding candidacy in these same patients with an ejection fraction between 31% and 35%, resulting from the different ejection fraction criteria in the primary prevention studies: MADIT II and SCD-HeFT. MADIT II studied patients with a history of a myocardial infarction at least 1 month prior to enrollment and an ejection fraction less than or equal to 30%; symptomatic heart failure was not a requirement for enrollment. Conversely, SCD-HeFT enrolled patients with symptoms (NYHA Class II or III heart failure) and had a higher ejection fraction criterion, less than or equal to 35%. The latest ACC/AHA/HRS guidelines on device-based therapy from 2008 updated ejection fraction criteria from the 2005 guidelines. The current recommendations have expanded Class I indications for primary prevention to now include an ejection fraction less than or equal to 35% for patients with symptomatic heart failure (NYHA Class II and III) and

---

| **Table 61-2 • ACC/AHA Classification of Recommendations and Level of Evidence** | | |
|---|---|---|
| **Classification** | | |
| Class I | condition for which there is evidence and/or general agreement that a given procedure or treatment is beneficial, useful, and effective | procedure/treatment should be performed |
| Class II | condition for which there is conflicting evidence and/or divergence of opinion about the usefulness/efficacy of a procedure/treatment | |
| Class IIa | weight of evidence/opinion is in favor of usefulness/efficacy | procedure/treatment is reasonable to perform |
| Class IIb | usefulness/efficacy is less well established by evidence/opinion | procedure/treatment may be considered |
| Class III | conditions for which there is evidence and/or general agreement that a procedure is not useful/effective and in some cases may be harmful | procedure/treatment should not be performed since it is not helpful and may be harmful |
| **Level of evidence** | | |
| A | Data derived from multiple randomized clinical trials or meta-analysis | |
| B | Data derived from a single randomized trial or nonrandomized studies | |
| C | Only consensus opinion of experts, case studies, or standard of care | |

*either ischemic or nonischemic disease.* A history of ischemic heart disease still includes those who are greater than 40 days out from a myocardial infarction and all candidates should be on chronic optimal medical therapy and have a reasonable expectation of survival with a good functional capacity for more than 1 year. Current recommendations also include NYHA Class I patients with ischemic disease with an ejection fraction less than or equal to 30% (based on MADIT II inclusion criteria). However, similar patients with nonischemic etiology do not have a Class I indication for prophylactic ICD therapy as SCD-HeFT did not include this functional class of patients. (Refer to **Table 61-3** for details on primary and secondary prevention indications.)

Concerning secondary prevention with ICD implantation, all guideline statements endorse the use of an ICD after an event of ventricular fibrillation, hemodynamically unstable ventricular tachycardia, or resuscitated cardiac arrest. **Table 61-3** reviews indications for ICD implantation in heart failure patients who have had ventricular tachyarrhythmias.

Electrophysiology study is reasonable in patients with left ventricular dysfunction (EF < 40%) secondary to coronary artery disease who present with nonsustained ventricular arrhythmias for risk stratification of SCD; however, it is not as informative in nonischemic heart disease due to low inducibility and poor replication of results.

In addition to reviewing indications for ICD implantation in chronic heart failure, it is also crucial to be familiar with contraindications in this patient population. Guidelines all clearly state that ICD implantation is not indicated in chronic, severe refractory heart failure where a reasonable life expectancy or expectation of improvement does not exist based on end-stage heart failure or comorbidities. Most of the landmark primary prevention trials excluded NYHA Class IV patients, with the exception of the Cardiac-Resynchronization Therapy With or Without an Implantable Defibrillator in Advanced Chronic Heart Failure (COMPANION) trial, which enrolled some Class IV patients. Current evidence did not include and therefore cannot be applied to this heart failure population.

| Table 61-3 • Recommendations for ICD Therapy in Chronic Heart Failure Based on ACC/AHA/HRS 2008 Guidelines | |
|---|---|
| **Recommendation** | **Level of Evidence** |
| **Class I (agreement on the benefit of ICD therapy)** | |
| 1. Patients with LVEF less than or equal to 35% due to a MI who are at least 40 days post-MI and are in NYHA functional Class II or III | A |
| 2. Patients with LVEF less than or equal to 35% with nonischemic dilated cardiomyopathy who are in NYHA functional Class II or III | B |
| 3. Patients with LV dysfunction due to prior MI with an LVEF less than or equal to 30% who are in NYHA Class I | A |
| 4. Patients with structural heart disease and spontaneous sustained VT, regardless if hemodynamically stable or unstable | B |
| 5. Patients with NSVT with prior MI, LVEF less than 40%, and inducible VF or sustained VT during EPS | B |
| **Class IIa (weight of evidence is in favor of usefulness of ICD therapy)** | |
| Patients with unexplained syncope, significant LV dysfunction, and nonischemic dilated cardiomyopathy | C |
| **Class IIb (efficacy of ICD is less well established)** | |
| Patients with nonischemic heart disease who have an LVEF less than or equal to 35% who are in NYHA functional Class I | C |
| **Class III (agreement that an ICD is not effective and may be harmful)** | |
| 1. Patients who do not have a reasonable expectation of survival with an acceptable functional status for at least 1 year, even if they meet specific ICD criteria specified in the Class I, IIa, and IIb recommendations listed above | C |
| 2. Incessant VT or VF | C |
| 3. NYHA functional Class IV patients with drug-refractory heart failure who are not candidates for heart transplantation or implantation of a CRT device | C |
| 4. Patients with significant psychiatric illnesses that may be aggravated by device implantation or may preclude follow-up | C |
| 5. Syncope of undetermined etiology without inducible VT or VF and without structural heart disease | C |
| 6. Ventricular tachyarrhythmias due to a completely reversible disorder in the absence of structural heart disease (e.g., electrolytes, drug, trauma) | B |

*Abbreviations: ICD, implantable cardioverter defibrillator; LVEF, left ventricular ejection fraction; MI, myocardial infarction; NYHA, New York Heart Association; LV, left ventricular; VT, ventricular tachycardia; NSVT, nonsustained ventricular tachycardia; VF, ventricular fibrillation; CRT, cardiac resynchronization therapy.*

## Other Issues Involving Defibrillator Therapy

The cost of a defibrillator implant along with follow-up (device interrogation, changeout of generator when the battery wears, lead revisions, etc.) is not inexpensive. Recommendations on such an intervention are based on the cost efficacy, meaning that the health benefits support the procedure. A combined CRT-ICD device costs around $30,000 in the United States, with additional costs from follow-up and repeat procedures for complications or generator change. Appropriate device candidates based on clinical trials have an estimated cost benefit per quality-adjusted life year of $34,900 in MADIT and $70,200 in SCD-HeFT.

Complications from a defibrillator implant include bleeding, infection, pneumothorax or hemothorax as a result of intravenous access, transient heart block from placing leads (usually in the setting of a left bundle branch block), perforation resulting in tamponade (from perforation of the myocardium or coronary sinus in a CRT implant), or arrhythmias such as ventricular tachycardia or supraventricular tachycardia from lead placement. Patients may require reoperation due to delayed perforation, noncapture from leads due to micro- or macro-dislodgement, and infection requiring extraction (from endocarditis, pocket infection, or erosion). Complications may also arise from conscious sedation resulting in hypoxia or defibrillation threshold testing after device implant. With the latter, patients may experience high thresholds requiring external rescue from induced ventricular fibrillation (VF), and induction of VF might not be well tolerated in advanced heart failure patients. Testing is usually not recommended in patients with critical aortic stenosis for this reason.

A concern with ICD therapy based on current guidelines is that many patients who meet criteria are lower risk and do not have lethal tachyarrhythmias. In fact, estimates of appropriate ICD therapies range from one-third to two-thirds of all ICD events in the first few years after implantation. This has led to controversy regarding the issue of risk assessment in these patients. Wider QRS complex has been associated with a higher cardiovascular risk in heart failure patients; on the other hand, some clinical trial data have not shown that QRS duration alone reliably predicts this mortality risk. Noninvasive testing with T wave alternans may be beneficial but is not well established with supportive data at this time.

## CARDIAC RESYNCHRONIZATION THERAPY

Cardiac resynchronization therapy is now a well-established treatment in chronic heart failure patients with moderate to severe symptoms, refractory to pharmacologic therapy. Lead

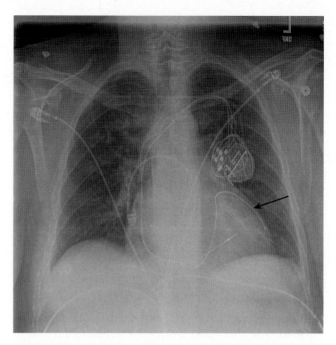

**Figure 61-2.** Chest radiograph of a cardiac resynchronization therapy system implanted in a patient with dilated cardiomyopathy. This is a pacing system only, as the right ventricular lead is not a defibrillator lead; it is also positioned on the septum. Arrow marks the left ventricular lead, which is in a lateral branch of the coronary sinus and is located on the epicardial surface of the heart. (*Chest radiograph obtained from the Ohio State University Medical Center.*)

placement is similar to dual chamber pacemakers and defibrillators, with the addition of a left ventricular (LV) lead. This lead is still implanted from the right sided chambers, with cannulation of the coronary sinus and placement of the LV lead in a lateral or posterior branch along the epicardial surface of the ventricle, opposed to the endocardial placement of the right ventricular (RV) and right atrial (RA) leads (**Figures 61-2 and 61-3**). Ideal placement is obtained with achievement of appropriate pacing thresholds, stable lead position, and avoidance of diaphragmatic stimulation. The concept behind biventricular pacing involves "resynchronization" of a dyssynchronous ventricular contraction. In a typical left bundle branch block or wide QRS, there is impaired contraction, related to delay in interventricular (between the right and left ventricles) and intraventricular (within the LV segments) timing. The end result is a dyssynchronous contraction and impaired cardiac output from reduced ventricular filling, prolonged mitral regurgitation (MR), and reduced LV dP/dt. Currently, we consider this dyssynchronous contraction as represented by the QRS width on ECG (or an electrical conduction delay); in fact, prolongation of QRS greater than 120 ms has been shown to be a significant predictor of LV systolic dysfunction and mortality in patients with heart failure. However, more evidence is emerging regarding mechanical dyssynchrony

# 62

# Hypertrophic Cardiomyopathy

Calum A. MacRae

## ● PRACTICAL POINTS

- The pathology of HCM is characterized hypertrophy of individual myocytes and extensive sarcomere disarray.

- The majority of inherited cases of HCM exhibit autosomal dominant transmission, but penetrance is variable and skipped generations are present.

- Molecular genetic studies have identified genes encoding sarcomeric contractile proteins as the causal mutation in the majority of cases.

- Symptoms: syncope, often with exercise or post exertion, atypical chest pain, exertional dyspnea, palpitations, asymptomatic.

- Physical exam findings: Bisferiens-type pulse, palpable S4, hyperdynamic apical impulse, dynamic (with maneuvers) outflow tract murmur with preserved A2, mitral regurgitation.

- LV outflow tract obstruction results from systolic anterior motion of the mitral valve apparatus as the anterior leaflet of the mitral valve is pulled into apposition with the septum by a Venturi effect.

- Prognosis of HCM is based on the risk of sudden cardiac death.

- High risk features requiring ICD: family history of sudden death, NSVT on 48-hour Holter, recurrent syncope, exertional syncope or exertional hypotension, severe LVH (>30 mm).

- Symptoms particularly in the presence of an outflow tract gradient are usually treated with beta-blockers or calcium channel blockers.

- Surgical myomectomy and mitral valve replacement/repair can be performed when there is significant mitral regurgitation with primary valvular abnormalities; controlled iatrogenic myocardial injury using alcohol septal ablation has been attempted in high risk surgical patients.

## DEFINITION AND DIAGNOSTIC CRITERIA

Idiopathic Left Ventricular Hypertrophy (LVH) or Right Ventricular Hypertrophy (RVH).

Hypertension, valve disease, infiltrative disorders, and athletic or endocrine stimuli to hypertrophy should be excluded during the initial evaluation (**Table 62-1**).

## Epidemiology

Estimates of the prevalence of hypertrophic cardiomyopathy (HCM) vary widely, but more recent studies suggest that the disorder may affect as many as 1 in every 1,000 individuals.

## Pathology

The pathology of HCM is characterized by sarcomere disarray and hypertrophy of individual myocytes. It is important to distinguish this from a range of rare storage disorders that also may cause increased ventricular wall thickness in the absence of true hypertrophy. In addition to this, there is also extensive myocyte disarray far beyond the focal areas of such disarray often seen in the septum of healthy individuals. Myocardial mass is typically greatly increased but in some instances may be completely normal. It is important

**Table 62-1 • Definition and Diagnostic Criteria**

| |
|---|
| **Primary diagnostic criterion** |
| Unexplained myocardial hypertrophy |
| **Secondary diagnostic criterion** |
| In context of a history of HCM in first-degree relative (with consequent a priori risk of 0.5), any unexplained cardiac abnormality should be treated with a high index of suspicion. It is recommended that family be formally evaluated. |
| **Exclusions** |
| Hypertension Pulmonary or aortic stenosis Extreme athletic activity Abnormalities of thyroid or pituitary function Infiltrative or storage disorders |

**Table 62-2 • Causal Genes in HCM**

| Protein | Gene | Typical Features |
|---|---|---|
| Cardiac β-myosin heavy chain | MYH7 | classic HCM |
| Cardiac troponin T | TNNT2 | less hypertrophy and more sudden death |
| Cardiac myosin binding protein C | MYBPC3 | general association with late onset LVH |
| Cardiac troponin I | TNNI3 | rare, less hypertrophy |
| α-tropomyosin | TPM1 | rare |
| Essential and regulatory myosin light chains | MYL2, MYL3 | mid-cavitary obstruction |
| Actin | ACTC | HCM and DCM overlap families |
| Titin | TTN | rare |
| α-myosin heavy chain | MYH6 | rare |
| AMP kinase (storage) | PRKAG2 | preexcitation, AV block, exercise hypotension |
| Lysosomal-associated membrane protein 2 (storage) | LAMP2 | massive wall thickening, sudden death |
| α-galactosidase A (storage) | GLA | other features of Fabry's disease |

HCM, hypertrophic cardiomyopathy; LVH, left ventricular hypertrophy; DCM dilated cardiomyopathy.

to remember that right ventricular as well as left ventricular involvement occurs.

Superimposed on chronic cases is myocardial fibrosis, which may be diffuse. There may be focal areas of endocardial thickening typically on the ventricular side of the anterior leaflet of the mitral valve and the region of the upper ventricular septum, where apposition results from dynamic outflow obstruction and systolic anterior motion of the mitral valve apparatus.

Abnormal insertion of individual chordae as well as distortion of the mitral valve itself are also seen in a subset of patients.

## ETIOLOGY

Some of the earliest descriptions of HCM recognized a substantial inherited contribution to the disease and a large proportion of those diagnosed with HCM (70-90%) have a family history of the disease. The vast majority of inherited cases of HCM exhibit autosomal dominant transmission, but penetrance can be quite variable and skipped generations are not uncommon.

Molecular genetic studies of large kindreds with multiple affected members led to the mapping and cloning of the causal mutations, the majority of which are in genes encoding sarcomeric contractile proteins (**Table 62-2**). These studies not only confirmed the genetic basis of the disease but also identified the sarcomere as a central regulator of myocardial mass. Subsequent studies have begun to explore the molecular mechanisms of HCM.

The manifestations of HCM are quite varied or pleiotropic even within each family, though certain phenotypic features are recognized to be most commonly associated with specific genes. There are also some clinical features that are common within specific families but rare or exceptional in HCM in general. These include massive left ventricular (LV) wall thickness (>30 mm), high-grade atrioventricular block,

and ventricular preexcitation. Molecular genetic studies in such families have identified mutations, not in sarcomeric contractile protein genes but rather in several metabolic pathways (**Table 62-2**). Clinical and basic studies of the mechanisms of disease in such kindreds suggest that while there may be a contribution from activation of myocyte hypertrophic pathways, much of the increase in myocyte size results from storage abnormalities. As our understanding of the molecular mechanisms grows, newer classifications of cardiomyopathy will emerge.

In all forms of HCM, there is expression of the mutant proteins outside the heart, for example, in skeletal muscle or even vascular smooth muscle. This may explain some of the exertional symptoms, vasomotor abnormalities, and other features of these disease entities.

## CLINICAL PRESENTATION

### History

Many of those with HCM will be completely asymptomatic, and as a result, the familial nature of the disease is often only identified after a clinical event in a family member. Syncope,

| Table 62-3 • Physical Exam |
| --- |
| Bisferiens-type pulse |
| Palpable $S_4$ |
| Hyperdynamic apex |
| Dynamic (with maneuvers) outflow tract murmur with preserved $A_2$ |
| Mitral regurgitation |

often with exercise or post exertion, atypical chest pain, exertional dyspnea, and palpitations all are common. Typically, these symptoms emerge during the pubertal growth spurt. Unfortunately, it is not uncommon for sudden death to be the initial presenting feature, and many individuals will present for reassurance after the loss of a relative. A history of a murmur during childhood or of recurrent bronchitis or pneumonia is sometimes seen. In view of the emerging evidence that Fabry's disease may present as isolated HCM, a history of acroparaesthesiae and renal impairment should be sought.

## Family History

The family history is a central component of the evaluation of anyone with unexplained myocardial disease but is particularly important in HCM. Affected relatives with sudden death or chest pain syndromes have often been labeled as suffering from myocardial infarction, and a careful assessment, ideally of primary clinical data from family members, can be very useful. In some instances, there is overlap with other forms of cardiomyopathy or valve disease diagnosed in first-degree relatives. Ultimately, a definitive diagnosis can sometimes only be made through evaluation of the entire family.

## Physical Examination

Late outflow tract obstruction results in a bisferiens-type pulse, which is often accompanied by a hyperdynamic apical impulse with similar biphasic features and a palpable $S_4$. A variable and provokable basal ejection systolic murmur with late systolic mitral regurgitation is typical for HCM, but less definitive findings are common. Indeed, this classic clinical exam (**Table 62-3**) associated with HCM is relatively unusual, especially in the context of an extended family. Many family members will exhibit only a fourth heart sound or a soft outflow tract murmur.

## INITIAL INVESTIGATION

### ECG

The ECG is often diffusely abnormal with widespread repolarization abnormalities that do not obey the patterns of coronary distribution. Voltage evidence of LVH is helpful but not uniform, while unusual conduction defects as well

as frank bundle branch blocks (often with very fractionated surface electrograms) are common. More subtle ECG abnormalities can also be useful, especially in the context of a family history of HCM, where the a priori probability of HCM is as high as 0.5 in every at-risk individual.

## Echo (Fig. 48-25)

The classical echocardiographic finding is asymmetric septal hypertrophy, but this is increasingly recognized to be the case in a minority of patients. More typical is concentric LVH, but the hypertrophic myocardium may be located anywhere including the apex, free wall, or right ventricle or even restricted to the papillary muscles. Systolic anterior motion of the mitral valve apparatus on M-mode correlates well with outflow tract obstruction as the anterior leaflet of the mitral valve is pulled into apposition with the septum by a Venturi effect. Areas of endocardial thickening on the leaflet and the septum reveal the chronicity of the physiology and can be helpful in differentiating this from the effects of volume depletion. Outflow tract obstruction usually occurs late in systole and correlates poorly with symptoms, signs, or objective hemodynamics. Primary mitral valve abnormalities are also visualized on echo.

## Laboratory Testing

There are no typical laboratory abnormalities in HCM. The presence of an elevated creatine kinase (CK) or creatine kinase myoglobin (CKMB) is suggestive of a nonsarcomeric variant of HCM, but systematic evaluation in broad cohorts under a range of conditions has not been performed.

## Holter

48-hour ECG monitoring has been used in the risk stratification of HCM patients for decades, and high levels of ventricular ectopy are an important determinant of possible therapy. It is also useful to define occult atrial fibrillation or other arrhythmias that may require intervention.

## Tomographic Imaging

Computed tomography (CT) and magnetic resonance (MR) are useful for the delineation of focal hypertrophy in locations that are poorly accessible from standard echocardiographic windows. Both techniques can assess for the anomalous coronary origins that are rarely found with HCM, but CT angiography is better suited for the evaluation of possible myocardial bridging, which should be specifically sought if there is a history of typical angina. MR offers insights into tissue characteristics including scarring, which may ultimately prove useful in risk stratification and also can be useful in the evaluation of those resuscitated from sudden death where there is still concern for other causes, including arrhythmogenic right ventricular cardiomyopathy (ARVC).

## Exercise Testing

Exercise performance is often normal; when there is limitation, it can be difficult to attribute the mechanism to myocardial dysfunction. On perfusion imaging, particularly with thallium, patchy defects are often seen but appear to represent regional metabolic abnormalities or scarring and are not associated with coronary disease. Some individuals with HCM exhibit profound abnormalities of the vasomotor response to exercise and display sudden onset of inappropriate vasorelaxation with hypotension and abrupt limitation of exertion. These individuals are at increased risk of sudden cardiac death.

## Cardiac Catheterization

In most instances, the diagnosis of HCM will have been made prior to invasive testing, though occasionally, in the context of chest pain, angiography will be performed acutely.

Interestingly, there is little correlation between hemodynamic findings and symptoms or exercise performance. Left heart catheterization ideally performed using an end-hole catheter may establish evidence of an intraventricular gradient at baseline or under provocation. Brockenborough's sign is typical but not pathognomonic for HCM. Left ventriculography classically describes a spade-shaped cavity distorted by mitral valve anterior motion or papillary muscle hypertrophy, while mitral regurgitation may be evident. Coronary angiography may reveal anomalous origins, in which case, the course of the coronaries with respect to the great vessels should be defined. Severe myocardial bridging may result in exertional chest pain or arrhythmias, but less significant bridging is not uncommon. Right ventricular biopsy is useful only in the context of potential storage disorders.

## SAECG

Signal averaged ECG has proven useful in the identification of subclinically affected family members. Hopes that it might prove useful in defining those at risk of sudden death have not been realized.

## Electrophysiology Studies

Electrophysiology input is often sought in making decisions regarding defibrillator implantation. Provokable arrhythmias in HCM do not predict the risk of sudden death. More recent efforts to characterize the arrhythmic substrate using multi-electrode arrays with systematic assessment of myocardial electrical heterogeneity have shown some promise. The presence of a bypass tract and the risk of associated conduction system abnormalities are an indication for an invasive electrophysiologic evaluation.

## PROGNOSIS AND NATURAL HISTORY

The main concern when evaluating a patient with HCM is the risk of sudden cardiac death. This risk is at its highest during the pubertal growth spurt but remains elevated throughout life. The majority of the risk factors thought to predict sudden death have been studied without regard for the familial nature of the disease, and it can be difficult to discriminate the family-specific risk from the disease-specific risk. In any event, currently accepted risk factors (**Table 62-4**) include ventricular ectopy and ventricular tachycardia on monitoring, extreme LVH (>30 mm), exercise hypotension, syncope, and a family history of sudden death. At present, the best predictor of sudden death in HCM patients is a personal history of cardiac arrest; 59% of individuals with one episode of cardiac arrest have a second one within 5 years. However, in the absence of a prior cardiac arrest, the criteria for risk prediction become less clear. A personal history of unexplained syncope or a family history of sudden cardiac death has modest additional predictive utility. Care is necessary in defining the true risk of sudden death within a family. In particular, it can be difficult to estimate the risk of sudden death if there is no reliable assessment of the denominator, i.e., the number of family members who actually have HCM.

Clinical symptoms with HCM will often progress with age, presumably as a result of worsening myocardial function as well as diminished pulmonary and peripheral compensation reserve. A small subset of HCM patients will develop progressive ventricular cavity enlargement, leading to dilated cardiomyopathy and overt heart failure. Interestingly, in families where this occurs, sarcomeric mutations are also seen supporting the clinical overlap of the major inherited myocardial syndromes (HCM, dilated cardiomyopathy, restrictive cardiomyopathy, and ARVC). Even more rare is a progressive restrictive cardiomyopathy with worsening bilateral heart failure. Very occasional kindreds exist where familial restrictive cardiomyopathy is associated with specific troponin mutations.

## CLINICAL AND GENETIC SCREENING

The allelic heterogeneity of HCM, which includes over 400 causal mutations, makes individualization of treatment and prognosis on the basis of genetics implausible. It

| Table 62-4 • Risk Factors for Sudden Death |
| --- |
| Family history of sudden death |
| Non-sustained ventricular tachycardia on 48-hour Holter |
| Recurrent syncope |
| Exertional syncope or exertional hypotension |
| Severe left ventricular hypertrophy (>30 mm) |

is unlikely that for any mutation, adequate samples will ever be assembled for a reliable estimate of risk. Furthermore, incomplete penetrance and variable expressivity within families erode confidence in the predictive utility of mutations. Attempts to prognosticate on the basis of genetic mutations have been difficult to replicate, and designations of mutations as "benign" or "malignant" are often the result of observational studies in small numbers of families. It is of course expected that some mutations will have a more deleterious impact on protein function than others, but extrapolation of the clinical impact of a single mutation from a small number of individuals to populations with different genetic and environmental backgrounds should be undertaken with caution.

Thus, at present, a genetic diagnosis is most useful for screening relatives in a family bearing a known mutation. A preclinical diagnosis of HCM, either through genetic or clinical screening, offers an opportunity to make therapeutic decisions prior to disease onset. Unfortunately, there are no clear options for treatment to alter the course of disease. Clinical screening also can be carried out using ECG and echocardiography and may be as useful in many instances. Echocardiography has greater specificity, although even subtle ECG abnormalities, even in the absence of LVH on echocardiography, are suggestive for affected status, given the high pretest probability of disease in first-degree relatives. As multiple HCM variants can show clinical onset late in life, it is unclear if screening can be stopped confidently at any age.

## THERAPY

The majority of those with HCM are asymptomatic and at low risk and do not require any therapeutic intervention. Substantial exertional symptoms particularly in the presence of an outflow tract gradient are usually treated with beta-blockers or calcium channel blockers in the first instance. Failure to respond to a combination of these drugs can be approached with the addition of disopyramide, but there must be monitoring for autonomic and proarrhythmic effects. These drugs are thought to reduce myocardial contractility and so diminish the outflow tract gradient and its physiologic consequences. Responses to these measures are difficult to predict but can be excellent.

In the presence of an outflow tract gradient, the failure of medical therapy has led to measures to address the gradient

mechanically. Especially if there is significant mitral regurgitation with primary valvular abnormalities, surgical myomectomy and mitral valve replacement or repair have been undertaken with some success. In those at high risk for surgery or those who do not desire surgery, controlled iatrogenic myocardial injury using alcohol septal ablation has been attempted. Results are not dissimilar to those seen with surgery, though with both modalities, randomized controlled trials are unlikely ever to be performed.

Atrial fibrillation can have a major impact on hemodynamics in those with HCM, and aggressive efforts are usually made to maintain sinus rhythm, usually with amiodarone. There are no studies of the utility of pulmonary vein isolation in HCM, but given the diffuse nature of the underlying myopathy, such interventions might be predicted to be of limited duration. Ablation of the AV node and permanent pacing can be used in extreme circumstances.

Implantable cardiac defibrillator (ICD) implantation is recommended for those who have any form of malignant arrhythmia or are at high risk for sudden death. Prediction of risk is unfortunately far from a perfect science, and the risks and benefits of chronic device implantation have to be carefully weighed with the patient. In those in whom ICD is not feasible or refused, long-term therapy with amiodarone has been used.

Endocarditis prophylaxis is no longer recommended for isolated HCM, though estimates of the incidence of endocarditis in HCM suggest it may be close to that seen in congenital heart disease.

## Suggested Readings

1. The Cardiomyopathies. J Wynne and E Braunwald. Braunwald's Heart Disease 8th Edition. Elsevier Saunders, *Phildelphia.*

2. Spirito P, Seidman CE, McKenna WJ, Maron BJ. The management of hypertrophic cardiomyopathy. *N Engl J Med.* 1997;336:775–785.

3. Elliott PM , Poloniecki J, Dickie S, et al. Sudden Death in Hypertrophic Cardiomyopathy: Identification of High Risk Patients. JACC 2000;36:2212–2218.

4. Ommen SR, Shah PM, Tajik AJ. Left ventricular outflow tract obstruction in hypertrophic cardiomyopathy: past, present and future. *Heart* 2008;94:1276-1281.

5. ACC/ESC Clinical Expert Consensus Document on Hypertrophic Cardiomyopathy. JACC 2003;42:1687-1713.

# .63

# Myocarditis

Manisha J. Shah

## ● PRACTICAL POINTS

- Myocarditis refers to inflammation that results from a distinct external agent.

- Currently, the Dallas criteria, based on a pathological sample from an endomyocardial biopsy, are considered the gold standard for the diagnosis of myocarditis.

- Infectious, pharmacologic, and autoimmune responses are the three main categories of causative agents.

- The most common etiology is viral, however, Chagas' disease (parasitic) is one of the most common etiologies worldwide, especially in endemic areas.

- Human immunodeficiency virus (HIV) may result in myocarditis and possibly, dilated cardiomyopathy.

- There are five main bacterial infections that should be considered for myocardial involvement: mycobacteria, chlamydia pneumoniae, streptococcus species, mycoplasma pneumoniae, and treponema pallidum.

- Giant cell myocarditis patients often have a progressive clinical course with significant congestive heart failure as well as arrhythmias and heart block.

- Indications for a biopsy include (a) rapidly progressive or refractory heart failure; (b) heart block or ventricular arrhythmias; (c) heart failure with rash, fever, or peripheral eosinophilia; (d) a history of collagen vascular disease or known infiltrative disorders; or (e) a high suspicion for giant cell myocarditis (young age and progressive heart failure).

- In terms of treatment, immunosuppressive therapy does not significantly improve mortality or left ventricular ejection fraction (LVEF) in acute myocarditis.

- Creatine kinase (CK) and CK-MB have a relatively poor predictive value and very low sensitivity, so troponin is clinically useful when myocarditis is suspected.

## INTRODUCTION

Myocarditis is a condition that results from direct injury to the heart and the concomitant immune and inflammatory host response. The injury often occurs as a result of exposure to a specific causative agent; however, there are many different possible agents that can incite the process. Perhaps the most common cause of cardiac inflammation is myocardial ischemia; however, myocarditis particularly refers to inflammation that results from a distinct external agent. Possible causative agents include viruses, bacteria, parasites, drugs, and autoimmune triggers. Currently, the Dallas criteria, based on a pathological sample from an endomyocardial biopsy, are considered the gold standard for the diagnosis of myocarditis. Determination of the actual inciting agent can often be elusive when based on common diagnostic techniques; however, there are new laboratory and imaging techniques that may improve the diagnostic yield. Therapeutic measures include not only the spectrum of management options for congestive heart failure but also the treatment of inflammatory response and specific etiologic agents.

## EPIDEMIOLOGY

The epidemiology of myocarditis is often a reflection of the diagnostic criteria as well as the examined population. The Dallas criteria of endomyocardial biopsy specimens are considered to be restrictive and incidence based on these criteria alone can be underestimated. Often, myocarditis is a diagnosis of exclusion, requiring exclusion of common conditions such as myocardial infarction secondary to epicardial coronary disease. Nevertheless, there are several studies that provide information about the incidence of myocarditis. Based on pathologic diagnosis, the incidence is estimated at 8 to 10 per 100,000. An early study of postmortem cases showed a prevalence of 1 to 9%. More recently, a large prospective trial of 1,278 patients with dilated cardiomyopathy (DCM) found that the incidence of myocarditis as the etiology of the DCM was 9% based on clinical and endomyocardial biopsy diagnosis. Postmortem data of young adults who died of sudden death found myocarditis as the probable cause in 8.6 to 12.0% of the group. In a similar evaluation of 25-year data of sudden death in military personnel, myocarditis was the probable cause in 20% of the group. The variability in incidence and prevalence may result from a disparity in timing of the initial insult and the resultant clinical presentation.

With the advent of new molecular and imaging techniques, the incidence and prevalence of probable myocarditis are found to be higher. Molecular presence (polymer chain reaction [PCR]) of a viral genome on biopsy was found in 67% of 245 patients with dilated cardiomyopathy, whereas there was no inflammatory infiltrate on these same biopsies. Another study found a lower but still elevated 38% viral positivity by PCR in 624 patients with biopsy-proven myocarditis. Advanced noninvasive imaging techniques, such as cardiac magnetic resonance imaging (MRI), may offer supportive evidence in conjunction with other diagnostic modalities that could increase accuracy of the true incidence and prevalence of the disease.

## ETIOLOGIC AGENTS

A variety of possible causative agents can induce myocarditis. Infectious, pharmacologic, and autoimmune response are the three main categories of causative agents. **Table 63-1** lists these possible etiologic agents according to category. Perhaps the most common agent is viral, and this has been supported with recent data from PCR detection of a viral genome in biopsies of those patients with suspected myocarditis or cardiomyopathy. However, global epidemiology indicates that Chagas' disease may be one of the most common etiologies of myocarditis and resultant cardiomyopathy, especially in endemic countries. Detection of other agents is usually based on supportive clinical or laboratory data. Understanding the etiology of myocarditis may be useful in the development of therapeutic options and monitoring methods.

| Table 63-1 • Etiologic Agents | | |
|---|---|---|
| **Category** | **Subcategory** | **Causative Agent** |
| Infectious | viral | adenovirus |
| | | coxsackie virus |
| | | enterovirus |
| | | cytomegalovirus |
| | | parvovirus B19 |
| | | hepatitis C virus |
| | | human deficiency virus |
| | | herpes virus |
| | | Epstein-Barr virus |
| | | mixed infection |
| | bacterial | mycobacteria |
| | | chlamydia pneumoniae |
| | | streptococcal species |
| | | mycoplasma pneumoniae |
| | | treponema pallidum |
| | fungal | aspergillus |
| | | candida |
| | | coccidioides |
| | | cryptococcus |
| | | histoplasma |
| | protozoal | trypanosoma cruzi |
| | parasitic | schistosomiasis |
| | | larva migrans |
| Drugs | | anthracyclines |
| | | cocaine |
| | | clozapine |
| | | sulfonamides |
| | | cephalosporins |
| | | penicillins |
| | | tricyclic antidepressants |
| Autoimmune | | giant cell myocarditis |
| | | Churg-Strauss |
| | | Sjögren's syndrome |
| | | sarcoidosis |
| | | systemic lupus erythematosus, rheumatoid arthritis, dermatomyositis, and polymyositis |
| | | Takayasu arteritis |
| | | Wegener's granulomatosis |
| | | small pox vaccination |
| | | inflammatory bowel disease |

### Viruses

A range of viral vectors has been implicated in myocarditis. Traditionally, the enteroviruses, especially the coxsackie virus, have been the most commonly diagnosed viral vector; however, there is growing evidence that there is a significant geographical variation to the viral etiology. Adenovirus, parvoviruses, hepatitis C, and cytomegalovirus have been seen in increasing frequency in endomyocardial biopsy specimens, primarily based on PCR diagnostic techniques. In a European study of 254 patients, 54% of patients tested positive for parvovirus, 21.6% for enteroviruses, and only 1.6% for adenovirus. In contrast, in a primarily North American sample, 22.8% of patients tested positive for adenovirus and 13.6% positive for enterovirus. Hepatitis C infection (HCV) seems to be most dominant in the Japanese population of myocarditis. It is interesting that the HCV infection was manifest in those patients as a hypertrophic cardiomyopathy.

Coxsackie B virus is a single-stranded ribonucleic acid (RNA) virus that primarily infects via the gastrointestinal or respiratory system. A coxsackie–adenoviral receptor (CAR) on the cell surface is utilized for cell entry, resulting in internalization of the virus and the subsequent inflammatory host response. In most cases, the virus is cleared within 1 to 2 weeks; however, it can persist longer and can lead to chronic inflammation and poor overall prognosis. Adenovirus is a DNA virus that utilizes the same CAR receptor for entry, primarily via mucosal surfaces. This virus is a common pathogen in the pediatric population and is significantly more virulent with a resultant increased cell death. Parvoviruses are single-stranded DNA viruses that also primarily infect a pediatric population and cause *fifth disease* with a presentation of fever and skin exanthem. Myocarditis can occur after this infection in some cases. Parvovirus has also been implicated in an adult population and is gaining strength as a possible etiological agent, especially in the European cohort studied to date. This virus also appears to infect endothelial cells, and the subsequent endothelial dysfunction may play a significant role in inflammation, vasospasm, and cardiac dysfunction. Hepatitis C is a RNA virus that appears to be a significant pathogen of myocarditis in Japan and other Asian countries, perhaps as a result of the overall greater incidence of the disease and/or the more aggressive myopathic course in this population. As noted earlier, more often, there is a hypertrophic response of the myocardium and this could result in dilated cardiomyopathy in the long term. Fulminant myocarditis is often seen after the 1st or 3rd week of the illness.

Cardiomyocytes are susceptible to the human immunodeficiency virus, resulting in myocarditis and possible dilated cardiomyopathy. Postmortem studies in HIV patients show a 67% infection rate. The incidence rate is 15.9 per 1000 cases in an asymptomatic HIV population, with high risk patients (CD4 counts <400) having a higher incidence (83% with histological evidence). HIV-related cardiomyopathy appears to have a poor prognosis compared to other etiologies. Of course, in HIV patients, reasons beyond the HIV infection could contribute to this presentation, including associated HIV medications, opportunistic infections, or immunological disarray. Influenza can be associated with cardiac symptoms, with symptoms occurring 4 days to 2 weeks after the onset of illness. Approximately 5 to 10% of patients during influenza epidemics are affected by cardiac symptoms; however, the actual incidence of myocarditis is unclear due to variable clinical presentation. Clinical manifestations can vary from asymptomatic electrocardiogram (ECG) changes to fulminant heart failure.

## Bacteria

Bacteria can cause myocarditis from the host inflammatory response, from direct invasion of the myocardium, or via bacterial toxins. Specifically, there are five main bacterial infections that should be considered for myocardial involvement. Group A Beta-hemolytic streptococcus may result in acute rheumatic fever (ARF) and is associated with acute carditis. Bacteria surface M-proteins mimic myocardium (myosin and tropomyosin) proteins and other associated cardiac structures (i.e., valves—laminin), with a resultant hyperantigenic response. Bacterial toxins may also play a role in the immunological response. Initially in acute carditis, there is significant inflammation, edema, and collagen degeneration, mainly in the valvular tissue, but it can also be seen in the endocardium. Approximately 40 to 60% of ARF episodes result in rheumatic heart disease, mainly presenting with acute valvular abnormalities (mitral regurgitation and less commonly, aortic regurgitation). In the following 6-month period, pathognomonic Aschoff bodies, which are granulomatous formations, manifest in all layers of the heart as well as in the valve tissue. Presence of the Aschoff bodies may or may not be associated with actual carditis. Both acute and chronic myocardial dysfunction can occur from acute rheumatic fever. The severity of the myocardial involvement appears to be primarily due to the valvulitis rather than the direct myocardial involvement, and repeated bouts of rheumatic fever are frequently associated with recurrence of carditis. Although steroids are utilized as empiric therapy for acute rheumatic carditis, the randomized clinical trials do not support the use of steroids. Otherwise, the treatment for cardiac involvement is based on guideline based management for valvular disease and heart failure.

Cardiac involvement occurs in approximately 10% of the patients affected with Lyme disease, caused by the tick-borne spirochete, Borrelia burgdorferi. The primary clinical manifestation is atrioventricular block. Patients with high-degree block require hospitalization, close monitoring, and possibly, temporary transvenous pacing. Direct spirochetal involvement (based on biopsy specimens) is likely responsible for the AV block. Antibiotics are utilized in treating cardiac manifestations; however, the actual efficacy of antibiotics is unclear. Although the ECG abnormalities are the main evidence of cardiac involvement, either cardiac biopsy or a gallium scan can be used to confirm the diagnosis. In general, Lyme disease associated myocarditis should be considered in patients who have traveled in endemic areas, especially if they have atrioventricular conduction problems.

Beyond rheumatic fever and perhaps Lyme disease, the prevalence of the bacterial manifestation is infrequent in the modern day. Systemic illness with Clostridium difficile can result in myocardial involvement and can result from a direct toxin effect on the myocardium, myocardial abscess formation, and associated purulent pericarditis. Diphtheria is not seen in the modern world due to standard vaccination programs. However, in half the cases of diphtheria infection, there can be myocardial involvement from toxin release, which, similar to Lyme disease, affects the conduction system. An antitoxin may be useful if administered immediately, however, complete AV block often results in death, despite transvenous pacing. In fact, cardiac involvement is the most common cause of death in this infection. Tuberculosis uncommonly effects the myocardium; however, when it does, it is usually by direct, lymphatic, or hematogenous spread and can result in a variety of abnormalities, including arrhythmias, heart failure, and sudden death. Most common, tuberculosis causes pericarditis and manifests as constrictive pericardial disease in later life. Finally, Whipple disease, primarily an intestinal disease, can be associated with myocardial involvement. This mainly occurs as a result of direct infection by the bacterium, Tropheryma whippelii, and the associated inflammation. A variety of cardiac manifestations, including valvular abnormalities (aortic regurgitation), heart block, and congestive heart failure (CHF), have been seen. Antibiotic therapy can be used to treat; however, relapses do occur.

## Parasites

### Protozoan Disease—Chagas' Disease

Chagas' disease is an important and common cause of acute myocarditis, chronic dilated cardiomyopathy, and other chronic cardiac problems. Worldwide, 18 million people are infected, with 5 million having symptomatic disease and South America being the primary endemic region being South America. During the acute phase of the disease, children and young adults are bitten by the reduviid bug. The causative agent, Trypanosoma cruzi, infects the GI tract of the bug and is transmitted during the reduviid bite. Parasites directly infect the myocardium with a marked cellular and antibody-mediated immunological reaction against the parasite antigens. Cardiac manifestation from the acute infection can be myocarditis with heart failure and pericardial effusion. Approximately 10% are symptomatic from the acute phase; however, death can occur in 10% of those clinically affected. Treatment during the acute phase improves both

acute and chronic outcomes in Chagas' disease. Chagas' has a latent phase that is often asymptomatic; however, ECG abnormalities occur and can portend increased morbidity and mortality in the chronic stage. Progressive cardiomyopathy can occur in 30% of the patients.

Chronic Chagas' disease has some unique pathological features with associated clinical manifestations. Cardiomyopathy usually involves all four chambers, however, right-sided involvement and heart failure are more common. Chagas' involvement in the conduction system results in parasympathetic denervation that can contribute to autonomic dysfunction. A variety of ECG abnormalities, including right bundle branch block, left anterior fascicular block, atrial fibrillation, and ventricular arrhythmias, can be present, with possible clinical sequelae including sudden death. Finally, the ventricular apex is markedly thinned, aneurysmal, and associated with bulky thrombus formation that has an increased risk of embolic phenomenon.

Diagnosis of Chagas' disease utilizes a serodiagnostic test (complement—fixation) with high sensitivity and specificity. In endemic areas, up to 50% of chronic Chagas' disease patients have persistent parasitemia, and xenodiagnosis is used for detection of the parasite. Essentially, patients are bitten by a noninfected reduviid insect and diagnosis is based on detection of the parasite in the GI tract of the insect. Treatment of Chagas' disease involves the following: (1) acute antiparasitic treatment with nifurtimox, benznidazole, or itraconazole that can reduce the parasitemia, (2) chronic antiparasitic treatment that may improve progression and outcomes, (3) traditional treatment of congestive heart failure, (4) amiodarone that may control arrhythmias, however, implantable cardioverter defibrillators (ICDs) are mainly utilized in life-threatening situations in most endemic areas, and (5) anticoagulation for left ventricular apical aneurysm with thrombus formation, atrial fibrillation, or recurrent thromboembolic events (i.e., stroke).

### Metazoal Parasites

Echinococcus and trichinosis can involve the myocardium, however, it is uncommon. Echinococcal infestation results in intramyocardial hydatid cyst formation and possible rupture. Depending on where the rupture occurs, the clinical manifestation can be acute or chronic pericardial disease, systemic embolic phenomenon, or pulmonary embolism and hypertension. Cardiac imaging with 2D echocardiography or MRI can aid in the diagnosis. Blood eosinophilia can be useful; however, the serological evaluation is usually not helpful in a cardiac diagnosis. Surgical excision of cysts is recommended, even in asymptomatic patients, to reduce the complication potential of cystic rupture. Trichinosis usually does not infest the heart; however, there can be an immunological response to the parasite in the myocardium with resultant dilated cardiomyopathy, clinical myocarditis, and heart failure. The cardiac involvement usually occurs in the 2nd or 3rd week of infection. ECG abnormalities can be seen primarily as depolarization or premature ventricular contractions (PVCs). A positive indirect immunofluorescence test in the appropriate clinical situation is diagnostic and treatment with anthelminthics and steroids can significantly improve the outcomes.

## Drugs

Hypersensitivity reactions to a number of different medications can induce myocarditis. The main drugs to consider as possible agents include penicillin, sulfonamides, cephalosporins, diuretics, digoxin, clozapine, and dobutamine. Symptoms can occur after the initial ingestion, or in the case of some drugs, it can be an idiosyncratic reaction. Clinically, patients may develop skin rash, fever, peripheral eosinophilia, and sinus tachycardia. A predominant eosinophilic infiltrate on biopsy may support the diagnosis, and in severe cases, there is a significant necrotic component on the biopsy that is associated with a rapidly deteriorating course. In most cases, drug cessation usually improves the situation. Use of steroids may improve the situation as well. There is approximately a 1% risk (10-year accrual) of myocarditis with clozapine, with the median age being 30 years and onset within 2 to 3 weeks of drug initiation.

## Autoimmune Disorders

Almost all of the autoimmune diseases listed in **Table 63-1** can be associated with active myocarditis. Myocarditis is the most common myocardial disease in systemic lupus erythematosus (SLE). Clinical presentation of myocarditis occurs in 3 to 15% of patients with SLE and 5 to 20% are noted to have echocardiographic evidence of global hypokinesis. Nonorgan-specific autoantibodies have been implicated in immune complex formation. Deposition of such antibodies is the initial trigger for the inflammatory processes responsible for Libman-Sacks verrucous endocarditis, myocarditis, and pericarditis in patients with SLE and associated disorders. Polymyositis and dermatomyositis have chronic inflammatory infiltration of the skeletal muscle. Similarly, cardiac involvement is primarily inflammatory with mononuclear cell infiltrates localized to the endomyosin and perivascular areas; however, there can also be degeneration of the cardiac myocytes. Chronic CHF is reported in 3 to 45% of this population. Left ventricular (LV) dysfunction has been reported in 12 to 42% of the population compared to 30% in an age-matched control group. Rheumatoid arthritis (RA) associated cardiomyopathy is seen in 3 to 30% of postmortem studies in RA patients, with histology showing either focal nonspecific, diffuse necrotizing, or granulomatous myocarditis. In a small case series, 37% of RA patients were found to have cardiomyopathy by echocardiography. Drugs such

as corticosteroids used in RA and other autoimmune disorders may be associated with cardiomyopathy. Smallpox vaccinations may cause myopericarditis, with cases usually identified 4 to 30 days after the vaccination. The reported incidence is 7.8 cases per 100,000. Eosinophilic myocarditis can result from systemic diseases, post-vaccination, and from certain drugs. Associated systemic diseases include the hypereosinophilic syndrome, Loeffler's endomyocardial fibrosis, and Churg-Strauss syndrome (CSS). Cancer as well as infectious causes such as helminthic, parasitic, or protozoal agents can lead to eosinophilic myocarditis. Clinically, the patient presents with congestive heart failure and on diagnostic evaluation will be found to have a predominant eosinophilic infiltrate, an endocardial and valvular fibrosis, and an endocardial thrombus formation. An acute necrotizing form of eosinophilic myocarditis often results in a high death rate. The most progressive and fulminant form of myocarditis, giant-cell myocarditis, is felt to be secondary to autoimmune causation and secondary to autoimmune disorders, thymoma, and drug hypersensitivity.

## Other Agents

A variety of physical agents can induce injury to the myocardium. Direct damage as well as an inflammatory reaction can be responsible for the myocardial changes, thus the clinical presentation can be acute myocarditis or chronic cardiomyopathy depending on the agent and the effect on the heart. Numerous chemicals, including arsenics, lithium, industrial agents, and medications, are associated with myocardial involvement. Radiation therapy can result in a variety of cardiac abnormalities, usually related to fibrotic changes in the myocardium and other structures. Radiation causes long-term effects on the capillary endothelial cells, which ultimately cause ischemia and chronic fibrosis. Epicardial coronary arteries can show radiation injury with chronic narrowing and focal ostial stenosis, resulting in ischemia induced cardiomyopathy. Clinical symptoms from radiation-related changes usually occur long after exposure. They are often related to the cumulative dose of radiation and the direct mass of heart irradiated. Acute myocardial involvement postradiation is infrequent; the patient often presents with acute pericarditis.

Significant variations in body temperature can also affect the heart and result in clinically important sequelae. Heat stroke patients can have a variety of cardiac involvement, including ECG abnormalities, transient right or left ventricular dysfunction, and frank decompensated heart failure. Pathological findings show hemorrhagic changes in the subendocardium and subepicardium, usually in the septum and posterior wall of the left ventricle. Hypothermia can also cause myocardial damage, with biopsy findings of microinfarcts in the myocardium, likely related to circulatory collapse, hemoconcentration, and depressed cellular metabolism from hypothermia. Supportive treatment and core warming may improve the clinical situation.

## PATHOPHYSIOLOGY

The development of the pathologic and clinical sequelae of myocarditis is a result of both the inciting agent and the host response. Viral myocarditis has been the most thoroughly investigated form of myocarditis from animal pathophysiologic models. It forms the basis of the understanding of the direct viral invasion as well as the host inflammatory and reparative processes in this disease. The first stage of viral myocarditis is the viral phase, which involves the direct viral effect by viral entry and proliferation, immune activation, and cell death. Many viruses, such as coxsackie, will initially invade the lymphoid organs, proliferate in the immune cells, and then enter the heart via transfer of the virus onto myocardial specific receptors (such as coxsackie-adenovirus receptor [CAR]). A cofactor or decay-accelerating factor (DAF) can aid in determining the virulence. Once in the myocyte, the RNA viruses will duplicate via a template that was formed from reverse-transcription of the initial viral strand. The virus affects the cell via the following mechanisms: (1) direct cell damage and death, (2) activation of various internal molecules, such as tyrosine kinase p56, that permit more viral entry and activate T-cells, (3) upregulation of the CAR and subsequent myocyte susceptibility as a result of the virus and associated inflammation, and (4) viral persistence that can lead to cleavage of the dystrophin and eukaryotic initiation factor-4, leading to myocardial dysfunction, chronic myocarditis, and dilated cardiomyopathy.

The immune system is intimately involved in the host response to the viral invasion in regard to defense as well as the damage to the cardiac myocyte. After the initial viral entry, there is often an inflammatory cell infiltration and ultimate release of proinflammatory cytokines and antiinflammatory interferons that will modulate the overall myocardial damage. Two forms of immunity are important—the innate and acquired immunity. Innate immunity is usually the first line of immune defense. The toll-receptors are cell surface receptors that recognize general molecular patterns, with myocardial toll receptors being able to recognize such entities as double-stranded RNA and bacterial liposaccharide. MyD88 is a key protein in the dendritic-cell toll-like receptor signaling that is required for the development of myocarditis. The viruses and other agents can be detected by the toll receptors and can lead to cytokine and interferon production. Cytokine production occurs via the transcription factor, Nuclear Factor-KappaB (NF-kB), and is generally detrimental to the cell. Cytokines, including interleukins, interferon-Y, and tumor necrosis factor (TNF), will induce further damage to the cell by recruiting inflammatory cells

and promoting production of additional cytokines. It is interesting that cytokines can induce nitric oxide (NO) synthase, which will decrease levels of nitric oxide and is apparently beneficial to cell survival by reducing viral replication and inflammation. Interferon is activated via interferon regulatory factors (IRFs) and is generally beneficial to the cell. The IRFs are also important in down-regulation of the NF-kB as well as the acquired immunity pathway. There are also other negative modulators of cytokine, such as the suppressors of cytokine signaling (SOCS). Imbalance in this system can also affect the host response.

In animal models of myocarditis, CD4+ T lymphocytes are stimulated by the large amount of circulating self-antigens and result in the release of both Th1 and Th2 cytokine release. Regulatory T cells influence the circulating CD4+ T cells and ultimately the course of autoimmune myocarditis. One subgroup of the regulatory T cells is known to express CD4, transcription factor forkhead box p3 (FOX P3), and a high level of corticosteroid-induced tumor necrosis factor receptors, all of which can prominently affect the inflammatory process. In an animal model of coxsackie B myocarditis, both CD4 and CD8 have been implicated in the inflammatory response. Associated CD4+CD25+FOXp3+ T cells are important negative regulatory T cells in the coxsackie virus B myocarditis. Th17 cells, a third group of T helper cells, can produce interleukin and have been implicated in myocarditis. Thus, T cells play an integral role in myocarditis, which supports the role of anti-T cell therapy in autoimmune myocarditis.

Acquired or cellular immunity plays an important role in the inflammatory response. Initially, the T-cell receptor recognizes a specific viral peptide pattern and then induces two main immune effects: (1) T-killer cell production to directly kill the viral antigen and (2) B-cell activation leading to production of specific antibodies to neutralize the antigen. It is unfortunate that, often, the viral protein mimics proteins in the heart and induces autoantibody action to such molecules as myosin, laminin, and so on. T-cell receptor activation may also be directly detrimental to the host. There is also cross-reactivity between cardiac myosin and the endogenous human cell-surface protein laminin, which could result in ongoing stimulus for chronic myocarditis. Recently, cross-reactivity between cardiac myosin and B1-adrenergic receptor has been noted and may contribute to cardiomyocyte apoptosis. For instance, T-cell receptor activation signals the tyrosine kinase p56, which permits greater viral entry and heightens the overall inflammatory response. P56 knock-out mice have essentially no inflammation and markedly reduced mortality. Activated T-cells also kill the infected cells via cytokines and perforins, which can worsen the overall inflammatory milieu. Thus, appropriate immune responsiveness likely modulates the overall viral clearance while keeping in check the overexuberant inflammatory response.

The description above essentially refers to most viral-mediated myocarditis processes; however, there are likely similar responses to other inciting agents. HIV likely infects in the same manner yet also can lead to significant endocardial fibrosis. Co-infection with opportunistic infections can result in direct invasion and contribute to myocardial damage. Giant cell myocarditis (GCM) is a unique type of myocarditis that appears to be autoimmune in nature as no particular inciting agent has been identified. Biopsy shows multinucleated giant cells with associated macrophage antigens and T-cell lymphocyte proliferation. The clinical course is often progressive and fatal.

Cardiac remodeling is important to the chronic outcome in myocarditis. Cytokines such as transforming growth factor lead to activation of pathologic fibrosis and contribute to chronic remodeling. Besides the cytokine and interferon balance for appropriate immune responsiveness, the immune system can activate the matrix metalloproteinases (MMPs) that affect collagen and elastin in the cardiac matrix and are important in chronic remodeling and myocardial function. Last, ongoing viral and inflammatory interchange as evidenced by a detection of viral RNA at both acute and chronic stages in both animal and human myocarditis affects the progression to cardiomyopathy and congestive heart failure.

## CLINICAL PRESENTATION

Clinical presentation of myocarditis is a wide spectrum including asymptomatic electrocardiographic and cardiac imaging abnormalities, acute and chronic heart failure, and frank acute hemodynamic collapse secondary to cardiogenic shock. Viral epidemics often have patients with transient ECG abnormalities but rarely with significant cardiac decompensation. Myocarditis usually has two patterns of manifestation—acute decompensation in children and young adults and chronic presentation of CHF in older adults. There are four possible clinical presentations: (1) acute myocarditis, (2) fulminant myocarditis, (3) giant cell myocarditis, and (4) chronic active myocarditis.

### Acute Myocarditis

Patients usually present with myocardial infarction, CHF symptoms, or arrhythmias. Symptoms in order of decreasing frequency can include fatigue, dyspnea on exertion, supraventricular and ventricular arrhythmias, and chest pain. Patients who present with frank chest pain often have other clinical features of myocardial infarction (focal ST elevation, elevated troponin, and wall motion abnormality on echo) that most likely require a cardiac catheterization to exclude coronary artery occlusion. The chest pain can occur from the associated pericarditis or coronary artery spasm. Report

of a viral prodrome is variable and has been reported 20 to 80% of the time; thus, diagnosis of myocarditis is essentially based on clinical presentation and diagnostic testing that is outlined later. In the European Study of Epidemiology and Treatment of Inflammatory Heart Disease (ESETCID), 3,055 patients with suspected myocarditis were screened and found to have the following symptom incidence of a viral prodrome: 72% with dyspnea, 32% with chest pain, and 18% with arrhythmias.

### Fulminant Myocarditis

Patients usually present with frank hemodynamic collapse secondary to cardiogenic shock. Also, in most cases, there is onset of viral prodrome symptoms 2 weeks prior to cardiac symptoms. Evaluation often reveals severe ventricular dysfunction with normal chamber size on echo. The inflammatory changes on biopsy are significant but do not necessarily match the clinical presentation. Likely secondary to overexuberant and acute cytokine response, the patients often present with hemodynamic collapse, rapid onset of symptoms, and fever. Aggressive supportive treatment with vasopressors, diuretic treatment, and mechanical cardiopulmonary support is key for survival as a majority of patients will recover.

### Giant Cell Myocarditis

Patients often have a progressive clinical course with significant congestive heart failure as well as arrhythmias and heart block. Endomyocardial biopsy can identify patients with the typical giant cell pathology, and treatment with immunosuppression may be temporarily effective. Although the onset of symptoms and hemodynamic status is often variable, the prognosis is usually worse than other types of myocarditis, more often leading to death and potential transplantation. The median survival is 6 months and selected patients are considered for a ventricular assist device (VAD) and transplantation.

### Chronic Active Myocarditis

This group essentially represents the majority of patients who are diagnosed with idiopathic dilated cardiomyopathy and congestive heart failure. The clinical presentation is of insidious CHF symptoms and biopsy usually shows chronic changes of fibrosis and myocyte necrosis. Myocyte viral positivity based on new PCR techniques may give supportive evidence of ongoing inflammatory effect.

## DIAGNOSTIC EVALUATION

Historically, the gold standard diagnosis of myocarditis has required the appropriate clinical presentation and a positive endomyocardial biopsy result based on the Dallas criteria.

However, because of difficulties with the biopsy-proven diagnosis, more recent, an expanded criterion for myocarditis diagnosis has been recommended (**Table 63-2**).

## Clinical Presentation

Features of the varying clinical presentation have been outlined above. ECG abnormalities are quite variable, including nonspecific T wave inversion, ST elevation, conduction abnormalities, and arrhythmias. The ECG changes have roughly 47% sensitivity but are generally nonspecific for myocarditis. In the appropriate clinical situation, they

will provide supportive evidence of myocardial damage and inflammation. ECG changes of pericarditis are not uncommon in the setting of myocarditis.

## Endomyocardial Biopsy

Histopathologic evidence of myocarditis based on the standardized Dallas criteria is the gold standard for diagnosis. Biopsy positivity is defined according to the presence of inflammatory infiltrate and myocyte necrosis (not due to ischemia). There are several reasons for the insensitivity of the biopsy and they include the following: (1) patchy inflammatory myocardial lesions not adequately sampled during the routine five biopsy samples obtained, (2) recent cardiovascular magnetic resonance imaging (CMRI) data that show the lateral wall as the most likely early area of inflammation in myocarditis—an area not usually sampled during biopsy, (3) moderate consensus by expert pathologists on repeated evaluations for confirmed diagnosis (64% in the National Institutes of Health [NIH] Myocarditis Treatment Trial biopsy diagnosis), and (4) risks of endomyocardial biopsy (2-5%), with 50% complications related to venous access (bleeding, pneumothorax, arterial puncture) and 50% related to the biopsy (arrhythmias, cardiac perforation, and death). Tamponade from perforation occurs rapidly, and without acute pericardiocentesis, patients can deteriorate due to hemodynamic collapse.

Diagnostic yield of the biopsy is estimated at 10 to 20%, with early timing (within weeks) more often having positive results. Sensitivity is 35 to 50% and specificity is 80 to 89%. A positive biopsy was found in only 10% of patients with idiopathic heart failure in the Myocarditis Treatment Trial and only 9% of idiopathic cardiomyopathy in a large (1,230 patients) case series. Level of evidence for support of an endomyocardial biopsy (EMB) is according to the patient presentation (2007 ACC/AHA) guidelines. Certain clinical presentations often require biopsy, including (a) rapidly progressive congestive heart failure, refractory to standard therapy; (b) cardiomyopathy associated heart block or ventricular arrhythmias; (c) heart failure with rash, fever, or peripheral eosinophilia; (d) history of collagen vascular disease or known infiltrative disorders; or (e) high suspicion for giant cell myocarditis (young age and progressive heart failure).

More recent, molecular techniques such as in situ hybridization or polymerase chain reaction to evaluate the viral genome in pathological specimens have improved the sensitivity of the biopsy sample. It is interesting that the presence of the viral genome is not associated with the inflammatory response on biopsy, but it does appear to correlate with clinical symptoms and outcome. Immunological approaches, including specific immunohistochemical staining, offer more precise characterization of lymphocytic infiltrates as well

### Table 63-2 • Diagnostic Scheme

| Diagnosis of Myocarditis | Positive Categories |
|---|---|
| Suspicious | 2 |
| Compatible | 3 |
| High probability | 4 |
| Category 1 | Clinical presentation clinical heart failure fever viral prodrome fatigue dyspnea on exertion chest pain palpitations presyncope/syncope |
| Category 2 | Myocardial damage and no regional cardiac ischemia 1. Echocardiography regional wall motion abnormality ventricular dilation regional hypertrophy 2. Troponin release (>0.1 ng/mL) 3. Positive Indium-111 antimyosin scintigraphy and 4. Normal coronary angiography or negative perfusion scan for regional defects |
| Category 3 | Cardiac magnetic resonance imaging 1. Increased myocardial T2 signal on inversion recovery sequence 2. Delayed contrast enhancement on gadolinium infusion |
| Category 4 | Myocardial biopsy 1. Positive biopsy based on Dallas criteria 2. Presence of viral genome by polymerase chain reaction or in situ hybridization |

as analyses of the upregulation of major histocompatibility (MHC) antigens in the tissue. Identification of cell surface antigens such as anti-CD3, anti-CD4, anti-CD20, and antihuman leukocyte antigen by immunoperoxidase staining can lead to increased sensitivity and prognostic utility. One small study showed that the upregulation of any MHC antigens on the biopsy specimen had increased sensitivity of 80% with specificity maintained at 85%, which is similar to sensitivity and specificity from using Dallas criteria alone. However, a larger independent study in a cohort of clinically suspected myocarditis found no correlation between MHC upregulation and Dallas criteria biopsy diagnosis. Despite this discordance between the trials, MHC expression has been utilized to guide immunosuppressive treatment in one clinical trial.

## Cardiac Biomarkers

Cardiac biomarkers can be useful to detect myocardial injury resulting from myocarditis. If there is reasonable clinical suspicion for myocarditis, there should be a routine evaluation of cardiac biomarkers including CK, CK-MB, and troponin. CK and CK-MB have a relatively poor predictive value and very low sensitivity (8%); therefore, troponin is usually more clinically useful. There have been two studies to evaluate the utility of troponin in myocarditis. In a cohort of 80 subjects with suspected myocarditis, troponin was positive only in 35% using a cutoff of >0.1 ng/mL. Furthermore, the sensitivity was 53%, specificity of 94%, positive predictive value of 93%, and negative predictive value of 56%. Hence, a positive troponin in the appropriate clinical presentation is predictive; however, a negative troponin does not exclude a diagnosis of myocarditis by biopsy. Low sensitivity (34%) and reasonable specificity (89%) for troponin were found in a subgroup of patients in the Multicenter Myocarditis Treatment Trial. The low sensitivity is likely related to timing of the biopsy—sensitivity usually increases if the biopsy is performed when there is a short duration of symptoms (closer to initial injury). The erythrocyte sedimentation rate has been studied in myocarditis, however, the sensitivity and specificity are very low. Other possible immune biomarkers, such as cytokines and so on, have not been validated in a biopsy-proven myocarditis; however, some such as Fas ligand and interleukin-10 may predict an increased risk of death.

## Myocardial Imaging

### Echocardiography

This imaging modality has been routinely utilized to evaluate patients with suspected myocarditis. Findings on echocardiography include possible chamber dilation as well as regional hypertrophy and wall motion abnormalities. However, the findings are not specific to myocarditis and can be seen in coronary artery induced ischemia/injury or in other etiologies of cardiomyopathy. The diagnosis of myocarditis can be generally suspected if there are echocardiographic changes, absence of matching coronary artery stenosis, and rapid recovery of ventricular dysfunction. In a cohort of 42 patients with biopsy-proven myocarditis, ventricular dysfunction was seen in only 69% and ventricular dilation was even more variable. Other echocardiographic findings in this cohort included right ventricular dysfunction (23%), segmental wall motion abnormalities (64%), and reversible left ventricular hypertrophy (15%). Compared to typical myocarditis or associated cardiomyopathy, the echocardiographic changes in fulminant myocarditis usually include significant ventricular dysfunction, increased septal thickness, and normal chamber size. It is apparent that loss of right ventricular function may be an important predictor of death as per a recent series of 23 patients with biopsy-proven myocarditis. In general, echocardiographic changes are variable in myocarditis and relatively nonspecific, however, echocardiographic evaluation (initial and serial) is useful in diagnosis and monitoring. Advanced echocardiographic techniques, including ultrasonic tissue characterization and tissue Doppler imaging, may provide supportive evidence for myocarditis. Ultrasonic tissue characterization is based on reflectivity of the tissue and depends on tissue density, elasticity, and acoustic impedance. In a cohort of 52 subjects with biopsy-proven myocarditis, ultrasonic characterization was found to be abnormal in myocarditis compared to normal controls, with sensitivity of 100% and specificity of 90%.

### Indium-111 Labeled Antimyosin Antibody Imaging

Monoclonal antibodies can bind to intracellular antimyosin once myocytes have been disrupted and there is loss of membrane integrity. Radioisotope linked antibodies can thus be imaged to evaluate areas of possible myocardial necrosis from myocarditis. In a large cohort of biopsy-proven myocarditis, the Indium-labeled imaging sensitivity was 83% and the specificity was 53%. The negative predictive value was high at 92%. The combination of a positive indium antimyosin scan and nonventricular dilation is significantly predictive of a positive myocardial biopsy. Gallium scanning can also be utilized in myocarditis, however, it only detects myocardial inflammation and is nonspecific for myocarditis.

### Cardiac Magnetic Resonance Imaging

Cardiac MRI is probably the most useful imaging technique to evaluate myocarditis. Similar to echocardiography, noncontrasted MRI gives information about anatomy, flow dynamics, and morphology. MRI evaluation allows for highly reproducible evaluation of left ventricular function. Identification of pericardial effusion, a marker of general inflammation, is reported in 32 to 57% of myocarditis patients. Standard steady-state free precession images provide inherent T2 sensitivity that shows pericardial fluid as a bright signal. Morphological changes in myocarditis include an increase in wall thickness, and LV volumes may also be seen. Myocardial tissue in myocarditis has a myriad of histopathological changes, including changes in membrane permeability, tissue edema and inflammation, and necrosis as well as fibrosis. Myocardial inflammation often leads to increased cellular membrane permeability. T2-weighted MRI imaging detects tissue edema as a bright signal and is useful in detecting either regional or global edema found in active myocarditis. Other imaging protocols such as double and triple inversion recovery turbo spin recovery sequences provide excellent contrast between regional edema and normal myocardium. Quantitative assessment of signal abnormality can be performed in comparison to adjacent normal myocardium or skeletal muscle (global edema). In those patients with active myocarditis, regional edema was found in 36% of the patients. In the absence of late gadolinium uptake, edema likely represents reversible myocardial injury. Tissue characterization is much more defined with MRI than echocardiography and is based on measuring MRI parameters of T1 and T2 relaxation times as well as spin densities. T1 weight fast spin-echo imaging with gadolinium infusion is useful in detecting tissue changes in myocarditis. Early gadolinium enhancement indicates hyperemia and capillary leakage that occurs in the active inflammatory state. The early gadolinium enhancement ratio (EGEr) allows for qualitative or quantitative detection of the normalized accumulation of gadolinium into the intravascular and interstitial space during the early washout period. In the abnormal milieu of myocarditis, gadolinium will persist in the myocardium, leading to changes in T1 relaxation that can be detected as delayed enhancement on late MRI T1-weighted imaging. Late gadolinium enhancement (LGE) gives evidence for irreversible changes of necrosis and fibrosis. An inversion pulse sequence is used to highlight the late gadolinium uptake as well as decrease the normal myocardial signal. Clinical and pathological studies give support to the use of late gadolinium enhancement as a gold standard for high specificity in the detection of irreversible myocardial injury. LGE does have the limitation of variable sensitivity to detect active versus chronic inflammation. This likely is related to the size of the inflammatory changes as well as the reversibility of some myocarditis lesions. Furthermore, there are a variety of MRI patterns that can be seen with active myocarditis. The subepicardium region is typically highlighted with gadolinium; however, this can have a transmural extension. Typical, subepicardial involvement is not isolated, thus distinguishing it from ischemia-mediated injury. Gadolinium uptake tends to localize in the inferolateral segments; however, anteroseptal areas can have involvement. Last, false-positive results can occur when LGE is detected in the basal septum, LV outflow tract, or membranous septum. Also, uptake in the

basal septum may represent fusion of the right ventricular moderator band to the intraventricular septum. There have been a few clinical studies evaluating the utility of CMRI in myocarditis. Friedrich et al found a specific pattern of MRI changes in patients with suspected myocarditis—focal patchy myocardial enhancement in early stage, global enhancement at 2 weeks, and normalization to baseline at 90 days. Roditi et al studied another cohort of 20 patients with suspected myocarditis who underwent spin-echo based MRI with contrast. It was found that focal myocardial enhancement in areas of regional wall motion abnormalities was present in 10 of 12 patients with suspected or biopsy proven myocarditis. Thus, these findings strongly support a diagnosis of myocarditis and can be utilized in clinical evaluation of myocarditis. Mahrholt et al have utilized new CMRI protocols (inversion recovery) with contrast administration to guide endomyocardial left and right ventricular biopsy in patients with suspected myocarditis. They were able to achieve a significantly improved positive (71%) and negative (100%) predictive value of MRI-guided biopsy in this cohort. Thus, MRI may not only be important in increasing the biopsy yield, but given the risks of endomyocardial biopsy, CMRI may be an important imaging tool that could aid in selecting patients for biopsy and, with typical MRI findings, could even offer independent support of the diagnosis. Comprehensive use of the cardiac MRI criteria (Lake Louise Criteria) is based on expert opinion and the data from available small clinical trials. It is generally recommended that at least two of the three findings be positive for the diagnosis of myocarditis: (1) regional or global increased signal intensity in T2 weighted images, (2) increased early gadolinium enhancement between myocardium over skeletal muscle in T1 weight images, and 3) at least one focal lesion with nonischemic regional distribution in inversion recovery-prepared late-gadolinium enhanced T1-weighted images. The initial MRI scan may have improved sensitivity if performed 7 days after the onset of disease. Follow-up of myocarditis by cardiac MRI is recommended 1 to 2 weeks after the initial study if no diagnostic MRI criteria are positive but there is strong clinical evidence for myocarditis.

## PROGNOSIS AND TREATMENT

### Prognosis

Prognosis in myocarditis is dependent on clinical presentation. Patients with a mild form of acute myocarditis and/or presentation of acute MI will generally recover without a long-term effect. For those with more significant ventricular dysfunction and moderate to severe congestive heart failure, the outcomes essentially include 25% who recover to normal function, 50% who have persistent ventricular dysfunction and CHF, and 25% who have a progressive course to a left ventricle assist device (LVAD)/transplantation/death. Patients with other forms of myocarditis have very different outcomes. It is interesting that if patients with fulminant myocarditis can recover from the initial insult of cytokine release and hemodynamic collapse, then the survival is ~90% at a decade. Giant cell myocarditis patients have the worst overall prognosis with medial survival of 6 months, and many are listed for transplantation. Chronic active myocarditis patients have a relatively poor prognosis with a mortality of 20% at 1 year and 56% at 4.3 years (NIH Myocarditis Treatment Trial). Five-year survival rates in the Mayo Clinic observational study were similar at 50%.

A variety of clinical markers have been evaluated for prediction of outcomes. In general, presentation with syncope, bundle branch block on ECG, and ejection fraction less than 40% are poor prognosticators. Also, in general, known predictors of CHF such as advanced New York Heart Association functional class, increased filling pressures, and pulmonary hypertension are associated with worse outcomes in patients with myocarditis and associated cardiomyopathy. Normal chamber size on echo, resolution of myocarditis on follow-up biopsy, and viral negative biopsy appear to predict a better outcome. The Intervention in Myocarditis and Acute Cardiomyopathy trial (IMAC-II) noted that increased levels of Fas ligand (cell apoptosis marker) and TNF receptor 1 were associated with poor recovery, indicating that ongoing markers of cell destruction and inflammation are important to outcome.

## Treatment

Treatment for myocarditis follows three main goals: (a) aggressive supportive treatment for initial presentation, (b) management of congestive heart failure based on ACC/AHA guidelines, and (3) possible immunosuppressive and antiviral therapy.

### Supportive Treatment

Aggressive treatment of acute decompensated CHF and cardiogenic shock may be necessary in some patients with acute myocarditis or fulminant myocarditis. Three main areas of support may be necessary, including (1) vasopressors for blood pressure and inotropic support, (2) IV diuretics and vasodilators such as nitroglycerin or nitroprusside for reduction of systemic vascular resistance and filling pressures, and (3) ventricular assist devices or, in some cases, extracorporeal membrane oxygenation (ECMO) to support patients refractory to medical therapy. Observational data support mechanical support in regard to benefit in the acute stage (improve wall stress and geometry and reduce cytokine burden) as well as long-term survival.

### Congestive Heart Failure Management

The standard evidence-based medical regimen should be initiated for CHF as per ACC/AHA guidelines. This would include pharmacologic treatment with angiotensin-converting enzyme inhibitor, beta receptor blocker, aldosterone antagonist, digoxin, and diuretics. Implantable cardiac defibrillator and biventricular pacemakers should generally be considered after optimization of medical management and reassessment of ventricular function and CHF status. There are no human clinical trials of clinical intervention in myocarditis. Animal data are available and suggest the following: (1) Aerobic exercise soon after onset of cardiac symptoms should be avoided based on exercise intervention in rats that had increased mortality, (2) use of candesartan improved survival in a murine model of myocarditis, and (3) pathologic data and ventricular dimensions improved after treatment with carteolol for coxsackie virus B myocarditis. Arrhythmias can be seen in patients with acute myocarditis; however, treatment is often supportive as they often resolve in the recovery phase. However, even in the setting of acute phase, management may need to be aggressive and could include temporary pacemakers for symptomatic bradycardia or complete heart block. Amiodarone or an implantable cardioverter defibrillator may be needed for symptomatic or sustained ventricular arrhythmias.

### Immunosuppressive and Antiviral Treatment

Treatment with immunosuppressive medications such as corticosteroids, cyclosporine, or immune globulin has been considered for the management of myocarditis and for the related cardiomyopathy. There have been a number of observational trials that have supported the immunosuppressive agents, however, the randomized trials performed to evaluate the actual utility and efficacy of these agents have yielded less than supportive evidence for these agents, including no significant change in mortality in most of these trials. The first trial of prednisone treatment (60 mg per day) in idiopathic cardiomyopathy (with biopsy and clinical evidence of inflammation), by Parillo et al in 1989, showed an initial improvement of greater that 5% in left ventricular ejection fraction (LVEF) at 3 months. However, this was not sustained over 6 to 9 months and there was no mortality benefit. The Myocarditis Treatment Trial randomized 111 patients with biopsy-verified myocarditis to placebo or prednisone plus cyclosporine or azathioprine. There was no change in mortality or LVEF improvement (24 to 36%) at 28 weeks between treatment groups and control. The Intervention in Myocarditis and Acute Cardiomyopathy Study (IMAC) was a double-blind, randomized, controlled trial of IV immune globulin (IVIG) in patients with recent onset (<6 months) heart failure and idiopathic cardiomyopathy. Again, there was no change in LVEF or mortality between the treatment group and placebo. Of note, only 16% of the patients were noted to have pathologic features of myocarditis on biopsy. Another small randomized study by Gullestad et al in chronic dilated cardiomyopathy showed that IVIG resulted in an increase in serum antiinflammatory markers and improvement in LVEF at 6 months.

It appears that inflammation in cardiomyopathy may be the marker for response from immunosuppressive therapy. A trial by Wojnicz et al focused on human leukocyte antigen (HLA) expression to identify possible responders. In this trial, 84 patients with increased HLA expression on biopsy and chronic dilated cardiomyopathy were randomized to placebo or 3 months of prednisone and azathioprine. There was no difference in mortality, readmission, or transplantation rate; however, LVEF did improve at 6 months and 2 years. Both interferon-alpha and interferon-beta have been independently studied in single clinical trials, again with no change in mortality but improvement in LVEF. It is interesting that a small study of lymphocytic myocarditis with all patients treated with either azathioprine or prednisone found that circulating cardiac autoantibodies were seen in responders and a biopsy-positive viral genome was seen in nonresponders at 1 year.

There are two possible approaches to immune therapy that involve physical modification. Immune adsorption therapy attempts to remove cardiac depressant factors (cytokines, antibodies, etc.) via plasmapheresis. Small trials have shown improvement in mortality, with one randomized study of 34 patients having an improvement in LVEF from 22% to 38%. Immune modulation therapy (IMT) is another physical therapy in which autologous whole blood is irradiated with ultraviolet radiation and injected back into the patient. The irradiation may induce apoptosis in the white blood cells and suppress activity of immune cells. After a promising reduction in mortality in a small, randomized trial, a larger randomized trial, ACCLAIM, of immune modulation therapy in chronic heart failure patients has since evaluated a primary endpoint of mortality. A total of 2,600 patients were enrolled and the IMT group was treated for at least 22 weeks. At a mean follow-up of 10 months, there was no significant difference in the two groups (placebo vs. IMT) in

regard to the primary endpoint. However, in two prespecified subgroups—those with no prior myocardial infarction and those with New York Heart Association (NYHA) Class II CHF—there did appear to be a significant difference in the primary outcome (26% mortality reduction in the no MI group and 39% reduction in NYHA Class II CHF). IMT is approved in Europe and is pending FDA approval in the United States for the two subgroups mentioned above.

In summary, it appears that immunosuppressive therapy does not significantly improve mortality or LVEF in acute myocarditis. However, in patients with chronic cardiomyopathy who have positive markers of inflammation (antibodies, HLA expression, etc.), immune therapy may be useful. Additional randomized, controlled trials will be needed to further examine the utility of inflammatory marker-guided therapy. Agents such as interferon appear promising but also need further supportive evidence. Immune modulation therapy may be useful in selected subgroups of nonischemic cardiomyopathy and NYHA Class II patients. As future trials will further explore immunosuppressive agents, it is important to remember that traditional CHF medications, such as ACE-I and beta-blockers, have an antiinflammatory effect that affects both myocarditis and idiopathic chronic cardiomyopathy.

Antiviral treatment has been mainly investigated in animal models and small human case series. The presence of a viral genome on biopsy has been associated with a progressive course of heart failure, death, and transplantation. Ribavirin and interferon alfa treatment reduced myocarditis severity and death in a murine myocarditis model. As the onset of symptoms is often delayed in acute myocarditis from initial viral infection, treatment would likely be less beneficial. However, in those patients with chronic, dilated cardiomyopathy, treatment with interferon resulted in viral clearance and improvement in left ventricular function. Additional treatment trials are needed in such patients to warrant recommendation of antiviral treatment in this setting.

# Heart Transplantation

MICHELLE M. KITTLESON AND JON A. KOBASHIGAWA

## ● PRACTICAL POINTS

- The 5-year mortality for patients with symptomatic heart failure approaches 50% and may be as high as 80% at 1 year for the end-stage patients.

- Improvements in surgical technique and posttransplant care have improved the success and quality of life of heart transplant patients, with a median survival of 10 years (up to 13 years for those surviving the 1st year posttransplant).

- The three major indications for heart transplantation are advanced heart failure (the most common), recurrent angina, and ventricular arrhythmias refractory to maximal medical therapy.

- There are two major areas of contraindication for heart transplantation: medical and social/psychological issues.

- Physiology of a transplanted heart includes a lack of innervation as both afferent and efferent nerve supply is lost; the loss of the afferent conduction results in a patient not experiencing angina.

- The loss of efferent nerves results in the loss of vagal tone (with higher resting heart rate) and the postganglionic direct release of norepinephrine stores in response to exercise (with blunting of the heart rate's response to exercise).

- Due to the lack of vagal tone, patients will not respond to rate controlling effects of digoxin or to the increase in heart rate expected from atropine.

- Triple drug therapy for immunosuppression most commonly consists of steroids, a calcineurin inhibitor (cyclosporine or tacrolimus), and an antimetabolite (azathioprine or mycophenolate mofetil).

- Transplant rejection remains one of the major causes of death after heart transplantation and is most frequent during the 1st month.

- Risk factors associated with early rejection (within 1 year after transplant) include younger age, female donor, female recipient, positive CMV serology, prior infections, and OKT3 induction therapy.

## INTRODUCTION

Despite advances in pharmacologic and device treatment of chronic heart failure, long-term morbidity and mortality remain unacceptably high with many patients progressing to end-stage heart failure. The 5-year mortality for patients with symptomatic heart failure approaches 50% and may be as high as 80% at 1 year for the end-stage patients. Over the past four decades, cardiac transplantation has become the preferred therapy for select patients with end-stage heart disease. Approximately 2,400 heart transplants are performed annually in the United States. According to the registry of the International Society of Heart and Lung Transplantation,

the median survival of patients posttransplantation is currently 10 years, up to 13 years for those surviving the 1st year posttransplant (**Figure 64-1**), a significant improvement over that of medical therapy for heart failure.

Critical to the success of heart transplantation are the continual investigational efforts to optimize immunosuppressive regimens. Improvements in immunosuppression, donor procurement, surgical techniques, and posttransplant care have resulted in a substantial decrease in acute allograft rejection, which had previously significantly limited survival of transplant recipients. Thus, heart transplant recipients can now expect excellent quantity and quality of life.

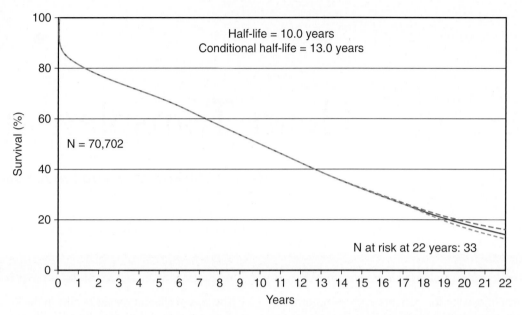

**Figure 64-1.** Kaplan–Meier survival data for adult and pediatric heart transplants performed between January 1982 and June 2005. Conditional half-life = time to 50% survival for those recipients surviving the 1st year posttransplantation. The transplant half-life (the time at which 50% of those transplanted remain alive, or median survival) for the entire cohort of adult and pediatric heart recipients is currently 10 years, with a half-life of 13 years for those surviving the 1st year. (Reproduced with permission from Taylor, et al. *J Heart Lung Transplant.* 2007;26:769–781.)

The purpose of this chapter is to provide an overview of heart transplantation in the current era, focusing on the evaluation process for heart transplantation, the physiology of the transplanted heart, immunosuppressive regimens, and early and long-term complications.

## EVALUATION FOR HEART TRANSPLANTATION

### Indications

The three major indications for heart transplantation are advanced heart failure, recurrent angina, and ventricular arrhythmias refractory to maximal medical therapy. The most common indication for heart transplantation is intractable heart failure. Angina alone is often not considered an indication for transplantation in the absence of heart failure, since it is not clear if the survival of such patients is improved with heart transplantation. Intractable ventricular arrhythmias, commonly referred to as "VT storm," may merit heart transplant evaluation and often urgent listing, given the association with hemodynamic compromise.

With advances in medical therapy, including ACE inhibitors, beta-blockers, implantable defibrillators, and cardiac resynchronization therapy, the long-term survival of patients with end-stage heart failure has dramatically improved. Thus,

it is essential to determine if patients are truly refractory to maximal medical therapy, which may require referral to an advanced heart failure center. At an advanced heart failure center, evaluation may include tailored therapy with pulmonary arterial catheterization for optimization of filling pressures and cardiac output, high-risk revascularization of coronary artery disease, or specialized therapies, such as ablation of ventricular tachycardia, before consideration of heart transplantation.

### Contraindications

There are two major areas of contraindication for heart transplantation: medical and social/psychological. Many of these factors are not absolute and need to be considered in the context of the severity of the patient's heart disease and the presence of associated comorbidities. The extensive evaluation process is designed to identify any contraindication, outlined in detail below and listed in **Table 64-1.**

#### Age
In general, patients should be considered for heart transplantation if they are 70 years of age or younger, since advances in posttransplant care have shown that survival in the older age group is comparable to that of younger transplant recipients. Patients older than 70 years have also been reported to have acceptable outcome, but careful consideration of associated comorbidities is essential.

| Table 64-1 • Recommended Tests for Baseline Evaluation for Heart Transplantation |
| --- |
| Weight/BMI |
| Immunocompatibility<br>  ABO typing<br>  HLA tissue typing<br>  Panel reactive antibodies and flow cytometry |
| Assessment of heart failure severity<br>  Cardiopulmonary exercise test<br>  Echocardiogram<br>  Right heart catheterization |
| Evaluation of multi-organ function<br>  Routine lab work (basic metabolic profile, complete blood count, liver function tests)<br>  Urinalysis<br>  24-hour urine collection for protein and creatinine<br>  Pulmonary function tests<br>  Chest radiograph<br>  Abdominal ultrasound<br>  Carotid Doppler (if >50 years or ischemic heart disease)<br>  Ankle-brachial indices (if >50 years or ischemic heart disease)<br>  Dental examination<br>  Ophthalmological examination (if diabetic) |
| Infectious serology and vaccination<br>  Hepatitis B surface Ag, Ab, core Ab<br>  Hepatitis C Ab<br>  HIV<br>  RPR<br>  IgG for HSV, CMV, toxoplasmosis, EBV, Varicella<br>  PPD<br>  Immunizations: Influenza, pneumovax, hepatitis B |
| Preventive and malignancy<br>  Stool for occult blood ×3<br>  Colonoscopy (if indicated or >50 years)<br>  Mammography (if indicated or >40 years)<br>  Pap smear<br>  Prostate-specific antigen and digital rectal exam (men >50 years) |
| General consultations<br>  Social work<br>  Psychiatry<br>  Financial<br>  As indicated: pulmonology, nephrology, infectious disease, endocrinology |

Source: Adapted with permission from Mehra et al., 2006.

## Obesity

Obese patients have a greater risk of poor wound healing, infections, and pulmonary complications after cardiac surgery, although the data for outcomes in heart transplant recipients are less clear. Nevertheless, it is recommended that weight loss be mandatory to achieve a body mass index (BMI) of less than 30 kg/m² before listing for heart transplantation.

## Malignancy

Active neoplasm excluding nonmelanoma skin cancer is an absolute contraindication to heart transplantation due to limited survival rates. In general, heart transplant recipients with cancers that have been in remission for more than 5 years or that are low-grade, such as prostate cancer, are often acceptable. These guidelines are arbitrary, since immunosuppressive therapy may reactivate a prior malignancy, and consultation with the patient's oncologist is essential in performing an accurate risk assessment.

## Pulmonary Hypertension

Right heart failure contributes to morbidity and mortality after heart transplantation, related to preoperative pulmonary hypertension. Thus, assessment of invasive hemodynamics is an essential part of the transplant evaluation. In general, contraindications to transplantation include (1) a transpulmonary gradient (mean pulmonary artery pressure minus the pulmonary capillary wedge pressure) above 15 mm Hg and calculated pulmonary vascular resistance (PVR) over 5 Woods units, (2) pulmonary artery systolic pressure over 60 mm Hg in conjunction with one of the above findings, and (3) the inability to reduce the PVR below 2.5 with vasodilator or inotropic therapy. In such patients, long-term unloading therapy with an intra-aortic balloon pump (IABP) or ventricular assist device may be required to achieve an acceptable PVR.

## Diabetes

Diabetes that is uncontrolled or associated with end-organ damage (proliferative retinopathy, severe neuropathy, nephropathy, peripheral vascular disease) is often considered a contraindication to transplantation. At our institution, patients will ideally achieve control with a hemoglobin A1c under 7.5% before listing for transplantation; ongoing collaboration with an endocrinologist is helpful in achieving this goal.

## Renal Dysfunction

Renal dysfunction is no longer considered an absolute contraindication to heart transplantation, unless the renal dysfunction is due solely to diabetes, since in this situation, it is a sign of poorly controlled diabetes with end-organ damage. If the renal dysfunction is related to poor cardiac function, it may improve posttransplant, and for some patients, dual heart-kidney transplantation is a consideration.

## Peripheral Vascular Disease

There is little consensus on the role of cerebrovascular and peripheral vascular disease in heart transplant candidates. It is clear that clinically severe disease that is not amenable to revascularization is an absolute contraindication. However, asymptomatic disease, which can be addressed prior to transplantation, may be considered in the overall context of other risk factors.

## Infections

It is understandable that active infection is an absolute contraindication to heart transplantation. Certain chronic infections are also considered contraindications in most centers, including human immunodeficiency virus (HIV) and hepatitis C. Chagas disease, although uncommon in the United Status, is a common indication for transplantation in South America, and reactivation of disease can occur. The decision to proceed with transplantation in these situations must be made in collaboration with an infectious disease specialist well-versed in transplantation.

## Substance Use

Active tobacco smoking is a relative contraindication to heart transplantation, and smoking during the previous 6 months before transplant is a risk factor for poor outcomes. At our institution, we require patients to achieve abstinence from tobacco smoking for 6 months, documented by urine cotinine screens, prior to listing for transplantation. Addiction to alcohol or illicit drugs is an absolute contraindication, as it suggests that these patients will have poor compliance after transplantation, and 6 months abstinence with participation in counseling programs is often required. This assessment may be difficult to make in the critically ill patient in whom transplantation cannot be delayed for 6 months. In this scenario, consultation with a social worker and psychiatric specialists is essential in gauging the patient's commitment to abstinence.

## Psychosocial Evaluation

Patients must be able to demonstrate the ability to comply with medications and follow-up after transplantation, which includes social support with a dedicated caregiver and transportation after transplant. This is a critical issue, and patients have been denied transplantation due to lack of demonstrated compliance and social support. Mental retardation and dementia are relative contraindications to heart transplantation—the former due to concerns of compliance and the latter due to overall poor prognosis.

## Listing for Heart Transplant

### Listing Status

A patient is deemed acceptable for heart transplantation after presentation of the case to a multidisciplinary selection committee composed of cardiologists, cardiothoracic surgeons, a psychiatrist, a social worker, and often other specialists including nephrologists, pulmonologists, and infectious disease physicians. At this point, a patient is listed for transplant. There are three tiers of listing based on medical urgency. The highest urgency is Status 1A, reserved for the following situations: (1) intubated patients, (2) patients on high doses of one or two continuous inotrope infusions with a pulmonary artery catheter in place, (3) patients with an intraaortic balloon pump, or (4) patients status post a ventricular assist device within the first 30 days or with a device-related complication. A Status 1AE exists for patients who require urgent listing but do not meet these criteria, for example, those patients with intractable ventricular arrhythmias in whom inotropes or pulmonary artery catheters are inadvisable. Status 1AE requires approval by a designated committee of the United Network of Organ Sharing. The next tier is Status 1B for the following situations: (1) continuous intravenous inotropic support with one agent and no pulmonary artery catheter in place or (2) a ventricular assist device beyond the first 30 days without a device-related complication. The rest of patients, essentially ambulatory end-stage patients, fall under Status 2 listing.

### Wait Time

The average wait time for a heart transplant varies by region, medical urgency status, blood type, and size. The shortest wait would be for a Status 1A patient who is small and non-O blood type, whereas the longest wait would be for a Status 2 patient who is large and blood type O. An assessment of the wait time to transplantation often factors into the decision to place a ventricular assist device as a bridge to transplant. For a failing patient, a ventricular assist device may be considered if the anticipated wait time is long.

### Alternate List

The major limiting factor in heart transplantation is supply of donor hearts. Based on this, our program began the use of nonstandard donor hearts often used for higher risk recipients, resulting in the creation of two recipient lists. The concept of the alternate list is to match donor and recipient risk, with a resulting expansion of both the donor and recipient pools.

Criteria for the alternate recipient list include those factors that would otherwise preclude transplant: advanced age (usually older than 70 years), moderate renal insufficiency, retransplantation, or peripheral vascular disease. Alternate, or nonstandard, donors are considered to be those with known coronary disease (often requiring revascularization before transplant), high-risk behavior, and hepatitis seropositivity and who are older than 55 years of age. The use of these donor hearts has increased the number of heart transplant operations being performed. In our program, older or nonstandard donor hearts have been used for alternate recipients for the past 15 years, with similar long-term survival and transplant coronary artery disease between older and younger donors.

# PHYSIOLOGY OF THE TRANSPLANTED HEART

## Lack of Innervation to the Transplanted Heart

When the donor heart is placed into the recipient, both afferent (from the heart to the central nervous system) and efferent (from the central nervous system to the heart) nerve supply is lost. The loss of afferent nerve supply means that the recipient will not experience angina. Therefore, chest discomfort in a heart transplant recipient, especially early after transplant, is likely not caused by coronary ischemia, and coronary ischemia will likely not present with chest discomfort. The standard practice of annual angiograms for surveillance of transplant coronary artery disease is a direct consequence of the lack of afferent nerves supplying the transplanted heart.

The consequences of the loss of efferent nerves are related to the loss of vagal tone and the postganglionic direct release of norepinephrine stores in response to exercise. With the loss of vagal tone, heart transplant recipients have a higher than normal resting heart rate of around 90 to 110 beats per minute. The lack of efferent nerves also means that the transplant recipient must rely on circulating catecholamines to respond to exercise, so there is a blunting of the heart rate's response to exercise. Similarly, after exercise, the heart rate returns to baseline more slowly because of the gradual decline of circulating catecholamine concentrations to baseline.

Heart transplant recipients lack the baroreceptor reflex, which relies on intact baroreceptors and sympathetic and parasympathetic innervation. Thus, heart transplant recipients are more susceptible to orthostasis and carotid sinus massage will not break a reentrant tachycardia in these patients.

Nevertheless, heart transplant recipients often experience renervation of the heart with return of angina, an improvement in exercise tolerance, and a decrease in resting heart rate. This process is inconsistent among patients yet tends to increase over time.

## Response to Medications

Some cardiac drugs are not effective in the denervated heart. Due to the lack of vagal tone, digoxin will have little effect on sinoatrial and atrioventricular conduction velocity and will not achieve rate control if the transplanted heart develops atrial fibrillation. However, the inotropic effects of digoxin persist after transplantation. Similarly, the parasympatholytic effect of atropine will not increase heart rate in transplanted hearts. Due to the lack of baroreceptor reflexes, vasodilators such as nifedipine and hydralazine will not cause reflex tachycardia.

The lack of postganglionic sympathetic nerves in the transplanted heart results in increased receptor density and, thus, more sensitivity to sympathetic agonists and antagonists. Clinically, this is most often seen with beta-blockers; heart transplant recipients will often have exaggerated fatigue in response to administration of beta-blockers, especially with exercise.

# IMMUNOSUPPRESSION

## Induction Therapy

### Purpose

The purpose of induction therapy was originally to induce tolerance in the graft. Although this goal has not been realized, induction therapy is still useful in reducing the risk of rejection early posttransplant, when the immune response may be the highest due to increased donor antigen expression from ischemia/reperfusion injury and surgical trauma. The benefits of induction therapy include a marked reduction in rejection in the first 4 to 6 weeks posttransplant and the ability to delay introduction of calcineurin inhibitors to prevent worsening renal dysfunction. The disadvantages of induction therapy include increased risk of infection, risk of malignancy, and rates of late rejection after therapy is completed.

### Regimens

Regimens for induction therapy include cytolytic agents and interleukin 2 receptor (IL-2R) antagonists (**Figure 64-2**). Cytolytic agents include polyclonal agents such as antithymocyte globulin and thymoglobulin and monoclonal agents such as OKT3. However, despite widespread use, no randomized trials of cytolytic agents as induction therapy have been performed in heart transplant recipients. Retrospective evaluations from a large, multiinstitutional database have suggested that cytolytic therapy reduces the risk of early rejection but increases the risk of infection. IL-2R antagonists such as dacluzimab and basiliximab may also be used for induction therapy. There has been a randomized trial of induction therapy with dacluzimab in heart transplant recipients. With dacluzimab, heart transplant recipients had less rejection but an increased risk of death from infection; due to the blinded nature of the study, some patients received both the IL-2R antagonist and cytolytic induction therapy.

Based on these results, induction therapy is not standard practice at our institution. Instead, induction therapy, most often with antithymocyte globulin, is reserved for those patients at the highest risk for rejection, including patients who are highly sensitized with donor-specific antibodies or those with significant renal dysfunction in whom delay of calcineurin inhibition is advisable.

## Rejection Therapy

Rejection therapy refers to immunosuppressive therapy given to reverse an episode of rejection. The type of rejection therapy depends upon whether it is T-cell mediated (cellular) or antibody mediated (humoral). The intensity of rejection therapy depends upon the clinical context: the presence of signs or symptoms of heart failure, reduced ejection fraction, or hemodynamic compromise. In general, therapy for cellular rejection may include an increase in oral

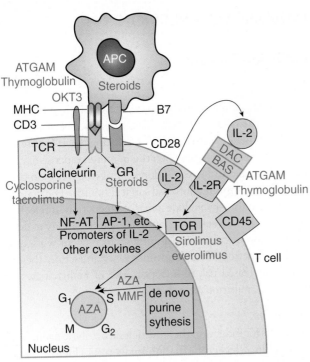

**Figure 64-2.** Immunologic mechanisms leading to graft rejection and sites of action of immunosuppressive drugs. Immunologic mechanisms are shown in blue; immunosuppressive drugs and their site of action are shown in red. Acute rejection begins with recognition of donor antigens that differ from those of recipient by recipient APCs (indirect allorecognition). Donor APCs (carried passively in graft) may also be recognized by recipient T cells (direct allorecognition). Alloantigens carried by APCs are recognized by TCR-CD3 complex on surface of T cell. When accompanied by costimulatory signals between APC and T cells such as B7-CD28, T cell activation occurs, resulting in activation of calcineurin. Calcineurin dephosphorylates transcription factor NF-AT, allowing it to enter nucleus and bind to promoters of IL-2 and other cytokines. IL-2 activates cell surface receptors (IL-2R), stimulating clonal expansion of T cells (T helper cells). IL-2, along with other cytokines produced by T helper cells, stimulates expansion of other cells of immune system. Activation of IL-2R stimulates TOR, which regulates translation of mRNAs to proteins that regulate cell cycle. Sites of action of individual drugs (highlighted in red) demonstrate multiple sites of action of these drugs, underscoring rationale for combination therapy. AZA indicates azathioprine; MMF, mycophenolate mofetil; GR, glucocorticoid receptor; DAC, daclizumab; BAS, basiliximab. (Reproduced with permission from Lindenfeld J, et al. *Circulation.* 2004;110:3734–3740.)

therapy, oral or intravenous pulse-dose steroids, a change in oral therapy, or monoclonal or polyclonal anti-lymphocyte agents (**Table 64-2**). Therapy for humoral rejection is less well-established but may include oral or intravenous pulse-dose steroids, intravenous immune globulin, plasmapheresis, photopheresis, or rituximab. Protocols differ by center, mainly due to the lack of randomized, controlled trials for rejection in heart transplant recipients.

**Table 64-2 • Treatment for Cellular and Humoral Rejection**

| | Cellular Rejection | Humoral Rejection |
|---|---|---|
| Asymptomatic | oral steroid bolus and taper | no treatment |
| Reduced ejection fraction | oral steroid bolus and taper or intravenous pulse steroids | oral steroid bolus and taper or intravenous pulse steroids +/− intravenous immune globulin |
| Hemodynamic compromise | intravenous pulse steroids, cytolytic therapy | intravenous pulse steroids, cytolytic therapy, plasmapheresis, intravenous immune globulin |

## Maintenance Therapy

The purpose of maintenance immunosuppressive therapy is to prevent rejection long term in transplant recipients. Triple drug therapy most commonly consists of steroids, a calcineurin inhibitor such as cyclosporine or tacrolimus, and an antimetabolite such as azathioprine or mycophenolate mofetil. In special situations, a proliferation signal inhibitor, such as sirolimus, may replace the calcineurin inhibitor or antimetabolite. Although the optimal maintenance immunosuppressive regimen has yet to be identified, there is evidence that regimens may be tailored to the individual patient, as detailed below.

## Steroid Therapy

### Mechanism of Action

Corticosteroids are potent immunosuppressive and anti-inflammatory agents (**Figure 64-2**). They diffuse freely across cell membranes and ultimately alter the expression of genes involved in the immune and inflammatory response, affecting the number, distribution, and function of all leukocytes.

### Administration

Corticosteroids are first given as a 500-mg intravenous bolus of methylprednisolone during the heart transplant surgery, followed by three doses of 125 mg intravenously at 12-hour intervals. Oral prednisone is then given in a standard taper, from 40 mg twice daily decreasing by 5-mg increments until the patient is on 10 mg twice daily. At 1 month post-transplant, the patient will start a slow prednisone wean so that by 3 months, the prednisone is reduced to 10 mg once daily and by 6 months, decreased to 5 mg once daily. In our program, patients with no rejection in the first 6 months are candidates to wean off prednisone completely at the

| Table 64-3 • Distinguishing Features of Cardiac Allograft Vasculopathy (CAV) from Nontransplant Atherosclerosis | |
|---|---|
| **Nontransplant Atherosclerosis** | **CAV** |
| Most epicardial disease | Panvascular disease (including microvasculature) |
| Slow progression | Rapid progression |
| Eccentic lesions | Concentric lesions (generally) |
| Lipid rich | Generally lipid poor |
| Early calcification | Late calcification |
| Compensatory remodeling with early dilation (Glagov phenomenon) | arterial constriction |

| Table 64-4 • Treatment Options for Cardiac Allograft Vasculopathy |
|---|
| **Prevention** |
| Aspirin |
| Control of hypertension (calcium channel blockers, ACE inhibitors) |
| HMG CoA reductase inhibitors |
| Control of diabetes |
| Mycophenolate mofetil |
| Proliferation signal inhibitors (sirolimus, everolimus) |
| **Treatment** |
| Drug-eluting stents |
| Proliferation signal inhibitors |
| Surgical revascularization |
| Retransplantation |

Glagov phenomenon) is inhibited and the artery may even undergo constriction, which may contribute to the earlier manifestation of clinically apparent disease. In some cases, subepicardial inflammatory infiltrates are noted even in the absence of myocardial interstitial inflammatory infiltrates and intravascular thrombus may be found at autopsy or following explant for retransplantation.

As CAV lesions are frequently concentric due to subintimal cellular proliferation, conventional coronary angiography generally underestimates the extent of disease. In contrast, intravascular ultrasound (IVUS) allows direct imaging of the vessel wall to determine the extent of intimal and medial disease (**Figure 64-4**). The technique has been useful in determining characteristics of donor-related lesions (conventional atherosclerosis) by examination early following transplant and comparing transplant-acquired lesions later on in the same regions. IVUS therefore is able to provide more detailed assessment of CAV with increased sensitivity. However, IVUS is not currently performed routinely at many centers but usually as part of research protocols.

### Treatment

Clinically apparent CAV is associated with a poor prognosis and therefore prevention is an important strategy (**Table 64-4**). Agents used in the treatment and prevention of conventional atherosclerosis are utilized for CAV. Aspirin is given due to its established role in nontransplant coronary disease. Control of hypertension and hyperlipidemia is paramount. HMG Co-A Reductase inhibitors are particularly important as they also prevent allograft rejection. Newer immunosuppressive agents, such as MMF and the proliferation signal inhibitors, also show significant promise in affecting the natural course of CAV, as discussed above.

Once clinically significant CAV is apparent, a number of approaches are available to relieve ischemia. For focal disease, percutaneous coronary intervention (PCI) with balloon angioplasty is successful, although restenosis is common in the transplant setting. Drug-eluting stents may help, but restenosis rates continue to be higher than for similar interventions in the nontransplant population. There is no evidence to date that PCI alters the prognosis of CAV and, since many patients with significant disease are asymptomatic, intervention often presents a dilemma. Patients with multivessel focal disease with adequate distal target vessels may be candidates for surgical revascularization with coronary artery bypass grafting (CABG). Efficacy is difficult to determine, as relatively small numbers have been reported, reflecting the many patients who do not have adequate targets and the preferential use of PCI.

Retransplantation may be a consideration for many patients with advanced CAV not amenable to PCI or CABG with

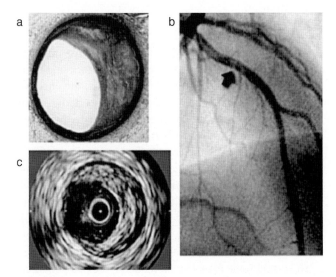

**Figure 64-4.** Concentric or eccentric subintimal proliferation in CAV seen histologically (a) are underestimated in lesion severity angiographically (b) but are better appreciated by IVUS (c). (Reproduced with permission from Kobashigawa JA, Patel JK. Chronica Allograft Failure: Natural History, Pathogenesis, Diagnosis and Management. *Landes Biosci.* 2007.)

comparable survival at our institution. The scarcity of donor hearts, however, creates an ethical dilemma. Some argue that it is better to maximally distribute organs rather than to allocate two organs to the same individual. Others contend that patients needing a second transplant should be considered on the same basis as those being evaluated for a first transplant.

## Malignancy

### Incidence

After CAV, malignancy is the second major impediment to long-term survival in heart transplant recipients, accounting for 24% of deaths 5 years after transplantation. The risk of malignancy from immunosuppressive agents is due to reduced immune surveillance for neoplasia. All immunosuppressive agents are believed to contribute to the cumulative risk of malignancy, with the possible exception of corticosteroids. In animal studies and renal transplantation, sirolimus may have antiproliferative properties that result in fewer malignancies.

### Clinical Presentation

Cutaneous malignancies are the most common type after heart transplantation, mainly squamous cell carcinomas. Posttransplant lymphoproliferative disorder (PTLD) can also occur. There is a strong association of PTLD with Epstein-Barr virus infection, and an increase in the total burden of immunosuppression increases the risk of developing lymphoma. Finally, neoplasms common in the general population also occur in heart transplant recipients, including breast, lung, and prostate.

### Treatment

The most critical point of treatment of malignancies is prevention. We encourage all heart transplant recipients at our institution to undergo routine health maintenance screenings with their primary care physicians, including mammograms, pap smears, prostate exams, and colonoscopies as indicated for nontransplant patients. In addition, patients are instructed to utilize sun protection and to have low threshold to establish care with a dermatologist for routine skin exams.

The initial approach to malignancy is reduction of immunosuppression, and this may be the only treatment required for some forms of PTLD. In our institution, we will consider switching patients with newly diagnosed malignancy to sirolimus, due to its possible protective effect in malignancies, in place of a calcineurin inhibitor or MMF.

## Other Long-term Complications

### Renal Dysfunction

Renal insufficiency is a common adverse effect of the calcineurin inhibitors and often worsens over time, such that up to 8% of transplant recipients will develop end-stage renal disease at 5 or more years posttransplant. Renal-sparing immunosuppressive regimens are often utilized in such patients, including a reduction in calcineurin inhibitor dose or substitution of the calcineurin inhibitor with sirolimus. To be successful, the timing is important; if the creatinine is too high, often above 2.5 mg/dL, the renal damage may be irreversible. When replacing calcineurin inhibitors with sirolimus, the key to preventing rejection is to withdraw calcineurin inhibitors gradually over a period of 2 to 4 weeks while awaiting therapeutic sirolimus levels and monitoring patients with a follow-up echocardiogram and biopsy at 1 month after complete withdrawal of the calcineurin inhibitor. Although randomized trial data of renal sparing regimens are not yet available, we have found that with these caveats, renal-sparing protocols appear efficacious, safe, and beneficial for select patients.

### Hypertension

Hypertension after cardiac transplantation is primarily a result of calcineurin inhibitor use and occurs in up to 80% of patients. Posttransplant hypertension is often difficult to control and often requires a combination of several antihypertensive agents. No agent has been shown to be superior, but beta-blockers are often avoided since the denervated heart relies on circulating catecholamines to maintain cardiac function during exercise and, thus, heart transplant recipients often experience significant fatigue with beta-blocker administration. ACE inhibitors and angiotensin receptor blockers may not be tolerated due to renal dysfunction or hyperkalemia. Dihydropyridine calcium channel blockers such as amlodipine and nifedipine are often effective but may result in troublesome dependent edema and will increase levels of calcineurin inhibitors (mainly diltiazem), which should be monitored after initiation.

### Dyslipidemia

Lipid abnormalities are common after heart transplantation due to the use of steroids, calcineurin inhibitors, and PSIs. The HMG-CoA reductase inhibitors (statins) are effective in reducing total and LDL cholesterol in heart transplant recipients. It is notable that treatment initiated within 2 weeks of transplantation with statins is associated with a lower frequency of hemodynamically compromising rejection episodes and improved survival over the first transplant year. These agents likely have an immunosuppressive effect in addition to their lipid-lowering activity. As hyperlipidemia is so common following transplantation, all cardiac transplant recipients should receive statin therapy. Pravastatin is the statin of choice, since it is not metabolized by the cytochrome 3A4 system, reducing the possible interactions with calcineurin inhibitors.

### Diabetes

Given that diabetes mellitus is a major cardiovascular risk factor leading to the development of end-stage heart disease, diabetes is common in patients pretransplant. Furthermore, the use of steroids and tacrolimus posttransplant may cause or worsen diabetes; up to 32% of heart transplant recipients are diabetic by 5 years posttransplant. Although diabetes is associated with poorer long-term survival, there are few data regarding the treatment of these patients. In general, since renal insufficiency in so common in these patients, metformin is often avoided. Furthermore, thiazoladinediones are not preferred due to the risk of fluid retention. Shorter-acting sulfonylureas may be the agents of choice for many heart transplant recipients.

## Osteoporosis

Osteoporosis resulting in vertebral compression fractures is a common and debilitating problem after heart transplantation, exacerbated by steroid use. At our institution, we recommend screening bone-density examinations by internists on an annual basis. To prevent osteoporosis, patients should receive supplemental calcium and vitamin D, engage in weight-bearing exercises, and receive biphosphonates as recommended by the primary care physician.

## Gout

Causes of gout after heart transplantation include calcineurin inhibitor use, diuretic use, and renal insufficiency. Nonsteroidal antiinflammatory agents are often avoided in heart transplant recipients due to the potential exacerbation of renal insufficiency. Colchicine may be used to treat acute attacks, although there is a risk of myoneuropathy when colchicine is given in conjunction with calcineurin inhibitors. Thus, for acute flares, systemic or intra-articular steroids are often the treatment of choice. Allopurinol is useful as suppressive therapy, as long as the patient is not receiving azathioprine, since the combination may result in severe myelosuppression. Given the potential for adverse effects and drug interactions, consultation with a rheumatologist is often helpful in management of gout in heart transplant recipients.

## SUMMARY

Over the past four decades, cardiac transplantation has become the preferred therapy for select patients with end-stage heart disease. Improvements in immunosuppression, donor procurement, surgical techniques, and posttransplant care have resulted in a substantial decrease in acute allograft rejection, which had previously significantly limited survival of transplant recipients. According to the registry of the International Society of Heart and Lung Transplantation, the median survival of patients posttransplantation is currently 10 years, up to 13 years for those surviving the 1st year posttransplant—far greater than would be expected for end-stage heart failure. However, major impediments to long-term allograft survival exist, including rejection, infection, cardiac allograft vasculopathy, and malignancy. Nevertheless, through careful balance of immunosuppressive therapy and vigilant surveillance for complications, we can expect further advances in the long-term outcomes of heart transplant recipients over the decades to come.

## Suggested Readings

1. Mehra MR, Kobashigawa J, Starling R, et al. Listing criteria for heart transplantation: International Society for Heart and Lung Transplantation guidelines for the care of cardiac transplant candidates. *J Heart Lung Transplant.* 2006;25: 1024–1042.

2. Taylor DO, Edwards LB, Boucek MM, et al. Registry of the International Society for Heart and Lung Transplantation: Twenty-fourth official adult heart transplant report. *J Heart Lung Transplant.* 2007;26:769–781.

3. Lindenfeld J, Miller GG, Shakar SF, et al. Drug therapy in the heart transplant recipient: Part I: Cardiac rejection and immunosuppressive drugs. *Circulation.* 2004a;110:3734–3740.

4. Lindenfeld J, Miller GG, Shakar SF, et al. Drug therapy in the heart transplant recipient: Part II: Immunosuppressive drugs. *Circulation.* 2004b;110:3858–3865.

5. Lindenfeld J, Page RL, Zolty R, et al. Drug therapy in the heart transplant recipient: Part III: Common medical problems. *Circulation.* 2005;111:113–117.

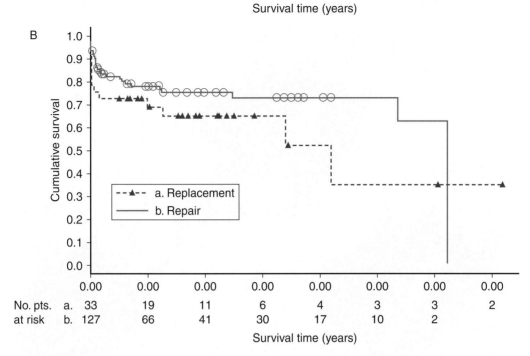

Survival time (years)

**Figure 65-4.** Survival is superior in mitral valve repair (solid line) compared to mitral valve replacement (interrupted line). (Source: Grossi, et al. *J Thorac Cardiovasc Surg.* 2001;122:1107–1124.)

Infarcted zones also contribute to the development of akinetic or dyskinetic segments of the left ventricular free wall. White et al. believe that left ventricular end-systolic volume is a major determinant of survival after recovery from myocardial resection and place a greater significance on this measurement than the ejection fraction. A left ventricular end-systolic volume index (LVESVI) greater than or equal to 40 mL/m$^2$ measured within 90 minutes of hospitalization was associated with a high incidence of congestive heart failure and poor long-term survival.

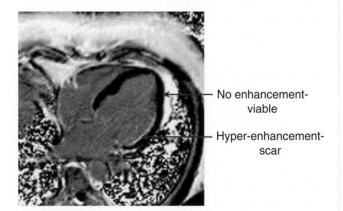

**Figure 65-5.** Cardiac MRI demonstration of myocardial viability. 50-year-old male with low ejection fraction. Cardiac MRI demonstrates subendocardial infarction along basal to mid-anterolateral wall. Remaining myocardium is viable.

## Surgical Ventricular Restoration

Surgical ventricular restoration (SVR) **(Figure 65-6)** aims to reshape the LV from a spherical shape to an elliptical shape and decrease the chamber volume. In the operation of surgical ventricular restoration, described by Vincent Dor, a coronary artery bypass procedure is initially performed along with addressing the mitral regurgitation by mitral valve repair or replacement, if necessary. Subsequently, a linear incision is made along the left ventricular free wall in the middle of the akinetic or dyskinetic segment. The anteroseptal, apical, and anterolateral akinetic or dyskinetic segments are identified and excluded by an intracardiac patch or direct closure. In an analysis of 1,198 postinfarction patients in the RESTORE registry who underwent SVR (previous anterior myocardial infarction, LVESVI ≥60 mL/m$^2$, and a regional noncontractile area of ≥35%), the investigators observed an overall 30-day mortality after SVR of 5.3%, a 5-year survival of 68.6±2.8%, and a significant improvement in the NYHA functional class (preoperatively 67% of patients were Class III or IV and postoperatively 85% were Class I or II). The results from the initial RESTORE studies led to the design of the STICH (Surgical Treatment of Ischemic Heart Disease) trial, which randomized patients with ischemic cardiomyopathy, Class II-IV HF, EF less than or equal to 35%, and an LV asynergic segment greater than or equal to 35% to different therapies. If the LVESVI was less than or equal to 60 mL/m$^2$, patients were

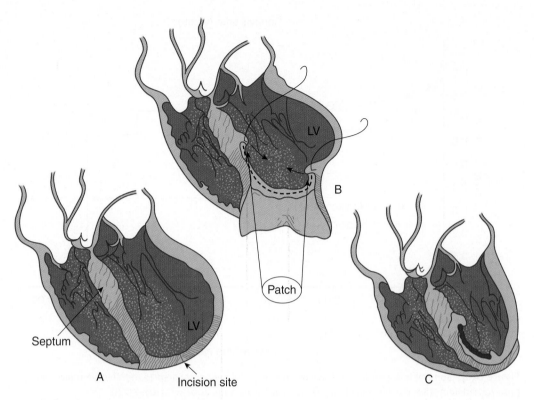

**Figure 65-6.** Surgical ventricular restoration.

randomized to medical therapy or coronary artery bypass grafting (CABG). However, if the LVESVI was greater than or equal to 60 mL/m², they were randomized to medical therapy, CABG, or CABG plus SVR. The STICH investigators have reported that adding SVR to coronary artery bypass grafting does not provide clinical benefit beyond that of CABG alone; both strategies provided similar short- and long-term relief of angina and heart failure and improvement in 6-minute walk test performance. Further subset analysis is pending to identify key features in patients who could benefit by the addition of SVR to CABG.

## Mitral Valve

Mitral valve apparatus consists of the mitral annulus, the valve leaflets, chordae tendinae, and the papillary muscles and their attachment to the left ventricular wall (left ventricle – mitral valve continuity). Mitral regurgitation (MR) in heart failure is multifactorial. The dilation of the left ventricle alters its geometry and causes incomplete leaflet coaptation, and this is further exacerbated by annular dilation. In addition, in ischemic cardiomyopathy, papillary muscle or segmental left ventricular wall motion abnormality causes tethering of the chordae tendinae and contributes to MR. Several techniques of mitral repair have been described **(Figures 65-7, 65-8,** and **65-9).** Ninety-two patients in NYHA Class III or IV heart failure underwent mitral valve

repair with an undersized flexible annuloplasty ring for severe mitral regurgitation and depressed ejection fraction (<25%). The overall mortality rate was 5%, and 1- and 2-year actuarial survival was 80% and 70%, respectively. At 24-month follow-up, all survivors had a subjective improvement in functional class, remained in NYHA Class I and II HF, and demonstrated improved LV ejection fraction, improved cardiac output, and a decrease in the sphericity index.

A number of retrospective studies have demonstrated improved LV function and survival in patients undergoing valve repair compared to valve replacement with or without subvalvular (chordal) preservation. If the anatomy is appropriate, mitral valve repair is preferred to maintain valve morphology.

## Heart Transplantation

Whereas the technique of heart transplantation was perfected by Norman Shumway and Richard Lower at Stanford University, the first human-to-human heart transplantation was performed by Christiaan Barnard in South Africa on December 3, 1961. This therapy is offered to patients in NYHA Class II, III, or IV who are failing maximal medical therapy with a severely depressed ejection fraction and a reduced functional capacity. Other indications include inoperable coronary artery disease with disabling angina or malignant ventricular arrhythmias, both of which are unresponsive to medical therapies.

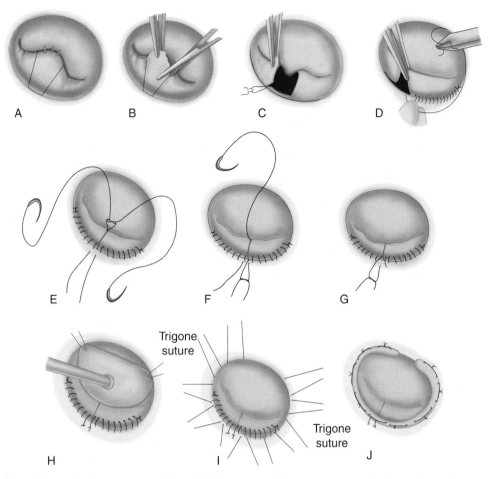

**Figure 65-7.** Quadrangular resection and sliding annuloplasty. (Source: Mitral Valve Repair, Chen FY, Cohn LH in Cardiac Surgery in Adult, Editor L H Cohn 3rd edition.)

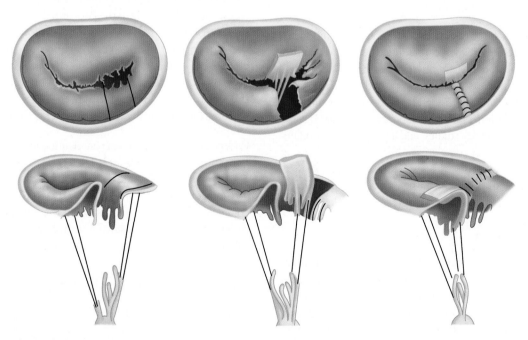

**Figure 65-8.** Chordal transfer. An isolated flair anterior leaflet is resected and replaced with an adjoining portion of the posterior leaflet. (Source: Chen FY, Cohn LH. Mitral valve repair. In: Cohn LH, ed. *Cardiac Surgery in Adult*. 3rd ed.)

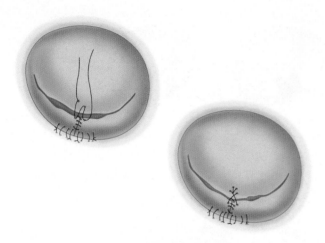

**Figure 65-9.** Alfieri stitch. The edges of middle portions of the anterior and posterior leaflet are brought together. (Source: Mitral Valve Repair, Chen FY, Cohn LH in Cardiac Surgery in Adult, Editor L H Cohn 3rd edition.)

**Contraindications:**

1. age >70 years (in most centers)
2. severe fixed pulmonary hypertension
3. end-organ damage due to diabetes
4. chronic debilitating illnesses
5. severe peripheral vascular disease
6. active infection
7. morbid obesity
8. substance abuse (current)
9. recent malignancy
10. HIV status
11. severe hepatic dysfunction
12. poor nutritional status

The evaluation for heart transplantation is a multidisciplinary approach involving heart failure cardiologists, cardiac surgeons, social workers, and physician extenders. Complete evaluation includes a detailed history and physical examination including an obstetric and gynecological evaluation, laboratory evaluation, pulmonary function tests, dental clearance, bone densitometry studies, and a psycho-social and nutritional assessment. A complete cardiac work-up includes an echocardiogram, exercise stress test with oxygen uptake measurements, right and left heart catheterization, and a myocardial biopsy, where the cause of heart failure is unclear.

## Donor Selection

The criteria for accepting a donor for heart transplantation include ABO blood group compatibility, donor weight within 30% of recipient weight, preferably an age younger than 55 years, an absence of the following: pre-existing cardiac disease, hemodynamic instability without high dose inotropic support, severe chest trauma, extracerebral malignancy, septicemia and positive serologies for human immunodeficiency virus, hepatitis B, or hepatitis C. With an increasing shortage of donor organs, marginal donors are currently being evaluated for organ retrieval. If the recipient's percentage of reactive antibodies (PRA) is greater than 10 to 15%, a T- and B-cell cross match is performed between the recipient and donor sera with a positive cross-match being an absolute contraindication to transplantation. Prior to accepting a donor heart, an echocardiogram is carefully evaluated for any valve pathologies or wall motion abnormalities. In addition, on occasion, a left heart catheterization is obtained to rule out coronary artery disease, usually based on donor age and risk factors. Moreover, at the time of surgery, the exterior of the heart is carefully palpated for thrills or areas of calcification along the coronary arteries and a visual assessment is made of the right ventricular function.

## Donor Heart Procurement

After a median sternotomy, the heart is evaluated. Careful dissection is carried out around the superior vena cava, the azygos vein and inferior vena cava, the aorta, and the main pulmonary artery. A cardioplegia cannula is placed in the aortic root. Once the abdominal team is ready, heparin is administered, snares are placed around the superior and inferior vena cava, and the cross clamp is applied across the ascending aorta, while one liter of cardioplegia solution is administered into the aortic root to obtain an efficient arrest of the heart. Care is taken to avoid distension of the left ventricle and the heart is vented by making a small incision in either the left atrial appendage or the right superior pulmonary vein. In addition, rapid cooling of the heart is achieved by throwing crushed ice into the pericardial well. Subsequently, the heart is excised by severing different locations: dividing the superior and inferior vena cava with a cuff, the aorta close to the innominate artery branch, the pulmonary artery at its bifurcation, and the pulmonary veins to leave a cuff at the left atrium. Following excision, the heart is examined for a patent foramen ovale, which, if present, is closed.

Preservation of the heart is of paramount importance and a safe ischemic period for the heart is 4 to 6 hours. The heart is generally transported in a sterile container immersed in a cardioplegic storage solution at a temperature of 4°C to 6°C. Various commercially available solutions exist that differ in their ionic composition and are classified as extracellular or intracellular solutions, each with its own protagonists and opponents.

## Orthotopic Heart Implantation

There are two different techniques for the right sided anastomosis: (1) the bicaval technique, in which the donor cavae are anastomosed to the recipient cavae, and (2) the biatrial technique, where the donor right atrium is attached to the recipient right atrium. The bicaval technique is preferred by some due to the reported decrease in the incidence of tricuspid regurgitation in the late post-transplant period, and this is the technique described below.

Under general anesthesia, the patient is laid supine on the operating room table and the chest and lower extremities are prepped and draped in a sterile fashion. A median sternotomy is performed and the patient is fully heparinized. Aortic and bicaval venous cannulation is carried out. Snares are passed along both the superior and inferior vena cava. The patient is placed on full cardiopulmonary bypass and the aortic cross clamp is applied. Following this, the native heart is excised to leave a cuff of the left atrium, superior and inferior vena cava, a cuff of the native aorta just proximal to the native aorta, and the main pulmonary artery just proximal to its bifurcation. The donor heart is prepared to match the native cuffs. It is brought into the field between small ice packs. Following completion of the left atrial and aortic anastomosis, adequate de-airing, and administration of steroids, the aortic cross clamp is removed. This minimizes the ischemic interval for the donor heart. Subsequently, the inferior vena caval, pulmonary arterial, and superior vena caval anastomoses are carried out and the patient is weaned off cardiopulmonary bypass. Protamine is administered to neutralize the effects of heparin and the cannulae are removed. Temporary pacing wires are placed on the epicardial surface of the right atrium and the right ventricle. Chest tubes are positioned in the mediastinum (and the pleural cavities as appropriate), followed by chest closure and transportation to the intensive care unit for observation. It is important to keep the heart rate around 110 beats per minute either by using isoproterenol or by pacing. This helps to prevent the distension of the donor right ventricle as it works against higher native pulmonary pressures than it is used to.

## Initial Immunosuppressive Therapy

Initial immunosuppression includes tacrolimus or cyclosporine, mycophenolate mofetil, and corticosteroids, but the specific regimen usually varies with the particular transplant center. Induction therapy with thymoglobulin or other agents is usually reserved for pretransplant renal insufficiency to avoid early exposure to calcineurin inhibitors or in high risk patients (e.g., elevated PRA, multiparous women, retransplant); however, again, this varies with the transplant center. The selection and modification of a particular regimen of immunosuppressive therapy are dependent on multiple factors including any evidence of rejection on surveillance heart biopsies, renal and liver dysfunction, and patient tolerance.

# Mechanical Circulatory Support Devices

The artificial heart program was initiated by the National Institutes of Health in 1964 to encourage the development of temporary mechanical circulatory support for end-stage heart failure. Subsequent research and development has led to the design of a plethora of devices intended to support patients in acute and chronic heart failure. The first total artificial heart, designed by Dr. Domingo Liotta in 1969, was implanted in a human being by Dr. Denton Cooley as a bridge to heart transplantation. The patient survived for almost 3 days with the artificial heart and a further 36 hours with a transplanted heart. In 1994, with further developments in the field, the U.S. Food and Drug Administration approved the use of left ventricular assist devices (LVAD) from Thermo Cardiosystems Inc. (TCI) for circulatory support in patients awaiting heart transplantation. In order to better understand the role of LVAD as an alternative to cardiac transplantation, the REMATCH (Randomized Evaluation of Mechanical Assistance for the Treatment of Congestive Heart Failure) was conducted. In this study, 129 patients in NYHA Class IV heart failure were randomized to maximal medical therapy (61 patients) or implantation of LVAD (68 patients). One- and 2-year survival for the medical arm was 25% and 8%, respectively, as compared to 53% and 23% survival in the surgical arm. A 48% mortality reduction favored the implantation of LVAD in theseis patients population with end-stage heart failure who were not transplant candidates.

Mechanical circulatory support devices (MCSD) are utilized in various clinical scenarios as a bridge to transplantation or recovery or as destination therapy. LVADs have been implanted in more than 4,000 patients as a bridge to heart transplantation. When a patient is deemed to be a suitable candidate for transplantation, the LVAD is implanted and the patient is discharged. Following adequate recovery and optimization of various parameters, including nutritional status, the patient is listed for heart transplantation. Upon the availability of a suitable donor, the LVAD and the native heart are explanted and the donor heart is implanted. In patients considered unsuitable for transplantation for a variety of reasons (smoking, obesity, recently diagnosed cancer, patient preference, severe pulmonary hypertension), LVADs are offered as destination therapy. A small cohort of patients (acute-onset fulminant myocarditis, postpartum cardiomyopathy, nonischemic dilated cardiomyopathy) may recover cardiac function while on LVAD support and the device can be successfully explanted. Our experience at Ohio State University Medical Center in the various categories is outlined in **Figure 65-10**.

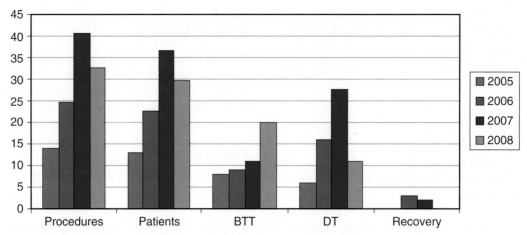

**Figure 65-10.** Categories of patients at Ohio State University Medical Center. BTT, bridge to transplantation; DT, destination therapy.

## Types of Devices

The devices can be classified depending on the duration of support or their flow characteristics **(Figure 65-11)**.

### Intra-aortic Balloon Pump (IABP)

The simplest of mechanical circulatory support, familiar in every hospital, is the percutaneously inserted intra-aortic counterpulsation balloon pump through the femoral artery with its tip positioned just distal to the origin of the left subclavian artery. The position of the tip of the balloon pump is confirmed either with a chest x-ray or by a trans-esophageal echocardiogram, if the patient is in the operating room. The intra-aortic balloon is programmed to rapidly inflate in early diastole when the aortic valve closes and rapidly deflate just before systole when the aortic valve opens and the left ventricle is ejecting. Coronary blood flow occurs during diastole and inflation of the balloon during diastole augments the coronary perfusion. In addition, the inflated balloon displaces blood and increases the mean blood flow to the periphery. Deflation of the balloon during systole, when the

aortic valve opens, decreases the afterload and augments the stroke volume. The main contraindications to the insertion of the IABP are aortic insufficiency, aortic dissection, and an extremely atheromatous and calcified aorta.

### Extracorporeal Membrane Oxygenation (ECMO)

The indications for placing a patient on ECMO can be broadly classified into cardiac and respiratory dysfunction. Some patients in cardiac failure, refractory to inotropic and IABP support, benefit from placement on ECMO; the categories include perioperative myocardial infarction, cardiac arrest in the catheterization laboratory, postcardiotomy cardiogenic shock, and cardiac allograft dysfunction or failure. In addition, ECMO is used to support patients in respiratory failure not responsive to conventional ventilation techniques (e.g., adult respiratory distress syndrome, acute lung injury). The circuit usually consists of a centrifugal pump, heat exchanger, membrane oxygenator, and cannulas (either inserted percutaneously into the vessels or central cannulation via a sternotomy). A veno-arterial ECMO supports both cardiac and respiratory function. The cannulas are inserted to drain the blood from the femoral vein, and after passage through the ECMO circuit, the blood is delivered into the femoral artery. If the chest is open, central cannulation can be carried out with a cannula in the right atrium for venous drainage and cannula in the aorta for delivery of the oxygenated blood. After a period of support and with recovery of cardiac and respiratory function, the patient is weaned off the ECMO support and decannulated. Venovenous ECMO is used for pure respiratory failure.

### Short-Term Mechanical Circulatory Support

The experience at Ohio State University Medical Center in providing short-term mechanical support for both the

| Short term support | Short term support |
|---|---|
| – Pulsatile | – Pulsatile |
| • Intra-aortic balloon pump | • Abiomed AB 5000 |
| • Abiomed BVS/AB 5000 | • Thoratec IVAD/PVAD |
| • Thoratec PVAD/IVAD | • Heartmate XVE |
| – Continuous flow | • Novacor |
| • Tandem heart | – Continuous flow |
| • Levotronix–centrimag | • Micromed |
| • Impella 2.5 | • Heartmate II |
| • Impella 5.0 | • Ventrassist |
| • Circulite | • Heartware |
| | • Duraheart |

**Figure 65-11.** Types of devices based on duration of support and flow characteristics.

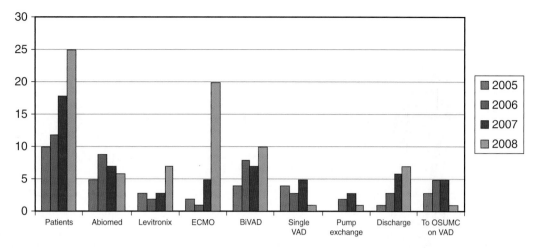

**Figure 65-12.** Ventricular assist devices—Short-term support at Ohio State University Medical Center.

left and right ventricle is illustrated in **Figure 65-12**. A wide variety of devices (**Figures 65-13** and **65-14**) are utilized as rescue therapy in patients in cardiogenic shock with right or left ventricular failure or biventricular failure. To provide support for the left side, the apex of the ventricle, the right superior pulmonary vein, or the left atrial appendage is cannulated and blood circulates through the pump and is delivered into the aorta. For right ventricular failure, a cannula is inserted into the right atrium to provide the venous drainage, and after circulating through the pump, the blood is delivered through a cannula in the pulmonary artery. Percutaneously inserted pumps of interest to the interventional cardiologists include the Tandem Heart and Impella 2.5 for use in high risk coronary interventions. The TandemHeart (**Figure 65-15**) consists of a percutaneously inserted cannula in the femoral vein, which is guided across the interatrial septum, and the tip is positioned in the left atrium. The blood is withdrawn from the left atrium and the magnetically driven centrifugal pump delivers the blood into the arterial circulation

**Figure 65-13.** A biomed AB ventricle.

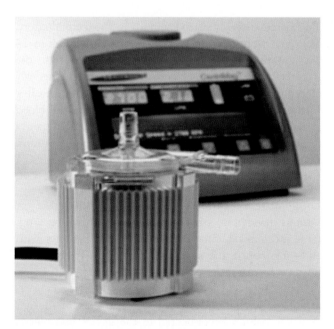

**Figure 65-14.** Levotronix centrimag.

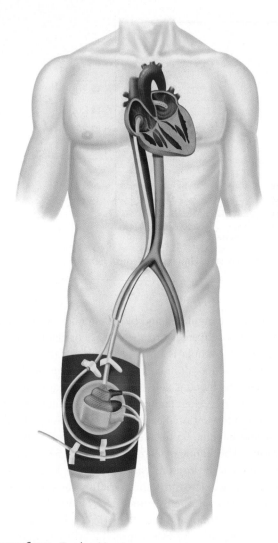

**Figure 65-15.** TandemHeart.

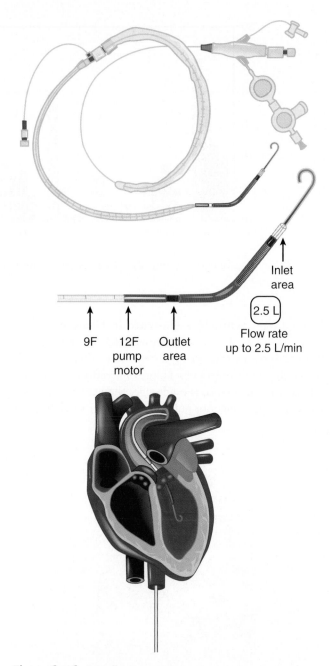

**Figure 65-16.** Impella 2.5 system.

via a percutaneously placed cannula in the femoral artery. The pump can provide support from a few hours to 14 days and help the left ventricle recover. In contrast, the Impella 2.5 heart pump (**Figure 65-16**) is percutaneously placed through the femoral artery, across the aortic valve with inlet tip in the left ventricle from where the blood is drawn, and is then delivered into the ascending aorta to provide safety during high risk coronary interventions. The safety and feasibility were studied in the PROTECT 1 trial.

### Long-Term Mechanical Circulatory Support

Various devices are currently in use for providing long-term mechanical circulatory support for patients with end-stage congestive heart failure, either as a bridge to heart transplantation, as recovery, or as destination therapy. A typical left ventricular assist device consists of an inflow cannula inserted into the apex of the left ventricle, which is connected to the device and placed in the left subcostal region in a pre-peritoneal pocket.

From the device, an outflow graft is anastomosed to the ascending aorta. The device is powered via a percutaneous lead connected to external rechargeable batteries and a power source. The devices have evolved from first-generation volume displacement pulsatile devices with valves (Heartmate XVE) to second-generation smaller axial flow pumps (Heartmate II;, **Figure 65-17**) and to the third-generation rotary pumps with noncontact magnetically levitated bearings pumps (VentrAssist™). Patients on the axial flow pumps and the rotary pumps need to be anticoagulated to minimize the risk of thromboembolic events. Whereas the above devices provide long-term support for the left ventricle, the Syncardia Cardiowest Total

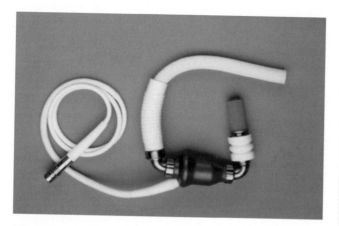

**Figure 65-17.** Heartmate II LVAD.

Artificial Heart **(Figure 65-18)**, approved by the Food and Drug Administration for bridge to cardiac transplantation in 2004, is indicated in patients with biventricular failure where the native heart is excised and the device is implanted within the mediastinum. The patient is subsequently transplanted when the device is removed and the donor heart is implanted. Our medical center's experience with long-term mechanical circulatory support is outlined in the graph **(Figure 65-19)**.

## SUMMARY

Congestive heart failure is a growing public health problem worldwide with significant morbidity and mortality. Optimization of medical therapy alleviates the symptoms and results in improved survival. Cardiac transplantation is epidemiologically trivial. With modifications and innovations

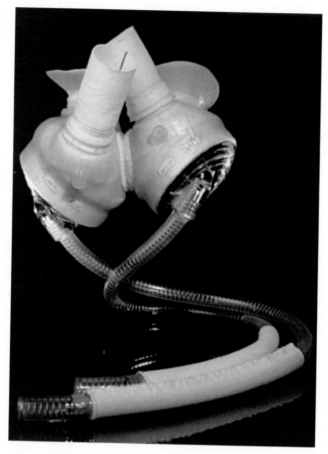

**Figure 65-18.** Syncardia Cardiowest Total Artificial Heart.

in the devices, long-term mechanical circulatory support appears to be a promising option in decreasing mortality from congestive heart failure and providing improved quality of life.

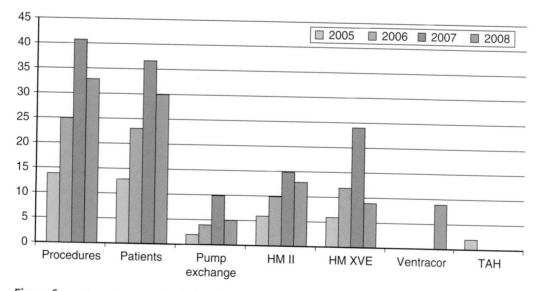

**Figure 65-19.** Long-term mechanical circulatory support at Ohio State University Medical Center. HM, HeartMate; TAH, Total Artificial Heart.

## Suggested Readings

1. Jones RH, Velazquez EJ, Michler RE, et al. Coronary bypass surgery with or without surgical ventricular reconstruction. *N Engl J Med.* 2009;360:1705–1717.

2. Bolling SF, Smolens IA, Pagani FD. Surgical alternatives for heart failure. *J Heart Lung Transplant.* 2001;20:729–733.

3. Rose EA, Gelijns AC, Moskowithz AJ, et al. Long-term mechanical left ventricular assistance for end stage heart failure. *N Engl J Med.* 2001;345:1435–1443.

4. Dixon SR, Henriques JP, Mauri L, et al. A prospective feasibility trial investigating the use of the Impella 2.5 system in patients undergoing high-risk percutaneous coronary intervention (The PROTECT I Trial). *J Am Coll Cardiol Intv.* 2009;2:91–96.

5. Chen FY, Cohn LH. Mitral valve repair. In: Cohn LH, ed. *Cardiac surgery in the adult.* 3rd ed. New York: McGraw-Hill; 2008:1013–1030.

# Electrophysiology

# 66

# Sudden Cardiac Death and Ventricular Arrhythmias

JOHN D. HUMMEL AND MACY C. SMITH

## ● PRACTICAL POINTS

- Sudden cardiac death is one of the leading causes of death in the United States with the absolute number of sudden cardiac deaths in the United States ranging between 200,000 and 450,000 per year.

- Ventricular fibrillation (VF) and ventricular tachycardia (VT) as well as premature ventricular contractions (PVCs), non-sustained VT, and accelerated idioventricular rhythms that occur during acute myocardial infarction or within the first 72 hours of the event are usually due to increased automaticity and generally do not have meaningful prognostic implications.

- Implantation of an implantable defibrillator for primary prevention of sudden death entails implantation in a patient at risk for sudden cardiac arrest who has never suffered such an event.

- Implantation of a defibrillator for primary prevention of sudden death is a Class I indication with an ischemic cardiomyopathy at least 40 days post-MI when patients have an LVEF ≤35% and are in NYHA class II or III; have an LVEF ≤ 30% and are in NYHA class I; or have non-sustained VT, LVEF≤40%, and inducible VF or sustained VT at electrophysiological testing.

- Implantation of an implantable defibrillator for secondary prevention of sudden death entails implantation of an ICD in a patient who has survived a sudden cardiac arrest or malignant ventricular arrhythmia.

- Patients have a class I indication for implantation of a defibrillator for secondary prevention of sudden death if they have hemodynamically stable (with structural heart disease) or unstable sustained VT or survive a cardiac arrest caused by VT/VF not due to reversible causes; or if they suffer syncope and have sustained VT or VF induced at electrophysiological study.

- Sudden cardiac death accounts for approximately 30% of the deaths that occur in irreversible cardiomyopathies unrelated to underlying coronary artery disease. If such a patient has a history of unheralded syncope, their incidence of sudden cardiac death can exceed 30%.

- The current recommendation for ICD implantation in patients with complex congenital heart disease qualifies as Class I only for those patients having suffered and survived a cardiac arrest or symptomatic sustained ventricular tachycardia not due to a reversible cause.

- Hypertrophic cardiomyopathic genetic polymorphisms affect approximately one out of every 500 persons in the general population and is the most common cause of cardiac arrest in people less than 40 years of age

- Patients with structurally normal hearts carry a low risk of sudden death as a whole, but there are populations of patients with congenital ion channelopathies that are an exception to this rule. The best characterized of these disorders are long QT syndrome, Brugada syndrome, catecholaminergic ventricular tachycardia, Short QT syndrome, and idiopathic ventricular fibrillation.

## INTRODUCTION

Sudden cardiac death (SCD) is one of the leading causes of death in the United States and its prevention remains a challenge. The absolute number of sudden cardiac deaths in the United States ranges between 200,000 and 450,000 per year. Although the death toll in patients with pre-existing coronary disease has declined dramatically over the years, sudden cardiac death rates have only modestly improved. Sudden cardiac death can either occur from cardiac mechanical failure (in the setting of an acute cardiac event or due to chronic disease of the myocardium) or result from malignant brady or tachyarrhythmias with tachyarrhythmic events representing the majority of these occurrences (**Figure 66-1**). Although sudden cardiac death occurs more frequently in patients with underlying coronary artery disease, these patients represent a minority of the total events per year in the general population (**Figure 66-2**). The objective of this chapter is to discuss the numerous causes of malignant ventricular arrhythmias that cause sudden cardiac death and to clarify the opportunities and recommendations for the primary and secondary prevention of these arrhythmias. Given that implantable defibrillators are the most often used tool in the primary or secondary prevention of sudden death in many populations, frequent reference will be made to the 2008 ACC/AHA/HRS Guidelines for Device-Based Therapy with regard to whether implantable defibrillator implantation should be performed. The guidelines' recommendations are categorized into Class I recommendations (should be performed), Class IIa recommendations (reasonable to perform), Class IIb recommendations (may be considered), and Class III recommendations (should not be performed).

## CORONARY ARTERY DISEASE AND SUDDEN DEATH

### Acute Myocardial Infarction

Ventricular fibrillation (VF) and ventricular tachycardia (VT) occur in approximately 10% of ST elevation and 2% of non-ST elevation acute myocardial infarctions (AMI) and usually occur within the first 24 hours of the event. Delayed phase arrhythmias such as premature ventricular contractions (PVCs), nonsustained VT, and accelerated idioventricular rhythms occur up to 72 hours post-MI and are due to increased automaticity of surviving Purkinje cells. Thrombolysis and acute coronary angioplasty recanalizes thrombotic coronary occlusions, which reperfuses the myocardium and reduces infarct size, reducing the risk of substrate for lethal ventricular arrhythmias. Reperfusion arrhythmias are similar to delayed phase arrhythmias but include transient sinus bradycardia after reperfusion of an inferior infarct. It is uncommon for reperfusion arrhythmias or delayed phase arrhythmias to require urgent treatment, and they generally do not have meaningful prognostic implications.

Coronary Care Units have significantly decreased the risk of death from VT/VF in AMI due to continuous cardiac rhythm monitoring by highly trained nurses. In this controlled setting, defibrillators, pacemakers, and emergent intravenous drugs are readily available in case of emergency. These units are also well equipped for intensive hemodynamic monitoring and intraaortic balloon counter pulsation to provide supportive care to hemodynamically compromised patients. Despite all the capabilities that these units provide, it is the rapid access to immediate defibrillation that appears to have had the greatest effect on acute survival. Beta-blockers initiated in the acute phase result in a 23% reduction in long-term mortality, whereas angiotensin converting enzyme inhibitors reduce SCD after an AMI, presumably from antiatherosclerotic effects and reverse myocardial remodeling. Often, despite an arrhythmic arrest in the setting of an acute myocardial infarction, further evaluation of the need for an implantable defibrillator to protect against future arrest is reserved until well after full recovery from the acute ischemic insult, when reverse remodeling is complete and the patient's long-term arrhythmogenic substrate is established.

An implantable cardioverter defibrillator (ICD) implantation has been found to be one of the most effective means of prevention of sudden cardiac arrest in populations at risk. ICDs are implanted for either primary or secondary prevention of sudden cardiac arrest. Primary prevention entails

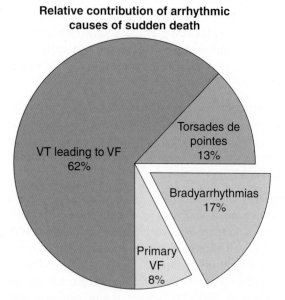

**Relative contribution of arrhythmic causes of sudden death**

VT leading to VF 62%

Torsades de pointes 13%

Bradyarrhythmias 17%

Primary VF 8%

Tachyarrhythmias 83%, Bradyarrhythmias 17%

**Figure 66-1.** Distribution of the arrhythmic events at the time of sudden cardiac arrest.

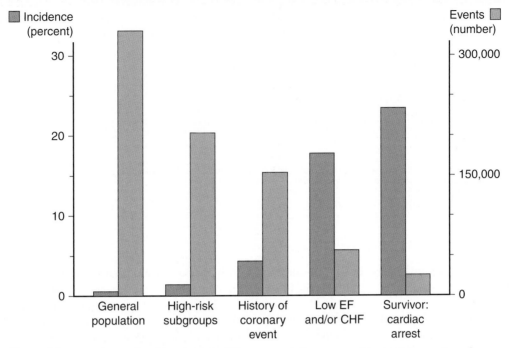

**Figure 66-2.** Incidence of sudden death in different populations versus the absolute number of deaths in the same populations. The general population has the lowest incidence of sudden death but the highest absolute number.

implantation in a patient at risk for sudden cardiac arrest who has never suffered such an event. Secondary prevention entails implantation of an ICD in a patient who has survived a sudden cardiac arrest or malignant ventricular arrhythmia. Despite the efficacy of ICD implantation, there is general agreement that there are populations in whom the implantation of ICDs may not prove beneficial and may even be deleterious. The 2008 ACC/AHA/HRS recommendations on device based therapies recommend against implantation of ICDs in the following populations:

1. Patients without a reasonable expectation of survival with an acceptable functional status for at least 1 year, even if they meet ICD implantation criteria in other respects.
2. Patients with incessant VT or VF.
3. Patients with significant psychiatric illnesses that may be aggravated by device implantation or that may preclude systematic follow-up.
4. Patients with NYHA Class IV heart failure who are not candidates for cardiac transplantation or cardiac resynchronization therapy.
5. Patients with syncope of undetermined cause without inducible ventricular tachyarrhythmias and without structural heart disease.
6. Patients in whom VT or VF is amenable to surgical or catheter ablation in the absence of structural heart disease.

7. Patients with ventricular tachyarrhythmias due to a completely reversible disorder (such as acute coronary ischemia) in the absence of structural heart disease.

## Ischemic Cardiomyopathy

Patients who have survived an acute myocardial infarction all develop some degree of myocardial scar and fibrosis from the ischemic insult. The amount of territory suffering the ischemic insult, the rapidity of reperfusion, and the pharmacologic agents employed postinfarction along with other factors all play a role in the severity of the resulting ischemic cardiomyopathy. The burden of scar and fibrosis on MRI and the chronic left ventricular ejection fraction resulting from the ischemic insult are among the best predictors of the patient's subsequent risk of sudden cardiac arrest. Implantable cardioverter defibrillator implantation is the most effective means of protecting certain populations from sudden death and exceeds the benefit of any membrane active antiarrhythmic medication. Multiple studies have proven the efficacy of secondary prevention use of ICDs and, subsequently, primary prevention use of ICDs. It is important to have a working knowledge of these studies and their seminal findings.

### Secondary Prevention

Cardiac Arrest Study Hamburg (CASH), Canadian Implantable Defibrillator Study (CIDS), and Antiarrhythmics Versus Implantable Defibrillators (AVID) were among the most

| | | Patients | | Inclusion | Other Inclu- | Hazard | 95% Confidence | |
|---|---|---|---|---|---|---|---|---|
| Trial | Year | (n) | Aim | Criterion LVEF ≤ to | sion Criterion | Ratio* | Interval | P |
| AVID | 1997 | 1016 | Antiarrhythmic treatment vs. ICD | 40 | Prior cardiac arrest | 0.62 | 0.43–0.82 | p=0.012 |
| CASH† | 2000 | 191 | ICD vs. antiarrhythmic agents | M: 45 ± 18 at baseline | Prior cardiac arrest | 0.77 | 1.112‡ | 0.081§ |
| CIDS | 2000 | 659 | ICD vs. Amiodarone | 35 | Prior Cardiac arrest | 0.82 | 0.60–1.10 | NS |

**Table 66-1 • Secondary Prevention Trials of Sudden Cardiac Dealth**

*Hazard ratios for death due to any cause in the implantable cardiaverter-defibrillator group compared with the non-implantable cardioverter-defibrillator group.
†Includes only implantable cardioverter-defibrillator and amiodarone patients from CASH.
‡Upper bound of 97.5% confidence incidence.
§One-tailed.

important prospective, randomized, multicenter trials evaluating strategies of secondary prevention of SCD (**Table 66-1**).

CASH, with 191 patients studied, compared treatment with an ICD versus metoprolol, propafenone, or amiodarone in cardiac arrest survivors. A nonsignificant reduction in the relative risk of mortality was found in the ICD group (23%, $p = 0.08$) compared to medication with a strong trend in favor of ICDs. However, the propafenone arm was discontinued early given its inferiority to the other three therapies.

CIDS, with 659 patients, compared total mortality in patients with cardiac arrest or hemodynamically significant VT receiving an ICD versus amiodarone. In this trial there was a nonsignificant reduction in mortality with ICD, which provided a relative risk reduction of 19.7% ($p = 0.14$).

However, the fact that CASH and CIDS, with an approximately 20% reduction in mortality, did not meet statistical significance was considered in the context of the AVID trial. AVID was the largest of these three secondary prevention trials enrolling 1,016 patients and following 4,595 patients in its registry. AVID randomized patients surviving cardiac arrest caused by VT/VF, patients with VT and a left ventricular ejection fraction ≤40%, or patients with VT and syncope to receive either an ICD, empiric amiodarone, or sotalol therapy. Enrollment was terminated early (18 months) due to a significant survival benefit in the ICD arm of the trial (39% reduction in mortality at 1 year). A later meta-analysis of secondary prevention trials found a significant 25% reduction in mortality with ICD therapy compared to amiodarone that was due to a 50% reduction in the risk of cardiac arrest in the ICD population.

Based on these studies and others, the recommendations are that patients surviving a cardiac arrest caused by VT/VF not due to reversible causes; patients with hemodynamically unstable sustained VT not due to reversible causes; patients

with sustained hemodynamically stable or unstable VT with structural heart disease; and patients with syncope with clinically relevant, hemodynamically significant sustained VT or VF induced at electrophysiological study have a Class I indication for ICD implantation.

## Primary Prevention

The Multicenter Automatic Defibrillator Trial I (MADIT I), Multicenter Automatic Defibrillator Trial II (MADIT II), and Sudden Cardiac Death in Heart Failure Trial (SCD-HeFT) were all trials comparing strategies for the primary prevention of SCD (**Table 66-2**). These trials were developed due to the difficulties encountered in accurately risk stratifying those patients known to be at high risk for sudden cardiac arrest. The trials implementing ICDs for secondary prevention defined those patients with reduced left ventricular systolic function (EF <40%) as the population at the highest risk for sudden death and heightened the need to determine if sudden cardiac death could be primarily prevented by preemptive ICD implantation.

MADIT I evaluated patients with a prior MI, LVEF <35%, and one episode of nonsustained VT. Patients who had inducible sustained monomorphic VT or VF at electrophysiologic testing that was nonsuppressible with IV procainamide were randomized to ICD versus medical therapy (amiodarone). A 54% reduction in mortality with ICDs prompted early termination of the trial.

MADIT II evaluated mortality in patients with ICDs whose sole risk factors were prior myocardial infarction and reduced left ventricular function. Patients required documentation of coronary artery disease, LVEF ≤30% of greater than 3 months' duration, and greater than 1 month since the most recent myocardial infarction. Of note, there was no requirement for NSVT or EPS. Patients were optimized medically including treatment with beta-blockers and ACE inhibitors.

| Table 66-2 • Primary Prevention Trials of Sudden Cardiac Death | | | | | | | | |
|---|---|---|---|---|---|---|---|---|
| Trial | Year | Patients (n) | Aim | Inclusion Criterion: LVEF ≤ to | Other Inclusion Criterion | Hazard Ratio* | 95% Confidence Interval | P |
| MADIT I | 1996 | 196 | ICD vs. standard medical treatment | 35 | NSVT and positive EP | 0.46 | 0.26–0.82 | 0.009 |
| MADIT II | 2002 | 1232 | Conventional therapy vs. ICD | 30 | Prior MI | 0.69 | 0.51–0.93 | 0.016 |
| SCD-HeFT | 2005 | 900 | Conventional therapy + placebo vs. conventional therapy + amiodarone vs. conventional therapy + ICD | 35 | Prior MI or NICM | 0.77 | 0.62–0.96 | 0.007 |

*Hazard ratios for death due to any cause in the implantable cardiaverter-defibrillator group compared with the non-implantable cardioverter-defibrillator group.

Randomization occurred in a 3:2 ratio with 742 patients receiving ICDs and 490 receiving conventional medical therapy. A significant 31% relative risk reduction for mortality was observed after a mean follow-up of 20 months.

SCD-HeFT compared amiodarone to shock-only ICDs with back-up single chamber pacing in patients with ischemic and nonischemic heart failure (NYHA Class II and III) and a LVEF ≤35%. Patients were randomized to receive an ICD versus amiodarone versus placebo along with standard heart failure medical therapy. At a median follow-up of 46 months, ICD implantation was associated with a significant reduction in mortality of 23% in comparison to the other arms of the trial. Amiodarone demonstrated no added benefit when compared to placebo.

Based on these and other trials, implantable defibrillators in addition to optimal medical therapy (beta-blockers, angiotensin converting enzyme inhibitors, and direct aldosterone inhibition) are the recommended interventions for primary prevention of sudden cardiac arrest in patients with underlying ischemic cardiomyopathies and congestive heart failure. The ACC/AHA/HRS guidelines for device based therapy in 2008 indicate that primary prevention implantation of an ICD in patients with an ischemic cardiomyopathy is warranted when:

1. Patients have an LVEF ≤35% due to prior MI, are at least 40 days post-MI, and are in NYHA Class II or III (Class I indication).
2. Patients have an LVEF ≤30% due to prior MI, are at least 40 days post-MI, and are in NYHA Class I (Class I indication).
3. Patients have nonsustained VT, prior MI, LVEF ≤40%, and inducible VF or sustained VT at electrophysiological testing (Class I indication).
4. Patients have sustained VT and normal or near-normal left ventricular function (Class IIa indication).

5. Patients are not hospitalized but are awaiting cardiac transplantation (Class IIa indication).
6. Patients have syncope and advanced structural heart disease without an identifiable cause of syncope (Class IIb indication).

## Risk Stratifying Techniques

The use of left ventricular ejection fraction alone as the sole major determinate for which patients receive an ICD is unappealing given that only 23% of the patients in the MADIT-II study received appropriate therapy from their devices. In an attempt to better define populations at risk for sudden cardiac arrest, several different techniques including signal averaged electrocardiography, heart rate variability analysis, baroreflex sensitivity, QRS duration, and electrophysiological testing have been employed in an effort to detect underlying substrate that predisposes patients to reentrant ventricular arrhythmias and an increased risk of sudden cardiac death. Most of these techniques have been developed and evaluated in patients with ischemic cardiomyopathies. Despite the fact that they can play a useful role in defining degree of risk around the edges when the patient's risk is less well defined, their overall usefulness in discriminating who is at highest risk of sudden death has been disappointing. Their role in nonischemic heart disease is even less clear.

Variations in the shape and amplitude of the T-wave (T-wave alternans) can be evaluated using a microvolt T-wave alternans (MTWA) technique. A negative microvolt T-wave alternans study appeared to confer a very low risk of sudden death in patients with ischemic cardiomyopathies, but this has not held up in clinical trials. The Microvolt T-Wave Alternans Testing for Risk Stratifications of Post MI Patients (MASTER I) trial included 654 patients who met the MADIT-II indication for ICD implantation. Patients underwent MTWA testing and then underwent ICD implantation with prespecified programming to minimize the likelihood of shocks for non-life-threatening arrhythmias. Results showed that the primary end point of life-threatening ventricular tachyarrhythmic events (as assessed by ICD shocks) was not significantly different between patients with negative and nonnegative MTWA tests. MTWA and Signal-Averaged ECG (SAECG) are reasonable for improving risk stratification in patients who are at risk for developing life-threatening ventricular arrhythmias without a clear indication for an ICD, such as those with borderline ejection fractions. Electrophysiologic (EP) testing has challenges in its positive predictive accuracy and, despite good negative predictive accuracy over a 2-year time horizon, has poor negative predictive accuracy over longer time periods. Despite these limitations, inducible sustained monomorphic VT in structurally abnormal hearts or in patients with symptoms suggestive of VT carries a very high risk of sudden death. EP testing is a Class I recommendation for evaluation of patients with remote MI and symptoms, such as syncope or symptomatic palpitations, suggesting ventricular tachyarrhythmia. EP testing is reasonable for risk stratification in patients with remote MI, NSVT, and LVEF <40%.

Thus, through multiple studies, the guidelines for management of the risk of sudden cardiac death are fairly well delineated in the population of patients with underlying coronary artery disease. This leaves open the question as to whether these same rules apply to those patients with cardiomyopathies unrelated to coronary artery disease.

## SUDDEN CARDIAC DEATH IN CARDIOMYOPATHIES UNRELATED TO CORONARY ARTERY DISEASE

### Nonischemic Cardiomyopathy

One population of patients with the highest risk of sudden cardiac arrest is those with irreversible cardiomyopathies unrelated to underlying coronary artery disease. Nonischemic dilated cardiomyopathies represent the final common pathway for many infectious, familial, and toxic causes of cardiomyopathy. Sudden cardiac death accounts for approximately 30% of the deaths that occur in this condition, and if such a patient has a history of unheralded syncope, his or her incidence of sudden cardiac death can exceed 30%. ICDs have been shown to be superior to antiarrhythmic medications (including amiodarone) and/or best medical therapy in the patients who have already endured and survived a potentially lethal arrhythmic event (secondary prevention). Primary prevention of sudden cardiac arrest in patients who are at risk for, but have not suffered, a cardiac arrest has also been proven to be best served by ICD implantation in this population. The Definite (Defibrillators in Non-Ischemic Cardiomyopathy Treatment Evaluation) trial randomized

459 patients with nonischemic cardiomyopathies, left ventricular ejection fraction less than or equal to 35%, and PVCs and/or nonsustained ventricular tachycardia to receive the best medical therapy with or without an ICD. There was a strong trend toward improved survival in the ICD arm of the trial. This was closely followed by the release of the SCD-HeFt trial, which was previously discussed. SCD-HeFt enrolled 2,521 patients with heart failure and LVEF ≤35% who were then randomized to placebo, amiodarone, or implantable defibrillator; 1,210 patients in this study had nonischemic cardiomyopathies and ICD therapy was associated with a significant reduction in all-cause mortality over and above both the amiodarone and placebo arms. The timing of defibrillator implantation should allow ample time to determine that optimal medical therapy will not significantly improve left ventricular dysfunction and ensure that reversible causes of cardiomyopathy have been excluded or addressed. However, the Definite trial demonstrated that patients with an early diagnosis of cardiomyopathy do not benefit less than those with long-standing cardiomyopathies.

Given these findings, the 2008 ACC/AHA/HRS indications for ICD implantation in patients with irreversible nonischemic cardiomyopathies include the following:

1. Patients surviving a cardiac arrest due to VF or hemodynamically unstable VT (Class I)
2. Patients with a left ventricular ejection fraction ≤35% who have NYHA Class II or III congestive heart failure (Class I)
3. Patients with unexplained syncope (Class IIa)
4. Patients awaiting cardiac transplantation (Class IIa)
5. Patients with a left ventricular ejection fraction ≤35% who have NYHA Class I congestive heart failure (Class IIb)

Outside the general categories of ischemic and nonischemic cardiomyopathies are specific forms of cardiomyopathy that carry an increased risk of sudden death, occasionally during the earliest stages. The most prominent of these are congenital heart disease and genetically based cardiomyopathies, such as hypertrophic cardiomyopathy, arrhythmogenic right ventricular dysplasia, noncompaction of the left ventricle, and familial cardiomyopathies. Extrinsic cardiomyopathies such as sarcoidosis, amyloidosis, giant cell myocarditis, Chagas disease, and those associated with neuromuscular disease also carry a significant risk of sudden death.

### Congenital Heart Disease

Sudden cardiac death in the pediatric population generally occurs in the setting of a genetic arrhythmia syndrome or cardiomyopathic process, both of which are discussed later in this chapter. Children and adolescents with complex congenital heart disease present a unique challenge in that there are no large, prospective, randomized trials to help one discern who would benefit from an ICD implant for primary prevention of sudden death. Indeed, the pediatric population as a whole accounts for less than 1% of all ICD implants. For this reason, the current recommendation for ICD implantation in patients with complex congenital heart disease qualifies as Class I only for those patients having suffered and survived a cardiac arrest or symptomatic sustained ventricular tachycardia not due to a reversible cause. If the patient has recurrent syncope of undetermined etiology, ventricular dysfunction, and/or inducible ventricular arrhythmias at electrophysiological testing, then there is a Class IIa recommendation for ICD implantation. Unexplained sudden death affects a large number of patients with transposition of the great arteries and congenital aortic stenosis as well as patients who have had successful surgical repair of Tetralogy of Fallot. ICD implantation can be considered on a Class IIb basis for patients with recurrent syncope with complex congenital heart disease and systemic ventricular dysfunction when studies have failed to reveal a cause. It is unfortunate that many of the patients at risk for sudden death have normal systemic ventricular function but remarkably abnormal ventricular function supporting the pulmonary circulation, which likely increases their risk of sudden death. Nevertheless, the ACC/AHA/HRS 2008 guidelines for device based therapy stipulate the above criteria, all of which require symptoms (in the form of syncope, VT, or cardiac arrest) in order for ICD therapy to be considered.

## Genetically Based Cardiomyopathies

Hypertrophic cardiomyopathic genetic polymorphisms affect approximately 1 out of every 500 persons in the general population and is the most common cause of cardiac arrest in people younger than 40 years of age. The annual mortality of patients with the phenotypic expression of this disorder ranges from 1 to 6% and, therefore, discrimination of those patients at greatest risk of sudden death is necessary to guide how aggressive a preventive strategy is needed. The major risk factors in this population include a history of syncope, a family history of sudden cardiac arrest, LV thickness greater than or equal to 30 mm, and a flat or hypotensive response to exercise in patients younger than 40 years of age. An ICD may be considered in these patients if they have one or more of the major risk factors listed above, but this is a Class IIa recommendation. If patients with hypertrophic cardiomyopathy suffer a cardiac arrest, have spontaneous sustained VT, or have syncope with inducible VT at EP testing, they have a Class I indication for ICD implantation.

Arrhythmogenic right ventricular dysplasia (ARVD) involves fibro-fatty infiltration of the right (and sometimes the left) ventricle and is genetically derived. Although difficult to diagnose, the right ventricular enlargement can be reflected by an epsilon wave on electrocardiogram (**Figure 66-3**). Right ventricular enlargement can also be identified at right

### Twelve-lead ECG in normal sinus rhythm with epsilon wave

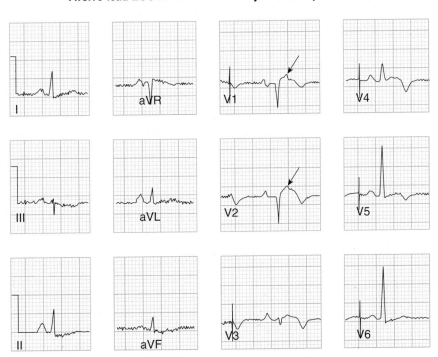

**Figure 66-3.** Note the presence of the epsilon wave as a late deflection at the terminal portion of the QRS in the early precordial leads. (Kenigsberg, D. N. et al. *Circulation.* 2007;115:e538–e539.)

ventriculography during cardiac catheterization, echocardiography, or cardiac MRI, which can also identify fibro-fatty infiltration of the myocardium. In addition, the majority of these patients will have an abnormal signal averaged electrocardiogram and often will have inducible ventricular tachycardia during EP testing. The major risk factors for sudden cardiac arrest in this population are inducibility of VT at EP testing, spontaneous nonsustained VT, male gender, young age at presentation (younger than 5 years), LV involvement, syncope, extensive RV involvement or RV dilation, or a genotype associated with a high risk of sudden death. A patient with any one of these major risk factors meets a Class IIa indication for ICD implantation. Prior cardiac arrest is a Class I indication for an ICD. ICDs are very effective in preventing arrhythmic death in this population.

Noncompaction of the left ventricle results in normal LV function but prominent trabeculae and intertrabecular recesses and a high risk of sudden cardiac arrest, which is the most common cause of death in this rare congenital condition. Implantation of an ICD is reasonable in these patients and qualifies as a Class IIb indication.

Familial cardiomyopathies have variable penetrance and transmission and have a varied risk of sudden cardiac arrest. Some familial cardiomyopathies have a strong family history of sudden death and these forms carry the highest risk for patients with this disorder. As with noncompaction of the left ventricle, patients with a familial cardiomyopathy in whom there is a family history of sudden death qualify for a Class IIb indication for an ICD.

Patients with some neuromuscular diseases (The Muscular Dystrophies, Friedreich Ataxia, and Mitochondrial Encephalopathies) have an increased risk of sudden cardiac arrest. The early cause is most commonly thought to be from complete heart block due to the high incidence of His-Purkinje conduction disease in this population, which carries a greater risk of complete heart block without a reliable escape rhythm. Many of these patients develop progressive cardiomyopathies that predispose them to lethal ventricular arrhythmias, and His-Purkinje disease predisposes this population to bundle branch reentrant ventricular tachycardia. Therapy needs to be individualized to the patient's particular problem and needs to be carefully considered in the context of the patient's overall prognosis.

## Extrinsically Induced Cardiomyopathies

Sarcoidosis, giant cell myocarditis, and Chagas disease create a scar within the myocardium and substrate for sudden cardiac arrest from ventricular tachyarrhythmia or bradarrhythmia that is somewhat unpredictable. For this reason, patients with these disorders receive a Class IIa indication for an ICD implantation in the 2008 ACC/AHA/ HRS guidelines for device based therapy. In amyloidosis, so far there has been little indication that ICDs affect survival due to the concomitant hemodynamic impairment or comorbidities, and pacing alone may be equally beneficial.

## SUDDEN DEATH IN STRUCTURALLY NORMAL HEARTS

Many patients who die suddenly without an identifiable cause at autopsy are victims of ventricular arrhythmias. Sudden death of unknown cause in a young patient with a structurally normal heart is devastating to the family and often leads to screening of first-degree relatives to determine if they carry an identifiable risk for the same fate. Chief causes in this population include ion channelopathies, coronary anomalies, Wolff-Parkinson-White syndrome, and medications.

### Ion Channelopathies

Patients with structurally normal hearts carry a low risk of sudden death as a whole, but there are populations of patients with congenital ion channelopathies that are an exception to this rule. The best characterized of these disorders are long QT syndrome, Brugada Syndrome, Catecholaminergic Ventricular Tachycardia, Short QT syndrome, and Idiopathic Ventricular Fibrillation. Genetic characterization of these different disorders is rapidly progressing and will certainly play an increasing role in helping identify patients at the highest risk of sudden cardiac arrest.

There are now more than 10 long QT syndromes identified. There are 3 major types of congenital long QT syndrome (in order of decreasing prevalence): Types 2, 1, and 3 with different clinical characteristics and different genotypes (**Figure 66-4**). All of these disorders adversely affect ventricular repolarization and are responsible for 3,000 to 4,000 sudden cardiac deaths in children annually in the United States. Patients are often asymptomatic and triggers for the arrhythmia vary with the genotype. Characteristically, polymorphic VT in LQTS Type 2 is triggered after being startled, in LQTS 1 by exercise, and in LQTS 3 by the bradycardia and hypervagotonia of sleep. The mutations are in genes that encode cardiac potassium or sodium ion channels except for LQTS 4, which encodes a plasma membrane protein. The risk of sudden death correlates with the severity of QT prolongation with a corrected QT interval greater than 500 msec conferring the highest risk. Treatment entails beta-blockade (generally ineffective in LQTS 3), antiarrhythmic treatment, potassium supplementation, dual chamber pacing, or implantable defibrillators. ICDs are recommended for secondary prevention of cardiac arrest and for patients with sustained ventricular arrhythmias, a strong family history of sudden cardiac arrest, or recurrent syncope despite beta-blocker treatment. Avoidance of agents with the potential to

**Typical ECG findings for different LQTS**

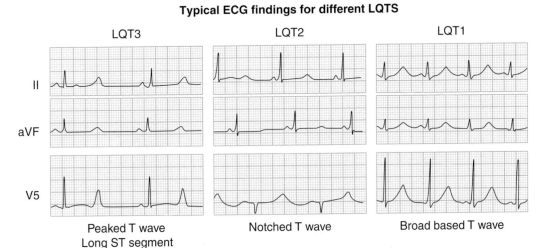

**Figure 66-4.** Examples of the surface electrocardiographic findings in the three major forms of long QT syndrome. (Strickberger, S. A. et at. *Circulation.* 2006;113:316–327.)

prolong the QT interval is recommended in this population; one can refer to the website www.qtdrugs.org to ensure the safety of the medication that he or she is initiating.

The Brugada syndromes make up a group of arrhythmias primarily caused by a mutation involving the cardiac sodium channel gene SCN5A. The syndrome is characterized by an autosomal dominant inheritance pattern, male predominance, and ST elevation in the right precordial ECG leads associated with an elevated risk of sudden cardiac arrest due to polymorphic VT or VF that often occurs at rest (**Figure 66-5**). Risk stratification is difficult as family history and specific mutations in the SCN5A gene are not necessarily predictive. Transient conditions such as fever can acutely increase the risk of a fatal ventricular arrhythmia. EP testing has a high negative predictive value and low positive predictive value. The Brugada ECG pattern can be elicited by infusion of sodium channel blocking agents such as procainamide for those patients with transient or borderline ECG findings. However, patients with a history of syncope and those with a spontaneous Brugada pattern on their ECG have a worse prognosis. ICDs are very effective in secondary prevention of sudden death in this cohort. Primary prevention ICD implantation is warranted in patients with Brugada syndrome and a history of syncope or spontaneous VT.

Catecholaminergic polymorphic ventricular tachycardia is a syndrome of polymorphic ventricular tachycardia temporally associated with exertion or emotional upset. The genetic abnormalities in both the autosomal dominant and recessive forms of this disease involve the modulation of calcium in the sarcoplasmic reticulum. Risk stratification is difficult and beta-blockers can limit occurrences and treat symptoms. If patients have an episode of sustained VT, syncope,

or hemodynamically unstable VT on beta-blockers, an ICD is generally indicated. In addition, patients with recurrent VF require ICD implantation.

The syndromes of polymorphic VT in the setting of short QT intervals and in other settings with no discernable cardiac abnormalities are limited to a small number of patients. The current recommendation is for ICD implantation in such patients for secondary prevention of sudden death.

## Sudden Death in Certain Populations

Outside of the inherited channelopathies, the most common cause of sudden death in structurally normal hearts becomes quite varied. These causes include commotio cordis, coronary anomalies, Wolff-Parkinson-White syndrome, physical and toxic agents, and medications (antiarrhythmic, chemotherapeutic, and various drug-drug interactions).

Commotio cordis occurs after a blow to the chest during the vulnerable period of cardiac repolarization, which precipitates polymorphic ventricular fibrillation (**Figure 66-6**). The mean age for this to occur is 13 years and is thought to be due to the greater pliability of the sternum in this young group of victims. Survival is very unusual (approximately 14%) but may be improved with the more widespread availability of automatic external defibrillators at high risk sporting events such as baseball, lacrosse, and ice hockey. A full cardiac evaluation of the survivors of these events rarely reveals any predisposition to cardiac arrest and, in general, the use of implantable defibrillators or restriction from athletic participation in this population is rare.

Coronary anomalies are most commonly present with cardiac arrest in the setting of athletic participation or

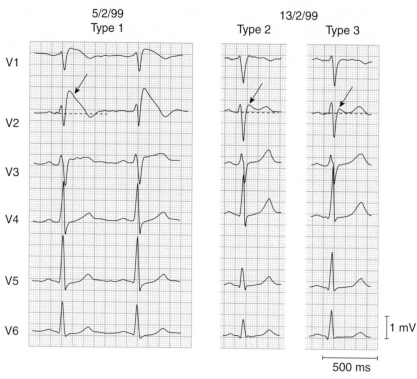

**ECG changes in the Brugada syndrome**

**Figure 66-5.** Changes in the surface electrocardiogram of a single patient with Brugada syndrome. Type I is much easier to distinguish as abnormal from Type II and III changes. (Strickberger, S. A. et al. *Circulation*. 2006;113:316–327.)

training. Only 12 to 30% of these patients will present with exertional dizziness, syncope, or chest pain. The lethality of the anomaly depends upon its course with the left main coronary artery arising from the right sinus of Valsalva and coursing between the aorta and pulmonary artery, causing sudden death before the age of 20 in approximately 75% of those afflicted. Electrocardiography and stress testing are often normal. The MRI angiogram is increasingly being used to exclude this anomaly due to the lack of ionizing radiation, the noninvasive nature of the imaging, and the lack of iodinated contrast. The treatment of choice is correction by open heart surgery.

Wolff-Parkinson-White syndrome rarely causes sudden death in asymptomatic patients. However, it can cause sudden death during athletic participation, which is thought to occur from uninhibited conduction of atrial fibrillation over the accessory pathway inducing ventricular fibrillation. The risk of sudden death appears to correlate with the refractory period of the accessory pathway, with refractory periods ≤ 250 msec carrying a greater risk. Treatment by radiofrequency ablation is low risk and curative.

## Medications

Congestive heart failure can be caused by chemotherapeutic agents such as anthracyclins as well as some interleukins and interferons. Coronary endothelial cell involvement can be induced by cyclophosphamide and coronary spasm by 5-FU

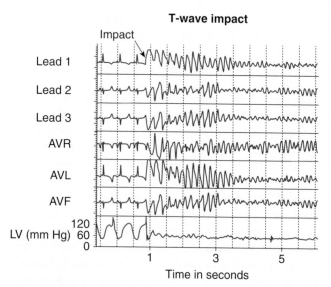

**Figure 66-6.** Six-Lead Electrocardiogram Showing the Electrophysiologic and Hemodynamic Consequences of an Impact to the Chest inducing Ventricular Fibrillation in a 9-kg Pig. (Link, M.S. et at. *N Engl J Med*. 1998;338:1805–1811.)

infusion. All of these effects can contribute to or directly cause sudden cardiac arrest.

The most common mechanism of sudden cardiac death from medications is polymorphic ventricular tachycardia caused by abnormal repolarization or "acquired long QT syndrome." The most common drug classes involved are tricyclic antidepressants, phenothiazine, antipsychotics, macrolide or flouroquinolone antibiotics, certain antihistamines, and antiarrhythmic agents. Antiarrhythmic agents account for 75% of the drug induced polymorphic ventricular tachycardia cases seen clinically. When initiating agents that can cause acquired LQTS if used in combination with other agents, it is probably prudent to have patients check any new medications on www.qtdrugs.org to decrease the chance of a lethal drug-drug interaction. Although most episodes of drug induced acquired long QT syndrome are due to interactions with other drugs, some of these events are due to the unmasking of a clinically apparent congenital LQTS gene. Thus, this consideration should be entertained when encountering sudden death in an acquired LQTS patient.

Last, toxic agents encountered during substance abuse such as inhalants, cocaine, and amphetamines carry the highest risk of sudden cardiac arrest.

## CONCLUSION

Sudden cardiac death is one of the leading causes of death in the United States. Despite all of the data presented in this chapter, the majority of people in this country who die suddenly do not fall into a high risk profile for which pre-emptive action can be taken. It is likely that, with further understanding of the genetic polymorphisms that predispose some people to sudden death over others, understanding of who is a risk in the general population will occur. Until then, more widespread use of automatic external defibrillators and broader training of CPR are the most likely ways to reduce the number of sudden cardiac deaths and allow the survivors to benefit from secondary prevention therapies.

## Suggested Readings

1. Zipes D, Camm AJ, Borggrefe M, et al. ACC/AHA/ESC 2006 guidelines for management of patients with ventricular arrhythmias and the prevention of sudden cardiac death – executive summary: A report of the American College of Cardiology/American Heart Association Task Force and the European Society of Cardiology Committee for Practice Guidelines (Writing Committee to Develop Guidelines for Management of Patients With Ventricular Arrhythmias and the Prevention of Sudden Cardiac Death) developed in collaboration with the European Heart Rhythm Association and the Heart Rhythm Society. JACC. 2006;48(5).

2. Epstein A, DiMarco J, Ellenbogen K, et al. ACC/AHA/ESC 2006 guidelines for device-based therapy of cardiac rhythm abnormalities: A report of the American College of Cardiology/American Heart Association Task Force on Practice Guidelines (Writing Committee to Revise the ACC/AHA/NASPE 2002 Guideline Update for Implantation of Cardiac Pacemakers and Antiarrhythmia Devices) developed in collaboration with the American Association for Thoracic Surgery and Society of Thoracic Surgeons. JACC. 2008;51:1–62.

3. Turakhia M, Tseng Z. Sudden cardiac death: Epidemiology, mechanisms, and therapy. *Curr Probl Cardiol.* 2007;32:501–546.

4. Lehnart S, Ackerman M, Benson DW Jr., et al. Inherited arrhythmias: A National Heart, Lung, and Blood Institute and Office of Rare Diseases workshop consensus report about the diagnosis, phenotyping, molecular mechanisms, and therapeutic approaches for primary cardiomyopathies of gene mutations affecting ion channel function. *Circulation.* 2007;116:2325–2345.

5. Santini M, Lavalle C, Ricci R. Primary and secondary prevention of sudden cardiac death: Who should get an ICD? *Heart.* 2007;93:1478–1483.

# 67

# Cardiac Electrophysiology Study: Basic Concepts and Techniques

ZHENGUO LIU AND JARET TYLER

## ● PRACTICAL POINTS

- Cardiac electrophysiology (EP) study is a comprehensive test to evaluate the cardiac electrophysiological properties including sinus node and conduction system function, arrhythmias, and their underlying mechanisms, and to guide therapies (medical, ablative, or surgical).

- It involves systematic and careful analysis of intracardiac electrical activities from different areas recorded at the basal state and during programmed electrical stimulation or drug challenges.

- For an optimal outcome, a systematic approach is recommended for EP study. However, the study protocol may be modified based on individual's specific situation.

- Basic measurements during an EP study include (but not limited to) cycle length, sinus node recovery time (SNRT) or corrected SNRT, atrial-His (AH) interval, His-ventricular (HV) interval, AV node, and ventricular effective refractory period. Other specific measurements may be obtained based on the specific needs for the study.

- EP study should be considered for patients with narrow and wide QRS tachycardia, and syncope or near-syncope of unknown etiology, for risk stratification of sudden cardiac death, and for evaluation of the efficacy of antiarrhythmic/interventional treatments and their associated prognosis.

- Cautions must be taken for EP study in patients with unstable angina, decompensated heart failure, bleeding disorders, severe PVD, sepsis, electrolyte imbalance, and severe aortic stenosis (especially if retrograde LV entry).

- Some drugs, especially beta-blockers, calcium channel blockers, and antiarrhythmics, may significantly affect the outcome of EP study. Therefore, cautions must be taken when EP study results are interpreted in the individuals who are taking these medications.

- EP study results should be interpreted in combination with the individual's clinical information due to the limitations of this test.

Cardiac electrophysiology (EP) study is a comprehensive test to evaluate the cardiac electrophysiological properties including the automaticity and conduction system (**Figure 67-1**) and to determine the mechanisms of arrhythmia. It involves systematic and careful analysis of intracardiac electrical activities from different areas recorded at the basal state and during programmed electrical stimulation or drug challenges. The EP study has tremendous potential to assess the heart's conduction system, to investigate the nature of arrhythmia and its underlying characteristics, and to guide therapies (medical, ablative, or surgical). To perform the test effectively and analyze the data correctly, one must first understand some general definitions and terminology used in EP studies.

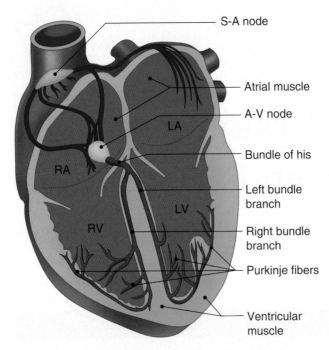

**Figure 67-1.** Schematic illustration of the electrical system in the heart. (Courtesy of Mr. Dennis E. Mathias at the Ohio State University Medical Center)

# DEFINITIONS AND TERMINOLOGY

*Excitability* is the ability of the cardiac tissue to depolarize in response to a stimulus.

*Conductivity* is the property of the muscle cell to conduct the depolarization wave to the next cell.

*Automaticity* is the ability to depolarize spontaneously.

*Cycle length* is the measured length of time (in msec) between subsequent heartbeats. The basic unit of time for EP study is millisecond (msec). Heart rates are typically referenced as cycle lengths (CL), not as beats per minute. To calculate a cycle length, one must first grasp that a heart rate (HR) of 60 beats per minute (bpm) corresponds to a CL of 1000 msecs (1 second); thus, the cycle length equals 60,000/HR. The cycle length and heart rate are inversely proportional, so that as the heart rate increases, the cycle length gets shorter. For example, an arrhythmia with a rate of 100 bpm has a cycle length of 600 msec (60,000 / 100 bpm = 600 msec), whereas a heart rate of 150 bpm equates to a cycle length of 400 msec (60,000 / 150 bpm = 400 msec). This can be confusing at first, but remember the simple relation that the shorter the cycle length, the faster the heart rate.

*Basic cycle length* is the interval between successive intracardiac A (or atrial) electrical signals as shown in **Figure 67-2**.

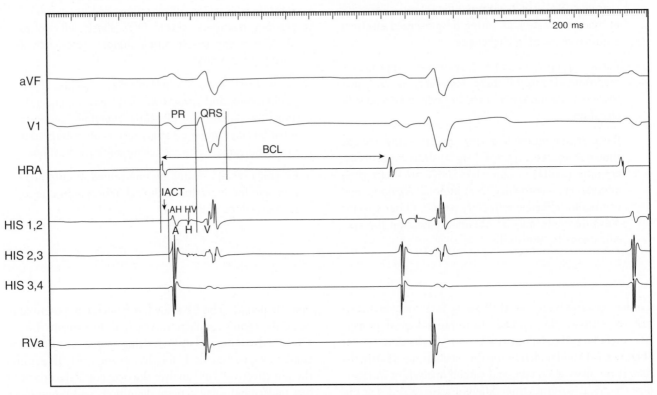

**Figure 67-2.** Baseline recordings and measurement of individual intervals during a typical electrophysiology study.
aVF and V1, surface ECG leads aVF and V1; HRA, recording of atrial activation at high right atrium close to SA node; HIS1-4, recording of electrical activities from His catheter from distal to proximal (1-4); RVa, recording of electrical activities at RV apex; A, atrial activation; H, His potential; V, ventricular activation.

**PR interval** is measured from the surface ECG and is the time from the beginning of the P wave to the beginning of the QRS, as demonstrated in **Figure 67-2**.

**QRS duration** is measured on the surface ECG and is the width of the QRS complex.

**Intraatrial conduction time (IACT)** is measured from the beginning of the surface P wave to the A deflection on the His bundle electrogram and represents the conduction interval from the sino-atrial (SA) node to atrioventricular (AV) node, typically 20 to 60 msec, as illustrated in **Figure 67-2**.

**Sinus node recovery time (SNRT)**—Maximal time (in msec) from the last paced atrial depolarization to the first sinus return cycle, at any paced cycle length, as shown

in **Figure 67-3a**. It is a measure of sinus node automaticity. Increased SNRT could be observed in sinus node dysfunction such as sick sinus syndrome, as demonstrated in **Figure 67-3b**.

**Corrected sinus node recovery time (CSNRT)**—It is a calculated time that equals sinus node recovery time minus sinus cycle length (**Figures 67-3a** and **67-3b**).

**Sino-atrial conduction time (SACT)** is a measure of tissue conduction in the SA node. It is usually not measured during a routine EP study. Abnormal values may indicate potential sinus exit block.

**Atrio-His (AH) interval** is defined as the time from the first rapid deflection of the atrial electrogram to the earliest onset of His bundle activation, as measured in the His catheter

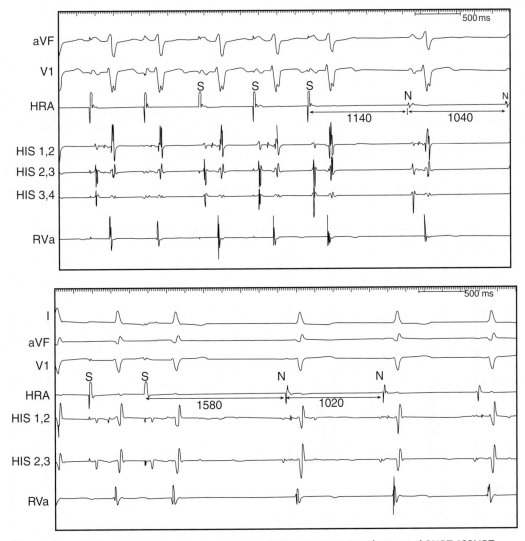

**Figure 67-3.** A. A normal sinus node recovery time (SNRT, 1140 msec) and corrected SNRT (CSNRT, 100 msec). S, atrial burst pacing at a cycle length of 500 msec; N, atrial activity during normal sinus rhythm with a cycle length of 1040. B. A prolonged (abnormal) SNRT (1580 msec) and corrected CSNRT (560 msec). S, atrial burst pacing at a cycle length of 500 msec; N, atrial activity during normal sinus rhythm with a cycle length of 1020.

electrograms (**Figure 67-2**). It represents the conduction time through the AV node and is usually less than 150 milliseconds. The AH interval varies dramatically with the patient's autonomic tone or some medications like beta-blockers.

***His-ventricular (HV) interval*** is defined as the time from the earliest His bundle deflection to the earliest onset of ventricular activation, measured in either intracardiac electrical recording or surface ECG (**Figure 67-2**). It represents the conduction time through the His-Purkinje system and is typically 35 to 55 milliseconds.

***Programmed electrical stimulation*** (PES) is the process of introducing electrical impulses in predetermined patterns and precise time intervals. This provides a powerful tool to assess the electrophysiological properties of the heart, such as tissue automaticity and refractory periods. Programmed stimulation also grants the ability to induce and terminate cardiac arrhythmias using pacing protocols, thereby allowing in-depth analysis of the mechanism of arrhythmia via electrogram patterns as well as risk stratification based on patients' response to induced arrhythmias. There are multiple programmed stimulation pacing protocols, often utilizing burst pacing, incremental pacing, and extrastimuli.

***Burst (or continuous) pacing*** is when a cardiac tissue is paced at a fixed cycle length continuously for a short period of time (usually less than 30 seconds). The baseline heart rate or particular conduction property being assessed will determine the drive train's duration and cycle length.

***Incremental pacing*** is burst pacing but with a continuous decrease in the pacing cycle length and, hence, an increase in the pacing rate. This protocol is often used when assessing Wenckebach properties of conducting tissue.

***Coupling interval*** is the length of time between a normal, or entrained, impulse and the ensuing premature impulse.

***Extrastimulus*** protocols occur when one or more premature paced stimuli are introduced at specific coupling intervals. Typically, a fixed drive train of 8 beats (usually referred as **S1**) is followed by 1 to 3 premature extrastimuli (usually referred as **S2**) at shorter cycle lengths. This protocol is typically used to induce reentrant arrhythmias like AV node reentry tachycardia and atrial flutter.

***Effective refractory period (ERP)***—The longest $S_1S_2$ coupling interval during pacing, at which extrastimulus $S_2$ is unable to result in a cardiac tissue depolarization. An example of ERP is presented in **Figure 67-4**.

***Relative refractory period (RRP)***—The longest $S_1S_2$ coupling interval at which an extrastimulus $S_2$ results in **slowed** conduction through that tissue. Because the cell is not fully repolarized, any stimulus during the RRP results in a blunted phase 0 upstroke of the cell's action potential resulting in a slowed conduction velocity. An example is shown in **Figure 67-5**.

***Functional refractory period (FRP)***—The shortest obtainable interval between two consecutive impulses that are conducted through any specified tissue at the recording site.

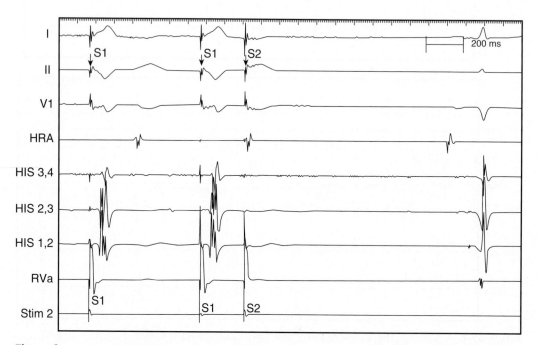

**Figure 67-4.** An example of right ventricular effective refractory period (ERP). The last pacing stimulation (S2) with coupling interval of 240 msec failed to depolarize the ventricle. S1, drive train of 8 beats at cycle length of 600 msec that depolarized the ventricle; I, II, V1, surface ECG leads I, II, and V1, respectively.

typically need no evaluation or treatment. Symptomatic sinus bradyarrhythmias can be treated with pacing or by addressing the reversible cause. An EP study can only help determine whether SA nodal dysfunction is present but typically cannot correlate the rhythm with symptoms. Therefore, the best method to diagnose SA nodal dysfunction is based on clinical information with documented symptomatic bradycardia. One indication for EP studies to assess SA nodal function is to further evaluate the patients with symptoms suggestive of bradyarrhythmias, such as syncope or near-syncope, but with no documented bradyarrhythmia on monitoring.

## ELECTROPHYSIOLOGICAL EVALUATION OF ATRIO-VENTRICULAR (AV) NODE AND HIS BUNDLE

The AV node serves to bridge the conduction of electrical impulses from the atria to the ventricles. The role of EP study in the evaluation of the AV node and His bundle is to help localize the site and degree of AV block. As a generalization, proximal block localized to the AV node is often a benign process and rarely requires definitive therapy like a permanent pacemaker implantation. Distal block below the level of AV node or in the His bundle, however, tends to be more progressive and malignant and is always an indication for a permanent pacemaker (PPM). The presence of symptoms (e.g., syncope or near-syncope) with any level of AV block is an indication for a pacemaker.

The key to assessing AV conduction is the His bundle intracardiac electrogram (**Figure 67-2**). With this, one can measure segmental AV node conduction times and their response to programmed electrical stimulation. As mentioned above in definitions, the AH interval represents the conduction time through the AV node (normal <150 msec) and the HV interval approximates the His-Purkinje conduction time (normal 35–55 msec).

Traditional AV nodal disease, as assessed by surface ECGs (i.e., 1° block, 2° block—Mobitz type I and II, and 3° block—complete heart block), can be accurately localized by performing an EP study. First-degree AV block, localized to the AV node, will show a prolonged AH interval on the His bundle electrogram and is typically a benign finding in itself. If presenting with a prolonged HV interval, however, the first degree AV block becomes more concerning, given its propensity to progress to higher degrees of AV block. Because of this propensity, most physicians agree that a PPM is indicated with distal first-degree block and an HV interval greater than 100 msec. Of note, a normal PR interval does not rule out an impaired conduction below the AV node or the His bundle. A patient who has a significantly prolonged HV interval and is at risk for complete heart block may have a normal PR interval on surface ECG.

On occasions, the level of slowed conduction can lie within the His bundle itself (normal <25 msec). If severe, splitting of the His deflection can be observed. AV block with a split His is an indication for PPM.

Defining the site of second-degree AV block (proximal versus distal) can determine the need for PPM. Mobitz Type I is a conduction delay of the AV node (proximal block) and is demonstrated on the His bundle electrogram by progressive prolongation of the AH interval immediately prior to a dropped atrial impulse as demonstrated in **Figure 67-10**. With the dropped beat, the A deflection is not followed by an "H" spike, indicating that the block is within the AV node. Mobitz Type II block always indicates distal AV block, located in the His-Purkinje system. Here, the AH and HV

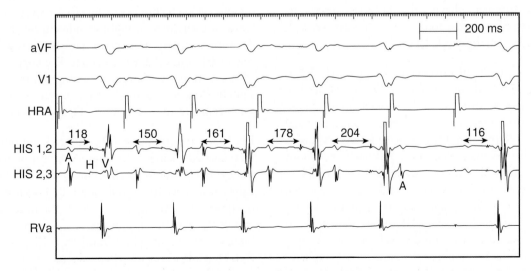

**Figure 67-10.** An example of AV Mobitz Type I block (Wenckebach) with progressive prolongation of AH interval until a blocked conduction of atrial impulse to the ventricle.

intervals remain constant for all conducted beats, with the dropped beat lacking a ventricular depolarization after the "H" spike.

Localizing the site of AV block can often be determined without an invasive EP study, thanks to the autonomic nervous system. We know that the AV node is richly innervated compared to the His-Purkinje network. Therefore, any maneuvers that decrease vagal or increase sympathetic tone, such as exercise, would be expected to improve proximal AV block. Valsalva and carotid sinus massage, on the other hand, would worsen proximal AV block. None of these maneuvers should affect distal AV block. If the site of AV block remains unclear, an EP study would answer the question.

## EVALUATION OF AV REFRACTORY PERIODS AND WENCKEBACH

When the degree and site of AV block is not definable by surface ECG and noninvasive maneuvers, incremental programmed electrical stimulation can be used to assess the integrity of the AV node. By applying burst pacing or extrastimuli protocols or in combination, one can assess the effective, relative, and functional refractory periods of the AV node and His-Purkinje systems. Wenckebach, an additional inherent conductive property, is assessed with incremental pacing.

Refractory periods give information about the conductive properties of tissue, with any abnormalities suggestive of conducting system disease not obvious at a baseline state. The refractory period of most cardiac tissue is directly proportional to the cycle length of one's rhythm, where shorter cycle lengths decrease refractory periods except the AV node. As discussed early, the AV node serves to regulate the electrical conduction from the atria to the ventricles. For the AV node, cycle length and refractory periods are inversely proportional, allowing the AV node to serve its purpose. The AV node has longer refractory periods with faster heart rates (shorter cycle lengths).

To assess the AV nodal effective refractory period, the RA is paced with an 8-beat drive train ($S_1$) of a fixed cycle length, followed by an extrastimulus ($S_2$) of a predetermined coupling interval. This series is repeated with a constant, fixed $S_1$ train (e.g., 500 msec) and progressively shortened $S_2$ coupling interval (450 msec, 400 msec, 350 msec, etc.) until AV block occurs. Observations are made of the coupling interval when AV block first occurs, of the ERP, and of the AH and HV intervals, thus pinpointing where in the conducting system it occurs (proximal or distal). One needs to know that about 20 to 30% of individuals may not develop AV node block during atrial pacing, since the AV node refractoriness in these patients is less than the atrial refractoriness at the pacing rates.

To determine FRP of the AV node and His bundle, the entire pacing sequence is assessed to obtain the shortest H1-H2 interval, indicating the FRP and measure of tissue output. Block in the His-Purkinje system at an H1-H2 interval of greater than 450 msec indicates significant distal conducting system disease. However, it is not performed routinely during EP study.

AV Wenckebach is assessed with incremental pacing of RA as shown in **Figure 67-10**. The pacing cycle length is gradually decreased with observations of AH and HV intervals made at each decrement. There is typically a progressively longer A-H interval and a stable H-V interval during incremental atrial pacing. The Wenckebach cycle length is when Mobitz Type I block occurs in the AV node and is normally less than 450 msec. Any block in HV conduction or lengthening in the HV interval occurring at a paced cycle length of greater than or equal to 400 msec indicates a diseased conducting system that may require a PPM. Of note, to accurately define the His-Purkinje conduction properties, it is important to use incremental atrial pacing instead of sudden onset of atrial pacing at various cycle lengths, since it may produce a physiologic block below the His bundle.

Incremental programmed ventricular pacing is routinely used in EP studies to characterize the retrograde conduction of the ventriculo-atrial system including the refractoriness of the VA conduction system and VA Wenckebach. It is also a very useful method to evaluate the conduction via accessory pathways.

## PROGRAMMED ELECTRICAL STIMULATION AND INITIATION OF ARRHYTHMIAS

One of the major purposes and endpoints for EP study is to induce arrhythmias, especially reentrant arrhythmia, with various pacing techniques. A reentrant arrhythmia requires a circuit with different limbs of different refractory periods. To initiate reentry, an impulse must be initially blocked in one limb but travel down the other. The impulse then propagates with retrograde conduction up the initially blocked limb (no longer refractory), thus completing the circuit and establishing reentry as shown in **Figures 67-11** and **67-12**.

Reentrant arrhythmias can be induced and terminated by programmed pacing techniques. A typical protocol for the induction of reentrant arrhythmias uses a drive train (typically 8 beats) of a fixed cycle length ($S_1$) to entrain the conducting tissue. An extrastimulus ($S_2$) is introduced to the end of the drive train and the coupling interval is slowly brought into refractoriness until the ERP is defined. The $S_1S_2$ coupling interval is then increased to just above ERP so that $S_2$ conducts. A second stimulus, $S_3$, is then added, and the $S_2S_3$ coupling interval is subsequently decreased

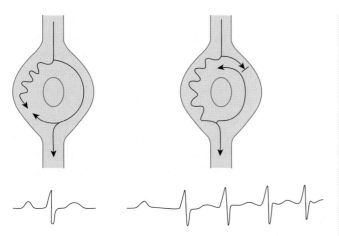

**Figure 67-11.** Schematic illustration of the initiation of AV node reentry tachycardia. A normal atrial impulse is conducted through both slow and fast pathways. The wave front in the slow pathway collides with the one from the fast pathway without initiation of arrhythmia (left). When a critically timed atrial premature impulse arrives in the circuit, it is blocked in the fast pathway, while conducting slowly in the slow pathway with long PR interval. It then turns around in the fast pathway to initiate AV node reentry tachycardia (right). (Courtesy of Mr. Dennis E. Mathias at the Ohio State University Medical Center)

until refractoriness is reached. The process continues with the addition of an $S_4$ stimulus until reentry is induced or the protocol ends. The initiating paced impulse must reach a reentrant circuit at just the right time to initiate and terminate the circuit. The timing of the impulse is dependent on the distance from the electrode as well as the refractoriness and conduction velocity of the surrounding tissue. This is why extrastimuli ($S_2 S_3 S_4$) are utilized. The short cycle lengths of the coupling intervals change the refractoriness of the tissue, increasing the chances of introducing the critically timed impulse to initiate reentrant arrhythmias. Because of this, multiple drive trains, pacing sites, and extrastimuli protocols are used in an attempt to initiate reentry. This pacing strategy may be used for both atrium and ventricule to initiate superventricular tachycardia or ventricular tachycardia.

## EFFECTS OF PHARMACOLOGICAL AGENTS ON EP STUDY

A variety of pharmacological agents may affect the outcome of the EP study due to their significant effect on the automaticity, refractory periods, and conduction velocity

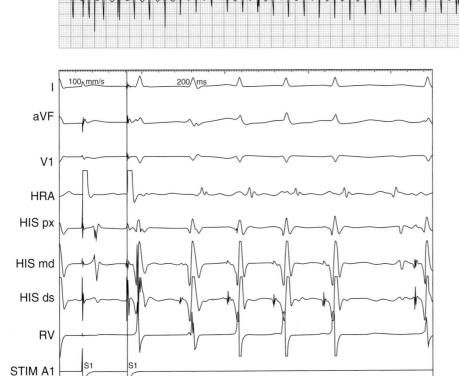

**Figure 67-12.** An example of typical AV node reentry tachycardia induced during EP study. The monitoring strip of arrhythmia is shown on the top. The intracardiac recordings show that both high right atrium and ventricle are activated almost the same time with very short VA time (lower panel). This is a characteristic finding for typical AV node reentry tachycardia.

of the cardiac tissues, especially SA node and AV node. A detailed review on this complex subject is beyond the scope of this chapter. For example, atropine dramatically reduces parasympathetic tone, thus increasing the heart rate with decreased cycle length. It also shortens the SNRT and CSNRT as well as the AV node ERP. Of note, atropine sometimes may result in a significant paradoxical prolongation of SNRT. On the other hand, isoproterenol enhances the sympathetic tone and, thus, increases cardiac automaticity and improves AV node conduction. Beta-blocker like propranolol prolongs SNRT, especially in patients with sick sinus syndrome, and slows AV node conduction. Calcium channel blockers like diltiazem and verapamil have minimal effects on SNRT and SACT in normal subjects but significantly slow AV node conduction with increased AV node ERP. Many antiarrhythmic agents including sotolol, amiodarone, ibutilide, procainamide, quinidine, lidocaine, mexiletine, flecainide, and propafenone may have significant effects on the sinus node and AV node electrophysiologically. Therefore, cautions must be taken when EP study results are interpreted in the individuals who are taking these medications.

# 68

# Supraventricular Tachycardia

Ashish Gangasani and Ralph Augostini

## ● PRACTICAL POINTS

- Atrial fibrillation is the most common sustained arrhythmia.

- Treatment of sinus tachycardia is directed at the underlying mechanism rather than the sinus rate for most cases.

- Digitalis toxicity is a well-known cause of triggered activity form of atrial tachycardia.

- Treatment of multifocal atrial tachycardia is directed toward lung disease.

- The presence of a terminal S wave or R' wave during PSVT, which is absent during sinus rhythm, is indicative of AV nodal reentry tachycardia.

- Asymptomatic pre-excitation on a 12-lead ECG does not require therapy.

- An irregular, wide complex tachycardia with varying appearance of the QRS should not be treated with AV nodal blocking agents as it may represent atrial fibrillation with WPW.

- A regular, narrow complex tachycardia in a patient with known WPW can be treated with AV nodal blocking agents.

- The preferred acute therapy for regular, narrow complex tachycardia is adenosine.

- Curative ablation therapy is the preferred chronic treatment for most regular PSVTs.

## INTRODUCTION

Supraventricular tachycardia (SVT) is a collective term referring to multiple forms of arrhythmia that incorporate the atria as part of the tachycardia circuit. It includes atrioventricular (AV) node dependent tachycardias such as atrioventricular node reentry tachycardia (AVNRT) and atrioventricular reentry tachycardia (AVRT) as well as the AV node independent tachycardias such as sinus tachycardia (ST), paroxysmal atrial tachycardia (PAT), atrial flutter (AFL), and atrial fibrillation (AF). Atrial flutter and atrial fibrillation will be addressed in another detailed chapter of this text.

Paroxysmal supraventricular tachycardia (PSVT) is described as a group of tachycardias that have sudden onset/offset of tachycardia often triggered by emotional or physical stress. They may be associated with chest pain, shortness of breath, lightheadedness, and for some patients, syncope. Additionally, many patients complain of anxiety and the PSVT may be

misdiagnosed as panic disorder. Tachycardia may also be triggered by consumption of stimulants such as caffeine, nicotine, or cocaine. These tachycardias are commonly regular and rapid in nature with pulse rates commonly in the 100-220 bpm range. PSVT with rates greater than 240 bpm are rare but significant. Additionally, the description of symptoms will sometimes give clues to the mechanism. For instance, AVNRT is commonly associated with neck pounding or discomfort in the throat.

Epidemiologic studies have shown that supraventricular arrhythmias are a frequent phenomenon. AF is known to be the most common sustained arrhythmia with reported incidence of 0.4-1.0% of the general population. The estimated prevalence of PSVT was 2.25 per 1,000 in a 3.5% sample of medical records in the Marshfield (Wisconsin, U.S.A.) Epidemiologic Study Area (MESA).[1] The incidence of PSVT in this survey was 35 per 100,000 person-years. Interestingly, the incidence rate of supraventricular arrhythmias among patients with CHF is 11.1%[2] with paroxysms more common in older patients, males, and those with longstanding CHF and radiographic evidence of cardiomegaly. Additionally, AF has increasing prevalence with age, affecting more than 10% of the population over the age of 80.

In the MESA population,[3] compared to those with other cardiovascular disease, "lone" (no cardiac structural disease) PSVT patients without associated structural heart disease were younger (mean age equals 37 vs. 69 years), had faster average heart rates (186 vs. 155 bpm), and were more likely to present first to an emergency room (69 vs. 30%). The age at tachycardia onset is higher for AVNRT (32 plus or minus 18 years) than for AVRT (23 plus or minus 14 years).[4] Gender also plays a role in the epidemiology of PSVT. Female residents in the MESA population had a twofold greater relative risk (RR) of PSVT (RR equals 2.0; 95% confidence interval equals 1.0 to 4.2) compared to males.

## SINUS TACHYCARDIA (ST)

The presentation of ST is most commonly observed as a secondary response. Commonly, there is an underlying process such as fever, dehydration, congestive heart failure, anemia, pain, anxiety, or hyperthyroid disease as factors contributing to elevated heart rate. Additionally, external factors such as stimulant use (caffeine, cocaine, nicotine) or withdrawal of drugs such as alcohol, morphine derivatives, and beta-blockers should be considered. In most cases, ST is found to be a secondary finding as an appropriate physiologic response to maintain cardiac output. Therefore, therapy should be focused on treating the underlying condition rather than the ST itself.

In some cases, ST is deemed inappropriate and the result of abnormal vagal or sympathetic tone. Often, this is found in association with position change as seen in the disorder of positional orthostatic tachycardia syndrome or POTS disease.

### ST Therapy

Treatment of sinus tachycardia is focused on addressing the underlying mechanism. Rarely, it may require an attempt to slow the sinus node with either beta-blocker or calcium channel blocker therapy. Sinoatrial node modification with radiofrequency ablation (RFA) may be considered for extreme cases of inappropriate ST.

## ATRIAL TACHYCARDIA (AT)

There are several different forms of AT, more commonly seen in patients with underlying structural heart disease. AT may be classified according to mechanisms that include interatrial reentry, automatic atrial tachycardia, triggered atrial tachycardia, and multifocal atrial tachycardia (MAT). Interatrial reentry as a mechanism for AT is seen in patients with prior congenital heart disease, ischemic heart disease, and valvular heart disease and particularly observed in the setting coexisting AF/AFL. Also, interatrial reentry is common after corrective surgery with tachycardia development related to reentry along surgically created atrial incisional scars.

Chronic obstructive pulmonary disease (COPD) is most commonly associated with MAT with characteristically at least three different P wave morphologies and irregular RR intervals as the diagnostic criteria. Treatment here is directed at the concurrent lung disease.

Triggered atrial tachycardia is the least common of the AT types. The mechanism is thought to be related to delayed afterdepolarizations seen with abnormal sympathetic discharge. The triggered form of atrial tachycardia presents in the setting of digitalis toxicity.

### AT Therapy

Adenosine and beta-blockers have had a variable response as therapy for interatrial reentry. Adenosine and verapamil have been effective in termination of triggered atrial tachycardias. RFA may be the preferred therapy for incessant forms of AT as most have a poor response to pharmacologic treatment. MAT therapy should be directed at addressing the underlying process with little benefit from antiarrhythmic medication or ablation therapies. If digitalis toxicity is evident, then withdrawal of the drug and use of Digibind, a binding agent, is indicated.

## ATRIOVENTRICULAR NODAL REENTRANT TACHYCARDIA (AVNRT)

Atrioventricular nodal reciprocating tachycardia is the most common form of PSVT and represents 65% of AVN dependent tachycardias. It is more common in females and usually not associated with structural heart disease. AVNRT involves a reentrant circuit that is formed by the slow and fast AV node pathways (see **Figure 68-1**). In most cases, the fast pathway appears to be located near the apex of Koch's triangle. This triangle is bounded by the tendon of Tadaro superiorly, and the tricuspid annulus is the base. The slow pathway extends inferoposterior to the compact AV node tissue and stretches along the septal margin of the tricuspid annulus at the level of, or slightly superior to, the coronary sinus.

The characteristic 12-lead ECG features include a regular narrow complex tachycardia with a rate typically between 140/min and 220/min. P waves are either entirely buried in

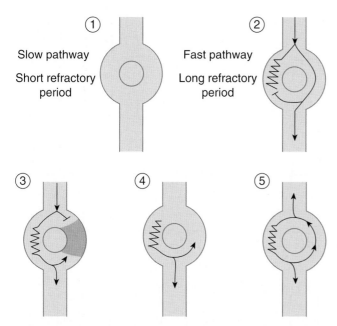

**Figure 68-1.** Schematic drawing showing dual atrioventricular (AV) nodal conduction. (1) The two AV nodal pathways, one with fast conduction and a relatively long refractory period and a second with slower conduction and a shorter refractory period. (2) During sinus rhythm, impulses are conducted over both pathways but reach the bundle of His through the fast pathway. (3) A premature atrial impulse finds the fast pathway still refractory and is conducted over the slow pathway. (4,5) If the fast pathway has enough time to recover excitability, the impulse may reenter the fast pathway retrogradely and establish reentry. (Source: Modified from Fogel RI, Prystowsky EN. Atrioventricularnodal reentry, In: Podrid PJ, Kowey PR, eds. Cardiac Arrhythmia: Mechanisms, Diagnosis and Management. New York: Lippincott Williams & Wilkins; 2001:436, with permission.)

the QRS complex and, therefore, absent on a 12-lead ECG or they occur at the end of the QRS complex, producing characteristic distortions known as a "pseudo-R" wave in lead V1 and "pseudo-S" wave in the inferior limb leads. The presence of a pseudo-R wave in lead V1 during PSVT, but absence during sinus rhythm, is highly correlated with AVNRT (see **Figure 68-2**).

AVNRT may occur as several different forms discerned through an invasive electrophysiology study. "Typical AVNRT" is the most common form (about 90%). It involves reentry with antegrade or forward conduction down the slow pathway and retrograde conduction up the fast pathway (slow-fast). This produces a short RP tachycardia on the surface ECG with RP interval characteristically less than 70 milliseconds (ms) (see **Figure 68-3**). "Atypical AVNRT" is much less common (10%) clinically. In atypical AVNRT, the circuit involves either antegrade conduction down the fast pathway and retrograde conduction up the slow pathway (fast-slow) or reentry involving multiple slow pathways (slow-slow). As a result of retrograde slow

conduction, atypical AVNRT results in a characteristically long RP tachycardia with an associated RP interval of more than 70 ms.

## AVNRT Treatment

AVNRT often can be terminated with vagal maneuvers (Valsalva or carotid sinus pressure). Nearly all cases can be terminated with escalating dosage of intravenous adenosine (6, 12, 18 mg) and adenosine is the preferred acute pharmacologic therapy due to its short half-life and lower risk in the setting of accessory pathways. Alternatively, intravenous calcium channel or beta-blocker therapy can be used with caution as well. Long-term pharmacological treatment includes oral beta-blocker (propranol, atenolol, or metoprolol) or calcium channel blocker (verapamil and diltiazem). These medications act by increasing AV nodal refractoriness and are generally well tolerated. However, they usually do not render patients asymptomatic and require lifelong administration.

Catheter ablation is the preferred treatment approach in patients with syncope, recurrent PSVT despite medical therapy or high risk occupation (firefighter, pilot, police officer). The procedure involves radiofrequency energy application (RFA) in the anatomic region of the slow pathway. The procedure is acutely successful in 97% of patients with less than 5% long-term recurrence rates. AV block as a complication occurs in only 0.5–1%.[15] Cryoablation may be considered when the operator deems the patient to be at high risk of AV block due to anatomical proximity to the His bundle. Ablation of the slow pathway may be performed in patients with documented SVT (which is morphologically consistent with AVNRT) but in whom only dual AV-nodal physiology (but not tachycardia) is demonstrated during electrophysiological study. Because drug efficacy is in the range of 30 to 50%, catheter ablation may be offered as first-line therapy for patients with frequent and disabling episodes of tachycardia. Patients considering RF ablation must be willing to accept the risk, albeit low, of AV block and pacemaker implantation.

## WOLFF-PARKINSON-WHITE SYNDROME (WPW) AND AVRT

These disorders are caused by an abnormal cardiac muscle bundle, called an accessory pathway or bypass tract, which provides a functional electrical connection between atrium and ventricle in a region outside the normal AV node. Delta waves detectable on an ECG have been reported to be present in 0.15 to 0.25% of the general population.[5,6] Pathway conduction may be intermittent. A higher prevalence of 0.55% has been reported in first-degree relatives of patients with accessory pathways.

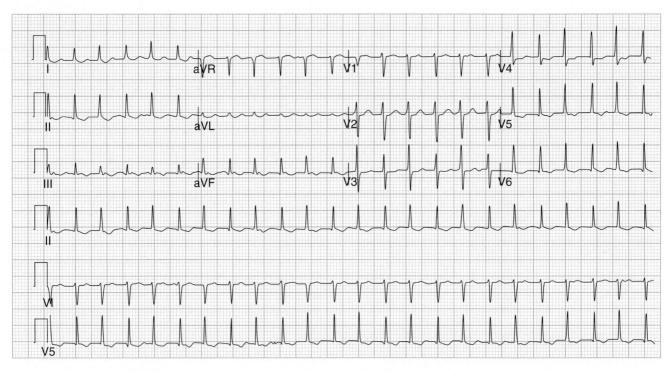

**Figure 68-2.** The 12-lead ECG demonstrates a narrow-complex tachycardia at 150 bpm. A close look at II, III, and aVF demonstrates pseudo S-waves as well as a pseudo R' wave in V1. These findings during tachycardia but absent in sinus rhythm suggest the typical form of atrioventricular nodal reentry (AVNRT).

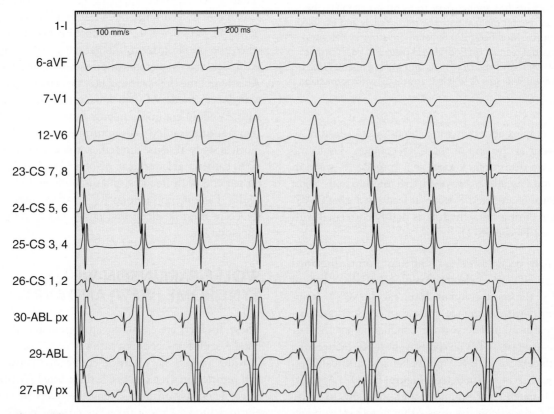

**Figure 68-3.** The intracardiac recordings obtained during an electrophysiology study are shown. Note the simultaneous activation of the left atrium (CS), His bundle recording (ABL), and the right ventricle (RV) with the activation occurring in a short RP fashion. All the EGMs "line up" in a vertical fashion over time. The RP interval during typical AVNRT is usually less than 65 msec.

There are many ways to classify the accessory pathways. They can be classified based on their position along the mitral or tricuspid annulus (left- or right-sided, respectively) or according to their conduction properties (decremental vs. nondecremental) Most accessory pathways are nondecremental (92%). Those that conduct in the anterograde direction only are uncommon, whereas those that conduct in the retrograde direction are common. Approximately 8% of accessory pathways display decremental anterograde or retrograde conduction.[7] Accessory pathways that are capable of only retrograde conduction are referred to as "concealed," whereas those capable of anterograde conduction are "manifest," as they demonstrate preexcitation on a standard ECG (see **Figure 68-4**). The appearance of a delta wave represents eccentric activation of ventricular myocardium across the accessory pathway (see **Figure 68-5**).

The diagnosis of WPW syndrome is reserved for patients who have both preexcitation and tachyarrhythmias. Among patients with WPW syndrome, AVRT is the most common

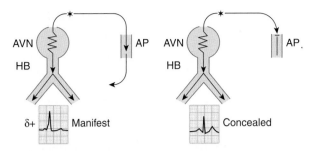

**Figure 68-4.** Atrioventricular conduction patterns and QRS morphologies during sinus rhythm for manifest and concealed accessory pathways. AP, accessory pathway; AVN, atrioventricular node; HB, His bundle. (Source: Modified from Cain ME, Luke RA, Lindsey BD. With permission.)

arrhythmia, accounting for 95% of reentrant tachycardias that occur in patients with an accessory pathway. AVRT is further classified into orthodromic and antidromic tachycardias (see **Figure 68-6**). In orthodromic tachycardia, the circuit is

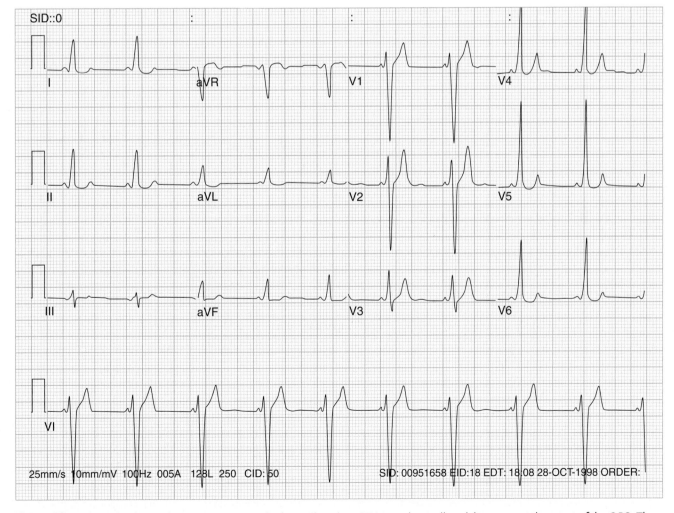

**Figure 68-5.** The 12-lead ECG demonstrates sinus rhythm with a short PR interval as well as delta waves at the onset of the QRS. The morphology of the QRS is an atypical LBBB pattern consistent with a manifest right-sided accessory pathway.

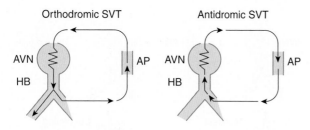

**Figure 68-6.** Schematic representation of the patterns of conduction through an accessory pathway (AP) and the normal conduction system (AVN-HB) during orthodromic AVRT and antidromic AVRT. AVN, atrioventricular node; AVRT, atrioventricular reciprocating tachycardia; HB, His bundle. (Source: Modified from Cain ME, Luke RA, Lindsey BD. With permission.)

composed of antegrade conduction down the AV node and retrograde conduction up the accessory pathway. In antidromic tachycardia, the antegrade conduction occurs down the accessory pathway and retrograde conduction up the AV node (see **Figure 68-7**). Antidromic AVRT occurs in only 5 to 10% of patients with WPW syndrome. Antidromic AVRT is always a wide complex tachycardia and may be difficult to discern from ventricular tachycardia on a standard ECG. Preexcited tachycardias can also occur in patients with AT, atrial flutter (AF), or AVNRT, with the accessory pathway acting as a bystander (i.e., not a critical part of the tachycardia circuit). Atrial fibrillation is a potentially life-threatening arrhythmia when it occurs in patients with WPW syndrome. If an accessory pathway has a short anterograde refractory period, then rapid repetitive conduction to the ventricles during AF can result in rapid ventricular response with subsequent degeneration to VF.[8] It has been estimated that one-third of patients with WPW syndrome also have AF. Accessory pathways appear to play a pathophysiological role in the development of AF in these patients, as most are young and do not have structural heart disease. Rapid AVRT may play a role in initiating AF in these patients. Additionally, AVRT is more commonly associated with the development of rate-related bundle branch block compared with AVNRT (see **Figure 68-8**). Surgical or catheter ablation of accessory pathways usually eliminates AF as well as AVRT.

It is unusual for cardiac arrest to be the first symptomatic manifestation of WPW syndrome. The incidence of sudden cardiac death in patients with WPW syndrome has been estimated to range from 0.15 to 0.39%[9] over 3- to 10-year follow-up.[11,12] Studies of WPW syndrome patients who have experienced cardiac arrest have retrospectively identified a number of markers that identify patients at increased risk.[12,13,14] These include (1) a shortest preexcited RR interval less than 250 ms during spontaneous or induced AF,

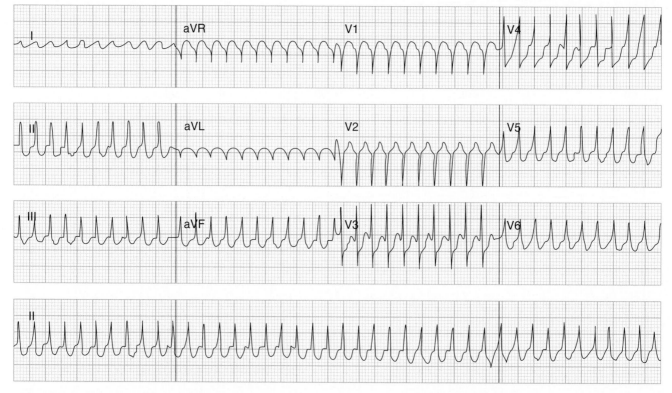

**Figure 68-7.** 12-lead ECG demonstrating narrow-complex tachycardia with P-waves identified in the terminal component of the ST segment and a long RP of 200 msec. The tachycardia proved to be related to orthodromic atrioventricular reentrant tachycardia (AVRT) incorporating a concealed left lateral accessory pathway.

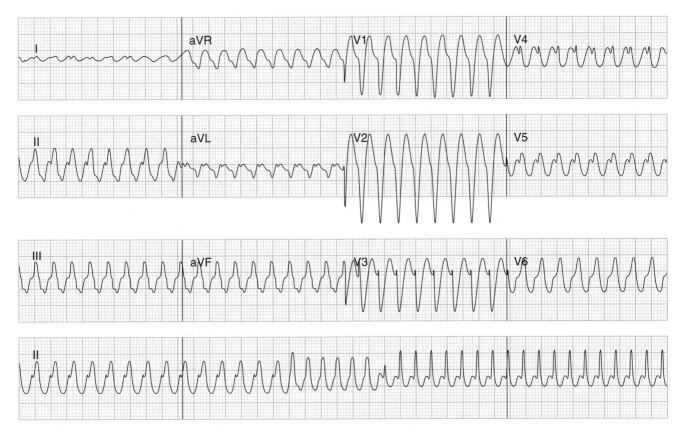

**Figure 68-8.** 12-lead ECG demonstrating orthodromic atrioventricular reentrant tachycardia (AVRT ) using the accessory pathway as the retrograde limb and the His bundle/AV node as the antegrade limb of reentry. Note the onset of tachycardia was wide with rate-related LBBB, which subsequently recovered conduction during tachycardia with sudden narrowing of the QRS observed best midway across the rhythm strip (lower pane).

(2) a history of symptomatic tachycardia, (3) multiple accessory pathways, and (4) Ebstein's anomaly. A high incidence of sudden death has been reported in familial WPW syndrome. This familial presentation is, however, exceedingly rare. The detection of intermittent preexcitation, which is characterized by an abrupt loss of the delta wave and normalization of the QRS complex, is evidence that an accessory pathway has a relatively long refractory period and is unlikely to precipitate VF.

## AVRT Treatment

In persons with hemodynamic stability, vagal maneuvers are a logical first step. Antiarrhythmic drugs represent another therapeutic option for acute management of accessory pathway mediated arrhythmias, but they have been increasingly replaced by catheter ablation for chronic treatment. Antiarrhythmic drugs that primarily modify conduction through the AV node include digoxin, adenosine, verapamil, diltiazem, and beta-blockers. Adenosine is the preferred agent for acute termination of AVRT. Antiarrhythmic drugs that depress conduction across the accessory pathway include Class I drugs such as procainamide, disopyramide, propafenone, and flecainide as well as

Class III antiarrhythmic drugs such as ibutilide, sotalol, and amiodarone.

Use of AV nodal blocking drugs during a preexcited tachycardia (secondary to atrial tachycardia or atrial fibrillation with rapid conduction down the accessory pathway) is contraindicated because of the possibility of worsening the tachycardia with rapid conduction down the accessory pathway following effective AV nodal blockage. If there is reasonable proof that a preexcited tachycardia is secondary to an AVRT with antegrade conduction down the accessory pathway and retrograde conduction up the AVN, then AV nodal blocking drugs can be effective since they will create a block in the AV node and modify the circuit.

The chronic treatment of choice is, however, a catheter based ablation procedure. The North American Society of Pacing and Electrophysiology (NASPE) registry of catheter ablations performed in 68 U.S. centers found an acute success rate of 93% for accessory pathway ablation. The success rate for catheter ablation of left free-wall accessory pathways is slightly higher than for catheter ablation of accessory pathways in other locations. After an initially successful procedure, resolution of the inflammation or edema associated with the initial injury allows recurrence of accessory pathway conduction in approximately 5% of patients. Accessory pathways that recur can usually be successfully ablated during a second session. The 1995 NASPE survey of 5,427 patients who underwent catheter ablation of an accessory pathway reported 1.82% of complications.

The role of electrophysiological testing and catheter ablation in asymptomatic patients with preexcitation is controversial. One-third of asymptomatic individuals younger than 40 years of age when preexcitation was identified eventually developed symptoms, whereas no patients in whom preexcitation was first uncovered after the age of 40 years developed symptoms.[10] Most patients with asymptomatic preexcitation have a good prognosis as cardiac arrest is rarely the first manifestation of the disease. The decision to ablate asymptomatic pathways in persons with high risk occupations, such as schoolbus drivers, pilots, firefighters, police officers, and scuba divers, is made on the basis of individual clinical considerations.

## Suggested Readings

1. Orejarena LA, Vidaillet H Jr, DeStefano F, et al. Paroxysmal supraventricular tachycardia in the general population. *J Am Coll Cardiol.* 1998;31:150–157.

2. Goyal R, Zivin A, Souza J, et al. Comparison of the ages of tachycardia onset in patients with atrioventricular nodal reentrant tachycardia and accessory pathway mediated tachycardia. *Am Heart J.* 1996;132:765–767.

3. Munger TM, Packer DL, Hammill SC, et al. A population study of the natural history of Wolff-Parkinson-White syndrome in Olmsted County, Minnesota, 1953-1989. *Circulation.* 1993;87:866–873.

4. Timmermans C, Smeets JL, Rodriguez LM, Vrouchos G, van den DA, Wellens HJ. Aborted sudden death in the Wolff-Parkinson-White syndrome. *Am J Cardiol.* 1995;76:492–494.

5. Beckman KJ, Gallastegui JL, Bauman JL, Hariman RJ. The predictive value of electrophysiologic studies in untreated patients with Wolff-Parkinson-White syndrome. *J Am Coll Cardiol.* 1990;15:640–647.

# 69

# Atrial Fibrillation and Atrial Flutter

EMILE G. DAOUD AND RAUL WEISS

## ● PRACTICAL POINTS

- The electrophysiologic feature of AFib is the simultaneous presence of multiple micro-reentrant loops (wavelets) randomly propagating throughout the right and left atria, while atrial flutter is due to a macro-reentrant circuit, often arising in the right atrium.

- There are four categories of AFib based on the response to therapy and the duration: paroxysmal AFib, persistent AFib, long-standing persistent AFib, and permanent AFib.

- There are two major categories of atrial flutter: isthmus-dependent and non-isthmus-dependent flutter. The most common variety is isthmus-dependent flutter, which has three types: counterclockwise isthmus-dependent flutter (typical atrial flutter); clockwise isthmus-dependent flutter (reverse typical atrial flutter); and lower loop flutter.

- Symptoms of AFib and atrial flutter include fatigue, weakness, palpitations, and chest discomfort, but many patients may be asymptomatic.

- In addition to evaluating for secondary causes of the atrial arrhythmias, management of patients with AFib or flutter must address a "triad of therapy":

controlling ventricular rate, prevention of thromboembolic events, and restoration and maintenance of sinus rhythm.

- One important clinical question is whether the goal of therapy for AFib is to control ventricular rate (rate control) or to restore sinus rhythm (rhythm control).

- Rate control is achieved either with medical therapy (e.g., beta-receptor or calcium channel antagonists) or with ablation of the AV junction.

- Methods to restore and maintain sinus rhythm typically begin with the use of a Class I or III antiarrhythmic drug, and if the response to this therapy is unsatisfactory, then patients are considered for AFib ablation.

- Because of a high success and low complication rate, ablation therapy is often considered as primary therapy for managing right atrial flutter.

- To prevent thromboembolic events, patients are often prescribed warfarin (INR range 2.0–3.0) or aspirin. The CHADS2 scoring system is one tool to aid physicians in deciding which therapy to initiate.

| Table 69-1 • Comparison of Atrial Fibrillation and Flutter | | |
|---|---|---|
| | **Atrial Fibrillation** | **Atrial Flutter** |
| **Epidemiology** | more common | less common |
| | similar risk factors: male gender, obesity, hypertension, atrial enlargement, valvular disease, coronary artery disease, cardiomyopathy/heart failure, cardiac surgery, pericardial disease, obstructive sleep apnea, thyrotoxicosis, alcohol consumption, and lung disease | |
| | simultaneous existing multiple micro-reentrant wavelets with random activation through both atria | single macro-reentrant arrhythmia with the wave of depolarization conducting repeatedly over a specific circuit |
| **Surface ECG pattern** | no organized fibrillatory wave on surface ECG | organized flutter waves on the surface ECG |
| | fibrillatory waves do not have similar morphology, amplitude, and timing | flutter waves have similar morphology, amplitude, and timing |
| **Ventricular activation** | irregularly irregular ventricular activation | often with 2:1 conduction with a ventricular rate of 150 bpm |
| **Classification** | based on if there is spontaneous conversion and duration: paroxysmal, persistent, longstanding persistent, & permanent | based on anatomical location of reentrant circuit:<br>—cavotricuspid isthmus-dependent, counterclockwise, clockwise, & lower loop<br>—noncavotricuspid isthmus-dependent incisional & left atrial |

# EPIDEMIOLOGY AND DEFINITION (TABLE 69-1)

## Atrial Fibrillation

Atrial fibrillation (AFib) is the most common arrhythmia and the prevalence increases with age, with >5% of people over the age of 70 experiencing AFib. Atrial fibrillation is also associated with male gender, obesity, hypertension, atrial enlargement, valvular disease, coronary artery disease, cardiomyopathy/heart failure, cardiac surgery, pericardial disease, obstructive sleep apnea, thyrotoxicosis, alcohol consumption ("holiday heart"), and lung disease (pneumonitis, pulmonary embolus, chronic obstructive disease) but can also occur in the absence of any of these features. It is estimated that the prevalence of AFib will more than double by 2050 to 5.6 million in the United States.

The electrophysiologic feature of AFib is the simultaneous presence of multiple micro-reentrant loops (wavelets) randomly propagating throughout the right and left atria. This irregularity of atrial activation accounts for the surface electrocardiogram (ECG) features: absence of uniform P waves and the presence of irregular fibrillatory waves. These waves are characterized by irregularity of morphology, amplitude, and timing often resulting in an irregularly irregular and rapid ventricular rate (**Figure 69-1A** and **B**). Often masquerading as AFib is multifocal atrial tachycardia, which is characterized by organized atrial activity, but with three or more different P wave morphologies, variable PR-interval, and presence of an isoelectric baseline.

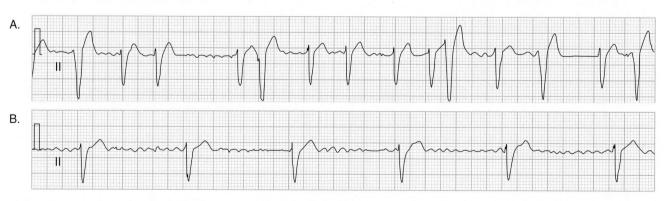

**Figure 69-1** A. A rhythm strip, lead II, of a patient with AFib and rapid ventricular rates. The hallmark features of AFib include the absence of P waves; irregularity of morphology, amplitude, and timing of the fibrillatory waves; and an irregularly irregular and rapid ventricular rate. B. The patient subsequently underwent ablation of the AV junction. This procedure results in permanent heart block, and the escape rhythm is from the junction, which explains the regular rhythm and slow rate. The fibrillatory waves are readily seen. The patient then underwent implantation of a pacemaker.

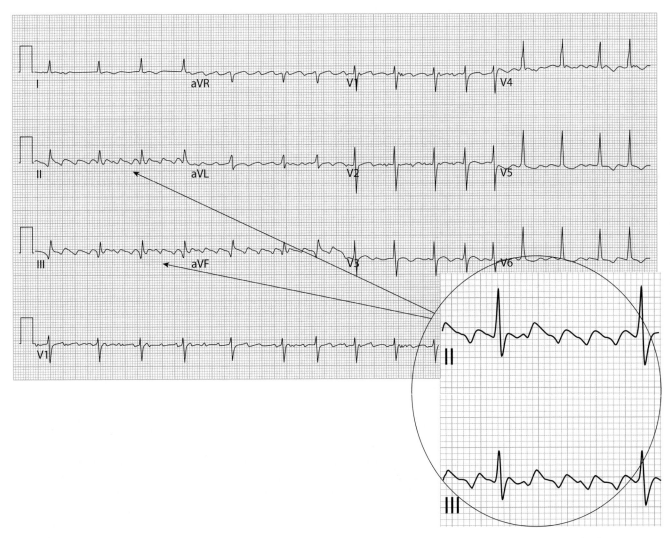

**Figure 69-2.** ECG of cavotricuspid isthmus-dependent AFlr with classical sawtooth flutter waves in leads II, III, aVF. The flutter waves (magnified in leads II and III on the right) have similar morphology, amplitude, and timing.

## Atrial Flutter

Atrial flutter (AFlr) is less common than AFib and the incidence is about 200,000 per year in the United States. Atrial flutter can coexist in patients with AFib. Clinical features that are associated with AFib (listed above) can also promote AFlr.

Atrial flutter is defined as a macro-reentrant arrhythmia with the wave of depolarization conducting repeatedly over a specific region of the atria. This repetitive activation of the right and left atria results in uniform activation of the atria and is reflected by organized flutter waves on the surface ECG (**Figure 69-2**). Unlike fibrillatory waves, flutter waves have similar morphology, amplitude, and timing. Although the *atrial* rate with AFlr is slower than with AFib, the ventricular rate in response to AFlr is often in a 2:1 pattern resulting in a faster ventricular rate of ≈150 bpm.

## CLASSIFICATION

### Atrial Fibrillation

Atrial fibrillation is classified as:

1. **Paroxysmal AFib**—recurrent AFib that terminates spontaneously within 7 days
2. **Persistent AFib**—AFib that is sustained beyond 7 days, or lasting <7 days but necessitating pharmacologic or electrical cardioversion
3. **Longstanding persistent AFib**—AFib that is continuous for >1 year, but attempts to restore sinus rhythm are pursued either with pharmacologic or electrical conversion radiofrequency ablation (RFA), percutaneous; or, surgical
4. **Permanent AFib**—AFib that is continuous and a decision has been made not to pursue restoration of sinus rhythm by any means

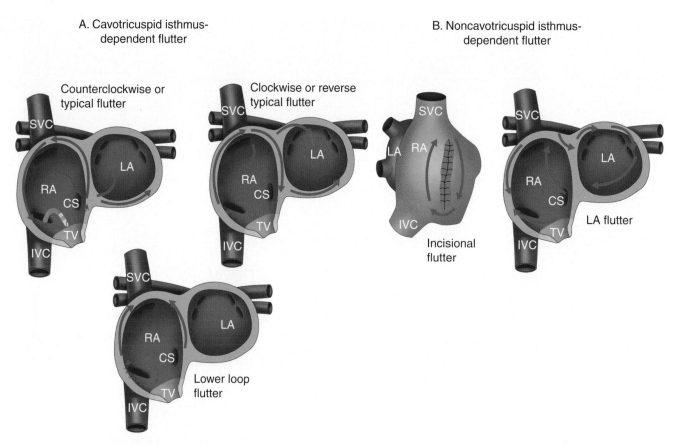

A. Cavotricuspid isthmus-dependent flutter

Counterclockwise or typical flutter

Clockwise or reverse typical flutter

Lower loop flutter

B. Noncavotricuspid isthmus-dependent flutter

Incisional flutter

LA flutter

**Figure 69-3** A. The three types of cavotricuspid isthmus-dependent flutter. In each of these macro-reentrant circuits, a critical zone of conduction is the isthmus region. As displayed in the image of counterclockwise or typical flutter, the goal of catheter ablation is to complete a line of bidirectional conduction block between the tricuspid valve (TV) and the inferior vena cava (IVC), thus interrupting conduction through the isthmus region. B. The two types of noncavotricuspid isthmus-dependent flutter. CS, coronary sinus; LA, left atrium; RA, right atrium; SVC, superior vena cava.

## Atrial Flutter (Figure 69-3)

Atrial flutter is classified according to the path of the macro-reentrant circuit. The most common form is[1] *cavotricuspid isthmus-dependent flutter*. The isthmus is a critical component of the circuit and is bounded anteriorly by the tricuspid valve and posteriorly by the inferior vena cava and the eustachian ridge. There are three forms of cavotricuspid isthmus-dependent flutter: (a) **counterclockwise isthmus-dependent flutter**, which is also referred to as typical atrial flutter, (b) **clockwise isthmus-dependent flutter**, which is also referred to as reverse typical atrial flutter, and (c) **lower loop**. The most common variety is counterclockwise flutter and is defined as the reentrant wave of depolarization traveling in a cranial-caudal activation along the right atrial free wall. This activation sequence results in the classic sawtooth flutter wave morphology in the inferior leads (**Figure 69-2A**). Clockwise flutter travels in the opposite direction. Lower loop flutter is the most uncommon form of cavotricuspid isthmus-dependent flutter and circulates around the inferior vena cava.

A second form of atrial flutter is[2] *noncavotricuspid isthmus-dependent flutter* and refers to any macro-reentrant atrial tachyarrhythmia that does not utilize the cavotricuspid isthmus as part of its circuit (**Figure 69-3B**). Examples include (a) **incisional flutters**, in which the reentrant circuit is around a line of scar tissue as a result of a prior atriotomy. Incisional flutters often present late after congenital heart surgery or valve surgery. A second type of noncavotricuspid isthmus-dependent flutter may occur after curative RFA of AFib. A proarrhythmic effect of the RFA lesions is the presence of incomplete RFA lines. The gaps in these lines are the substrate for (b) **left atrial flutter**. Left atrial flutters due to a gap in a linear ablation can also occur after epicardial surgical ablation for AFib, i.e., surgical maze procedure.

One final variety of atrial flutter is as a result of a proarrhythmic effect of Class IC antiarrhythmic drugs (AAD), flecainide and propafenone, or amiodarone. When these AAD are prescribed for management of AFib, the patient may then present with new-onset cavotricuspid isthmus dependent AFlr. This response is likely due to sodium channel blockade, which slows and organizes AFib into the macro-reentrant AFlr. This can occur in about 15 to 20% of patients and the approach to managing the AFlr is often catheter ablation. In this manner, hybrid therapy

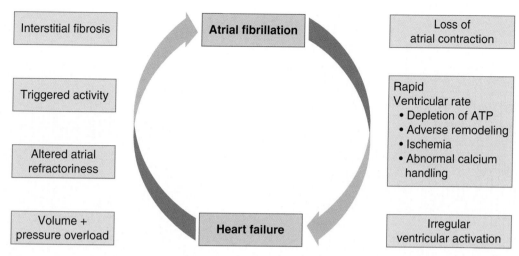

**Figure 69-4.** Adverse interplay between AFib and congestive heart failure that promotes worsening heart failure and perpetuation of AFib.

(AAD + catheter ablation of AFlr) results in a more successful management of the AFlr than just medical therapy alone.

## CLINICAL PRESENTATION AND MANAGEMENT

### General Features & Initial Evaluation

#### Symptoms

Symptoms associated with AFib and AFlr are most often due to rapid ventricular rates as well as to the loss of atrial contractility. Patients present with complaints of palpitations, fatigue, shortness of breath, exercise intolerance, and chest discomfort. Once AFib begins, it can result in a downward cascade of adverse hemodynamics that precipitate congestive heart failure. The heart failure results in further changes in the atria that can promote perpetuation of AFib (**Figure 69-4**).

Patients may present with AFib and near-syncope/syncope. The latter may be due to excessive bradycardia following conversion to sinus rhythm (termed tachy-brady syndrome or sick sinus syndrome), due to rapid ventricular rates during the tachycardia or rarely due to the presence of a manifest accessory pathway. When AFib occurs in the setting of Wolff-Parkinson-White Syndrome (WPW), rapid and unimpeded conduction to the ventricle over the accessory pathway can precipitate ventricular fibrillation and death (**Figure 69-5**).

Patients with AFib/AFlr can also present with symptoms that are more consistent with heart failure. In these patients, the newly diagnosed cardiomyopathy is often due to the rapid ventricular rates and, typically, patients are unaware of the atrial arrhythmia. Prolonged rapid ventricular rates can result in a tachycardia-induced cardiomyopathy. If the ventricular rate is controlled or if sinus rhythm is restored, the myopathy will likely reverse.

For some asymptomatic patients, the diagnosis of AFib and AFlr is an incidental finding on a routine examination. The ventricular rate in these patients is usually controlled.

#### Secondary Causes

Each new diagnosis of AFib/AFlr should have a thorough evaluation to rule out secondary causes of AFib/AFlr. This evaluation should entail a history/physical exam (with attention to presence of hypertension, lung or pericardial disease, and sleep apnea), 12-lead ECG, transthoracic echocardiography, laboratory studies including thyroid function studies, and often stress testing. Potentially reversible causes of AFib/AFlr include acute pericarditis, recent myocardial infarction, severe mitral regurgitation, atrial septal defect, presence of an accessory pathway, cardiac tumors, pneumonitis, pulmonary embolus, thyrotoxicosis, and excessive alcohol use ("holiday heart"). Management of these other comorbidities (e.g., thyrotoxicosis, severe mitral regurgitation) may eliminate the atrial arrhythmias, however, even when managed appropriately (e.g., hypertension, sleep apnea) AFib/AFlr may continue.

The incidence of new onset AFib/AFlr after cardiac surgery can be as high as 40% but is generally considered a reversible cause of AFib. Risk factors for AFib after heart surgery are elderly age, valvular surgery, and the arrhythmia most often occurs during postoperative days 2-4. The exact pathophysiology is unclear, but typically, a few weeks after surgery, the factors promoting the AFib have resolved and it rarely becomes a chronic clinical problem. However, even though it usually resolves, the strategy for managing recurring episodes of postoperative AFib is the same as managing clinical AFib episodes with attention to rate control, anticoagulation, and restoration of sinus rhythm.

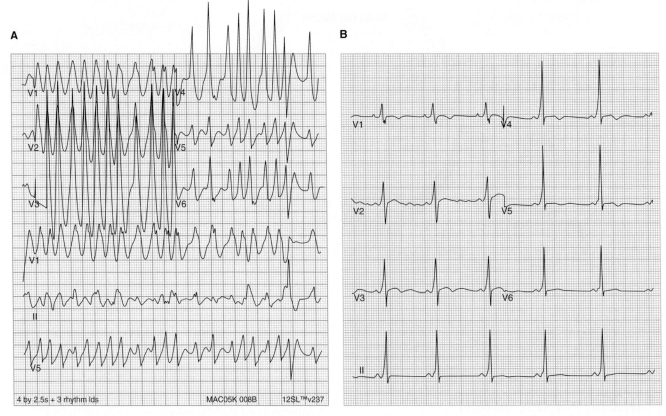

**Figure 69-5.** Example of a young patient who presented with an irregular wide complex tachycardia with varied QRS morphologies. A. The precordial tracings (V1-V6) and the rhythm strips below (V1, II, V5) represent AFib with conduction over an accessory pathway. B. After cardioversion, the precordial leads reveal sinus rhythm with preexcitation/WPW.

Since the incidence of post open heart surgery is high, prophylactic beta-blocker therapy is favored and has been demonstrated to reduce the incidence of postoperative AFib. Sotalol, amiodarone, and biatrial pacing have also been reported to significantly reduce postoperative AFib.

## GOALS OF MANAGING AFIB/AFLR

The current strategy for managing recurrent episodes of AFib/AFlr focuses on a "triad of therapy": control of ventricular rate, prevention of thromboembolic events (TE), and restoration and maintenance of sinus rhythm. Each clinical decision requires a separate management strategy that is based on patient-specific features.

### Rate Control

As described above, the bulk of symptoms related to AFib/AFlr is due to rapid ventricular rates. The ventricular rate in response to AFib/AFlr is altered by electrophysiologic properties of the AV node, autonomic tone, and medical therapies (such as beta-blockers) that blunt AV node conduction.

An initial therapy should be prompt rate control through the use of intravenous or oral beta-receptor or calcium channel

antagonists. Calcium channel blockers (Class IV agents), such as diltiazem or verapamil, and beta-blockers (Class II agents), such as metoprolol or atenolol, reduce ventricular rate because of slowing of conduction through the AV node and are not likely to promote conversion to sinus rhythm. Intravenous diltiazem is often a first-line therapy for rate control during an emergency room evaluation with patients subsequently being transitioned over to oral medical therapy. When used alone, digoxin rarely provides adequate rate control. Digoxin is beneficial when used as adjunctive therapy with beta- or calcium channel blockers.

Rate control is important not only for managing symptoms but also to prevent a tachycardia-induced cardiomyopathy (see above).

One caveat regarding rate control is in the patient with WPW. These patients may present with an irregular wide complex tachycardia attributable to AFib conducting over the accessory pathway (**Figure 69-5**). The use of AV blocking agents in this situation should be avoided, since blunting AV node conduction may facilitate more rapid conduction over the accessory pathway and result in ventricular fibrillation. The best approach is cardioversion or intravenous procainamide, ibutilide or amiodarone.

In certain circumstances, medical therapy for rate control can be challenging. For example, side effects may preclude adequate dosing of beta-blockers in patients with obstructive lung disease. Sometimes, rate control may only be achievable through RFA of the AV junction, which results in permanent complete heart block and mandates implantation of a pacemaker (**Figure 69-1B**). Obviously, RFA of the AV junction and implantation of a pacemaker do not correct the AFib and, thus, do not alter the risk of TE or the need for anticoagulation.

## Anticoagulation

### Medical Therapy

Perhaps the most important aspect of managing a patient with AFib/AFlr is to prevent TE, the most severe being ischemic stroke. A few important features regarding the use of anticoagulation therapy need to be remembered. First, the risk of TE does not correlate with the type of AFib. In other words, patients with paroxysmal AFib seem to be at the same risk as persistent AFib. Second, even if sinus rhythm is restored, the risk of TE may not be adequately reduced to recommend discontinuation of anticoagulation therapy. An explanation for these two points is that many patients are not aware of recurrent AFib ("silent" AFib), thus the absence of symptoms does not equate to freedom of AFib.

From pooled data of several anticoagulation trials in patients with nonvalvular AFib, the annual risk of TE for the unanticoagulated/control group of patients with AFib was 4.5%, but warfarin therapy (INR 2.0-3.0) reduced the risk to 1.5% (a relative risk reduction of ≈65%). Anticoagulation therapy is about 50% more effective than aspirin for the prevention of TE. The concern with anticoagulation therapy is the rate of major hemorrhage. The rate was 1% in the control group, 1% in the aspirin group, and 1.3% in the warfarin group. The most severe complication, intracranial hemorrhage, is associated with excessive anticoagulation, poorly controlled hypertension, and elderly age. The optimal dosage of aspirin is not defined and 81-325 mg daily can be prescribed. For warfarin, the target INR of 2.0–3.0 is recommended, since the risk of TE increases for an INR <2.0 and the risk of hemorrhage increases for an INR >3.0. To reduce bleeding complications/intracranial hemorrhage, some trials suggest an INR range of 1.7-2.5 for patients >75 years. If TE occurs in a patient even though the INR is 2.0-3.0, the target range of INR can be increased to 3.0-3.5. If warfarin therapy needs to be interrupted, anticoagulation should be bridged with either unfractionated or low-molecular-weight heparin. To date, no trials suggest a role for other therapies that inhibit platelet function such as IIb/IIIa inhibitors (i.e., Plavix) to reduce TE without increasing hemorrhagic complications.

| Table 69-2 • Summary of CHADS2 Scoring System and Associated Annual Stroke Risk | | |
|---|---|---|
| **CHADS2 risk criteria** | **score** | |
| Congestive heart failure | 1 | |
| Hypertension | 1 | |
| Age ≥75 years | 1 | |
| Diabetes mellitus | 1 | |
| Prior Stroke or transient ischemic attack | 2 | |
| **Patients (n = 1733)** | **CHADS2 score** | **Adjusted stroke rate, %/year (95% confidence intervals)** |
| 120 | 0 | 1.9 (1.2-3.0) |
| 463 | 1 | 2.8 (2.0-3.8) |
| 523 | 2 | 4.0 (3.1-5.1) |
| 337 | 3 | 5.9 (4.6-7.3) |
| 220 | 4 | 8.5 (6.3-11.1) |
| 65 | 5 | 12.5 (8.2-17.5) |
| 5 | 6 | 18.2 (10.5-27.4) |

A challenging clinical question is which patients with *nonvalvular* AFib should be treated with warfarin versus aspirin. For recurrent episodes of AFib, a widely accepted scoring method has been proposed through the mnemonic, CHADS2. This scoring method was developed as a result of a study of 1,733 Medicare patients older than 65 years. With this method, 1 point is assigned for the presence of Congestive heart failure, Hypertension, Age ≥ 75 years, or Diabetes, and 2 points are assigned for prior transient ischemic attack or Stroke (represented by S2). The estimated annual risk of stroke associated with each score of the CHADS2 is summarized in **Table 69-2**. In general, patients with a CHADS2 score of 0 are treated with aspirin. A score of 1 can be managed with either aspirin or warfarin, and warfarin is recommended for scores >1.

The CHADS2 scoring system is only applicable to patients with nonvalvular AFib. Patients who have AFib and mitral stenosis or a prosthetic heart valve should be prescribed warfarin. Other patient populations at increased risk for TE and in whom anticoagulation therapy is recommended are patients with hyperthyroidism and hypertrophic cardiomyopathy. High and moderate risk features for TE with AFib and the suggested method to reduce risk of TE are summarized in **Table 69-3**.

Although not as thoroughly investigated, the risk of TE in patients with AFlr is considered similar to AFib and so recommendations for use of aspirin or warfarin in patients with AFib are extended to patients with AFlr, especially since the arrhythmias can coexist in up to 50% of patients.

Whether patients who have undergone curative RFA of AFib require continuation of anticoagulation is an area

**Table 69-3 • Moderate and High Risk Features of Thromboembolism in Atrial Fibrillation and Recommended Prophylaxis for Thromboembolism**

| Moderate risk factors | High risk factors |
|---|---|
| Age ≥75 years | previous stroke, transient |
| Hypertension | ischemic attack, or systemic |
| Diabetes mellitus | thromboembolism |
| Heart failure | mitral stenosis |
| Left ventricular ejection fraction ≤35% | prosthetic heart valve |

| Assessment of risk | Recommended prophylaxis therapy |
|---|---|
| No risk factors (none of the above) | aspirin, 81–325 mg daily |
| Only 1 moderate risk factor | aspirin, 81–325 mg daily, or warfarin, INR 2.0-3.0 |
| More than 1 moderate risk factor | warfarin, INR 2.0-3.0 |
| Any high risk factor | warfarin, INR 2.0-3.0 |

of ongoing research. The most recent HRS/AHA/ACC/EHRA/STS recommendations of 2007 state the following:

1. Warfarin is recommended for all patients for at least 2 months following RFA of AFib.
2. Decisions regarding the use of warfarin beyond 2 months postprocedure should be based on the patient's stroke risk factors and not based on the absence, presence, or type of AFib.
3. Warfarin should not be discontinued in patients postablation who have a CHADS2 score > = 2.

### Device Therapy

Nonpharmacologic therapy to prevent TE complications of AFib/AFlr is quite compelling, since it would eliminate the inconvenience and cost of chronic warfarin therapy as well as the potential bleeding complications and systemic side effects. Implantable devices have been designed to occlude the left atrial appendage and thus may eliminate the need for warfarin. The strategy of these devices is that all AFib-related TE are due to left atrial thrombi that arise from the appendage and that occlusion of the appendage will adequately reduce the risk of TE when compared to warfarin. Ongoing noninferiority trials are comparing occlusion devices to warfarin.

## Rhythm Control: Conversion & Maintenance of Sinus Rhythm

### Electrical Cardioversion

Electrical cardioversion is perhaps the most expedient and safe method to restore sinus rhythm, however, it is essential to perform cardioversion when the risk of TE is low. The risk is considered low if the onset of AFib/AFlr is within 48 hours from starting fractionated or unfractionated low-molecular weight heparin or if transesophageal echocardiography excludes the presence of a left atrial thrombus. In both scenarios, patients can undergo immediate electrical cardioversion, but it is important to note that the patient will require anticoagulation (heparin bridge to warfarin therapy, INR 2.0-3.0) from the time of cardioversion until at least 4 weeks postcardioversion. Even in the absence of a left atrial thrombus on transesophageal echocardiography, the left atrial contractile function may take a few weeks to recover (known as atrial stunning), even with restoration of sinus rhythm.

If the onset of AFib/AFlr is unknown or if a transesophageal echocardiogram is not performed, then the patient can proceed with electrical cardioversion once the INR is ≥2.0 for 3 consecutive weeks; anticoagulation is then continued for at least 4 weeks postcardioversion.

These recommendations for anticoagulation around the time of cardioversion are not only for electrical cardioversion, but also for pharmacologic conversion, and these recommendations are distinct from recommendations for anticoagulation as chronic therapy to prevent TE (discussed earlier).

### Antiarrhythmic Medications

When considering antiarrhythmic drug (AAD) therapy, there are two key questions: (1) Does the risk/benefit ratio favor the use of AAD? (2) If yes, which AAD should be prescribed?

Antiarrhythmic medications are utilized to prevent recurrences of AFib/AFlr and to maintain sinus rhythm. The primary benefit of sinus rhythm is to eliminate symptoms associated with irregularity of AFib/AFlr and with rapid ventricular rates. To date, there are no prospective studies that demonstrate that maintaining sinus rhythm with an AAD reduces mortality.

Although demonstrated to reduce frequency of AFib/AFlr in comparison to placebo, the long-term success of AAD is, at best, modest. In the Canadian Trial of Atrial Fibrillation, patients were randomly assigned to amiodarone or to either sotalol or propafenone for maintenance of sinus rhythm after conversion of AFib. The freedom from AFib/AFlr was ≈50% for sotalol and propafenone and ≈70% for amiodarone at 1 year, with a progressive decline in efficacy over time. However, 18% of patients assigned to amiodarone and 11% of patients assigned to sotalol or propafenone stopped the medication due to side effects.

The Canadian trial and other AAD trials have demonstrated that since drug efficacy is not significantly different among the AAD, the primary criterion for selecting an AAD is to minimize the risk of side effects, in particular,

| Table 69-4 • Proarrhythmic Complications of Antiarrhythmic Medications | | |
|---|---|---|
| **Antiarrhythmic Medication** | **Type of Proarrhythmia** | **Increased Risk Profile** |
| Class IA (procainamide, quinidine, disopyramide) | Long QT/torsade, bradycardia | heart failure/low ejection fraction, renal insufficiency, preexisting long QT interval, preexisting bradycardia |
| Class IC (flecainide, propafenone) | Exercise-induced ventricular arrhythmias, AFlr 1:1 AV conduction, ventricular arrhythmias/sudden cardiac death, bradycardia | coronary artery disease, heart failure/low ejection fraction, preexisting bradycardia |
| Class III (dofetilide, ibutilide, sotalol, dronedarone) | Long QT/torsade, bradycardia (sotalol and dronedarone) | heart failure/low ejection fraction, renal insufficiency, preexisting long QT interval, female gender |
| Amiodarone | rare cardiac proarrhythmia (torsade, bradycardia), but potentially serious end-organ toxicity (liver, lung, or thyroid) | preexisting bradycardia |

proarrhythmia. Proarrhythmia is the occurrence of a potentially serious arrhythmia attributable to the initiation of an AAD. The more common proarrhythmic complications for the AAD classes are outlined in **Table 69-4**. In general, the risk of proarrhythmia is about 0.8% for amiodarone, and about 1.5-2% for Class I or other Class III AAD, and the risk of proarrhythmia is highest among patients with structural heart disease/heart failure. Because of the potential for life-threatening proarrhythmia, AADs are often initiated in a monitored setting, except perhaps amiodarone.

The risk/benefit profile, therefore, for an AAD includes the benefit of maintaining sinus rhythm (eliminate symptoms and reduce recurrences of AFib/AFlr), with an expected drug efficacy of about 50-70% at 1 year and a serious risk profile of about 1-2%.

### Curative Catheter Ablation

#### Atrial Fibrillation

Catheter RFA of AFib is based on two mechanisms of AFib. One mechanism is that a rapidly firing focal trigger encroaches on the refractory period of the surrounding atrial myocardium and, thus, conduction through the atria is not uniform but, rather, fibrillatory. These focal triggers often arise from sleeves of atrial myocardium that extend from the left atrium into the pulmonary veins (PVs) and display abnormal automaticity. Once a focal driver initiates AFib, even brief episodes of fibrillatory conduction can trigger adverse changes in the atria that perpetuate AFib. The perpetuation and maintenance of AFib is related to the existence of multiple wandering reentrant circuits called wavelets. Catheter ablation therapies for AFib either target the focal trigger arising from the PV or attempt to modify the atrial myocardium to interrupt and prevent the reentrant atrial wavelets.

Empiric segmental ostial PV isolation is one of the first techniques that targeted triggers originating from PV musculature responsible for initiating AF. A circular mapping catheter, positioned at the PV-left atrium junction, is used to record PV potentials for empiric RFA. Segmental PV isolation is performed for all PVs and thus the procedure is based on an anatomical identification of PV potentials rather than attempting to ablate only specific focal triggers. Segmental PV isolation is best suited for curative therapy of paroxysmal AFib.

For persistent or longstanding persistent AFib, segmental PV isolation provides a lower success rate compared to the technique of wide area circumferential RFA (**Figure 69-6**). The intent of this procedure is to create circumferential lesions in the atrial myocardium around each PV ostium, and some centers also favor the addition of linear ablation, such as from the mitral valve to the left inferior PV (i.e., the mitral isthmus). Compartmentalizing the left atrium improves procedural efficacy by interrupting atrial wavelets of reentry that perpetuate AFib and prevent focal triggers that may still exist from initiating sustained AF. Also, wide area circumferential ablation can modify cardiac autonomic inputs and atrial rotors that also contribute to AFib.

Clinical trials have demonstrated moderate long-term freedom from AFib following segmental PV isolation, ≈65 to 70% for all patients. However, the success rate is considerably higher for patients with paroxysmal AFib (≈70%) in comparison to patients with persistent/longstanding persistent AFib (≈35%). With the circumferential ablation technique, the freedom from paroxysmal AFib is ≈75% and freedom from persistent and permanent AFib is ≈60% with the first RFA procedure. Complications related to curative RFA of AFib have been reported to be 2 to 6% and include pericardial tamponade, stroke, PV stenosis, injury to the phrenic nerve, pericardial-esophageal fistula, and rarely, death.

#### Atrial Flutter

Since the macro-reentrant circuit of cavotricuspid isthmus-dependent AFlr is well-defined (bounded anteriorly by the tricuspid valve and posteriorly by the inferior vena

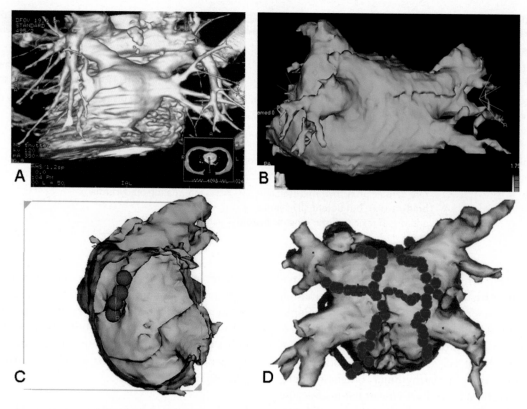

**Figure 69-6.** Imaging techniques to assist with three-dimensional reconstruction of the left atrium at the time of catheter ablation of AFib. A. Prior to the RFA procedure, a CT image of the left atrium and PVs is completed and reconstructed. B. The CT three-dimensional image is then downloaded into the mapping computer that is used in the electrophysiology laboratory during the RFA procedure. C. When a RFA lesion is applied, a red dot is placed on the image to denote the site. In this example, the virtual shell of the left atrium and PVs can be manipulated to reveal a virtual image of the left atrial chamber. This image reveals that four overlapping RFA lesions (red dots) have been delivered at the os of the left superior PV. D. With completion of the procedure, RFA lesions were delivered in a circumferential manner around each PV.

cava and the eustachian ridge), successful curative RFA is rather straightforward with excellent first procedure success (>90%) and minimal complications (<1%), and RFA is often considered as primary therapy (Class I indication). The goal of the RFA procedure is to create a line of overlapping ablation lesions connecting the tricuspid valve to the inferior vena cava, thus creating a line of bidirectional conduction across the cavotricuspid isthmus region. This complete ablation line transects the isthmus region, which is critical to sustaining the AFlr.

Successful RFA of noncavotricuspid isthmus-dependent AFlr is more challenging. Incisional flutters are often located along the site of an atriotomy and atypical left atrial flutters are usually due to gaps in a prior surgical or percutaneous RFA procedure for management of AFib. In these procedures, the circuit is defined by detailed 3D mapping and the response to pacing maneuvers. Once the circuit is defined, often the goal of the RFA procedure is to create a line of ablation from one nonconducting anatomical structure (e.g., mitral valve) to another (e.g., left

inferior PV), thus transecting the intervening atrial myocardium that is critical to sustaining the AFlr (e.g., mitral valve isthmus). In some circumstances, the AFlr is due to the presence of an excitable gap from a prior circumferential ablation for AFib, and RFA at this area will terminate the tachycardia.

## Rate Control vs. Rhythm Control

When managing patients with AFib/AFlr, in addition to managing the risk of TE, an essential decision is whether the focus of the management will be either rate control (prevent rapid ventricular rates during AFib/AFlr, but not attempt to maintain/restore sinus rhythm) or rhythm control (prevent recurrences of AFib/AFlr). To date, since there is no mortality benefit that favors one approach, this decision is often based on a patient-specific assessment of risk/benefit profile that considers symptoms, frequency of the arrhythmia, structural heart disease, and other comorbidities.

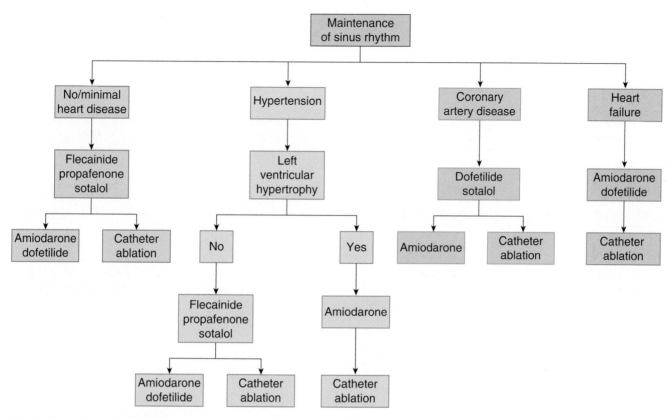

**Figure 69-7.** Algorithm for rhythm control. First-line therapy is AAD. Second-line therapy can be catheter ablation.

## Rate Control for AFib/AFlr

The AFFIRM trial (Atrial Fibrillation Follow-up Investigation of Rhythm Management) was a large trial that randomized 4,060 patients >65 years, with AFib and risk factors for stroke or death, to either rate control or rhythm control. In this population, there was no difference in mortality, stroke, quality of life, or heart failure between the two groups. Rhythm control was associated with a trend toward higher mortality, perhaps due to increased mortality related to the use of AAD and the underuse of anticoagulation. These adverse effects may have masked the benefits of sinus rhythm. In elderly patients with asymptomatic AFib/AFlr, rate control is an acceptable method and is often preferred due to simplicity and minimization of expenses.

## Rhythm Control for AFib

The algorithm for rhythm control has been outlined in the 2006 ACC/AHA/ESC Consensus Statement and is summarized in **Figure 69-7**. In general, the first-line therapy for managing recurrent episodes of AFib is AAD therapy. As discussed earlier, the selection of the AAD is primarily directed by the presence/absence of structural heart disease (heart failure) and other comorbidities (renal insufficiency/lung disease). If AAD therapy is unsuccessful, a second AAD trial or curative catheter ablation is recommended as second-line therapy. Strategies for managing paroxysmal,

persistent/longstanding persistent, and permanent AFib are outlined in **Figure 69-8**. It should be recalled that, by definition, permanent AFib is continuous and a decision has been made not to pursue restoration of sinus rhythm by any means.

## Rhythm Control for AFlr

The strategy of managing AFlr varies based on the mechanism of AFlr. Since RFA for cavotricuspid isthmus-dependent AFlr has high success, low recurrence, and low complications and since AAD therapy has moderate success and requires chronic therapy, many centers favor RFA as primary therapy for cavotricuspid isthmus-dependent AFlr.

Many patients with noncavotricuspid isthmus-dependent AFlr develop the AFlr as a result of curative RFA for AFib. In these patients (those who have tried and failed AAD and have a preference for nonpharmacologic therapy), a repeat RFA procedure is often recommended. Another patient population with noncavotricuspid isthmus-dependent AFlr are patients who have had a prior atriotomy for valvular or congenital heart disease. Certainly, AAD therapy is an option, however, considering the extensive structural changes in the atria, AAD therapy has lower-than-usual success in this population and often RFA is required. The RFA procedure for both these patient populations is associated

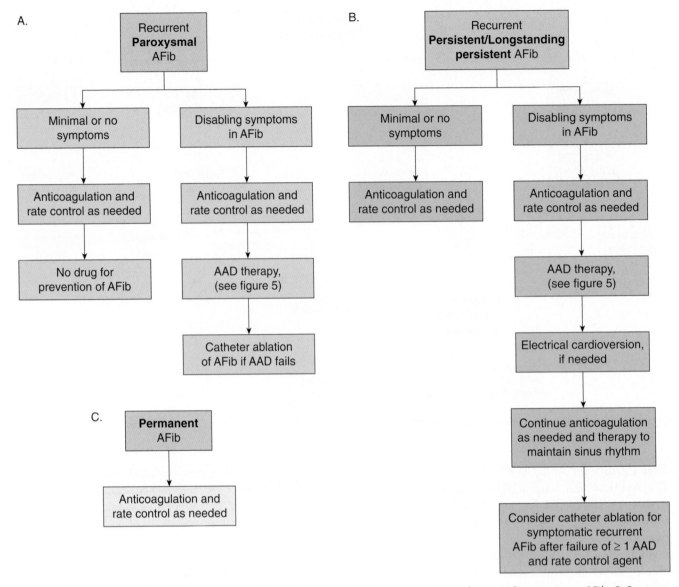

**Figure 69-8** A. Strategy for managing paroxysmal AFib. B. Strategy for managing persistent/longstanding persistent AFib. C. Strategy for managing permanent AFib.

with a lower success and increased risk for procedural complications in comparison to cavotricuspid isthmus-dependent AFlr.

## Future Therapies

Future investigations in AFib/AFlr will be to further evaluate the role of inhibition of the renin-angiotensin system and the impact of statin therapy to reduce episodes of atrial arrhythmias. Preliminary studies suggest that these therapies reduce AFib independent of their primary effect (blood pressure control and lipid reduction). One study, the NIH CABANA trial, is evaluating whether maintenance of sinus rhythm through curative RFA of AFib without the use of AAD will reduce mortality. New antithrombotic drugs

include both parenteral agents (e.g., a long-acting factor Xa inhibitor idraparinux) and oral anticoagulants, such as oral factor Xa inhibitors and direct oral thrombin inhibitors (e.g., dabigatran), that may replace warfarin therapy due to simplicity of dosing and monitoring.

| Abbreviations |
| --- |
| AAD = antiarrhythmic drug |
| AFib = atrial fibrillation |
| AFlr = atrial flutter |
| ECG = electrocardiogram |
| PV = pulmonary vein |
| RFA = radiofrequency ablation |
| WPW = Wolff-Parkinson-White |

## Suggested Readings

1. Fuster V, Rydén LE, Cannom DS, et al. ACC/AHA/ESC 2006 guidelines for the management of patients with atrial fibrillation. *Circulation*. 2006;114:e257–354.

   This is an extensive discussion regarding management of all aspects of atrial fibrillation and also discusses atrial flutter.

2. Calkins H, Brugada J, Packer DL, et al. HRS/EHRA/ECAS expert consensus statement on catheter and surgical ablation of atrial fibrillation: Recommendations for personnel, policy, procedures and follow-up. A report of the Heart Rhythm Society (HRS) Task Force on catheter and surgical ablation of atrial fibrillation. *Heart Rhythm*. 2007;4:816–861.

   This is an extensive discussion regarding management of all aspects of the role of catheter ablation for atrial fibrillation.

3. Rienstra M, Van Gelder IC. Who, when and how to rate control for atrial fibrillation. *Curr Opin Cardiol*. 2008;23: 23–27.

   A summary of rate control trials for atrial fibrillation.

4. Waldo AL. Anticoagulation: Stroke prevention in patients with atrial fibrillation. *Med Clin North Am*. 2008;92:143–159, xi

   A summary of anticoagulation trials for atrial fibrillation.

# 70

# Wide Complex Tachycardia: Ventricular Versus Supraventricular Tachycardia

Steven J. Kalbfleisch

## ● PRACTICAL POINTS

- A wide complex tachycardia is typically defined as having a rate of > 100 bpm and a QRS duration of ≥ 120 ms.

- Tachycardias are categorized by the direction of the dominant deflection in lead V1 as either a right bundle morphology (positive) or left bundle morphology (negative) tachycardia. This categorization allows the interpreter to know which morphology criteria to apply to the ECG to help differentiate between ventricular tachycardia and supraventricular tachycardia with aberration.

- An understanding of normal His-Purkinje conduction and the morphology criteria to diagnosis a right and left bundle branch block greatly aids the interpreter by appropriately diagnosing a wide complex tachycardia.

- During conduction with either a right or left bundle branch block, the initial 40 to 60 ms of the QRS complex is activated via a portion of the His-Purkinje system and therefore inscribes a sharp deflection during this portion of the ECG; the terminal portion of the QRS occurs as a result of myocardial conduction and this portion of the QRS complex often has a much more rounded appearance.

- In patients with a right bundle morphology tachycardia, a monophasic, biphasic, or atypical triphasic QRS complex in lead V1 is most consistent with ventricular tachycardia. In patients with a left bundle morphology tachycardia, if the initial down stoke in lead V1 is notched or has a time to the nadir of >60 ms this is most consistent with ventricular tachycardia.

- The Brugada criteria for differentiation of wide complex tachycardias are applicable regardless of the morphology of the tachycardia in lead V1.

- The only QRS axis deviation that is truly indicative of ventricular tachycardia is extreme left axis deviation (axis between –90 and –180 degrees).

- The simple fact that a patient has a history of prior myocardial infarction makes the likelihood that a wide complex tachycardia is ventricular tachycardia approximately 95%.

- A wide complex tachycardia that is irregularly irregular is most likely due to atrial fibrillation with aberration.

- Ventriculo-atrial dissociation or ventriculo-atrial block during a wide complex tachycardia is essentially diagnostic of ventricular tachycardia. This feature, however, is difficult to detect and is reported in only 20 to 25% percent of cases of ventricular tachycardia.

# INTRODUCTION

A wide complex tachycardia (WCT) is typically defined as having a rate greater than or equal to 100 bpm and a QRS duration greater than 120 ms. QRS prolongation to this degree can be the result of either ventricular tachycardia (VT) or supraventricular tachycardia (SVT) with aberrant conduction down the His-Purkinje system or over an accessory pathway. Wide complex tachycardias as a result of antegrade conduction down an accessory pathway are rare, and therefore, the major differential of a WCT is between SVT with either left bundle branch block (LBBB) or right bundle branch block (RBBB) aberration and VT. There are a number of criteria that have been described over the years to help in differentiating these two entities. Simply memorizing these criteria as a list and then trying to apply them can make the process confusing. The thing to remember is that the principle goal of most of the criteria developed is to try to help answer the question, Is this a typical right bundle or left bundle branch block pattern? If it is a typical bundle branch block pattern, SVT is more likely, and if it is not, then VT is more likely. It is, therefore, important to understand the basics of His-Purkinje conduction and the features of right and left bundle branch block conduction patterns. This section will outline the major criteria used to differentiate wide complex tachycardias with an emphasis on specific ECG features.

# NORMAL HIS-PURKINJE CONDUCTION AND BUNDLE BRANCH BLOCKS

Normal His-Purkinje conduction proceeds from the His bundle to the right and left bundles and then to the Purkinje network. This allows for rapid and nearly simultaneous activation of the right and left ventricles, resulting in a QRS duration on the order of 80 ms. With normal conduction, the initial activation of the ventricles starts on the left ventricular side of the septum and due to the orientation of the septum proceeds in an anterior and rightward direction. This results in the inscription of a *septal* Q wave in the left-sided limb leads (I and aVL) and lateral precordial leads (V5 and V6) (**Figure 70-1**). These normal septal Q waves are small and short in duration (<30 ms). After the initial septal activation, the right and left ventricles are activated. Because the mass of the left ventricle is so much larger than the right and their activation occurs nearly simultaneously, the majority of right ventricular activation is masked by the left ventricle and the resultant QRS complex primarily reflects left ventricular depolarization.

During atrioventricular (AV) conduction with a bundle branch block, the normal sequence of ventricular activation is altered and the duration of ventricular activation is

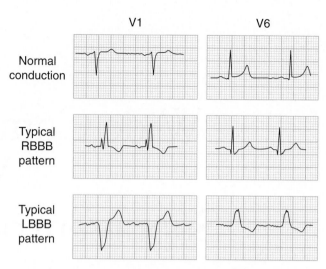

**Figure 70-1. Normal conduction and typical right and left bundle branch block conduction patterns.** On the left side of the figure is lead V1 and on the right is lead V6. During normal conduction, there is a small but perceptible Q wave in lead V6. In some cases, such as this one, the Q wave is very small and appears as almost a pinpoint. The Q wave is a result of early septal activation via the left bundle branch. During conduction with a right bundle branch block (RBBB), the QRS in lead V1 has a triphasic pattern, with the initial R wave smaller than the terminal R wave, and in lead V6, the septal Q wave is preserved. During left bundle branch block (LBBB) in the case shown, the QRS configuration appears almost monophasic in both leads V1 and V6, with some notching on the top of the QRS complex. Notice the loss of the normal septal Q wave in lead V6 as a result of loss of early septal activation from the left bundle branch.

prolonged. With either a right or left bundle branch block, the initial activation of the ventricles is via part of the His-Purkinje system and is therefore very rapid. This is reflected in the QRS morphology as very sharply inscribed initial forces that are typically less than 40 to 60 ms in duration. With RBBB, normal septal activation is maintained and left ventricular activation is still rapid. The primary abnormality in RBBB is delayed and unmasked activation of the right ventricle. Right ventricular activation occurs through myocardial cellular conduction, which is relatively slow and proceeds in an anterior and rightward direction from the left ventricle. This pattern of conduction results in broad terminal S waves in the QRS in the left-sided limb and lateral precordial leads (I, aVL, V5, and V6) and a triphasic RSR' QRS in lead V1 (**Figure 70-1**). During the typical triphasic pattern of a RBBB, the initial R wave is smaller than the terminal R wave in lead V1.

With left bundle branch block (LBBB), ventricular activation is more disturbed. With complete LBBB, normal septal activation is altered and activation of the right ventricle occurs before the septum and left ventricle. After right ventricular activation via the right bundle, the septum and left ventricle are activated through myocardial cellular conduction in a leftward and posterior direction. This pattern of conduction results in loss of the normal septal Q waves in the left-sided limb and lateral precordial leads. Because of the posterior and leftward direction of conduction during activation of the left ventricle, the QRS complex is negative in lead V1 and positive in the left-sided limb and lateral precordial leads. The QRS morphology in these leads is typically either monophasic or biphasic but may have some degree of notching on the peak of the QRS complex (**Figure 70-1**).

## ECG CRITERIA FOR DIFFERENTIATING VT AND SVT BASED UPON TACHYCARDIA MORPHOLOGY

Wide complex tachycardias are usually categorized based upon their morphology in lead V1 and their axis. This allows for very broad groupings and invokes certain rules for differentiating between tachycardia types. The differential diagnosis and ECG rules applied to a left bundle inferior axis morphology tachycardia are different from those of a right bundle superior axis tachycardia. The tachycardia morphology is categorized based on the major deflection of the QRS complex in V1; if the deflection is predominantly negative, it is a left bundle morphology, and if it is positive, it is a right bundle morphology tachycardia. Once a tachycardia has been broadly categorized as either a right or left bundle morphology, the QRS morphology features of leads V1 and V6 are the most helpful in differentiating whether it is a typical right or left bundle morphology and, therefore, it is consistent with SVT and aberration, or it is an atypical morphology and consistent with VT. Ventricular arrhythmias that arise in the ventricular myocardium, that don't involve the His-Purkinje system as part of their circuit, conduct through the myocardium relatively slowly. They, therefore, tend to have very long QRS durations and don't have the initial rapid deflections and sharp onset to the QRS complex that are seen with right and left bundle branch block conduction patterns. It is unfortunate that there are exceptions to every rule. Some VTs that arise in the ventricular septum can have relatively narrow QRS durations as a result of a simultaneous spread to the right and left ventricles. They may also have sharp initial deflections as a result of the utilization of the His-Purkinje system as part of their tachycardia circuit. In these cases, differentiating SVT from VT based upon ECG criteria can be very difficult. The next part of this section will highlight the ECG features that help to differentiate SVT from VT based upon QRS morphology.

Approximately 60% of ventricular tachycardias have a right bundle morphology configuration. Early studies by Wellens et al helped establish the value of evaluating the QRS morphology in leads V1 and V6 for differentiating right bundle morphology tachycardias.[1] A monophasic or biphasic complex

in lead V1 strongly favors VT as the diagnosis. A typical triphasic complex in lead V1 (where the initial R wave is smaller than the terminal R wave) favors SVT, especially when the ECG also demonstrates normal septal Q waves in leads I and V6 as a result of the preservation of the normal His–Purkinje activation of the septum. In patients in whom the diagnosis is not clear from the morphology in lead V1, an R:S ratio less than 1 in V6 is more consistent with VT, and this can be used as a secondary criteria to the lead V1 QRS morphology (**Figure 70-2**). Some patients have an atypical triphasic complex in lead V1, in which the initial R wave is taller than the terminal R wave. An atypical triphasic morphology strongly favors VT as the diagnosis (**Figure 70-3**). Lead V1 QRS morphologies that favor VT are shown in **Figure 70-4**.

Some notable exceptions to these rules need to be highlighted. In patients with a RBBB and an old anterior MI, Q waves may be seen throughout the anterior precordial leads (V1 to V4), which can give the appearance of a biphasic QRS morphology in lead V1 during sinus rhythm and SVTs. Patients with a preexisting RBBB and left anterior fascicular block often have an R:S less than 1 in V6, making the R:S ratio criterion unreliable in cases of a right bundle morphology tachycardia when left axis deviation is present.[1]

Later studies by Kindwall et al specifically evaluated the morphology of the QRS complex in leads V1, V2, and V6 for differentiating left bundle morphology tachycardias.[2] Four principle morphologic criteria were described to favor VT as the diagnosis (**Figure 70-5**). Three of these criteria involve the morphology in leads V1 or V2 and are (1) an initial R wave in lead V1 or V2 of greater than 30 ms in duration, (2) R wave onset to S wave nadir in V1 or V2 of greater than 60 ms, and (3) any notching on the down stroke of the S wave in V1 or V2 (**Figure 70-6**). The fact that these criteria favor VT is not surprising because they simply reflect the fact that during VT there is a relatively slow and possibly irregular conduction through the myocardium even during the early phases of the QRS complex. This is opposed to the rapid initial conduction seen during left bundle aberration as a result of myocardial activation via the right bundle. The fourth criterion that favored VT in their study is the presence of any Q wave in lead V6. This criterion makes sense when one remembers that with a true LBBB, septal activation is altered and the normal septal Q waves should be eliminated. Although the sensitivity of any one of these criteria was relatively low, ranging from 35 to 60%, the specificities were found to be high (>95%).[2]

## THE BRUGADA CRITERIA

In 1991, Brugada et al reported on one of the largest series evaluating new criteria for differentiating wide complex tachycardias.[3] Their criteria did not depend on whether

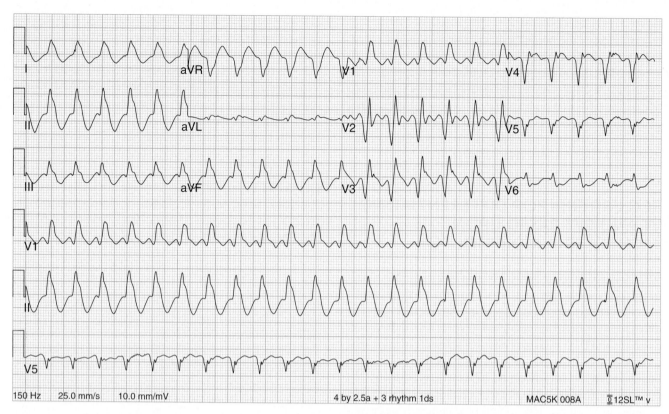

**Figure 70-2. Right bundle morphology ventricular tachycardia.** During this tachycardia, the QRS morphology in lead V1 is difficult to classify as either biphasic or triphasic, and the QRS axis is normal (between 0 and 90 degrees). In this situation, lead V6 can be used to help discriminate between ventricular tachycardia and supraventricular tachycardia. The R:S ratio in lead V6 is <1 and therefore indicative of ventricular tachycardia. When the axis is either normal or rightward during a right bundle morphology tachycardia, the R:S ratio criterion in lead V6 can be used to help discriminate ventricular from supraventricular tachycardia; however, when left axis deviation is present, this criterion is not valid. Another feature that is consistent with ventricular tachycardia on this ECG is the QRS duration. When measured at the widest QRS complex in either the limb or precordial leads, the QRS is 160 ms. A QRS complex >140 ms during a right bundle morphology tachycardia is indicative of ventricular tachycardia (see text for discussion).

the tachycardia was of a specific morphology type, but some of their concepts were extensions of the observations made by Kindwall et al regarding left bundle morphology tachycardias.[2] Their major observations were that patients with aberrant conduction due to a bundle branch block (whether right or left) had an RS complex in at least one precordial lead (V1 to V6) on their ECG and that in the leads with an RS complex, the time from the onset of the R wave to the nadir of the S wave was less than or equal to 100 ms. The relatively short time from the onset of the R wave to the nadir of the S wave during bundle branch aberration is a result of the initial activation of the ventricle via the His-Purkinje system. Their observations led to the addition of two new criteria favoring the diagnosis of VT during a WCT: (1) the absence of an RS complex in all precordial leads and (2) a time of greater than 100 ms from the onset of the R wave to the nadir of the S wave when an RS complex is present in the precordial leads (**Figure 70-7**). In their study, the absence

of an RS complex was noted in 21% of VTs and an RS complex with an RS interval of greater than 100 ms in at least one precordial lead was seen in 52% of the remaining VTs.[3] Brugada et al recommended using a hierarchal systematic approach for differentiating WCTs, combining their new criteria with other previously described criteria. The approach recommended is as follows: (1) Look for the presence of an RS complex in the leads V1 to V6, and if none is found, then VT is diagnosed. (2) If an RS complex is present, measure the time from the onset of the R wave to the nadir of the S wave in the lead with the longest measurement, and if this measurement is greater than 100 ms, then VT is diagnosed. (3) Evaluate for atrioventricular dissociation, and if this is present, then VT is diagnosed. (4) Evaluate the QRS morphology in leads V1 and V6, and if both of these fulfill the criteria for VT as outlined previously, then VT is diagnosed. Using this step-wise approach in more than 500 wide complex tachycardias leads to a correct diagnosis in 98% of cases.[3]

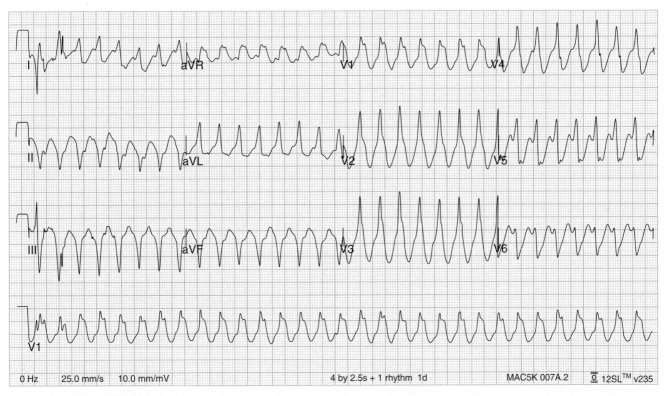

**Figure 70-3. Atypical right bundle morphology.** During this case of a wide complex tachycardia, the QRS morphology in lead V1 is triphasic. This is an example of an atypical triphasic V1 morphology where the initial R wave is larger than the terminal R wave. This pattern is strongly suggestive of ventricular tachycardia as the diagnosis. Notice also that there is a left-superior axis. Because of the left axis deviation, the R:S ratio criterion in lead V6 is not helpful for diagnosing ventricular tachycardia, but in this case, it is not needed. The QRS duration of 160 ms is also suggestive of ventricular tachycardia.

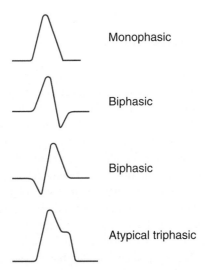

**Figure 70-4. QRS morphologies in lead V1 indicative of ventricular tachycardia.** Any deviation from the typical triphasic QRS morphology of a right bundle branch block where the initial R wave is smaller than the terminal R wave is suggestive of ventricular tachycardia. With a biphasic QRS morphology, the initial or terminal portion of the QRS in V1 may be either positive or negative, but in either case, the positive deflection in the lead needs to be the dominant deflection to classify it as a right bundle morphology. With an atypical triphasic QRS, the initial R wave is larger than the terminal R wave.

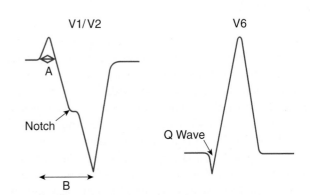

**Figure 70-5. QRS morphology features in leads V1/V2 and V6 indicative of ventricular tachycardia.** In leads V1 or V2, the presence of an R wave of long duration (A > 30 ms), long duration from the onset of the R wave to the nadir of the S wave (B > 60 ms), or any notching on the down stroke of the S wave is suggestive of ventricular tachycardia. In lead V6, the presence of a Q wave is indicative of ventricular tachycardia.

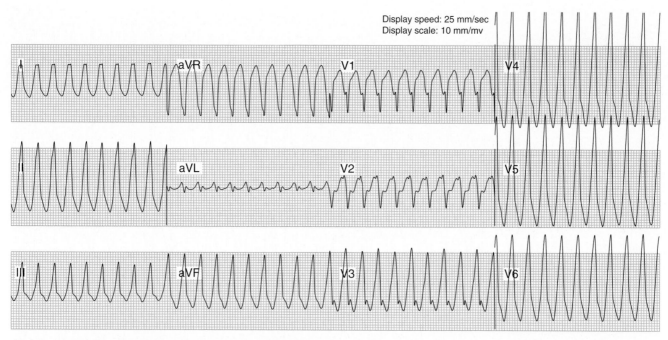

Display speed: 25 mm/sec
Display scale: 10 mm/mv

**Figure 70-6. Left bundle morphology ventricular tachycardia.** This ECG is an example of a left bundle inferior axis morphology tachycardia. The QRS duration is relatively narrow and measures approximately 120 ms. The onset of the QRS in lead V1 is difficult to discern, but in lead V2, an R wave is present with a duration of <30 ms. The R wave onset to the nadir of the S wave measures approximately 50 ms. All of the above features are more consistent with a supraventricular tachycardia. In this case, however, there is clear notching on the down slope of the S wave in V1, which is highly suggestive of ventricular tachycardia. Indeed, this was a case of idiopathic ventricular tachycardia arising from the left ventricular outflow tract tachycardia. In patients with idiopathic ventricular tachycardias without structural heart disease, myocardial conduction can be fairly rapid. Many of these tachycardias can be located more centrally near the septum and conduct to the right ventricle and left ventricle nearly simultaneously. These two features of a central location with fairly rapid conduction can lead to a relatively narrow QRS complex with the appearance of sharp initial deflections. In these cases, other morphologic features besides QRS timing may be needed to differentiate supraventricular from ventricular tachycardias.

## ADDITIONAL CRITERIA USED TO DIAGNOSIS A WIDE COMPLEX TACHYCARDIA

A number of previous studies have evaluated other clinical and ECG variables for their usefulness in differentiating WCTs. Akhtar et al reported on a series of 150 consecutive patients referred for evaluation of a wide complex tachycardia and looked at the usefulness of clinical variables such as the presence of known structural heart disease and age as well as traditional ECG criteria, including rate, axis, atrioventricular relationship, and QRS morphology and duration.[4] In their series, the diagnosis of VT was far more common than SVT and represented roughly 80% of the tachycardias. Their data showed that knowing a few simple pieces of clinical information can significantly change the probability of whether the tachycardia is an SVT or VT. Young patients without structural heart disease are more likely to have an SVT with aberration or ventricular activation via an accessory pathway. More important is the fact that if a patient has a history of structural heart disease, especially a history of prior myocardial infarction, the likelihood that the tachycardia is VT is approximately 95%.[4]

## QRS DURATION

The general rule is that the wider the QRS complex, the more likely the diagnosis of VT. In patients with a VT focus in the free wall of either the RV or LV, the impulse has to conduct to the rest of the ventricle via myocardial cellular conduction, which is relatively slow compared to the His-Purkinje system. This results in significant QRS prolongation, especially in patients with underlying cardiac disease and myocardial scaring. Early studies used a QRS duration cutoff of 140 ms to discriminate between VT and SVT. This seemed to be reasonable for right bundle morphology tachycardias but did not work well for tachycardias with a left bundle morphology, and later studies have shown that a cutoff of 160 ms is better in these cases.[1,4]

There can be a number of exceptions to these rules. In patients with a VT focus located in or near the septum, the QRS may be quite narrow because the spread of activation occurs nearly simultaneously toward the right and left ventricles. Although a very wide QRS complex is indicative of VT, a narrow complex (<140 ms) does not rule out VT. There are also a number of examples where patients

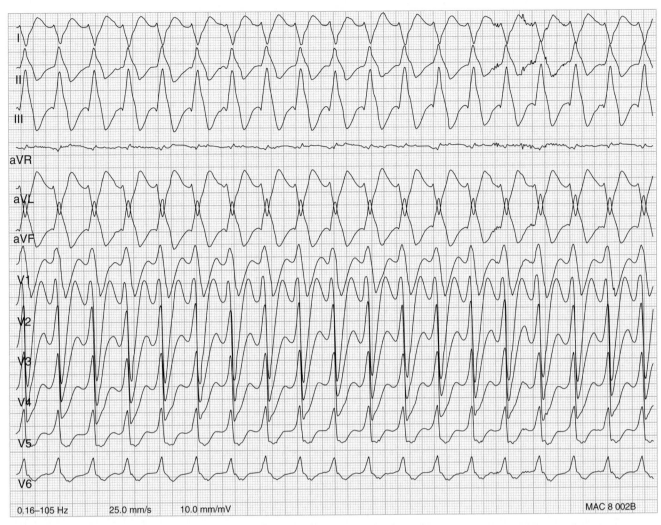

**Figure 70-7. Brugada criteria.** On this ECG, there are clear RS complexes across the anterior precordial leads from V1 to V4. The longest duration of the R onset to S nadir is seen in lead V1 and measures 160 ms. The presence of an RS interval >100 ms in a precordial lead is essentially diagnostic of ventricular tachycardia. Other features on this ECG that are indicative of ventricular tachycardia are a QRS duration of 280 ms in lead V1 and a right axis deviation associated with a left bundle morphology tachycardia.

with aberration can have significant QRS prolongation (>160 ms); this is especially true in patients with significant structural heart disease and extensive myocardial scarring or patients taking antiarrhythmic drugs with conduction slowing effects such as the Class 1A and 1C drugs. Despite these exceptions, QRS durations of greater than 140 ms for right bundle and greater than 160 ms for left bundle morphology tachycardias are fairly good predictors of ventricular tachycardia with specificities of approximately 95%.[1,4]

## QRS AXIS

Much was initially written regarding QRS axis abnormalities as being indicative of ventricular tachycardia. Some early studies indicated that left axis deviation during a WCT was highly suggestive of VT.[1] The study by Akhtar et al showed that although left axis deviation was more frequent during

VT compared to SVT, there were too many exceptions to this rule to make this a useful criterion.[4] There are two instances where an abnormal QRS axis seems to be helpful: (1) finding an axis between –90 and ±180 degrees, i.e., extreme left axis deviation (**Figure 70-8**) and (2) right axis deviation in combination with a left bundle morphology tachycardia. If either of these is found, VT is the probable diagnosis (**Figure 70-7**).

## PRECORDIAL CONCORDANCE

Concordance is defined as the QRS morphology being either all positive or all negative in the precordial leads and is seen in approximately 10% of WCTs.[4] Positive concordance, although uncommon, is strongly indicative of VT.[4] Positive concordance can also be seen in cases of antegrade conduction across a left posterior accessory pathway, but these cases

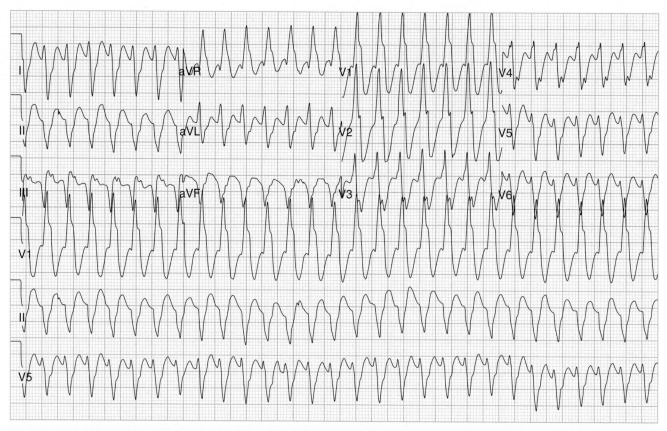

**Figure 70-8. Extreme left axis deviation.** With negative deflections in the inferior limb leads (II, III, and aVF) and predominantly negative deflections in the left limb leads (I and aVL), the axis is between −90 and ±180 degrees. This extreme left axis deviation is essentially diagnostic of ventricular tachycardia. Other ECG features consistent with ventricular tachycardia on this ECG are the monophasic right bundle QRS morphology in lead V1 and a QRS duration of 200 ms.

are significantly less common than VT. Negative concordance is less specific for VT than positive concordance, and in the series described by Akhtar et al, negative concordance was seen in 3 out of 10 cases of SVT with left bundle aberration.[4,5] Therefore, if negative concordance is seen, other criteria will need to be used to reliably distinguish VT from SVT.

## ATRIOVENTRICULAR RELATIONSHIP

Essentially any atrioventricular (AV) relationship, in which there are more ventricular events than atrial events is diagnostic of VT. During VT, any of a number of AV relationships can exist, from complete AV dissociation to 1:1 VA conduction and every degree of VA conduction block in between. During VT, the status of the AV relationship is dependent on the retrograde conduction characteristics of both the His-Purkinje system and the AV node. VA conduction block can occur at any level of the conduction system and result in a non 1:1 relationship. Many SVTs are dependent on the atrium for maintenance of the tachycardia and therefore cannot exist without a 1:1 AV relationship. In order for a SVT not dependent on the atrium, such as AV node reentrant tachycardia, to have VA block or AV

dissociation, there would have to be a conduction block between the proximal AV node and the atrium. Although this has been reported, it is extremely rare.

AV relationships are easy to see during invasive electrophysiologic testing but can be very difficult to recognize on the surface ECG, especially during a wide complex tachycardia where the QRS complex takes up a substantial part of the R to R interval. One of the most reliable criteria used for diagnosing VT, if it can be recognized, is the presence AV dissociation. This has been reported to be seen in 20 to 25% of VTs in most series, but it must be remembered that in these series, the ECGs were often read by expert observers who would tend to maximize the percentage of time that this was found.[3,4] AV dissociation is recognized by finding atrial activity independent of ventricular activity that is seen marching through the ST/T wave segment of the ECG. The faster the VT, the more likely AV dissociation will be present but the more difficult it is to recognize. If P waves appear to be seen on the ECG, attempts should be made to confirm them in other leads and see if there is a common interval that can be used to march out some of the P wave activity. AV dissociation is often best seen on the longer rhythm strips where enough time is given to see a

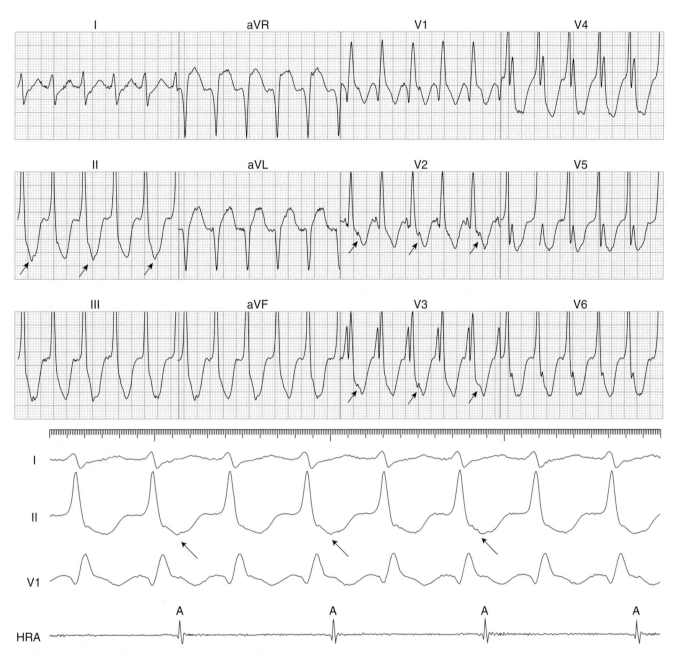

**Figure 70-9. A and B. 2:1 VA block during ventricular tachycardia.** The tachycardia shown in A is a right bundle morphology tachycardia with a QRS duration of 140 ms and a rightward inferior axis. The morphology in lead V1 appears biphasic in the first two complexes, but there is a suggestion of an initial R wave in the third, fourth, and fifth complexes, indicating the presence of a triphasic QRS morphology. Probable triphasic morphology in V1 is supported by the clear triphasic morphology in lead V2. The QRS morphology is consistent with the typical triphasic pattern seen with a right bundle branch block where the initial R wave is smaller than the terminal R wave. The R:S ratio in V6 is >1 and the R onset to S nadir in V5 and V6 is <100 ms. All of the features listed above indicate that this ECG is consistent with a supraventricular tachycardia. In these situations, evaluating the VA relationship becomes even more important for differentiating the tachycardia types. On the 12-lead ECG, there is evidence of 2:1 VA conduction seen best in leads II, V2, and V3 (arrows). Although difficult to see on the 12 lead, it is very easy to recognize during EP testing as shown in B. In this recording made at 50 mm/sec, speed surface leads I, II, and V1 are shown along with intracardiac recordings from the high right atrium (HRA). There is a clear pattern of 2:1 VA conduction. The atrial electrogram (A) is seen on the HRA recording and the P waves on surface lead II are denoted by the arrows. This non 1:1 VA relationship is essentially diagnostic of ventricular tachycardia.

pattern in the AV relationship. Fixed or variable degrees of VA block during VT can be even more difficult to recognize than AV dissociation. For VA conduction (and block) to be recognized, the VA conduction time must be such that the P wave occurs after the QRS complex so it can be seen in the ST/T wave segment. An attempt should be made to confirm the presence of P waves in multiple leads to help ensure that true conduction is occurring (**Figure 70-9**).

Other indicators that a 1:1 relationship may not exist between the atrium and ventricle are the presence of capture and fusion beats during the tachycardia. These beats are the result of antegrade conduction from the atrium to the ventricle across the His-Purkinje system occurring during ventricular tachycardia. In the case of a capture beat, the entire QRS complex is the result of ventricular activation via the His-Purkinje system, and in the case of a fusion beat, the complex is a blend of native conduction and the VT beat. If the AV conduction is normal, a narrower complex beat will be seen. A couple of areas of caution need to be mentioned. In patients with SVTs, the occurrence of ventricular ectopy can also result in *fusion* beats, which can appear narrower than the tachycardia beat and give the appearance of a capture beat leading to the erroneous diagnosis of VT (**Figure 70-10**). In patients with atrial arrhythmias such as atrial fibrillation or flutter with conduction across an accessory pathway, intermittent conduction across the normal His-Purkinje system will also create capture beats and might lead to a misdiagnosis of VT if the reader is not careful. Like

AV dissociation and various degrees of VA block, capture and fusion beats may be best appreciated on longer rhythm strips.

## TACHYCARDIA RATE AND HEMODYNAMIC STABILITY

The most important statement regarding these two features of a wide complex tachycardia is that neither of these can be used to help discriminate the tachycardia type.[4] The rate range is of absolutely no value for differentiating SVT from VT. Both of these tachycardia types encompass the same rate ranges, and although in some series the average rate of SVTs was greater than VTs, there is too much overlap to make it a useful discriminator. Morady et al showed that it is a common misconception among physicians that hemodynamic stability during tachycardia favors SVT.[6] Although it may be true that at any particular rate, a ventricular tachycardia is more likely to be hemodynamically unstable, there are

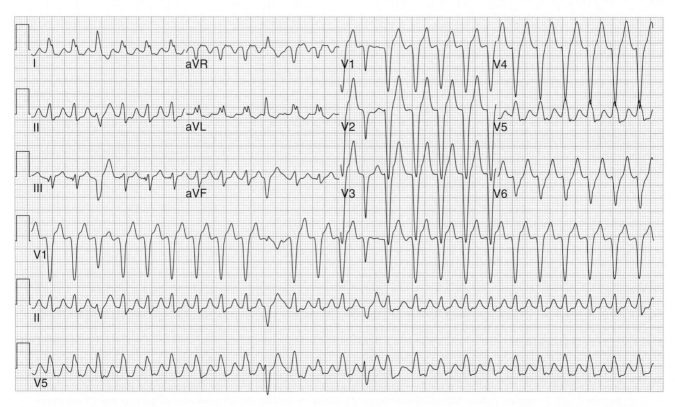

**Figure 70-10. Capture and fusion beats.** This ECG shows a left bundle morphology tachycardia with a QRS duration of 140 ms. The R onset to S nadir in lead V1 and V2 is <60 ms; no Q wave is seen in lead V6 and the QRS axis is normal. All of these features point to a supraventricular tachycardia with left bundle aberration as the cause of the tachycardia. The one feature that is against this is fusion beats and what appears to be a capture beat, which are marked with arrows on the 12-lead ECG. The first two beats marked look consistent with fusion beats, but the last beat marked looks like a capture beat with significant narrowing and near normalization of the QRS morphology in leads V1 to V3. If this were a true capture beat, it would indicate that the tachycardia was due to ventricular tachycardia (see text for discussion). In fact, all of these beats were fusion beats as a result of ventricular ectopy occurring during the tachycardia. This patient has a baseline left bundle branch block and, even at slower rates, had a QRS duration of 140 ms. The tachycardia was secondary to an atrial tachycardia and ventricular ectopy could be seen as the cause of the fusion beats during real-time recordings from the patient's ICD. This example was given to show that the ECG reader has to be careful in interpreting fusion beats because they can be the result of ventricular ectopy fusing with supraventricular beats and, therefore, not diagnostic of ventricular tachycardia.

# 71

# Pacemakers and Defibrillators

MAHMOUD HOUMSSE AND CHARLES LOVE

## ● PRACTICAL POINTS

- Understanding the 5-position permanent pacemaker code is essential to comprehend the pacing function.

- Medications could increase or decrease the pacing threshold, which becomes very important in a pacemaker-dependent patient. This could result in a loss of pacing activity if drugs increase pacing threshold.

- Electromagnetic interference (EMI) could result in oversensing and inhibition of pacing, which could be serious in pacemaker-dependent patient.

- Symptomatic sinus node dysfunction, acquired complete and advanced second-degree atrioventricular (AV) block, and chronic bifasicular block are the main indications for permanent pacemaker.

- Biventricular pacemaker is indicated in patients with low left ventricular ejection fraction (LVEF) <35%, electrical dyssynchrony (QRS duration more than 120 ms), and NYHA function class III/IV stage C heart failure symptoms while on optimal medical therapy.

- Symptomatic permanent pacemaker malfunction requires urgent restoration of stable cardiac rhythm, which could require temporary pacing.

- Pacemaker syndrome results from loss of atrial contribution to ventricular filling, which results in drop of cardiac output especially in patients with diastolic dysfunction and pericardial disease. This causes fatigue and palpitation.

- Pacemaker-mediated tachycardia (PMT) is usually initiated with premature ventricular beat, which travels retrograde up the bundle of His to the AV node then atrium, which could conduct down the AV node to restart another cycle over.

- Secondary ICD prevention is indicated in survivors of cardiac arrest due to ventricular fibrillation (VF), unstable ventricular tachycardia (VT), or syncope with inducible VT or VF during electrophysiology study.

- Primary ICD prevention is indicated if patient has LVEF <35%, NYHA function class II/III, and ischemic or non-ischemic cardiomyopathies.

- Primary ICD prevention is indicated if patient has LVEF <30%, NYHA function class I, and ischemic cardiomyopathy

- Primary ICD prevention is indicated if patient has LVEF <40%, non-sustained VT due to prior myocardial infarction, and inducible VT or VF during electrophysiology study.

- Inappropriate ICD shock occurs due to supraventricular tachycardia (SVT), oversensing of EMI or lead fracture, as well as insulation failure.

# MODE CODE FOR PERMANENT PACING

In order to understand the "language" of pacing, it is necessary to comprehend the coding system. The code has undergone a number of revisions over the past several decades. The current system consists of a five-position system using a letter in each position to describe the programmed function of a pacing system (**Table 71-1**). For standard pacing devices, only the first three or four positions are routinely used. The first position designates the chamber or chambers paced. It is useful to remember that the primary purpose of a pacemaker is to pace, and thus the first letter of the code represents this first function of the device. The letters used are V, A, D, and O to designate Ventricle, Atrium, Dual chamber, or Off.

The secondary function of a modern device is to sense the native heart rhythm. The letters used to designate the chambers being sensed are identical to those used for the chambers being paced; V, A, D, and O, with the same meanings. The third letter of the code describes how the pacemaker will respond to a sensed event. The letters used are I, T, D, and O to designate Inhibited, Triggered/Tracking, Dual response, or Off (no response). A device programmed to the VVI mode would therefore pace the ventricle and sense the ventricle, and if a sensed QRS occurred before the pacemaker stimulus was due, it would withhold the stimulus (i.e., be inhibited) and reset for another cycle. The triggered mode is often a source of confusion, as it had not been used in single chamber pacing applications very often until biventricular pacing became

common. Instead of inhibiting the output when the device senses an intrinsic event, a pace output is delivered when the sensed event occurs. While programmed to the VVT mode (or if the "pace on sensed QRS" feature is activated resulting in the same function), the device will pace at the programmed rate. However, if a sensed QRS occurs (or any electrical event is detected by the pacing lead) before the next pacing pulse is due to occur, the device will immediately deliver a pace output. The appearance will be a pacemaker pulse somewhere within the native QRS. AAT performs in the same fashion, except it is triggered by a sensed event on the atrial lead (usually a P wave) and paces immediately into the atrium.

In a device programmed to the DDD mode (dual chamber pacing, dual chamber sensing, and dual mode of response) the operation of the pacemaker is much more complex, as the atrial and ventricular channels must work together. If an atrial event is sensed, the atrial output is inhibited and a ventricular output will be triggered after a programmed interval: the AV delay or AV interval. Similar to the VVI mode, any sensed ventricular event will inhibit the output to the ventricle. However, if a ventricular sensed event occurs before the next atrial event is due (e.g., PVC), both atrial and ventricular outputs are inhibited and the device is reset for the next timing cycle. This combined inhibited and triggered/tracking response is represented by the third "D" in the dual response designation of the code.

The fourth letter is only used when a rate modulation sensor is present. Thus, a device programmed to the VVIR, AAIR, or DDDR mode would have the capability to regulate the rate based on its own sensor, whereas those programmed VVI or AAI would only be able to pace at a fixed rate. A device programmed to DDD could increase the pacing rate based on tracking the intrinsic atrial rate but could not increase the pacing rate independently (such as in a patient with sick sinus syndrome or sinus node arrest).

The fifth position has undergone several iterations of change and is currently used to designate multisite pacing function. In a similar fashion to the fourth position, it is used only when the feature is present and is otherwise omitted. The codes O, A, V, and D are used once again. These describe nO multichamber pacing, multisite Atrial pacing, multisite Ventricular pacing, and Dual chamber multisite pacing.

## BASIC CONCEPTS OF PACING

### Pacemaker Components

#### Battery

The primary power source for permanent pacemakers has evolved from short lived and unreliable chemistries to the long-lasting and durable ones that we use today. Lithium

---

**Table 71-1 • Pacemaker Mode Code**

**First position indicates the chamber paced:**
V = ventricle
A = atrium
D = dual
O = no pacing

**Second position indicates the chamber sensed:**
V = ventricle
A = atrium
D = dual
O = no sensing

**Third position indicates the response to a sensed event:**
I = inhibited
T = triggered/tracking
D = dual
O = no response

**Fourth position indicates programmability and rate response:**
R = rate responsive feature active

**Fifth position indicates multisite pacing activation:**
O = none
A = atrium
V = ventricle
D = dual

iodine is currently the power source being used in virtually all pacemakers (but not defibrillators) today. Lithium iodine has two other characteristics that make it an excellent power source. First, the self-discharge rate is very low, resulting in a long shelf life. Second, it has a stable voltage through much of the useful life, which then tapers down in a gradual and predictable manner. The latter makes determining the elective replacement time safe and predictable.

### Circuitry

New devices are now highly complex and integrated microprocessor based systems. The newest devices have the ability to store intracardiac electrograms and function as implantable event monitors, these are essentially computers, are software based, and have the ability to download new features or "bug" fixes.

### Connector Block

The connector block (also referred to as the "header") is the means by which the pacemaker wire is connected to the pacemaker circuitry. Most pacemakers use set screws or a combination of set screws and automatic connectors to attach the lead to the pacemaker and make the electrical connections. Proper placement of the lead(s) into the connector block is critical.

### Leads: Lead Components

Pacemaker leads are far more than simple "wires." They are complex and highly engineered devices that consist of many components. Most pacing leads are unipolar, bipolar parallel, bipolar coaxial, and bipolar coated coil (coradial) in design. Newer leads have up to four pacing electrodes to allow more flexibility for multisite pacing applications. Leads remain the "weak link" in any pacing or ICD system, with lead failure being the most common cause of system failure.

### Electrode

The purpose of the electrode is to deliver an electrical stimulus and to detect intrinsic cardiac electrical activity. Many modern electrodes used for pacing are designed to deliver an antiinflammatory drug such as the steroid dexamethasone sodium phosphate during the initial weeks postimplant. Eluting such a drug at the electrode surface has been shown to reduce the amount of acute inflammation and thus the amount of fibrosis at the electrode myocardial interface. Less fibrosis allows the electrode to remain in closer contact with the excitable myocardial cells. This provides a greater charge density at the site of stimulation and has the effect of reducing the amount of electrical current required to stimulate the muscle. The result is lower battery drain and increased longevity of the pacemaker by allowing the pacemaker output to be reduced.

### Insulation

One of the most important components of any lead system is the insulation. The insulation prevents electrical shorting between the conductor coils within the lead, prevents stimulation of tissues other than the heart, and allows smooth passage of the lead into the vein. Failure of the insulation may result in a number of different problems, the most important of which is failure to pace due to a short circuit. ICD leads that have this type of insulation failure may exhibit either failure to sense a tachycardia or may generate false signals that are misinterpreted as a tachycardia and therefore result in an unnecessary shock to the patient.

### Conductor

The metal portion of the wire that carries the electrical impulse from the pacemaker to the heart and the signal from the heart back to the pacemaker is the conductor coil.

### Fixation

Once the lead is placed, there is usually some type of fixation mechanism present to prevent the lead from dislodging. Leads have either a passive mechanism that entangles the lead into the trabeculae (or for cardiac vein leads, allows them to wedge into the vessel) or a helix that can be screwed into the myocardium. The helix may be extendible and retractable or may be fixed to the end of the lead. Over the past decade, there has been a steady shift to the use of active fixation leads for sites other than the cardiac veins. Cardiac vein leads often have complex shapes added to the distal portion of the lead body to help prevent dislodgement.

### Connector

The portion of the lead that connects it to the pacemaker is known as the connector. Currently, all manufacturers have agreed upon the International Standard-1 (IS-1) for pacing leads. This allows one or two connections (unipolar and bipolar; see **Figure 71-1**) on a single lead. The standard assures that leads from one manufacturer will fit properly in a device made by any manufacturer, assuming that the lead and the device are both made to the IS-1 standard. The standard became necessary due to the presence of nearly a dozen proprietary (and generally incompatible) connection designs on the market. An even newer standard now being deployed is known as IS-4. This connector allows up to four conductors to be attached via a single connector (e.g., quadrapolar leads). The IS-4 design simplifies the connections and minimizes the size of the connector block on the device for multipolar pacing leads as well as ICD leads.

### Unipolar and Bipolar Pacing Systems

All functioning electrical circuits must have a cathode (negative pole) and an anode (positive pole). In general, there are two types of pacing systems with reference to where the anode is located. One type of system (as shown in **Figure 71-2a**) uses the metal can of the pacemaker as the anode (+) and the distal electrode of the wire as the cathode (−). This is referred to as a **unipolar** system, as the lead has only one electrical pole. **Figure 71-2b** shows the other

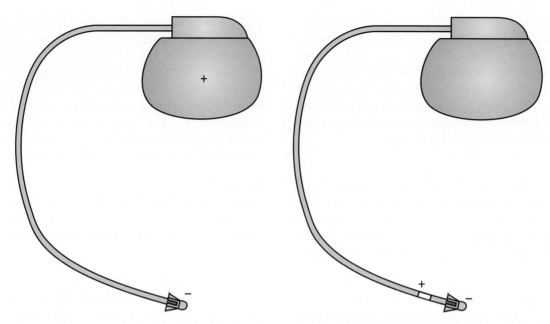

**Figure 71-1.** A. Unipolar pacing. The heart is captured or paced via negative electrode at the tip of the unipolar lead (cathode). The device is positive (anode). B. Typical pacing in bipolar pacing system. The heart is captured or paced via negative electrode at the tip of the bipolar lead (cathode). The ring next to the tip of the lead is positive (anode).

type of system where both the anode (+) and the cathode (−) are on the pacing lead. This is referred to as a **bipolar** system. With rare exceptions, pacing systems use the distal pole that is in contact with the heart muscle as negative.

Unipolar systems have the advantage of a more simple and (many insist) more reliable single coil lead construction. It is also much easier to see the pace artifact with a unipolar system as the distance between the two poles is long and the electrical path is closer to the skin surface. However, bipolar systems have several characteristics that have made this polarity choice increasingly popular. Because the distance between the electrodes is small (short antenna) and because both of the electrodes are located deep within the body, these devices are much more resistant to electrical interference caused by skeletal muscle activity or electromagnetic interference (EMI) relative to unipolar systems. Also, at higher output settings, one may have stimulation of the pocket around the pacemaker in a unipolar system. This is virtually unknown in normally functioning bipolar systems. The one complaint that is often heard about the bipolar pacing polarity is that the pace artifact is very small on the electrocardiogram. This makes determination of function and malfunction more difficult. Note that in most pacemakers, a bipolar lead may be programmed to function in the unipolar polarity, but due to physical limitations, a unipolar lead is only functional in the unipolar polarity.

## Basic Concepts and Terms

### Pacing Threshold
This is the minimum amount of energy required to consistently cause depolarization and, therefore, contraction of the heart. Note that the threshold may be somewhat dynamic. There is typically a rise and then a plateau of threshold after the initial implant. This has been largely blunted or eliminated with the use of steroid eluting leads, however, it is sometimes still significant. Some changes may occur gradually over time as the lead/myocardial interface matures. Finally, there may be transient changes to the threshold during periods of significant metabolic or physiologic abnormalities at the lead myocardial interface that will acutely affect the capture threshold (e.g., hypoxemia, hyperkalemia, and acidemia). Some medications may also affect the threshold for capture (**Table 71-2**).

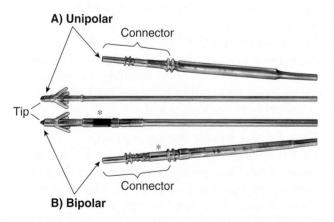

**Figure 71-2.** Unipolar and bipolar IS-1 leads are 3.2 mm with sealing rings on the connector. A) Unipolar lead. The cathode is at the tip of the lead and the lead header. B) Bipolar lead. The cathode is at the tip of the lead and the anode is at the ring (*).

| Table 71-3 • Causes of Pacemaker Failure |
| --- |
| i. Battery depletion |
| ii. Defibrillation near or over the device |
| iii. Use of electrocautery near or on the device |
| iv. Random component failure |
| v. Severe direct trauma to the device |
| vi. Therapeutic radiation directed at or near the device |
| vii. Known modes of failure for devices on recall or alert |

| Table 71-4 • Common Causes of Noncapture |
| --- |
| i. Exit block (high capture threshold) |
| ii. Inappropriate programming to a low output or pulse width |
| iii. Malfunction or inappropriate programming of automatic capture output algorithms |
| iv. Lead dislodgment |
| v. Lead fracture |
| vi. Lead insulation failure |
| vii. Loose lead connection to pacemaker |
| viii. Low battery output |
| ix. Severe metabolic imbalance |
| x. Threshold rise due to drug effect |
| xi. "Pseudo-noncapture" (pacing during the myocardial refractory period due to undersensing of the preceding complex) |

appropriate chamber following the impulse (**Figure 71-3**). Causes of noncapture are listed in **Table 71-4**.

## Undersensing

Undersensing is recognized by the presence of a pulse artifact occurring after an intrinsic event that occurs, without resetting the escape interval (**Figure 71-4**). The pace output may or may not capture depending on where in the cardiac cycle the pace output falls. Causes of undersensing (thus "overpacing") are listed in **Table 71-5**.

## Oversensing

In a single chamber pacing system, oversensing is recognized by inappropriate inhibition of the pacemaker. Note that in an ICD, oversensing may cause a therapy to be delivered as well as pacing inhibition. Oversensing may be seen as total inhibition of output or as prolongation of the escape interval (**Figure 71-5**). Myopotentials are a common cause of oversensing and are seen predominately in unipolar pacemakers and in ICDs using extended bipolar configuration (sensing from tip to coil). These are electrical signals caused by skeletal muscle activity (e.g., the pectoralis muscle or the diaphragm and abdominal rectus muscles), which is sensed by the device. Myopotentials are

typically caused by arm movements or lifting for pectoral implants and by sitting up or straining during defecation for abdominal implants. Oversensing may also be caused by the ventricular lead sensing the T wave or the atrial lead sensing the QRS. Although electromagnetic interference (EMI) in our environment has been increasing over the years, pacemakers continue to get more resistant to this omnipresent challenge by design improvements. Sensing of any of these intrinsic or extraneous signals "fools" the device into believing a cardiac event has occurred. Pacemaker output is therefore inhibited as long as these signals continue. Dual chamber systems may exhibit tracking of electrical signals such as myopotentials. This is caused by the same mechanisms as inhibition and, as just discussed, inhibition may occur in the atrium, ventricle, or both with a dual chamber pacemaker. However, rapid pacing may be the result of oversensing of electrical signals on the atrial channel, when those same signals are not strong enough to be sensed and thus inhibit the

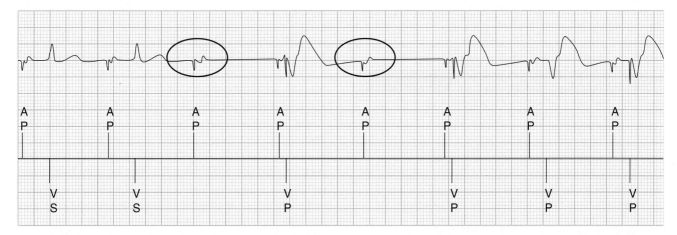

**Figure 71-3.** Loss of ventricular capture. Circles show no ventricular output. It's important to note that there are no markers following this atrial pace, so you know the device did not oversense as with the case with crosstalk. It also shows that there is no ventricular pace, which is indicative of a fractured lead.

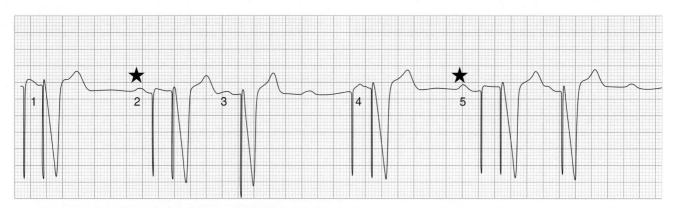

**Figure 71-4.** Intermittent atrial undersensing. Note that the 2nd and 5th atrial complexes are under-sensed. There is also functional noncapture due to atria being in the absolute refractory period.

ventricular channel. The atrial channel is usually set to a more sensitive value than the ventricular one. When the events are sensed on the atrial channel, an AV interval (AVI) is started each time oversensing occurs, triggering a ventricular output at a rate up to the programmed upper rate limit (URL). This is demonstrated by tracking of myopotentials on a unipolar system. Additional causes of oversensing are listed in **Table 71-6**.

## Diaphragm Pacing and Extracardiac Stimulation

Until the widespread use of lateral cardiac veins for pacing, this was relatively unusual. It may be caused either by an atrial or coronary vein lead stimulating the phrenic nerve or by direct stimulation of the diaphragm or chest wall muscle by the ventricular lead or cardiac vein lead. Extracardiac stimulation occurs due to poor lead placement and/or high output setting of the pacemaker. Occasionally, perforation by the lead through the ventricular myocardium may cause this as well. Unipolar pacemakers and leads with failed outer insulation may also cause tissue stimulation at the site of the exposed conductor coil, typically in the device pocket.

| Table 71-5 • Causes of Undersensing |
| --- |
| 1. Poor lead position with poor R wave or P wave amplitude |
| 2. Lead dislodgment |
| 3. Lead conductor fracture |
| 4. Lead insulation failure |
| 5. Severe metabolic disturbance |
| 6. Defibrillation near pacemaker |
| 7. Myocardial infarction of tissue near electrode |
| 8. Ectopic beats of poor intracardiac amplitude |
| 9. Safety pacing |
| 10. Inappropriate programming |
| 11. Magnet application |

## Pacemaker Syndrome

Pacemaker syndrome can occur in patients with sinus rhythm who receive VVI pacing systems or in patients with dual chamber devices where the atrial lead does not properly capture or sense. When the atrial contribution to ventricular filling is lost by pacing the ventricle alone, the cardiac output drops and the patient feels fatigued and uncomfortable whenever the pacemaker is pacing. They may have palpitations or chest pulsations due to the "cannon A waves" caused by the atrium contracting against the closed mitral and tricuspid valves. The classic patient to develop pacemaker syndrome is one with retrograde AV node conduction. The latter occurs when the ventricle is paced and contracts. The depolarization impulse travels in a retrograde manner up the bundle of His through the AV node to the atrium. The atrium then contracts against the mitral and tricuspid valves, which are closed due to the ventricular contraction. The late atrial contraction causes retrograde blood flow in the venous system with "cannon A waves," dyspnea, hypotension, fatigue, and even syncope. Clues to this phenomenon can be seen on the surface ECG.

In many cases, an inverted P wave can be seen in the T wave (**Figure 71-7**). This represents the retrograde conduction and the ineffective (as well as detrimental) atrial contraction. Patients without retrograde conduction may also have a form of pacemaker syndrome due to loss of consistent atrioventricular synchrony. Patients with diastolic dysfunction, pericardial disease, or other reason for loss of ventricular compliance are more likely than others to experience pacemaker syndrome. The latter is seen in patients with hypertension, ischemic disease, hypertrophic disease, and those who are elderly. On occasion, programming of the device such that very long PR intervals are possible may allow for a type of pacemaker syndrome, even in the setting of intact AV conduction. With the trend toward programming extremely long AV intervals and with algorithms that

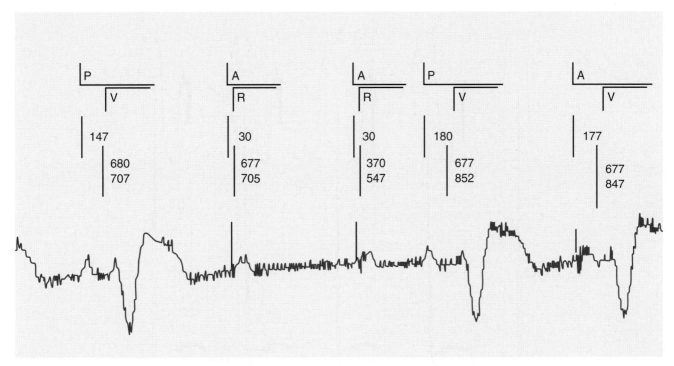

**Figure 71-5.** Oversensing. Crosstalk is a form of ventricular oversensing. The ventricular output is inhibited due to sensing atrial signal as a native QRS resulting in no ventricular output.

encourage intrinsic AV conduction at any interval, this is becoming an increasingly common problem.

## Dual Chamber Pacing

Many pacing problems are shared between single and dual chamber systems. However, there are a number of behaviors and malfunctions that are unique to the dual chamber pacemakers. These will now be discussed.

### Pacemaker Mediated Tachycardia (PMT)

PMT (also referred to as endless loop tachycardia or ELT) is an abnormal state caused by the presence of an accessory pathway (the pacemaker). It is essentially identical to the tachycardia seen in patients with Wolff-Parkinson-White syndrome. PMT often begins with a premature ventricular beat that is either spontaneous or pacemaker induced (**Figure 71-8**). The electrical impulse travels retrograde up the bundle of His to the AV node and then to the atrium.

| Table 71-6 • Causes of Oversensing |
| --- |
| 1. Myopotentials |
| 2. Electromagnetic interference |
| 3. T wave sensing (ventricular lead) |
| 5. Far-field R wave sensing (atrial lead) |
| 6. Lead insulation failure |
| 7. Lead fracture |
| 8. Loose fixation screw "chatter" |
| 9. Crosstalk (ventricle sensing atrial pacing output) |

If this retrograde P wave occurs after the postventricular atrial refractory period (PVARP) has ended, it will be sensed by the pacemaker. This will start an AV interval, after which the pacemaker will deliver an impulse into the ventricle. This starts the cycle over again. It will continue until one of the following occurs:

1. The retrograde P wave blocks at the AV node
2. The retrograde P wave falls within PVARP
3. A magnet is applied to the pacemaker (disabling sensing)
4. The device is reprogrammed to a longer PVARP or nontracking mode

The patient may also attempt to cause transient AV block by using standard vagal maneuvers to block the AV node, terminating the tachycardia. Although not commonly used, adenosine may be given intravenously to break the tachycardia. PMT may be initiated or restarted by anything that causes a ventricular beat to occur before an atrial beat. This includes a PVC, PJC, loss of atrial sensing or capture, and myopotential tracking or inhibition in the atrium.

PMT may be prevented by appropriate programming of the PVARP, such that any retrograde P waves will fall within this interval and therefore not be sensed by the atrial channel.

### Crosstalk

This is a potentially dangerous or lethal problem in patients who are pacemaker dependent. Crosstalk occurs when the

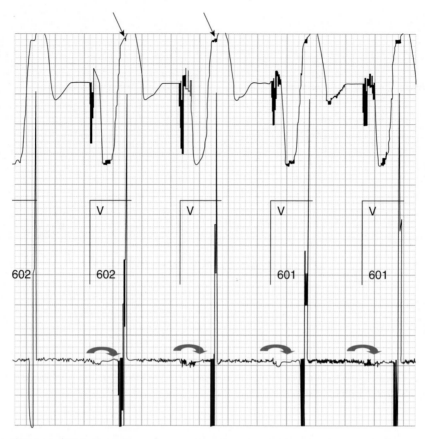

**Figure 71-6.** Retrograde conduction. Note the P wave (arrow) in the T wave after each paced ventricular beat.

ventricular sensing amplifier senses the atrial pacing impulse and interprets the atrial pace as an intrinsic ventricular beat. The ventricular output is then inhibited and, if the patient has no ventricular escape, asystole occurs (**Figure 71-5**). This is seen on the ECG strip as paced atrial P waves without a ventricular output. Typically, the atrial pacing interval is equal to the atrial escape interval (AEI). This is because the AVI is

terminated by the ventricular sensing of the atrial pacing pulse, resetting the pacemaker for the next cycle (ventricular based timing device). However, in an atrial based timing system, the AVI will be allowed to complete before the next AEI starts, thus maintaining the programmed pacing rate. Crosstalk is most likely to occur when the atrial output is set very high and the ventricular channel is set to be very sensitive.

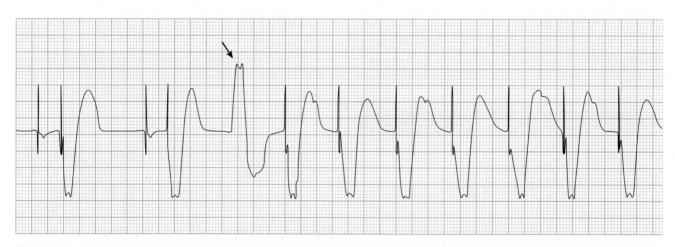

**Figure 71-7.** Pacemaker mediated tachycardia (PMT). PMT often begins with a premature ventricular beat that is either spontaneous or pacemaker induced. Retrograde P-waves (arrows) are noticed in the T-wave.

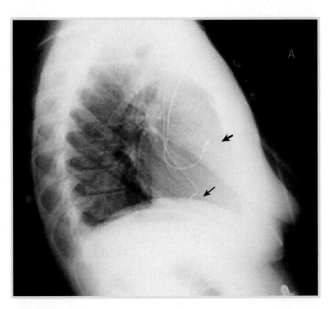 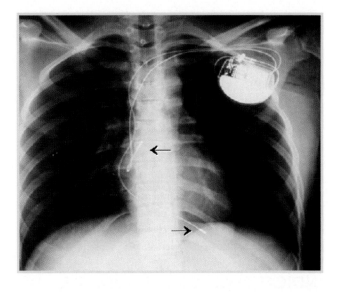

**Figure 71-8.** Lateral (A) and posteroanterior (B) CXR of dual chamber pacemaker. A. Lateral CXR: Note anterior position (A) of the RV lead (small arrow) and RA lead in the RA appendage (large arrow).

## BASIC CONCEPTS OF IMPLANTABLE CARDIOVERTER DEFIBRILLATORS

### Basic Concepts

#### Sensing

In addition to normal pacing function, sensing the heart rate is very important as this is the primary method for the ICD to determine if a tachycardia is present or not.

#### Detection

The common tachycardia detection criteria are listed in **Table 71-7**. The simplest method of determining if an arrhythmia is present is to use a simple rate criterion. If the ventricular rate exceeds a given rate for a given duration, therapy is delivered. The rate stability criterion is useful when a patient has atrial fibrillation with a rapid ventricular response at times. If the ventricular tachycardia detection rate and the ventricular rate when the patient is in atrial fibrillation overlap, then the patient could get an unnecessary shock or series of shocks. Ventricular tachycardia (VT) tends to be very regular in its rate, whereas the ventricular response to atrial fibrillation tends to be irregular. The rate stability criterion allows the programming of a minimal beat to beat variability (in milliseconds) that is acceptable for VT detection. If the cycle lengths of the ventricular beats varies more than this amount, it is classified as not being ventricular tachycardia and therapy is withheld. The shortcomings of this methodology would be the presence of a polymorphic ventricular tachycardia, which would not be regular like monomorphic ventricular tachycardia. However, polymorphic VT tends to be faster in rate and is thus less likely to overlap with the ventricular rates as seen in atrial fibrillation.

In order to avoid shocking the patient when the ventricular rate enters the detection zone due to normal physical activity, a sudden onset criterion may be used. VT tends to occur suddenly, whereas faster rates that occur in conjunction with exertion gradually rise to the higher rate. The device can be programmed to withhold therapy if entry into the VT zone is gradual rather than abrupt, as defined by a percentage of the cycle length measured beat-to-beat.

Note that some highly sophisticated algorithms also use atrial rhythm to identify VT. The presence of AV dissociation (ventricular rate faster than atrial rate) is a powerful discrimination technique. Also, the relationship of the P wave to the QRS, in terms of timing of AV and VA conduction (when present), may be helpful as well. Atrial rates faster than ventricular rates (as in atrial flutter or fibrillation) can assist in correctly indentifying these rhythms.

Wide complex beats are most often ventricular and narrow complex beats are usually supraventricular in origin. The ICD may use a morphology criterion to determine whether a beat is wide or narrow. More sophisticated algorithms now save a template of the "normal" QRS morphology and compare the QRS of the fast beats to those at baseline. Identical QRS morphology is categorized as supraventricular tachycardia (SVT), whereas those that deviate by a significant percentage are dealt with as VT.

Finally, since none of the discrimination criteria are foolproof, a sustained high rate or "time-out" feature is often available. This will allow therapy for VT to be delivered if the heart rate remains in the VT detection zone for a specified period of time, even if some or all of the discrimination criteria noted

## Table 71-7 • Detection Criteria

i. Rate only
ii. Rate stability
iii. Sudden rate onset
iv. Sustained high rate
v. Morphology
vi. Atrial rhythm discrimination

above are enabled. Note that VT may initiate during atrial fibrillation with rapid ventricular response, sinus tachycardia with exertion, or even have similar morphology of the QRS to VT. This time-out feature provides a safety mechanism should a fast heart rate be misclassified or VT occur after a non-VT rhythm is correctly identified.

# INDICATIONS FOR IMPLANTABLE CARDIOVERTER DEFIBRILLATORS

The current guidelines as published by the American College of Cardiology and the American Heart Association are as follows:

## Class I

Survivors of

1. cardiac arrest due to ventricular fibrillation or hemodynamically unstable sustained VT after evaluation to define the cause of the event and to exclude any completely reversible causes
2. structural heart disease and spontaneous sustained VT, whether hemodynamically stable or unstable
3. syncope of undetermined origin with clinically relevant, hemodynamically significant sustained VT, or ventricular fibrillation induced at electrophysiological study
4. LVEF less than 35% due to prior myocardial infarction, who are at least 40 days postmyocardial infarction and are in NYHA functional Class II or III
5. nonischemic dilated cardiomyopathy who have an LVEF less than or equal to 35% and who are in NYHA functional Class II or III
6. LV dysfunction due to prior myocardial infarction who are at least 40 days postmyocardial infarction, have an LVEF less than 30%, and are in NYHA functional Class I
7. nonsustained VT due to prior myocardial infarction, LVEF less than 40%, and inducible ventricular fibrillation or sustained VT at electrophysiological study

## Class IIa

Patients with

1. unexplained syncope, significant LV dysfunction, and nonischemic dilated cardiomyopathy

2. sustained VT and normal or near-normal ventricular function
3. hypertrophic cardiomyopathy with one or more major risk factors for SCD
4. arrhythmogenic right ventricular dysplasia/cardiomyopathy with one or more risk factors for SCD
5. long-QT syndrome who are experiencing syncope and/or VT while receiving beta-blockers
6. nonhospitalized patients awaiting transplantation
7. Brugada syndrome with syncope
8. Brugada syndrome with documented VT that has not resulted in cardiac arrest
9. catecholaminergic polymorphic VT with syncope and/or documented sustained VT while receiving beta-blockers
10. cardiac sarcoidosis, giant cell myocarditis, or Chagas disease

## Class IIb

Patients with

1. nonischemic heart disease with an LVEF of less than or equal to 35% and in NYHA functional Class I
2. long-QT syndrome and risk factors for SCD
3. syncope and advanced structural heart disease in which thorough invasive and noninvasive investigations have failed to define a cause
4. familial cardiomyopathy associated with sudden death
5. LV noncompaction

## Class III

Patients

1. who do not have a reasonable expectation of survival with an acceptable functional status for at least 1 year, even if they meet ICD implantation criteria specified in the Class I, IIa, and IIb recommendations above
2. who have incessant VT or ventricular fibrillation
3. with significant psychiatric illnesses that may be aggravated by device implantation or that may preclude systematic follow-up
4. who are NYHA Class IV with drug-refractory congestive heart failure and are not candidates for cardiac transplantation or implantation of a CRT device that incorporates both pacing and defibrillation capabilities
5. with syncope of undetermined cause without inducible ventricular tachyarrhythmias and without structural heart disease
6. with ventricular fibrillation or VT that is amenable to surgical or catheter ablation (e.g., atrial arrhythmias associated with Wolff-Parkinson-White syndrome, right ventricular or LV outflow tract VT, idiopathic VT, or fascicular VT in the absence of structural heart disease)

7. with ventricular tachyarrhythmias due to a completely reversible disorder in the absence of structural heart disease (e.g., electrolyte imbalance, drugs, or trauma)

# EVALUATION OF DEFIBRILLATOR MALFUNCTION

Failure to shock or deliver anti-tachycardia pacing: The failure of an ICD to deliver antitachycardia therapy can be lethal. The reasons for failure to shock are listed in **Table 71-8a**

Failure to convert arrhythmia: **Table 71-8b** lists many of the problems that result in delivered therapy that fails to restore normal rhythm.

## Inappropriate Delivery of Therapy

**Table 71-9** lists the major causes of inappropriate therapy delivered by ICDs. The most common cause of inappropriate shock is the presence of an atrial arrhythmia and has already been discussed above. Atrial fibrillation is, by far, the most common arrhythmia leading to spurious shock. Many patients who receive ICD implants have enlarged atria, predisposing them to atrial arrhythmias. Oversensing may also

### Table 71-8a • Failure to Shock

i. Undersensing
 1. Lead malposition
 2. Lead dislodgment
 3. Lead perforation
 4. Lead fracture
 5. Lead insulation failure
 6. Lead to device connector problem
 7. Device set to an insensitive value
 8. Poor electrogram amplitude due to change in myocardial substrate:
  a. Myocardial infarction
  b. Drug therapy
  c. Metabolic imbalance
 9. "Fine" ventricular fibrillation
ii. Primary circuit failure
iii. Battery failure
iv. Shock therapy turned off (by programming or magnet)
v. Magnet placed over the device
vi. Strong magnetic field present
vii. Detection rate set too high
viii. Failure to meet additional detection criteria
 1. Rate stability
 2. Sudden onset
 3. Morphology criteria
ix. Slowing of tachycardia below detection rate
 1. Substrate changes
 2. Metabolic changes
 3. Electrolyte changes
 4. Drug therapy changes
x. Interaction with permanent pacemaker

### Table 71-8b • Failure to Convert the Arrhythmia

i. High defibrillation threshold
 1. Poor cardiac substrate
 2. Acute myocardial infarction
 3. Metabolic abnormality
 4. Electrolyte abnormality
 5. Drug therapy (e.g., amiodarone)
ii. Drug proarrhythmia
iii. High voltage lead fracture
iv. High voltage lead insulation failure
v. High voltage lead migration
vi. Inappropriate device programming
 1. Low shock energy
 2. Ineffective polarity
 3. Suboptimal "tilt" or pulse-width
 4. Ineffective antitachycardia pacing sequence
vii. Pacemaker polarity switch (from bipolar to unipolar)
viii. Atrial arrhythmias

lead to inappropriate detections, often caused by strong electromagnetic interference, myopotentials, or by over-sensing T-waves. A fractured lead or one with failed insulation is a common source of false signals. These leads produce large spurious signals that can be easily sensed by the ICD.

# RADIOGRAPHIC EVALUATION OF PACEMAKER AND ICD

Either prior to discharge when the pacing system is known to be functioning properly or when the patient enters your practice, obtain a baseline posteroanterior (PA) and lateral chest X-ray for future comparison. When examining the chest X-ray,
- Do NOT ignore the rest of the chest X-ray while focusing on the lead(s) and pulse generator.
- If possible, obtain a slightly overpenetrated PA and lateral chest X-ray to provide better definition of the pacing components.

### Table 71-9 • Inappropriate Delivery of Therapy

i. Oversensing
 1. Electromagnetic interference
 2. Interaction with another implanted device
 3. Lead fracture
 4. Lead insulation failure
 5. Loose connections
 6. Myopotentials
 7. Permanent pacemaker
ii. Detection rate set too low
iii. Supraventricular arrhythmias
 1. Paroxysmal supraventricular tachycardia
 2. Atrial fibrillation
 3. Atrial flutter
 4. Sinus tachycardia

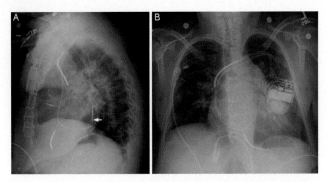

**Figure 71-9.** Lateral (A), note the posterior orientation of the LV lead (arrow), and posteroanterior (B), the CXR of biventricular ICD.

- PA and lateral film will fully evaluate the lead position in the cardiac chambers.
- A portable chest X-ray may be ordered immediately postimplant if complications are suspected to have occurred.

The right ventricle is an anterior and retrosternal structure, whereas the left ventricle is a posterior structure close to the spinal column (**Figure 71-8** for a dual chamber pacer and **Figure 71-9** for a biventricular pacer/ICD device). A lead placed into the coronary sinus and cardiac vein (intentionally or not) will take a posterior course on the lateral X-ray. The PA X-ray will not demonstrate this fact, thus the need for the lateral view as well.

Complications of subclavian venipuncture can be acute, including pneumothorax, hemothorax, and chylothorax.

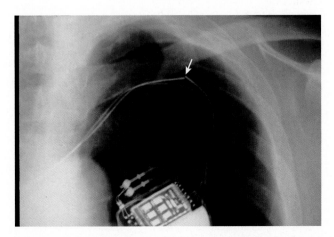

**Figure 71-10.** Lead fracture (arrow) due to rib-clavicle crush in dual chamber pacemaker.

| Table 71-10 • Acute and Chronic Complications of Device Implantations |
| --- |
| 1. Acute |
|   a. Pneumothorax |
|   b. Hemothorax |
|   c. Hemopneumothorax |
|   d. Brachial plexus injury |
|   e. Arterial puncture or tear |
|   f. Cardiac perforation with tamponade |
|   g. Chylothorax |
| 2. Chronic |
|   a. Rib-clavicle crush (Figure 71-10) |
|   b. Conductor fracture |
|   c. Damaged insulation |
|     i. External |
|     ii. Internal |

Although these problems are not common, they can be catastrophic and even fatal.

Leads will commonly be damaged at points of physical stress. A common mode of failure is "subclavian crush," caused by pressure on the lead when it is placed by a medial subclavian stick (**Figure 71-10**). Another is caused at the site of the suturing sleeve on the lead should the physician tie the ligature too tightly, or if an anchoring sleeve is not used at all when attaching the lead to the pectoral fascia. **Table 71-10** summarizes the acute and chronic complications of device implantation.

## Suggested Readings

1. Epstein et al. ACC/AHA/HRS 2008 guidelines for device-based therapy of cardiac rhythm abnormalities: executive summary. A report of the American College of Cardiology/American Heart Association Task Force on Practice Guidelines (Writing Committee to Revise the ACC/AHA/NASPE 2002 Guideline Update for Implantation of Cardiac Pacemakers and Antiarrhythmia Devices): Developed in collaboration with the American Association for Thoracic Surgery and Society of Thoracic Surgeons. *Circulation.* 2008;117:2820–2840.

2. Ellenbogen, Kay, Lau, Wilkoff. *Clinical Cardiac Pacing, Defibrillation and Resynchronization Therapy.* 3rd ed. Philadelphia: Saunders/Elsevier; 2007.

3. Love CJ. *Cardiac Pacemakers and Defibrillators.* 2nd ed. Georgetown, TX: Landes Bioscience; 2006.

4. Kenny T. *The Nuts and Bolts of ICD Therapy.* Malden, MA: Blackwell; 2006.

5. Kenny T. *The Nuts and Bolts of Cardiac Pacing.* Malden, MA: Blackwell; 2005.

# • 72

# Syncope

AMIT A. DOSHI AND DAVID T. HART

## ● PRACTICAL POINTS

- Cerebral hypoperfusion and systemic hypotension differentiate syncope from other causes of transient loss of consciousness such as trauma, seizure, and psychiatric disorders.

- Patients with syncope and underlying structural heart disease have a much higher mortality rate.

- The initial evaluation of the syncope patient must include a very thorough history and physical examination as well as a standard 12-lead ECG.

- The presence of myoclonic jerks and upward eye deviation does not imply seizure activity, and is a consequence of cerebral hypoperfusion.

- The echocardiogram is a very useful tool to help risk stratify syncope patients, patients with structural heart disease having a much higher mortality rate.

- Head CT/MRI scans have very little diagnostic yield in the work-up of syncope in patients without focal neurological deficits.

- When the history of a single syncopal spell is consistent with neurocardiogenic cause for syncope, tilt table testing is not indicated.

- Serial tilt table tests to evaluate the efficacy of pharmacologic therapy have not been shown to be clinically advantageous.

- Initial treatment for vasovagal/neurocardiogenic syncope is increased salt and water intake and avoidance of triggering stimuli if possible.

- Syncopal spells in the elderly should always prompt a systematic review of medications, especially vasoactive drugs such as diuretics, nitrates, and ACE inhibitors.

Syncope in its simplest form is defined as a transient loss of consciousness (TLOC) with associated loss of postural tone and subsequent spontaneous recovery. Global cerebral hypoperfusion and systemic hypotension differentiate syncope from other causes of TLOC such as trauma, seizure, and psychiatric disorders. Cardiovascular disorders (including neurocardiogenic syncope) are the most common causes of syncope, and the subset of patients with underlying structural heart disease and/or myocardial ischemia is associated with the highest mortality rates.

Approximately one third of all adults will experience one episode of syncope in their lifetime, accounting for approximately 3% of all emergency room visits and 6% of all hospital admissions in the United States. An episode of syncope can imply a benign episode in most cases, to an aborted sudden cardiac death in those fortunate to survive this ill fate. The vast majority of cases fall in between these two extremes. Therefore, in evaluating a patient with syncope, the clinician must initially discern whether there is a life-threatening etiology. If this is found not to be the case, subsequent evaluation and treatment should be guided toward improving the patient's quality of life and preventing injury.

There is significant heterogeneity in regard to the etiology of most syncope cases as documented by previous studies (**Figure 72-1**). It is unfortunate that despite extensive investigation on the part of the clinician, more than one third of the cases fall under the realm of unexplained or idiopathic syncope. However, a thorough initial evaluation can help exclude the vast majority of etiologies and allows a focused and cost-saving investigation as to the specific cause of the syncopal spell (**Table 72-1**).

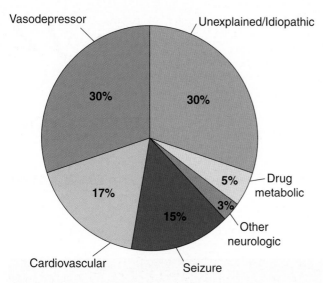

**Figure 72-1.** The most common etiologies of syncope and the respective prevalence among the general population.

| Table 72-1 • Causes of Syncope and Nonsyncope |
|---|
| **Syncope** |
| **Neurocardiogenic** |
| • Vasovagal (common faint)<br>• Carotid sinus hypersensitivity<br>• Situational syncope<br>    Cough<br>    Defecation<br>    Micturition<br>    Postexercise |
| **Orthostatic** |
| • Autonomic failure<br>    Primary or secondary (diabetic neuropathy)<br>• Volume depletion<br>    Acute blood loss<br>    Diarrhea<br>• Drug induced<br>    Diuretics<br>    Nitrates<br>    ACE inhibitors/ARBs |
| **Cardiac arrhythmias** |
| • Bradycardia<br>• Supraventricular tachycardia (WPW with atrial fibrillation)<br>• Ventricular tachycardia<br>• Drug induced Torsades de Pointes<br>• Inherited ion-channelopathies (Brugada syndrome, long QT) |
| **Structural heart disease** |
| • Hypertrophic obstructive cardiomyopathy<br>• Severe valvular stenosis<br>• Myocardial infarction/ischemia<br>• Intracardiac tumors<br>• Acute aortic dissection<br>• Pericardial tamponade<br>• Arrhythmogenic right ventricular dysplasia/cardiomyopathy (ARVD/C) |
| **Noncardiac etiologies** |
| • Pulmonary embolism<br>• Cerebrovascular steal syndromes |
| **Nonsyncopal episodes**<br>  **No transient loss of consciousness** |
| • Falls<br>• Cataplexy<br>• Conversion disorder<br>• Cerebrovascular events |
| **Partial or complete loss of consciousness** |
| • Hypoglycemia<br>• Hypocapnia due to hyperventilation<br>• Epilepsy |

The initial evaluation of the patient must include a thorough history, physical examination (including orthostatic blood pressures), and a standard 12-lead electrocardiogram (ECG). Two important aspects that tend to be trivialized but are of paramount importance include the patient's age and the degree of detail surrounding the syncopal episode. A patient's age is very helpful in isolating possible etiologies of syncope (**Table 72-2**).

## HISTORY AND PHYSICAL EXAMINATION

A detailed history is paramount in evaluating the syncopal patient. While obtaining a detailed history of the events surrounding a witnessed syncopal event, it's often useful to question family members and bystanders who may have seen the event. Onlookers may be able to provide useful information about whether the patient exhibited any prodrome or seizure-like activity. It is important to note that myoclonic jerks and upward eye deviation do not necessarily equate to seizure-like activity but are generally related to a state of impaired cerebral perfusion. In addition, a thorough family history, with attention to unexpected sudden cardiac death, will often provide clues for pursuing other testing modalities such as an echocardiogram or cardiac magnetic resonance (CMR) imaging study, if indicated. Particularly in the elderly population, a comprehensive medication list is also important. This can provide insight into potential culprits that may cause orthostasis as well as drug-induced proarrhythmias.

Many patients will often complain of visual changes and gastrointestinal symptoms preceding the syncopal event. The visual prodromal symptoms are due to a reduction in blood flow to the retina via the ophthalmic arteries, whereas the excessive vagal stimulation that can occur is known to release pancreatic polypeptides resulting in gastrointestinal distress.

The physical exam must start with a careful examination of the vitals with orthostatic blood pressures. This, in conjunction with careful cardiac auscultation, will frequently reveal the etiology if due to valvular heart disease,

| Table 72-2 • Age Predominant Causes of Syncope |
| --- |
| **Pediatric** |
| • Neurocardiogenic syncope |
| • Reflex anoxic seizure (breath holding spells) |
| • Psychiatric causes (conversion reactions) |
| • Long QT syndrome |
| • Wolff-Parkinson-White syndrome |
| **Middle age** |
| • Neurocardiogenic syncope |
| • Situational syncope (cough, micturition) |
| • Orthostasis |
| **Elderly** |
| • Valvular heart disease (aortic stenosis) |
| • Arrhythmias |
| • Pulmonary embolus |
| • Orthostasis (predominantly drug induced) |

hypertrophic cardiomyopathy, orthostatic hypotension, pulmonary hypertension, or autonomic dysfunction. The neurological examination, including assessment of gait, speech, and motor and sensory function, can also provide clues to a neurological disorder. Carotid sinus massage to evaluate for carotid hypersensitivity as an etiology will be discussed separately.

## DIAGNOSTIC WORKUP

In general, the diagnostic evaluation should begin with the patient's history and physical exam, as outlined above, and a 12-lead ECG. Unless indicated, routine laboratory studies, including a toxicology screen, should not be obtained for a single episode of syncope, particularly if the history is suggestive of a neurocardiogenic cause (**Figure 72-2**).

**Suggested approach to the diagnostic workup in a patient with syncope**

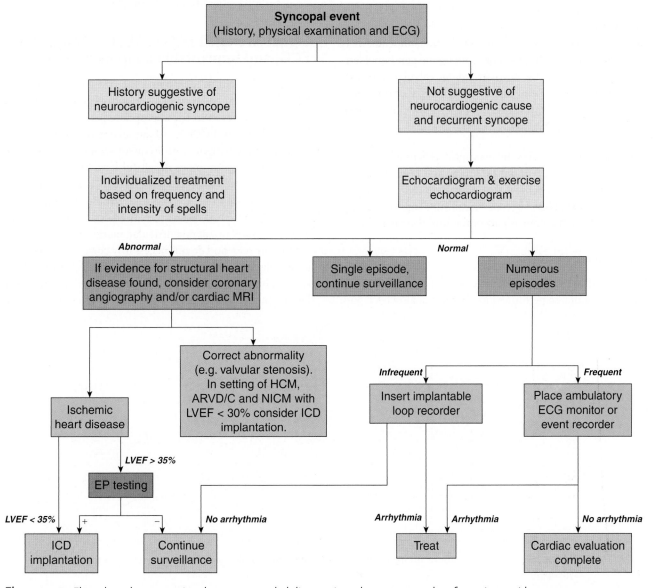

**Figure 72-2.** Flow-chart demonstrating the recommended diagnostic and treatment workup for patients with syncope.

## Electrocardiogram

The ECG, by itself, has little utility in the diagnosis of syncope but is helpful when coupled with the history and physical exam, being able to identify the etiology in approximately 35 to 45% of the cases. The ECG does provide important information regarding intra-atrial conduction, AV node conduction, bundle-branch block, and ventricular arrhythmias. The presence of a delta wave may assist with the diagnosis of WPW syndrome, whereas T wave inversion in the right precordial leads and an incomplete RBBB pattern may be suggestive of arrhythmogenic right ventricular dysplasia/cardiomyopathy (ARVD/C). In addition, inherited channelopathies associated with Brugada syndrome and long QT syndome can be identified by ECG.

## Echocardiogram

There should be very little hesitation in obtaining an echocardiogram if the history, physical exam, and ECG do not provide the diagnosis. However, the overall diagnostic yield with an echocardiogram is relatively low in the setting of a normal physical exam and electrocardiogram. It is important, though, that the echocardiogram can help identify structural heart disease (particularly valvular stenosis), pulmonary hypertension, and gross RV dysfunction and is a key tool in the identification of hypertrophic obstructive cardiomyopathy (HOCM).

Malignant syncope, a specific descriptor, is defined as syncopal spells that occur without prodrome and result in severe injury. The authors believe that all patients with recurrent syncope or malignant syncope should undergo evaluation with an echocardiogram as part of the initial evaluation.

## Ischemia Evaluation

Exercise stress testing (preferable with echocardiographic imaging) should be performed in all individuals who report exertional syncope. In addition, exercise stress testing should be done in those patients with a history of ischemic heart disease or those with significant coronary artery disease risk factors. Aside from the evaluation of significant coronary disease and structural heart disease, stress testing may help unmask syndromes such as profound autonomic failure and catecholaminergic ventricular tachycardia. For example, a hypotensive response to exercise may indicate high risk for sudden cardiac death in patients with HOCM. Heart rate response to increased exercise also allows evaluation of sinus node chronotropic function in those patients with suspected sinus node dysfunction.

## Neurological Evaluation

If the history and/or witnessed accounts are suggestive of seizure type activity, then an EEG should be considered. However, the diagnostic yield of brain CT and MRI in the absence of any focal neurological deficit is marginal and should not be ordered indiscriminately.

## Signal Averaged ECG (SAECG), Ambulatory ECG, and Implantable Loop Recorders

The overall yield in identifying the cause of syncope with SAECG and ambulatory ECG monitors has been historically low. However, in the appropriate patient, a 24- to 48-hour ambulatory ECG or 30-day event recording may be useful in those patients with frequent symptoms. In general, these recordings are more insightful if symptoms are occurring with bradycardia related spells such as prolonged sinus pauses with symptoms (>3 seconds) and/or high-grade AV block (**Figure 72-3**). Premature atrial contractions (PACs) and brief runs of supraventricular tachycardia (SVT) are commonly seen and do not necessarily corroborate with any symptoms. Ventricular premature contractions (VPCs) and short salvos are also frequently seen in the general population. In the lack of underlying structural cardiac disease,

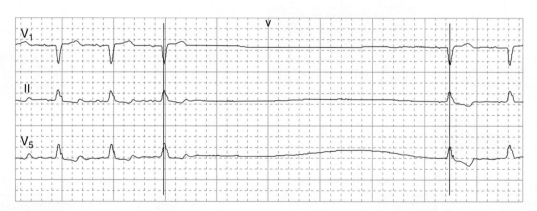

**Figure 72-3.** Holter monitor recording from a patient displaying a prolonged sinus pause with resultant syncope.

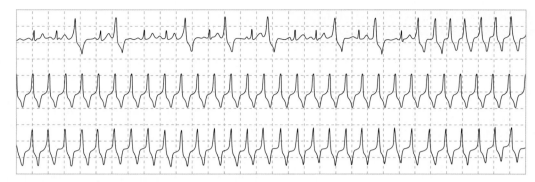

**Figure 72-4.** Event recorder tracing during a syncopal event in a patient with underlying ischemic LV dysfunction and unexplained syncope. Tracing displays frequent ventricular ectopy, which degenerates into sustained monomorphic ventricular tachycardia.

there is no significant association with increased mortality. However, in those patients with structural heart disease and greater than 10 VPCs/hr, there is an increased risk for sudden cardiac death, which may warrant a further workup including placement of an implantable cardioverter defibrillator (ICD). Hence, in the proper patient population, noninvasive ambulatory ECG monitoring does serve as an adjunct tool for risk stratification for patients with syncope (**Figure 72-4**).

The introduction of implantable loop recorders (ILRs) has assisted in identifying the etiology of recurrent syncope in many cases. There are now several manufacturers of ILRs, all of which are implanted under a surgical sterile field. These recorders provide bipolar ECG signals with higher signal fidelity compared to surface ECG recordings and are either automatically triggered by an event or patient triggered, based on symptoms. Most ILRs can be left in for greater than 12 months in duration, especially beneficial to the patient with less frequent spells. In patients with recurrent unexplained syncope, an ILR for 1 year has identified diagnostic information on more than 90% of patients. In addition to being more cost-effective, the use of ILRs is also likely to be associated with increased diagnostic yield, compared to traditional ambulatory ECG monitors and event recorders.

The use of T wave alternans and SAECG to help risk stratify those patients at increased risk of sudden cardiac death with underlying structural disease has been well established. It is unfortunate that the current level of data does not support the use of these modalities in the diagnostic workup of those patients with syncopal events.

## Tilt Table Testing

When the history of a single syncopal event is consistent with a neurocardiogenic cause, there is no indication to perform a tilt table test (TTT). Tilt table testing may be advocated in those with malignant syncope or those in a high risk occupation (e.g., pilots). There can be significant differences in operator protocol for a TTT and this may explain the poor reproducibility and variation in both the sensitivity (26–80%) and specificity (90%) based on any one study.

Tilt table testing is based on the idea that prolonged upright posture can result in venous pooling and provide a stimulus for syncope in predisposed individuals. The general protocol will have a patient tilted head up on a table between an angle of 60° and 80° for up to 45 minutes. The angulation of the TTT prevents the skeletal muscle of the lower extremities from assisting in venous return and thus relies only on the autonomic nervous system (ANS) to compensate. If this passive portion of the test is negative, a provocative agent such as isoproterenol or sublingual nitroglycerin may be used. The addition of a provocative maneuver can increase the yield by approximately 25%. Approximately 30% of patients who have a positive TTT will have a syncopal event within 2 years. Neither age, TTT outcome, hypotension, nor bradycardia during the test is a useful predictor of recurrent syncope. Only the frequency of episodes prior to TTT is correlated with posttest syncopal events. It should be noted that TTT is absolutely contraindicated in patients with known aortic/mitral valvular stenosis, high-grade left main disease, severe left ventricular outflow obstruction, and severe cerebrovascular disease. In addition, it has been shown that the mechanism of syncope during TTT does not always correlate with episodes occurring in the clinical setting in which there appears to be more profound bradycardia spells.

Abnormal responses to TTT can be grouped into five basic types, which are summarized in **Table 72-3**.

There may be a role for TTT, especially in those patients with a first episode of malignant syncope; however, in patients who have a normal initial evaluation and a single episode of syncope, the TTT is likely to offer very little additional

---

**Table 72-3 • Abnormal Responses to Tilt Table Testing with Resultant Syncope Epression**

**Neurocardiogenic**
- Rapid drop in blood pressure, usually with bradycardia

**Dysautonomic**
- Gradual fall in blood pressure
- No significant change in heart rate
- Usually seen in autonomic syndromes

**Postural tachycardia syndrome (POTS)**
- Greater than 30 bpm increase in HR
  OR
- HR greater than 120 bpm during the first 10 minutes of passive TTT

**Cerebral syncope**
- Syncope without systemic hypotension
- Severe cerebral vasoconstriction—by transcranial Doppler
- Cerebral hypoxia—measured by electroencephalogram

**Psychogenic**
- Syncope without hypotension
- No evidence of cerebral vasoconstriction or hypoxia
- Seen with conversion disorders and major depression

---

diagnostic information as most cases will predominantly be of a neurocardiogenic origin (**Figure 72-2**). In addition, serial TTT to evaluate efficacy of pharmacologic therapy has not been shown to be clinically advantageous. Although there are no formal guidelines for the use of TTT in syncope, a summary of indications and contraindications, as recommended by an American College of Cardiology consensus panel, is shown in **Table 72-4**.

---

**Table 72-4 • Indications and Contraindications for Tilt Table Testing with Syncope**

**Tilt table testing is indicated:**
- Recurrent syncope or single syncopal episode in high risk patient and/or
  1. No evidence of structural cardiac disease
  2. Structural disease is present, but other causes of syncope have been excluded by appropriate testing
- Further evaluation in patients where an apparent cause of syncope has been established, but in whom demonstration of susceptibility to neurally mediated syncope would affect treatment plans
- Evaluation of exercise-induced or exercise-associated syncope

**Tilt table testing not warranted:**
- Single syncopal episode without injury and not in a high risk setting with clear-cut vasovagal clinical features
- Syncope where an alternative cause has been established and in which additional demonstration of neurally mediated susceptibility would not alter treatment plans

*Extracted from ACC Expert Consensus Document, Benditt DG et al, 1996.*

---

## Electrophysiology Testing

The utility of an electrophysiology study (EPS) is greatest in those patients with underlying structural heart disease and/or an abnormal ECG. The diagnostic yield of an EPS in patients with an otherwise normal evaluation is between 1 and 3%. In those patients with a structurally normal heart, the EPS does not exclude an arrhythmogenic cause for syncope. The EPS has a particularly poor predictive value for future events in those with structurally normal hearts and in those with profound systolic LV dysfunction (particularly if nonischemic in etiology). The majority of patients who would benefit from EPS would be between these two patient groups.

However, given the low procedural risk, EP testing can be considered in those with recurrent syncope and structural heart disease as well as those with malignant syncope in a high risk occupation. In particular, it can help identify those patients with sick sinus syndrome, abnormal AV node conduction, infra-Hisian block, SVT, and ventricular tachycardia (VT) (**Figure 72-5**). A summary of Class I and Class III indications for the role of EPS in the evaluation of syncope are shown in **Table 72-5**.

## SPECIFIC SUBGROUPS OF SYNCOPE

### Neurocardiogenic Syncope

Neurocardiogenic syncope (NCS) represents the most common type of syncope in the adult population. It is the dysfunction of the ANS that plays a common central role. The ANS provides the primary mechanism for compensation in relation to short- and long-term responses for positional changes. Upon standing, in the normal individual, there is approximately a 30% decrease in blood volume returning to the right heart. Respectively, this causes an equal reduction in cardiac stroke volume. The skeletal musculature of the leg, venous valve system, and peripheral autonomic tone, as determined by the ANS, work together to actively pump blood back to the right heart.

Neurocardiogenic syncope is usually associated with a prodrome of lightheadedness, nausea, visual changes, and diaphoresis followed by a transient loss of consciousness. The triggering event in most cases is not clear, but certain events such as an emotional crisis and pain are associated with NCS. The primary mechanism for NCS is thought to involve significant venous pooling in the lower extremities, especially in the upright position with a decrease in the venous return to the heart. This subsequently leads to increased cardiac inotropy, stretch via mechanoreceptors in the heart, which then stimulates the medulla and causes a paradoxical withdrawal of sympathetic tone that results in hypotension, bradycardia, and the syncopal event. In patients with both

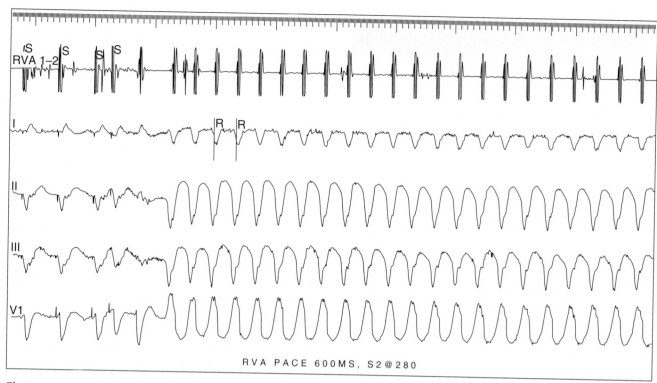

RVA PACE 600MS, S2@280

**Figure 72-5.** Intracardiac electrocardiogram during electrophysiologic testing in a patient with known ischemic LV dysfunction and recurrent syncope. Electrocardiogram displays ventricular pacing from the RV apex at a programmed rate of 600 ms, followed by a premature impulse (S2), which is introduced at 280 ms after the last paced beat. This initiates sustained monomorphic ventricular tachycardia, which was subsequently terminated with rapid ventricular pacing.

carotid hypersensitivity syndrome and NCS, there are often marked initial hypotensive responses with TTT or carotid sinus massage, respectively. This response is frequently accompanied by bradycardia and occasionally asystolic spells. In addition, other forms of reflex syncope such as those associated with cough, micturition, or defecation are also the result of local mechanoreceptor activation and subsequent loss of autonomic tone.

Treatment options for NCS must be tailored on an individual basis. Initial measures should concentrate on avoidance of triggering stimuli and staying exceedingly well hydrated. Subsequently, nonpharmacological treatments should be encouraged. These can include resistance exercise training and aerobic activity. In addition, if the patient is agreeable, the use of high pressure (>30 mm Hg), waist level, elastic support hose can be useful in those patients with significant autonomic disorders. Another useful, noninvasive measure for patients without significant baseline hypertension is liberalization of salt in the diet, which can sometimes make a dramatic improvement at a very low cost. For patients who are refractory to conservative measures or for those who suffer significant injury during syncopal spells, preventive pharmacotherapy is indicated.

Beta-blockers have long been the initial mainstay of pharmacotherapy. The exact mechanism of their action on limiting spells of NCS is unclear. However, it is felt to be largely due to their negative inotropic effects on the cardiac stretch mechanoreceptors, which are triggered during insufficient venous return. Large randomized studies have provided mixed results in comparing beta-blockers to placebo for the treatment of NCS. In those patients who continue to be symptomatic despite beta-blocker therapy, several second-line agents such as fludrocortisone, midodrine, and serotonin specific reuptake inhibitors (SSRI) are available.

As a mineralcorticoid, fludrocortisone works by increasing overall plasma volume and peripheral alpha-receptor sensitivity, leading to peripheral vasoconstriction. Fludrocortisone has been shown to be effective in the treatment of orthostatic hypotension. Midodrine is a peripheral α-1 receptor stimulant that also promotes peripheral vasoconstriction. It has been shown in two randomized trials to be beneficial in the prevention of NCS. Serotonin has been thought to play a central role in regulating heart rate and blood pressure through the central nervous system. In patients with both NCS and other forms of reflex syncope, there appears to be an imbalance in serotonin production and receptor hypersensitivity, which may contribute to sympathetic withdrawal. Several studies have shown that SSRI therapy can be effective in preventing episodes of NCS. Other agents that have shown limited clinical utility include subcutaneous erythropoietin, pyridostigmine, theophylline, and disopyramide.

The most extreme therapy for the treatment of NCS is permanent cardiac pacing. As mentioned previously, bradycardia frequently accompanies hypotension and syncope in these patients. However, it is important to understand that the primary mechanism and inciting event is that of venous pooling and poor venous return to the heart. Thus, providing intracardiac pacing in the setting of inadequate cardiac venous return does nothing to rectify the initial problem. Thus, as studies have shown, there is no conclusive evidence

that intracardiac pacing is of benefit in patients with NCS. This therapy can be recommended only as a last line for those patients with recurrent malignant syncope who have failed all other therapeutic measures.

## Orthostatic Syncope

There are two primary sources of orthostatic dysfunction leading to syncope. The first is dysfunction of the ANS (primary autonomic failure or secondary autonomic failure). The second major cause of orthostatic syncope is medication related.

An in-depth evaluation of autonomic failure is beyond the scope of this focused review; however, of the disorders of autonomic function, one in particular, postural tachycardia syndrome (POTS), should be noted. In the typical presentation of POTS, the hallmark of the syndrome is persistent tachycardia in an upright position. Patients can often reach heart rates greater than 160 bpm and tend to complain of several associated symptoms such as fatigue, palpitations, lightheadedness, and even syncope. During TTT, these patients develop a significant increase in their HR (>30 bpm) within the first 10 minutes with only a mild decline in their blood pressure (**Figure 72-6**). Patients with POTS do have a predisposition toward developing total autonomic failure and this disorder does appear to have a genetic component. The treatment of POTS is notoriously difficult and patients may require several medication changes in conjunction with nonpharmacological measures.

Secondary causes of autonomic dysfunction include diabetes mellitus, amyloidosis, and paraneoplastic syndromes. Aside from systemic involvement with these secondary causes, a key distinguishing factor is that in dysautonomic syncope, there is usually no associated bradycardia or diaphoresis. In addition, patients with substantial autonomic dysfunction may have a combination of upright hypotension and supine hypertension, which is thought to be due to an inability to vasoconstrict when upright or vasodilate when prone.

It is clear that the most common cause of orthostatic syncope in the elderly is medication induced. Diuretics, in particular, play a key role in volume depletion and, with the addition of peripheral vasodilators such as nitrates and ACE inhibitors, provide a milieu for frequent syncopal spells. Therapy revolves around slow withdrawal and introduction of medications until orthostatic equilibration is achieved.

## Syncope and Coronary Artery Disease

Syncope in patients with underlying coronary artery disease (CAD) is directly correlated with left ventricular function. In patients with CAD and syncopal spells, an evaluation

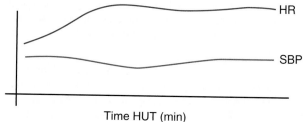

A. Inappropriate sinus tachycardia (IST)

HR

SBP

Time HUT (min)

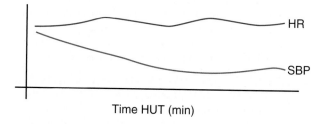

B. Autonomic failure: Primary or secondary

HR

SBP

Time HUT (min)

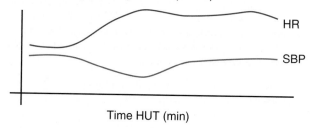

C. Postural tachycardia syndrome (POTS)

HR

SBP

Time HUT (min)

**Figure 72-6.** Heart rate and blood pressure response to tilt table testing for (A) inappropriate sinus tachycardia, (B) autonomic failure syndromes, and (C) POTS.

of underlying ischemia and arrhythmias must be performed. If testing indicates that a patient with a past history of myocardial infarction needs repeat revascularization, this should not preclude arrhythmia evaluation as the substrate (myocardial scar) has not been removed.

Once the need for any additional revascularization is gone, patients with CAD, LVEF >35%, and syncope should undergo evaluation with an electrophysiology study. Although the ability to induce sustained monomorphic ventricular tachycardia in patients with an LVEF >35% is relatively low, a positive finding carries a very poor prognosis. These patients, regardless of their LVEF, should be treated with an implantable cardioverter defibrillator (ICD).

In those patients with CAD and an LVEF <35%, an electrophysiology study may be indicated; however, in the absence of syncope, these patients have been shown to receive substantial survival benefit when implanted with an ICD and, therefore, an electrophysiology study would not necessarily be indicated.

## Syncope and Nonischemic Dilated Cardiomyopathy

The overall frequency of syncopal spells in this group is poorly defined. However, syncope is associated with an increased mortality rate among patients with nonischemic dilated cardiomyopathy (NIDCM), since it is likely due to frequent self-terminating bouts of nonsustained ventricular tachycardia.

Data do not support routine electrophysiology studies in patients with NIDCM as programmed ventricular stimulation has been shown to have a relatively low predictive value in this population. Several large studies including SCD-HeFT and DEFINITE have shown a significant survival benefit in patients with NIDCM and no preceding syncopal event. Based on these data and the fact that syncope increases the risk of sudden cardiac death, appropriate ICD implantation is warranted in this population.

## Syncope in Hypertrophic Cardiomyopathy

Among young patients, HOCM remains a predominant cause of sudden cardiac death, ranging from 0.6 to 1%. Episodic syncope, with and without exertion, has a very high positive predictive value for sudden cardiac death in this population. Although the predominant cause of syncope in this population is likely ventricular tachycardia, other clinical scenarios such as NCS with or without bradycardia and LV outflow tract obstruction can contribute.

There is no role for electrophysiology testing in patients with HOCM. Risk stratification to define a patient as high risk is based on past syncopal events, family history of sudden cardiac death, and if needed, genetic analysis of the mutation involved. In addition, although patients with HOCM have a higher likelihood of inappropriate shocks, ICD therapy has been well proven to improve survival in the high risk patient.

## Syncope and Inherited Ion Channel Abnormalities

Long QT (LQT) syndrome and Brugada syndrome are the two ion channel abnormalities most likely to be associated with syncope and sudden cardiac death. Past syncopal events, family history, and evaluation of the ECG all play an important role in the diagnosis and subsequent treatment strategy.

LQT syndrome is defined as prolongation of the corrected QT interval, $QT_C$ >450 ms (a slight variation can exist based on gender). Both LQT1 and LQT2 involve genetic defects of the cardiac potassium channels, whereas LQT3 involves defects of the sodium channels. Although there are several risk factors that determine the likelihood of a cardiac event (e.g., gender, age), the single most important determinant is the degree of QT prolongation. Syncopal events and a family history of sudden cardiac death are poor prognostic indicators. Most patients can be initially treated with beta-blocker therapy, however, ICD implantation is appropriate if a patient is deemed to be high risk.

Brugada syndrome is an inherited disorder involving the cardiac sodium channels. There are several different Brugada patterns, however, they all involve ST elevation to some degree in the anterior precordial leads ($V_1$ and $V_2$). Syncopal events in patients with Brugada syndrome are associated with a very high incidence of future sudden cardiac death and ICD implantation is warranted in these patients.

## Suggested Readings

1. Benditt DG, et al. Tilt table testing for assessing syncope. American College of Cardiology. *J Am Coll Cardiol.* 1996;28(1):263–275. *Provides an excellent review of the physiology seen in neurocardiogenic syncope and the role of a tilt table test.*

2. Strickberger SA, et al. AHA/ACCF scientific statement on the evaluation of syncope: From the American Heart Association Councils on Clinical Cardiology, Cardiovascular Nursing, Cardiovascular Disease in the Young, and Stroke, and the Quality of Care and Outcomes Research Interdisciplinary Working Group; and the American College of Cardiology Foundation: In collaboration with the Heart Rhythm Society: Endorsed by the American Autonomic Society. *Circulation.* 2006;113(2):316–327. *The most recent guidelines as published by the AHA/ACC/HRS. Served as the backbone of this review manuscript.*

3. Kapoor WN, et al. A prospective evaluation and follow-up of patients with syncope. *N Engl J Med.* 1983;309(4):197–204. *Timeless article. Provides key information regarding the varied presentation of syncope and the appropriate diagnostic workup.*

4. Brignole M, et al. Guidelines on management (diagnosis and treatment) of syncope-update 2004. Executive Summary. *Eur Heart J,* 2004;25(22):2054–2072. *ESC consensus statement on the workup and treatment of syncope. Provides differing opinions compared to the AHA/ACC/HRS statement in 2006 and therefore is a very thought provoking article, especially in regard to diagnostic workup and treatment of neurocardiogenic syncope.*

5. Abedin Z. *Essential Cardiac Electrophysiology.* Chennai: Blackwell Publishing; 2007. *Highly recommended reading. Provides a great concise summary of the differential diagnosis and workup for syncope. Particularly helpful for those individuals wishing to pursue a career in clinical electrophysiology.*

6. Grubb BP. Neurocardiogenic syncope and related disorders of orthostatic intolerance. *Circulation,* 2005;111(22):2997–3006. *Now a classic article from the foremost authority on neurocardiogenic syncope. Provides great detail about various reflex syncopes as well as the autonomic syndromes.*

7. Zipes D, et al. Guidelines for clinical intracardiac EP studies. *Circulation.* 1989;80(6):1925–1939.

# Valvular Heart Disease

SECTION XI

# Valvular Heart Disease

# 73

# Valvular Stenosis

LUIS M. MOURA AND NALINI M. RAJAMANNAN

## AORTIC STENOSIS

Aortic stenosis (AS) is the obstruction to outflow of blood from the left ventricle to the aorta. Over time, this obstruction progresses as the valve becomes more stenosed and the symptoms of chest pain, shortness of breath, and syncope develop. If the valve is not replaced at the onset of symptoms, the time to increased morbidity and mortality is rapid in these patients. The causes of outflow obstruction can occur at three levels within the heart. Left ventricular outflow obstruction in adults is most often due to aortic valve stenosis; less common causes are subvalvular or supravalvular disease.

## VALVULAR AORTIC STENOSIS

Valvular aortic stenosis is the most common level of aortic stenosis. The etiologies of aortic stenosis are congenital aortic stenosis (most commonly bicuspid and less commonly unicuspid, and quadricuspid), rheumatic aortic stenosis, and calcific aortic stenosis. Diagnosis of the cause of aortic stenosis can be performed by two-dimensional echocardiography and Doppler echocardiography, which define the level of stenosis and severity of obstruction.

## SUBVALVULAR AORTIC STENOSIS

Subvalvular AS can result from a variety of fixed lesions. These include a thin membrane (the most common lesion), thick fibromuscular ridge, diffuse tunnel-like obstruction, abnormal mitral valve attachments, and occasionally, accessory endocardial cushion tissue. Subvalvular AS also may have a dynamic component due to systolic anterior motion of the anterior mitral valve leaflet that is primarily seen in the genetic disease hypertrophic cardiomyopathy. Diagnosis of discrete subvalvular aortic stenosis presents with a high Doppler velocity across the aortic outflow tract and a structurally normal aortic valve on two-dimensional echocardiography.

## SUPRAVALVULAR AORTIC STENOSIS

There are at least two anatomic forms of supravalvar AS. The majority of patients (60-75%) have a discrete constriction in the ascending aorta at the superior aspect of the sinuses of Valsalva (the "hourglass deformity"). More diffuse narrowing for a variable distance along the ascending aorta

| Table 73-1 • Causes of Valvular Aortic Stenosis |
| --- |
| • Congenitally bicuspid valve with superimposed calcification (unicuspid or bicuspid) |
| • Calcific disease of a trileaflet valve |
| • Rheumatic valve disease |
| • Rare causes: metabolic diseases (e.g., Fabry's disease), systemic lupus erythematosus, Paget's disease, alkaptonuria, chronic kidney disease |

is seen in the remaining patients. There is a high frequency of supravalvular AS in patients with Williams syndrome, which is due to a mutation in the elastin gene. Other associate phenotypical findings include elfin facies, hypercalcemia, and peripheral pulmonic stenosis. Supravalvular AS is also common in patients with homozygous familial hypercholesterolemia and occurs infrequently in heterozygotes. Physical exam demonstrates an isolated thrill along the right carotid artery secondary to obstruction directed toward the left innominate artery. Diagnosis can be made with two-dimensional echocardiography and doppler echocardiography. Aortic root angiography, computed tomography (CT) of the aorta, or magnetic resonance angiography may be necessary to demonstrate the anatomic definition of the extent of the disease (see **Table 73-1**).

## RELATIVE FREQUENCY

Valvular aortic stenosis is the most common type of valvular heart disease in the world. The etiology and frequency depend on the location and age of the patient. In the United States and Europe, calcific aortic stenosis is the most common etiology. In developing countries, rheumatic valve disease is the most common cause. The age of the patient population is also important in the diagnosis. Patients who are in their 40s to 60s have bicuspid aortic stenosis causing their disease, but also present earlier or later with this specific abnormality. In older patients, calcific aortic stenosis is the most common cause of trileaflet aortic valve disease.

## CELLULAR MECHANISMS OF DISEASE

Calcific aortic valve disease is characterized by leaflet thickening and calcification in patients with a congenital bicuspid valve or an anatomically normal trileaflet valve. The cellular abnormalities characteristic of calcific aortic valve disease are characterized by three primary processes: lipid accumulation, inflammation, and calcification. For years, this disease was thought to be due to degeneration, but current evidence shows that it has an active cellular biology. Many of the risk factors for atherosclerosis are also associated with aortic valve sclerosis (believed to be an early form of stenosis), which has led to the suggestion that calcific aortic

valve disease is an atherosclerotic-like process. Randomized clinical trials of statin use have failed to demonstrate significant slowing in the progression of aortic stenosis.

## PATHOPHYSIOLOGY

Individuals with normal aortic valves have an effective area of valve opening that equals the cross-sectional area of the left ventricular outflow tract (3.0 to 4.0 cm$^2$ in adults). As AS progresses, there is a minimal valve gradient until the orifice area reaches less than half of normal. Calcific aortic valve disease without a significant gradient (defined as an aortic jet velocity ≤2.5 m/sec) is defined as aortic valve sclerosis. Advancement to stenosis occurs when the antegrade velocity across an abnormal valve rises to ≥2.6 m/sec. Stenosis severity is based upon echocardiographic estimation of the aortic jet velocity, mean transvalvular gradient, and calculated aortic valve area.

As outflow obstruction becomes hemodynamically significant, it results in obstruction to left ventricular ejection. Because the process is gradual in onset and progression, it results in adaptive changes in the left ventricle. The increased systolic pressure in the ventricular chamber leads to concentric hypertrophy as a mechanism to maintain normal wall stress. In most patients with a compensated ventricle, the cardiac output and left ventricular end-diastolic volume are maintained for a prolonged period despite a systolic pressure gradient between the left ventricle and aorta.

As the stenosis severity and hypertrophy continue to progress, the left ventricle becomes less compliant and left ventricular end-diastolic pressure can become elevated, even as the ventricular size remains normal. Abnormal diastolic function contributes to symptom onset and may continue after relief of stenosis due to interstitial myocardial fibrosis. The pathophysiology of aortic stenosis, characterized by an increase in afterload, a decrease in systemic and coronary blood flow, and progressive hypertrophy, leads to the development of angina, shortness of breath, and syncope. Angina develops in these patients secondary to a mismatch of myocardial oxygen supply and demand resulting from an increase in myocardial mass and high diastolic pressure. Dyspnea is initially secondary to diastolic dysfunction in the presence of normal systolic function, but increased left ventricular filling pressures eventually drive an increase in pulmonary pressure that further exacerbates symptoms. Finally, the etiology of syncope can be multifactorial, with decreased cardiac output, arrhythmias, and abnormal vasodepressor reflexes potentially playing a role.

In general, symptoms in patients with aortic stenosis and normal left ventricular systolic function rarely occur until the valve area is <1.0 cm$^2$, the jet velocity is over 4.0 m/sec,

| Table 73-2 • Three Classic Symptoms Associated with Aortic Stenosis |
| --- |
| • Heart failure (HF)<br>• Syncope or dizziness<br>• Angina |

and/or the mean transvalvular gradient exceeds 50 mm Hg. However, disease severity and symptoms may not always correlate, particularly if there is coexisting aortic regurgitation. Most patients with AS develop symptoms before the onset of left ventricular systolic dysfunction. Associated symptoms include palpitations from arrhythmias, gastrointestinal (GI) bleeding, secondary systemic emboli, and worsening mitral regurgitation.

## CLINICAL PRESENTATION

The patient with AS is asymptomatic for a prolonged period despite the obstruction and increased pressure load on the left ventricle. There is wide variability in the degree of outflow obstruction that causes symptoms, depending in part upon patient size and level of physical activity. As a result, there is no single value that defines severe valve obstruction (see **Table 73-2**).

However, in patients with known AS who are followed prospectively, the most common symptoms are decreased exercise tolerance and dyspnea on exertion. Once symptoms develop, even when mild, prompt surgical intervention is needed because average survival without valve replacement is only 2 to 3 years and carries a significant risk of sudden death.

## PHYSICAL EXAMINATION

The physical examination often provides the first clue to the presence of aortic stenosis. The most common findings are a low amplitude and slowly rising carotid pulse (parvus and tardus). The systolic ejection murmur may also radiate to the apex of the heart, where it may have a different quality (musical due to high frequency vibrations) and be louder, suggesting that the patient also has mitral regurgitation (Gallavardin phenomenon). S2 is soft and single, since A2, which is due to aortic valve closure, is delayed and tends to occur simultaneously with P2, which is due to pulmonary valve closure. The S2 may become paradoxically split when the stenosis is severe and associated with left ventricular dysfunction. With increasingly severe, fixed AS, the A2 closing sound disappears.

The presence of a normal split S2 is the most reliable finding to exclude severe AS in adults. In severe aortic stenosis, patients may have a palpable and audible fourth heart sound (S4) due to vigorous left atrial contraction into the noncompliant ventricle. In addition, a systolic thrill may be felt at the base of the heart (second intercostal space) or at the sternal notch, especially during full expiration with the patient leaning forward, which indicates the presence of severe stenosis (> 50 mm Hg). The murmur must be differentiated from that of hypertrophic cardiomyopathy or mitral regurgitation.

## DIAGNOSTIC STUDIES

A number of tests can help to document the presence and to assess the severity of valvular AS. The 2008 American College of Cardiology/American Heart Association (ACC/AHA) focused update of the guidelines on the management of valvular heart disease includes recommendations for the diagnostic evaluation of adolescents and young adults with congenital AS and for the evaluation and monitoring of older patients with known AS. The utility of echocardiography has largely eliminated the need for cardiac catheterization for hemodynamic assessment. Echocardiography is necessary for the diagnosis and assessment of the aortic valve, LV size, function, and hemodynamics. Reevaluation is necessary for patients with known AS who describe worsening symptoms and for patients with severe AS.

### Electrocardiogram

The primary electrocardiographic findings in AS are related to the presence of left ventricular hypertrophy. Most patients are in normal sinus rhythm. The voltage of the QRS complex can be markedly increased with associated ST-T wave changes and left atrial enlargement. However, the absence of hypertrophy on the ECG does not exclude the presence of severe AS. Atrial fibrillation is usually a late arrhythmia, primarily occurring in association with heart failure.

### Chest X-ray (Fig. 46-10)

The routine chest radiograph is usually normal when AS is mild to moderate. There are, however, a number of findings that may be seen (**Table 73-3**).

| Table 73-3 • Classic Chest X-ray Findings |
| --- |
| • A rounding of the left ventricular apex suggests left ventricular hypertrophy and poststenotic dilation of the ascending aorta secondary to a bicuspid aortic valve.<br>• Calcification of the aortic leaflets and aortic root is present in most adults with hemodynamically significant AS. |

## Echocardiography (Table 48-6, Fig. 48-20)

The 2008 American College of Cardiology/American Heart Association (ACC/AHA) focused update of the guidelines on the management of valvular heart disease recommends the use of echocardiography for the evaluation and monitoring of patients with AS. The location of obstruction can be identified (supravalvular, valvular, or subvalvular) and the cause of the lesion may be assessed.

Doppler echocardiography is excellent for assessing the severity of aortic stenosis. Maximum peak and mean aortic valve gradients can be derived from the continuous wave Doppler across the aortic valve. Reproducible echo measurements of the aortic valve gradient require detailed and accurate measurements using multiple sites of interrogation to optimize acquisition of the maximum peak velocity. Calculation of the aortic valve area is performed by calculating the continuity equation. Parameters used to assess severity of aortic stenosis as measured by the ACC/AHA guidelines are listed in **Table 73-4**.

## Cardiac Catheterization

The increased use of echocardiography in AS has reduced the importance of hemodynamic measurements obtained at the time of cardiac catheterization and left ventricular contrast angiography. The 2008 ACC/AHA focused update of the guidelines on the management of valvular heart disease recommends cardiac catheterization for hemodynamic assessment in only one setting in adults: symptomatic patients in

### Table 73-4 • Definition of the Severity of Aortic Stenosis in Adults

| | Aortic Jet Velocity | Mean Gradient | Valve Area |
|---|---|---|---|
| Normal | ≤1.5 | <5 | 3.0-4.0 |
| Mild | <3.0 | <25 | >1.5 |
| Moderate | 3.0-4.0 | 25-40 | 1.0-1.5 |
| Severe* | >4.0 | >40 | <1.0 |

*Critical aortic stenosis has been defined hemodynamically as a valve area <0.75 cm² and/or an aortic jet velocity >5.0 m/sec. However, the decision about valve replacement is not based solely on hemodynamics, as some patients who meet these criteria are asymptomatic, whereas others with less severe measurements are symptomatic.*
*Severe aortic stenosis is also considered to be present if the valve area index is <0.6 cm²/m². However, in patients with severe aortic stenosis who also have a low cardiac output state, the aortic jet velocity and mean gradient may be lower (low-gradient aortic stenosis).*
*Adapted from Bonow RO, Carabello BA, Chatterjee K, et al. ACC/AHA 2008 focused update incorporated into the guidelines for the management of patients with valvular heart disease. A report of the American College of Cardiology/American Heart Association Task Force on Practice Guidelines. J Am Coll Cardiol. 2008.*
*The recommended frequency of echocardiographic monitoring in adults varies with the severity of aortic stenosis: every year for severe aortic stenosis, every 1 to 2 years for moderate aortic stenosis, and every 3 to 5 years for mild aortic stenosis. The rationale for monitoring is provided by the marked variability in the rate of disease progression.*

whom noninvasive tests are inconclusive or provide discrepant results from clinical findings regarding the severity of aortic stenosis. There is some risk of cerebral embolization associated with crossing the aortic valve in patients with severe calcific aortic stenosis. As a result, this approach should be avoided in such patients whenever possible. Coronary angiography is also recommended in patients with mild to moderate AS who have progressive angina, objective evidence of ischemia, or either asymptomatic or symptomatic left ventricular dysfunction. Aortic valve gradients by cardiac catheterization depend not only on the severity of obstruction but also on flow. To measure the aortic valve area, a formula has been derived by Gorlin and Gorlin (as shown in the cardiac catheterization hemodynamics chapter).

## Computed Tomography

Both electron beam and rapid multislice chest tomography can provide quantitative evaluation of the amount of valve calcification. The degree of calcification correlates both with stenosis severity by echocardiography and with clinical outcomes. However, the role of quantitation of valve calcium in clinical decision making has not been defined.

## Magnetic Resonance Imaging (MRI)

MRI can detect the presence of AS and the anatomic valve area can be measured from short axis views of the valve. In addition, velocity-encoded MRI can accurately measure the antegrade velocity through the stenotic valve. MRI evaluation of AS severity is not yet widely accepted, in part due to limited experience and availability.

# TREATMENT OF PATIENTS WITH AORTIC STENOSIS

## Natural History

Angina, dizziness or syncope, and heart failure (e.g., dyspnea) are the primary manifestations of AS, usually occurring with exertion. Average survival after the onset of these symptoms is only 2 to 3 years with a high risk of sudden death. As a result, symptomatic AS is an indication for valve replacement. Although randomized trials comparing surgery to continued medical therapy have not been performed, observational studies have found that corrective surgery in this setting is almost always followed by symptomatic improvement and a substantial increase in survival with a low mortality of less than 1 to 2%. In older patients, the incidence of this disease is increasing, and progression may be more rapid. After valve replacement in older patients, survival is similar to that of age- and gender-matched populations.

Coronary angiography should be performed in all patients with cardiovascular risk factors, but it is not officially required in men younger than 40 years and women younger than 50 years as their risk of obstructive coronary disease is generally lower. It is a Class I indication for symptomatic patients with isolated AS should undergo aortic valve replacement.

## ALTERNATIVE APPROACHES TO SURGICAL VALVE REPLACEMENT

Percutaneous aortic balloon valvuloplasty was introduced in the 1980s as an alternative to valve replacement, avoiding a high operative mortality in elderly patients. This approach has evolved as a therapy for patients who are critically ill and not candidates for surgery and as a "bridge" in critically ill patients before aortic valve replacement. It is important for short-term interventions, as the device has a high risk of restenosis and often creates or worsens insufficiency. The most recent advance in the field is percutaneous aortic valve stents. Investigation of this procedure is ongoing in a number of clinical trials in the United States and Europe. These devices are currently not FDA approved, but the technique is in rapid evolution.

### Low Gradient Aortic Stenosis

Patients with AS and left ventricular dysfunction may have a low transvalvular pressure gradient despite significant valve narrowing. Such patients are said to have low gradient AS, which is defined as a transaortic pressure gradient of less than 30 mm Hg and a calculated aortic valve area $<1.0$ cm$^2$ in association with low flow. Some patients with low gradient AS have true severe AS, whereas others have "pseudostenosis," with a low transvalvular pressure gradient because of the combination of moderate AS and low cardiac output. The distinction between true stenosis and pseudostenosis is made by evaluation of characteristic changes in hemodynamic and structural measurements in response to pharmacologic interventions that augment cardiac output. Patients with low-gradient true AS have a high perioperative and postoperative mortality. Nonetheless, surgery is still reasonable in most patients because valve replacement is associated with better outcomes than continued medical therapy. Dobutamine echocardiography is helpful in differentiating patients with severe true AS from those with pseudostenosis and determining the appropriate therapy. Patients with contractile reserve in response to dobutamine have a much better outcome after surgery.

### Asymptomatic Severe Aortic Stenosis

With infrequent exceptions, such as patients undergoing coronary artery bypass graft surgery or surgery on the aorta or other heart valves, the 2008 ACC/AHA focused update to the guidelines on the management of valvular heart disease concludes that valve replacement should not be routinely performed for isolated severe AS in asymptomatic patients.

However, careful monitoring is required, since asymptomatic patients with severe AS have a low rate of survival free from valve replacement. This is associated with a progressive reduction in aortic valve area that averages 0.1 cm$^2$/year and a progressive increase in aortic jet velocity that averages 0.3 m/sec per year. Risk factors for progression include small valve area, left ventricular hypertrophy, and moderate to severe valve calcification.

### Surgical Versus Medical Therapy

Consideration of surgery in an asymptomatic patient with severe AS requires an appreciation of the relative risks of surgical and medical therapy. The surgical mortality of aortic valve replacement varies widely. If it is not well under 2 to 3% at a particular center, then the operative risk clearly exceeds the risk of sudden death in an asymptomatic patient who does not undergo surgery. Furthermore, valve replacement does not abolish the risk of sudden death. Insertion of a prosthetic heart valve is also associated with appreciable morbidity. Among the complications of prosthetic heart valves are prosthesis dysfunction, paravalvular leak, thrombus formation, arterial embolism, endocarditis, and problems associated with anticoagulation. The incidence of serious complications depends upon the type of valve and a number of clinical variables, but significant complications occur at a frequency of at least 3% per year, and death due directly to the valve occurs at the rate of approximately 1% per year. Thus, even if surgical mortality can be minimized, the combined risk of valve replacement and the late complications of a prosthetic valve exceed the possibility of preventing sudden death in a truly asymptomatic patient.

## MITRAL STENOSIS

Mitral stenosis is an obstruction to blood flow between the left atrium (LA) and the left ventricle (LV) and is caused by abnormal mitral valve function. In virtually all adult patients with mitral stenosis, the cause is rheumatic valve carditis. However, almost 60% of patients with rheumatic heart disease do not give a history of rheumatic fever. Other causes of mitral stenosis are uncommon or extremely rare. Mitral stenosis in association with an atrial septal defect is called Lutembacher's syndrome. Other causes of obstruction to flow across the mitral valve include LA myxoma, massive LA ball thrombus, and cor triatriatum in which a congenital membrane is present in the left atrium leading to an anatomic obstruction (see **Table 73-5**).

## PATHOLOGY

Acute rheumatic carditis is a pancarditis involving the pericardium, myocardium, and endocardium. In temperate climates and developed countries, there are usually long

| Table 73-5 • Causes of Mitral Stenosis |
| --- |
| • Rheumatic fever |
| • Congenital |
| • Active infective endocarditis |
| • Neoplasm |
| • Massive annular calcification |
| • Rare causes: systemic lupus erythematosus, carcinoid, methysergide therapy, Hunter-Hurler syndromes, Fabry's disease, Whipple's disease, rheumatoid arthritis |

intervals (averaging 10 to 20 years) between an episode and the clinical presentation of symptomatic mitral stenosis. In tropical and subtropical countries, the latent period is shorter, and MS may occur during childhood or adolescence. The pathologic hallmark is an Aschoff's nodule, inflammatory cells, bone formation, and angiogenesis. The most common lesion of acute rheumatic carditis is mitral valvulitis. In this condition, the mitral valve has vegetations along the line of closure and the chordea tendinaea. Mitral regurgitation may be present during an acute episode of rheumatic carditis.

The most critical aspect of the pathophysiology is that mitral stenosis usually results after repeated episodes of carditis alternating with healing and is characterized by the deposition of fibrous tissue. This process results in fusion of the commissures, cusps, or chordae. This disease progression causes obstruction to the flow of blood between the left atrium and the left ventricle. The time to severe stenosis may depend on the number of episodes of repeated bouts of rheumatic valvulitis. Many times, the repeat episodes of rheumatic heart disease are not clinically apparent to the patient. It is critical to understand that the course of this disease is a slow progression occuring over decades.

## PATHOPHYSIOLOGY

The pathophysiologic features of this disease manifest from the obstruction of blood flow between the LA and LV due to a pressure gradient across the stenotic valve. The relationship between the valve area, flow period, and average diastolic gradient between the LA and LV is defined by the formula of Gorlin and Gorlin (please see the cardiac catheterization chapter).

Complications of mitral stenosis include atrial arrhythmias and systemic emboli. The chronic elevation in LA pressure leads to left atrium enlargement, sometimes creating pressure on the laryngeal nerve with secondary hoarseness (Ortner's syndrome). Right heart disease eventually develops, manifesting as increased pulmonary artery pressures, right ventricular hypertrophy, and tricuspid regurgitation. Patients are also at risk for infective endocarditis due to their abnormal mitral valve.

## PHYSICAL EXAM

The clinical presentation of mitral stenosis is progressive dyspnea secondary to increased left atrial pressure over time. The physical exam is manifested as a prominent A wave (secondary to RV hypertrophy) or a prominent V wave (secondary to triscuspid regurgitation). Cardiac auscultation demonstrates an accentuated S1, which is caused by flexible valve leaflets with a wide closing excursion. The loud first heart sound is followed by an opening snap and a diastolic rumble. The interval between aortic valve closure and the opening snap (A2-OS interval) is related to left atrial pressure and, therefore, can be used to determine the severity of mitral stenosis. Patients with severe mitral stenosis have A2-OS intervals shorter than 60 to 70 ms and those with mild mitral stenosis have A2-OS intervals longer than 100 to 110 ms. As right heart manifestations become significant, P2 increases with rising pulmonary pressure. Finally, two key pearls are to be sure the patient is examined in the left lateral position (as the subtle sounds of mitral stenosis can easily be missed) and to be aware that exercise may bring out a diastolic rumble, so a patient may be asked to do sit-ups or walk briskly in the hallways to increase his or her heart rate before reexamination.

## DIAGNOSTIC STUDIES

### Chest X-ray (Fig. 46-19)

The PA and lateral CXR have classic findings important in the diagnosis of mitral stenosis. Lung fields demonstrate evidence of elevated pulmonary venous pressure, with accumulation of fluid into the interlobular septa, producing linear streaks that extend into the pleura (Kerley B lines). Pulmonary artery hypertension results in enlargement of the main pulmonary artery or right and left main artery silhouettes. The LA is enlarged and manifests as a density behind the RA and elevation of the PA artery. The RV may be enlarged if PA hypertension is present.

### Electrocardiogram

The ECG often demonstrates sinus rhythm signs of LA enlargement, specifically appearing as broad and notched in lead II and biphasic in lead V1. Atrial fibrillation is common and RV hypertrophy is present if PA hypertension is marked.

### Echocardiography (Fig. 48-1, Fig. 48-18)

Two-dimensional echocardiography demonstrates valve thickening, fused commissures, and a small valve orifice on the short axis view of the mitral valve. The parasternal long axis demonstrates the classic "hockey stick" appearance of the anterior mitral valve leaflet as it opens during diastole. Doppler echocardiography can calculate the severity of the mitral stenosis using the pressure half-time equation. It is important to reevaluate patients who have changing symptoms, but is not necessary in patients who are asymptomatic, have mild mitral stenosis, or have stable clinical findings.

An echocardiographic grading system (Table 48-3) has been established to determine the suitability for mitral valve valvotomy based on the two-dimensional features of the following: (1) leaflet thickening, (2) leaflet calcification, (3) leaflet mobility, and (4) subvalvular thickening/fusion. Each of these features is assigned a score from 1 to 4, with 1 being the least involvement and 4 being the most severe. A score of less than 8 is suitable for balloon valvuloplasty or commissurotomy, and a score of 12 or greater would be appropriate for valve replacement. Determining the severity of the mitral valve area by Doppler echocardiography is also important. A valve area less than 1.0 cm$^2$ indicates severe stenosis, an area of 1.0-1.5 cm$^2$ indicates moderate stenosis, and greater than 1.5 cm$^2$ indicates mild stenosis. A gradient of less than 5 mm Hg is mild, 5.0-10.0 mm Hg is moderate, and greater than 10.0 mm Hg is severe. PA pressure greater than 60 mm Hg is severe pulmonary hypertension.

## NATURAL HISTORY

The 10-year survival for asymptomatic patients with MS is approximately 84%, and 34% to 42% in those with mild symptoms. The 10-year survival of patients who are moderately or severely symptomatic is ≤40% with no therapy and ≤10% at 20 years. Patients with NYHA functional Class IV have a poor survival without treatment.

## MANAGEMENT

Rheumatic carditis needs to be detected and managed rapidly by diagnosing streptococcal infections and treating properly. All patients with acute rheumatic fever/rheumatic carditis, with or without obvious valve disease, should receive appropriate antibiotic prophylaxis against recurrent streptococcal infection. Years later, when patients develop symptoms from valvular obstruction, medical therapy may provide some benefit from tachyarrhythmias and fluid overload. Beta-adrenergic blocking agents, calcium channel blockers, and digitalis can control the ventricular rate in patients with atrial fibrillation and amiodarone can reduce the occurrence of atrial arrhythmias. Anticoagulation is especially necessary in patients with atrial fibrillation secondary to mitral stenosis, as embolization risk is higher than in those with a "nonvalvular" etiology.

Patients who are carefully selected can undergo percutaneous mitral balloon valvuloplasty provided that they have less than moderate concomitant regurgitation. This procedure requires expertise and should be performed at a center with sufficient volume. Potential complications included systemic emboli, severe mitral regurgitation, and left ventricular perforation. Careful preoperative assessment of the mitral valve is necessary to ensure safety in performing this procedure.

# 74

# Valvular Regurgitation

QIONG ZHAO AND VERA H. RIGOLIN

## ● PRACTICAL POINTS

- Aortic regurgitation may result from an intrinsic structural abnormality of the aortic valve or from an abnormality of the aortic root.

- Acute AR may lead to emergent decompensation and have an underwhelming cardiac auscultatory exam.

- Two-dimensional echocardiography is the principal diagnostic tool for patients with AR.

- The benefits of chronic vasodilator therapy in asymptomatic patients with severe AR and normal ejection fraction remain controversial.

- Mitral regurgitation may result from disorders of the valve leaflets themselves or any of the supporting structures.

- The cardiac auscultatory exam can be misleading in acute MR.

- The echocardiogram is an indispensable tool for the evaluation of the patient with suspected MR.

- Mitral valve prolapse usually occurs as a primary problem that is not associated with other diseases.

- The most common cause of tricuspid regurgitation is dilation of the right ventricle and tricuspid annulus secondary to the left-sided valvular disease or heart failure.

- Tricuspid regurgitation does not require treatment unless right ventricular dysfunction or right-sided heart failure develops.

## OVERVIEW OF REGURGITANT VALVULAR DISEASE

Regurgitant valvular diseases, especially mitral regurgitation, are among the most frequently encountered valvular heart diseases in clinical practice. Valvular regurgitation may result from the primary valvular diseases or from the dysfunction of the surrounding supporting structures.

## AORTIC REGURGITATION

### Etiology and Pathophysiology

Aortic regurgitation may result from an intrinsic structural abnormality of the aortic valve or from an abnormality of the aortic root. Primary disorders of the aortic valve include

- calcific aortic stenosis (some degree of AI is present in 75%)

- infective endocarditis
- trauma
- congenital abnormalities of the aortic valve (bicuspid, unicuspid, quadricuspid valves, or rupture of congenitally fenestrated valve)
- other congenital defects that may indirectly result in AI (large ventricular septal defects and subaortic membranes)
- rheumatic
- myxomatous
- other systemic disorders (Lupus, giant cell arteritis, Takayasu's arteritis, ankylosing spondylitis, Jaccoud's arthropathy, Whipples disease, and Chron's disease)
- anorectic drugs (prior to their removal from the market)

Aortic regurgitation due to aortic root disease is now more common than primary valve disease. Acute destruction of the aortic root, such as in the case of aortic dissection, disrupts the supporting structures of the valve and results in regurgitation. In aortic dissection, the aortic intima and media are longitudinally separated by a column of blood. Patients at most risk for aortic dissection include those with

- idiopathic dilation of the ascending aorta
- bicuspid aortic valve
- hypertension
- Marfan's syndrome
- pregnancy
- blunt chest trauma
- acute aortitis, complicating infective endocarditis

Many diseases cause chronic dilation of the aortic root, which leads to AR due to annular dilation. This results in leaflet separation and loss of coaptation. Tension on the leaflets from the regurgitation may also result in scarring that diminishes coaptation by shortening the leaflets. The most common causes of root enlargement include

- age related (degenerative) dilation
- degeneration of the extracellular matrix (as an isolated condition, associated with Marfan syndrome, or congenital bicuspid aortic valve)
- aortic dissection
- systemic hypertension
- osteogenesis imperfecta
- syphilitic aortitis
- ankylosing spondylitis
- giant cell arteritis
- the Behçet syndrome
- psoriatic arthritis
- other forms of arthritis associated with ulcerative colitis, relapsing polychondritis, and Reiter syndrome

In AR, the total LV stroke volume is the sum of the forward plus the regurgitant stroke volume. Normal forward cardiac output is maintained by an increase in total stroke volume. In acute or subacute AR, a large volume of blood is introduced into a noncompliant left ventricle (LV), which results in elevated LV filling pressure and pulmonary venous pressures leading to dyspnea or pulmonary edema. Thus, acute severe AR is characterized by normal LV size and hyperdynamic LV systolic function. Acute AR usually is due to aortic dissection or infective endocarditis and the clinical presentation of the underlying process predominates. The patient usually develops significant dyspnea. The murmur may be minimal because of the abrupt and rapid increase in the LV end-diastolic pressure and diminishing aortic-left ventricular diastolic pressure gradient. Peripheral vascular manifestations may also be absent.

In chronic AR, compensatory remodeling of the left ventricle occurs. The chronic excessive volume overload causes progressive dilation of the left ventricle with increased end-diastolic and end-systolic volumes. In addition, LV afterload is also increased since the elevated end-diastolic volume increases LV wall stress. The increased stroke volume ejected into the high-impedance aorta often creates systolic hypertension, which further increases ventricular afterload. Thus, chronic AR represents a combination of elevated preload and elevated afterload. The volume overload associated with AR results in compensatory eccentric hypertrophy, whereas the pressure overload results in superimposed concentric hypertrophy. Preload is normalized due to eccentric hypertrophy and the addition of new sarcomeres. Increased systolic wall stress and afterload is a stimulus for further concentric hypertrophy. These compensatory mechanisms allow patients to remain asymptomatic for years. Since left atrial pressure increases late in the course of the disease, symptoms develop slowly and late when AR is chronic. However, when preload reserve or compensatory hypertrophy is insufficient, afterload mismatch will occur, eventually resulting in systolic dysfunction. The most common initial symptom is shortness of breath with exercise, then later at rest. Patients often notice an uncomfortable awareness of overactivity of the heart and neck vessels because of the forceful, pounding heartbeat associated with the high pulse pressure. Palpitations may also result from supraventricular or ventricular premature beats. Syncope may occur due to diminished diastolic blood pressure. Angina may also result in the absence of coronary artery disease.

## Physical Examination

The findings, upon physical examination in patients with chronic AR, are mainly related to the increased stroke volume and widened pulse pressure. In severe AR, the pulse pressure may increase to more than 100 mm Hg. However, the pulse pressure does not reflect the severity of the aortic regurgitation in young people with compliant vessels or in patients with congestive heart failure and elevated LV filling pressure. Because the LV is enlarged, the apical impulse is diffuse, hyperdynamic, and laterally and inferiorly displaced. A rapid ventricular filling wave (diastolic thrill) can often be palpated at the apex and there may also be systolic retraction of the parasternal region. A systolic thrill may be heard at the base of the heart, the suprasternal notch, and the carotid arteries. At times, a carotid shudder is palpable. The carotid pulse is usually bounding with a pronounced upstroke followed by a rapid run-off (waterhammer or Corrigan's pulse). There may be a bifid systolic pulse (bisferiens pulse) that can be appreciated in the brachial and femoral arteries in addition to the carotid arteries.

The S1 is often normal. However, in severe AR, there may be partial diastolic closure of the mitral valve, which decreases the intensity of the S1. The S2 may be increased or decreased depending on the etiology of the AR. A loud closure sound is associated with a dilated aortic root. A soft S2 is found when the AR is due to abnormally thickened and retracted leaflets. An early systolic ejection click can be heard in young patients with bicuspid valves. It may also signify a large stroke volume entering a dilated aortic root. An S3 may be found in the presence of a failing left ventricle.

The classic murmur of AR is that of a high-pitched decrescendo diastolic murmur along the left sternal border. The murmur is best heard in left sternal border (3-4 intercostal spaces), if the cause of the AR is related to diseased valves. On the other hand, if it is most audible at the right sternal border, significant aortic root dilation is suggested. The murmur is best heard with the diaphragm of the stethoscope when the patient is sitting up and leaning forward with held exhalation. The murmur is increased by maneuvers that increase blood pressure such as squatting or isometric exercise. The murmur decreases with maneuvers that decrease blood pressure such as standing, amyl nitrate inhalation, or the strain phase of the Valsalva maneuver. The duration of the murmur, rather than its loudness, correlates best with the severity of the regurgitation. A systolic outflow murmur radiating to the carotids, resulting from the increased stroke volume, is also common. A coexisting aortic systolic murmur may be a functional flow murmur due to the increased flow across the aortic valve and does not always imply aortic stenosis.

Mild degrees of AR result in a murmur only in early diastole. As the severity of AR increases, the murmur becomes more holodiastolic. However, when the left ventricle decompensates, there is a diminished gradient between the left ventricle and the aorta, which then shortens the murmur.

Patients with severe AR may also demonstrate a second diastolic murmur, which is low pitched and heard best at the apex (Austin-Flint murmur). This diastolic rumble, similar to that of mitral stenosis in pitch and intensity, has been postulated to represent physiological mitral stenosis caused by the rapid increase in LV diastolic pressure and by the jet of AR hitting the mitral valve. Others have concluded that this murmur is related to the AR jet directed at the anterior leaflet of the mitral valve and the LV free wall causing vibrations that are appreciated on auscultation as a diastolic rumble. Other peripheral signs of AR related to the widened pulse pressure and increased stroke volume are as follows:

- De Musset's sign:
    Head bobbing in synch with arterial pulse
- Quinke's pulse:
    Pulsation of nail beds when mild pressure is placed on the nail
- Duroziez's sign:
    Systolic and diastolic bruit heard over the femoral artery with gentle compression of the stethoscope
- Traube sign (also known as "pistol shot sounds"):
    Booming systolic and diastolic sounds heard over the femoral artery

- Müller sign:
    Systolic pulsations of the uvula
- Hill's sign:
    Increase in lower extremity systolic blood pressure > 40 mm Hg compared to the brachial artery

Acute AR is often a catastrophic illness. Since the ventricle has not had time to compensate, diagnosis is often difficult. Patients are usually tachypneic, tachycardiac, and in pulmonary edema. The precordium is usually quiet. There is a soft first heart sound due to early closure of the mitral valve and a short diastolic murmur. Early closure of the mitral valve noted on echo is a poor prognostic sign and should prompt rapid surgical correction. The importance of rapid surgical correction for acute severe AR is imperative, since medical therapy can often worsen the hemodynamics.

## Diagnostic Testing

### Chest Radiograph
The chest X-ray demonstrates an enlarged cardiac silhouette as well as enlargement of the aorta, if present. Pulmonary congestion is noted when heart failure has developed. An example of a chest X-ray from a patient with bicuspid aortic valve and severe AR is shown in **Figure 74-1**.

### Electrocardiogram (ECG)
Acute, subacute, or mild chronic aortic regurgitation may not display ECG abnormalities. In chronic moderate or severe

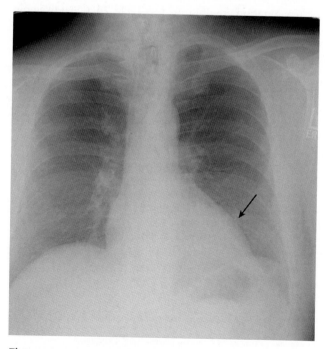

**Figure 74-1.** ECG from a patient with a bicuspid aortic valve and severe aortic regurgitation. Note the left atrial enlargement (arrow) and left ventricular hypertrophy.

aortic regurgitation, the ECG may show LV hypertrophy with or without associated repolarization abnormalities. Left axis deviation may also be present. With early LV volume overload, there are prominent Q waves in Leads I, aVL, and V3 through V6. As the disease progresses, the prominent initial forces decrease, but the total QRS amplitude increases.

## Echocardiography (Table 48-7, Fig. 48-21)

Two-dimensional (2D) echocardiography is the principal diagnostic tool for patients with AR. The echocardiogram demonstrates the size and function of the left ventricle as well as the morphology of the aortic valve and ascending aorta. Color and spectral Doppler are then used to further quantify the severity of AR and to identify lesions in the other valves. Semiquantitative echocardiographic measures of AR severity include the size of the left ventricle, the AR jet width measured by color Doppler in the LV outflow tract, measurement of the vena contracta width using color Doppler, assessment of flow reversal in the descending aorta by spectral Doppler, and measurement of pressure half-time by spectral Doppler. Quantitative measures of AR severity include proximal flow convergence (PISA) and calculation of regurgitant volume and fraction using stroke volume determinations across the mitral and aortic valves. When used in the correct clinical setting, transesophageal echocardiography enables a more thorough evaluation of the thoracic aorta and is more sensitive in identifying valvular vegetations and other infectious processes. It is also helpful in determining the severity of the aortic regurgitation and morphology of the aortic valve when the transthoracic echocardiogram is technically limited. The Doppler indicators of severe aortic regurgitation are illustrated in **Table 74-1**. An example of echo findings from a patient with bicuspid aortic valve and severe aortic regurgitation is shown in **Figure 74-2**.

### Table 74-1 • Doppler Indicators of Severe Aortic Regurgitation

AR color jet diameter/LVOT diameter in parasternal long-axis view (>65%)

AR color jet area/LVOT area in parasternal short-axis view (>60%)

AR pressure half-time by CW Doppler (<200 ms)

Transmitral PW Doppler diastolic profile (restrictive or premature flow cessation)

Flow reversal by PW Doppler in proximal descending thoracic aorta (holodiastolic)

CW Doppler signal intensity (dense)

Regurgitant volume (>60 mL)[a]

Regurgitant fraction (>50%)[a]

*AR, aortic regurgitation; CW, continuous-wave; LVOT, left ventricular outflow tract; PW, pulsed wave.*

*\*Measurements indicative of severe regurgitation are in parentheses.*

*[a]Can be measured by volumetric Doppler, proximal isovelocity surface area method, or a combination of these, including two-dimensional measures.*

*Adapted from reference 3 with permission.*

## Cardiac Catheterization

Cardiac catheterization is usually needed to identify the presence of coronary artery disease (CAD) in patients who require aortic valve replacement surgery. This procedure may also be needed in the uncommon situation when noninvasive imaging is inconclusive.

## Radionuclide Imaging

Radionuclide imaging is able to provide information about the LV ejection fraction, measurement of the LV/ right ventricular (RV) stroke volume ratio to help quantify the AR, and the assessment of LV function before and during exercise. However, this technique is generally only used when echo images are technically difficult or when there is a discrepancy between clinical and echo findings.

## Magnetic Resonance Imaging (MRI)

Velocity encoded cine magnetic resonance imaging provides a direct measurement of forward and regurgitant flow across the aortic valve. Magnetic resonance imaging can also measure LV volumes and ejection fraction and can assess the size and structure of the aorta. Currently, this technique is used when the echo images are suboptimal or when imaging of the full extent of the aorta is needed.

## Treatment

In patients with significant acute AR, dyspnea and heart failure usually develop rapidly. Mortality is high without surgical intervention. Early surgical replacement of the aortic valve is usually required.

Patients with chronic AR may remain asymptomatic for many years. Published data suggest that the rate of progression to symptoms or LV dysfunction in patients with chronic, severe AR averages 4.3% per year. The rate of sudden death is less than 0.2% per year and the rate of development of LV dysfunction without symptoms is 1.2% per year. However, significant LV dysfunction may develop in the absence of symptoms, emphasizing the importance of close follow-up of these patients.

Asymptomatic patients with severe AR and normal LV size and function should undergo clinical exams and echocardiography yearly unless symptoms arise beforehand. Patients with significant LV dilation (end-diastolic dimension >60 mm) require clinical evaluation every 6 months and echocardiographic imaging every 6 to 12 months. Patients with very severe LV dilation (end-diastolic dimension >70 mm or end-systolic dimension >50 mm) may require serial echoes every 4 to 6 months.

The benefits of chronic vasodilator therapy in asymptomatic patients with severe AR and normal ejection fraction remain controversial. Vasodilators may be helpful

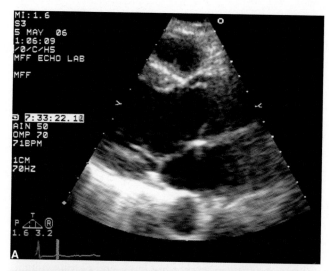

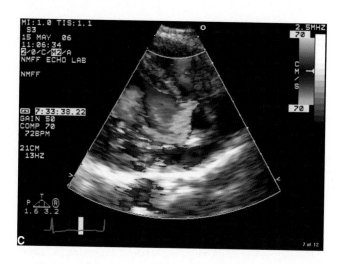

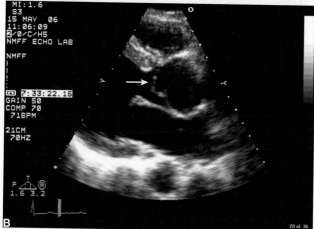

**Figure 74-2.** Echo from the patient in Figure 74-1 with a bicuspid aortic valve and severe aortic regurgitation. Panel A shows the parasternal long axis view; note the doming of the aortic valve during systole. Panel B shows the aortic valve during diastole (arrow); note the prolapse of the aortic valve. Panel C shows a Color Doppler image that demonstrates an eccentric jet of aortic regurgitation that is directed toward the anterior leaflet of the mitral valve.

in patients who have symptoms and/or LV dysfunction but are not surgical candidates. They may also be helpful for improving the hemodynamic profile of patients with severe heart failure prior to undergoing aortic valve surgery.

The most important predictor of outcome after aortic valve replacement is preoperative resting left ventricular systolic function. Patients should be referred for aortic valve replacement when symptoms develop or when there is severe LV dilation or a decline in ejection fraction. The specific criteria defining the timing of surgical referral are outlined in **Table 74-2**.

# MITRAL REGURGITATION (MR)

## Etiology and Pathophysiology

The mitral apparatus is a complex structure. The normal function of the mitral valve is dependent on normal functioning of the valve leaflets, valve commissures, mitral annulus, papillary muscles, chordae tendineae, and left

ventricle. Mitral regurgitation may result from disorders of the valve leaflets themselves or from any of these surrounding structures. Causes of leaflet dysfunction, often described as *organic* MR, include

- rheumatic heart disease
- mitral valve prolapse
- mitral annulus calcification
- endocarditis
- drugs, i.e., ergotamine toxicity
- collagen vascular diseases
- congenital cleft of the anterior mitral leaflet
- radiation therapy
- trauma

Mitral regurgitation can also result from dilation of the mitral valve annulus or from myocardial infarction usually involving the inferolateral wall and the posteromedial papillary muscle. This type of MR is often referred to as *functional* MR, since the valve leaflets themselves are normal. Identifying the cause of MR is crucial to understanding the natural history of the disorder and defining the appropriate therapy.

**Table 74-2 • Indications for Surgery in Patients with Aortic Insufficiency**

**Class I**

1. AVR is indicated for symptomatic patients with severe AR irrespective of LV systolic function (*Level of Evidence: B*)
2. AVR is indicated for asymptomatic patients with chronic severe AR and LV systolic dysfunction (ejection fraction 0.50 or less) at rest (*Level of Evidence: B*)
3. AVR is indicated for patients with chronic severe AR while undergoing CABG or surgery on the aorta or other heart valves (*Level of Evidence: C*)

**Class IIa**

AVR is reasonable for asymptomatic patients with severe AR with normal LV systolic function (ejection fraction >0.50) but with severe LV dilation (end-diastolic dimension > 75 mm or end systolic dimension > 55 mm)[a] (*Level of Evidence: B*)

**Class IIb**

1. AVR may be considered in patients with moderate AR while undergoing surgery on the ascending aorta (*Level of Evidence: C*)
2. AVR may be considered in patients with moderate AR while undergoing CABG (*Level of Evidence: C*)
3. AVR may be considered for asymptomatic patients with severe AR and normal LV systolic function at rest (ejection fraction > 0.50) when the degree of LV dilation exceeds an end-diastolic dimension of 70 mm or end-systolic dimension of 50 mm, when there is evidence of progressive LV dilation, declining exercise tolerance, or abnormal hemodynamic responses to exercise[a] (*Level of Evidence: C*)

**Class III**

AVR is not indicated for asymptomatic patients with mild, moderate, or severe AR and normal LV systolic function at rest (ejection fraction >0.50) when degree of dilation is not moderate or severe (end-diastolic dimension < 70 mm, end systolic dimension < 50 mm)[a] (*Level of Evidence: B*)

[a]*Consider lower threshold values for patients of small stature of either gender. Adapted from reference 3 with permission.*

In acute severe MR, there is sudden volume overload in the left atrium and left ventricle. The left ventricle accommodates this increased volume by sarcomere stretch and increase of stroke volume. However, because of the opening of the low pressure pathway across the incompetent mitral valve, left ventricular afterload decreases. Although the total LV stroke volume increases, the forward stroke volume drops. The combined effect of this increased preload, decreased afterload, and increased LV contractility leads to hyperdynamic LV systolic function with the ejection fraction usually increased to 60 to 75%. In the acute stage of MR, the left atrial size and compliance are usually unaltered. Thus, the left atrial pressure can increase significantly, leading to dyspnea and/or pulmonary edema.

In patients with slow, progressive, mitral valve disease or in patients who survive the acute episode, the LV is able to develop compensatory changes. The adaptive and compensatory changes that occur in the LV include the addition of sarcomeres in a series, resulting in an increase in the overall length of individual cardiomyocytes. The resultant LV dilation and eccentric hypertrophy cause an increase in LV end-diastolic volume. Afterload (wall stress) increases from subnormal to normal, according to La Place's law (Wall stress = Pressure × Radius / Thickness × 2). The left atrium also enlarges, thus allowing accommodation of the regurgitant volume at a lower pressure.

Patients with compensated MR may remain asymptomatic for many years. However, if the regurgitation is severe enough, decompensation may eventually result. The LV eventually weakens and can no longer eject the excess volume, resulting in an increase in LV end systolic volume. Forward stroke volume is decreased and LV filling pressure and left atrial pressure are increased. Ejection fraction in all phases, however, may be greater than normal due to the increase in preload and the afterload-reducing effect of ejection into the low-impedance left atrium. Thus, ejection fraction can be misleading as a measure of compensation in this disorder, and advanced myocardial dysfunction may occur while LV ejection fraction is still well in the normal range.

## Physical Exam

In acute severe mitral regurgitation, a third and fourth heart sound is usually heard, consistent with high left atrial pressure and LV diastolic pressure. The systolic murmur of MR may be short, soft, or completely absent when the left ventricular to atrial gradient is minimal. Physical findings of severe pulmonary congestion are expected.

The examination of the patient with chronic, severe MR varies according to the degree of decompensation. The carotid upstroke is sharp, as opposed to delayed in aortic stenosis. The volume of the carotid pulse is reduced in the presence of advanced heart failure. The apical impulse is usually brisk and hyperdynamic. However, it may be enlarged and displaced in patients with cardiac enlargement. A diastolic rumble or third heart sound may be present and does not necessarily indicate LV dysfunction. S1 is usually soft. A widely split S2 is common. The systolic murmur of MR varies according to the etiology of the regurgitation. Such murmurs may be early systolic, holosystolic, or late systolic. Early systolic murmurs are typical for acute MR. Late systolic murmurs are typical of mitral valve prolapse or papillary muscle dysfunction. The systolic murmur is usually heard best at the apex in the left lateral decubitus position. Signs of pulmonary hypertension, such as a loud P2, are usually ominous and represent advanced disease.

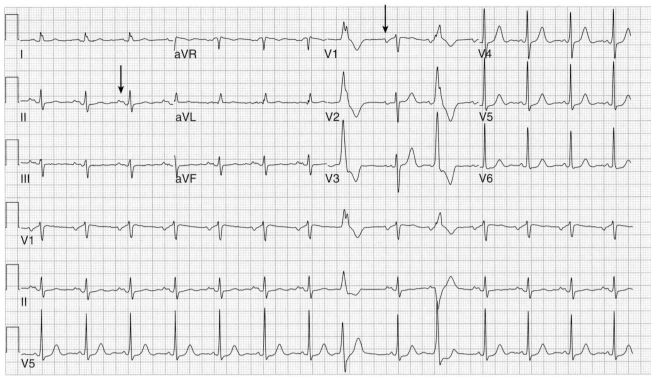

25mm/s 10mm/mV 100Hz 005E 12SL 235 CID: 16

**Figure 74-3.** ECG from a patient with severe mitral regurgitation. Note the left atrial enlargement (arrows).

## Diagnostic Testing

### Electrocardiogram

The most common findings on the ECG in patients with MR are those of left atrial enlargement (**Figure 74-3**) or atrial fibrillation. Left ventricular enlargement is noted in approximately one third of patients and right ventricular hypertrophy in 15%.

### Chest Radiograph

Cardiomegaly due to LV and LA enlargement is commonly seen in patients with chronic MR. Left atrial enlargement is recognized by straightening of the left border of the heart, an atrial double density, or elevation of the left main-stem bronchus. Right-sided chamber enlargement may also be present in patients with pulmonary hypertension. Kerley B lines and interstitial edema are often seen in patients with acute MR or progressive LV failure. An example of a chest X-ray from a patient with severe MR is shown in **Figure 74-4**.

### Echocardiogram (Table 48-5, Fig. 48-19)

The echocardiogram is an indispensable tool for the evaluation of the patient with suspected MR. The echo provides information about the mechanism and severity of MR, size and function of the LV and right ventricle, size of the left atrium, degree of pulmonary hypertension, and the presence of other associated valve lesions. The indications

for transthoracic echocardiography in MR are listed in **Table 74-3**. The indications for transesophageal echo are listed in **Table 74-4**. The Doppler indicator of severe mitral regurgitation is listed in **Table 74-5**. An example of the

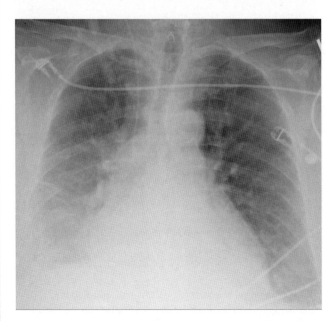

**Figure 74-4.** CXR from the patient in Figure 74-3 with severe mitral regurgitation. Note the cardiomegaly, pulmonary edema, and bilateral pleural effusions.

## Table 74-3 • Indications for Transthoracic Echocardiography in Patients with Mitral Regurgitation

**Class I**

1. Transthoracic echocardiography is indicated for baseline evaluation of LV size and function, RV and left atrial size, pulmonary artery pressure, and severity of MR (Table 74-4) in any patient suspected of having MR. *(Level of Evidence: C)*
2. Transthoracic echocardiography is indicated for delineation of the mechanism of MR. *(Level of Evidence: B)*
3. Transthoracic echocardiography is indicated for annual or semiannual surveillance of LV function (estimated by ejection fraction and end-systolic dimension) in asymptomatic patients with moderate to severe MR. *(Level of Evidence: C)*
4. Transthoracic echocardiography is indicated in patients with MR to evaluate the MV and LV function after a change in signs or symptoms. *(Level of Evidence: C)*
5. Transthoracic echocardiography is indicated to evaluate LV size and function and MV hemodynamics in the initial evaluation after MV replacement or MV repair. *(Level of Evidence: C)*

**Class IIa**

Exercise Doppler echocardiography is reasonable in asymptomatic patients with severe MR to assess exercise tolerance and the effects of exercise on pulmonary artery pressure and MR severity. *(Level of Evidence: C)*

**Class III**

*Transthoracic echocardiography is not indicated for routine follow-up evaluation of asymptomatic patients with mild MR and normal LV size and systolic function. (Level of Evidence: C)*

*Adapted from reference 3 with permission.*

## Table 74-4 • Indications for Transesophageal Echocardiography

**Class I**

1. Preoperative or intraoperative transesophageal echocardiography is indicated to establish the anatomic basis for severe MR in patients in whom surgery is recommended to assess feasibility of repair and to guide repair. *(Level of Evidence: B)*
2. Transesophageal echocardiography is indicated for evaluation of MR patients in whom transthoracic echocardiography provides nondiagnostic information regarding severity of MR, mechanism of MR, and/or status of LV function. *(Level of Evidence: B)*

**Class IIa**

Preoperative transesophageal echocardiography is reasonable in asymptomatic patients with severe MR who are considered for surgery to assess feasibility of repair. *(Level of Evidence: C)*

**Class III**

Transesophageal echocardiography is not indicated for routine follow-up or surveillance of asymptomatic patients with native valve MR. *(Level of Evidence: C)*

*Adapted from reference 3 with permission.*

## Table 74-5 • Doppler Indicators of Severe Mitral Regurgitation

Color jet area (jet area > 40% of LA area)
Wide vena contracta (0.7 cm)
Regurgitant volume (>60 mL)[a]
Regurgitant fraction (>50%)[a]
ERO (>0.4 cm²)[†]
Pulmonary vein PW Doppler flow profile
  (systolic flow reversal)
CW Doppler signal intensity (dense)
*Transmitral PW flow velocity (E > 1.2 m/s)*

*CW, continuous-wave; E, early transmitral flow; ERO, effective regurgitant orifice area; LA, left atrium; PW, pulsed-wave.*
*\*Measurements indicative of severe regurgitation are in parentheses.*
*[a]Can be measured by volumetric Doppler, proximal isovelocity surface area method, or a combination of these, including two-dimensional measures.*
*Adapted from reference 3 with permission.*

echo findings in a patient with severe mitral valve prolapse and severe mitral regurgitation is shown in **Figures 74-5, 74-6,** and **74-7.**

### Cardiac Catheterization

Cardiac catheterization is generally performed to assess the hemodynamic severity of MR when noninvasive testing is inconclusive or there is a discrepancy between clinical and noninvasive findings. Angiographic grading of mitral regurgitation is also dependent on the volume and injection rate of the contrast agent, catheter position, and volume of the left atrium; thus, the accuracy of the assessment is limited by the above factors. Coronary angiography is indicated for patients who are planning to undergo surgery and are at risk for coronary artery disease.

## Treatment

Patients with acute severe MR require rapid evaluation and therapy with intravenous inotropes, intravenous vasodilators, or intraaortic balloon counterpulsation. Patients with hemodynamic instability usually require surgical intervention.

Patients with chronic MR can remain asymptomatic for years. However, since LV dysfunction can develop in the absence of symptoms, serial clinical exams and noninvasive testing are warranted. Patients with mild MR and an otherwise normal heart may be followed with clinical exams yearly and echocardiographic imaging only if there has been a change in clinical status. In patients with moderate MR, clinical examination and echocardiography should be performed yearly or sooner if symptoms develop. Asymptomatic patients with severe MR should be followed with clinical exam and echocardiography every 6 to 12 months to assess for changes in symptoms and/or LV function.

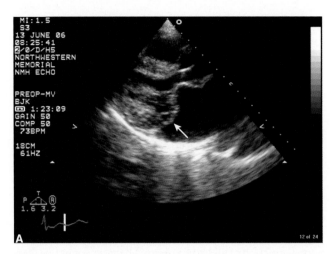
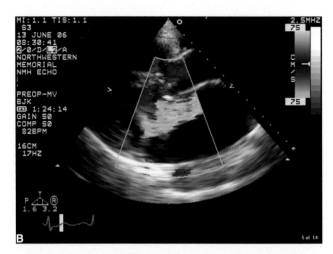

**Figure 74-5.** Echo from a patient with prolapse of the posterior leaflet of the mitral valve. Panel A shows the marked prolapse of the posterior leaflet during systole (arrow). Panel B shows the eccentric jet of severe mitral regurgitation that is directed anteriorly.

For patients with asymptomatic MR, there is no accepted medical therapy. However, in patients with associated LV dysfunction, treatment with angiotensin-converting enzyme inhibitors, beta-blockers, and biventricular pacing has been shown to be beneficial. Such treatments have often resulted in a reduction in the severity of functional MR. Patients with severe MR who develop symptoms or LV dysfunction should be referred for surgical correction. The indications for surgery in severe MR are listed in **Table 74-6**.

The timing of surgical correction depends on the estimated perioperative risk, the presence of LV dysfunction, the dilation of the LV, and the long-term morbidity associated with valvular prostheses. With increasing experience in valve repair surgery, patients with chronic, severe MR may be referred for surgical correction earlier in their disease course, often before the onset of symptoms of LV dysfunction. The

other two factors that predict poor postoperative outcome and reduced long-term survival include increased end-systolic internal dimension and atrial fibrillation. It is critical that such patients are referred to high volume surgical centers where the success rate of valve repair is high.

*Mitral valve prolapse:* Mitral valve prolapse usually occurs as a primary problem that is not associated with other diseases less commonly it is associated with connective tissue disorder such as Maltan's. It can be familial or nonfamilial. The natural history of mitral valve prolapse in the majority of cases is benign. However, complications may develop, so close follow-up is warranted. The systolic billowing of the mitral leaflet(s) into the left atrium may cause an audible click followed by a systolic murmur. The systolic murmur from mitral valve prolapse needs to be differentiated from the murmur of aortic stenosis and hypertrophic cardiomyopathy. The physical exam maneuvers that can be implemented to differentiate these murmurs are listed in

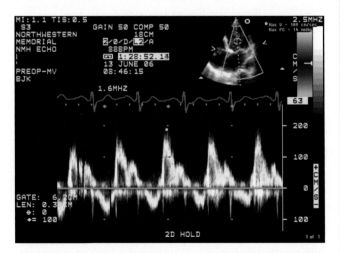

**Figure 74-6.** Spectral Doppler image from the echo of the patient in Figure 74-3 with prolapse of the posterior leaflet of the mitral valve. The Doppler signal of mitral inflow shows an increased E velocity to 1.9 m/sec that is suggestive of severe mitral regurgitation.

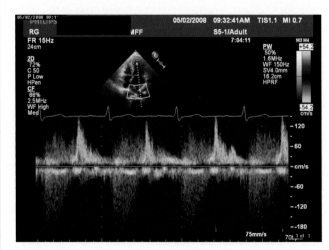

**Figure 74-7.** Echo from another patient with severe mitral regurgitation. There is systolic reversal in the pulmonary veins.

| Table 74-6 • Indications for Mitral Valve Operation |
|---|
| **Class I** |
| 1. MV surgery is recommended for the symptomatic patient with acute severe MR.* (*Level of Evidence: B*) |
| 2. MV surgery is beneficial for patient with chronic severe MR* and NYHA functional class II, III, or IV symptoms in the absence of severe LV dysfunction (severe LV dysfunction is defined as ejection fraction <0.30) and/or end-systolic dimensions > 55 mm. (*Level of Evidence: B*) |
| 3. MV surgery is beneficial for asymptomatic patients with chronic severe MR* and mild to moderate LV dysfunction, ejection fraction 0.30 to 0.60, and/or end systolic dimension greater than or equal to 40 mm. (*Level of Evidence: B*) |
| 4. MV repair is recommended over MV replacement in the majority of patients with severe chronic MR* who require surgery, and patients should be referred to surgical centers experienced in MV repair. (*Level of Evidence: C*) |
| **Class IIa** |
| 1. MV repair is reasonable in experienced surgical centers for asymptomatic patients with chronic severe MR* with preserved LV function (ejection fraction >0.60 and end-systolic dimension < 40 mm) in whom the likelihood of successful repair without residual MR is greater than 90%. (*Level of Evidence: B*) |
| 2. MV surgery is reasonable for asymptomatic patients with chronic severe MR,* preserved LV function, and new onset of atrial fibrillation. (*Level of Evidence: C*) |
| 3. MV surgery is reasonable for asymptomatic patients with chronic severe MR,* preserved LV function, and pulmonary hypertension (pulmonary artery systolic pressure > 50 mm Hg at rest or >60 mm Hg with exercise). (*Level of Evidence: C*) |
| 4. MV surgery is reasonable for patients with chronic severe MR* due to a primary abnormality of the mitral apparatus and NYHA functional Class III-IV symptoms and severe LV dysfunction (ejection fraction <0.30 and/or end-systolic dimension > 55 mm) in whom MV repair is highly likely. (*Level of Evidence: C*) |
| **Class IIb** |
| MV repair may be considered for patients with chronic, severe, secondary MR* due to severe LV dysfunction (ejection fraction <0.30) who have persistent NYHA functional Class III-IV symptoms despite optimal therapy for heart failure, including biventricular pacing. (*Level of Evidence: C*) |
| **Class III** |
| 1. MV surgery is not indicated for asymptomatic patients with MR and preserved LV function (ejection fraction >0.60 and end-systolic dimension < 40 mm) in whom significant doubt about the feasibility of repair exists. (*Level of Evidence: C*) |
| 2. Isolated MV surgery is not indicated for patients with mild or moderate MR. (*Level of Evidence: C*) |
| *Adapted from reference 3 with permission.* |

**Table 74-7.** Patients with mitral valve prolapse and severe mitral regurgitation are managed similarly to other individuals with severe mitral regurgitation. Mitral valve repair is usually the choice of surgical intervention when MR is severe. Patients with mitral valve prolapse sometimes develop palpitations, atypical chest pain, anxiety, or fatigue, which are usually associated with increased adrenergic tone. These patients should avoid exogenous stimulants and may benefit from beta-adrenergic blocker therapy.

# TRICUSPID REGURGITATION

## Etiology and Pathophysiology

The tricuspid apparatus consists of six parts including the leaflets, chordae, papillary muscles, annulus, right ventricle, and right atrium. Proper functioning of the tricuspid valve requires normal function of all of these parts. The most common cause of tricuspid regurgitation is dilation of the right ventricle and tricuspid annulus secondary to the left sided valvular disease or heart failure. Other less common causes include cor pulmonale, right ventricular myocardial infarction, and pulmonary hypertension. Isolated diseases of the tricuspid valve are unusual and include congenital abnormalities, i.e., Ebstein's anomaly, tricuspid valve prolapse, rheumatic valvulitis, infective endocarditis, and carcinoid syndrome. Iatrogenic causes include trauma from transvenous pacemakers, catheters, or repetitive right ventricular biopsy.

Tricuspid regurgitation decreases the blood returning from the venae cavae to the right atrium, thus decreasing the cardiac output. In severe TR, the venous pressure in the circulation increases significantly and leads to fluid extravasation. Tricuspid regurgitation is usually well tolerated in the absence of pulmonary hypertension. With the presence of pulmonary hypertension, right heart failure often occurs. The clinical presentation of TR varies depending on the underlying mechanism of the regurgitation. The patients usually develop dyspnea on exertion, malaise, ascites, and edema. Atrial fibrillation is common.

## Physical Examination

Patients with right-sided heart failure usually have increased jugular venous pressure (JVP) with a prominent CV wave, a right ventricular heave, liver enlargement, ascites, and edema. A holosystolic murmur is best heard at the left sternal border or the subxiphoid region. The intensity of the murmur increases with inspiration. The coexisting diastolic rumble may be due to the increased flow across the tricuspid valve due to severe TR or due to coexisting tricuspid stenosis.

## Diagnostic Testing

### Electrocardiography
The ECG may show right or bi-atrial enlargement, incomplete right bundle branch block, and right ventricular hypertrophy and dilation. Atrial fibrillation is common.

| | **Table 74-7 • Effect of Various Interventions on Systolic Murmurs** | | | |
| **Intervention** | **Hypertrophic Obstructive Cardiomyopathy** | **Aortic Stenosis** | **Mitral Regurgitation** | **Mitral Valve Prolapse** |
|---|---|---|---|---|
| Valsalva | ↑ | ↓ | ↓ | ↑ or ↓ |
| Standing | ↑ | ↑ or unchanged | ↓ | ↑ |
| Handgrip or squatting | ↓ | ↓ or unchanged | ↑ | ↓ |
| Supine position with legs elevated | ↓ | ↑ or unchanged | unchanged | ↓ |
| Exercise | ↑ | ↑ or unchanged | ↓ | ↑ |
| Amyl nitrite | ↑↑ | ↑ | ↓ | ↑ |
| Isoproterenol | ↑↑ | ↑ | ↓ | ↑ |

*Modified from Paraskos JA. Combined valvular disease. In: Dalen JE, Alpert JS, Rahimtoola SH, eds. Valvular Heart Disease. 3rd ed. Philadelphia: Lippincott Williams & Wilkins; 2000:332. ↑↑ = markedly increased.*
*Adapted from reference 1 with permission.*

### Chest X-ray

The chest X-ray usually shows right atrial enlargement and right ventricular enlargement.

### Echocardiography

Echocardiography is the most commonly used imaging study for the assessment of TR. Combined with Doppler interrogation, echo can identify the etiology and severity of the tricuspid diseases as well as the structure and function of the right and left heart. An example of echo findings in a patient with flail anterior leaflet of tricuspid valve and severe tricuspid regurgitation is shown in **Figure 74-8**.

### Treatment

Tricuspid regurgitation does not require treatment unless right ventricular dysfunction or right-sided heart failure develops. Medical management includes sodium and water restriction. Significant tricuspid regurgitation with pulmonary

hypertension is usually secondary to the left-sided heart disease or pulmonary disease; thus, treating the primary disease is the aim of management. Surgical correction depends on the mechanism of the regurgitation. Annuloplasty is indicated when TR is caused by annular dilation. Organic tricuspid diseases that cause severe tricuspid regurgitation are treated either with tricuspid valve repair or replacement.

## PULMONARY REGURGITATION (PR)

Pulmonary valve regurgitation is a common finding in adults. A small amount of PR is often seen in normal individuals. Isolated, severe PR is uncommon. Common causes of significant PR include

- pulmonary annular dilation
- ectasia of the main pulmonary artery
- infective endocarditis

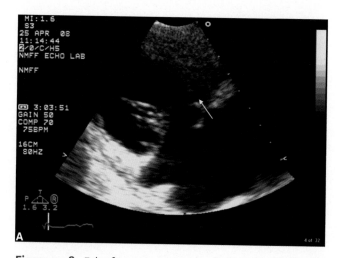
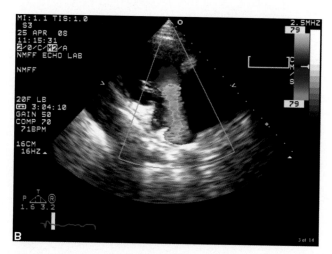

**Figure 74-8.** Echo from a patient with a flail anterior leaflet of the tricuspid valve. Panel A shows parasternal view of the right-sided chambers showing the flail anterior leaflet of the tricuspid valve (arrow). In Panel B, there is severe tricuspid regurgitation with an eccentric jet of tricuspid regurgitation that is directed in the posterior direction.

- collagen vascular diseases
- carcinoid
- trauma
- congenital abnormalities

Chronic, severe PR may cause volume overload of the right ventricle, which leads to right-sided heart failure. The clinical presentation of PR usually is related to the underlying disease process. Patients may develop fatigue, shortness of breath, edema, ascitis, and passive enteric congestion when right-sided heart failure develops. Physical examination may reveal a loud P2 when there is pulmonary hypertension; a widened splitting of the second heart sound; and a low-pitched, brief, and diamond-shaped murmur in diastole. The intensity of the murmur increases with inspiration or inhalation of the amyl nitrate. Primary pulmonary valve diseases that lead to severe PR and right ventricular dysfunction require surgical correction.

## Suggested Readings

1. Bonow RO. Mitral regurgitation. In: Libby P, Bonow RO, Mann DL, Zipes DP, eds. *Braunwald's Heart Disease: A Text Book of Cardiovascular Medicine*. 8th ed. Philadelphia: WB Saunders; 2007:1657–1668.

2. Bonow RO. Aortic regurgitation. In: Libby P, Bonow RO, Mann DL, Zipes DP, eds. *Braunwald's Heart Disease: A Text Book of Cardiovascular Medicine*. 8th ed. Philadelphia: WB Saunders; 2007:1635–1645.

3. Bonow RO, Carabello BA, Chatterjee K, et al. ACC/AHA 2006 guidelines for the management of patients with valvular heart disease: A report of the American College of Cardiology/American Heart Association Task Force on Practice Guidelines (writing committee to revise the 1998 Guidelines for the Management of Patients With Valvular Heart Disease): Developed in collaboration with the Society of Cardiovascular Anesthesiologists: Endorsed by the Society for Cardiovascular Angiography and Interventions and the Society of Thoracic Surgeons. *Circulation*. 2006;114(5):e84–231.

4. Otto CM. Aortic regurgitation. In: Otto CM, ed. *Valvular Heart Disease*, 2nd ed. Philadelphia: WB Saunders; 2004: 302–335.

5. Zoghbi WA, Enriquez-Sarano M, Foster E, et al. Recommendations for evaluation of the severity of native valvular regurgitation with two-dimensional and Doppler echocardiography. *J Am Soc Echocardiogr*. 2003;16:777.

# 75

# Prosthetic Valve Evaluation and Management

MANISHA J. SHAH

- Selection of a prosthetic valve depends on two primary issues: durability of the valve and the risk and benefit profile of long-term anticoagulation.

- Thrombogenesis and bleeding complications are the main long-term complications of mechanical valves.

- Structural changes in bioprosthetic valves such as cuspal tears, fibrosis, and calcification lead to degeneration and failure of the valve.

- It is important to choose a valve that is appropriate for the underlying native valve size, leading to optimum hemodynamics.

- Mechanical prosthetic valves in pregnant women merit specialized attention to a strict anticoagulation regimen to lower the risk for both mother and fetus.

- Echocardiography is a mainstay in the evaluation of prosthetic valve function.

## INTRODUCTION

Prosthetic cardiac valves are utilized as replacements for underlying valvular abnormalities. The first successful replacement of a cardiac valve was accomplished in 1960 by Nina Braunwald and colleagues. There are two main types of prosthetic valves: mechanical prostheses and bioprostheses (tissue) valves. There is a variety of both types of valves and selection of the appropriate heart valve for each patient takes valve durability, thrombogenic potential, and the particular underlying valve to be replaced into consideration. Monitoring for several important prosthetic valve-related complications is key in the proper management of patients with prosthetic valves.

## PROSTHETIC VALVE CLASSIFICATION

Prosthetic valves can be classified as either mechanical or bioprosthetic. Each has its own advantages and problems, which will be considered in further detail. **Table 75-1** gives a list of the common cardiac valves for replacement in adults. Of note, each valve is available in a range of sizes from 19 to 33 mm and it is important to choose the most appropriate size for the valve to be replaced

| Table 75-1 • Common Replacement Prosthetic Valves | | |
|---|---|---|
| **Type** | | **Model** |
| Mechanical | Ball-cage | Starr-Edwards (Figure 75-1) |
| | Tilting disk | Medtronic-Hall |
| | | Omniscience |
| | | Monostrut |
| | Bileaflet | St. Jude (Figure 75-2A) |
| | | Duromedics |
| | | Carbomedics (Figure 75-2B) |
| Biological | Porcine | Hancock Standard |
| | | Hancock MO |
| | | Carpentier Edwards (CE) Standard |
| | | CE SupraAnnular |
| | | Toronto Stentless (TSP) (Figure 75-3A) |
| | | Free Style (Stentless) (Figure 75-2B) |
| | Pericardial | CE (Figure 75-4) |
| | Homograft | |
| | Autologous | Pulmonary autograft |

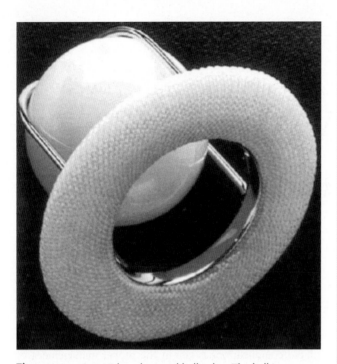

**Figure 75-1.** Starr-Edwards caged ball valve. The ball is a silicone rubber polymer, impregnated with barium sulfate for radiopacity, which oscillates in a cage of cobalt-chromium alloy. When the valve opens, blood flows through the circular primary orifice and a secondary orifice between the ball and the housing. In the aortic position, there is a tertiary orifice between the ball and the aortic wall.

in order to obtain the most optimal postoperative flow hemodynamics.

## Mechanical Valves

Mechanical prosthetic valves can be classified into three main categories: ball-cage, bileaflet, and tilting disc. Each valve has specific flow characteristics based on the valve mechanics, implanted size, and particular valve position. The St. Jude valve is a bileaflet valve and is currently the most common mechanical valve utilized, primarily because of its favorable hemodynamics.

### Ball-cage Mechanical Valve

The ball-cage valve was the first mechanical valve to be used for valve replacement. The valve is composed of a ball (silicone rubber), cage (Stellite alloy of cobalt and chromium), and sewing ring (Teflon). The silicone rubber ball also has barium sulfate that allows for opacification. The Starr-Edwards ball-cage valve has been available since 1965 and is the only surviving ball-cage valve available. The valve has a bulky design that can be associated with obstructive flow, especially in patients with either small left-ventricular cavity (mitral position) or small aortic annulus. Increased incidence of hemolysis and thromboembolism has been associated with this particular valve.

### Tilting Disc Mechanical Valve

The tilting disc valve is composed of a disc occluder (graphite with pyrolytic carbon) and housing (titanium or stainless

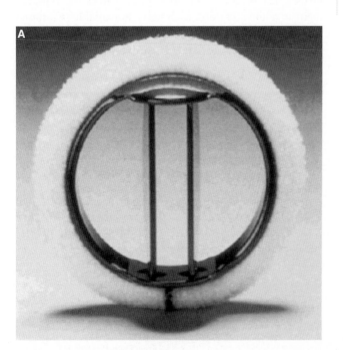

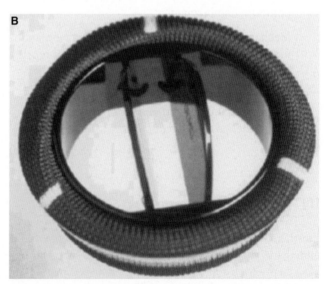

**Figure 75-2.** Bileaflet valves. The St. Jude Medical valve (A) has leaflets that open to an angle of 85 degrees from the plane of the orifice and travel from 55 to 60 degrees to the fully closed position, depending on valve size. The original version, whose housing did not rotate within the sewing ring, has been supplemented by a model that does rotate for intraoperative adjustment. The Carbomedics valve (B) has flat leaflets that open to 78 to 80 degrees and close at an angle of 25 degrees with the horizontal and has a carbon-coated surface on the sewing ring to inhibit thrombus formation.

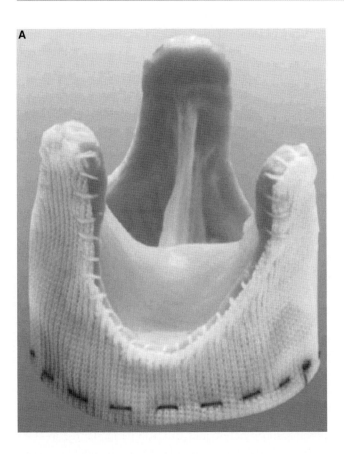

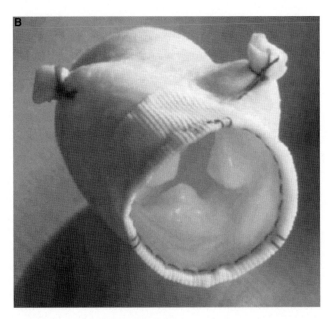

**Figure 75-3.** St. Jude Toronto SPV (**A**) and Medtronic Freestyle (**B**) stentless porcine valves. The Toronto SPV is designed to be used as a subcoronary valve replacement. The Freestyle can be impanted using any of the methods of implantation used for homografts: subcoronary implantation of the valve alone, aortic root replacement, or cylinder (root) inclusion.

steel). The housing is a valve ring with a strut that projects into the center of the ring and passes through the hole of the disk. The first available tilting disk valve, the Bjork-Shiley valve, has been available since 1969. However, it has been discontinued in the United States due to occurrences of strut failure. A modified version, the Monostrut, is available. The

Medtronic-Hall tilting disk valve is the most common utilized tilting disk valve and the main design improvement is that the occluder has a perforation that allows for improved hemodynamics. The Omniscience tilting disk valve is similar to the Medtronic-Hall valve, however, is not used as frequently. Both valves have low thrombogenicity and good performance over the long term. The opening angle of both of these valves is approximately 70 to 75 degrees.

### Bileaflet Mechanical Valve

The bileaflet valve was first introduced in 1977 by St. Jude Medical and is currently the most common mechanical valve. Made entirely of pyrolytic carbon, the valve is composed of a housing and two leaflets (semi-circular disks). The leaflets do not require struts and are connected to the valve ring with a butterfly hinge mechanism. The leaflets open and close with both sliding and tilting motions, achieving a near parallel open angle of 85 degrees. The bileaflet valve is considered to have the most favorable hemodynamic profile and possibly lower thrombogenicity than the other two valve types. The other two available bileaflet valves include the Duromedics and Carbomedics.

## Bioprosthetic Valves

Tissue or bioprosthetic valves are widely used and primarily considered for implantation when anticoagulation

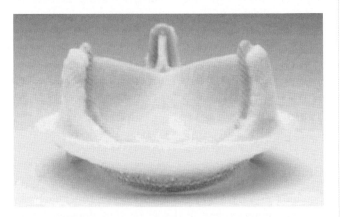

**Figure 75-4.** The Carpentier-Edwards Perimount pericardial bioprosthesis uses a method of mounting the leaflets to the stent, which does not depend on retaining stitches passed through the pericardium—a design weakness of previous pericardial valves. Instead, the leaflets are anchored behind the stent pillars.

is an unfavorable option for the patient. The main problem is the reduced durability associated with these valves. Bioprosthetic valves are available in three different tissue options: (a) autografts or autologous valves, (b) homografts, and (c) heterografts.

### Autografts or Autologous Valves

There are two main types of autografts: pericardial autologous valve or pulmonary autograft. The pericardial autologous valve is composed of patient's pericardium that is excised in the operating room and then mounted onto a frame and reinserted during the same operation. Long-term durability is very good with 85 to 94% free of replacement at 14 years. The pulmonary autograft or the Ross procedure consists of replacing the aortic valve with the patient's own pulmonary valve and then a homograft is implanted into the pulmonary position. The valve seems desirable in children and adults (especially child-bearing age women) in whom anticoagulation would be disadvantageous. Furthermore, in children, there is the potential advantage of in vivo growth of the valve with the child's development. There is also a low incidence of infection and favorable overall valve hemodynamics. However, the disadvantages include a more difficult operative procedure and early valve failure of both the aortic valve as well as the pulmonic homograft. A variety of comparative trials shows no major outcome benefit between the autograft procedure and aortic homografts.

### Homograft (Allograft) Valves

Valvular tissue from donor human cadavers is referred to as homograft or allograft. Most commonly the homograft tissue is used for replacement in the aortic position, especially if there is associated aortic vessel disease. There are three main methods of implantation: subcoronary valve replacement, complete aortic root replacement with reimplantation of the coronary arteries, or miniroot replacement with donor valve and aorta inserted below the coronary ostia. The hemodynamics of the homograft is excellent and it is generally preferred in younger patients who would otherwise not be ideal candidates for anticoagulation. Homografts are also used commonly in the treatment of complex aortic valve endocarditis, although there is no reported long-term benefit in randomized studies. Other common problems include a higher incidence of severe calcification of valve and root as well as increased risk of regurgitation with the subcoronary technique. Stentless homografts are also considered a reasonable choice for those patients with small aortic size who may be at risk for patient-prosthesis mismatch. Of note, a randomized clinical trial of homograft versus stentless bioprosthetic valves showed no significant difference in hemodynamics or outcomes at 1 year. Furthermore, as with stentless prostheses, there is an increased risk for

aortic regurgitation, especially for those younger than age 40. Overall, the advantages of the homograft include decreased rates of thromboembolism and excellent hemodynamics in smaller sizes, however, the main disadvantage is the increased complexity of the initial operation and the difficulty with reoperation because of significant homograft calcification.

### Porcine Heterograft (Xenograft) Valves

Heterografts are composed of tissue from other species, with the current available valves being the porcine valve or the bovine pericardial valve. Several different companies manufacture the porcine valve and it is by far the most commonly used biological prosthesis. In preparation for human implantation, the heterograft tissue is treated with glutaraldehyde, which not only sterilizes the tissue but makes it bioacceptable by destroying the antigenicity. Porcine valves are usually mounted to a stent, which is then attached to the sewing ring. There are also nonstented versions that are available that may improve durability and hemodynamics. However, current data indicate that stentless heterografts have a 20% failure rate by 10 years and often require reoperation. Mitral and aortic porcine heterografts are available. The porcine aortic heterograft can also be implanted in association with the aorta, similar to the homograft valves. Limited durability is the main problem with the porcine homograft. The bovine pericardial valve is sewn onto a stented frame. The initial pericardial valves were associated with an increased risk of structural deterioration, however, the current generation valves are felt to have better hemodynamics and durability than porcine valves. Failure for mitral heterografts appears to be greater than that for aortic heterografts, however, second-generation porcine valves and bovine pericardial valves appear to have improved durability compared to first-generation porcine valves.

## VALVE SELECTION

Selection of the valve depends on two primary issues: durability of the valve and the risk and benefit profile of the patient in regard to anticoagulation.

### Bioprosthesis

Porcine valves have limited durability, with structural problems becoming evident in the 4th or 5th postoperative year and the 15-year failure rate being 30 to 60%. Structural changes including cuspal tears, fibrosis, and calcification result in degeneration and failure. The failure appears to be greater in aortic versus mitral valve position, possibly secondary to higher pressures. Bioprosthetic structural degeneration and failure is age-dependent. In children and young adults (<35-40 years old), there is a high rate of failure. In those older than 65 years, the rate is less than 10% at 10 years and is considered to be rare in those having first implantation older than 70 years.

## Mechanical Valves

Mechanical valves have an excellent record of durability with up to 40 years for Starr-Edwards and 25 years for the St. Jude valve. Because of the risk of thromboembolism, all mechanical valves require long-term anticoagulation and possibly aspirin. Without these agents, the risk of thromboembolism is 3 to 6 times higher. The overall risk is greater for the mitral position than the aortic position, hence it is suggested that the International Normalized Ratio (INR) be 2.0 to 3.0 for aortic and 2.5 to 3.5 for mitral mechanical prostheses. Despite anticoagulation, the risk is 0.2 fatal complications and 1.0 to 2.0 nonfatal complications per 100 patient-years for aortic valve and 2.0 to 3.0 for mitral valves. Valve thrombosis occurs at the rate of 0.1% per year for the aortic position and 0.35% in the mitral position. Rates are even higher in the tricuspid position due to low flow and so on, and it is usually recommended that bioprostheses be used in this position. Warfarin therapy is associated with greater bleeding risk, with serious hemorrhage occurring at 0.2 to 2.2 episodes per 100 patient years. Thrombogenicity and bleeding complications are the main long-term complications of mechanical valves.

## Hemodynamic Profile

Another issue to take into consideration is the hemodynamic profile of the implanted valve. Mechanical and stented bioprosthesis have smaller effective orifice areas than the normal native valve. Other bioprostheses have slightly better orifice areas, however, all artificial valves are felt to be stenotic compared to a normal native valve. It is therefore important to choose a valve that is appropriate for the underlying native valve size. One common problem is that of patient-prosthesis mismatch, which tends to be more common in aortic valve replacements for aortic stenosis (AS). Valve size is based on the aortic annulus and proper sizing can be hindered by heavy calcification and thickening around the diseased native valve. Thus, careful evaluation of annular size and patient's body size should be taken into consideration to avoid mismatch. The hemodynamics of the prosthetic valve based on size and type, location of insertion (i.e., effect of mitral valve prosthetic struts), and other issues (aortic size, LV function, etc.) should be taken into consideration when evaluating the resultant hemodynamics of the prosthetic valve.

## Comparison

In the first 5 years, both bioprostheses and mechanical valves appeared to have similar outcomes in regard to both morbidity (endocarditis, reoperation, etc.) and mortality. There are two randomized trials that have evaluated long-term outcomes in a comparison of bioprostheses and mechanical valves, The Veterans Affairs Cooperative Study on Valvular Heart Disease and the Edinburgh Heart Trial. The VA study compared Bjork-Shiley tilting disc valve with the Hancock porcine valve in 575 men. At 11 years of follow-up, the bleeding risk was higher for the mechanical prosthesis in both the aortic and mitral position, however, the porcine valve had a higher number of structural failures and need for reoperation. The risk of reoperation is estimated to be twice that of initial operation and can reach 10 to 15% surgical mortality in many patients due to increased age, associated coronary artery disease (requiring bypass grafting), and comorbidities at reoperation. Fifteen-year survival in the VA study was 34% for mechanical valves compared to 23% for bioprostheses. Patients younger than 65 years appeared to have an increased rate of structural deterioration and those with mechanical aortic valve replacement (AVR) did better than those with bioprostheses. The Edinburgh trial compared the Bjork-Shiley standard valve with the porcine valve. Similar to the VA study, there was a higher risk of reoperation in bioprostheses and a higher risk of bleeding in those with the mechanical prostheses. The survival was better in those with a mechanical valve than those with the bioprosthesis (72% vs 52%, P = 0.08), with a significant effect for those with a mechanical valve in the mitral position (42% vs. 24%, P < 0.05). The trials also found that there were no significant differences in endocarditis, valve thrombosis, or systemic embolism.

Since the above trials, additional clinical data have been published that give further insight into appropriate valve selection. There are lower rates of structural valve deterioration in the current second-generation bioprosthetic valves currently utilized, with an associated drop in the need for reoperation in those patients older than age 65. AVR is occurring in a more elderly population with reasonable success rates. Large nonrandomized comparative trials have shown a benefit of bioprosthetic AVR, particularly for those older than age 65.

## Special Situations

Women and pregnancy pose special circumstances for which specific management should be considered. The main issue during pregnancy is that of anticoagulation. Pregnancy is associated with a hypercoagulable state. In a pregnant female with a mechanical valve, there are

| Table 75-2 • Management of Antithrombotic Therapy during Pregnancy | |
|---|---|
| **Time period** | **Options** |
| Weeks 1-36 | 1. Continued warfarin therapy<br>2. Replacement with heparin for weeks 6-12 (when highest risk for fetal defects)<br>3. Heparin for entire time (weeks 1-36) with frequent monitoring of anticoagulant<br>   a. I.V. or SQ heparin (PTT)<br>   b. Low molecular weight heparin (anti-Xa level) |
| Weeks 36 onward | I.V. unfractionated heparin |

several risks, including (a) risk for warfarin-related teratogenic effects, (b) potential fetal hemorrhage with any anticoagulation, and (c) risk of valve-related thrombosis due to inadequate anticoagulation. Thus, women with a mechanical valve should be counseled and they should strongly consider not getting pregnant. For women with mechanical valves who do become pregnant, issues related to anticoagulation become even more important to consider carefully. **Table 75-2** outlines the possible anticoagulation strategies in this situation.

Women often present with signs and symptoms of cardiac valve abnormalities during pregnancy. In women with significant valvular abnormalities, valve replacement should be undertaken after childbirth if possible. For critical aortic stenosis or mitral stenosis (MS), balloon valvuloplasty should be considered. Often, valvular regurgitation is able to be medically managed, however, for those women with hemodynamically significant mitral regurgitation, mitral valve repair can be considered.

There are a few other special situations that should also be considered. Patients on chronic hemodialysis have problems with both types of valves (bioprosthetic and mechanical). There is a higher risk of deterioration with bioprosthetic valves and a higher risk of bleeding and stroke with mechanical valves (and the need for anticoagulation). As a result of these issues, the survival in patients with chronic kidney disease (CKD) and an artificial valve are lower compared with healthier patients without kidney disease, but with no difference between the two valve types. In general, bioprosthetic valves are preferred because of the increased risk of anticoagulation problems with mechanical prosthesis in this population.

Tricuspid valves have an increased risk for thrombosis, probably due to the lower flow velocities and pressures on the right side. Primarily because of this increased risk,

patients who have tricuspid valve abnormalities should be considered for a bioprosthesis or valve repair/annuloplasty ring.

Children have an increased risk for bioprosthetic deterioration, therefore, a mechanical prosthesis should often be considered with increased caution in using anticoagulation. Another option is pulmonary autograft, however, the long-term risk/benefit should be considered.

## COMPLICATIONS

There are several possible complications of valve replacement. The American Association for Thoracic Surgery and Society of Thoracic Surgeons guidelines give the greatest clinical importance to the following: structural valvular deterioration, nonstructural dysfunction (patient-prosthesis mismatch), valve thrombosis, embolism, bleeding, and valve endocarditis. Consequences include reoperation, valve-related morbidity (congestive heart failure), and death. Valve deterioration could lead to either stenosis or regurgitation. Stenosis often occurs chronically, secondary to patient-prosthetic mismatch, pannus formation, or leaflet deterioration (thickening and calcification of bioprosthesis). Acute stenosis or flow obstruction can occur secondary to thrombus formation and can result in overt congestive heart failure and/or hemodynamic collapse. Regurgitation can occur secondary to leaflet destruction from endocarditis and resultant central or paravalvular destruction, surgical complications, or leaflet deterioration (bioprosthesis).

## CLINICAL EVALUATION

Evaluation of the postsurgical prosthetic valve should include a clinical history and physical exam, ECG, and echocardiography. **Table 75-3** outlines the timetable for follow-up according to the clinical situation.

### History and Physical Exam

The clinical history should include evaluation for symptoms of shortness of breath, chest pain, syncope, and palpitations. A baseline evaluation in 3 to 4 weeks postoperation should include an estimation of functional capacity and NYHA classification. It is also important to document the basic operative details, including reason for surgery, extent of surgery, and type and size of prosthetic valve. New cardiac symptoms could point toward the possibility of significant complications, especially if the symptoms are abrupt or significant (such as new onset congestive heart failure). Physical examination should be

**Table 75-3 • Clinical Evaluation for Short- and Long-term Follow-up**

| Follow-up | Evaluation and Management Considerations |
|---|---|
| **First postoperative visit** | |
| 3-4 weeks after surgery | Complete H & P<br>ECG, Chest X-ray<br>2D and Doppler echocardiography<br>Labs–CBC, serum chemistry, and INR |
| **Long-term with no complications** | |
| Asymptomatic | Yearly–Complete H & P and labs<br>Consider echocardiogram (2D and Doppler) |
| New murmur, CHF, or change in sx | Echocardiogram |
| **Long-term with complications** | |
| No improvement after surgery or deterioration of functional capacity | 2D and Doppler echocardiogram<br>Consider transesophageal echocardiogram and/or cardiac catheterization for diagnosis |
| **Significant complication** | |
| Moderate-severe prosthetic dysfunction<br>Dehiscence<br>Prosthesis endocarditis<br>Recurrent thromboembolism<br>Severe intravascular hemolysis<br>Severe bleeding from anticoagulant Rx<br>Thrombosed prosthetic valve<br>Prosthetic valve-patient mismatch | Reoperation should be considered |

focused on evaluation of CHF and valve function. During auscultation of the mechanical prosthesis, one should hear a crisp click during valve closure; this would be S1 for mitral valve and S2 for aortic valve. Abnormal or new heart sounds should be possible markers of possible valve dysfunction, complications, or a new onset of congestive heart failure related to the valve.

## Echocardiography

Echocardiography is the mainstay of both short-term and long-term monitoring of artificial heart valve structure and function. An echocardiographic examination of a prosthetic valve should include assessment of the underlying valve structure and a unique hemodynamic profile, depending on type, size, and location of valve, while taking into consideration the potential challenges/complications of imaging prosthetic valves. The echocardiographic evaluation of a prosthetic valve should include the two-dimensional (2D) evaluation of the structure, paying particular attention to the valve housing stability and leaflet motion. Doppler evaluation allows for hemodynamic assessment of the valve and should include evaluation of peak flow velocity, mean gradient, and evaluation of possible stenosis or regurgitation. Reference values for the hemodynamic profile of various prosthetic valves are available in the literature and are based on valve type and size as well as valve position. These reference values should be taken into consideration when evaluating a valve for stenosis or regurgitation. Aortic valve obstruction or stenosis can be ascertained by using the continuity equation; however, more common, the left ventricular outflow tract time-velocity integral (LVOT TVI)/aortic valve TVI ratio is utilized for aortic valve evaluation because often the LVOT diameter cannot be well-visualized. Regurgitation can be evaluated for native valves, using various Doppler techniques, however, it is important to pay close attention to physiologic versus pathologic regurgitation. Complications of prosthetic valves can often be visualized or considered based on Doppler evaluation. These include thrombus formation, dehiscence, vegetation, pannus formation, or frank valve dysfunction.

## Other Options

There are limitations of transthoracic echocardiography and often transesophageal echocardiography may offer the benefits of better leaflet visualization, improved hemodynamic assessment, and more thorough evaluation for complications such as paravalvular regurgitation, dehiscence, vegetation, and thrombus. For those patients with possible hemodynamically important valve obstruction due to leaflet immobility (dysfunction or thrombus), fluoroscopy can be utilized for visualization of leaflet motion. Of course, in certain cases where it is clinically important to further evaluate valve-related complications, cardiac catheterization for hemodynamics can be utilized as appropriate to the clinical situation.

## MANAGEMENT

### Endocarditis Prophylaxis

As per recent ACC/AHA guideline statements, patients with prosthetic valves and or with prosthetic material are still considered to be high risk and should be given antibiotic

**Table 75-4 • Antithrombotic Therapy**

| Mechanical Valve | Anticoagulation |
|---|---|
| **Aortic position** | |
| Bileaflet | Warfarin INR–2.0–3.0 |
| Tilting disc and Starr-Edwards | Warfarin INR–2.5–3.5 |
| Higher risk of TE* (afib, prior TE, hypercoag state, and severe LV dysfunction) | Warfarin INR–2.5–3.5 and consider ASA 81-100 mg |
| **Mitral valves** | |
| All Valves | Warfarin INR–2.5–3.5 |
| Higher risk of TE* (afib, prior TE, hypercoag state, and severe LV dysfunction) *TE–thromboembolism | Warfarin INR–2.5–3.5 and consider ASA 81-100 mg |
| **Biological valves** | |
| Higher risk of TE* (afib, prior TE, hypercoag state, and severe LV dysfunction) | Initially heparin goal PTT of 55–70 First 3 months–Warfarin INR–2.0-3.0 and ASA 81-100 mg Chronic Warfarin INR–2.0-3.0 |

**Table 75-5 • Modification of Antithrombotic Therapy for Those Patients with Thromboembolism**

| Current Anticoagulation | Modification |
|---|---|
| Warfarin INR 2.0-3.0 | Increase warfarin with goal INR of 2.5-3.5 |
| Warfarin INR 2.5-3.5 | Increase warfarin with goal INR of 3.5-4.5 |
| Warfarin INR 3.5-4.5 | Add ASA 80-100 mg per day |
| Warfarin INR 3.5-4.5 and ASA 80-100 mg/day | Increase ASA to 325 mgqd |

## Difficult Situations

There are several potential clinical situations in which anticoagulation must be modified to assure both safety of the patient and the valve. Embolic events can occur despite appropriate anticoagulation and require changing the INR threshold and adding aspirin (**Table 75-5**). Excessive bleeding can also occur on anticoagulant therapy, especially if the INR is excessively elevated. Usually, the warfarin can be held and the INR will self-correct. In emergency situations where there is significant bleeding, fresh frozen plasma is desirable over intravenous vitamin K, given the risk of overcorrection with vitamin K. **Table 75-6** outlines the adjustment protocol for excessive anticoagulation. Patients who undergo dental or surgical procedures should have their anticoagulant therapy adjusted according to the details in **Table 75-7**. Patients at high risk of thromboembolism should be considered for bridging with heparin and close monitoring of anticoagulation.

Last, perhaps one of the most concerning difficult situations is thrombus formation on the prosthetic valve. Depending on the severity of the clinical situation, options include reoperation, thrombolytics, and/or additional anticoagulation options. **Table 75-8** outlines the management strategy for the conditions of large or small thrombus on the prosthetic valve.

prophylaxis for dental procedures that involve manipulation of gingival tissue. Prophylaxis is not necessarily needed for nondental procedures such as transesophageal echocardiography, diagnostic bronchoscopy, esophagogastroscopy, or colonoscopy (in the absence of known active infection).

## Antithrombotic Therapy

All mechanical valves require anticoagulation therapy, primarily with warfarin, for the patient's lifetime. With warfarin, the risk for thromboembolism is reduced but is still 1 to 2% per year. The risk is greatest in the initial postoperative and recovery periods. **Table 75-4** gives the ACC/AHA guideline targets for anticoagulation for mechanical valves. Given the increased potential for mitral valve thromboembolism, the warfarin INR targets are higher. Aspirin can be added for those patients with increased risk of thromboembolism, and concomitant use for those with known vascular disease is warranted at the 81- to 100-mg dose without significant increase in bleeding.

Biological valves pose a 0.7% risk for thromboembolic events without warfarin use. The highest risk is during the initial 3 months; thus, heparin/warfarin therapy, especially for the mitral valve, is recommended soon after the operation. Once surgical bleeding risk is reduced (24-48 hours), warfarin should be initated and a heparin bridge with a goal partial thromboplastin time (PTT) of 55 to 70 seconds should be continued until the warfarin therapy INR reaches goal of 2.0 to 3.0.

**Table 75-6 • Modification of Antithrombotic Therapy for Patients with Excessive Anticoagulation**

| Excessive Anticoagulation | Recommendation |
|---|---|
| INR 5-10 and not bleeding | Withhold warfarin and give 2.5 mg of vitamin K. Determine INR after 24 hours and restart warfarin if appropriate. |
| Emergency situation | Fresh frozen plasma is preferred over IV vitamin K because of overcorrection concern. |

### Table 75-7 • Antithrombotic Therapy in Patients Requiring Noncardiac Surgery/Dental Care

| Situation | Details | Management Plan |
|---|---|---|
| **Very low risk for bleeding** | Local skin surgery<br>Teeth cleaning<br>Dental care treatment<br>Eye surgery (glaucoma or cataracts) | Continue current antithrombotic therapy |
| **On aspirin** | | Hold 1 week prior to procedure<br>Restart within 24 hours of procedure |
| **On warfarin** | | Stop 72 hours before procedure<br>Aim for INR <1.5<br>Restart within 24 hours of procedure |
| **High risk of thromboembolism (TE)**<br>Any one of below<br>1. Recent TE<br>2. Bjork-Shiley valve<br>3. 3 risk factors<br>   (nonmitral position)<br>4. Mechanical MVR<br>   and one risk factor<br>5. Cardiac cath and<br>   ≥1 risk factor | Risk factors:<br>Atrial fibrillation, Previous TE, etc.<br>Hypercoagulable<br>Mechanic prosthesis<br>LV dysfunction | Stop warfarin 72 hours prior to procedure<br>Start heparin when INR falls below 2.0<br>Hold heparin 4-6 hours prior to surgery<br>Restart warfarin soon as possible after<br>surgery and aim for PTT of 55–70 sec. |
| **Special**—cardiac cath with transeptal or LV puncture | | Same as previous category, except INR < 1.2 and restart heparin 4 hours after procedure without a bolus after sheath removed |

### Table 75-8 • Management Strategy for Prosthetic Valve Thrombosis

| Presentation | Plan |
|---|---|
| **Large thrombus with Evidence of obstruction NYHA Class III/IV CHF** | 1. Early reoperation<br>2. If high surgical risk, then consider thrombolytic therapy –duration 24 hours if no improvement Partial or complete improvement–stop at 72 hours<br>3. If #2 successful –I.V. heparin until INR of 3.0–4.0 for AVR or 3.5–4.5 for MVR<br>4. Partial success–Subcutaneous heparin (PTT 55–80) and warfarin INR of 2.5-3.5) for 3 months. |
| **Small thrombus with NYHA Class I or II CHF LV dysfunction** | 1. Short-term I.V. heparin therapy<br>2. If #1 unsuccessful, then continuous infusion of thrombolytics (48–72 hours) or SQ heparin (2× daily for PTT of 55–80) and warfarin (INR 2.5–3.5) for 3 months<br>3. If #2 unsuccessful, then consider reoperation<br>4. Long-term warfarin increased to 3.0–4.0 for AVR and 3.5–2.4 for MVR and add ASA 80-100 mg per day |

## CONCLUSION

Prosthetic valves are an important and useful replacement technology for a variety of human valvular abnormalities. In considering the type of replacement valve, there should be an understanding of the valve hemodynamics, disadvantages of particular valve types, and complexity of the operation. Also important to take into consideration is the specific underlying valve to be replaced, anticoagulation issues, and special clinical situations. Valve replacement often does not give back normal native valve function, however, it does offer significant benefits and improves natural history of progressive valve disease. Management of a prosthetic valve is a lifelong issue and must include close monitoring of anticoagulation (for mechanical valves), clinical suspicion for valve complications, and an understanding of their management.

# • 76

# Drug-Related Valvular Heart Disease

AHMAD A. ZANKAR

## • PRACTICAL POINTS

- Most drugs associated with valvular heart disease either have a structural similarity to serotonin or interfere with its metabolism.
- Migraine headaches, obesity and Parkinson's disease are the most common indications for use of specific drugs that carry risk of drug-related valvular heart disease.
- Symptoms suggesting valvular heart disease or a pathologic murmur require further diagnostic testing.

## INTRODUCTION

Drugs and toxins are uncommon causes of valvular heart disease. Certain drug categories especially drugs used for the treatment of obesity, Parkinson's disease, and migraine headaches have been implicated. Given the epidemiologic importance of the problems of obesity and Parkinson's disease, valvular heart disease related to these agents has been highly publicized. The evidence incriminating some of these drugs has been mostly derived from retrospective and observational studies. Few randomized or prospective studies have been done regarding the relationship of some of these agents to valvular heart disease. As will be described later, pathways involving the neurotransmitter serotonin play a key role in the pathogenesis.

## PATHOGENESIS

Most drugs associated with valvular heart disease either have a structural similarity to serotonin or interfere with its metabolism (**Figure 76-1**). Major categories are drugs used for the treatment of obesity, Parkinson's disease, and migraine headaches. Valvular heart disease related to these drugs has similar pathologic and echocardiographic features to carcinoid valvular heart disease. The neurotransmitter serotonin plays an important role in the pathogenesis of carcinoid heart disease as well. Animal studies have demonstrated that excess serotonin can lead to valvular abnormalities that are histologically similar to those found in

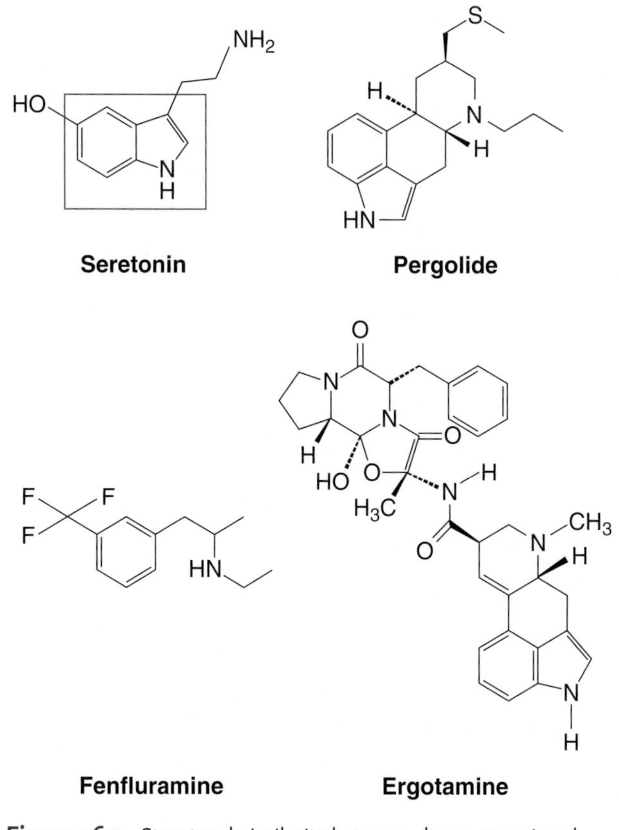


**Figure 76-1.** Structural similarity between drugs associated with valvular heart disease and serotonin.

carcinoid heart disease. Fibroblast growth and fibrogenesis resulting from excess serotonin appear to underlie the valve pathology seen in carcinoid and drug-related valvular heart disease.

## DRUGS USED FOR THE TREATMENT OF HEADACHES

Ergot alkaloids such as ergotamine and methysergide are used in the treatment of headaches, especially migraine headaches. Both compounds have a similar chemical structure to serotonin, a neurotransmitter that is involved in the pathogenesis of vascular headaches. Methylsergide, for example, is a partially synthetic ergot alkaloid that is a specific serotonin (5HT2) receptor antagonist. It is commonly used for migraine prophylaxis.

### Epidemiology

The association between ergot alkaloids and cardiac valve dysfunction dates back to the 1970s. The incidence is low, and has been reported to be approximately 3.6% in those patients who are on a continuous regimen. Valvular disease seems to occur in patients who have taken the medications chronically over years. In 1992 Redfield et al. reported five patients who were treated either with ergotamine suppositories or methylsergide tablets. All subjects took the medication for at least 6 years. All patients underwent aortic, mitral or tricuspid valve replacements. Three of five of these patients exceeded recommended doses of ergot alkaloids. On the other hand, there are multiple reports of valvular disease even with doses that did not exceed the recommended doses over a relatively brief duration. This suggests that the pathologic process is not necessarily dose-dependent.

### Pathology and Echocardiography

The gross appearance of ergot alkaloid-related valvular disease is indistinguishable from that of chronic rheumatic valvular disease. Unlike rheumatic heart disease, however, there is a lack of calcifications. Histologically, there is fibrotic thickening on the surface of what appears to be normal valve tissue ("stuck-on" plaques) (**Figure 76-2**). These lesions resemble lesions of carcinoid valve disease that result from stimulation of fibroblast growth and proliferation by serotonin agonist effects. In contrast, rheumatic involvement of the valve leaflets causes disruption of the leaflet tissue architecture with fibrosis, neovascularization, and calcification (**Table 76-1**). On echocardiography there is usually thickening of one or more valves, especially the mitral and/or the aortic, with resultant regurgitation and sometimes stenosis. Rarely, isolated tricuspid and pulmonic valve disease have been reported.

**Photomicrograph of Resected Mitral Valve**

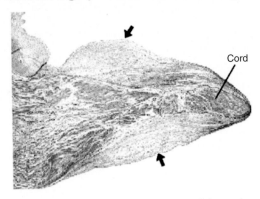

**Figure 76-2.** Histopathological examination of drug-related valvular heart disease demonstrates intact valve architecture and plaque-like lesions ("stuck-on" plaques). (Connolly H, et al. *N Engl J Med.* 1997;337:581–588.)

### Course

The true natural history of ergot-induced valvular disease is unknown. There have been no published studies in the echocardiography literature confirming resolution of valvular dysfunction following the termination of therapy. Bana et al. reported regression of murmurs in some patients after discontinuation of methylsergide for approximately 20 to 40 months. Some cases, however, may go on to require surgical intervention. Most have undergone aortic and/or mitral valve replacements. Few patients have also had proximal coronary artery involvement, presumably secondary to the underlying fibrotic process.

## DRUGS USED IN THE TREATMENT OF OBESITY

The proportion of obese people in the United States has increased at an alarming rate of approximately 50% per decade throughout the 1980s and 1990s. Two-thirds of American adults are now either obese or overweight. Pharmacologic options for the treatment of obesity are being sought to fight

| Table 76-1 • Features of Drug Related Valvular Disease Versus those of Chronic Rheumatic Valvular Disease and those of Carcinoid Valve Disease | | | |
|---|---|---|---|
| | Rheumatic Heart Disease | Carcinoid Heart Disease | Drug Related Valve Disease |
| Intact leaflet architecture | No | Yes | Yes |
| Calcification | Yes | No | No |
| Right or left sided lesions | Usually left | Usually right | Usually left |

this epidemic. Fenfluramine, dexfenfluramine, and phentermine, among others, have been used as pharmacotherapy for this problem. Fenfluramine, a sympathomimetic amine that promotes the release of serotonin and prevents its neuronal uptake, was approved by the FDA as a short-term adjunct therapy for obesity in 1973. Dexfenfluramine, which is an isomer of fenfluramine, acts in a similar way. Phentermine, on the other hand, is a nonadrenergic stimulant that was approved in 1959 by the FDA as an adjunct short-term therapy for obesity. In itself, phentermine has not been shown to cause valvular pathology, but its combination with fenfluramine (Fen-Fen) has been associated with valvular heart disease.

## Epidemiology

The use of these medications surged in the mid 1990s, and it is estimated that close to 18 million prescriptions have been written for these drugs. It is likely that several million Americans have been exposed. In 1997, 24 female patients (mean age ±SD, 44 ±8 years) with cardiac symptoms and/or a heart murmur, who had been treated with the combination of fenfluramine and phentermine, were found to have aortic or mitral regurgitation or both. Twelve patients also had tricuspid regurgitation. The patients were evaluated a mean (±SD) of 12.3 (±7.1) months after the initiation of fenfluramine–phentermine treatment. Five patients required valve replacement. Additional cases were subsequently reported by physicians from the Food and Drug Administration (FDA) and by other non-FDA providers. Valvulopathy was associated with the use of fenfluramine or dexfenfluramine, alone or in combination with phentermine. There were no cases involving the use of phentermine alone. As a result of these observations, the manufacturer withdrew fenfluramine and dexfenfluramine from the market (September 1997).

The FDA describes a case of appetite suppressant-induced valve disease as a patient with no previously known valve disease who had used appetite suppressants and presented with mild or greater aortic regurgitation or moderate or greater mitral regurgitation (The prevalence of mild or greater aortic regurgitation and moderate or greater mitral regurgitation is less than 1% in healthy subjects). The prevalence of valve disease meeting the case definition was similar across many echocardiography surveys ranging from 30 to 38%. The prevalence of valve disease is higher with the combination therapy compared with single therapy, and with longer durations of treatment. The prevalence in most surveys is greater than 15%, except in studies when the duration of treatment is short. Subsequent randomized and case-controlled studies provided additional information. In their study Gardin et al. demonstrated that the duration of therapy was a predictive factor of disease. Among patients who took these agents for 3 months or less, there was no statistically significant difference in prevalence of valve

regurgitation by FDA criteria compared with untreated subjects. A study by Jick et al. showed that the risk of developing valvular regurgitation was low in those who had received 3 or fewer 1-month prescriptions for dexfenfluramine or fenfluramine (7.1 per 10,000 exposed subjects over a 5-year period), whereas the risk for those who had received the drugs for 4 or more months was substantially higher (35.0 per 10,000 exposed subjects over a 5-year period). The disparity between reported prevalence of valve regurgitation reflects differences in methods, single-agent versus combination of therapy, and duration of drug exposure. Initial reports suggested a higher prevalence of cardiac valvular abnormalities among patients. These reports involved small groups of patients and lacked baseline data, blinded echocardiography readings, and an untreated cohort. Subsequent randomized and controlled prospective studies showed lower incidence of valvular regurgitation (5-15%).

Gardin et al. demonstrated in their study that dexfenfluramine-treated patients with FDA-positive valvular regurgitation were more likely to have had a history of heart murmur, rheumatic fever, myocardial infarction, ventricular arrhythmia, or other cardiovascular history or to have had an echocardiogram or cardiac catheterization prior to anorexigen therapy. Shively et al. addressed the question of whether other factors contribute to valve regurgitation and found that age and diastolic blood pressure may affect the prevalence of regurgitation. Concomitant therapy with a selective serotonin reuptake inhibitor for depression or panic disorder does not appear to confer incremental risk. Fewer patients are now presenting for initial evaluation since the drugs were removed from the market in 1997.

## Pathology

Grossly, the valve leaflets of patients treated with anorexigens look tethered and the chordae appear shortened. The valves appear glistening white, have no rheumatic calcification or yellowish discoloration, and resemble valves affected by carcinoid valve disease. Unlike rheumatic involvement, histopathological examination demonstrates intact valve architecture and plaque-like lesions ("stuck-on" plaques) of apparent myofibroblasts in an abundant extracellular matrix.

## Echocardiography

The echocardiographic features of the valvulopathy related to anorexigen therapy are similar to those seen in some patients with rheumatic heart disease, but valve obstruction is absent. For the mitral valve there is an echocardiographic appearance that consists of thickening and immobility of the posterior mitral valve leaflet and doming with preserved mobility of the anterior leaflet. Similar to rheumatic valve disease, there is also thickening and shortening of the subvalvular apparatus. The combination of abnormalities results in malcoaptation of valve leaflets and mitral regurgitation. As for the aortic valve, the cusps are usually thickened, resulting in malcoaptation and central regurgitation. Also, tricuspid valve leaflets exhibit the same echocardiographic features with variable degree of thickening and immobility, resulting in tricuspid regurgitation.

## Course

Echocardiography has been used to evaluate the course of valvular heart disease associated with anorectic drugs. The valvular lesions stabilize or improve in the great majority of patients after the cessation of these drugs .The development or progression of valvular disease is unlikely after the cessation of therapy. The potential for stabilization or improvement must be considered in the counseling of patients about the possible need for eventual valve replacement. The 2003 Guidelines from the American College of Cardiology, the American Heart Association, and the American Society of Echocardiography (ACC/AHA/ASE) recommend echocardiography to assess valve morphology and regurgitation in patients with a history of use of anorectic drugs or any other drug known to be associated with valvular heart disease who are symptomatic, have a cardiac murmur, or have an inadequate or technically difficult cardiac examination. Routine screening of all patients who have taken anorectic drugs is not recommended.

## DRUGS USED FOR THE TREATMENT OF PARKINSON'S DISEASE

Ergot-derived dopamine receptor agonists, often used in the treatment of Parkinson's disease, have been associated with an increased risk of valvular heart disease. Evidence from population studies of patients with Parkinson's disease and nonparkinsonian controls suggests a 5-6 times increased risk of substantial valve regurgitation in patients with Parkinson's disease treated with cabergoline or pergolide. The findings are consistent across studies, despite differences in echocardiographic techniques and definitions of abnormality.

## Epidemiology

Studies of similar designs have demonstrated that the frequency of moderate-to-severe regurgitation in at least one heart valve is higher in patients receiving cabergoline or pergolide than in patients taking non-ergot agonists or controls, and the incidence of new-onset valvulopathy is also higher in patients taking these drugs. These adverse events do not occur in all patients, however, and no clear susceptibility factors have been identified in patients. Thus, individual vulnerability seems to have a role in the process. The majority of patients who have been exposed to these agents did not develop valvulopathy, despite

several years' exposure. An echocardiographic prevalence study by Zannetti et al. included 155 patients taking dopamine agonists for Parkinson's disease (pergolide, 64 patients; cabergoline, 49; and non-ergot-derived dopamine agonists, 42) and 90 control subjects. The relative risk for moderate or severe valve regurgitation in the pergolide group was 6.3 for mitral regurgitation (P = 0.008), 4.2 for aortic regurgitation (P = 0.01), and 5.6 for tricuspid regurgitation (P = 0.16). The relative risks in the cabergoline group were 4.6 (P = 0.09), 7.3 (P < 0.001), and 5.5 (P = 0.12) respectively. Patients treated with ergot derivatives who had higher grades of regurgitation of any valve had received a significantly higher mean cumulative dose of pergolide or cabergoline than had patients with lower grades. Another study analyzed data from the United Kingdom General Practice Research Database. A population-based cohort comprising 11,417 subjects 40 to 80 years of age who were prescribed antiparkinsonian drugs between 1988 and 2005 was identified. A nested case–control analysis within this cohort was done. Each patient with newly diagnosed cardiac valve regurgitation was matched with up to 25 control subjects according to age, sex, and year of entry into the cohort. There were 31 case patients with newly diagnosed cardiac-valve regurgitation, 6 were exposed to pergolide, 6 were exposed to cabergoline, and 19 had not been exposed to any dopamine agonist within the previous year. The rate of cardiac valve regurgitation was increased with current use of pergolide (incidence rate ratio, 7.1; 95% confidence interval, 2.3 to 22.3) and cabergoline (incidence rate ratio, 4.9; 95% CI, 1.5 to 15.6), but not with current use of other dopamine agonists. The risk of cardiac valve regurgitation was increased only for patients taking pergolide or cabergoline for 6 months or longer, and was particularly increased for both medications at doses higher than 3 mg daily.

In the United States, pergolide was voluntarily withdrawn from the market in March 2007 due to the potential risk of heart valve damage.

## Pathology and Echocardiography

The exact pathway leading to valvulopathy is unknown. Pergolide and cabergoline have a high affinity for the serotonin (5-hydroxytryptamine [5-HT]) receptor subtype $5\text{-HT}_{2B}$, which are expressed in heart valves and have been shown to mediate fibroblast growth and proliferation. Other ergot-derived dopamine agonists, such as lisuride, and non-ergot dopamine agonists are devoid of this agonistic activity and their use has not been shown to induce fibrotic changes in heart valves. The fibrotic changes cause thickening, retraction, and stiffening of valves, which result in incomplete leaflet coaptation and clinically significant regurgitation. This has necessitated surgical valve replacement in some patients.

## Course

It is unknown whether the valve pathology resulting from the use of pergolide and cabergoline is reversible. Further prospective studies are needed. Such studies should also clarify the clinical course of mild-to-moderate echocardiographic changes, their natural history and optimal follow-up schedules. For now follow-up clinical and echocardiographic monitoring is advisable in all patients with Parkinson's disease who are treated with these agents. This is based on the ACC/AHA/ASE recommendations discussed below.

# ACC/AHA/ASE RECOMMENDATIONS

Fenfluramine and dexfenfluramine were withdrawn from the market (September 1997). For patients who have been exposed to these agents, recommendations were made by the 2003 ACC/AHA/ASE Guidelines. A similar approach may be adopted in the case of other agents with similar pathogenesis. A cardiac history and physical examination is indicated in all exposed patients. Symptoms of valvular heart disease or a pathologic murmur necessitate further work up. The absence of a murmur predicts absence of mild or worse regurgitation of any valve. Therefore, cardiac examination is the screening method of choice for detecting valvular regurgitation in patients with suspected drug-related valvular heart disease. Echocardiography is indicated in patients with a heart murmur, symptoms of valvular heart disease, or physical characteristics that preclude adequate cardiac examination. The optimal timing of follow-up echocardiography to determine the progression, regression, or stabilization of valvular lesions is not known. Depending on the severity of the lesion(s) a period of 6 to 12 months seems to be reasonable. Routine follow-up echocardiography is not recommended with previously normal studies or known trivial valvular abnormalities.

## Suggested Readings

1. Cheitlin MD, Armstrong WF, Aurigemma GP, et al. ACC/AHA/ASE 2003 Guideline Update for the Clinical Application of Echocardiography: summary article: A Report of the American College of Cardiology/American Heart Association Task Force on Practice Guidelines (ACC/AHA/ASE Committee to Update the 1997 Guidelines for the Clinical Application of Echocardiography). *Circulation.* 2003; 108(9):1146–1162.

2. Connolly HM, Crary JL, McGoon MD, et al. Valvular heart disease associated with fenfluramine-phentermine. *N Engl J Med.* 1997;337:581.

3. Khan MA, Herzog CA, St. Peter JV, et al. The prevalence of cardiac valvular insufficiency assessed by transthoracic echocardiography in obese patients treated with appetite-suppressant drugs. *N Engl J Med.* 1998;339:713.

4. US Food and Drug Administration Center for Drug Evaluation and Research, and Center for Disease Control and Prevention. Cardiac valvulopathy associated with exposure to fenfluramine or dexfenfluramine. *MMWR Morb Mortal Wkly Rep.* 1997;46:1061–1066.

5. Weissman NJ, Tighe JF, Gottdiener JS, et al. for the Sustained-Release Dexfenfluramine Study Group. An assessment of heart-valve abnormalities in obese patients taking dexfenfluramine, sustained-release dexfenfluramine, or placebo. *N Engl J Med.* 1998;339:725.

# 77

# Carcinoid Heart Disease

FRANK SEGHATOL-ESLAMI

## ● PRACTICAL POINTS

- Carcinoid tumors are rare malignant digestive tumors derived from enterochromaffin cells of GI tract usually the ileum.

- Carcinoid heart disease is characterized by the deposition of a white plaque-like material on the endocardium of right-sided valves as well as the right atrium and right ventricle.

- A major advance in the treatment of carcinoid syndrome was achieved with the discovery of somatostatin analogues, especially octreotide and its long-acting formulation.

- Tricuspid valve replacement provides good palliation in selected patients.

- Pulmonary valve replacement is advised in some cases to prevent RV remodeling. However, it has not been shown to prolong survival.

## OVERVIEW

Carcinoid tumors are rare malignancies of the neuroendocrine system. Carcinoid heart disease has been reported in more than half of patients with carcinoid syndrome and is related to vasoactive substances secreted by these tumors. Serotonin is implicated in the development of tricuspid and pulmonary valve lesions. Valves appear retracted and encased in a white material. The resultant tricuspid regurgitation and pulmonary stenosis may become severe with signs of right heart failure. The survival of patients with carcinoid heart disease has been improved over the past decade with combination of pharmacologic and surgical intervention. A multidisciplinary approach is needed for optimal management of these patients.

## DEFINITION AND PREVALENCE

- Carcinoid tumors are rare malignant digestive tumors derived from enterochromaffin cells of the GI tract, usually the ileum.
- Their incidence is 1 in 100,000 of the general population.
- The neurosecretory granules of enterochromaffin cells contain vasoactive substances such as 5--hydroxytryptamin (serotonin) and tachykinins (substance P) responsible for cutaneous flushing and secretory diarrhea.

## PATHOPHYSIOLOGY

- Carcinoid heart disease is thought to relate to the vasoactive substances secreted by the metastatic carcinoid tumor cells in the liver, reaching the right heart.
- Several series have reported carcinoid heart disease in up to 70% of cases of carcinoid syndrome.
- The pathogenesis of carcinoid heart disease is incompletely understood. However, many studies support a key role for serotonin (5-HT) in the development of cardiac lesions.
- Robiolo et al. have shown in patients with carcinoid heart disease a correlation between the serum level of serotonin and the extent of valvular involvement.
- Long-term exposure to 5-HT in animal models induces valvular fibrosis similar to those seen in human CHD.
- Similar valvular lesions have been caused by the appetite suppressants fenfluramine and phentermine, now withdrawn from the market in the United States.

## CLINICAL PRESENTATION

- The classical symptoms of carcinoid tumor are cutaneous flushing, secretory diarrhea, and bronchospasm. At the time of diagnosis, 50% of patients have clinical cardiac pathology manifesting with symptoms such as fatigue and dyspnea on exertion.

- Physical exam shows signs of right heart failure, including murmur of tricuspid regurgitation and pulmonary stenosis, and hepatomegaly with pulsatile liver due to severe tricuspid regurgitation.

## BIOCHEMICAL MARKERS

- Carcinoid tumor cells contain many different peptides and vasoactive substances.
- One of the main secretory products is serotonin or 5-hydroxytryptamine. Following its release from the tumor, serotonin is inactivated in the liver. The final byproduct of serotonin is 5-hydroxy-indolacetic acid (5-HIAA), which is excreted into the urine.

## ECHOCARDIOGRAPHIC FEATURES

- Carcinoid heart disease is characterized by the deposition of a white plaque-like material on the endocardium of right-sided valves as well as the right atrium and right ventricle. Left-sided valve involvement may rarely occur via a patent foramen ovale.

2-D echocardiography reveals the tricuspid valve to be thickened and retracted. The leaflets become shortened and less mobile with a great degree of non coaptation, leaving a large regurgitant orifice (**Figure 77-1**).

- With progression of the disease, the septal and the anterior leaflets become more retracted and immobile, whereas the posterior leaflet may exhibit a relatively preserved mobility. In advanced stages, the tricuspid valve leaflets become fixed in a semi-open position as-

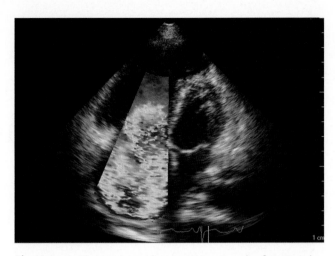

**Figure 77-2.** Severe tricuspid regurgitation on color-flow Doppler. (Courtesy of Dr. Navin Nanada.)

sociated with severe tricuspid regurgitation and some degree of stenosis.

- On color-flow Doppler, the regurgitation appears severe or torrential (**Figure 77-2**), with systolic flow reversal into the hepatic veins.
- Continuous-wave Doppler across the tricuspid valve shows a dagger-shaped spectral envelope with early peak and rapid decline, consistent with equalization of pressures between the right atrium and ventricle.
- The pulmonary valve cusps appear thick and retracted as well, although they are more difficult to visualize by 2-D imaging. They exhibit both stenosis and regurgitation with increased peak systolic velocity due to stenosis and dense spectral signal with rapid P1/2 time secondary to significant regurgitation. Often, by the time the patient presents with carcinoid heart, the right chambers are dilated due to volume overload.
- Echocardiography is the technique of choice for making the diagnosis of carcinoid heart disease.
- In one study involving 74 patients, tricuspid valve disease was present in 97% of patients by 2-D echocardiography, and pulmonary valve was present in 49%.

## PROGNOSIS AND FACTORS ASSOCIATED WITH PROGRESSION OF CARCINOID HEART DISEASE

- Some studies have looked at factors associated with the progression of carcinoid heart.
- In one study, patients who had higher urinary 5-HIAA exhibited an increased risk of progressive heart disease.
- In another study, it was demonstrated that left-side valve involvement occurs only if there is an associated PFO. The authors recommend that a PFO should be systematically searched in all patients with carcinoid syndrome.

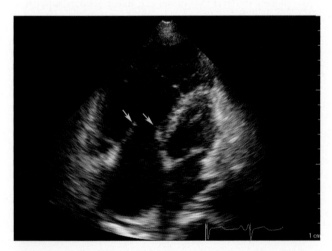

**Figure 77-1.** 2-D echocardiography of a tricuspid valve. In real-time one can note that the valve is immobile in a semi-open position with non coaptation of leaflets.

# DIAGNOSIS OF CARCINOID SYNDROME AND CARCINOID HEART DISEASE

- When all clinical features of carcinoid syndrome are present, a diagnosis is easy to establish. This diagnosis also should be considered when any one of its clinical manifestations is present.
- The diagnosis of carcinoid syndrome is confirmed when 24-hour urinary excretion of 5-HIAA is elevated (>25 mg/24h; normal < 9 mg/24h). Carcinoid heart disease is diagnosed primarily by echocardiography performed initially or during the clinical course.
- Patients with cardiac involvement tend to have higher circulating concentrations of 5-HIAA.

## NATURAL HISTORY

- Carcinoid tumors are slow-growing tumors.
- However, the development of carcinoid heart disease heralds a decline in clinical outcome. In one study, the mean survival in patients with carcinoid heart disease was 1.6 years from the time of diagnosis, compared to 4.6 years in those without cardiac involvement.

## TREATMENT

- The treatment of carcinoid syndrome and of carcinoid heart disease has evolved during the past decade. It has two objectives: 1- pharmacologic therapy directed toward reducing the secretory function of the tumor, and 2- surgical therapy to reduce the tumor mass and to replace cardiac valve(s).

### Pharmacologic treatment

- A major advance in the treatment of carcinoid syndrome has been achieved with the discovery of somatostatin analogues, especially octreotide and its long-acting formulation.
- Octreotides decrease blood level and urinary excretion of 5-HIAA and other tachykinins improving cutaneous flushing and other endocrine manifestations of carcinoid syndrome.
- Octreotides can also slow down the progression of the tumor mass and carcinoid heart disease.

- Common side effects of octreotides are hypoglycemia as a result of inhibition of glucagon and growth hormone secretion, and rarely steatorrhea and cholelithiasis.

### Surgical treatment

- In selected patients with unilateral liver metastases, hemihepatectomy and removal of the primary tumor and affected lymph nodes has led to complete surgical cure.
- Hepatic resection results in improved outcome (62% survival at 5 years) in those who are amenable to surgical resection. Hepatic artery embolization performed preoperatively may reduce the tumor mass.
- However, the recurrence rate after tumor resection is high (82% at 5 years).
- Tricuspid valve replacement provides good palliation in selected patients.
- Pulmonary valve replacement is advised in some cases to prevent RV remodeling. However, it has not been shown to prolong survival.
- Indications for cardiac valve replacement surgery are right heart failure with RV enlargement and RV systolic dysfunction, as survival of these patients is poor (median survival 11 months).

## Suggested Readings

1. Bhattacharyya S, Davar J, Dreyfus G, et al. Carcinoid heart disease. *Circulation*. 2007;116;2860–2865.

2. Bernheim AM, Connolly HM, Hobday TJ, et al. Carcinoid heart disease. *Prog Cardiovasc Dis*. 2007;49:439–451.

3. Connolly HM, Schaff HV, Mullany CJ, et al. Carcinoid heart disease: impact of pulmonary valve replacement in right ventricular function and remodeling. *Circulation*. 2002;106[supplI]:51–56.

4. Møller JE, Pellika PA, Bernheim AM, et al. Prognosis of carcinoid heart disease: analysis of 200 cases over two decades; *Circulation*. 2005;112:3320–3327.

5. Pellika PA, Tajik AJ, Khandheria BK, et al. Carcinoid heart disease: clinical and echocardiographic spectrum in 74 patients. *Circulation*. 1993;87:1188–1196.

6. Robiolio P, Rigolin V, Wilson J. Carcinoid heart disease: correlation of high serotonin levels with valvular abnormalities detected by cardiac catheterization and echocardiography. *Circulation*. 1995;92:790–795.

# 78

# Surgeon's Perspective on Aortic and Mitral Valves

Paul Vesco, Yazhini Ravi, and Chittoor B. Sai-Sudhakar

## ● PRACTICAL POINTS

- Symptomatic Aortic Stenosis is associated with angina, syncope or dyspenea with exertion.

- Patients with symptomatic critical AS benefit from surgery. Asymptomatic patients with critical AS need further evaluation including exercise testing.

- LV dimensions are an important criteria in evaluating patients with chronic aortic regurgitation.

- Aortic Root enlargement procedures are occasionally necessary to insert an adequately sized valve to avoid patient-prosthetic mismatch.

- Indications for surgery in patients with mitral stenosis depends on their functional class.

- Chronic mitral regurgitation is well tolerated. Specific guidelines have been developed for the timing of surgery.

- Systolic anterior motion (SAM) of the anterior leaflet of the mitral valve results in significant left ventricular outflow tract obstruction and a low cardiac output state. Treatment options include beta-blockade and volume loading.

- Acute aortic or mitral regurgitation are considered to be surgical emergencies.

- Bioprosthetic valves in the aortic position have more durability than in the mitral position likely due to the transvalvular gradients encountered.

- Robotic assisted mitral valve surgery is gaining favor in some highly specialized centers.

Aortic valve pathology can result in stenosis or regurgitation. Degenerative valve disease is the most common cause of aortic stenosis (AS) and includes calcific aortic stenosis observed in congenital bicuspid valves and senile calcific stenosis. In addition, rheumatic heart disease causes thickened leaflets and fused commissures resulting in aortic stenosis. In contrast, common causes of aortic regurgitation include rheumatic heart disease, aortic dissection, chronic aortic aneurysm, or destruction of the valve leaflets by infective endocarditis.

Indications for surgery for aortic stenosis include symptomatic disease, left ventricular dysfunction and, in some cases, hemodynamic severity observed on echocardiography.

Symptomatic aortic stenosis is associated with angina, syncope, and dyspnea. Asymptomatic patients require consideration of surgery when the valve area is $\leq 1$ cm$^2$ or mean transvalvular gradient is $\geq 40$ mm Hg. Patients with moderate aortic stenosis have a relative indication for aortic valve replacement if they are undergoing a concomitant cardiac procedure. (**Figure 78-1**) Patients requiring aortic valve replacement for stenosis will almost always benefit from an operation regardless of the ejection fraction. Perioperative risk is elevated in patients with a low transvalvular gradient, low ejection fraction, and a calcified ascending aorta. It is recommended that patients over the age of 40 should undergo cardiac catheterization prior to aortic valve replacement to rule out significant coronary artery disease.

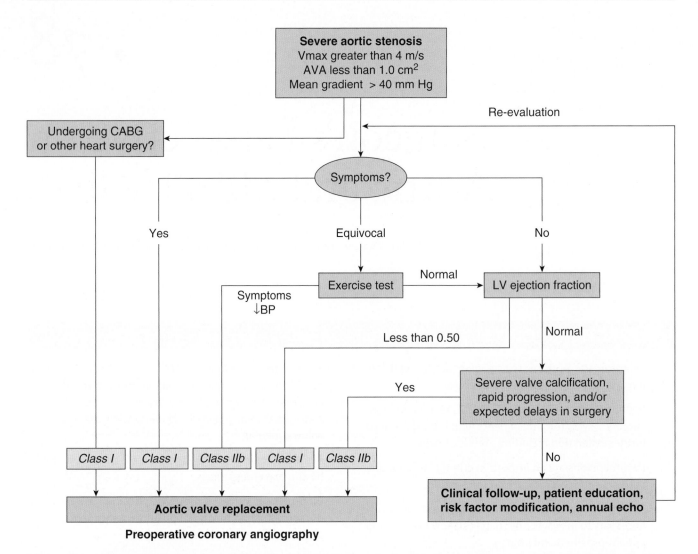

**Figure 78-1.** Management strategy for patients with severe aortic stenosis. Preoperative coronary angiography should be performed routinely as determined by age, symptoms, and coronary risk factors. Cardiac catheterization and angiography may also be helpful when there is discordance between clinical findings and echocardiography. (Modified from Otto. *J Am Coll Cardiol.* 2006;47. AVA, aortic valve area; BP, blood pressure; CABG, coronary artery bypass graft surgery; echo, echocardiography; LV, left ventricular; Vmax, maximal velocity across aortic valve by Doppler echocardiography.)

Indications for surgery in patients with aortic regurgitation are NYHA Class III or IV heart failure in the presence of preserved left ventricular function. However, in patients in NYHA Class I or II heart failure, surgery is indicated if LVEF is <50%, ventricular function worsens with a stress test, left ventricular end-systolic dimension is >55 mm, or left ventricular end-diastolic dimension is >75 mm (**Figure 78-2**). Aortic regurgitation is significantly insidious and onset of symptoms indicates advanced stage of the disease process. Patients with severely depressed ejection fraction may not benefit from aortic valve replacement. Aortic regurgitation secondary to annular ectasia requires a valve sparing aortic root reconstruction or an aortic root replacement, and in this situation, the timing of surgery should take into account the concomitant aortic root and the ascending aortic pathology. Acute aortic regurgitation caused by infective

endocarditis necessitates operative intervention in the presence of intractable heart failure, persistent sepsis, embolic events, heart block, or extension of the infection into adjacent cardiac structures.

## AORTIC VALVE SURGERY

Standard open aortic valve replacement is performed via a median sternotomy. Partial sternotomy incisions or small right anterior thoracotomy can also be utilized. Currently, aortic valve surgery requires placement of the patient on full cardiopulmonary bypass (CPB). The choice of sites for arterial cannulation include the ascending aorta, axillary artery or femoral artery and is based on several factors such as the degree of calcification or atheromatous involvement of

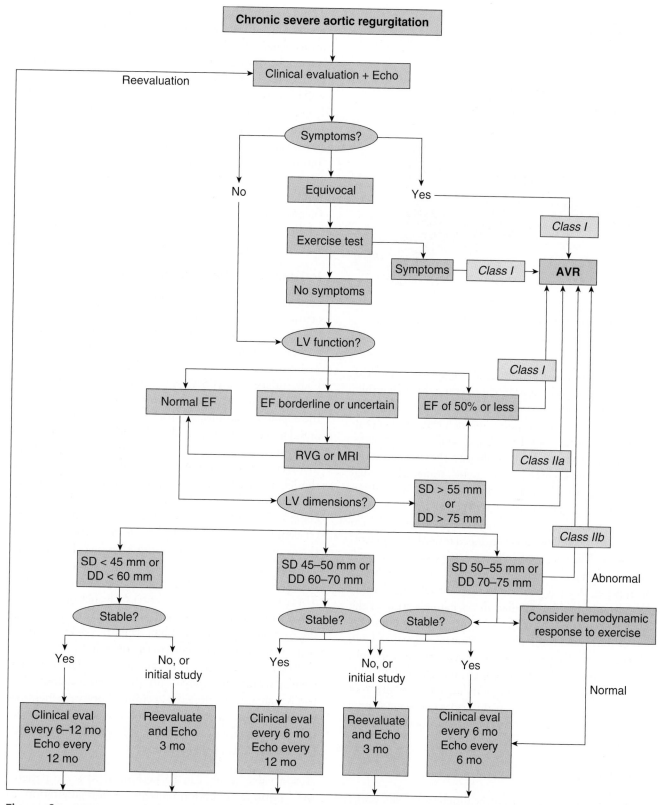

**Figure 78-2.** Management strategy for patients with chronic severe aortic regurgitation. Preoperative coronary angiography should be performed routinely as determined by age, symptoms, and coronary risk factors. Cardiac catheterization and angiography may also be helpful when there is discordance between clinical findings and echocardiography. "Stable" refers to stable echocardiographic measurements. In some centers, serial follow-up may be performed with radionuclide ventriculography (RVG) or magnetic resonance imaging (MRI) rather than echocardiography (Echo) to assess left ventricular (LV) volume and systolic function. AVR indicates aortic valve replacement; DD, end-diastolic dimension; EF, ejection fraction; eval, evaluation; and SD, end-systolic dimension.

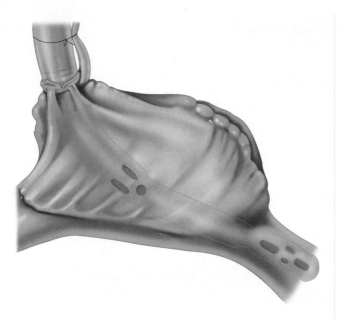

**Figure 78-3.** Right atrial cannulation with a dual-staged cannula through the right atrial appendage.

the ascending aorta, or if mini-access surgery is considered. Venous drainage is obtained by cannulating the right atrium (**Figure 78-3**) and after cross-clamping the aorta, the heart is arrested by infusion of a potassium-rich cardioplegia solution into the aortic root. In addition, some surgeons prefer retrograde delivery of cardioplegia into the coronary sinus through a cannula placed in the right atrium. Myocardial protection is crucial for successful outcomes, especially in the presence of left ventricular hypertrophy. The aortic valve is approached via an oblique aortotomy created 2 cm proximal to the annulus and continued towards the noncoronary sinus. The valve is then excised. For calcific processes, the aortic annulus is then mechanically debrided, with care taken not to lose any debris into the ventricle. Removal of the calcium from the annulus allows better seating of the valve. Forceful flushing of the left ventricle and administration of retrograde cardioplegia facilitates removal of loose debris from the ventricle and coronary ostia, respectively. The annulus is sized with valve sizers, the appropriate valve is chosen and sutured to the annulus. Occasionally, root enlargement procedures are performed to accommodate a larger-sized valve and to avoid patient–prosthetic valve size mismatch.

## Valve Choice

Life expectancy of the patient, willingness to take warfarin, and the ability to undergo another open heart surgery are factors in the decision-making process involving the choice of valves. In general, a mechanical valve has excellent durability and should be expected to last the patient's lifetime. Lifelong anticoagulation with warfarin is necessary for mechanical valves so thrombosis is avoided.

The 5-year mechanical valve complication rate includes about a 5% thromboembolism rate and a 3% risk of an anticoagulation-related issue. The bioprosthetic valves have low thrombotic rates and do not require anticoagulation. In all comers, 50% of patients will need valve replacement by 15 years. Tissue valves deteriorate by becoming calcified and stenotic; or, the leaflet could tear in the region of the strut. Paradoxically, younger patients have a faster rate of deterioration of a prosthetic valve. Yet, a 65-year-old patient would have a 15-year freedom from structural deterioration of 85% and a 75-year-old would have a 93% chance of freedom from reoperation. Bioprosthetic valves in the aortic position have more durability then in the mitral position likely due to the transvalvular gradients encountered.

## Patient–prosthetic Mismatch

Patient prosthesis mismatch occurs when the orifice area of the prosthesis is inadequate, as compared to the body surface area of the patient. A 23-mm or larger valve should be hemodynamically appropriate for an adult patient. A 21-mm valve may be used in a sedentary adult or with a body surface area (BSA) <1.5. Root enlargement procedures are performed for small aortic annuli in addition to the supra-annular placement of the aortic valve. A supra-annular patch can be placed in the middle of the noncoronary sinus to upsize by 2 mm. A Manouguian procedure involves cutting into the noncoronary sinus and entering the left atrium laterally. An extension can be made into the anterior leaflet of the mitral valve, but it will need to be curved to the midpoint of the leaflet, as the incision starts off center. A patch is used to reconstruct the leaflet and the atrium. An upsize of 1-2 valve sizes or 2-4 mm can be accomplished. A Nicks procedure involves cutting between the noncoronary and left coronary cusp into the annulus. This can be extended to the anterior leaflet of the mitral valve with reconstruction with a patch. This can enlarge the root one valve size or 2 mm. (**Figure 78-4**). A Konno aorto-ventriculoplasty opens to the right of the commissure between the right and left coronary cusp. The interventricular septum and right ventricle are both incised. Two patches are used to close the openings. Survival benefit has not been shown with a larger sized valve. Exercise capacity may be improved and quality of life made better with a larger valve in younger patients.

Aortic valve repair can be performed in some patients with aortic regurgitation. Patients with regurgitation associated with a bicuspid valve are more amendable to a repair, while a valve with three leaflets would need to be replaced. Occasionally, regurgitation associated with dilation of the annulus or sinus of Valsalva can be corrected with a valve-sparing procedure or resuspension of the leaflets.

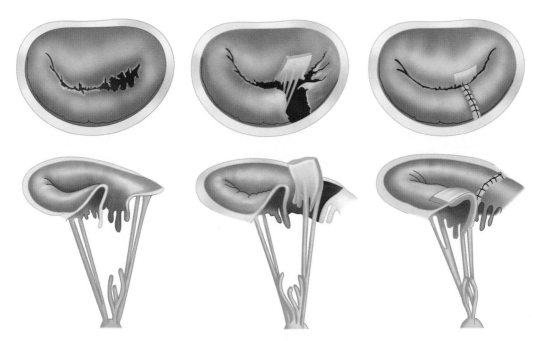

**Figure 78-10.** Chordal transposition from posterior leaflet with attached viable chordae to the anterior leaflet with ruptured chordae.

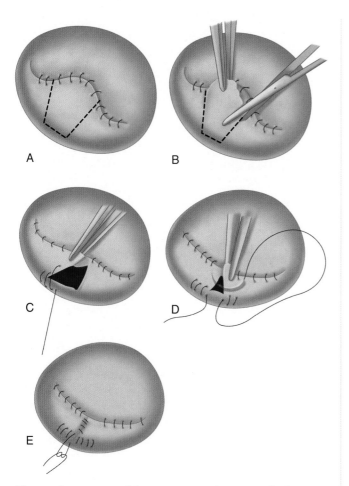

**Figure 78-11.** Repair of the myxomatous floppy mitral valve using the leaflet advancement technique. This depicts a valve with ruptured chordae from the middle segment (P2) of the posterior leaflet.

anterior leaflet toward the septum during systole. In addition, SAM can also lead to severe mitral regurgitation. A redundant posterior leaflet leads to the coaptation point at the middle of the anterior leaflet, which forces it toward the ventricular septum. A small and hyperdynamic ventricle is an additional contributory factor. Inotropes or afterload reduction with an intraaortic balloon pump make the condition worse. Treatment options include beta-blockade and volume-loading. Surgical maneuvers consist of reducing the height of the posterior leaflet with a larger quadrangular resection and sliding annuloplasty. A valve replacement should be considered in patients with refractory SAM.

With improvements in alternate cannulation methods, different approaches to the mitral valve have evolved. Partial sternotomy, right thoracotomy, robotic assisted, and robotic closed chest mitral repair and replacement are current options. The robotic assisted and robotic closed chest mitral procedures utilize a series of small ports and a working port to perform the replacement or repair. The robotic endowrist instruments provide 7 degrees of freedom for the manipulation of the instruments within the chest and provide superb three-dimensional vision and unparalleled precision for the conduct of the operation. Tremor modulation, movement scaling, and significant magnification (up to 10 times) are further refinements to improve the operative efficiency. The robot-assisted procedures have been shown to be cost effective, and in addition to a quicker postoperative recovery and decreased hospital stay, provide a better cosmetic outcome than a standard median sternotomy with its attendant risk of wound infection.

# Congenital Heart Disease

# 79

# Cardiovascular Genetics

Luke Kim, Konstantinos Charitakis, and Craig T. Basson

---

## ● PRACTICAL POINTS

- Hypertrophic cardiomyopathy (HCM) is one of the most common causes of sudden cardiac death in young people (with an estimated prevalence of 1:500) and is the leading cause of death in competitive athletes in the United States.

- Considering the variable onset of disease and the phenotypic expression of ARVC, genetic testing can have an important role allowing presymptomatic diagnosis in order to monitor the development of disease in the affected family members.

- Aortic root involvement is the leading cause of deaths in patients with Marfan syndrome and they should be routinely followed up with echocardiography. All first-degree relatives of a patient should also have screening echocardiography.

- Bicuspid aortic valve is one of the most common congenital cardiac disorders with a frequency of 1–2% in general population. Bicuspid aortic valve is associated with many other cardiac disorders including coarctation of the aorta and aortic dilatation/aneurysm.

- Implantable cardioverter-defibrillator remains the therapy of choice in high-risk patients with long QT syndrome. High-risk features include cardiac arrest, extremely prolonged QT, history of recurrent syncope, and genotypes associated with high risk of sudden cardiac death.

- Carney complex is an autosomal dominant disorder in which cardiac myxomas occur in the setting of spotty pigmentation of the skin, extracardiac myxomas, rare nonmyxomatous tumors, and endocrinopathy. Affected individuals should have annual echocardiography, and first-degree relatives need to be screened not only with echocardiography but also with physical exam including careful evaluation for skin findings.

- Tetralogy of Fallot represents approximately 10% of congenital heart diseases, and is characterized by subaortic ventricular septal defect, right ventricular infundibular stenosis, overriding aorta, and right ventricular hypertrophy.

- Aorta and pulmonary arteries arise as a single vessel from the heart in truncus arteriosus, resulting in cyanosis at birth along with poor feeding and tachypnea. Diagnosis is confirmed with echocardiography, and the treatment is operative repair.

---

## CARDIOMYOPATHIES

### Dilated Cardiomyopathy

Idiopathic dilated cardiomyopathy (IDC) is characterized by left ventricular dilation and systolic dysfunction in the absence of secondary etiologies, such as coronary ischemia, myocarditis, excessive alcohol exposure, severe hypertension, or other toxic/metabolic causes. It is more frequently observed in male patients. The annual incidence is approximately 5 to 8 cases per 100,000 population, and IDC is responsible for more than 10,000 deaths per year. 25% to 50% of patients with IDC have an inherited form of the disease. Familial dilated cardiomyopathy (FDC) is defined by the presence of two or more family members with IDC. No particular clinical or morphologic features of individual patients can distinguish FDC from IDC. More challenging is the screening of asymptomatic relatives and determining

**Table 79-1 • Autosomal Dominant Genes in Familial Dilated Cardiomyopathy**

| Gene | Category |
|------|----------|
| ACTC (cardiac actin) | sarcomeric proteins with role in muscle contraction |
| MYH7 (beta-myosin heavy chain) | |
| TNNT-2 (cardiac troponin T) | |
| TPM1 (alpha-tropomyosin) | |
| MYBPC (myosin binding protein C) | |
| MYH6 (alpha-myosin heavy chain) | |
| TTN (titin) | sarcomeric structural protein |
| VCL (vinculin) | |
| ACTN2 (alpha-actinin-2) | |
| DES (desmin) | dystrophin associated glycoprotein complex |
| SGCD (delta-sarcoglycan) | |
| PLN (phospholamban) | regulator of Kir6.2 |
| LMNA (lamin A/C) | associated with conduction defects |
| ABCC (sulfonylurea receptor 2A protein) | regulatory subunit of Kir6.2 |

whether subtle findings represent early signs of FDC. Left ventricular enlargement has been suggested as the most useful indication of preclinical disease, but patients should also be classified based on the presence or absence of atrioventricular block and other electrocardiographic abnormalities.

Approximately 90% of FDC is inherited in an autosomal dominant pattern. Sixteen autosomal genes have been identified so far, and discovery of more genes will likely ensue. Mutations in the beta-myosin heavy chain and lamin A/C genes appear to be the most common and are responsible for 5 to 10% of FDC cases, but other mutations in genes encoding for structural proteins had been reported (**Table 79-1**). X-linked FDC also accounts for 5 to 10% of FDC, and the most common causes are mutations in the dystrophin gene. Mutations in the dystrophin gene are associated with cardiomyopathy in conjunction with Duchenne or Becker's muscular dystrophy. Autosomal recessive FDC has been reported as mutations in cardiac troponin I. FDC appears to be genetically heterogeneous, and the role of additional genes will likely be discovered.

FDC demonstrates incomplete penetrance and variable expressivity; therefore, families usually demonstrate a wide range of mild to severe disease across generations, underlying the importance of careful family history and pedigree analysis in the care of patients with IDC. Diagnostically, electrocardiography and echocardiography allow a safe and noninvasive risk assessment. It is recommended that all first-degree relatives of patients with IDC undergo electrocardiography and echocardiography screening. It

has been shown that such clinical screening in association with family history has a greater sensitivity than family history alone. Second-degree relatives should be screened in X-linked FDC. Presence of atrioventricular block should suggest the potential for lamin A/C mutation. The recent American College of Cardiology/American Heart Association HF guidelines suggest that for a highly positive family history of DCM, referral to a cardiovascular genetics center is indicated.

FDC is clinically managed the same way as IDC with supportive care for cardiac dysfunction, atrioventricular block, and atrial/ventricular dysrhythmia. Genetic counseling can be beneficial for patients with FDC and their family members. Genetic testing is not currently widely available because of the genetic and locus heterogeneity and the given insensitivity due to the number of genes that have not been discovered yet. Genetic testing is still useful in screening family members of patients with mutations in identified genes. However, vigilant clinical screening will still be the keystone of disease monitoring in mutation positive individuals.

## Hypertrophic Cardiomyopathy

Hypertrophic cardiomyopathy (HCM) is a relatively common genetic cardiovascular disorder with an estimated prevalence of 1:500 in the United States. HCM is one of the most frequent causes of sudden cardiac death in young people and the leading cause of death in competitive athletes. It is characterized by ventricular hypertrophy with markedly variable clinical manifestations. Histopathologically, this disorder is characterized by myocyte hypertrophy with myocardial disarray and increased fibrosis. The age of onset varies from early childhood to late adulthood and can present with dyspnea, chest pain, and exercise intolerance. The disorder may also be an incidental finding during an investigation of an asymptomatic murmur. Symptoms may arise from either diastolic dysfunction or left ventricular outflow tract (LVOT) obstruction. LVOT obstruction occurs at rest in about 25% of patients, and more than half of these patients without obstruction at rest can generate significant obstruction with exercise.

HCM is mainly caused by autosomal dominant mutations in sarcomeric genes that encode myocardial contractile proteins, and numerous mutations have been identified to date in 12 different genes (**Table 79-2**). Hypertrophy in the context of Noonan syndrome (particularly important in the pediatric population) has been associated with mutations in the PTPN11 and related genes. (See Section Noonan syndrome below.) Although many attempts have been made to predict the genotype-phenotype correlation, a clear association of specific genes and their severity has been difficult to establish due to variable penetrance and expressivity

| Table 79-2 • Genes Associated with Hypertrophic Cardiomyopathy | |
|---|---|
| beta-MHC (beta-myosin heavy chain) | sarcomeric proteins |
| alpha-MHC (alpha-myosin heavy chain) | |
| cMYBPC (cardiac myosin binding protein C) | |
| cTnT (cardiac troponin T) | |
| cTnI (cardiac troponin I) | |
| cTnC (cardiac troponin C) | |
| alpha-TM (alpha-tropomyosin) | |
| MLC-1 (myosin essential light chain) | |
| MLC-2 (myosin essential light chain) | |
| Actin | |
| Titin | |
| PRKAG2 (protein kinase, AMP-activated, gamma-2 subunit) | metabolic cardiomyopathies |
| LAMP2 (linked lysosome-associated membrane protein-2) | |

of these genes. Different genetic forms of HCM, associated with WPW syndrome and other conduction anomalies, have been associated with mutations in the PRKAG2 (the gene encoding for the gamma2 regulatory subunit of AMP-activated protein kinase) or the LAMP2 gene (encoding for the lysosome-associated membrane protein). It is important to distinguish "pseudo" hypertrophy due to glycogen storage disease in the setting of PRKAG2 or LAMP2 mutations from true sarcomeric gene derived primary hypertrophic cardiomyopathy. Glycogen storage disease derived hypertrophy may have some therapeutic response to treatment of the underlying disorder.

The screening of HCM includes physical examination, electrocardiogram, and echocardiography. First-degree relatives of HCM patients younger than 12 years of age should be screened every 5 years. In patients age 12 to 22 years, screening should be repeated every 12 to 24 months, and if patients are older than 23 years, it should be repeated every 5 years or until genetic testing confirms the diagnosis. It is unfortunate that currently available genetic testing has a detection rate of less than 70%. Nevertheless, the identification of a gene mutation provides a definitive diagnosis of HCM in affected individuals and identifies carriers at risk for developing HCM. These carriers should be counseled, since there is a 50% probability of transmitting the mutation to their offspring. Thus, genetic testing is most often useful in determining risk in relatives of an affected individual, rather than in establishing the primary diagnosis of HCM in a given family.

HCM is typically diagnosed by asymmetric, marked left ventricular hypertrophy (LVH) on echocardiography. Athlete's heart can mimic HCM with significant LVH. It is important to carefully distinguish these two separate entities, as these conditions require different management. Temporary deconditioning with regression of LVH can aid in the diagnosis of athlete's heart. Mortality from HCM is primarily attributed to stroke, heart failure, and sudden cardiac death (SCD). Some of the risk factors for SCD include family history of SCD, unexplained syncope, abnormal blood pressure response to exercise, ventricular tachycardia on Holter monitoring, and massive (30 mm) LVH. Patients with two or more risk factors should be referred for implantable cardioverter-defibrillator placement. In terms of symptoms from LVOT obstruction, medical treatment consists of beta-blockers, verapamil, and disopyramide. In patients with marked intracavitary gradients and NYHA class III/IV symptoms refractory to maximal medical therapy, invasive therapy including surgical myectomy and alcohol septal ablation can be considered.

## Arrhythmogenic Right Ventricular Cardiomyopathy (ARVC)

ARVC is characterized by replacement of the ventricular myocardium with fatty and fibrous elements, preferentially involving the right ventricular (RV) free wall. This disorder has a frequency of 1:5000 in the general population. ARVC is more common in men and often diagnosed between the second and fourth decades of life. Phenotypic expressions can range from palpitations and syncope to sudden cardiac death. ARVC is one of the main, and increasingly more recognized, causes of ventricular tachyarrhythmias leading to sudden cardiac death. Familial disorders account for about 50% of the cases, mostly in an autosomal dominant pattern. Ten different genes and two different loci have been associated with the development of ARVD, including mutations of TGFß3, RYR2, and components of the cardiac desmosomes (i.e., PKP2, DSP, DSG2, and DSC2). Considering variable phenotypic expressions of the disorder, genetic analysis is very important in families with ARVD as it allows a presymptomatic diagnosis in order to monitor the development of disease in the affected family members.

Diagnostic criteria are based on characteristic structural abnormalities, tissue characterization, electrocardiographic changes, arrhythmias, and family history. This is accomplished utilizing multiple diagnostic modalities including ECG, echocardiography, cardiac MRI (CMR) and CT, and endomyocardial biopsy. Advances in CMR have improved diagnosis of ARVC. Major criteria for the diagnosis of ARVD by CMR are severe global RV dilation, global RV systolic dysfunction, RV wall thickening, and localized aneurisms of RV and RVOT. Although a point scoring scheme has been frequently used to establish the diagnosis of ARVC, it has more recently become clear that there is only a moderate correlation between this scheme and the molecular genetic diagnosis of ARVC. The clinical implications of carrying an ARVC mutation without fully meeting the consensus point scoring scheme cutoffs are unclear.

The therapeutic aim is to detect the patients at high risk and prevent sudden cardiac death. Patients diagnosed with ARVC should be counseled to minimize vigorous activity. Although low risk patients may be managed with beta-blockers, patients with high risk factors need to be evaluated for ICD along with antiarrhythmics. In patients with end stage ARVC, transplant can be considered.

## Noncompaction of the Left Ventricle (NCLV)

NCLV is an anatomical condition of the myocardial wall characterized by prominent LV trabeculae and deep inter-trabecular recesses. It can present as an isolated cardiac feature or in association with other cardiac conditions such as HCM, DCM, Barth syndrome, or Ebstein anomaly. It may also be a feature of mitochondrial or metabolic diseases and neuromuscular disorders. NCLV usually manifests itself with ventricular arrhythmias, systemic embolization, or heart failure. The diagnosis of NCLV is typically made by echocardiography, cardiac MRI, and 64-slice CT.

NCLV may be either sporadic or familial with an autosomal dominant or recessive inheritance. As with other cardiomyopathies, NCLV demonstrates genetic heterogeneity. Several genes have been implicated in the pathogenesis including the TAZ gene encoding for the G4.5 protein, which plays a role in the biosynthesis of the mitochondrial inner membrane, cardiolipin. Mutations of other genes encoding muscle proteins like α-dystrobrevin and LIM domain binding protein 3/ZASP have been reported in some familial or sporadic cases. Recently, sarcomeric protein genes, namely, β-myosin heavy chain, α-cardiac actin, and cardiac troponin T, have been proposed to be associated with NCLV, possibly adding NCLV to a broad spectrum of cardiac disorders caused by sarcomeric gene mutations.

## Restrictive Cardiomyopathy (RCM)

Restrictive cardiomyopathy is characterized by impaired diastolic filling with normal or mildly abnormal systolic function. Idiopathic restrictive cardiomyopathy is a diagnosis of exclusion when secondary causes such as amyloidosis, sarcoidosis, and hemochromatosis have been excluded. Familial restrictive cardiomyopathy is extremely rare in the absence of the above secondary causes. However, sarcomeric gene mutations also have been implicated in RCM including in genes encoding cardiac troponin T, cardiac troponin I, and α-cardiac actin.

# CONNECTIVE TISSUE DISORDERS

## Marfan Syndrome

Marfan syndrome is a systemic connective tissue disorder with a frequency of 2 to 3 in 10,000. The disorder is characterized by manifestations involving the cardiovascular, skeletal, and ocular systems. Current diagnostic criteria are based on involvement of above organ systems and family history. Cardiovascular manifestations include mitral valve prolapse, progressive aortic root enlargement, and ascending aortic aneurisms, possibly leading to aortic regurgitation, dissection, or rupture. Some characteristic skeletal manifestations of this syndrome include disproportional increase of linear bone growth resulting in malformations of the digits (arachnodactyly), craniofacial abnormalities, pectus excavatum/carinatum, and scoliosis. A common ocular involvement is severe myopia and lens dislocation in one or both eyes (ectopia lentis).

Marfan syndrome is an autosomal dominant disorder caused by fibrillin-1 gene mutations encoding for the extracellular matrix protein fibrillin (Fbn-1). Fibrillin is an integral component of both elastic and nonelastic connective tissue. The mechanism of fibrillin mutation in Marfan syndrome remains unclear. However, animal models of Fbn-1 have demonstrated a role of TGF-beta signaling. In some patients with phenotypes similar to Marfan syndrome but without fibrillin-1 gene mutations, TGF-beta receptor mutations have been identified, suggesting a significant role of TGF-beta pathway in the pathogenesis of Marfan syndrome features.

Aortic root involvement remains the leading cause of death in patients with Marfan syndrome. Echocardiography is recommended to routinely screen and to follow aortic root dilation. In addition, all first-degree relatives of the family should have screening echocardiography. Patients should be advised against strenuous exercises. Medical therapy for Marfan syndrome includes beta-blockers to reduce myocardial contractility and pulse pressure. Animal models of Marfan syndrome have demonstrated a possible benefit of losartan in preventing progression of the disease by inhibiting the TGF-beta pathway, and this therapy is the subject of an active clinical trial. Elective aortic root replacement remains the therapy of choice once the aortic root becomes significantly enlarged. Marfan patients who become pregnant need to be counseled not only about the 50% chance of transmitting the disease but also the substantially increased risk of aortic rupture/dissection during and after pregnancy. Important components of Marfan syndrome counseling are consideration of contraception and pregnancy management.

usually ostium secundum (the most common type of atrial septal defect [ASD]) or muscular VSDs. A careful clinical examination alone is not enough to make the diagnosis of HOS and to distinguish it from other heart-hand syndromes. However, genetic testing is useful in establishing diagnosis for family members of a patient with HOS and a *TBX5* mutation. When invitro fertilization (IVF) is used as a reproductive strategy in a *TBX5* positive mother with HOS, the blastocysts can be genetically tested for *TBX5* mutations before their transfer to uterus.

## Familial ASD with or Without Progressive Atrioventricular Block

Atrial septal defects occur in about 1 in 1,500 live births. There are four different types of ASD, and they include ostium primum, ostium secundum, sinus venosus, and coronary sinus septal defect. The clinical effects of isolated ASDs are usually related to the degree of left-to-right shunting and the resulting changes in the pulmonary and systemic circulation. Children with ASDs are typically asymptomatic and only diagnosed after a characteristic widely split, fixed S2 is detected during a routine examination. If ASD is unrecognized until late childhood, patients may develop arrhythmias, pulmonary hypertension, or heart failure. Diagnosis is made with two-dimensional and Doppler echocardiography, demonstrating both the extent of the defect and the degree of left-to-right shunting. However, a transesophageal echocardiogram or cardiac MR may be necessary to detect sinus venosus or coronary sinus defects.

Although most cases of ASD are sporadic, ASD may also be related to different genetic syndromes. Familial ASD with progressive AV block is an autosomal dominant syndrome associated with mutations of the homeodomain-containing transcription factor Nkx2.5. It is characterized by variable degrees of AV conduction abnormality and can present along with other abnormalities, such as VSD and Tetralogy of Fallot (TOF). Familial ASD without progressive AV block, on the other hand, has been associated with mutations in GATA4, a key transcription factor in cardiac development. Diagnosis of familial ASD can be made with the mutational analyses of *NKX2.5* and *GATA4* genes, respectively.

## CONOTRUNCAL DEFECTS

### Tetralogy of Fallot

TOF is a complex of anatomic abnormalities arising from the maldevelopment of the right ventricular infundibulum. The disorder consists of a subaortic ventricular septal defect, a right ventricular infundibular stenosis, an overriding aorta, and a right ventricular hypertrophy. TOF represents approximately 10% of congenital heart diseases, and it occurs at a frequency of 3 to 6 infants for every 10,000 births. The physiologic consequences of TOF are largely dependent upon the degree of right ventricular outflow obstruction. Most children will present in the immediate newborn period with cyanosis. Squatting can help with the symptoms by increasing the peripheral vascular resistance and decreasing the magnitude of the right-to-left shunt across the VSD. Infants frequently suffer from hypoxic spells, which are characterized by unpredictable episodes of bluish pale skin during crying or feeding. Without treatment, mortality rates gradually increase, ranging from 30% at the age of 2 years to 50% by the age of 6 years. Rarely, 5 to 10% of patients may remain marginally cyanotic or even acyanotic into adult life, developing congestive heart failure by the age of 30 years. The diagnosis is typically made with color-flow Doppler echocardiography or cardiac MRI, which provides anatomical information including delineation of the aorta, right ventricular outflow tract, VSDs, right ventricular hypertrophy, and the pulmonary artery. Furthermore, the above studies also provide physiologic data including intracardiac pressures and gradients. Cardiac catheterization complements noninvasive imaging modalities by providing definitive anatomical and physiologic data. Almost all patients undergo intracardiac repair consisting of patch closure of the ventricular septal defect and the enlargement of the right ventricular outflow tract. The outcome of surgical repair is excellent with minimal morbidity and mortality. Some of the early postoperative complications include heart blocks and residual VSDs.

TOF can be associated with fetal alcohol syndrome and sometimes drugs such as phenytoin and carbamazepine. Furthermore, several genetic syndromes have been associated with TOF. So-called 22q11 deletion syndrome has been associated with conotruncal defects, such as TOF, truncus arteriosus, and transposition of the great arteries. Genetic tests, such as FISH for the detection of 22q11 deletion, and chromosome analyses for 22q rearrangement can aid in diagnosis. Cat-eye syndrome is associated with duplication of the chromosomal region 22pter22q11 and has variable clinical presentation, including TOF, anal atresia, coloboma, cleft palate, microphthalmia, and facial dysmorphia. Alagille syndrome is also associated with TOF. Its manifestations include cardiac features, such as TOF and pulmonary artery brunch stenosis, and noncardiac features like characteristic facies, growth retardation, cholestasis, and vertebral anomalies.

### Truncus Arteriosus

Truncus arteriosus is a congenital anomaly resulting from incomplete or failed septation of the embryonic truncus arteriosus. Aorta and pulmonary arteries arise as a single vessel from the heart by means of a single semilunar valve. This in turn results in cyanosis and systemic ventricular volume overload. Because the mixing of left and right ventricular output occurs at the level of the common arterial trunk, systemic arterial oxygen saturation is usually low. Cyanosis is usually present at birth along with poor feeding and tachypnea. Symptoms of heart failure manifest as pulmonary vascular resistance falls and pulmonary overcirculation increases. Other associated cardiac abnormalities include structural abnormalities of the truncal valve with resultant regurgitation, interruption of the right aortic arch, a left superior caval vein, an aberrant subclavian artery, and an atrial septal defect. Truncus arteriosus occurs in approximately 5 to 15 per 100,000 live births. The median age at death ranges from 2 weeks to 3 months with mortality reaching close to 100% by 1 year without surgical repair. For patients undergoing complete repair in the neonatal or early infant periods, early postoperative mortality is generally less than 10%. As mentioned above, patients with truncus arteriosus have a higher incidence of association with band 22q11 deletion and with trisomy of chromosome 8. Echocardiography with cross-sectional and Doppler flow analysis is usually sufficient to confirm diagnosis of truncus arteriosus and fully characterize the various anatomic features. Truncus arteriosus invariably requires operative repair by closing the ventricular septal defect, committing the common arterial trunk to the left ventricle, and reconstructing the right ventricular outflow tract.

## Transposition of Great Arteries

Transposition of great arteries (TGA) involves placement of the great vessels across the plane of the interventricular septum, so that the aorta arises from the right ventricle and the pulmonary artery from the left ventricle, with resultant cyanosis apparent within hours of birth. Usually, the origin of the aorta is anterior and rightward to the origin of the pulmonary artery along with concomitant VSD, PFO, or PDA. It is the most common cyanotic congenital heart disease in neonates, and the overall annual incidence is 20 to 30 per 100,000 live births. This disorder is associated with a poor prognosis with mortality reaching 90% by the end of the 1st year if untreated. As mentioned above, TGA is associated with 22q11 deletion syndrome and with trisomies 18 and 21.

There are four different anatomic subtypes: TGA with intact ventricular septum, TGA with ventricular septal defect, TGA with ventricular septal defect and left ventricular outflow tract obstruction, and TGA with ventricular septal defect and pulmonary vascular obstructive disease. Echocardiography is usually diagnostic of TGA by demonstrating the characteristic anatomical presentations. Initial treatment consists of maintaining ductal patency with continuous intravenous (IV) prostaglandin E1

infusion to promote left-to-right intercirculatory mixing at the atrial level. Most full-term neonates with uncomplicated TGA can undergo an arterial switch procedure with good prognosis.

## DiGeorge Syndrome

DiGeorge syndrome is a relatively rare disorder associated with aplasia/hypoplasia of the thymus and parathyroid along with cardiac malformations and characteristic facial features. Most of the cases are due to microdeletion of chromosome 22q11 and are detectable by FISH. Common cardiac defects include VSD, Tetralogy of Fallot, truncus arteriosus, and aortic arch anomalies. Considering the variable expressivity of the microdeletion, FISH should be offered to patients with suspected DiGeorge's syndrome to aid with diagnosis. The cardinal cardiac features of DiGeorge syndrome are recapitulated by missense mutation of the *TBX1* gene, which is usually included within DiGeorge syndrome 22q11 deletions.

## Chromosomal Aberration

Many of the common chromosomal aberrations are associated with cardiac anomalies. Trisomy 21, or Down syndrome, is the most common cause of an ostium primum ASD, produced as a failure of fusion of the superior and inferior endocardial cushions around the 5th week of gestation. Commonly, ASDs coexist with a cleft in the anterior leaflet of the mitral valve. Other cardiac defects include aortic valve stenosis and transposition of the great arteries. More than 90% of the infants with Trisomy 18, or Edwards syndrome, have cardiac manifestations including atrial and ventricular septal defects with polyvalvular heart disease (pulmonary and aortic valve defects), patent ductus arteriosus, overriding aorta, coarctation of aorta, hypoplastic left heart syndrome, Tetralogy of Fallot, and transposition of the great arteries. Trisomy 13, Patau syndrome, is the most severe of the viable autosomal trisomies with a median survival of less than 3 days. It is expressed prenatally and is fully evident at birth. Cardiac manifestations occur in 80% of the cases and include ASD, VSD, dextrocardia, and bicuspid semilunar valves. Therefore, in patients with chromosomal aberration, caution needs to be taken to rule out associated cardiac anomalies. Management will depend on the associated abnormality and the hemodynamic effect of the anomaly.

## Suggested Readings

1. Wang Q, Pyeritz RE, Seidman CE, Basson CT. Genetic studies of myocardial and vascular disease. In: *Textbook of Cardiovascular Medicine*. Philadelphia: Lippincott Williams & Wilkins; 2007.

2. Lehnart SE, Ackerman MJ, Benson DW Jr, et al. Inherited arrhythmias: A National Heart, Lung, and Blood Institute

and Office of Rare Diseases workshop consensus report about the diagnosis, phenotyping, molecular mechanisms, and therapeutic approaches for primary cardiomyopathies of gene mutations affecting ion channel function. *Circulation.* 2007 Nov 13;116(20):2325–2345.

3. Pierpont ME, Basson CT, Benson DW Jr, et al. American Heart Association Congenital Cardiac Defects Committee, Council on Cardiovascular Disease in the Young. Genetic basis for congenital heart defects: Current knowledge: A scientific statement from the American Heart Association Congenital Cardiac Defects Committee, Council on Cardiovascular Disease in the Young: Endorsed by the American Academy of Pediatrics. *Circulation.* 2007 Jun 12;115(23):3015–3038.

4. Maron BJ, Towbin JA, Thiene G, et al. American Heart Association; Council on Clinical Cardiology, Heart Failure and Transplantation Committee; Quality of Care and Outcomes Research and Functional Genomics and Translational Biology Interdisciplinary Working Groups; Council on Epidemiology and Prevention. Contemporary definitions and classification of the cardiomyopathies: An American Heart Association Scientific Statement from the Council on Clinical Cardiology, Heart Failure and Transplantation Committee; Quality of Care and Outcomes Research and Functional Genomics and Translational Biology Interdisciplinary Working Groups; and Council on Epidemiology and Prevention. *Circulation.* 2006 Apr 11;113(14):1807–1816.

# 80

# Essential Echocardiographic Images in Adult Congenital Heart Disease

Alexander R. Opotowsky and Martin St. John Sutton

## ● PRACTICAL POINTS

- Bicuspid aortic valve is the most common type of congenial heart defect, present in ~1–2% of the population. Bicuspid aortic valve predisposes to aortic valve stenosis and regurgitation, aortic valve endocarditis, and proximal aortic dilation.

- Coarctation of the aorta is associated with bicuspid aortic valve. Approximately 50% of patients with coarctation have bicuspid aortic valve.

- Perimembranous (also called membranous) ventricular septal defects (VSD), the most common type of VSD, often close spontaneously.

- Transthoracic echocardiography with color Doppler flow imaging is highly sensitive for the detection of VSD. The type (location) of VSD can be well defined by transthoracic echocardiography.

- Ostium secundum atrial septal defect (ASD) is the most common type of ASD. It is the only type of ASD amenable to percutaneous closure.

- Patients with unexplained right atrial and right ventricular dilatation on transthoracic echocardiogram should have further evaluation with transesophageal echocardiogram, CT, or MRI for sinus venosus defect or partial anomalous pulmonary venous drainage.

- Pulmonary regurgitation is a common sequela of intracardiac repair of tetralogy of Fallot and can lead to progressive right ventricular dilation and dysfunction.

- Down syndrome is highly associated with congenital heart disease, most typically endocardial cushion (AV canal) defects.

- Ebstein anomaly is characterized by apical displacement of the septal +/− posterior tricuspid valve leaflets resulting in a portion of atrialized right ventricle and is highly associated with the presence of patent foramen ovale or ASD and with accessory pathways (i.e., Wolf–Parkinson–White syndrome)

- The 20th century saw dramatic advances in surgical treatment of congenital heart disease, from palliative shunts aimed at increasing pulmonary blood flow (systemic arterial-to-pulmonary arterial: Blalock-Taussig, Waterston, Potts; systemic venous-to-pulmonary arterial: Glenn) to intracardiac repair of certain lesions to Fontan procedures that result in an acyanotic single ventricle circulation with essentially passive pulmonary blood flow.

# INTRODUCTION

Congenital heart disease (CHD), defined as structural heart disease present at birth, occurs in approximately 0.8% of live births (excluding common simple lesions such as bicuspid aortic valve and mitral valve prolapse). Simple defects, such as small atrial septal defects (ASDs), may be asymptomatic during childhood with symptoms developing later in life. However, many children with complex congenital heart defects previously fatal early in life are now living to adulthood after surgical and catheter-based interventions.

Echocardiographic assessment of adults with CHD includes the evaluation of the intracardiac anatomy of both uncorrected and corrected congenital defects. In addition, not only must the primary lesion or surgical correction be defined, but there must also be a thorough evaluation of long-term structural and hemodynamic sequelae.

# GENERAL PRINCIPLES

## Special Echocardiographic Techniques in CHD

The echocardiographic modalities (e.g., 2D Doppler) and basic principles (e.g., modified Bernoulli equation) used for CHD are the same as for acquired heart disease. However, a "*standard protocol*" for performing and interpreting the data is often inadequate.

### 2-Dimensional (2D) Echocardiography

- Orientation to patient anatomy precedes the full evaluation in patients with adult congenital heart disease (ACHD).
- Atypical views may be needed to define certain defects.
- Knowledge of specific anatomy (native and postsurgical) is required to correctly interpret images.
- Contrast echocardiography can provide better endocardial definition and precise determination of shunt location. This technology is especially useful for shunt locations that are difficult to visualize directly (e.g., sinus venosus defect) or those with a modest pressure gradient across the defect (e.g., any ASD).

### Doppler Echocardiography

- Pressure gradients are estimated using the modified Bernoulli equation. Off-axis imaging and color flow velocity mapping are often required to align the ultrasound beam parallel to blood flow.
- Shunt quantification is often a critical determinant of patient management. 2D and Doppler echocardiography can provide an estimate of shunt flow: and can be accurately estimated using 2D and Doppler echocardiography:
  - Blood flow through the right ventricular outflow tract (RVOT) at the pulmonary annulus is estimated by multiplying the velocity time integral (VTI) by the cross-sectional area ($\pi r^2$) of the flow stream at the level of the pulmonary annulus.
  - Blood flow through the left ventricular outflow tract (LVOT) is estimated by multiplying the VTI by the cross-sectional area ($\pi r^2$) at the level of the LVOT.
  - The ratio of pulmonary to systemic flow (Qp:Qs) is calculated (**Figure 80-1**).
  - Any right- and left-sided locations can theoretically be used to define right- and left-sided flow, but the outflow tracts are usually best because of their circular shape and relatively stable cross-sectional area throughout systole.
  - The reliability of this technique depends on the accurate estimation of VTI and cross-sectional diameter (especially important, because this term is raised to the second power).

## Orientation

Proper orientation is an essential first step in interpreting congenital echocardiograms. Unlike standard echocardiography in acquired heart disease, the echocardiographer cannot assume normal apical position, atrial situs, atrioventricular relationship, or ventriculoarterial relationship. The *segmental approach* to the diagnosis of congenital heart disease is described below.

## Apical Position

A standard subcostal view demonstrates whether the apex is directed to the left (levocardia, normal), middle (mesocardia), or right (dextrocardia).

## Atrial Situs

Atrial situs is determined using specific morphologic criteria (**Table 80-1**). Atrial situs is usually the same as abdominal situs (IVC/aortic relationship, side of liver, stomach and spleen, etc.) and is classified as situs solitus (right atrium on right side, normal), situs inversus, or situs ambiguous, or there can be right or left atrial isomerism (both atria have the same morphologic characteristics).

## Ventricular Morphology and Atrioventricular Connection

As with the atria, the right and left ventricles are defined by morphologic criteria (**Table 80-1**). Atrioventricular concordance is present when the morphologic right atrium (RA) empties into the morphologic right ventricle (RV) and the morphologic left atrium (LA) empties into the morphologic left ventricle (LV). Atrioventricular discordance is present when the morphologic RA empties into the morphologic LV

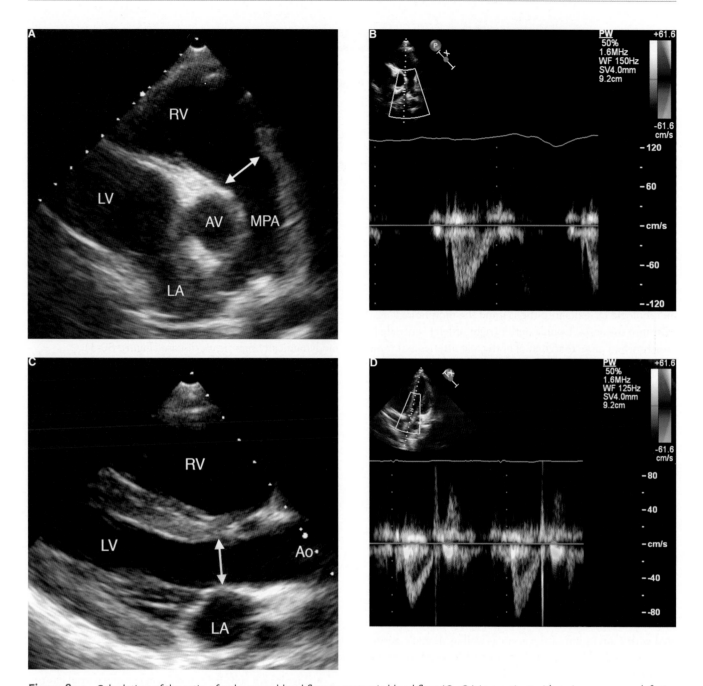

**Figure 80-1.** Calculation of the ratio of pulmonary blood flow to systemic blood flow ($Q_p$:$Q_s$) in a patient with a sinus venosus defect and partial anomalous pulmonary venous return. The RVOT diameter measures 2.1 cm (a), with an RVOT VTI of 26 cm (b). The LVOT diameter smeasures 1.8 cm (arrow, c), with an LVOT VTI of 13 cm (d). The estimated RV stroke volume is 90 mL ($\pi * 1.05^2 \times 26$), as compared with an LV stroke volume of 33 mL ($\pi * 0.9^2 \times 13$). Using these numbers, the $Q_p$:$Q_s$ is approximately 2.7:1. LA, left atrium; LV, left ventricle; RV, right ventricle; MPA, main pulmonary artery; AV, aortic valve; Ao, aorta.

and the morphologic LA empties into the morphologic RV. Double inlet (right or left) ventricle is present when both atria empty into one ventricle (right or left, respectively).

## Ventriculoarterial Relationship

The pulmonary artery (PA) and aorta differ in several ways:

- The PA bifurcates soon after its origin into equal primary branches.

- The aorta gives origin to the coronary arteries and the aortic arch with its candy cane shape and major branches supplying the upper extremities, head, and neck (brachiocephalic, carotid, and subclavian arteries).

Ventriculoarterial concordance is present when the morphologic RV exits into the PA and the morphologic LV exits into the aorta. Ventriculoarterial discordance is present when the

| Table 80-1 • Determination of Atrial and Ventricular Morphology | | | |
|---|---|---|---|
| **Atria** | | **Ventricles** | |
| **Right** | **Left** | **Right** | **Left** |
| Broad-based appendage | Narrow-based appendage | Heavily trabeculated apex | Smooth apex |
| Usually on same side of liver | Usually on opposite side from liver | More apical AV valve insertion | More basal AV valve insertion |
| Lateral wall with pectinate muscles* | Smooth wall* | Septal attachment of AV valve (tricuspid) | No septal attachment of AV valve (mitral) |
| Muscular ring surrounding fossa ovalis* | Thin (*flap valve*) septal tissue* | Moderator band | No moderator band |

*Transthoracic echocardiography usually does not provide adequate images to define these characteristics. AV, atrioventricular.

morphologic LV exits into the PA and the morphologic RV exits into the aorta. Double outlet (right or left) ventricle is present when more than half of both great arteries exit from a single right or left ventricle, respectively.

# SPECIFIC LESIONS

## Bicuspid Aortic Valve and other Congenital Aortic Valve Defects

Bicuspid aortic valve is the most common form of CHD (1-2% of the general population), and is often found in multiple members of a kindred. Aortic regurgitation (AR), as the result of inadequate coaptation of the leaflets and prolapse of the fused leaflet, usually precedes the development of aortic stenosis (AS). AR, on average, develops in the fourth and fifth decades, whereas AS, a more common sequala of bicuspid valve, resulting from accelerated calcification develops later in life. Bicuspid aortic valve is associated with coarctation of the aorta as well as thoracic aortic aneurysm and other left-sided obstructive lesions (see below for discussion of the Shone complex).

Echocardiographic characteristics of bicuspid aortic valve include (**Figure 80-2**):
- Parasternal long axis view demonstrates doming of the leaflets during systole and asymmetric diastolic closure.
- The parasternal short axis view at the level of the aortic valve may clearly demonstrate a bicuspid valve, but there is often a ridge of tissue (raphe) at the location of leaflet fusion suggestive of an incomplete commissure. During systole, the aortic valve orifice is oval-shaped (fish mouth) instead of the usual triangular orifice.
- With fusion of left and right coronary cusps, the most common form of bicuspid aortic valve, the AR jet is o posteriorly directed due to the prolapse of the anterior fused leaflet.

Unicuspid, quadricuspid, and dysplastic aortic valves are less common and associated with earlier development of hemodynamically significant disease (**Figure 80-3**).

## Left Ventricular Outflow Tract and Nonvalvular Aortic Obstruction

### Subaortic stenosis
Discrete subaortic stenosis due to obstruction to flow by a fibrous membrane across the LVOT (often attaching to the anterior mitral valve leaflet) just below the aortic valve is the most common cause of congenital subaortic stenosis (**Figure 80-4**). Because of the close proximity of the membrane to the aortic valve, damage to the valve can result from the turbulent systolic jet and lead to AR.
- The membrane may be difficult to visualize by 2D echocardiography, especially in the parasternal long axis view when the transducer is parallel to the membrane.
- Estimation of the peak gradient across the subaortic membrane provides an accurate assessment of the severity of the stenosis in the absence of other levels of LVOT obstruction.
- Significant subaortic stenosis may cause partial closure of the aortic valve leaflets in mid systole, which may be documented with 2D or M-Mode echocardiography.

A thicker fibromuscular ridge and tunnel type subaortic obstructions are less common causes of subaortic stenosis and usually present in childhood. Subaortic stenosis is usually isolated but may be associated with a wide array of other defects.

Hypertrophic cardiomyopathy, usually with systolic anterior motion of the mitral valve, is a more common cause of subaortic obstruction.

### Supravalvular Aortic Stenosis (SVAS)
Supravalvular aortic stenosis usually consists of fibromuscular thickening at the sinotubular junction but can also

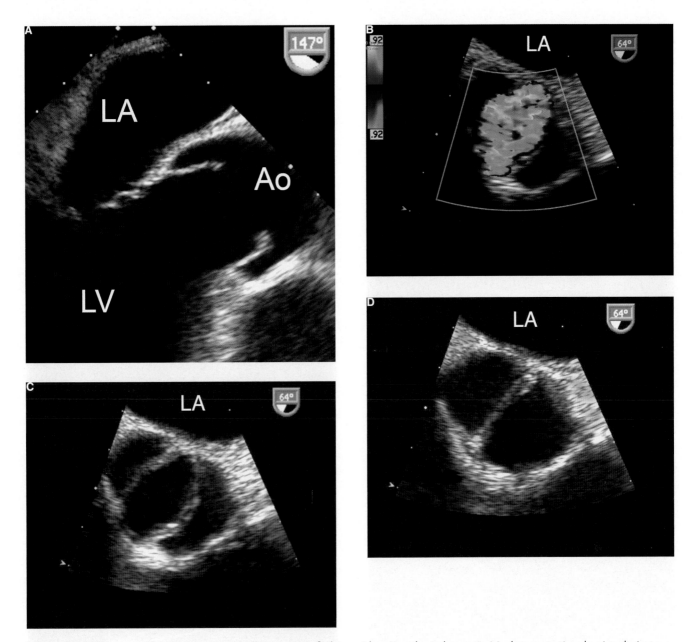

**Figure 80-2.** Transesophageal echocardiographic images of a bicuspid aortic valve in long axis (a), demonstrating doming during systole. A systolic short axis image with (b) and without (c) color Doppler demonstrates the "fish-mouth" orifice. The two leaflets are well shown in this diastolic frame (d). LA, left atrium; LV, left ventricle; Ao, aorta.

comprise thin fibrous membranes or more diffuse aortic hypoplasia. It is associated with thickened aortic cusps, coronary ostial obstruction, and dilation of the coronary arteries as is often seen in Williams syndrome, which also includes elfin facies, muscular peripheral pulmonary artery stenoses, and mental retardation (**Table 80-5**).

## Coarctation of the Aorta

Coarctation of the aorta accounts for 5 to 8% of congenital heart disease, and adults may present with either corrected or uncorrected lesions. Most commonly, there is a discrete band of tissue just distal to the take-off of the left subclavian artery opposite the aortic insertion of the ligamentum arteriosum.

Less commonly, the coarctation may be tubular or diffuse and may be in other locations including the abdominal aorta.

Symptoms and signs include:
- Systemic arterial hypertension (proximal to obstruction)
- Blood pressure discrepancy between upper and lower extremities, often with lower extremity pulse delay
- Left ventricular hypertrophy
- Bilateral lower extremity claudication

Aortic coarctation is associated with:
- Bicuspid aortic valve (~20-85%)
- Turner syndrome (**Table 80-5**)

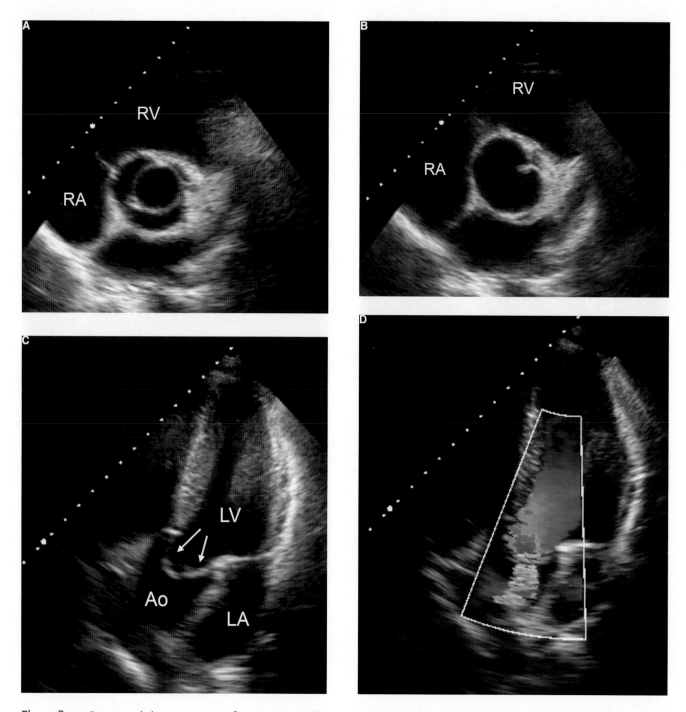

**Figure 80-3.** Parasternal short-axis images from a patient with a unicuspid aortic valve during systole (a) and diastole (b). The apical three-chamber view shows abnormal opening (doming) of the valve (c), and turbulence and aliasing at the level of the valve is demonstrated with color Doppler flow mapping (d). LA, left atrium; LV, left ventricle; RA, right atrium; RV, right ventricle; Ao, aorta.

- Berry aneurysms of the Circle of Willis and intracranial hemorrhage
- Endarteritis

Echocardiographic findings in coarctation of the aorta include (**Figure 80-5**):
- A discrete stenosis may be present on suprasternal notch images, but off-axis images often falsely suggest coarctation and 2D images must be confirmed by Doppler evidence of obstruction.
- The modified Bernoulli equation may be used to estimate the pressure gradient across a suspected coarctation. The suprasternal notch location usually allows ultrasound interrogation almost parallel to the direction of flow.
- An expanded version of the modified Bernoulli equation [$4 \times (V^2_{distal} - V^2_{proximal})$] should be used if the

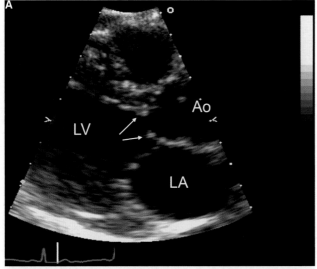

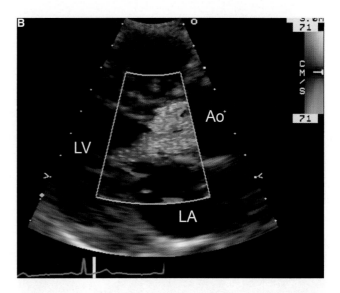

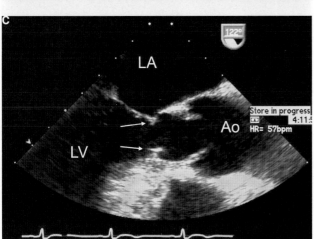

**Figure 80-4.** A parasternal long-axis view in a patient with a discrete subaortic membrane (arrows, a). Color Doppler (b) demonstrates increased velocity and turbulence during systole originating below the level of the aortic valve. A TEE image (c) from the same patient provides a clear view of the membrane (arrows). The patient also had a bicuspid aortic valve, as suggested by the doming of the aortic valve during systole. LA, left atrium; LV, left ventricle; Ao, aorta.

proximal aortic velocity is >1 m/s in order to prevent overestimation of the pressure gradient.

- With severe coarctation, the pressure gradient across the lesion persists beyond systole, resulting in continued antegrade flow during diastole. Diastolic runoff is a specific finding for hemodynamically important aortic coarctation.

## Patent Ductus Arteriosus (PDA)

The ductus arteriosus is a normal fetal connection between the descending aorta and pulmonary circulation. The ductus arteriosus usually closes soon after birth to become the ligamentum arteriosum. When persistent, it is termed a patent ductus arteriosus and permits blood flow from the systemic circulation to the pulmonary circulation. Over time, the left-to-right flow results in pulmonary arterial hypertension as well as left atrial and ventricular volume overload. The ductus arteriosus' pulmonary insertion is immediately to the left of the main pulmonary trunk at the takeoff of the left pulmonary artery. The systemic side

inserts into the descending aorta opposite the left subclavian artery.

Echocardiographic features of PDA include (**Figures 80-6 & 80-7**):

- PDA is usually best imaged in the adult from a slightly off axis (clockwise rotation) parasternal short axis view.
- A sagittal suprasternal notch view may also demonstrate PDA, but this view is often difficult to obtain in adults.
- Color Doppler imaging demonstrates continuous flow from the insertion of the ductus to the PA from the distal to the pulmonary valve.
- In the absence of severely elevated pulmonary pressures, spectral Doppler demonstrates continuous left-to-right flow with a peak velocity in late systole.
- With elevated pulmonary arterial pressure, there may be bidirectional flow across the PDA with right-to-left flow in early systole.
- The presence of left atrial and left ventricular dilation suggests a significant shunt causing left-sided volume overload.

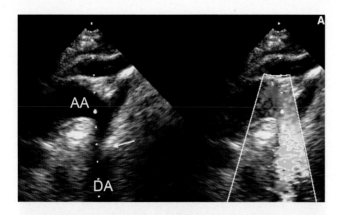

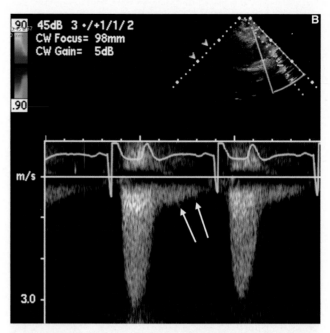

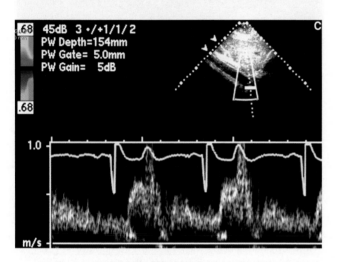

**Figure 80-5.** A transthoracic suprasternal notch view in a patient with coarctation of the aorta, suggesting stenosis distal to the left subclavian artery (arrows, a). There is turbulent blood flow with aliasing on color Doppler (a). Continuous-wave spectral Doppler across the coarctation demonstrates a peak velocity over 3 meters per second with continued antegrade flow across the defect through diastole (b). Likewise, pulsed wave spectral Doppler of the abdominal aorta shows pandiastolic antegrade aortic flow (c). AA, aortic arch; DA, descending aorta.

## Left Atrial Anomalies

The two main congenital malformations of the left atrium, cor triatriatum and supravalvular stenosing ring, are rare. The physiology of these obstructive lesions is similar to mitral stenosis.

Cor triatriatum describes a three-chamber left heart with a residual membrane resulting from incomplete incorporation of the pulmonary venous confluence into the left atrium. The degree of obstruction is variable, depending on the size of the perforation(s) in the membrane. A supravalvular stenosing ring is a similar thin membrane positioned just proximal to the mitral valve and may even be adherent to the mitral leaflets. Both cor triatriatum and supravalvular stenosing ring can often be seen using 2D echocardiography. The perforation(s) are usually not visible with 2D imaging but can be demonstrated with color Doppler echocardiography (**Figure 80-8**). These defects are associated with other left-sided obstructive lesions such as parachute mitral valve, subaortic stenosis, and aortic coarctation. The presence of multiple levels of left-sided stenoses is termed the Shone complex (note: this term has several definitions).

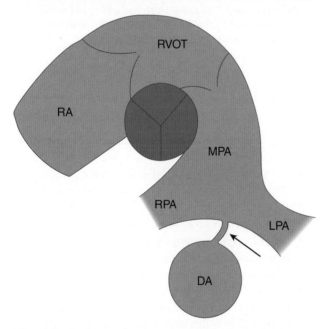

**Figure 80-6.** A diagram of the parasternal short-axis view at the aortic valve level. The ductus arteriosus (arrow) travels between the pulmonary trunk at the takeoff of the left pulmonary artery and the descending aorta opposite the left subclavian artery. DA, descending aorta; RA, right atrium; RVOT, right ventricular outflow tract; MPA, main pulmonary artery; RPA, right pulmonary artery; LPA, left pulmonary artery.

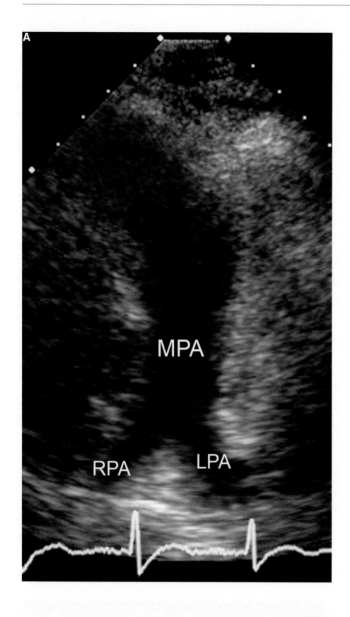

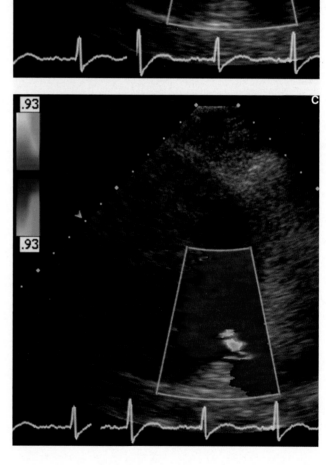

**Figure 80-7.** A parasternal view showing the main pulmonary artery branching into the left and right pulmonary arteries (a). Color Doppler demonstrates flow into the pulmonary artery at the level of the bifurcation during diastole (b) and systole (c). MPA, main pulmonary artery; RPA, right pulmonary artery; LPA, left pulmonary artery.

## Mitral Valve Defects

### Cleft Mitral Valve

A *cleft* mitral valve refers to a malformed mitral valve with an apparent cleft dividing the anterior mitral leaflet. Cleft mitral valve is usually associated with complete and partial atrioventricular canal (alternatively termed endocardial cushion) defects, although it can exist as an isolated lesion.

It reflects failure of complete fusion of the left aspect of the inferior and superior bridging leaflets.

Echocardiographic features of cleft mitral valve include (**Figure 80-9**):

- A divided anterior mitral valve leaflet (a trileaflet mitral valve), best seen in the parasternal short axis view.

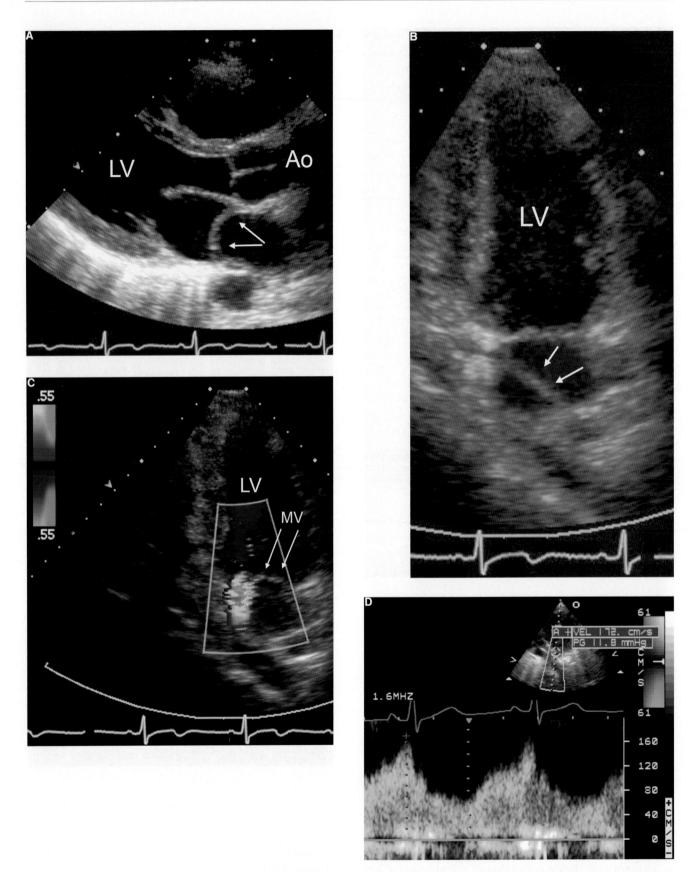

**Figure 80-8.** A parasternal long-axis view in a patient with cor triatriatum shows a membrane (arrows) dividing the left atrium (a). This can also be seen in this apical four-chamber image (arrows, b), and flow acceleration above the mitral valve is apparent with the addition of color Doppler flow mapping (c). There was a mild gradient across the membrane in this asymptomatic patient, as demonstrated by spectral Doppler (d). LV, left ventricle; MV, mitral valve; Ao, aorta.

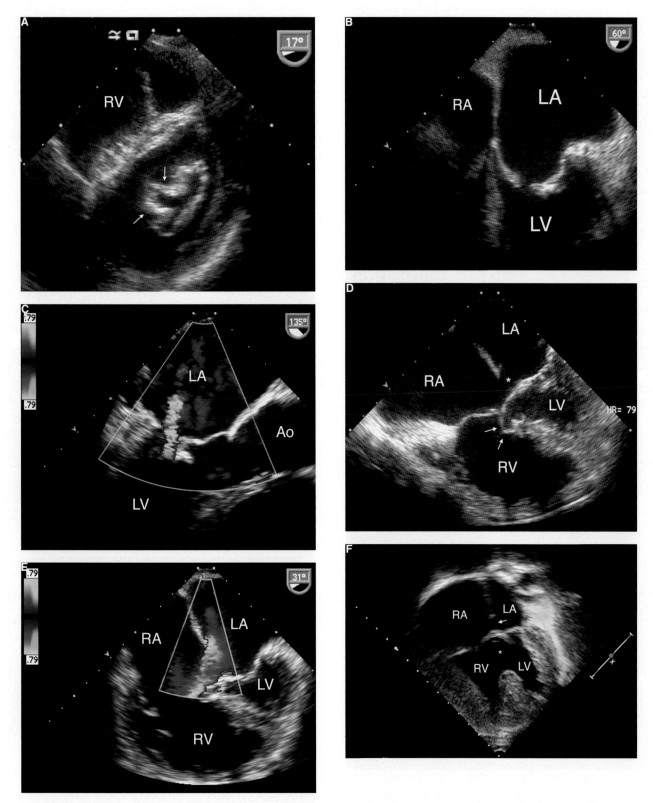

**Figure 80-9.** These transesophageal images from a patient with a partial atrioventricular canal defect demonstrate a "cleft" in the "anterior" leaflet of the mitral valve (arrows, a). As described in the text, the mitral valve is more accurately described as trileaflet. The abnormal architecture of the valve can lead to restricted opening (b), and occasionally causes hemodynamically significant mitral stenosis. More commonly, there is mitral regurgitation, often eccentric and posteriorly directed (c). Of note, the patient may have had a ventricular septal defect earlier in life, which is no longer patent. A "ventricular septal aneurysm," likely consisting of tricuspid valve tissue can be seen (arrows, d). Color flow mapping shows left-to-right flow across the primum atrial septal defect (e). A ventricular septal defect (asterisk) in conjunction with a primum atrial septal defect (arrows) is shown in another patient with a complete atrioventricular canal defect (f). LA, left atrium; LV, left ventricle; RA, right atrium; RV, right ventricle; Ao, aorta.

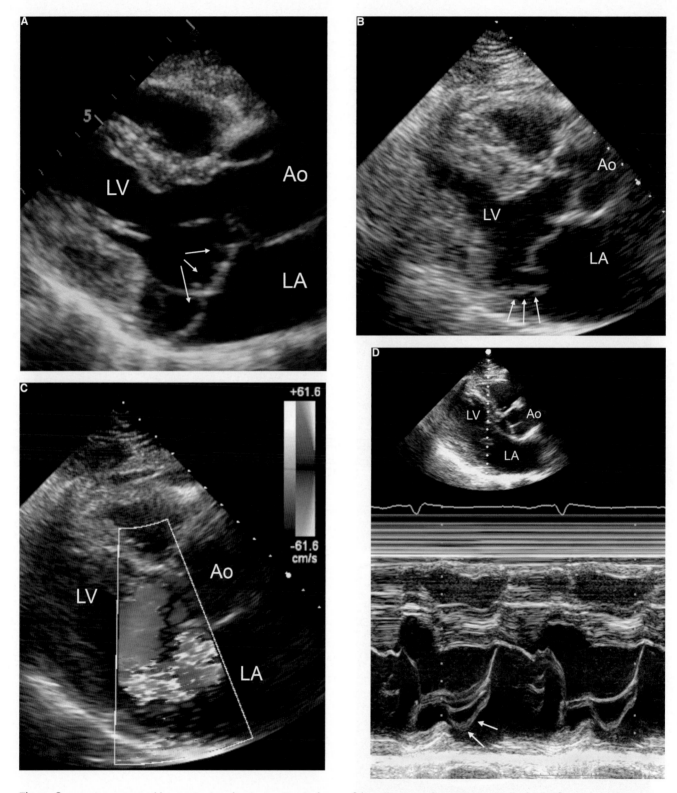

**Figure 80-10.** A parasternal long-axis view demonstrating prolapse of the anterior and posterior mitral valve leaflets (arrows) >2 mm beyond the mitral annulus (a). This parasternal long-axis image is from a patient with posterior mitral leaflet prolapse (arrows, b). As a result, there is anteriorly directed mitral regurgitation (c). M-Mode echocardiography demonstrates prolapse of the posterior leaflet into the left atrium in mid- to late-diastole (arrows, d). Apical four-chamber views also demonstrate the posterior leaflet prolapse (arrows, e) and eccentric mitral regurgitation (f). LA, left atrium; LV, left ventricle; Ao, aorta.

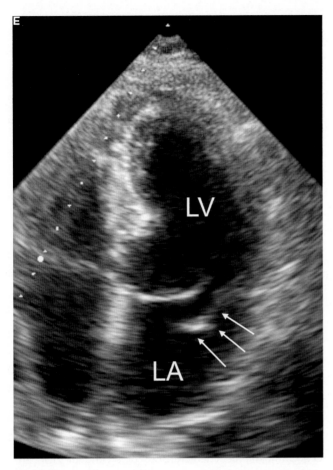

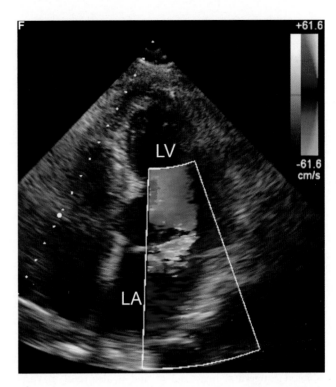

**Figure 80-10.** (continued)

- There is often eccentric posteriorly directed mitral regurgitation.
- It is important to look for associated lesions, especially those related to endocardial cushion defects (e.g., primum ASD, inlet ventricular septal defect [VSD]).

### Congenital Mitral Stenosis

Parachute mitral valve results when all the chordae tendinae insert onto a single, papillary muscle. Demonstration of the single papillary muscle with 2D imaging in the parasternal short axis view differentiates this lesion from rheumatic mitral stenosis as does the lack of commissural fusion. Double orifice mitral valve and anomalous mitral arcade are rare causes of congenital mitral stenosis.

### Mitral Valve Prolapse (MVP)

Mitral valve prolapse is seen in 2 to 4% of subjects with widely varying clinical significance. Prolapse of the mitral valve leaflets greater than 2 mm beyond the plane of the mitral annulus occurs frequently in healthy young women and usually has an excellent prognosis. The form of MVP related to progressive myxomatous mitral leaflet thickening, usually seen in older patients, is more commonly associated with significant mitral regurgitation.

The main echocardiographic features of MVP are (**Figure 80-10**):

- Prolapse of either or both of the mitral valve leaflets greater than 2 mm past the plane of the mitral annulus, best seen in the parasternal long axis view, defines MVP.
- M-Mode can also be used to demonstrate leaflet thickening and prolapse, when the cursor is directed just to the left atrial aspect of the mitral annulus in the parasternal long axis view.
- Myxomatous degeneration is frequently associated with ruptured chordae that may result in flail mitral leaflets.
- The mitral annulus is saddle-shaped so that apical views tend to overestimate the degree of prolapse and should not be used to make the diagnosis.
- Mitral regurgitation due to MVP is often mid-to-late systolic.
- The severity of associated mitral regurgitation is the main prognostic feature.

## Right Ventricular Outflow Obstruction

Right ventricular outflow obstruction can be divided anatomically into subvalvular, valvular, and supravalvular obstruction.

## Subvalvular Stenosis

Subvalvular stenosis is usually due either to fibromuscular stenosis or to right ventricular hypertrophy (RVH), causing dynamic obstruction of the right ventricular outflow tract.

- RVH often develops in patients with valvular pulmonary stenosis. Obstruction due to this hypertrophied muscle can complicate surgical or percutaneous treatment of the valvular lesion.
- Pulmonary atresia refers to complete obstruction of blood flow from the right ventricle to the pulmonary circulation via the right ventricular outflow tract (RVOT) and can occur at the subvalvar or valvar level. This complex and heterogeneous disease is relatively uncommon, and survival to adulthood with an intact ventricular septum without early intervention is very rare, although, it can occur in the presence of a VSD and with collateral flow to the pulmonary vasculature.

## Valvular Pulmonic Stenosis

Valvular pulmonic stenosis (PS) is a relatively common isolated congenital heart defect and is also seen in various syndromes including Noonan and Williams syndromes (**Table 80-5**). Mild pulmonary stenosis is usually well tolerated and does not require intervention. The most common treatment for moderate or severe pulmonary stenosis is balloon valvuloplasty.

Echocardiographic features of valvular pulmonic stenosis include (**Figure 80-11**):

- Thickened valve leaflets, which dome in systole (similar to bicuspid aortic valve).
- The modified Bernoulli equation is used to determine peak and mean gradients but is less accurate in the presence of multiple sequential stenoses (e.g., valvular and subvalvular obstruction) or with a long stenotic lesion.
- The modified Bernoulli equation can be used to determine right ventricular systolic pressure from the velocity of the tricuspid regurgitant jet. This can provide a general estimate of the maximal severity of the RVOT/valvular obstruction.
- M-Mode may demonstrate late diastolic opening of the pulmonary valve with atrial contraction in the setting of a noncompliant (restrictive) hypertrophied RV.

## Supravalvular Stenosis

Supravalvular stenosis may be due to proximal pulmonary artery stenosis or more distal branch pulmonary artery stenoses. Patients with congenital rubella syndrome often have pulmonary artery stenosis, and multiple distal muscular pulmonary artery stenoses are associated with Williams syndrome (**Table 80-5**).

## Atrial Septal Defects

ASDs comprise approximately 20% of ACHD. In general, they are associated with left-to-right shunts, which can be characterized echocardiographically by:

- Elevated Qp:Qs (a *significant* shunt is often defined by a Qp:Qs $\geq$ 1.5-2).
- Right atrial and right ventricular dilation.
- Paradoxical interventricular septal (IVS) motion, with the IVS bowing toward the left during diastole (a D-shaped IVS, **Figure 80-12**).
- In some cases, patients develop increased elevated pulmonary vascular resistance and consequent pulmonary artery hypertension. When severe, this can lead to a persistent D-shaped IVS during systole, **Figure 80-13**.

There are four major types of ASD (**Table 80-2**).

### Ostium Secundum ASD

Ostium secundum ASD is a defect of the septum primum and is located in the area of the fossa ovalis. It is the most common type of ASD (~70-80%), and it's the only ASD currently appropriate for percutaneous closure. The electrocardiogram usually demonstrates incomplete or complete right bundle branch block (RBBB) with normal or right axis deviation.

Echocardiographic characteristics of secundum ASD include the following (**Figure 80-14**):

- There is often echo dropout in the mid-septum at the level of the fossa ovalis, but because this structure is normally so thin, dependence on this finding in isolation (without evidence of right-sided volume overload or elevated Qp:Qs) may produce false positive results.
- Best seen from the subcostal view because the interatrial septum is in the near field (relative to an apical view) and is perpendicular to the ultrasound beam.
- Color and spectral Doppler flow across suspected defects (especially from the subcostal view) confirms the presence and direction of flow across a defect. Velocities are usually low because there is only a small pressure gradient between the right and left atria, especially in the setting of chronic left-to-right shunt.

### Ostium Primum ASD

Ostium primum ASD (primum, partial atrioventricular septal defect, partial atrioventricular canal defect) makes up ~15 to 20% of ASD and is associated with Trisomy 21 (Down syndrome, **Table 80-5**). This defect reflects abnormalities in endocardial cushion development. The electrocardiogram usually presents an incomplete or complete RBBB but can be differentiated by the presence of left axis deviation and an increased prevalence of first degree AV block. Primum ASD may be isolated but is often associated with

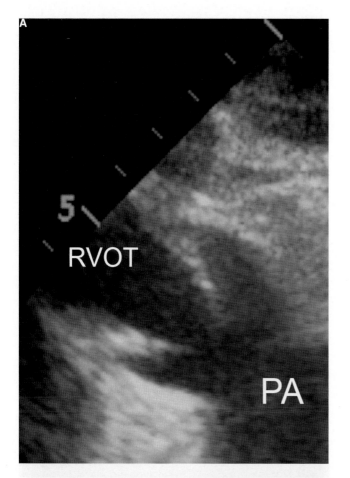

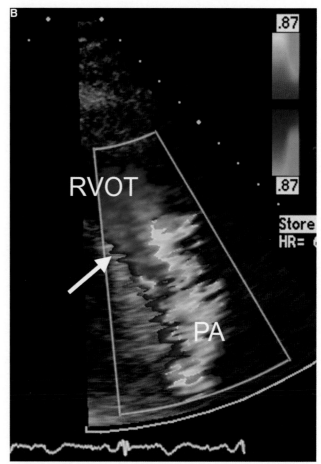

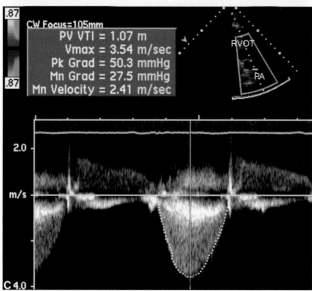

**Figure 80-11.** A parasternal view demonstrates doming of the pulmonary valve in this patient with valvular pulmonic stenosis (a). Color Doppler demonstrates systolic flow acceleration with aliasing and turbulent flow at the level of the valve (arrow, b). Spectral Doppler allows accurate estimation of the pressure gradient across the valve (c); in this case the peak gradient is just over 50 mm Hg, consistent with moderate pulmonary stenosis. RVOT, right ventricular outflow tract; PA, pulmonary artery.

other endocardial cushion abnormalities (**Figure 80-9**). The endocardial cushions contribute to adult cardiac structures including the lower atrial septum, the inlet ventricular septum, and most portions of mitral (anterior leaflet) and tricuspid (septal and anterior leaflets) valves. A complete atrioventricular canal defect is defined by the presence of a

primum ASD and an inlet VSD. It is also often associated with:

- Cleft mitral valve, with a defect of the A2 segment of the anterior mitral valve, permitting mitral regurgitation, which is often eccentric and directed posteriorly

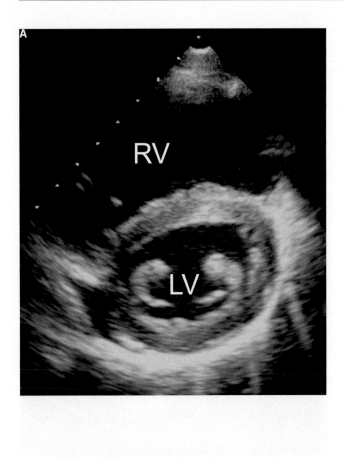

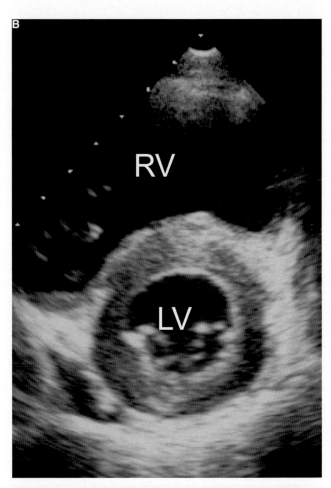

**Figure 80-12.** Parasternal short-axis images from a patient with right ventricular volume overload due to a sinus venosus defect. In diastole, the intraventricular septum is flattened (a), but returns to the normal configuration during systole (b). LV, left ventricle; RV, right ventricle.

- Widened commissure between the anterior and septal tricuspid leaflets

### Sinus Venosus Defects

Sinus venosus defects accounts for 5 to 10% of ASDs. They usually occur in the posterosuperior aspect of the atrium at the junction of the superior vena cava (SVC) and RA (superior sinus venosus defects, **Figure 80-15**), and thus are not truly defects of the atrial septum. Characteristics of sinus venosus defects include:

- Frequent association of superior sinus venosus defects with partial anomalous pulmonary venous return (usually the right superior and middle pulmonary veins draining to SVC/RA).
- Difficult to diagnose with transthoracic echocardiography (TTE) because of the posterosuperior location of defect. You should have a high index of suspicion in a patient with dilated right-sided chambers without other etiology.
- Contrast injection can help demonstrate shunt, but anatomic diagnosis often requires a transesophageal echocardiogram (TEE), computed tomography (CT), or magnetic resonance imaging (MRI).

### Unroofed Coronary Sinus Defect

Unroofed coronary sinus defects result in a communication between the LA and coronary sinus and are not truly defects of the atrial septum but they permit similar hemodynamic physiology and sequelae.

## Ventricular Septal Defects

VSDs are the most common congenital heart defects overall, but are less common among adults. Small defects often close spontaneously (50-80%) through several mechanisms including adherence of the tricuspid valve leaflets or subvalvular apparatus, myocardial hypertrophy, and fibrous ingrowth, whereas larger defects are often corrected in childhood. VSDs are classified by their physiology (degree of restriction to interventricular flow) and anatomic location.

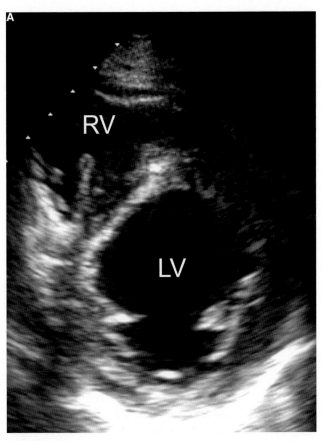 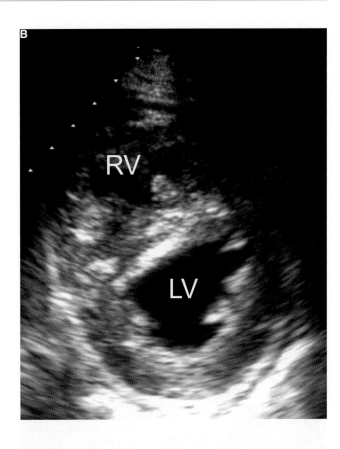

**Figure 80-13.** Parasternal short-axis images from a patient with right ventricular pressure overload. In diastole, the intraventricular septum is normal (a), but flattens (bows toward the left ventricle) during systole (b). LV, left ventricle; RV, right ventricle.

Physiologic classification is based on the size and resulting amount of flow between the left and right ventricles.

- Restrictive VSD
  - Small defect (less than one third the size of the aortic root)
  - High pressure gradient between left and right ventricles (usually >4 m/s or 64 mm Hg)
  - Not associated with elevations in right ventricular pressure or pulmonary arterial resistance

| Table 80-2 • Atrial Septal Defects | | | | | |
|---|---|---|---|---|---|
| **Type of ASD** | **% of ASD** | **Percutaneous Closure?** | **Other Names and Subtypes** | **Risk Factors** | **Associated Features and Syndromes** |
| Secundum | 70-80 | yes, with favorable anatomy | ostium secundum, fossa type | female (~60%) Trisomy 21 (less than primum) maternal alcohol use | Holt-Oram syndrome RBBB with normal or right axis of QRS |
| Primum | 15-20 | no | partial AV canal defect | Trisomy 21 | other endocardial cushion issues: -Inlet VSD -*Cleft* mitral valve -Wide anteroseptal tricuspid commissure RBBB with left axis deviation of QRS |
| Sinus venosus | 5-10 | no | superior inferior (rare) | | PAPVR (esp. with superior form) Atrial ectopic pacemaker |

*AV, atrioventricular; RBBB, right bundle branch block; VSD, ventricular septal defect; PAPVR, partial anomalous pulmonary venous return.*

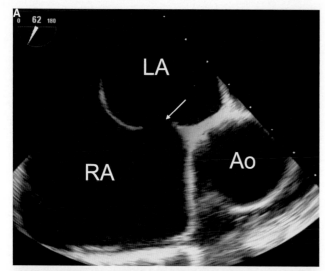

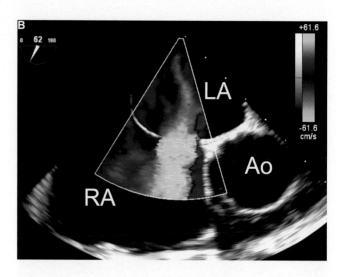

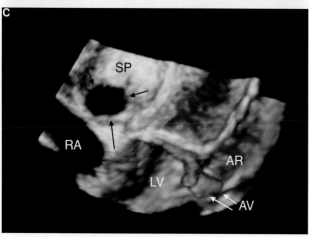

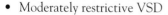

**Figure 80-14.** These transesophageal echocardiographic images demonstrate a secundum atrial septal defect (arrow, a), and color Doppler reveals left-to-right flow through the defect (b). Three-dimensional echocardiography shows the relationship between the defect and aortic valve (c). LA, left atrium; LV, left ventricle; RA, right atrium; RV, right ventricle; SP, septum primum; AR, aortic root; AV, aortic valve.

- Moderately restrictive VSD
  - Defect approximately half the size of aortic root
  - Moderate pressure gradient between left and right ventricles (~3 m/s or 36 mm Hg)
  - May be associated with right ventricular systolic hypertension, and patients may develop elevated pulmonary arterial resistance
- Nonrestrictive VSD
  - Large defect (larger than half the size of the aortic root)
  - Minimal pressure gradient between the left and right ventricles
  - Right ventricular systolic hypertension is universally present, and elevated pulmonary arterial resistance develops over time

Anatomic classification (**Table 80-3**, **Figure 80-16**) is based on the location of the VSD.

- Perimembranous VSD, also referred to as membranous VSD, is the most common type (~80%) of VSD. These VSDs are associated with a high rate of spontaneous closure (**Figure 80-17**).

- Muscular VSD accounts for ~10 to 15% of VSDs. Muscular VSD is further categorized by its location:
  - The inlet septum is derived from the endocardial cushions. The inlet septum divides the mitral and tricuspid valves.
  - The trabecular septum is created by the muscular invagination of the embryologic ventricle and is bordered by the apex, tricuspid insertions, and crista supraventricularis. Muscular VSDs are often multiple (*Swiss-cheese*) defects, especially trabecular VSD (**Figure 80-18**).
  - The outlet is the smooth-walled ventricular septum superior to the crista supraventricularis, derived from the conotruncal septum. Separates the RVOT and LVOT.
- Doubly committed subarterial or supracristal VSD is less common (~5-8%, also called infundibular), although it accounts for a higher proportion among East Asian patients (upwards of 25% of VSD in this population). Supracristal VSD are located between the LVOT and RVOT adjacent to the fibrous continuity between the pulmonary and aortic valves.

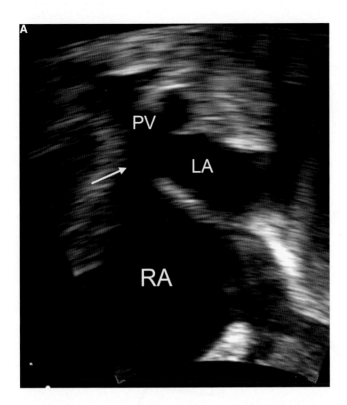

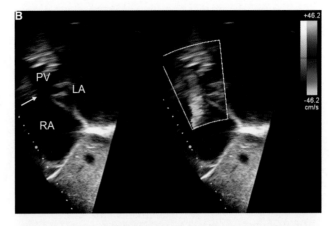

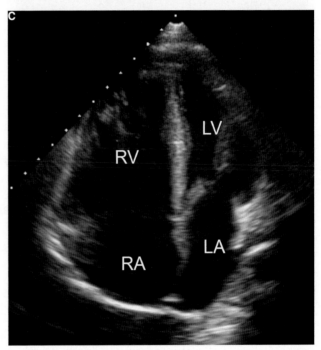

**Figure 80-15.** A sinus venosus atrial defect with partial anomalous venous return is demonstrated in these transthoracic echocardiographic images. There is a defect (arrow) in the superoposterior aspect of the atrial septum; the right upper and right middle pulmonary veins (PV) straddle the defect (a). Color Doppler demonstrates flow through the pulmonary veins and left-to-right flow through the ASD (b). The chronic right-sided volume overload leads to right atrial and right ventricular dilation (c). LA, left atrium; LV, left ventricle; RA, right atrium; RV, right ventricle; PV, pulmonary veins.

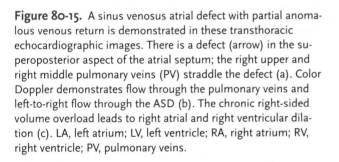

| Table 80-3 • Ventricular Septal Defects | | | |
|---|---|---|---|
| Type of VSD | % of VSD | Other Names or Subtypes | Associated Features and Syndromes |
| Perimembranous | 75-80 | membranous | |
| Muscular | 10-15 | inlet | AV canal defects |
| | | trabecular outlet | often multiple (*Swiss Cheese*) |
| Doubly committed, subarterial | 5-8 | supracristal, conoseptal | more common in East Asians |

*VSD, ventricular septal defect; AV, atrioventricular.*

Complications of VSD include:
- Elevated right ventricular pressure
- Elevated pulmonary arterial resistance
  - Eisenmenger physiology is near-equalization of right and left ventricular pressures due to markedly elevated pulmonary vascular resistance as the result of chronic left-to-right shunting.
- Left atrial and left ventricular volume overload
- Atrial arrhythmia, most commonly atrial fibrillation
- Bacterial endocarditis
  - Classically, endocarditis develops in locations with turbulent flow from the VSD. This often results in lesions on the tricuspid or pulmonary valves.
- Aortic regurgitation, most commonly with outlet muscular and doubly committed subarterial defects due to lack of support for the aortic annulus

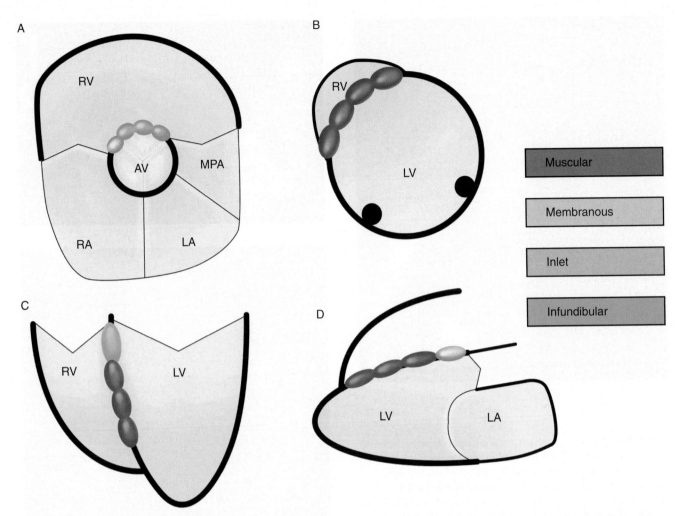

**Figure 80-16.** Diagrams showing the location of several anatomic types of ventricular septal defect in four common echocardiographic views: A- parasternal short-axis view at the level of the aortic valve. Well seen are membranous (perimembranous) and infundibular (supracristal) defects. B- parasternal short-axis view at the level of the left ventricular papillary muscles demonstrates muscular defects. C- apical four-chamber view allows visualization of inlet (canal-type) and muscular defects. D- parasternal long-axis view shows both membranous and muscular defects. RV, right ventricle; LV, left ventricle; RA, right atrium; LA, left atrium; MPA, main pulmonary artery; AV, aortic valve.

Other echocardiographic features of VSD include:

- With elevated right ventricular pressure, there may be bidirectional flow across the VSD.
- Left atrial and ventricular dilation reflect a significant shunt causing left-sided volume overload.
- Remember, there can be *less* flow across larger defects because of equalization of right and left ventricular pressure. This is shown by color flow Doppler as nonturbulent flow without aliasing.

## D-Transposition of the Great Arteries (D-TGA)

D-transposition of the great arteries involves ventriculoarterial transposition with the aorta arising from the morphologic right ventricle and the pulmonary artery from the morphologic left ventricle. There must be an associated lesion to allow mixing of deoxygenated systemic venous blood and oxygenated pulmonary venous blood. Otherwise, the cardiovascular system would comprise two entirely separate parallel circuits, a configuration that is incompatible with life. Possible shunt locations include ASD, VSD, and PDA. Other associated lesions include coarctation of the aorta and pulmonic stenosis.

The echocardiographic assessment of adults with D-TGA depends on the surgery performed to repair the defect. Surgical approaches include:

- The Mustard and Senning procedures involve baffling (redirecting) systemic venous blood to the left atrium (**Table 80-4**). These are often referred to as *atrial switch* operations. The morphologic right ventricle is the systemic ventricle with long-term complications (systemic tricuspid regurgitation, and systemic right

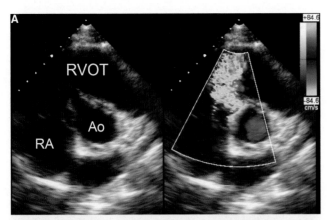

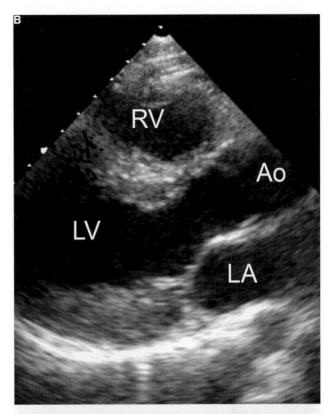

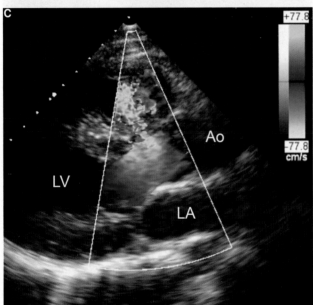

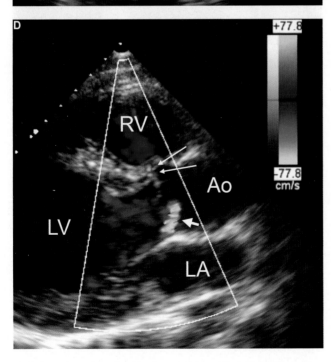

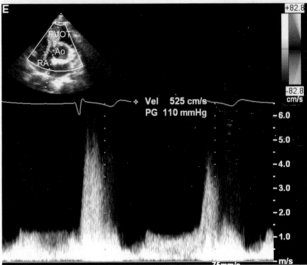

**Figure 80-17.** A perimembranous ventricular septal defect (VSD) is demonstrated with 2D and color Doppler flow mapping in the parasternal short-axis view at the level of the aortic valve (a). The defect is not seen on 2D parasternal long-axis images (b), but the likely presence of a VSD is suggested by color Doppler imaging during systole (c). In this diastolic parasternal long-axis image, there is diastolic left-to-right flow across the defect (black arrow, d). Also noted is the associated posteriorly directed aortic regurgitation (white arrow, d). Spectral Doppler reveals a high gradient across this restrictive perimembranous VSD (e). LA, left atrium; LV, left ventricle; RA, right atrium; RV, right ventricle; RVOT, right ventricular outflow tract; Ao, aorta.

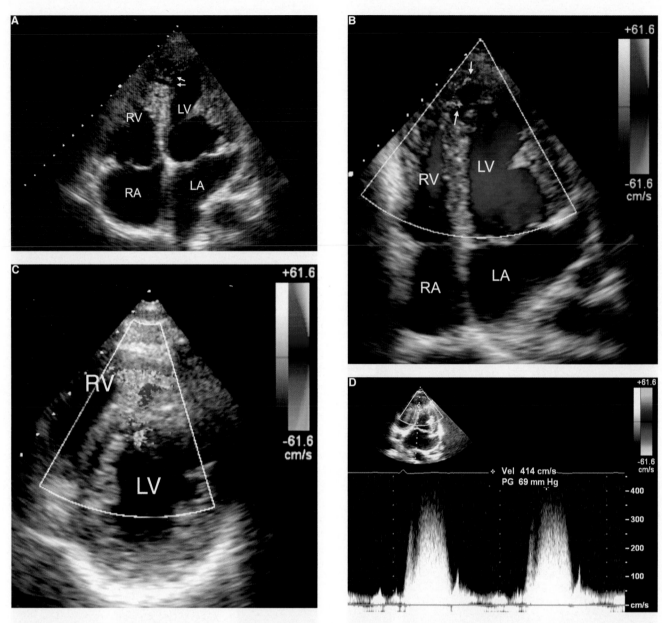

**Figure 80-18.** An apical four-chamber image suggests several small, muscular ventricular septal defects (VSD) near the apex (a), and color Doppler flow mapping confirms multiple left-to-right jets (arrows, b). The left-to-right flow across the defects is also seen in parasternal short axis with color Doppler (c). Spectral Doppler (d) demonstrates a high-velocity jet between the left and right ventricles in the setting of these small restrictive apical muscular VSD. LA, left atrium; LV, left ventricle; RA, right atrium; RV, right ventricle.

ventricular dysfunction) as outlined below for congenitally corrected transposition of the great arteries (ccTGA). Baffle leaks and stenoses are increasingly common with aging.

- The arterial switch procedure involves transposing the aorta and pulmonary artery (**Table 80-4**). This is the currently favored procedure because it results in a systemic left ventricle. The most technically challenging aspect of this operation, which prevented its widespread use for decades, is transferring the very small coronary arteries from the aorta to the neo-aorta (native pulmonary artery root).

Echocardiographic features of D-TGA include (**Figure 80-19**):

- The morphologic right ventricle receives blood from the morphologic right atrium and pumps blood to the aorta (**Table 80-1**).
- The aortic valve is usually anterior and right of the pulmonary valve (opposite normal configuration).
- The mitral and pulmonary valves share a fibrous continuity (similar to the normal aortomitral continuity).
- The aorta and pulmonary artery have a common parallel course.

| Table 80-4 • Basic Operations and Interventional Procedures for Palliation or Correction of Congenital Heart Defects | | | | | |
|---|---|---|---|---|---|
| **Operation or Procedure** | **Year Introduced** | **Common Diseases or Physiology** | **Description** | **Physiology** | **Long-term Issues** |
| Ligation of PDA | 1938 | PDA | First CHD surgery | | |
| Blalock-Taussig shunt | 1944 | TOF, other diseases with low pulmonary blood flow | Right subclavian artery to right PA shunt. Left-sided if the aortic arch is on right. Modified B-T shunt uses graft material to connect subclavian artery to PA. | Increase pulmonary blood flow | Pulmonary hypertension (if flow too great) stenosis or occlusion of shunt systemic ventricular volume overload |
| Potts/ Waterston shunts | 1946/1962 | TOF, other diseases with low pulmonary blood flow | Descending aorta to left PA/ascending aorta to right PA with side-to-side anastomosis | Increase pulmonary blood flow | Pulmonary hypertension (if flow too great) stenosis or occlusion of shunt distortion of PA anatomy systemic ventricular volume overload |
| Mustard/ Senning | 1964/1959 | D-TGA | Baffle systemic venous blood to left atrium and pulmonic venous blood to right atrium. Mustard uses pericardium or graft material and Senning uses native atrial tissue. | Create venoatrial discordance so systemic RV will receive oxygenated blood | Atrial arrhythmias systemic RV dysfunction systemic TV regurgitation |
| Glenn | 1958 | Single ventricle | SVC to PA shunt (~half-Fontan) | Increase pulmonary blood flow | |
| Rashkind | 1967 | D-TGA | Balloon atrial septostomy (percutaneous) | Allows mixing of oxygenated & deoxygenated atrial blood | |
| Fontan | 1971 | Single ventricle such as tricuspid atresia or (HLHS) | Diverts systemic venous return (SVC and IVC) to pulmonary artery | Single systemic ventricle with passive flow to pulmonary circulation | Atrial flutter and fibrillation protein losing enteropathy cirrhosis |
| Arterial switch | 1975 | D-TGA | Anatomic correction of D-TGA | | Great vessel dilation/ stenosis neo-aortic regurgitation coronary artery abnormalities |

PDA, patent ductus arteriosus; CHD, congenital heart disease; TOF, Tetralogy of Fallot; PA, pulmonary artery; D-TGA, D-transposition of the great arteries; RV, right ventricular; TV, tricuspid valve; SVC, superior vena cava; HLHS, hypoplastic left heart syndrome; IVC, inferior vena cava.

## Congenitally Corrected Transposition of the Great Arteries (ccTGA or L-TGA)

Congenitally corrected transposition of the great arteries occurs when the atria are in their normal position (situs solitus), but there is both atrioventricular and ventriculoarterial discordance. Thus, systemic venous blood returns to the morphologic right atrium and then flows to the morphologic left ventricle and on via the pulmonary artery to the lungs. The blood returns via the pulmonary veins to the morphologic left atrium, to the morphologic right ventricle, and out via the aorta to the systemic circulation. Patients with isolated ccTGA may be asymptomatic well into adulthood. Associated lesions, to a large degree, determine the clinical course of ccTGA. These include:

- VSD (60-80%), most often perimembranous.
- Pulmonic stenosis (30-50%).
- Ebstein-like tricuspid malformation (20-40%).
- Abnormal AV nodal position and the course of conduction system, often with dual AV nodes. There is a high incidence of complete heart block that increases with age.

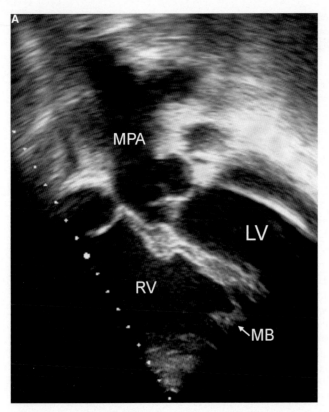

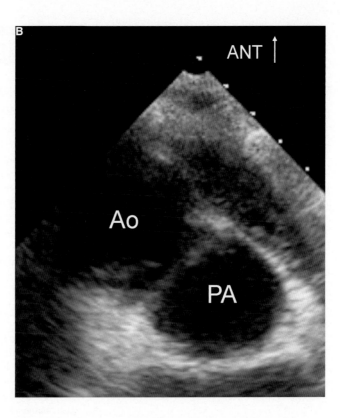

**Figure 80-19.** A transthoracic echocardiographic image from a patient with D-transposition of the great arteries demonstrating a connection between the morphologic left ventricle and the pulmonary artery (a). The aorta is positioned anterior and to the right of the pulmonary artery (b). LA, left atrium; LV, left ventricle; RV, right ventricle; MB, moderator band; MPA, main pulmonary artery; PA, pulmonary artery; Ao, aorta.

- Other associated lesions are less common including ASD, subaortic stenosis, and pulmonary atresia.
- Dextrocardia is present in 20%.

Surgical approaches to ccTGA include the classic approach and the double-switch operation. The classic approach addresses associated lesions such as VSD and outflow obstruction, but retains the right ventricle as the systemic ventricle. The double-switch operation involves both a Mustard or a Senning procedure (to redirect systemic venous blood to the left atrium and pulmonary venous blood to the right atrium) and an arterial switch (transposing the pulmonary artery and aorta).

Long-term issues for patients with ccTGA include:
- Heart block (see above)
- Systemic right ventricular dysfunction and secondary systemic tricuspid regurgitation leading to systemic right ventricular failure
- Bacterial endocarditis, especially with associated VSD or regurgitant valvular lesions
- Atrial arrhythmias are more common than ventricular arrhythmias and are associated with systemic right ventricular dysfunction and systemic tricuspid regurgitation.

Echocardiographic characteristics of ccTGA include (**Figure 80-20**):
- The morphologic right ventricle receives blood from the morphologic left atrium and pumps blood to the aorta. See **Table 80-1** for criteria to define the morphology of each structure.
- The aortic valve is anterior and left of the pulmonary valve.

## Ebstein's Anomaly

Ebstein's anomaly involves apical displacement of one or more leaflets of the tricuspid valve. Most common, the septal (+/− the inferior/posterior) leaflet attachment is apically displaced, whereas the anterosuperior leaflet is large and abnormally tethered to the free wall of the right ventricle. This results in a significant distance between the tricuspid annulus and the tricuspid valve orifice. This portion of the right side of the heart is referred to as the *atrialized* portion of the right ventricle. There is a wide spectrum of clinical severity mainly related to the size of the right ventricle (small ventricles have worse outcomes) and the degree of tricuspid regurgitation. The prognosis is poor in patients with a functional right ventricle less than one-third the size of the area below the tricuspid annulus. There are several associated lesions. Approximately

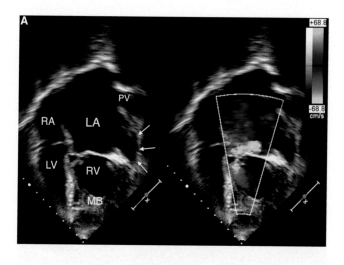

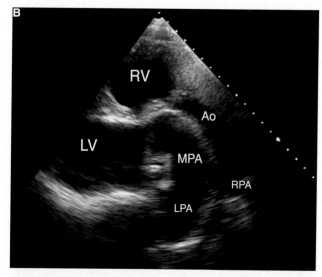

**Figure 80-20.** An apical four-chamber image from a patient with congenitally corrected transposition of the great arteries (a). The left atrium is identified by the presence of draining pulmonary veins as well as the narrow-based left atrial appendage (arrows). The right ventricle is characterized by an apically displaced valve and the presence of the moderator band. Color flow mapping demonstrates at least moderate systemic tricuspid regurgitation. A modified parasternal long-axis image demonstrates the posteriorly positioned left ventricle ejecting into the pulmonary artery, which is characterized by an early bifurcation into the left and right pulmonary arteries (b). LA, left atrium; LV, left ventricle; RA, right atrium; RV, right ventricle; MB, moderator band; PV, pulmonary vein; MPA, main pulmonary artery; RPA, right pulmonary artery; LPA, left pulmonary artery; Ao, aorta.

one half of patients have either an ASD or stretched patent foramen ovale (PFO) allowing interatrial shunting. There is also a high prevalence of accessory conduction pathways (e.g., Wolff-Parkinson-White), with the potential for 1:1 conduction of supraventricular tachycardia. This takes on increased significance given the high incidence of atrial tachyarrhythmias due to abnormal right atrial structure, right ventricular dysfunction, and tricuspid regurgitation.

Other associated lesions include:
- ccTGA
- Pulmonary stenosis or atresia
- Left ventricular dysfunction and mitral valve prolapse

Echocardiographic features include (**Figure 80-21**):
- The hallmark is a marked apical displacement of the septal tricuspid leaflet. The tricuspid valve is usually more apical than the mitral valve, but the difference is usually ≤8 mm/m² body surface area (BSA) or ≤20 mm.
- Variable degree of tricuspid regurgitation and, much less common, tricuspid stenosis
- It is important to determine the presence or absence of an atrial level communication such as a PFO or ASD.

## Tetralogy of Fallot (TOF)

Tetralogy of Fallot consists of four associated defects, which derive directly from anterior deviation of the infundibular septum. The four components of TOF are infundibular pulmonary stenosis, a large nonrestrictive VSD as a result of

septal malalignment, aorta overriding the right ventricular outflow tract, and right ventricular hypertrophy. The clinical presentation depends on the degree of pulmonary stenosis; the diagnosis can be delayed until adulthood in patients with very mild pulmonary stenosis and trivial right-to-left shunting.

The surgical approach to TOF can be divided into palliation and repair. Palliative surgical approaches include the Blalock-Taussig shunt and the Potts and Waterston shunts (**Table 80-4**). The goal of these operations is to increase pulmonary blood flow. The current surgical approach is early primary repair (alleviation of pulmonary stenosis and closure of VSD) without palliation, but most current adult patients with TOF will have had a palliative procedure prior to repair.

Early surgical approaches emphasized the importance of total alleviation of pulmonary stenosis with little concern about subsequent pulmonary regurgitation (PR). As a result, many adult patients have severe PR. This eventually leads to progressive RV dilation and dysfunction. As such, severe PR is the most common indication for reoperation in patients with repaired TOF.

Echocardiographic features of repaired TOF include (**Figure 80-22**):
- Severe PR is common, and the findings parallel those for severe AR.
  - Wide vena contracta

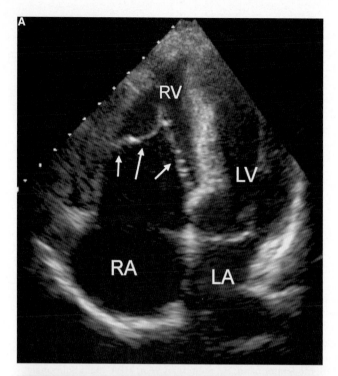

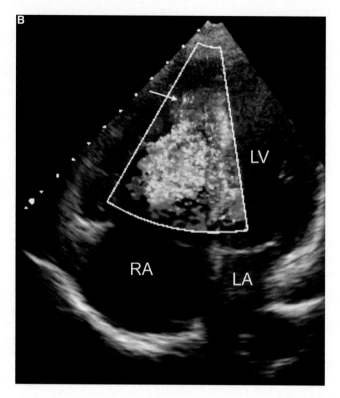

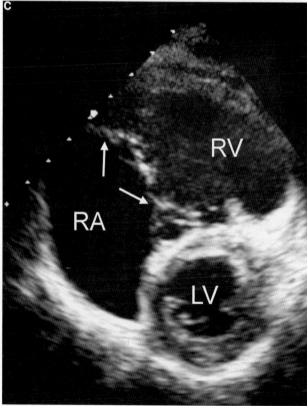

**Figure 80-21.** An apical four-chamber image from a patient with Ebstein's anomaly (a). There is marked apical displacement of the tricuspid valve (arrows), and a large right atrium inclusive of an 'atrialized' right ventricle. Color Doppler demonstrates significant tricuspid regurgitation (b). This parasternal short-axis image shows the tricuspid valve (arrows) insertion at the level of the left ventricular papillary muscles, as well as the presence of a dilated right ventricle (c). LA, left atrium; LV, left ventricle; RA, right atrium; RV, right ventricle.

- ○ Rapid deceleration time (pressure half-time <100 msec) of the pulmonary regurgitant flow velocity signal
- ○ Branch pulmonary artery diastolic flow reversal
- RVH is less common than RV dilation, because surgical approaches trade the PS for PR.

- Tricuspid regurgitation is also common, as a result of RV dilation.

Echocardiographic features of palliated or unoperated TOF include the four components of TOF and findings specific to a given palliative procedure (**Figure 80-23**).

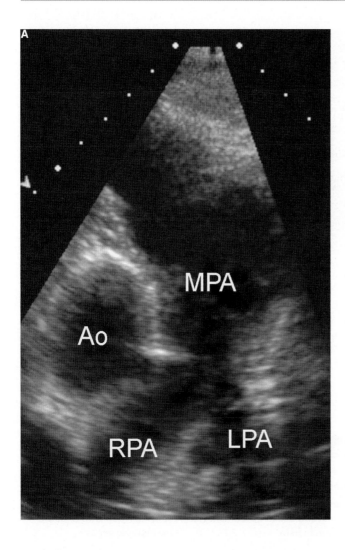

**Figure 80-22.** A parasternal image of the pulmonary artery in a patient with repaired tetralogy of Fallot (a). Color Doppler demonstrates a broad regurgitant jet (black arrow), as well as retrograde flow in the branch pulmonary arteries in this early diastolic frame. Severe pulmonary regurgitation is also suggested by the steep slope (short pressure half-time) of the regurgitant jet as measured by spectral Doppler (c). MPA, main pulmonary artery; RPA, right pulmonary artery; LPA, left pulmonary artery; Ao, aorta.

Other lesions associated with TOF include:

- Right-sided aorta in ~25%, often in patients with a 22q11 mutation (CATCH-22 syndrome, **Table 80-5**).
- Atrioventricular septal defect (AVSD) can be seen with TOF, especially with Trisomy 21 (**Table 80-5**).
- Approximately 3 to 5% have an aberrant left anterior descending coronary artery arising from the right coronary artery that crosses the RVOT anteriorly. In

this setting, incision of the RVOT (an approach to alleviate infundibular PS) can cause catastrophic anterior myocardial infarction.

## Arrhythmogenic Right Ventricular Cardiomyopathy/Dysplasia and Hypertrophic Cardiomyopathy

Although usually not clinically significant at birth, arrhythmogenic right ventricular cardiomyopathy/dysplasia

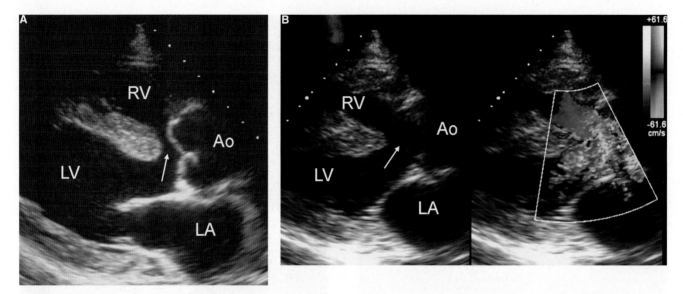

**Figure 80-23.** This parasternal long-axis image demonstrates a large ventricular septal defect (arrow) and overriding aorta (a portion of the aorta is positioned over the right ventricle), in an adult with unrepaired tetralogy of Fallot (a). Color Doppler during systole demonstrates flow from both the right and left ventricle toward the aorta. There is no predominant direction of flow across the nonrestrictive VSD, since the right and left ventricular pressures are equal.

## Table 80-5 • Heritable Syndromes Associated with Congenital Heart Disease

| Syndrome | Associated Congenital Heart Defects* | Other Associated Lesions | Genetic Defect |
|---|---|---|---|
| Noonan syndrome (OMIM 163950) | **PA stenosis, dysplastic PV with PS**, ASD, TOF, HCM | Short stature, webbed neck, sternal and ocular abnormalities, cryptorchidism | Autosomal dominant, abnormality on chromosome 12q, multiple genes |
| Williams syndrome (OMIM 194050) | **Supravalvular AS**, distal PA stenoses | Elfin facies, *cocktail* personality, hypercalcemia, elastin abnormality, cognitive impairment | Autosomal dominant, elastin gene and others (7q11.2) |
| Turner syndrome | Left-sided obstructive lesions especially **coarctation of the aorta (CoA)**, bicuspid AV, PAPVR | Short stature, webbed neck, sterility | 45 Xo karyotype |
| Down syndrome (OMIM 190685) | **AVSD**, VSD, ASD | Cognitive issues, single palmar crease, epicanthic fold of eyelid, Brushfield spots | Trisomy 21, ~50% have a congenital heart defect |
| Ellis-van Creveld syndrome (OMIM 225500) | Primum ASD, common atrium, partial AVSD | short limb dwarfism, polydactyly | Autosomal recessive (4p16) |
| Holt-Oram syndrome (OMIM 142900) | **Secundum ASD**, VSD | Abnormalities of radial aspect of forearms and hands | Autosomal dominant, TBX5 gene (12q21.4) |
| Multiple lentigines syndrome (Leopard syndrome) (OMIM 151100) | **Pulmonic stenosis**, conduction abnormalities | Multiple lentigines, hypertelorism, sternal malformation | Autosomal dominant, multiple genes |
| DiGeorge syndrome (CATCH-22, velocardiofacial syndrome) (OMIM 188400) | **Conotruncal abnormalities** (e.g., TOF), right-sided aortic arch | Hypocalcemia (parathyroid hypoplasia), thymic hypoplasia, cleft palate, abnormal facies | 22q11.2 deletion |

*The strongest associations are presented in bold font. AV, aortic valve; ASD, atrial septal defects; VSD, ventricular septal defect; AVSD, atrioventricular septal defect; TOF, Tetralogy of Fallot; PA, pulmonary artery; PV, pulmonary valve; PS, pulmonary stenosis.

(ARVC/D) is a rare heritable cardiomyopathy with significant importance to the adult cardiologist and echocardiographer. The most common presentation is of a young or middle-aged person with left bundle branch pattern ventricular ectopy. Electrographic findings include right precordial T wave inversions, prolonged ventricular depolarization in V1 to V3 out of proportion to V4 to V6, and Epsilon waves, usually seen in V1 and V2. Histopathologically, there is fibrous and fatty infiltration of the right ventricle and sometimes the left ventricle. Echocardiography has limited specificity for ARVC/D (MRI may provide more specific diagnostic information), because many diseases can cause echocardiographic findings similar to ARVC/D. These include:

- Dilated right ventricle with poor systolic function
- Thin RV free wall and apical RV aneurysms

Echocardiographic features of HCM include:

- LV hypertrophy, classically asymmetric septal hypertrophy
- Systolic anterior motion of the mitral valve, leading to LVOT obstruction
- Increased LVOT gradient with Valsalva maneuver

## Other Miscellaneous Lesions

### Left Superior Vena Cava (LSVC)

LSVC is present in approximately 0.5% of the general population and 10% of patients with congenital heart disease. The left anterior cardinal vein regresses to form the remnant ligament of Marshall. Failure of regression results in a persistent LSVC, which usually drains via the coronary sinus if there is no bridging vein between the left and right brachiocephalic veins, resulting in normal drainage of systemic venous blood to the right atrium. A dilated coronary sinus, reflecting increased flow, should raise suspicion for a left LSVC. The diagnosis can be confirmed with injection of agitated saline into a left upper extremity vein, causing opacification of the coronary sinus.

### Total and Partial Anomalous Pulmonary Venous Return (TAPVR, PAPVR)

TAPVR is almost universally fatal early in life if not surgically repaired. PAPVR, on the other hand, is often asymptomatic and presents in adulthood. PAPVR is associated with ASD, especially sinus venosus defects (**Figure 80-16**). More than 90% of patients with sinus venosus defects have PAPVR, most frequently a superior sinus venosus defect with anomalous return of the superior or middle pulmonary vein to the right atrium. Up to 10% of patients with secundum ASD have PAPVR.

The *scimitar syndrome* is a subtype of PAPVR where the inferior right pulmonary veins (+/– the middle and superior right pulmonary veins) course below the diaphragm to the IVC.

- The portion of the lung associated with the anomalous venous drainage is often hypoplastic, as is the pulmonary artery supplying the territory (a phenomenon not usually associated with other forms of PAPVR).
- The name derives from the appearance of the lesion on chest radiography (like a scimitar, or Turkish sword).
- On echocardiography, the main diagnostic finding is a "*hepatic*" vein (the anomalous pulmonary vein) bridging the diaphragm. The Qp:Qs is mildly elevated.

## Suggested Readings

1. Gatzoulis MA, Webb GD, Daubeney PEF. Diagnosis and management of adult congenital heart disease. *Churchill Livingstone.* 2003.

2. Feigenbaum H, Armstrong WF, Ryan T. Feigenbaum's echocardiography, 6th ed. *Lippincott Williams & Wilkins.* 2005.

3. Care of the adult with congenital heart disease. Presented at the 32nd Bethesda Conference, Bethesda, Maryland, October 2—3, 2000. *J Am Coll Cardiol.* 2001;37:1161–1198.

4. Gersony WM, Rosenbaum MS. Congenital heart disease in the adult. *McGraw-Hill.* 2002.

5. Brickner ME, Hillis LD, Lange RA. Congenital heart disease in adults. Two parts: *N Engl J Med.* Jan 2000, Jan 27;342:256, and *N Engl J Med.* Feb 2000, Feb 3;342:334.

# 81

# Catheter Closure of Intracardiac Shunts

Joseph D. Kay

## ● PRACTICAL POINTS

- Atrial septal defects cause primary left-to-right intracardiac shunts, which lead to right atrial and right ventricular dilation, and late atrial arrhythmias. Many patients with these defects will be minimally symptomatic in childhood and early adulthood, but progress to have symptoms by the fourth to fifth decade of late, in part secondary to an increased magnitude of left-to-right shunting with increased left atrial pressure with age.

- Only secundum atrial septal defects with adequate surrounding rims are appropriate for transcatheter device closure.

- Patent foramen ovale is a transient connection between the right and left atria, which usually does not allow for significant shunting at rest, but at times maneuvers such as valsalva, which increases right atrial pressures, can cause right-to-left shunting. Potential indications to close these defects include hypoxemia caused by shunting through these defects, cryptogenic strokes believed to occur through paradoxical embolism through the defect, and severe migraine headaches, although further research is needed to clearly define indications for closure of these common defects.

- Ventricular septal defects cause predominantly left atrial and left ventricular dilation secondary to volume overload, but can occasionally lead to right ventricular dilation and hypertrophy in the case of larger shunts and with the development of pulmonary hypertension.

- Ventricular septal defects are heterogeneous, with four types. Although there is experience with transcatheter closure of perimembranous defects, the higher rate of heart block compared with surgical closure has thus far precluded routine use of this technique. Outlet ventricular septal defects are close to the aortic and pulmonary valves, and this makes them rare candidates for device closure. Muscular defects can frequently be closed via a transcatheter route, although it is technically much more challenging than closure of secundum atrial septal defects.

- Patent ductus arteriosus causes left heart enlargement, and can lead to pulmonary hypertension. Transcatheter occlusion has become the preferred method of choice outside the neonatal period, with high success rate.

Physicians involved with the closure of cardiac shunts, whether at the atrial, ventricular, or great arterial level, need to understand the pathophysiologic consequences of each lesion in order to understand the risk/benefit ratio of closure, whether surgical or via catheterization. Pretricuspid level left–to-right shunts cause right atrial and ventricular volume overload and dilation. This occasionally causes symptoms such as failure to thrive or recurrent pulmonary infections in early childhood but frequently does not lead to symptoms such as atrial arrhythmias and right heart failure until the fourth or fifth decade of life. With aging, especially with comorbid conditions such as hypertension, left atrial pressure increases, leading to increased left-to-right shunting through an atrial level shunt and therefore increased shunting and right ventricular volume loading with time. Persistence of the patent foramen ovale (PFO) is common, with an incidence of 20 to 30% of the population, and should only be considered pathologic in certain circumstances, as will be discussed later. Although closure of such defects carries a low risk, an approach to close all defects detected noninvasively would invariably lead to iatrogenic complications in patients who may never have otherwise encountered problems related to this variance of the normal anatomy. Whereas none of the pretricuspid level shunts place the patient at risk for endocarditis (provided they are not associated with other cardiac defects), closure to prevent such a problem is unwarranted. Ventricular septal defects (VSDs) lead primarily to volume loading of the left ventricle, although the right ventricle is affected as well with larger defects. Other late complications can occur with VSDs such as late right or left ventricular outflow tract obstruction, pulmonary hypertension, endocarditis, damage to either the aortic or tricuspid valves, and mitral annular dilation with secondary regurgitation. In childhood, this lesion is less likely to be missed secondary to the loud systolic murmur. Patency of the ductus arteriosus (PDA), like VSDs, leads to volume loading of the left ventricle and secondary left ventricular dilation, pulmonary hypertension of varying degrees, as well as risk of endarteritis during periods of bacteremia.

## ATRIAL LEVEL SHUNTS

Catheter closure of atrial level shunts was among the earliest therapies for catheter-based devices for cardiac defects, first described in humans in 1976. It took more than 2½ decades, however, for improved devices to be approved by the U.S. Food and Drug Administration (FDA) for the closure of cardiac septal defects. In 2001, the FDA approved the CardioSEAL® device (NMT, Boston, MA) for closure of VSDs felt to be at high risk for surgical closure and the Amplatzer atrial septal occluder (AGA, Golden Valley, MN) for closure of secundum atrial septal defects measuring 4 to 38 mm in diameter. In 2006, the FDA approved a second device called the HELEX® septal occluder (Gore, Flagstaff, AZ) for closure of small to moderate-sized secundum atrial septal defects no larger than 20 mm. In 2008, the Amplatzer cribriform atrial septal occluder was approved for closure of multifenestrated atrial septal defects (**Figure 81-1**). A number of other devices are currently in trials for closure of PFOs. These trials are studying the efficacy of a PFO closure compared to medical therapy of the prevention of recurrent systemic thromboembolic events for the treatment of severe migraine headaches.

### Secundum Atrial Septal Defects (ASDs)

As stated above, there are currently three devices that have received FDA approval for closure of secundum atrial

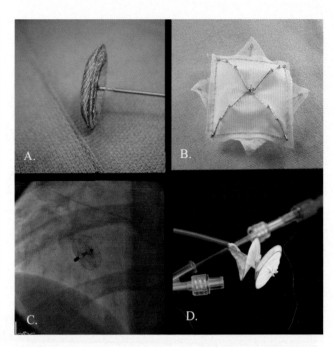

**Figure 81-1.** The four devices approved by the FDA and used for closure of secundum atrial septal defects. (A) The Amplatzer septal occluder (ASO) attached to the delivery cable. The cable is attached to the smaller right atrial disc, with the left atrial disc slightly larger. The size of the middle waist, not well seen in this photograph, is chosen to correspond to the ASD size during balloon sizing. The device consists of 54 Nitinol wires welded together with three Dacron sheets sewn into each of the three discs. (B) The CardioSEAL occluder, made from two polyester sheets attached to two flexible hinged metal frames. Each frame is of identical size. (C) An implanted 18-mm Amplatzer cribriform occluder in a **left anterior oblique** (LAO) projection. Note the central waist is a thin pole, allowing it to be placed through the central most defect in the fenestrated septum, regardless of size. The right and left atrial discs are of identical size for all three sizes of this device. (D) HELEX atrial septal occluder as it is packaged, preloaded in this case with the right atrial disc partially retrieved within the delivery sheath. The thin white thread is the retrieval cord that allows retrieval of the device even after deployment of the locking loop. The device consists of a single Nitinol wire, which forms both the right and left atrial discs, as well as the locking loop. The device is covered by a polytetrafluoroethylene (PTFA) membrane to allow for defect closure. This device is the most flexible of the four devices.

septal defects, with many practitioners having used the CardioSEAL device off label for this purpose (**Table 81-1**). The multicenter trial performed to assess the success and risk of ASD occlusion with the Amplatzer atrial septal occluder (ASO) had an overall success rate of more than 97%,[1] with few complications, making catheter closure of appropriate ASDs preferred over surgery in most centers throughout the developed world. Because these defects may coexist with other congenital cardiac defects that are not always readily apparent on transthoracic echo, care must be taken to ensure that no such defects exist, which would require surgical

| Table 81-1 • List of Available FDA Approved Devices that have been Used for Closure of Secundum Atrial Septal Defects. Although the CardioSEAL Device Received FDA Approval for VSD Closure, It has Also been Used Extensively for ASD Occlusion. | | | | |
| --- | --- | --- | --- | --- |
| **Device** | **Manufacturer** | **Year of Approval** | **Available Device Sizes** | **Closable Sizes of Defects** |
| Amplatzer septal occluder (ASO) | AGA Medical (Golden Valley, MN) | 2001 | 4-20 mm (by increments of 1 mm) 20-38 (by increments of 2 mm) | 4-38 mm (40 mm device available under HDE) |
| Amplatzer cribriform septal occluder | AGA Medical (Golden Valley, MN) | 2008 | 18, 25, 35 mm | multiple small and large defects |
| HELEX septal occluder | Gore (Flagstaff, AZ) | 2006 | 15, 20, 25, 30, 35 mm | defects up to 20 mm |
| CardioSEAL | NMT Medical (Boston, MA) | 2001 (for VSDs) | 17, 23, 28, 33 mm | defects up to 20 mm |

intervention. Therefore, most centers perform a careful transesophageal echocardiogram (TEE) in adults prior to attempted closure, a careful TEE, or an intracardiac echo (ICE) at the time of closure in children. Although some experienced structural interventionalists report closure without ultrasound guidance, this is not recommended in routine practice, because deficient septal rims can lead to device prolapse into either the right or left atrium, leading to device failure and embolization. Therefore, TEE or ICE guidance for successful closure is recommended to ensure adequate positioning of the device and stability, for which fluoroscopy is not always adequate.

Patients felt to be candidates for device closure should be pretreated with aspirin prior to catheterization. Prior to crossing the defect, the patient is systemically anticoagulated to maintain a minimum activated clotting time of 200 seconds in order to prevent systemic thromboembolism. It is currently recommended to balloon size the defect under ultrasound and X-ray guidance in order to most accurately size the diameter of the defect (**Figure 81-1**). A device of the same size (central waist), or only slightly larger than the balloon-sized measurement of the defect, is recommended for the ASO. Oversizing of the device has been suggested to be the cause of rare late erosion.[2] If choosing the HELEX device for closure, it is recommended that the device diameter be a minimum of 1.8 times the balloon stretched diameter. Failure to size as such has been shown to lead to incomplete closure.[3] As shown in **Table 81-1**, the HELEX device is manufactured in diameters of 15, 20, 25, 30, and 35 mm and, therefore, the largest defect size appropriate for the HELEX device is one that has a balloon stretched diameter of ≤20 mm.

Each of the devices has its own advantages and disadvantages. The choice of closure device should depend upon the patient, the anatomy of the defect, and the operator's experience. The Amplatzer device is technically a little simpler to deploy and is designed to close a larger spectrum of defects. The HELEX device, although slightly more technically

demanding to deploy with a more complex locking loops system, offers the advantage of a much more flexible device with less Nitinol wire. This offers the theoretical advantage of fewer, longer term complications. This may be more important if the position of the defect is such that the device's edges lie immediately adjacent to the atrial free wall or the mitral valve, particularly in smaller children or in more posterior/inferior defects. In addition to adequate heparinization, judicial flushing of the lines and delivery systems is required during catheter exchanges and device loading to avoid air embolization into the systemic circulation. In preparation for the insertion of the ASO, the delivery sheath is advanced into the left atrium over a stiff guidewire stabilized in a pulmonary vein (usually the left upper vein). The guidewire is removed while paying careful attention to eliminating all of the air from the sheath. With a continuous saline flush system, the device is advanced to the tip of the sheath, after which the delivery system and sheath are withdrawn back into the body of the left atrium. Under both echo and fluoroscopic guidance, the sheath is pulled back while fixing the delivery system in place, exposing the left atrial disc. This disc is then carefully pulled back to the left atrial surface of the atrial septum with careful attention being paid to ensure that portions of the disc do not prolapse into the right atrium. The delivery cable is then fixed in place and the sheath is withdrawn, allowing expansion of both the central and right atrial discs. Careful attention is then paid to the device positioning to ensure that neither disc has prolapsed into the other chamber and the device is not interfering with the mitral valve function or obstructing the pulmonary vein flow. The stability of the device is tested within the septum with a gentle push pull. Until this point, the device can be withdrawn back into the delivery sheath easily and removed if the sizing was inappropriate or the defect anatomy does not allow for stable device insertion (**Figure 81-2**). The delivery cable is then unscrewed, releasing the device. Potential problems that may occur include misalignment of the device with embolization, right or left

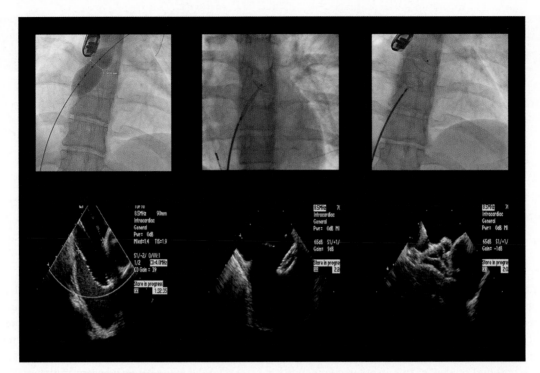

**Figure 81-2.** This panel shows the individual steps of ASD occlusion. The far left panel shows balloon occlusion of the defect to assess its size, as seen on fluoroscopy in the upper panel, and intracardiac echo (ICE) in the lower panel. The middle panels show left atrial disc deployment of an ASO, in fluoroscopy in the upper panel, and ICE in the lower panel. The two panels on the far right show the fluoroscopy and ICE images of the device after right atrial disc expansion, prior to device release. The ICE more clearly confirms appropriate positioning of the two sides of the device, without prolapsing into either chamber.

atrial injury, heart block (rare but seen more commonly in young children), atrial arrhythmias, thrombus formation on the delivery equipment of the device with systemic embolization, and vascular injury.

The Amplatzer fenestrated occluder is available for closure of the more rare atrial septal anatomy consisting of multiple fenestrations. This device comes in three sizes—18 mm, 25 mm, and 35 mm—with the right and left atrial discs identical in size. The central waist is narrow, allowing for placement of the defect through the most central defect, no matter what size, to allow the discs to cover all of the other defects as well. Delivery is otherwise identical to the Amplatzer atrial septal occluder.

The HELEX device comes preloaded within the delivery sheath (**Figure 81-1**). The device is withdrawn into the sheath, and the sheath can be advanced directly through the defect or advanced over a guidewire in the pulmonary vein, similar to the Amplatzer device. The left atrial disc is then advanced into the left atrium. Once the central locking loop portion of the device is outside the sheath, the device is pulled back to engage the atrial septum. If the operator is comfortable and there is adequate positioning within the left atrium, the right atrial disc is pushed out of the sheath. After adequate positioning of both discs is confirmed with

fluoroscopy and echo, the most proximal portion of the Nitinol frame is released. This proximal end of the wire serves as the locking loop that springs forward and secures the right and left atrial discs together. The confirmation of the proper closure of this locking mechanism by fluoroscopy is important, otherwise device withdrawal is required. The device can easily be withdrawn back into the delivery sheath and redeployed at any point prior to the release of the locking loop. After the release of the locking loop, the device can still be retrieved but cannot be redeployed. Discussion of the technique for CardioSEAL deployment in the atrial septum will not be discussed, as it is not formally FDA approved for this indication.

Each of these devices has been reported to have more than a 93% initial success rate in premarketing trials for closure of defects, with closer to 100% closure rate at 6 months if preselection of patients is done carefully. Long-term studies on the safety of these FDA approved devices are lacking at the time of this writing, but excellent long-term safety has been reported with older experimental devices. Follow-up for these patients should include postprocedure echocardiogram, with a follow-up within the 1st month after closure, as well as 6 months, 12 months, and periodically thereafter to screen for late device malfunction. A few rare complications include device fracture or erosion, the later of which has been reported for the Amplatzer device even more than 1 year after implant. Antiplatelet therapy is recommended with full dose aspirin and spontaneous subacute bacterial endocarditis (SBE) for 6 months after device insertion.

## Patent Foramen Ovale

Because of their ease of access, the devices listed above have been used by many physicians for closure of the PFO off label for various clinical scenarios. Potential indications for closure of the PFO include the prevention of recurrent systemic thromboembolic events, platypnea-orthodeoxia (right-to-left shunting through the atrial level shunt leading to systemic hypoxemia with activity), the prevention of paradoxical embolism and decompression illness in divers, and the treatment of severe recurrent migraine headaches. Because the incidence of PFO is believed to be as high as 25 to 30%, indications for closure for this device must be carefully defined. Although device closure is associated with a low incidence of complications, large-scale closure will invariably lead to complications in patients who may not clinically benefit from the procedure. Where as most clinicians would agree that closure is warranted for patients with right-to-left shunting through an atrial level defect resulting in systemic hypoxemia in the absence of severe pulmonary hypertension, for prevention of recurrent cryptogenic strokes and as a treatment for migraines, it has not been proven to be superior or equivalent to medical therapy. Hence, routine practices of doing so may be exposing the patients to increased risk. Young adults who have suffered from cryptogenic strokes have been shown to have a higher incidence of PFOs, believed to be the route for a venous thromboembolism to reach the cerebral circulation. It has been shown in a retrospective case series that defect closure has decreased the incidence of recurrent neurological events compared to historic controls on medical therapy alone, but prospective randomized trials have yet to be completed as proof of efficacy. In fact, enrollment in these randomized trials has been slow, partly due to a large number of closures being performed off label based upon patient and referral provider preference rather than enrollment in the prospective randomized trials. At the time of this writing, there are currently three trials under way in the United States and two abroad looking at the efficacy of PFO closure versus the best medical therapy in prevention of recurrent cryptogenic strokes. The RESPECT trial, sponsored by AGA Medical, randomizes patients with image-proven cryptogenic stroke to closure with their investigational PFO device versus the best medical therapy. Their PFO device is similar to the cribriform ASD device in that it comes in three sizes—18 mm, 25 mm, and 35 mm. The difference and potential advantage of the PFO device are that all three device sizes have a small left atrial disc—size 18 mm—providing less foreign material in the left atrium as a potential nidus for thrombus formation prior to device endothelialization. The CLOSURE I, sponsored by NMT Medical (manufacturers of the CardioSEAL device), randomized patients with a transient ischemic attack (TIA) or cryptogenic stroke to the best medical therapy versus their investigational STARFlex® device, which represents modifications of the CardioSEAL. Enrollment began in 2003, with patient enrollment complete as of this writing. The third trial is REDUCE, sponsored by Gore, which randomizes patients with proven TIA or cryptogenic stroke to the best medical therapy or closure of the PFO with the HELEX atrial septal occluder, with enrollment having started in 2008. Until data from these trials are available, the current American Heart Association/American Stroke Association (AHA/ASA) guidelines[4] and American College of Chest Physicians guidelines (ACCP)[5] recommend antiplatelet therapy for TIA or ischemic stroke in the setting of PFO unless a condition exists suggesting the need for vitamin K antagonists (Class IIa recommendation, Level of evidence C). They mention that as insignificant data exist to recommend PFO closure, after a first neurological event for patients not previously on medical therapy, PFO occlusion should only be considered for patients with recurrent cryptogenic stroke on medical therapy (Class IIb recommendation, Level of evidence C).

Clinical trials for PFO device occlusion in the treatment of migraine headaches are complicated by the subjective nature of the migraine reporting and the large potential for bias. The first randomized trial evaluating the efficacy of PFO closure in the treatment of migraines, MIST I,[6] failed to show a significant benefit for those randomized to closure with the STARFlex device, although many critics feel the trial was flawed, with a low complete occlusion rate. A follow-up trial, MIST II, has been performed using the same device, with recruitment at or near completion. A recent trial conducted by St. Jude Medical (ESCAPE), in which patients were randomized to catheterization with or without closure with their novel PFO device (patient blinded to randomization assignment with all patients receiving a catheterization), discontinued enrollment early secondary to poor enrollment. An ongoing trial by AGA (PREMIUM) is attempting to answer this question with a similar trial design using their PFO device, with results hopefully available within the next couple of years.

The anatomy of the PFO can be very heterogeneous, some with long narrow tunnels and some with large, floppy, atrial septal aneurysms. This makes it impossible for one size device to fit all defects and achieve complete occlusion. Although closure of PFOs is possible with fluoroscopic and angiographic guidance alone, with a low incidence of complications such as embolization, such a practice may lead to a higher incidence of residual shunting through the defect with ongoing potential risk to the patient. This is particularly likely in defects with large "stretched defects," which may require a larger device to fix the septum primum and secundum together or a large central disc to fill the defect such as the AGA atrial septal occluders. Therefore, care should be taken to carefully assess the atrial septal anatomy pre- and postclosure and assess the efficacy of the closure. Although many defects with small persistent shunts seen with contrast echo will close after device endothelialization, some will not, and the operator must decide, based on device position and septal anatomy, whether a larger or different device is needed to eventually achieve a complete closure.

## VENTRICULAR SEPTAL DEFECTS

The first approved device for a transcatheter closure of VSDs was the CardioSEAL device by NMT (**Figure 81-1**) that was approved in 2001. This was approved for closure of congenital VSDs located in the muscular septum, which were felt to be at high risk for surgical closure, or recurrent defects after attempted surgical closure. Surgical closure of these defects is particularly challenging, even in the congenital variants, because of the difficulty in identifying the defect in the operating room through the dense trabeculations in the right ventricle. A disadvantage of this device is its square shape that occasionally makes it difficult to conform to the surrounding anatomy. More recent, in September 2007, a newer device developed by AGA Medical called the muscular VSD device was approved for closure of congenital muscular VSDs. Closure of VSDs is technically more challenging than ASD closure, secondary to the tortuous course needed for the delivery system due to the dense trabeculations frequently covering the right ventricular side of the defect, adjacent tricuspid valve choral attachments, and the heterogeneous nature of muscular VSD anatomy.

Because of the difficulty in crossing muscular VSDs from the densely trabeculated right ventricle, the defect is usually crossed from a retrograde approach through the left ventricle. The wire is advanced into the main pulmonary artery where it is snared by a catheter advanced through either the internal jugular vein (IJ) or femoral vein. Access via the IJ gives the straightest route for the delivery sheath to the more apical VSDs, whereas the femoral venous approach may be more appropriate for defects located in the basil ventricular septum. The tip of the guide wire is then externalized through the venous sheath, creating an arterial to venous loop (**Figure 81-3**). When using the AGA devices, a device is chosen in which the central waist is at least 2 mm larger than the defect size as measured in end diastole. The CardioSEAL device should be approximately twice the size of the defect. Sizing of the VSD is done via both cineangiography and transesophageal assessment. In our practice, CT angiography has been helpful in sizing and reprocedure planning as well (**Figure 81-4**). The short venous sheath

is then removed, and the delivery sheath is advanced over this wire into the left ventricle across the VSD. As the device is loaded through the sheath, the guidewire is slowly pulled back through the arterial sheath, with the device "chasing" the tip of the guidewire through the sheath (sometimes referred to as chasing the dragon). Failure to utilize this technique may lead to kinking of the sheath and an inability to advance the device through the sheath, requiring restarting the entire process. This technique may no longer be required with the newer braided delivery sheaths that are more "kink" resistant, although this remains to be seen. This technique is not required if the operator is able to easily cross the defect prograde from the right ventricle. Similar to atrial septal defects, the left ventricular disc is exposed by withdrawal of the sheath over the delivery cable, and the device is pulled into the defect. After exposing the right ventricular disc, a left ventricular angiogram is performed to assess for adequate device positioning and the amount of residual shunting. Similar to ASD closure, the ACT should be carefully monitored to keep the ACT at least greater than 200, and saline flushes should be carefully used to avoid systemic air embolization. In the multicenter trial that first reported the use of this defect for muscular VSD closure, the initial complete closure rate was only 47%, which improved to 96% at 6 months postimplantation.[7]

Multiple centers have also reported experience with the percutaneous closure of post myocardial infarction induced ventricular septal defects, although the results are not as good as for congenital muscular VSDs. Although our experience with closure of the VSD early after the myocardial infarction may stabilize or improve the patient initially in the catheterization lab with little to no residual shunting, enlargement of the VSD and clinical deterioration within the first few days after closure has been seen. What is not clear is whether the self-expanding central waist of these defects leads to further expansion of the defect because of the surrounding necrotic boarders. Case series and registry data, however, have reported a much more favorable outcome when closure is performed more than 3 weeks following the infarction. Another challenge that these defects pose to percutaneous closure is the frequent proximity of the defect to the posterior, anterior, or distal apical septum, making it more difficult for the device to completely expand secondary to the adjacent ventricular free wall. Mortality, however, is high with and without surgery, so ongoing refinement of technology will be useful in improving closure success for these frequently critically ill patients. A device slightly more specific for closure of post myocardial infarction VSDs has also been developed by AGA Medical that is similar to the muscular VSD occluder and available with a longer and larger central waist, with the hope of fitting into some more complex defects, which are occasionally seen

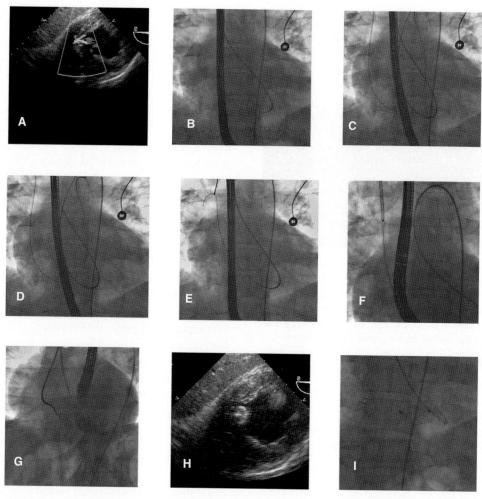

**Figure 81-3.** This series of images walks the reader through the steps involved with muscular VSD occlusion. (A) First, there is careful assessment of the defect size, with echocardiography frequently being the modality most heavily relied upon. (B) At this stage, the VSD has been crossed via a retrograde approach. (C) The guidewire is now advanced up into the main pulmonary artery. (D) A snare catheter has been advanced into the pulmonary artery to snare the retrograde placed guidewire. (E) The wire is withdrawn back into the superior vena cava (SVC) to create a venous to arterial loop. (F) The device is being inserted through the delivery sheath now placed in the internal jugular (IJ) and through the VSD. The device is "chasing the wire" to avoid kinking of the delivery sheath. (G) Repeat left ventricular (LV) angiography demonstrating device positioning after expansion, but prior to release. (H) Confirmation of an adequate device position on a transgastric TEE. (I) Final release of the VSD device. The right ventricular (RV) disc has not fully expanded secondary to the longer nature of this VSD tunnel and its posterior nature, although the device remains stable.

post myocardial infarction. However, this device remains investigational.

A similar device had been designed for perimembranous ventricular septal defects with a novel left ventricular retention skirt designed to minimize risk to the adjacent aortic valve. Initial trials showed a similarly high success rate in complete closure but a high incidence (close to 10%) risk of heart block, some of which occurred weeks to months following the device closure.[8] With a low surgical risk of heart block and mortality (<1%) for VSDs within the perimembranous septum, further plans to market this device in the United States were abandoned.

## PATENT DUCTUS ARTERIOSUS

The physiologic effects of a patent ductus arteriosus (PDA), similar to VSD, correlate to its size and degree of shunting. Small inaudible PDAs have little clinical significance in most people, aside from case reports of endarteritis. Larger PDAs lead to left ventricular dilation that frequently leads to congestive heart failure and poor growth in early childhood. If untreated, this large aortic to pulmonary artery shunt may lead to pulmonary vascular occlusive disease and the eventual development of Eisenmenger's physiology with right to left shunting. The classic clinical picture is exercise intolerance with clubbing and cyanosis isolated to the lower

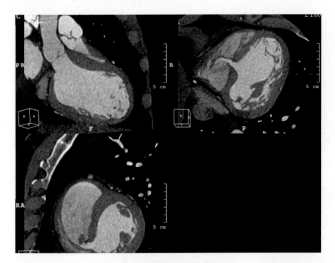

**Figure 81-4.** Computed tomography (CT) angiography of the previous muscular VSD prior to closure. The 3D nature of this imaging modality allows for a better appreciation of the location within the heart and surrounding structures. Although the four-chamber view seen in the upper right hand panel suggests that the defect is in the middle of the septum, the lower left image shows the posterior nature of the defect, predicting that the right ventricular disc may not fully expand secondary to its close proximity to the posterior wall.

extremities. With the equalization of the pulmonary and aortic pressures, the murmur becomes inaudible and potentially undetectable on Doppler echo.

The closure of the PDA by Gross and Hubbard in 1938 is among the first documented cardiac surgery performed. For a long time, cardiologists have tried to identify a less invasive approach to closing these defects. Although surgical ligation is simple with a low risk in children, this is not the case for the adult. With age, the PDA often becomes fibrotic and calcified, requiring cardiopulmonary bypass for safe closure. Although many different devices have been developed for PDA closure since the initial report by Portsman et al in 1967, wide spectrum PDA closure with any of these devices was not adopted until

Cambier reported the first successful use of the transcatheter occlusion of small PDAs with Gianturco coils in 1992. These coils are stainless steel with Dacron fibers attached along its length to promote fibrin deposition and clotting of the vessel. They were initially designed for nonsurgical control of hemorrhage. Since then, thousands of patients have undergone transcatheter coil embolization of PDAs, which have become the procedure of choice except for most PDAs. Exceptions include small neonates and older patients with PDAs larger than 5 to 6 mm at minimal diameter. Standard Gianturco coils are available in wire diameters of 0.025", 0.035", 0.038", and 0.052". Because of a higher rate of coil embolization when these are used to occlude moderate and larger PDAs, detachable coils have been developed. These allow for repositioning of the coil in the event of inadequate initial positioning. The diameter of the coil loop chosen for closure should be greater than 2 times the minimum diameter of the PDA to ensure coil stability. Depending upon the PDA size, multiple coils can be implanted if residual shunting remains. Although many interventionalists still prefer the Gianturco coils because of their low cost and size, citing higher rates of immediate PDA occlusion than the smaller 0.035-inch detachable coils, these larger stainless steel coils are not MRI compatible. Insertion of these coils in young patients would prohibit this imaging modality if needed in the future for other medical conditions that may develop. More recent, the FDA has approved platinum detachable "Flipper" coils, which would not preclude future MRI imaging of the mediastinum.

A significant advancement in occlusion of moderate to large PDAs occurred in the United States in 2003 with the FDA approval of the MRI compatible Amplatzer ductal occluder (ADO). Approval was based on a pivotal trial performed showing a 1-year successful occlusion rate of 98% with few complications.[9] Device sizes are based upon the aortic and pulmonary ends of the device, with the aortic side 2 mm larger in diameter than the pulmonary side (aside from the smallest device with the aortic side only 1 mm larger) (**Figure 81-5**). Devices available in the United States range

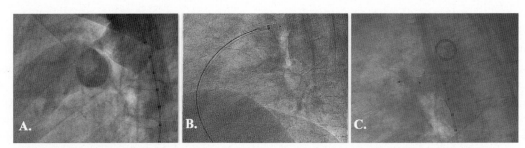

**Figure 81-5.** Catheter occlusion of a moderate sized PDA. (A) Lateral aortic angiography showing a conical shaped ductus with the smallest dimension measuring 3.5 mm. (B) Fluoroscopy showing the appropriate positioning of this 8 × 6 mm Amplatzer ductal occluder (ADO) fitting within the defect. Of note, the aortic retention skirt is 4 mm larger (12 mm) than the 8 mm aortic side of the occluder, with the PA side measuring 6 mm. (C) Following release, there is complete occlusion of the PDA.

from 5/4 to the largest of 12/10, allowing for PDAs up to 11 mm. The larger 14/12 and 16/14 devices are available only outside the United States. The aortic retention skirt is 4 to 6 mm larger than the aortic side of the device. Release of this device has allowed operators to relatively easily occlude PDAs up to 11 mm, with coil occlusion usually reserved for defects less than or equal to 2 mm in their smallest dimension. The occlusion of larger defects in the United States still requires more innovative approaches such as the use of an ASO or muscular VSD device off label, which has a good success rate at our center.

The first step in PDA occlusion is an aortic angiogram performed in the straight lateral projection. After proper measurements of the PDA are made, a right heart catheterization is performed to assess the magnitude of the shunt as well as pulmonary pressures and resistance (PVR). Our preference is to reserve this until after the angiogram in order to prevent a catheter induced spasm of the PDA during inadvertent trauma from the right heart sweep. Underestimation of the PDA size secondary to transient vasospasm could lead to device undersizing and possible late device embolization. Closing a PDA is not recommended in a patient whose PVR is 8 Woods Units or greater or with a pulmonary to systemic resistance ratio of greater than or equal to 0.5, although it remains to be seen if treatment with newer medical therapies for pulmonary hypertension will eventually make these patients candidates for device closure. Our general approach is that if the smallest dimension of the PDA is less than or equal to 2 mm, then an occlusion is performed with a detachable coil (**Figure 81-6**). The defect can be easily crossed retrograde with a 4 or 5 French Judkins right coronary catheter or a more flexible angled glide catheter and a soft tipped guidewire. With the catheter and wire across the defect, the wire is retracted and the coil is loaded into the catheter. On the pulmonary side of the PDA, three quarters

of the loop is extruded and pulled back until contact is made with the coil and PDA. The delivery cable is fixated and the catheter withdrawn, allowing the rest of the coil loops to form in the aortic side of the ductus. The length of the coil selected depends upon length and anatomy of the ductus, but the largest number of coil loops that will fit within in the ductus is preferred to ensure occlusion. If adequate initial positioning is not achieved with this coil, it can easily be retracted back into the catheter and redeployed. Some operators prefer to deploy coils from the pulmonary side in order to better test how the coils sit within the ductus as well as allow for aortic angiography prior to coil deployment. If complete PDA occlusion is not seen on an aortic angiography 10 minutes after coil insertion, the procedure can be repeated with additional coil(s) inserted and interlocking with the initial coil.

If the PDA is greater than 2 mm, the Amplatzer ductal occluder usually allows for straight forward closure. The PDA is crossed from the pulmonary side with a guidewire that is advanced into the descending aorta. If crossing the PDA is difficult from the pulmonary artery, which is sometimes the case in the smaller PDAs, then it can easily be crossed retrograde as described above. The wire is then snared within the pulmonary artery, and the snare and pulmonary artery catheter are pulled through the PDA into the descending aorta. The snare is then exchanged for an extra stiff or super stiff J-tipped 260-cm wire. The catheter is then exchanged for a 180° curved delivery sheath. Care must be taken in younger children during this maneuver, because passage of the sheath over this stiff wire may cause bradycardia or hypotension by tenting open the tricuspid valve. Continuous arterial pressure should therefore be monitored. With the delivery sheath in the descending aorta, the dilator and wire are removed and the device advanced to the end of the sheath. The sheath and device are withdrawn until the tip of the sheath is adjacent to the aortic ampulla of the PDA.

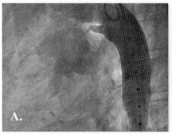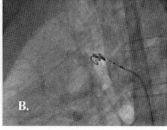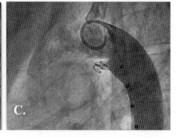

**Figure 81-6.** Patent ductus arteriosus (PDA) closure with a detachable coil. (A) Straight lateral angiography showing a moderately sized aortic ampulla that tapers to a small PDA measuring 1.8 mm at its smallest dimension. Note a marker pigtail being used for angiography to allow for accurate calibration and measurement of the defect size. Catheter lumen size is not sufficiently accurate for calibration. (B) Ideal coil insertion with three-quarters of a loop positioned within the pulmonary size and the rest packed into the ampulla of the PDA. Note the coil remains attached and can be easily retrieved if it's felt to be necessary. (C) Repeat angiography shows complete PDA occlusion.

The aortic retention disc is then exposed, with care not to injure the posterior aortic wall. The sheath and device are withdrawn into the PDA, and the sheath is further withdrawn allowing expansion of the device within the PDA. A repeat aortic angiogram is performed prior to the release of the device to ensure adequate positioning. The delivery cable is then unscrewed with the careful withdrawal of this sharp wire into the delivery sheath. Repeat aortic angiography is performed to ensure closure of the defect. The 98% 1-year complete occlusion rate[9] represents a significant improvement from the 86 to 94% success rate with coil occlusion of these larger defects, with fewer device embolizations.

In addition to the usual complications that can be seen with vascular access, residual shunting can lead to hemolysis, occasionally leading to renal insufficiency if severe enough. If clinically significant hemolysis occurs, device removal is needed if the simple placement of additional coils is not successful in occluding any residual shunt. Late embolization in the first 24 to 48 hours is possible, particularly with elevated PA pressures or initial undersizing of the PDA. No antiplatelet therapy is needed, and 6 months of SBE prophylaxis is indicated until endothelialization is complete

## SUMMARY

The last decade and a half has seen a dramatic improvement in our ability to close many cardiac septal defects in the catheterization lab, avoiding surgery. The question of "can we close a particular defect" no longer remains, but should we? This is a particularly important question we need to ask with smaller defects, with minimal to no apparent hemodynamic effects, or in the case of PFOs where data are still lacking to support the risk benefit ratio of most people. In addition, although the short- and mid-term results seem excellent for all the above procedures, data are lacking on the longer term safety and efficacy. This needs to be discussed with the patients when entertaining a transcatheter route for defect closure.

## References

1. Omeish A, Hijazi ZM. Transcatheter closure of atrial septal defects in children & adults using the Amplatzer Septal Occluder. *J Interv Cardiol.* 2001;14:37–44.

2. Amin Z, Hijazi ZM, Bass JL, et al. Erosion of Amplatzer septal occluder device after closure of secundum atrial septal defects: Review of registry of complications and recommendations to minimize future risk. *Catheter Cardiovasc Interv.* 2004;63: 496–502.

3. Jones TK, Latson LA, Zahn E, et al. Results of the U.S. multicenter pivotal study of the HELEX septal occluder for percutaneous closure of secundum atrial septal defects. *J Am Coll Cardiol.* 2007;49:2215–2221.

4. Sacco RL, Adams R, Albers G, et al. Guidelines for prevention of stroke in patients with ischemic stroke or transient ischemic attack: A statement for healthcare professionals from the American Heart Association/American Stroke Association Council on Stroke: Co-sponsored by the Council on Cardiovascular Radiology and Intervention: The American Academy of Neurology affirms the value of this guideline. *Circulation.* 2006;113:e409–e449.

5. Salem DN, O'Gara PT, Madias C, Pauker SG. Valvular and structural heart disease: American College of Chest Physicians Evidence-Based Clinical Practice Guidelines (8th Edition). *Chest.* 2008;133:593S–629S.

6. Dowson A, Mullen MJ, Peatfield R, et al. Migraine Intervention With STARFlex Technology (MIST) trial: A prospective, multicenter, double-blind, sham-controlled trial to evaluate the effectiveness of patent foramen ovale closure with STARFlex septal repair implant to resolve refractory migraine headache. *Circulation.* 2008;117:1397–1404.

7. Chessa M, Carminati M, Cao QL, et al. Transcatheter closure of congenital and acquired muscular ventricular septal defects using the Amplatzer device. *J Invasive Cardiol.* 2002;14:322–327.

8. Fu YC, Bass J, Amin Z, et al. Transcatheter closure of perimembranous ventricular septal defects using the new Amplatzer membranous VSD occluder: Results of the U.S. phase I trial. *J Am Coll Cardiol.* 2006;47:319–325.

9. Pass RH, Hijazi Z, Hsu DT, Lewis V, Hellenbrand WE. Multicenter USA Amplatzer patent ductus arteriosus occlusion device trial: Initial and 1-year results. *J Am Coll Cardiol.* 2004;44:513–519.

# Aorta and Vascular Disease

# 82

# Diseases of Aorta

ANISH K. AMIN AND ALEX J. AUSEON

## ● PRACTICAL POINTS

- Any patient with a known aortic aneurysm presenting with a change in the quality of pain or new discomfort should be considered as a possible rupture or dissection.

- Consideration for surgical management of abdominal or thoracic aneurysmal disease should be given to aneurysms expanding at greater than 0.5 cm per year or those with dimensions greater than 5.5 cm in men and 5.0 cm in women.

- When aortic dissection patients are appropriately selected, medical management can result in a 30-day

survival of 92%. Patients leaving the hospital have actuarial survival rates similar to those persons having never had dissection.

- The goal of medical therapy in aortic dissection is to reduce shear stress by controlling the rate of systolic pressure rise in the aorta (dP/dt) effectively, which is done by beta-blockade prior to or simultaneous with afterload reduction.

- Of patients with symptoms suggesting aortic dissection, 5-20% were found to have intramural hematoma or a penetrating atherosclerotic ulcer.

## ANEURYSMAL DISEASE

### Introduction

Aortic aneurysms represent a continuum of disease from benign to lethal. Rupture of an aortic aneurysm in the outpatient setting confers mortality in excess of 60-80%, and nearly 50% in a hospital setting. Appropriate treatment depends on rapid assessment of patients and accurate risk stratification.

### Abdominal Aneurysms

#### Clinical Presentation

The diagnosis of abdominal aortic aneurysm (AAA) confers localized enlargement of the abdominal aorta greater than 3.0 cm. The incidence is approximately 1.7% of women and 5% of men by age 65. They may be discovered on routine physical examination, but sensitivity is poor. More often, they are revealed incidentally during imaging for another clinical indication. Symptoms are infrequent and ambiguous, with patients describing "gnawing" hypogastric or low

back pain which does not improve with position. Diligence on the part of the physician is crucial in identifying at-risk patients (Table 82-1). Common risk factors include male sex (which confers a 5- to 10-fold increased risk), cigarette smoking (increasing risk is dependent on the duration of exposure and not necessarily amount), age (with particular risk conferred for men greater than 50 years and women greater than 70 years), hypertension, and atherosclerosis. The most common pathophysiology is degenerative atherosclerosis, with other etiologies including connective tissue disease, inflammation, or infection. Recent data suggest altered production of matrix metalloproteinases leading to remodeling of the extracellular matrix and vessel media. Fewer than 33% of patients with aneurysm rupture present with the classic triad of low back or abdominal pain, pulsatile mass, and hypotension. Surgical repair in the setting of acute rupture carries an operative risk greater than 40%. However, only 10% of patients reach the operating room alive after rupturing. Therefore, any patient with a known aneurysm presenting with a change in the quality of pain or new discomfort should be considered as a possible rupture or dissection (Figure 82-1). The acute nature demands

## Table 82-1 • ACC/AHA Guidelines for Management of Abdominal Aortic Aneurysms (AAA)

**Class I**

1. Patients with infrarenal or juxtarenal AAAs measuring 5.5 cm or larger should undergo repair to eliminate the risk of rupture. *(Level of Evidence: B)*
2. Patients with infrarenal or juxtarenal AAAs measuring 4.0 to 5.4 cm in diameter should be monitored by ultrasound or computed tomographic scans every 6 to 12 months to detect expansion. *(Level of Evidence: A)*

**Class IIa**

1. Repair can be beneficial in patients with infrarenal or juxtarenal AAAs 5.0 to 5.4 cm in diameter. *(Level of Evidence: B)*
2. Repair is probably indicated in patients with suprarenal or type IV thoracoabdominal aortic aneurysms larger than 5.5–6.0 cm. *(Level of Evidence: B)*
3. In patients with AAAs smaller than 4.0 cm in diameter, monitoring by ultrasound examination every 2 to 3 years is reasonable. *(Level of Evidence: B)*

**Class III**

Intervention is not recommended for asymptomatic infrarenal or juxtarenal AAAs if they measure less than 5.0 cm in diameter in men or less than 4.5 cm in diameter in women. *(Level of Evidence: A)*

## Table 82-2 • Natural History of Abdominal Aortic Aneurysms

| Aneurysm Size (Diameter) | Average Annual Rate of Expansion | Annual Rate of Rupture |
| --- | --- | --- |
| Small (<4.0 cm) | 1–4 mm | Very low |
| Moderate (4.0–5.9 cm) | 4–5 mm | 7% |
| Large (>6.0 cm) | Up to 7–8 mm | 20% |

accurate and efficient evaluation to facilitate appropriate surgical management.

### Diagnostic Testing

Imaging should focus on precise depiction of an aneurysm and be available in a timely manner to augment patient care. Aortography has traditionally been the gold standard for evaluation of aneurysms, but has been supplanted by ultrasound (US), computed tomography (CT), and magnetic resonance (MR). Abdominal US is used primarily for screening purposes in patients at risk for developing AAA. Current United States Preventative Services Task Force recommendations are for every male patient 60-75 years of age with a history of smoking to receive a one-time ultrasound evaluation. The probability of aneurysm rupture is based on size at presentation (**Table 82-2**). Patients found to have intermediate-sized AAA (4.0-5.0 cm between 4.0 and 5.4 cm) should undergo US surveillance every six months. In women and nonsmoking men, no current recommendations exist, as the perceived benefit from screening is small. Acute diagnosis requires a more definitive imaging modality with widespread availability and the ability to quickly acquire accurate images. CT angiography satisfies all of these criteria, while also allowing three-dimensional reconstruction capabilities and providing valuable data about other causes for abdominal pain. MR angiography (MRA) is neither preferred for screening nor acute diagnosis when AAA rupture is suspected. This is primarily due to its expense and the time required for obtaining images from various scanning sequences that make up a comprehensive angiogram. However, MRA does present an excellent alternative to CT in patients with contraindications to iodinated contrast or radiation exposure.

### Treatment

The timing of nonurgent intervention is dependent not only on aneurysm size but also rate of expansion. Consideration should be given to aneurysms expanding at >0.5 cm per year or those with dimensions >5.5 cm in men and 5.0 cm in women. Older patients may benefit from a nonsurgical percutaneous approach, using endovascular repair instead of a more traditional open surgery (**Figure 82-2**). This is feasible only in patients with specific arterial anatomy, allowing for proper fixation of the proximal and distal portions of the endograft, distance of the aneurysm from the renal artery ostia and the length and condition of the iliac arteries. Recent evaluations in the Dutch Randomized Endovascular Aneurysm Management (DREAM) and Endovascular Aneurysm Repair (EVAR) 1 and 2 study groups demonstrated decreased immediate mortality with

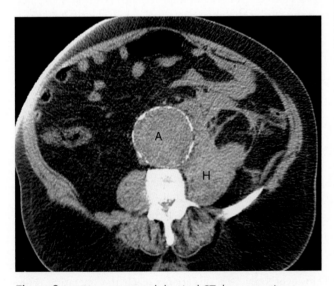

**Figure 82-1.** Non-contrast abdominal CT demonstrating a large ruptured infrarenal abdominal aortic aneurysm (A) with vessel wall calcification. Hemorrhaging is noted in the left perirenal space (H). (Reproduced from *Braunwald's Heart Disease, A Textbook of Cardiovascular Medicine,* 7ᵗʰ ed.)

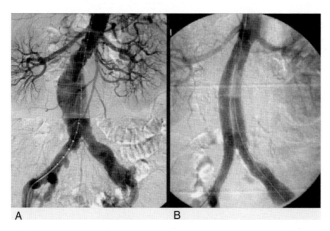

**Figure 82-2.** Angiographic views of an infrarenal abdominal aortic aneurysm treated by endovascular stent grafting before (A) and after device deployment (B). (Reproduced from *Braunwald's Heart Disease, A Textbook of Cardiovascular Medicine*, 7th ed.)

comparable long-term survival. Combined mortality was 5.8% for open surgical procedures and 1.9% in endovascular procedures in these studies, conferring a risk ratio of 3.1 in favor of endovascular techniques. Early enthusiasm has been blunted by longitudinal studies demonstrating increased endograft failure rates of 3% annually, compared to 0.3% for open repair, and complications with endoleaks and or tension may ultimately require open conversion after discovery. The American College of Cardiology (ACC) and American Heart Association (AHA) 2005 Guidelines for Peripheral Arterial Disease (**Table 82-3**) give a Class IIa

---

### Table 82-3 • ACC/AHA Guidelines for Surgical or Endovascular Interventions for Abdominal Aortic Aneurysms (AAA)

**Class I**

1. Open repair of infrarenal AAAs and/or common iliac aneurysms is indicated in patients who are good or average surgical candidates. *(Level of Evidence: B)*
2. Periodic long-term surveillance imaging should be performed to monitor for an endoleak, to document shrinkage or stability of the excluded aneurysm sac, and to determine the need for further intervention in patients who have undergone endovascular repair of infrarenal aortic and/or iliac aneurysms. *(Level of Evidence: B)*

**Class IIa**

Endovascular repair of infrarenal aortic and/or common iliac aneurysms is reasonable in patients at high risk of complications from open operations because of cardiopulmonary or other associated diseases. *(Level of Evidence: B)*

**Class IIb**

Endovascular repair of infrarenal aortic and/or common iliac aneurysms may be considered in patients at low or average surgical risk. *(Level of Evidence: B)*

---

recommendation to endovascular repair in patients at high surgical risk and a Class IIb recommendation in patients at low or average surgical risk.

## Thoracic Aneurysms

### Clinical Presentation

As in abdominal aneurysms, evaluation of thoracic aneurysms focuses on early recognition and management guiding elective repair to reduce the mortality associated with rupture or dissection. As many as 50% of patients are asymptomatic at the time of diagnosis, with the remainder diagnosed as a consequence of aortic insufficiency or compression of adjacent mediastinal structures. Overall, thoracic aneurysms occur primarily in individuals in the sixth and seventh decade with an incidence of 6 per 100,000 per year. However, there are distinct subgroups within this cohort based on specific pathophysiology. Ascending aneurysms account for 60% of disease and are of greater importance due to the potential to cause aortic insufficiency or be complicated by proximal aortic dissection. Additionally, as pathogenesis of ascending aneurysms is most commonly cystic medial degeneration associated with bicuspid aortic valve and connective tissue disease, affected individuals tend to be younger than those with descending aneurysms. The classic older, hypertensive patient with atherosclerosis often has descending disease in association with other cardiovascular disease and in as much as 20% of cases can have aneurysms which transcend anatomic descriptions and involve portions of both the thoracic and abdominal aorta. The natural history of thoracic aneurysms is unknown, largely due to varying rates of expansion and stability based on location and etiology (**Table 82-4**). Recent longitudinal studies have established predictors of rupture or dissection, with associated relative risks as described in **Table 82-5**. Not surprisingly, larger aneurysms and connective tissue disorders conferred greater risk. Likewise, these same studies demonstrated more rapidly expanding aneurysms in patients with connective tissue disorders.

### Diagnostic Testing

Accurate diagnosis again requires appropriate imaging. A widened mediastinal silhouette on chest radiography can suggest aneurysmal disease, but is a rare and nonspecific

---

### Table 82-4 • Natural History of Thoracic Aortic Aneurysms

| Aneurysm Size (Diameter) | Average Annual Rate of Expansion | Five-year Cumulative Risk of Rupture |
|---|---|---|
| Small (<4.0 cm) | | Very low |
| Moderate (4.0–5.9 cm) | Range 0.1–0.25 cm/year | 16% |
| Large (>6.0 cm) | | 31% |

| Table 82-5 • Risk Conditions for Aortic Dissection |
| --- |
| Long-standing arterial hypertension |
|   Smoking, dyslipidemia, cocaine use |
| Connective tissue disease |
|   Marfan syndrome |
|   Ehlers–Danlos syndrome type 4 |
|   Bicuspid aortic valve |
|   Coarctation of the aorta |
|   Hereditary aortopathy |
| Vascular inflammation |
|   Takayasu arteritis |
|   Giant cell arteritis |
|   Behcet's disease |
|   Syphilis |
| Iatrogenic factors |
|   Catheter/instrument intervention |
|   Valvular/aortic surgery |
| Deceleration trauma |
|   Motor vehicle accident |
|   Fall from height |

*Adapted from Tsai et al. Circulation. 2005;112.*

finding. Both CT and MR are highly accurate when diagnosing thoracic aortic aneurysms in non-emergencies. In the acute setting where rupture is suspected, CT and transesophageal echocardiography (TEE) are considered the most appropriate modalities. The choice of diagnostic imaging depends on the expertise and availability at each medical center. CT angiography is most widely available and has been proved accurate. Emergent TEE requires on-call cardiology staff, sedation in a potentially unstable patient, and is less sensitive when the junction of the distal ascending and aortic arch is imaged.

### Treatment

Medical management of established aneurysms focuses on controlling risk factors with strict blood pressure and lipid control as well as smoking cessation. Appropriate surveillance with serial imaging is necessary in all patients with asymptomatic thoracic aortic aneurysms, and intervals commonly start at 6 months. Surgical indications are similar to abdominal disease, namely, size and rate of expansion. Aneurysms of >5.5 cm in the ascending position, >6.0 cm in the descending position, and rates of expansion >0.5 cm/year should be considered for surgery. In patients with known connective tissue disease, smaller aneurysms may be corrected, given the increased risk of rupture in these individuals. Similarly, if aortic valve replacement is indicated, a threshold as low as 4.0 cm is appropriate to consider simultaneous aneurysmal repair. Elective surgery is preferred, as data confirms 10-fold greater mortality in the setting of emergent procedures. While endovascular techniques are available, utilization is commonly restricted to isolated descending disease, given the technical demands of ascending and arch lesions.

# ACUTE AORTIC SYNDROMES

## Introduction

These syndromes share a common pathophysiology where a weakened aortic medial layer leads to vessel dilation and aneurysm formation. The final manifestation of intramural hemorrhage or dissection depends upon the extent of tearing and separation of the intima from the vessel media. All forms of acute aortic syndromes share a high morbidity and mortality, placing high importance on early diagnosis and management.

## Aortic Dissection

### Clinical Presentation

Aortic dissection is classically defined as a tear in the aortic intima, allowing blood to occupy the space and create a false lumen that propagates along varying lengths of the artery. It occurs with an incidence of approximately 2.9 per 100,000 per year, equating to roughly 7000 cases annually in the United States. Common risk factors include age, male sex, hypertension, Marfan syndrome, and aortopathy associated with a bicuspid aortic valve, with the latter two accounting for 10% of all cases. Traditionally classified according to the DeBakey or Stanford classifications, plans of care are determined by the pathophysiology and anatomy of each individual's presentation. The Stanford classification labels all dissections involving the ascending aorta as type A, regardless of the site of origin, while all others are type B. The DeBakey classification organizes into type I (originating in the ascending aorta and propagating at least to, and sometimes beyond, the arch), type II (originates and is confined to the ascending aorta) and type III (originates in the descending aorta, extending distally) (**Figure 82-3**). Symptoms are variable, and can be much more dramatic than those associated with acute myocardial infarction (AMI). Most commonly, patients will describe "tearing" or "ripping" pain that can migrate as the dissection extends. Interestingly, distribution of symptoms can sometimes localize lesions, with anterior pain indicating ascending dissection and back or abdominal pain reflecting descending disease. Because dissection can involve any aspect of the aorta, clinical presentation can vary. Initial evaluation should focus on stabilizing the patient and localizing the intimal defect. It is not uncommon for patients to present with complicated dissections, with multiple tears that spiral along the length of the vessel lumen. The poor blood flow or thrombus formation within the false lumen can lead to secondary ischemic complications as it potentially obstructs flow into critical structures along the path of the artery. These include interruption of aortic valve leaflet coaptation causing acute aortic insufficiency (AI) with or without heart failure; obstruction of coronary ostia

Type I          Type II          Type III

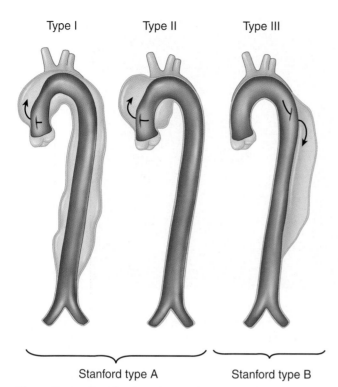

Stanford type A          Stanford type B

**Figure 82-3.** Classification of aortic dissection. Types I, II and III designate the DeBakey system. Stanford Type A describes any dissection involving the proximal aorta, while Type B refers only to those occurring beyond the aortic arch. (Reproduced from *Braunwald's Heart Disease, A Textbook of Cardiovascular Medicine*, 7th ed.)

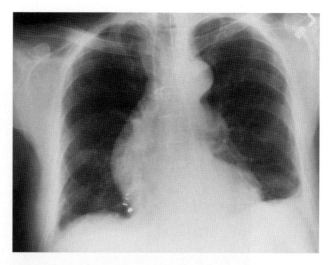

**Figure 82-4.** Chest radiograph demonstrating a large ascending thoracic aortic aneurysm. A widened mediastinum with an abnormal aortic contour is clearly evident. (Reproduced from *Braunwald's Heart Disease, A Textbook of Cardiovascular Medicine*, 7th ed.)

leading to AMI; or disruption of the major branch vessels with neurologic, limb or visceral compromise. In addition, aortic root dissection leading to acute accumulation of a bloody pericardial effusion can result in pericardial tamponade and death.

## Diagnostic Testing

Mediastinal widening on chest radiography can have sensitivity approaching 80-90% (**Figure 82-4**), particularly when occurring in the presence of the "Calcium Sign," when separation of intimal calcification from the outer aortic soft tissue border exceeds 1 cm. However, this is rarely the first test of choice in patients with a high suspicion for acute dissection. Electrocardiogram (ECG) findings can include left ventricular hypertrophy (LVH) secondary to longstanding hypertension or ischemic changes if the dissection flap occludes a coronary ostium. Most dissections that involve the coronaries arise from the right sinus of Valsalva and therefore present as inferoposterior MIs.

Definitive imaging is chosen on an individual basis, taking into account the chronicity of the dissection and the stability of the patient. Invasive angiography, CT, MR, and echocardiography have benefits and disadvantages. Invasive catheter-based angiography, formerly considered the gold standard, is treacherous, carrying a risk of perforation or propagating the dissection, and is generally considered contraindicated. CT and MR provide noninvasive modalities to visualize the aorta without risk of disturbing the dissection flap. MR provides excellent visualization (**Figure 82-5**) and does not expose the patient to iodinated contrast or radiation, but typically has longer image acquisition times and is not suited for unstable patients. CT, despite requiring iodinated contrast and radiation exposure, has near-universal availability and can provide accurate three-dimensional images in a very short time. However, because it cannot be completed at the bedside, it has reduced utility in unstable patients. As a result, TEE is considered ideal for unstable patients, as it can be completed at the bedside or in the operating room. As a diagnostic modality, TEE has 98-99% sensitivity for dissection (**Figure 82-6**) and 100% sensitivity for AI or pericardial effusion complicating proximal dissection.

## Treatment

Overall management is summarized in **Table 82-6**. Collective untreated mortality of acute aortic dissection approaches 25% in the first 24 hours and 50% in seven days. Treatment is driven by location and extent of dissection, with emergent medical therapy focused around halting progression of the dissection by reducing systolic blood pressure and the force of left ventricular contraction **Table 82-7**. Systolic blood pressure goals are less than 100-120 mm Hg or the lowest level tolerated without development of symptoms. Surgical treatment includes the removal of the intimal tear, excision of the diseased aorta, and replacement with a graft. Surgical indications include acute proximal and complicated dissections as well as Marfanoid patients.

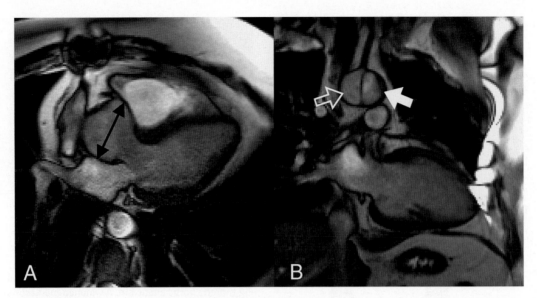

**Figure 82-5.** Magnetic resonance imaging of a patient with a dilated aortic root (double head arrow), aortic regurgitation (A) and a chronic aortic arch dissection (B). The true lumen (open white arrow) includes the ostium of a branch vessel and the false lumen (solid white arrow) is nearly the same diameter.

Surgery remains the standard of care for proximal, ascending dissections (Stanford type A and DeBakey type I and II), but complications can include disruption of the anterior vertebral and intercostal arteries, leading to spinal cord ischemia and possible paralysis. As a result, endovascular options are under investigation, but are currently limited to therapy for distal dissections. For those cases where a dissection flap disrupts aortic valve coaptation or coronary flow, consideration should be applied to aortic valve replacement and coronary artery bypass grafting (CABG). While ascending dissections can result in aortic insufficiency, aortic valve replacement carries long-term consequences of anticoagulation and prophylaxis, and thought should be given as to whether correction of the dissection can correct the AI. Diagnostic coronary angiography is not typically recommended prior to surgical repair of the aorta, primarily due to limited data supporting its use, technical difficulty of completing the study through an often tortuous and diseased aorta, and

the consequences of delaying surgery. In cases where coronary anatomy must be known prior to aortic surgery, CT coronary angiography is very useful, particularly if it can be performed during the aortic CT scan. Alternatively, once there has been confirmation by TEE or CT that the ascending aorta is not involved, coronary angiography can be performed via upper extremity, avoiding the need to have to instrument the descending aorta.

When patients are appropriately selected, medical management can result in a 30-day survival of 92%. The ultimate

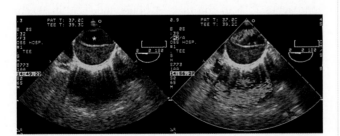

**Figure 82-6.** Transesophageal echocardiogram images of a type B dissection in the descending thoracic aorta. A dissection flap is seen separating the true lumen (asterisk) from the false lumen, and normal color flow is evident.

| Table 82-6 • Indications for Definitive Surgical and Medical Therapy in Aortic Dissection |
|---|
| **Surgical** |
| Treatment of choice for acute proximal dissection |
| Treatment for acute distal dissection complicated by the following: |
|   Progression with vital organ compromise |
|   Rupture or impending rupture (e.g., saccular aneurysm formation) |
|   Retrograde extension into the ascending aorta |
|   Dissection in the Marfan syndrome |
| **Medical** |
| Treatment of choice for uncomplicated distal dissection |
|   Treatment for stable, isolated arch dissection |
|   Treatment of choice for stable chronic dissection (uncomplicated dissection presenting 2 weeks or later after onset) |

*Reproduced from Braunwald's Heart Disease, A Textbook of Cardiovascular Medicine, 7th ed.*

| Table 82-7 • ACC/AHA Guidelines for Initial Management of Acute Thoracic Aortic Dissection | | |
|---|---|---|
| **Medication** | **Dosing** | **Comment** |
| Propanolol | 1 mg intravenous push (i.v.p.) every 2–5 min to a heart rate of 60–80 bpm; Maximum dose 10 mg | Commonly used due to being one of the first available beta-blockers |
| Labetalol | 20 mg i.v.p. followed by doses of 40–80 mg every 10 min for a maximal dose of 300 mg. Also as continuous infusion. | |
| Esmolol | 500mg/kg/min bolus followed by continuous infusion of 50–200 mg/kg/min | Ultra short-acting, making it suitable for patients with labile hemodynamics or those going to surgery |
| Enalaprilat | 0.625–1.25 mg i.v.p. every 6 h with a maximum dose of 5 mg every 6 h | Particularly useful in patients whose dissections involve one or both of the renal arteries, counteracting large secondary renin release |
| Nitroprusside | Intravenous (i.v.) infusion of 20 mg/min-800 mg/min | Can adversely increase aortic shear stress when infused in absence of beta-blocker |

goal in these patients is to reduce shear stress by controlling the rate of systolic pressure rise in the aorta (dP/dt) effectively, as late complications are 10 times more likely in hypertensive patients. Patients leaving the hospital have actuarial survival rates similar to those persons having never had dissection. CT evaluation at 1, 3, 6, 12 months, and annually thereafter is considered for surveillance. The primary concern in these patients is not only for recurrence or rupture, but also for postoperative aneurysm formation at surgical graft sites.

## Intramural Hematoma and Penetrating Atherosclerotic Ulcer

### Clinical Presentation

The pathophysiology of intramural hematoma (IMH) is incompletely understood and is considered either a variant or precursor of aortic dissection. The hallmark of IMH differentiation from simple dissection is an absence of false luminal flow with varying degrees of extension. The aortic lesion may be secondary to vasa vasorum rupture with medial hematoma development or due to intimal tears too small to visualize. Deep ulceration from a penetrating atherosclerotic plaque (**Figure 82-7**) is also associated with aortic injury, resulting in either IMH or complete dissection of the intima. Risk factors are shared for all acute aortic syndromes, with the exception of Marfan syndrome, which is associated with dissection alone. Of patients with symptoms suggesting aortic dissection, 5-20% were found to have IMH.

### Diagnostic Testing

Because of the similarity in symptoms among acute aortic syndromes, the diagnostic approach to identify specific pathophysiology is universal. After history and physical examination leads to adequate suspicion, testing consists of an electrocardiogram, chest radiograph, and aortic imaging study—either CT/MR angiography or TEE, depending on availability and patient stability.

### Treatment

As with aortic dissection, descending aortic lesions are generally treated with beta-blockade and afterload reduction to aggressively control systolic blood pressure and reduce aortic

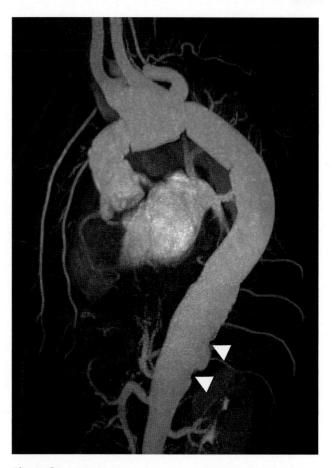

**Figure 82-7.** Magnetic resonance imaging of the length of the aorta. Diffuse aneurysmal dilation is seen with areas of atherosclerotic ulcerations noted in the abdominal aorta (arrowheads).

shear stress. Patients with ascending lesions have an overall lower mortality with surgery than they have with medical treatment (14 versus 36%, respectively). However, there is evidence that both IMH and penetrating atherosclerotic ulcers (PAU) differ somewhat from classic aortic dissection because of a lack of continuous flow communication into a false lumen. As a result, each patient and their aortic lesion should be assessed individually, as some ascending cases of IMH and PAU may have lower morbidity and mortality with a medical approach.

## OTHER ETIOLOGIES OF AORTIC DISEASE

### Infectious Aortitis

While aortitis and mycotic aneurysms are known entities, they tend to be rare and are not confined specifically to the aorta. In one series, 31% were found in the abdominal aorta, with the other sites being femoral, superior mesenteric, carotid, iliac, and brachial arteries. The majority are bacterial, with Staphylococcus, Salmonella, and Streptococcus species being most common. Historically, most cases were due to late-stage syphilis (Treponema pallidum) and, less frequently, Mycobacterium tuberculosis. Risks for development of infectious aortitis include age, local infection, immunosuppression, infective endocarditis, and arterial trauma.

### Aortic Vasculitis

Takayasu arteritis is the most frequent cause of large vessel vasculitis, affecting the aorta and its primary branches. Inflammatory thickening of the vessel wall is the hallmark pathological change, and may be accompanied by luminal narrowing, dilation, or even occlusion. Symptoms and presentation are dependent on the specific arterial branches involved. Systemic complaints and signs may include fever, weight loss, hypertension, myalgias, joint synovitis, arthralgias, chest pain, dyspnea, hemoptysis, abdominal pain, headache, and visual changes. The diagnosis is made by history, physical examination and imaging of the aorta. Both MR and CT angiography are highly accurate and reliable. They also have the additional advantage of vessel wall visualization, where conventional invasive angiography can only demonstrate the vessel lumen in two dimensions.

### Aortic Trauma

Aortic trauma can occur secondary to any number of penetrating or blunt causes. Because of the diversity in etiology, the exact incidence is unknown, but it remains the most common cause of sudden death following a motor vehicle accident or fall. Tearing or rupture of the vessel occurs most commonly at the aortic isthmus, aortic root, or the diaphragmatic annulus. Hemorrhagic decompensation leads to early mortality, most often occurring in the field prior to medical evaluation. As such diagnosis and evaluation is guided by patient stability, imaging focuses on localizing the extent of injury prior to proceeding with surgery. Bedside TEE is the most appropriate assessment for unstable patients as it can rapidly assess relevant anatomy if there is a high suspicion of isolated aortic injury , but CT is far more comprehensive for evaluation of general thoracic and abdominal trauma.

### Aortic Occlusion

Acute aortic occlusion is a surgical emergency requiring immediate diagnostic evaluation to guide intervention. Classic symptoms and signs include levido reticularis, diminished peripheral pulses, cold and mottled skin distal to the occlusion, and ischemic neuropathy. Further evidence includes laboratory changes indicative of visceral organ injury, depending on the level of occlusion. Consideration should also be given to differential diagnosis of systemic embolization, and a thorough evaluation for a cardiac source of embolus should be completed. Primary thrombus, while rare, can form through a variety of mechanisms including infectious involvement of the cardiac valves or aorta, aortitis, or primary malignancy leading to a hypercoaguable state. Aortography is the gold standard in diagnosis, but CT angiography is a reliable alternative. Surgical treatment is often associated with a high mortality.

### References

1. ACC/AHA 2005 Guidelines for the Management of Patients with Peripheral Arterial Disease. *J Am Coll Cardiol.* 2006;47:1–192.

2. ACC/AHA 2010 Guidelines for the Diagnosis and Management of Patients with Thoracic Aortic Disease. *J Am Coll Cardiol.* 2010;55:e27–129.

3. Greenhalgh RM, Powell JT. Endovascular repair of an abdominal aortic aneurysm. *New Engl J Med.* 2008;358:494–501.

4. Patel HJ, Deeb GM. Ascending and arch aorta. Pathology, natural history, and treatment. *Circulation.* 2008;118: 188–195.

5. Tsai TT, Niebaurer CA, Eagle KA. Acute aortic syndromes. *Circulation.* 2005;112:3802–3813.

6. Hagan PG, Nienaber CA, Isselbacher EM, et al. International Registry of Acute Aortic Dissection (IRAD): New insights into an old disease. *JAMA.* 2000;283:897–903.

# 83

# Atherosclerotic Renal Artery Stenosis

QUINN CAPERS, IV

## ● PRACTICAL POINTS

- Atherosclerotic renal artery stenosis is associated with renal insufficiency, hypertension, and an increased risk for myocardial infarction, stroke, and cardiovascular and all-cause mortality.

- Angiotensin II stimulates oxidase activity in cultured vascular cells, in animals infused with angiotensin II, and in patients with renovascular hypertension, imparting an oxidative stress on the vascular wall.

- Experimentally, angiotensin II induces proinflammatory gene products via a redox-sensitive mechanism.

- Multiple drugs are now available to block the renin-angiotensin system at different locations, from distal to proximal.

- Percutaneous stenting is a safe, effective treatment for ostial atherosclerotic renal artery stenosis.

- Although theoretically intriguing, it is unclear whether mechanical correction of renal artery stenosis offers sustained cardiovascular protection.

- Current trials are ongoing to determine if renal artery stent placement reduces cardiovascular complications in patients with renal artery stenosis

Atherosclerotic stenosis of the renal artery is a common disorder in the United States, with prevalence estimates that vary by demographic descriptors. It is present in 4% of the general population, 20 to 30% of all patients on dialysis, 30% of patients with coronary artery disease undergoing cardiac catheterization, and 50% of patients undergoing peripheral angiography.

Atherosclerotic renal artery stenosis occurs when atherosclerotic plaque deposition in the renal arteries results in a critical narrowing, which restricts blood flow to the renal parenchyma. It is often associated with significant atheromatous disease of the abdominal aorta. Although many cases are asymptomatic, atherosclerotic renal artery stenosis (ARAS) can have very definite clinical consequences. It is associated with renal insufficiency, hypertension, and an increased risk for myocardial infarction, stroke, and cardiovascular and all-cause mortality.[1] Although the mere presence of RAS identifies a population at high risk for cardiovascular and renal events, a causal link has not been firmly established. Whether ARAS is a mediator of the increased vascular risk or simply a marker for the presence of systemic atherosclerosis is not clear. Thus, the treatment of this condition is controversial. It seems intuitive that patients with ARAS are best treated with the same measures that reduce cardiovascular risk in patients with atherosclerosis in any location. These measures include regular physical activity; medications such as statins, ACE inhibitors, and antiplatelet drugs; and tobacco avoidance. What is unclear is whether mechanical correction of the renal artery stenosis offers additional cardiovascular protection. Important clinical trials are currently under way, which should help answer this question.

# CLINICAL CONSEQUENCES OF ATHEROSCLEROTIC RENAL ARTERY STENOSIS

## Hypertension

As first noted by Dr. Harry Goldblatt in the 1930s, a stenosis in the renal artery, leading to ischemia of the kidney, produces a severe elevation of blood pressure. Subsequently, it was discovered that the ischemic kidney releases renin, which, through a series of steps, leads to the production of the small peptide, angiotensin II. In addition to being a potent vasoconstrictor, recent evidence reveals that angiotensin II also stimulates the production of oxygen derived free radicals, which inactivate the ubiquitous vasodilator substance, nitric oxide (NO). In addition to being the most potent vasodilator known to man, NO has antiinflammatory and antiproliferative properties, and the relative lack of effective NO is thought to play a permissive role in the development of atherosclerosis. (**Figure 83-1** outlines the pathophysiology of renovascular hypertension.) Atherosclerotic renal artery stenosis is the most common

### 1. FORMATION OF ANGIOTENSIN I

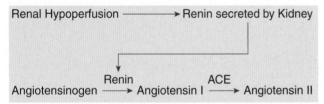

### 2. ACTIONS OF ANGIOTENSIN II

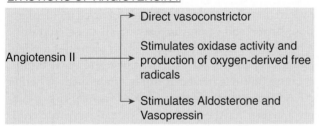

**Figure 83-1.** Renal hypoperfusion from a variety of causes (low cardiac output, renal artery stenosis, hypovolemia) stimulates the kidney to secrete renin, an enzyme which acts on the constitutively secreted protein angiotensinogen, cleaving it to yield angiotensin I. Angiotensin I is transformed to Angiotensin II most commonly by the angiotensin converting enzyme (ACE), though other enzymes have been discovered that can catalyse this reaction. Angiotensin II then stimulates a variety of actions which ultimately result in volume and salt retention and vasoconstriction.

cause of secondary hypertension and is often present as a bystander in patients with primary hypertension, particularly the elderly and those with severe coronary or peripheral atherosclerosis. Differentiating between renal artery stenosis that is the cause of the renovascular hypertension (RVH) and "bystander" renal artery stenosis (RAS) that simply accompanies primary hypertension can be challenging. (**Table 83-1** lists useful clues in trying to differentiate RVH from bystander RAS.) Renovascular hypertension is often quite severe and accompanied by evidence of hypertensive end-organ damage, such as left ventricular hypertrophy, hypertensive retinopathy, and so on.

## Ischemic Nephropathy

Chronically reduced blood flow to the kidney leads to renal atrophy and a diminished glomerular filtration rate. Severe renal artery stenosis has been identified in 15 to 25% of patients receiving hemodialysis. Although not proof of a cause and effect relationship, renal artery stenosis is considered an important reversible cause of renal failure. Some have reported that percutaneous renal artery stenting in selected dialysis patients can salvage renal function and obviate the need for dialysis.[2]

## Cardiovascular Events

The most common cause of death in patients with ARAS is ischemic heart disease and its complications. This is true of patients with atherosclerosis in any location of the body. However, patients with ARAS carry the additional vascular burdens of severe hypertension, supraphysiologic levels of the proatherogenic prothrombotic vasoconstrictor angiotensin II, and possibly diminished renal function with its cardiovascular consequences. Conlon et al found that in patients undergoing coronary angiography, the presence of renal artery stenosis is an independent risk factor for cardiovascular and all-cause mortality during 5 years of follow up. These investigators demonstrated a "dose-dependent" effect, with a graded increase in mortality in patients with severe compared to moderate narrowing of the renal arteries.[1]

# PATHOPHYSIOLOGY OF RENOVASCULAR HYPERTENSION

Much of our understanding of the pathophysiology of renovascular hypertension comes from a series of elegant animal experiments carried out in the 1930s, 1950s, and 1970s by Drs. Goldblatt, Braun-Menendez, Barger, Gavras, and others. Experimental renal artery stenosis results in hypertension that is characterized by three separate phases, with variable responsiveness to renin-angiotensin blockade or relief of the renal artery stenosis.

**Table 83-1 • Clinical Clues to Differentiate True Renovascular Hypertension from Primary Hypertension with "Bystander" Renal Artery Stenosis**

| | Renovascular Hypertension | Primary Hypertension with "Bystander" Renal Artery Stenosis |
|---|---|---|
| Blood pressure levels | Very severe, usually relatively refractory to medications | From mild to severe, usually responds to medications |
| Metabolic clues | Unexplained hypokalemia may be present | Unexplained hypokalemia not present |
| Evidence for hypertensive end-organ damage | Usually present, especially left ventricular hypertrophy | May or may not be present |
| Acute ACE inhibitor- or ARB-induced hyperkalemia or azotemia | When this occurs, a strong clue to the presence of bilateral renal artery stenosis | Usually does not occur |

## RVH Phase I

In this initial phase of "two kidney, one clip" RVH (analogous to human unilateral renal artery stenosis), the ischemic kidney secretes large amounts of renin, which results in the formation of large amounts of angiotensin I. Angiotensin I is cleaved by angiotensin converting enzyme (ACE) to angiotensin II, a powerful vasoconstrictor that has other important vascular effects. The stenosed kidney is underperfused while the nonstenosed kidney, exposed to hypertension, experiences intraglomerular hypertension. This causes a pressure induced natriuresis, resulting in no overall increase in volume. This phase of RVH is responsive to the relief of the stenosis or ACE inhibitors.

## RVH Phase II

Persistent renovascular hypertension enters another phase, in which intravascular volume is expanded, shutting down or slowing renin production. In the experimental models, this is seen in either the "one kidney, one clip" model or the "two kidney, two clip" model—in other words, global renal ischemia. The analogous situation in humans would be bilateral critical renal artery stenosis or unilateral renal artery stenosis in a patient with only one functioning kidney. In this situation, pressure natriuresis cannot occur, because all of the renal mass is hypoperfused and unable to increase sodium and water excretion. The expanded volume is a strong stimulus to shut down or slow renin secretion, thus renin and angiotensin II levels decrease toward normal in this phase. This phase of RVH is responsive to the relief of the stenosis or stenoses but not as responsive to ACE inhibitors.

## RVH Phase III

Persistent, chronic RVH leads to renal parenchymal damage secondary to the chronic hypertension. Typical hypertensive nephrosclerosis results in irreversible loss of renal function, volume expansion, lower renin and angiotensin II levels, and less responsiveness to renin-angiotensin blockade. This

phase of RVH is not responsive to the relief of the stenosis and is not very responsive to ACE inhibitors.

## ANGIOTENSIN II

From vasoconstrictor to promoter of inflammation and atherosclerotic plaque rupture.

Early studies of angiotensin II attempted to study its role in homeostasis to characterize its cell surface receptors and to block its powerful vasoconstrictive action. It was not until the 1990s, some 60 years after Goldblatt's first experiments, that investigators began dissecting the mechanism of angiotensin II-induced blood pressure elevation, which was to shed light on a possible link between atherosclerosis and angiotensin II. In 1994, Griendling et al[3] discovered that cultured vascular smooth muscle cells exposed to angiotensin II produce oxygen derived free radicals, with the source likely to be the membrane bound NADH/NADPH oxidase system. That this occurs in vivo, via the coupling of angiotensin II to its AT1 receptor, was demonstrated by the same group in 1996 on a series of experiments in rats.[4] In this important paper, Rajagopalan et al hypothesized that the hypertensive response to angiotensin II is, in part, a result of the inactivation of nitric oxide by oxygen free radicals produced when angiotensin II stimulates its AT1 receptor. In a study of hypertensive patients, some with renal artery stenosis and some with essential hypertension, indices of oxidative stress were higher in those with renovascular disease.[5] It is now well accepted that angiotensin II stimulates oxidase activity in cultured vascular cells, in animals infused with angiotensin II, and in patients with renovascular hypertension.

It has subsequently been shown that NADPH oxidase produces a superoxide radical in atherosclerotic human coronary arteries and that this is inhibited by pharmacologic blockade of the AT1 type angiotensin II receptor.[6] Parallel with these findings was a growing body of evidence that oxidative stress in the vascular wall is an important stimulus for the upregulation of gene products believed to play a role in atherosclerosis. For instance, in 1998, we found that angiotensin II induced hypertension in rats and was unique for its ability to stimulate the upregulation of the mRNA for the thrombin receptor (now called protease activated receptor-1, or PAR-1) and for the chemokine monocyte chemotactic protein-1 (MCP-1).[7,8] Both of these gene products are present in human atherosclerotic plaques, with a putative role for MCP-1 in recruiting monocytes to the vascular lesion ultimately resulting in plaque rupture. Both of these gene products are redox-sensitive, and their in vivo upregulation in the presence of angiotensin II proceeds via redox-sensitive mechanisms. Thus, angiotensin II stimulates oxidase activity in animals and humans. Gene products known to be associated with the maintenance and progression of human atherosclerotic plaques are induced by angiotensin II via the production of oxygen-derived free radicals. Taken together, these findings potentially provide a mechanistic basis for the findings of increased clinical events driven by atherosclerotic plaque rupture (acute myocardial infarction, stroke) in patients with renal artery stenosis[1] or in those with high plasma renin activity without renal artery stenosis.

# MANAGEMENT OF RENAL ARTERY STENOSIS

## Medical Therapy

Patients with renal artery stenosis have clinical sequelae secondary to hyperreninemia. These can include elevated levels of the prooxidant, proinflammatory angiotensin II and secondary severe or malignant hypertension, hypervolemia, and possibly increased clinical events characterized by atherosclerotic plaque rupture. It is fortunate that there are now pharmacologic agents that inhibit most facets of an activated renin-angiotensin-aldosterone system. From distal in the pathway to proximal, agents are available that antagonize the aldosterone receptor (Spironolactone and Eplerenone), the angiotensin II receptor (ARBs), and the vasopressin receptor (vaptans). More proximal, one can inhibit the formation of angiotensin II with angiotensin converting enzyme (ACE) inhibitors. More proximal still is the new agent Aliskiren, which inhibits renin by mimicking its substrate, angiotensinogen, and irreversibly binding the renin molecule (site of effect of various drug classes in RAS shown schematically in **Figure 83-2**). Although these agents are not used in patients with uncorrected severe bilateral

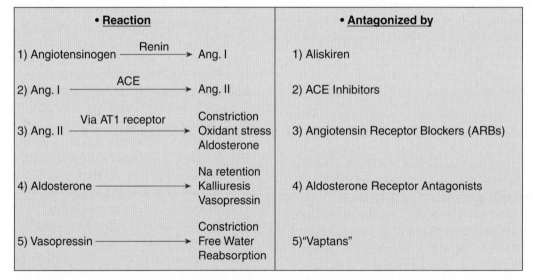

**Figure 83-2.** Reactions in the renin-angiotensin-aldosterone axis and pharmacologic inhibitors. Angiotensinogen is acted upon by the enzyme renin to give angiotensin I. The direct renin inhibitor, aliskiren, blocks this reaction by irreversibly binding renin. Angiotensin I (Ang. I) serves as the substrate for the angiotensin converting enzyme (ACE), and this reaction produces the multifunctional protein angiotensin II (Ang. II). Angiotensin converting enzyme inhibitors block this enzymatic pathway and prevent the formation of angiotensin II. Most known effects of Ang. II proceed after the small peptide couples with the AT1 receptor on vascular and other cells, and can be blocked by antagonizing this receptor with angiotensin receptor blockers (ARBs). In addition to promoting vasoconstriction and the production of oxygen-derived free radicals, Ang. II stimulates the adrenal cortex to produce aldosterone, which in turn stimulates the kidney to reabsorb sodium and excrete potassium (kalliuresis). Aldosterone stimulates the secretion of vasopressin, which has pressor properties and also increases free water reabsorption by the kidney. The effects of aldosterone and vasopressin can be blocked by aldosterone receptor antagonists and vasopressin antagonists or "vaptans", respectively. Ang. I, angiotensin I; ACE, angiotensin converting enzyme; Ang. II, angiotensin II; Na retention, sodium retention.

renal artery stenosis, as they can precipitate acute renal failure and hyperkalemia in such patients, ACE inhibitors and ARBs in particular are quite useful in the management of renovascular hypertension secondary to severe unilateral hypertension. More data are needed on the use of Aliskiren, the vaptans, and aldosterone blockers in RAS.

It is usually recommended that medications that inhibit the renin angiotensin system be used with caution in patients with known renal artery stenosis as well as unilateral renal artery stenosis. If used chronically, these can lead to a medical nephrectomy, which was once a sought-after endpoint in the management of patients with refractory hypertension secondary to renal artery stenosis.

## Renal Artery Revascularization

Mechanical treatment of renal artery stenosis has evolved through several distinct stages: from surgeries such as nephrectomy and renal endarterectomy, to balloon angioplasty, to percutaneous stent placement with or without distal embolic protection devices. The progressive evolution has been fueled by the strong personal conviction of operators and other clinicians that patients benefit from these procedures. However, objective data have been controversial. Many registries have reported improved outcomes in groups of patients with renal artery stenosis treated with mechanical revascularization. The evidence from prospective, randomized trials has been less robust. Three randomized studies of balloon angioplasty versus medical therapy for the treatment of renal artery stenosis conducted in 1998 and 2000 were sobering; balloon angioplasty was no better or only slightly better than maximal medical therapy at improving blood pressure control in hypertensive patients with renal artery stenosis. These studies have been criticized, with the most cited flaw being that stents were rarely used in one study and not at all in the other two. Balloon angioplasty is not an effective therapy for aorto-ostial atherosclerotic renal artery stenosis. Elastic recoil of ostial lesions is often evident immediately after balloon deflation. In a 1999 study comparing balloon angioplasty with stent placement to stand-alone balloon angioplasty in patients with renal artery stenosis, the differences between balloon angioplasty and stenting were striking. The primary success rate of stent placement was 88% compared to 57% for balloon angioplasty alone. The restenosis rate at 6 months was 71% in the balloon group and 25% in the stent group.[13] These studies, and many early studies and registries, concentrated on endpoints of blood pressure control and renal function. These are important endpoints, for sure. Yet, given the scientific discussion above, one is intrigued by the possibility that renal artery stenting might decrease cardiovascular complications such as MI and stroke.

The first completed randomized evaluation of stenting versus medical therapy in patients with "incident" renal artery stenosis was reported at the major cardiology meetings and nephrology meetings of 2008. At the Angioplasty and Stent for Renal Artery Lesions (ASTRAL) trial, investigators found no difference in blood pressure, renal outcomes, cardiovascular outcomes, or overall mortality in more than 800 patients randomized to stent placement or maximal medical therapy and followed for 5 years. The published manuscript is eagerly awaited as of this writing. The multicenter, NIH sponsored Cardiovascular Outcomes in Renal Atherosclerotic Lesions (CORAL) trial will randomize 1,080 patients with atherosclerotic renal artery stenosis to maximal medical therapy based on an angiotensin receptor blocker or maximal medical therapy plus stenting. Entry criteria include renal artery stenosis of greater than or equal to 60% and either chronic renal insufficiency or hypertension on two or more antihypertensive drugs. Enrollment is anticipated to close in late 2009 or early 2010. When both the CORAL and ASTRAL trials are completed and published in full length manuscript form, physicians may finally have some hard evidence on which to base management decisions in their renal artery stenosis patients.

## CONCLUSION

Atherosclerotic renal artery stenosis is a disease that harkens back to the very beginning of endocrinology as a discipline of study, and classical physiology experiments taught us much about endocrine function, blood pressure regulation, and regulation of volume. This disease with potential deadly consequences will become more frequent in the United States as the population continues to age and peripheral atherosclerosis becomes more prevalent. Although the presence of ARAS identifies patients at high risk for cardiovascular events such as MI and stroke, it is not clear as of this writing if mechanical correction of renal artery stenosis reduces that risk. There is a scientific rationale to expect that such would be the case, and it is clear that individuals can be found who do respond to renal artery interventions in terms of blood pressure control and renal function. In the case of the patient with severe bilateral renal artery stenoses and recurrent bouts of "flash" pulmonary edema, one would be hard pressed to find a clinician who would not recommend renal artery intervention. However, beyond the short term, it is controversial whether there is a sustained cardiovascular benefit to be gained from renal artery interventions. Forthcoming randomized trial data should help settle this long-standing controversy.

## References

1. Conlon PJ, Little MA, Pieper K, Mark DB. Severity of renal vascular disease predicts mortality in patients undergoing coronary angiography. *Kidney Int.* 2001 Oct;60(4):1490–1497.

2. Thatipelli M, Misra S, Johnson CM, et al. Renal artery stent placement for restoration of renal function in hemodialysis recipients with renal artery stenosis. *J Vasc Interv Radiol.* 2008 Nov;19(11):1563–1568.

3. Griendling KK, Minieri CA, Ollerenshaw JD, Alexander RW. Angiotensin II stimulates NADH and NADPH oxidase activity in cultured vascular smooth muscle cells. *Circ Res.* 1994 Jun;74(6):1141–1148.

4. Rajagopalan S, Kurz S, Münzel T, et al. Angiotensin II-mediated hypertension in the rat increases vascular superoxide production via membrane NADH/NADPH oxidase activation. Contribution to alterations of vasomotor tone. *J Clin Invest.* 1996 Apr 15;97(8):1916–1923.

5. Minuz P, Patrignani P, Gaino S, et al. Increased oxidative stress and platelet activation in patients with hypertension and renovascular disease. *Circulation.* 2002 Nov 26;106(22): 2800–2805.

6. Guzik TJ, Sadowski J, Guzik B, et al. Coronary artery superoxide production and nox isoform expression in human coronary artery disease. *Arterioscler Thromb Vasc Biol.* 2006 Feb;26(2):333-339. Epub 2005 Nov 17.

7. Capers Q 4th, Laursen JB, Fukui T, et al. Vascular thrombin receptor regulation in hypertensive rats. *Circ Res.* 1997 Jun;80(6):838–844.

8. Capers Q 4th, Alexander RW, Lou P, et al. Monocyte chemoattractant protein-1 expression in aortic tissues of hypertensive rats. *Hypertension.* 1997 Dec;30(6):1397–1402.

9. Blumenfeld JD, Sealey JE, Alderman MH, et al. Plasma renin activity in the emergency department and its independent association with acute myocardial infarction. *Am J Hypertens.* 2000 Aug;13(8):855–863.

10. van Jaarsveld BC, Krijnen P, Pieterman H, et al. The effect of balloon angioplasty on hypertension in atherosclerotic renal-artery stenosis. Dutch Renal Artery Stenosis Intervention Cooperative Study Group. *N Engl J Med.* 2000 Apr 6;342(14):1007–1014.

11. A van de Ven PJ, Kaatee R, Beutler JJ, et al. Arterial stenting and balloon angioplasty in ostial atherosclerotic renovascular disease: A randomised trial. *Lancet.* 1999 Jan 23;353(9149):282–286.

# 84

# Peripheral Arterial Disease

FADI SHAMOUN AND GEORGE S. ABELA

## ● PRACTICAL POINTS

- PAD is more prevalent in elderly and smokers.

- Most patients with PAD are asymptomatic or have atypical leg symptoms.

- PAD is a cardiovascular risk equivalent.

- Treatment goals are:
  - improve functional status
  - treat the underlying atherosclerosis.

- Endovascular procedures are indicated for individuals with:
  - lifestyle-limiting disability
  - reasonable likelihood of symptomatic improvement
  - inadequate response to exercise or pharmacologic therapy
  - favorable risk-benefit ratio

- Supervised exercise 3 times/week for 3-6 months is safe, efficacious, and cost effective therapy.

- Patients who complete a supervised exercise program have 100% improvement in their symptoms compared to 50% improvement with cilostazol and 12% improvement with pentoxifylline.

- Surgical versus percutaneous intervention for the superficial femoral artery disease seems to be comparable.

- Patients with acute limb ischemia (ALI) should undergo an emergent evaluation, the goal of which is to lead to prompt endovascular or surgical intervention.

- Statins improve pain-free walking distance (PFWD), quality of life (QOL), and limb salvage in patients, post-revascularization.

## PERIPHERAL ARTERIAL DISEASE (PAD)

Peripheral artery disease (PAD) defined by an ankle brachial index (ABI) of less than 0.9 affects 8.5-10 million adults in the United States. It is more prevalent in older patients (>70years) (**Figure 84-1**), in diabetic patients, or in those who smoke (>50 years), especially if atherosclerotic risk factors are present. It affects 25% of those over the age of 70 and is found in 33% of patients in the primary care office. Black ethnicity is a strong and independent risk factor for PAD independent of diabetes, hypertension, and BMI.

Most patients with PAD are asymptomatic (**Figure 84-2**). These patients have an abnormal ABI of less than 0.9 but have no walking limitations. Others could present with atypical symptoms such as leg fatigue or cramps. Patients with typical claudication (pain that is brought by walking and relieved after few minutes of rest) account for about 11% of those with PAD.

Patients with PAD have metabolic abnormalities stemming from reduced blood flow and $O_2$ delivery to the lower extremity muscles. There is reduction in muscle fibers by up to 50% compared with controls, smaller type I, and II muscle fibers. It is associated with hyperplastic mitochondria and demyelination of nerve fibers.

Two-thirds of patients with PAD can walk one-half a block with maximal walking speed at 1-2 mph and a peak $VO_2$ at 50% (similar to patients with heart failure NYHA III) in comparison to unlimited distance at 3-4 mph for normal patients.

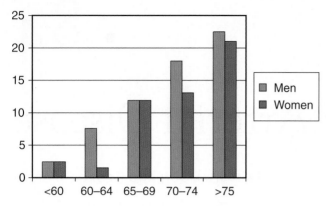

**Figure 84-1.** Prevalence of PAD by age. (Criqui et al. *Circulation.* 1985;71.)

## Physical Examination and Diagnosis

With a high index of suspicion for PAD, a thorough physical examination is done utilizing the vascular diagnostic laboratory (**Figure 84-3**).

Patients with any exertional limitation of the lower extremity or any history of walking impairment (fatigue, numbness, aching, or pain), ulcers of the legs or feet that heal poorly or not at all, and pain at rest localized in the lower leg or foot and its association with the upright or recumbent positions (**Figure 84-4**).

Measuring the ABI during the initial office visit is an easy but vital diagnostic and prognostic tool. Therefore, it is recommended for patients with the following characteristics:

1. Exertional leg symptoms
2. Non-healing wounds
3. Age 70 years or older
4. Age 50 years and older with history of smoking or diabetes.

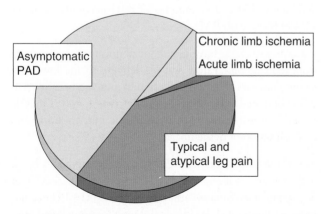

**Figure 84-2.** The clinical manifestations of PAD. (Hirsch. *Fam Pract Recertific.* 2000;15(suppl).)

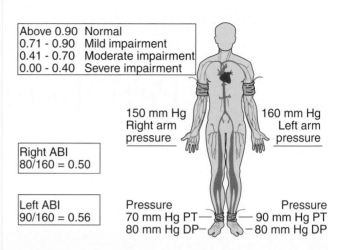

PT = posterior tibial; DP = dorsalis pedis.

**Figure 84-3.** Measuring ABI is a simple but vital diagnostic and prognostic tool. It should be performed on every high risk patient during his or her initial visit to the office. This figure also presents the correlation of ABI with the severity of PAD.

There is strong correlation between the ABI and cardiovascular mortality.

It is important to differentiate between claudication and pseudo-claudication. Claudication is characterized by recurring burning, aching, fatigue, or heaviness in the leg muscles with predictable level of walking, that resolves with a predictable duration of rest. It is not:

- pain at rest;
- pain while standing, lying, or sitting;
- pain that improves with walking or by leaning (e.g., on a shopping cart).

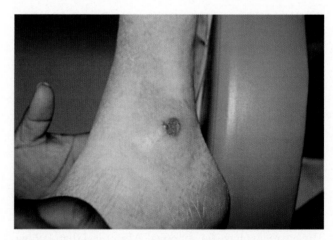

**Figure 84-4.** Arterial ulcer on the interior aspect of the ankle in a patient with severe PAD. (Modified from *Peripheral Vascular Disease: Basic Diagnostic and Therapeutic Approaches.* Abela et al.)

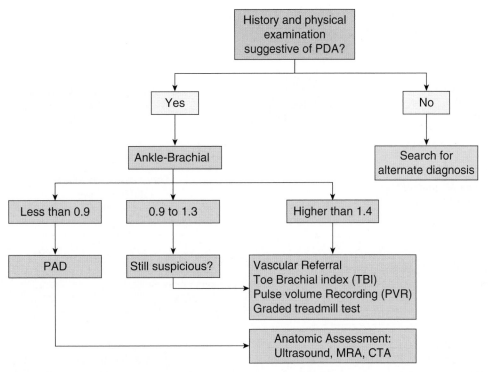

**Figure 84-5.** Approach to patient with leg pain.

Measuring ABI before and immediately after exercising the patient for 5 minutes on a 12.5% incline at a speed of 2 mph (stress ABI) helps to reveal those patients who have with PAD whose resting ABI is otherwise normal. For those who cannot exercise, reactive hyperemia testing (transient increase in organ blood flow that occurs following a brief period of ischemia) might be the alternative.

Smoking is the most important risk factor for developing PAD; it is followed by diabetes. The toe-brachial index (TBI) is used to establish the lower extremity PAD diagnosis in patients in whom lower extremity PAD is clinically suspected, but in whom the ABI test is not reliable due to calcified noncompressible vessels (advance age or diabetes) with normal TBI > 0.8.

Leg segmental pressure measurements are useful to establish the lower extremity PAD diagnosis when anatomic localization of lower extremity PAD is required to create a therapeutic plan.

Ultrasound is useful toward assessing PAD anatomy and presence of significant stenoses and to select patients who are candidates for endovascular or surgical revascularization. We suggest the following evaluation algorithm for patients with suspected PAD (see **Figure 84-5**):

- TBI should be checked in patients with an ABI >1.4.
- Walking stress test should be ordered in patients with lower extremity symptoms and normal ABI.

- A drop in ABI immediately after exercise indicates a positive stress test.
- A significant change from normal ABI pre-exercise to low ABI post-exercise may signify inflow disease involving the external iliac or common femoral arteries.

### Clinical Outcome
Patients with an ABI less than 0.9 (even without symptoms) have 3-5 times higher cardiovascular mortality, and those with an ABI of more than 1.4 have a similar increase in mortality. Also, the more abnormal the ABI the worse the prognosis. Diabetics and smokers are expected to have more amputations (**Figure 84-6**).

### Goals of Therapy and Revascularization
The goal of therapy is to improve the quality of life and functional status, identify and treat established systemic atherosclerosis, prolong survival, prevent progression of atherosclerosis, aggressively intervene where risk factors are present, and preserve or salvage limbs. According to the ACC/AHA PAD Guidelines, the indications for revascularization are:

1. non-healing ulcers
2. ischemic rest pain
3. claudication causing lifestyle limitations refractory to pharmacologic intervention and behavioral modification.

The following algorithm explains treatment targets in patients with PAD (see **Figure 84-7**).

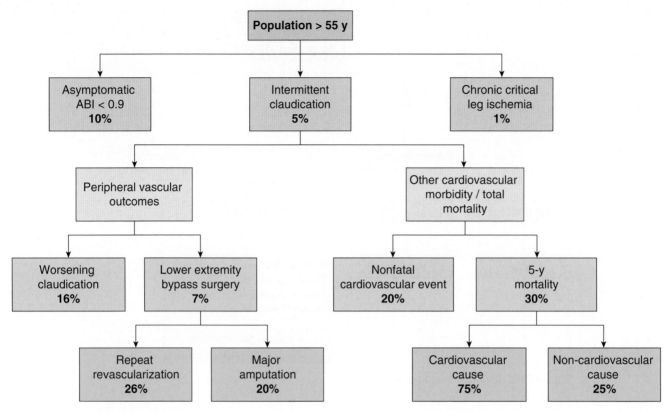

**Figure 84-6.** Outcome of patients with PAD. (From Weitz et al *Circulation* 1996;94(11):3026–3049 with permission)

Treatment of Symptomatic Lower Extremity Atherosclerotic Occlusive Disease

Medical management
- Risk factor modification
- Exercise
- Medications

Endovascular management
- Transluminal angioplasty
- Endovascular stents
- Intra-arterial thrombolytic therapy

Surgery
- Endarterectomy
- Bypass grafting
- Autogenous prosthetic
- Amputation
- Skin grafting (see **Figure 84-8**)

## Claudication Exercise Programs

Supervision of claudication exercise program 3 times/week for 3-6 months is effective for improving exercise performance, walking ability, and physical functioning. Patients should be encouraged to exercise until symptoms in the

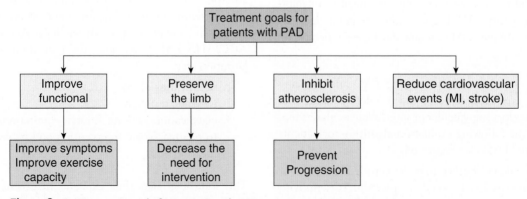

**Figure 84-7.** Treatment goals for patients with PAD.

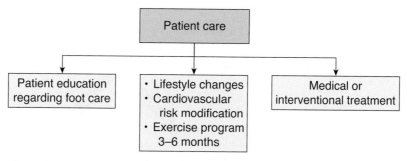

**Figure 84-8.** Comprehensive care for patients with PAD.

lower extremities are reproduced. However, although supervision is safe and cost effective, availability of supervised programs is limited; the patient who is on such a program requires discipline and motivation. Moreover, the benefits dissipate unless the exercise regimen is maintained. Also, education concerning risk factor modification is important.

Exercise therapy enlarges the radius of the supply vessels, enhances collateral vascular growth, increases type I muscle fibers, improves oxygen affinity by hemoglobin, and improves endothelial function.

## Pharmacotherapy for PAD

### FDA-Approved Medications
The following medications are approved by the U.S. Food and Drug Administration in the treatment of peripheral artery disease:

- Pentoxifylline
- Cilostazol

The following are medications that are under investigation:

- Statins
- Propionyl-L-carnitine
- L-arginine
- Prostaglandins
- Angiogenic factors: VEGF, bFGF

### Cilostazol
Cilostazol is the most effective drug therapy for claudication. It is a phosphodiesterase III inhibitor with vasodilator, metabolic, and antiplatelet activity; it inhibits platelet aggregation, arterial thrombosis, and vascular smooth muscle proliferation. The most common side effects include headache, diarrhea, and palpitations. The phosphodiesterase III inhibitor class of agents should not be given to patients with any evidence of congestive heart failure, because of a concern for increased risk of mortality as shown for other phosphodiesterase inhibitors. This agent has shown the best overall evidence for treatment benefit in patients with claudication. According to the ACC/AHA Guidelines, a course of cilostazol for 3-6 months should be first-line pharmacotherapy for the relief of claudication

symptoms, as evidence shows such a regimen results in both improved treadmill exercise performance and quality of life.

Thus:

- Cilostazol is the first-line of pharmacotherapy

### Lipid Lowering Agents
It is recommended that patients with PAD and LDL cholesterol of 100 mg/dL or greater be treated usually with a HMG Co-A reductase inhibitor (statins), but when the risk is very high (i.e., prior MI or stroke) the LDL cholesterol goal of less than 70 mg/dL is desirable. Statins have been shown to play an important role in the treatment of patients with PAD. There is evidence that statins:

- slow the progression of atherosclerosis in the lower extremities.
- improve cardiovascular risk morbidity and mortality in these patients.
- improve pain-free walking distance (PFWD) and quality of life (QOL).
- improve limb salvage in patients, post-revascularization.

### Antithrombotic Agents
Aspirin is effective in maintaining vascular-graft patency and may prevent thrombotic complications of PAD. However, if patients have severe disease, other precluding risk factors, or intolerance to aspirin, clopidogrel is recommended for the prevention of ischemic events in PAD patients.

### Endovascular Treatment
Endovascular procedures are indicated for individuals with lifestyle-limiting disability due to intermittent claudication when clinical features suggest a reasonable likelihood of symptomatic improvement, along with inadequate response to exercise or pharmacologic therapy and favorable risk-benefit ratio (i.e., focal aortoiliac occlusive disease). Endovascular intervention is recommended for TASC type A iliac and femoropopliteal lesions (for more in-depth information see recommended readings *The Trans-Atlantic Society Consensus*) (see **Figure 84-9**).

Endovascular intervention is not indicated if there is no significant pressure gradient across a stenosis, despite flow augmentation with vasodilators. Primary stent placement is not recommended in the femoral, popliteal, or tibial arteries. Endovascular intervention is not indicated as prophylactic therapy in an asymptomatic patient with lower extremity PAD.

### Surgical Treatment

A preoperative cardiovascular risk evaluation is important in patients with lower extremity PAD in whom a major vascular surgical intervention is planned. Bypasses to above-knee, below-knee popliteal, or the femoral-tibial arteries should be constructed with autogenous vein when possible. Prosthetic material can be used effectively for bypasses to the below-knee popliteal artery when no autogenous vein is available. Surgical intervention is not indicated to prevent progression from intermittent claudication to limb-threatening ischemia. In patients with combined inflow and outflow disease

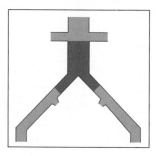
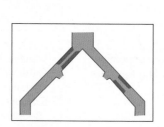

**Figure 84-9.** An example of TASC type A lesion (left) in the common iliac artery best treated with endovascular intervention. Type D lesion, (right) where open surgical revascularization is the preferred approach. (TASC II. *Eur J Vasc Endovasc Surg.* 33;2007.)

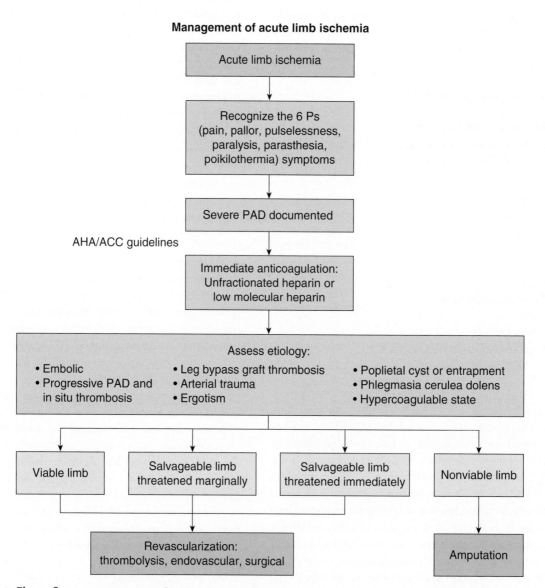

**Figure 84-10.** Management of acute limb ischemia.

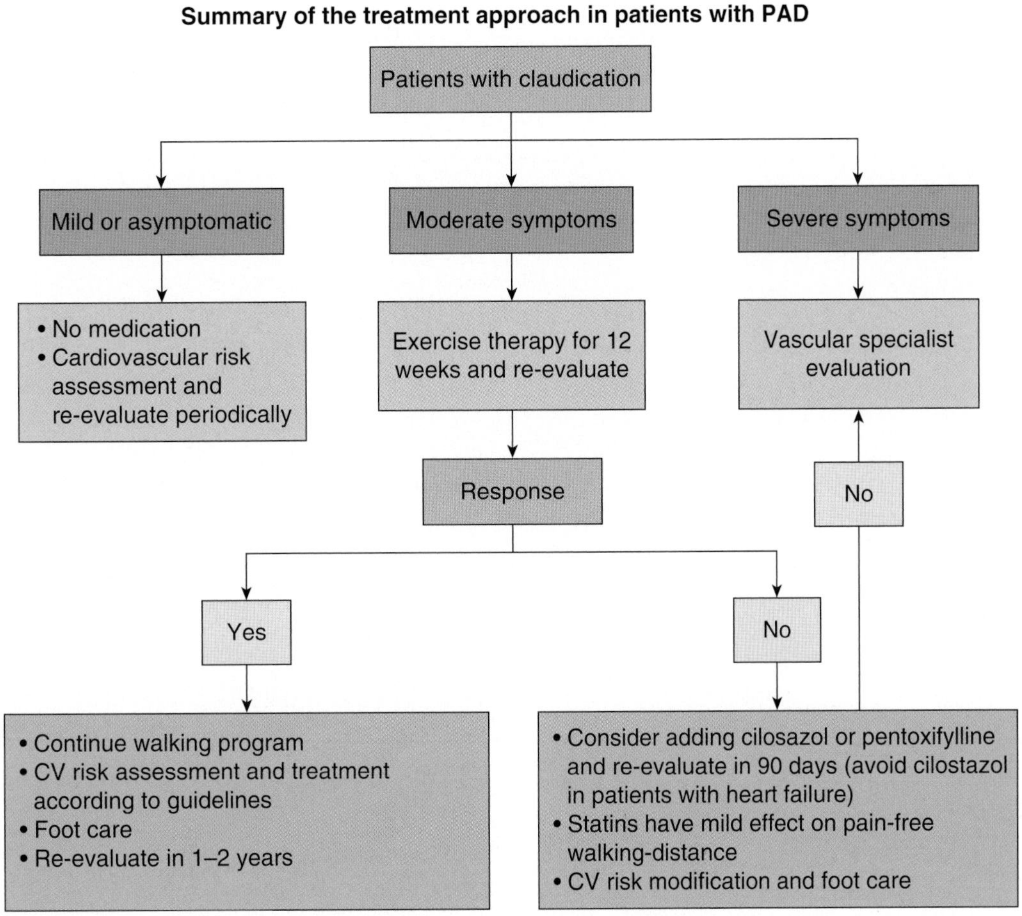

**Summary of the treatment approach in patients with PAD**

Figure 84-11. Summary of the treatment approach in patients with PAD.

with chronic limb ischemia (CLI), the inflow lesions should be addressed first. The outflow revascularization procedure should be performed in those with combined inflow and outflow disease when symptoms of CLI or infection persist after inflow revascularization. Patients with acute limb ischemia (ALI) and a salvageable extremity should undergo an emergent evaluation in order to define level of occlusion, which leads to prompt endovascular or surgical intervention. The risk of complications associated with lower extremity bypass surgery include: myocardial infarction (1.9-3.4%), death (1.3-6%), wound infection (10-30%), and scar-related neuropathic pain (23%). Thirty percent of grafts will require revision sometime during their lifetime.

## Management of Acute Limb Ischemia
The following flow chart (AHA/ACC Guidelines) outlines the management of acute limb ischemia (see **Figure 84-10** and **84-11**).

## Suggested Readings

1. ACC/AHA Guidelines for the Management of Patients with Peripheral Arterial Disease (lower extremity, renal, mesenteric, and abdominal aortic). *J Vasc Interv Radiol.* 2006 Sep;17(9):1383–1397.

2. Abela GS. *Peripheral Vascular Disease: Basic Diagnostic and Therapeutic Approaches.*

3. Inter-Society Consensus for the Management of Peripheral Arterial Disease (TASC II). *Eur J Vasc Endovasc Surg.* 2007;33(Suppl 1):S1–S75.

4. Creager M, Dzau V, Loscalzo J. *Vascular Medicine—A Companion to Braunwald's Heart Disease.*

5. William Hiatt. Medical treatment of peripheral arterial disease and claudication. *N Engl J Med.* 2001 May 24;344(21): 1608–1621.

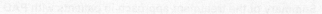

# 85

# Carotid Artery Disease

Justin E. Trivax and Robert D. Safian

- In contrast to the pathophysiology of acute coronary artery syndromes where symptoms are secondary to plaque rupture/erosion leading to in situ occlusive thrombus, embolization is the most frequent cause of symptomatic carotid artery disease (CAD).

- Patients undergoing coronary artery bypass graft surgery (CABG) have a high incidence of asymptomatic carotid stenosis, and 30% of postoperative strokes are due to severe carotid artery stenosis.

- Preoperative carotid screening is recommended in CABG patients with age >65 years, left main stenosis, known peripheral arterial disease, or any history of smoking, TIA, or stroke.

- Both NASCET and ECST established that symptomatic patients with carotid stenosis >70% derive the most benefit from carotid endarterectomy (CEA) compared to medical therapy.

- Carotid artery stenting is a reasonable alternative to CEA in patients with carotid artery stenosis who are at high risk for complications with traditional CEA.

## BACKGROUND

The public health and economic impact of cerebrovascular disease in the United States is staggering: Approximately 780,000 people per year experience a cerebrovascular accident (CVA), including 600,000 (77%) with a first stroke and 180,000 (23%) with recurrent stroke. Stroke remains the third leading cause of death despite aggressive medical therapy, counseling on healthy lifestyles, and revascularization. One stroke occurs every 40 seconds and 1 fatal stroke occurs every 3 to 4 minutes. Most stroke victims endure significant functional impairment, and the total cost of stroke care was estimated to be 65 billion dollars in 2008.

## ETIOLOGY OF STROKE

Stroke is a heterogeneous group of diseases with multiple etiologies and clinical presentations, including ischemic stroke in 85% and hemorrhagic stroke in 15% (**Table 85-1**). Ischemic stroke results from in situ thrombosis of a preexisting stenosis (50%), atheroembolism originating from the heart, aortic arch, or carotid arteries (20%), or lacunar infarction and thrombotic occlusion associated with hypertension (15%). Atherosclerosis alone accounts for one-third of all ischemic strokes. Cardioembolic sources of stroke are due to thrombi originating from the left atrium (left atrial appendage clot associated with atrial fibrillation), or from the left ventricle (mural thrombus associated with acute myocardial infarction or dilated cardiomyopathy); or from thrombi transiting through the heart (paradoxical embolism through a patent foramen ovale). Uncommon causes of ischemic stroke include endocarditis, hereditary thrombophilia, vasculitis, cerebral artery vasospasm, and venous thrombosis.

| Table 85-1 • Causes of Stroke | |
| --- | --- |
| Ischemic | 85% |
| Atherothrombotic | 50% |
| Embolic | 20% |
| Lacunar | 15% |
| Hemorrhagic | 15% |
| Subarachnoid | 10% |
| Intracerebral | 5% |

## ANATOMY OF THE CERVICOCEREBRAL CIRCULATION

The cervicocerebral circulation includes the aortic arch, great vessels, and intracranial arteries. Aortic arch types are arbitrarily defined by the spatial relationship of the great vessels to an imaginary line representing the apex of the superior curvature of the arch in a standard left anterior oblique (LAO) projection (**Figure 85-1**). In Type I aortic arch, the great vessels arise at or above the horizontal plane of the superior curvature of the aortic arch. In Type II aortic arch, the innominate artery (IA) originates below this line, and in Type III aortic arch, all three great vessels arise below this line. Selective angiography and intervention are more difficult in patients with arch Types II and III.

The arch configuration refers to the order of origin of the great vessels from the aortic arch and is generally classified as usual or anomalous configuration. In the usual configuration (65%), the order of origin from proximal to distal is the IA, the left common carotid artery (CCA) and the left subclavian artery (SCA). Usually, the IA gives rise to the right CCA and right SCA, and the right SCA gives rise to the right vertebral artery (VA). The right CCA bifurcates into the right internal (ICA) and external (ECA) carotid arteries, and the left CCA bifurcates into the left ICA and ECA. The left SCA arises from the distal aortic arch and gives rise to the left VA. Although anomalous configurations of the aortic arch are rarely associated with pathologic disease states, they are important to recognize for diagnostic and therapeutic purposes. The most common anomalies are shared origin of the IA and left CCA (bovine configuration, 27%) and origin of the left CCA from the proximal IA (7%). Other anomalies include origin of left VA directly from the arch (0.5%), aberrant right SCA and left-sided arch origin (arteria lusoria <0.5%), and common origin of the left CCA and left SCA from a left IA (1-2%).

Both ICA extend superiorly to the base of the skull and course intracranially as they enter the petrous bone. The ICA

bifurcates into the anterior cerebral artery (ACA) and middle cerebral arteries (MCA). In the posterior circulation, the left and right VA merge into the basilar artery which ascends inferior to the pons and divides into the posterior cerebral arteries (PCA) and superior cerebellar arteries. The left and right posterior circulation connect via the posterior communicating arteries (PCOM) and the left and right anterior circulation connect via the anterior communicating artery (ACOM).

## PATHOPHYSIOLOGY OF CAROTID ARTERY DISEASE

Atherosclerosis of the carotid artery is histologically similar to atherosclerosis in other arterial beds. Approximately 90% of carotid atherosclerotic lesions involve the cervical portion of the ICA within 2 cm of the carotid bulb, whereas 10% of lesions are located in the intrathoracic or intracranial carotid artery. Despite histologic similarities, there are many pathophysiologic differences between coronary and carotid artery disease (CAD) (**Table 85-2**). Clinical consequences of chronic ischemic heart disease are generally related to progressive coronary artery stenosis, and the mismatch between myocardial blood flow and demand is usually manifested as exertional angina. Anginal symptoms often progress to angina at rest when stenosis severity impairs resting myocardial blood flow. Acute coronary syndromes (UA-NSTEMI) are associated with unstable plaque and vessel thrombosis. ST elevation myocardial infarction is most often due to in situ thrombosis of a coronary artery, and the extent of myocardial damage and resultant disability are closely related to the location of the thrombus and to the size and distribution of the occluded artery. In contrast, while progressive stenosis and in situ thrombosis are the most frequent causes of coronary artery disease, embolization is the most frequent cause of symptomatic CAD, which manifests as transient ischemic attack (TIA) or stroke. In the absence of embolization, progressive carotid stenosis leading to occlusion is often clinically silent because of the

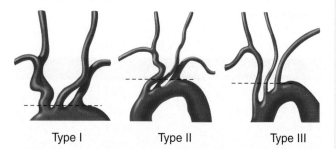

**Figure 85-1.** Aortic arch types. (Reprinted with permission from Casserly IP, Yadav JS. Carotid intervention. In: Casserly IP, Sachar R, Yadav JS, eds. *Manual of Peripheral Vascular Intervention.* Philadelphia, PA: Lippincott Williams & Wilkins; 2005:83–109.)

| Table 85-2 • Comparison of Coronary and Carotid Artery Disease | | |
| --- | --- | --- |
| **Factor** | **Coronary** | **Carotid** |
| Pathophysiology | Atherosclerosis | Atherosclerosis |
| Symptoms due to: | Progressive stenosis | Embolization |
| MI or CVA due to: | In situ thrombosis | Embolization |
| MI/CVA: | Nonhemorrhagic | Hemorrhagic (20%) |
| Injury and disability | Closely related | Variable |
| *MI, myocardial infarction; CVA, cerebrovascular accident* | | |

integrity of the ACOM and PCOM. Acute carotid artery occlusion is a less common cause of acute stroke, and generally suggests incomplete development of the Circle of Willis and the communicating arteries. The extent of disability after a stroke is variable. While large strokes are often disabling, small strokes in strategic locations, particularly the brain stem, can lead to devastating disabilities. Finally, hemorrhagic transformation of ischemic infarction is rarely observed in the heart (unless thrombolytic therapy is used), but occurs in 20% of ischemic strokes.

## CLINICAL SYNDROMES OF CAROTID ARTERY DISEASE

Symptomatic extracranial carotid artery disease is usually due to embolization leading to retinal, hemispheric, and global cerebral syndromes. Monocular retinal syndromes (transient visual loss and permanent retinal infarction) are highly suggestive of ipsilateral carotid disease. Transient retinal ischemia or amaurosis fugax is classically described as a shade coming down over one eye. Symptoms may last seconds to minutes and may not be associated with motor or sensory deficits, aphasia, or neglect. Retinal artery occlusion presents as an acute, painless loss of vision; complete monocular visual loss is usually due to central retinal artery occlusion, whereas loss of segments of the visual field are usually due to branch occlusion.

Unilateral motor or sensory loss, and aphasia or neglect, are the cardinal hemispheric manifestations of contralateral carotid stenosis. Patients presenting with global cerebral ischemia often have cerebellar (ataxia) or brainstem signs (dysarthria, diplopia, dysphagia) and unilateral or bilateral visual, motor, and/or sensory impairment. Most global ischemic syndromes are due to disease in the posterior circulation (vertebrobasilar system) rather than unilateral CAD. However, patients with critical bilateral carotid stenosis may experience simultaneous or alternating bilateral hemispheric symptoms, which may be confused with vertebrobasilar insufficiency.

## SCREENING FOR CAROTID ARTERY DISEASE

The purpose of screening for extracranial carotid artery disease is stroke prevention. Indications for screening in the general population of asymptomatic patients include age >65 years and at least 3 cardiovascular risk factors (hypertension, coronary artery disease, current cigarette smoking, and hyperlipidemia) (**Table 85-3**). Asymptomatic carotid bruits may be heard in 50% of patients with carotid stenosis ≥75%, but may be absent in patients with critical stenosis. Patients undergoing coronary artery bypass graft surgery

**Table 85-3 • Indications for Screening for Asymptomatic Carotid Artery Disease**

| General population of asymptomatic patient |
| --- |
| Age >65 years and >3 risk factors, including: |
|   Hypertension |
|   Coronary artery disease |
|   Current smoking |
|   Hyperlipidemia |
|   Carotid bruit |
| **Patients undergoing coronary artery bypass surgery (CABG)** |
| Age >65 years and having: |
|   Left main coronary stenosis |
|   Peripheral arterial disease |
|   History of smoking |
|   History of transient ischemic attack or stroke |

(CABG) have a high incidence of asymptomatic carotid stenosis. In fact, 20% have carotid stenosis >50%, 12% have carotid stenosis >80%, and 30% of postoperative strokes are due to severe carotid artery stenosis. Accordingly, preoperative carotid screening is recommended in CABG patients with age >65 years, left main stenosis, known peripheral arterial disease, or any history of smoking, TIA, or stroke.

## DIAGNOSIS OF CAROTID ARTERY DISEASE

The standard method for the noninvasive evaluation of carotid artery disease is carotid duplex ultrasound (CDU). CDU relies on a transverse two-dimensional grayscale ultrasound to localize the carotid bifurcation and to characterize the extent and location of plaque. Longitudinal scans are performed to delineate the layers of the vessel wall, plaque composition, and to guide Doppler interrogation (spectral waveform analysis and velocity). The most reliable measurement for assessment of stenosis severity is the ICA peak systolic velocity (PSV), although end-diastolic velocity (EDV) and internal carotid to common carotid artery velocity ratio add to the assessment (**Table 85-4**). CDU has a sensitivity and specificity of 89% and 84%, respectively, for carotid

**Table 85-4 • Duplex Ultrasound Criteria for Carotid Stenosis**

| Stenosis (%) | PSV (cm/sec) | EDV (cm/sec) | ICA/CCA |
| --- | --- | --- | --- |
| <50 | <125 | <40 | <2 |
| 50-69 | 125-230 | 40-110 | 2-4 |
| 70-99 | >230 | >110 | >4 |

*PSV, peak systolic velocity in internal carotid artery; EDV, end-diastolic velocity in internal carotid artery; ICA/CCA, ratio of peak systolic velocities in internal and common carotid arteries*

**Table 85-5 • Advantages and Disadvantages of Imaging Modalities for Carotid Artery Disease**

|  | Advantages | Disadvantages |
|---|---|---|
| CDU | Easy<br>Inexpensive<br>Plaque characterization | Differentiate subtotal occlusion from total occlusion<br>Complex lesions (kinked, calcified)<br>Aortic arch and intracranial evaluation |
| CTA | Calcified lesions<br>Plaque characterization<br>Aortic arch and intracranial evaluation | Iodinated contrast<br>Radiation exposure |
| MRA | Aortic arch and intracranial evaluation<br>No iodinated contrast or radiation | Expensive<br>Calcified lesions<br>Overestimates stenosis |

CDU, carotid duplex ultrasound; CTA, computed tomography angiography; MRA, magnetic resonance angiography

stenosis 70-99%, as compared to carotid angiography. CDU is more limited in the presence of heavy calcification, arterial kinking, and differentiation of complete occlusion from near-total occlusion. Velocity profiles may be more difficult to interpret in the presence of frequent arrhythmia, aortic insufficiency, contralateral carotid occlusion, and in patients with intrathoracic or intracranial stenosis.

In contrast, computed tomographic angiography (CTA) and magnetic resonance angiography (MRA) permit reliable imaging of the arch and intrathoracic great vessels, cervical portion of the carotid and vertebral arteries, and the intracranial circulation. CTA is especially useful for assessment of calcified lesions and is better than CDU for differentiating high-grade stenosis from complete occlusion. Limitations of CTA include patient exposure to ionizing radiation and iodinated contrast. MRA avoids exposure to radiation and iodinated contrast, but gadolinium should be used with caution in patients with advanced renal insufficiency because of a small risk of nephrogenic systemic fibrosis. MRA correlates well with angiography, but may overestimate stenosis severity. In general, CTA and MRA are not recommended for screening purposes or for evaluation of an asymptomatic bruit, and they are not recommended to "confirm" CDU finding, unless there is something ambiguous about the results (**Table 85-5**).

## CAROTID ANGIOGRAPHY

Catheter-based carotid angiography is rarely necessary to establish a diagnosis of carotid stenosis, but may be recommended prior to carotid revascularization and in ambiguous situations. The purpose of angiography is to define the aortic arch type, configuration of the great vessels, condition of the intracranial circulation, and stenosis severity. Potential complications of carotid angiography include contrast nephropathy, anaphylactoid reactions, atheroembolism, vascular injury, stroke, and rarely death. There is a slightly increased risk of stroke and transient ischemic attack in symptomatic patients compared to asymptomatic patients. Major complication rates have declined with improvements in operator technique and equipment, occurring now in <1% of patients. Three angiographic methods have been used to assess stenosis severity, and each result in different estimates (**Figure 85-2**). The North American Symptomatic Carotid Endarterectomy Trial (NASCET) method is the most widely accepted, and uses the normal internal carotid artery distal to the stenosis as the reference segment. The European Carotid Surgery Trial (ECST) method and the common carotid method may overestimate stenosis severity compared to the NASCET method, as they rely on the larger carotid bulb and common carotid artery, respectively, as the reference segments.

## MEDICAL TREATMENT

### Risk Factor Modification

Risk factors for atherosclerosis include modifiable (hypertension, dyslipidemia, diabetes mellitus, smoking, obesity, and physical inactivity) and nonmodifiable risk factors (age >65 years, male gender, African-American race, and family history of vascular disease); risk factor modification is essential for reducing cardiovascular morbidity, including stroke. More than 50 million people in the United States have hypertension, which is the strongest risk factor for ischemic and hemorrhagic stroke. Even small reductions in systolic and diastolic blood pressure (5-10 mm Hg) can decrease risk of stroke by almost 40%. Angiotensin-converting enzyme inhibitors (ACEI) and angiotensin receptor blockers are ideal agents for hypertension, and are associated with beneficial effects on stroke and cardiovascular morbidity and mortality compared to beta-blockers and diuretics.

The relationship between hyperlipidemia and the overall risk of stroke is ambiguous, but there appears to be a stronger relationship between hyperlipidemia and ischemic stroke than hemorrhagic stroke. There is also a strong relationship between total- and LDL-cholesterol and carotid atherosclerosis. The Heart Protection Study demonstrated a 30% reduction in first ischemic stroke (primary prevention) in patients with cardiac and vascular disease treated with simvastatin versus placebo. The Stroke Prevention by Aggressive Reduction in Cholesterol Levels (SPARCL) Trial demonstrated that patients with recent stroke or TIA had a 21% reduction in stroke (secondary prevention) after treatment with atorvastatin versus placebo. The benefits of statins for primary and secondary

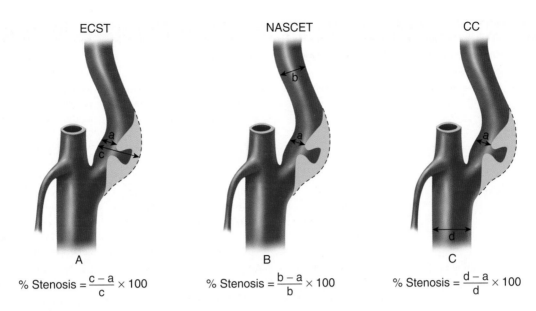

**Figure 85-2.** Angiographic methods for assessment of carotid stenosis severity. (Reprinted with permission from Osborn AG. *Diagnostic Cerebral Angiography*. 2nd ed. Philadelphia, PA: Williams & Wilkins; 1999. Abbreviations: CC= common carotid; ECST= European Carotid Surgery Trial; NASCET= North American Symptomatic Carotid Endarterectomy Trial.)

prevention of stroke appear to be multifactorial, and may be due to reduction in LDL-cholesterol, plaque stabilization, less inflammation, and improvement in endothelial function. These data support current guidelines for the use of statins in patients with carotid stenosis >50% and those with prior TIA or stroke, although statins have not been studied for stroke prevention in patients with carotid disease. Current recommendations are for patients to achieve LDL <100 mg/dL (<70 mg/dL if IHD is present) and non-HDL-cholesterol <130 mg/dL.

Diabetes mellitus is strongly associated with ischemic stroke, imparting a two- to fivefold higher risk than that experienced by nondiabetics. The risk of stroke is increased by the duration of diabetes and the presence of hypertension. Even though tight glycemic control has not been proven to reduce the risk of stroke, the American Diabetes Association recommends A1C level <7.0% and fasting glucose levels 90-130 mg/dL.

Cigarette smoking is a strong risk factor for ischemic and hemorrhagic stroke, and heavy smokers (>40 cigarettes per day) have a two- to fourfold higher risk of stroke than light smokers (<10 cigarettes per day). Patients who quit smoking for 5 years have the same risk of stroke as nonsmokers. Smoking cessation and avoidance of secondhand smoke are recommended in all patients with carotid artery disease, and should be accomplished by pharmacological agents, nicotine replacement, or formal smoking cessation programs.

Physical inactivity and obesity are considered important risk factors for stroke. Inactivity may contribute to premature carotid artery disease, and truncal obesity may increase the risk of stroke by its strong association with hypertension, hyperlipidemia, and insulin resistance. The beneficial effects of physical fitness and weight reduction are probably related to effects on blood pressure, lipid metabolism, insulin sensitivity, and inflammation. A body mass index 18.5-24.9 kg/m² is recommended, including a waist circumference <40 inches in men and <35 inches in women.

## Antiplatelet Therapy

While patients with acute coronary syndrome and those undergoing percutaneous coronary intervention benefit from combination antiplatelet therapy, regimens for myocardial protection may increase the risk of bleeding without reducing the risk of stroke. Four antiplatelet agents have been evaluated for primary or secondary prevention of stroke (aspirin (ASA), clopidogrel, ticlopidine, dipyridamole) (**Table 85-6**), leading to treatment guidelines from the American Heart Association and American Stroke Association. The Framingham Risk Score may be used to assess the 10-year risk of stroke, and aspirin (81-325 mg) is recommended for primary prevention in patients with stroke risk >6%. In a large primary prevention trial in women, aspirin decreased the risk of TIA or stroke by 9%, but did not impact the risk of myocardial infarction or cardiovascular death. In contrast, aspirin decreased overall cardiovascular risk in men, but did not prevent TIA or stroke. Aspirin is recommended for secondary prevention of TIA or stroke, providing a relative risk reduction of 16% and 28% for fatal and nonfatal stroke, respectively. Aspirin doses >325 mg daily do not provide additional benefit.

**Table 85-6 • Summary of Antiplatelet Therapy and Stroke Prevention**

| Drug | Stroke: Primary Prevention | Stroke: Secondary Prevention | Cardiovascular Morbidity and Mortality | Comment |
|---|---|---|---|---|
| Aspirin | Effective in women, not men | Effective in men, not women | Effective for primary prevention in men and secondary prevention in men and women | Recommended for primary prevention of all cardiovascular (coronary or stroke) events in patients with 5-year coronary heart risk >3%; does not reduce the risk of stroke in low risk patients. |
| Ticlopidine | Not studied | Effective in men and women as an alternative to aspirin | Reduces the incidence of MI, need for vascular surgery for PAD, and vascular morbidity | Effective in the secondary prevention of stroke, MI, vascular events. Side effects include TTP, neutropenia and gastrointestinal symptoms |
| Clopidogrel | Not studied | Effective in men and women as an alternative to aspirin | Alternative to aspirin for prevention of cardiac events in PAD patients | Dual therapy with ASA is not recommended for primary or secondary prevention of TIA or stroke, and causes increased bleeding. Dual antiplatelet therapy is recommended in patients with ACS and after recent PCI |
| Dipyridamole | Not studied | Dual therapy with ASA is superior to ASA alone | Not recommended | Only therapy better than ASA alone for secondary prevention of stroke |

*MI, myocardial infarction; PAD, peripheral arterial disease; TTP, thrombotic thrombocytopenic purpura; ASA, aspirin; TIA, transient ischemic attack; ACS, acute coronary syndrome; PCI, percutaneous coronary intervention*

The thienopyridines (ticlopidine and clopidogrel) have not been studied for primary prevention of TIA and stroke. For secondary prevention, ticlopidine resulted in a 23% reduction in cardiovascular events compared to placebo and fewer cerebrovascular events and bleeding complications than effected by aspirin. However, long-term use of ticlopidine is limited by neutropenia, so it has been replaced by clopidogrel. When prescribed alone, aspirin and clopidogrel have similar benefits for secondary prevention of stroke. The combination of aspirin and clopidogrel does not provide incremental risk reduction compared to aspirin alone, increases the risk of systemic and intracranial bleeding, and is not routinely recommended.

Extended-release dipyridamole (ER-DP) is not recommended for primary prevention of TIA, stroke, or cardiovascular disease. For secondary prevention, ER-DP is superior to placebo and similar to aspirin. Although one study suggested that the combination of aspirin and ER-DP was not superior to aspirin alone, another study suggested that the combined therapy resulted in less myocardial infarction (MI), stroke, and vascular death. In fact, aspirin plus ER-DP is the only approved combination therapy for secondary prevention of stroke. Ongoing studies are evaluating the combination of ER-DP plus aspirin compared to clopidogrel alone for secondary prevention of stroke.

# CAROTID ARTERY REVASCULARIZATION

In all patients with coronary or peripheral arterial disease (PAD), risk factor modification and antiplatelet therapy are recommended for prevention of stroke and cardiovascular events. Decisions about carotid artery revascularization are based on symptoms, stenosis severity, and the procedural risk of revascularization. Symptomatic status is based on the presence of TIA or stroke within 6 months; patients with remote neurological events are considered asymptomatic. In addition, patients with symptomatic carotid artery disease are considered to have retinal and/or hemispheric symptoms in the distribution of the ipsilateral carotid stenosis; nonfocal symptoms such as generalized weakness or dizziness are not typical for symptomatic carotid stenosis. Symptomatic status is important, since the presence of symptoms imparts >twofold increase in the risk of subsequent stroke compared to asymptomatic patients. The risk of revascularization is generally considered in the context of the risk of carotid endarterectomy (CEA), which is widely accepted as the gold standard for carotid revascularization. Major clinical trials of CEA and medical therapy included patients with a relatively low risk of perioperative cardiovascular complications (<3-6%), and patients at high risk were uniformly excluded.

In the contemporary assessment of the risk of CEA, it is generally accepted that some patients have a high risk of perioperative cardiovascular complication (>6-10%), including the presence of one or more complex anatomical conditions or medical comorbidities.

Early randomized trials of CEA failed to show any benefit compared to medical therapy, suggesting that CEA was a "sham" procedure. These early trials were limited by poor design, operator inexperience, and unexpectedly high perioperative morbidity, and have been mostly rejected. Subsequently, five large randomized clinical trials were published, confirming the benefits of CEA. The studies for symptomatic patients were NASCET, ECST, Veterans Affairs Cooperative Studies Program 309 Trial (VA); for asymptomatic patients, the studies were Asymptomatic Carotid Atherosclerosis Study (ACAS) and Asymptomatic Carotid Surgery Trial (ACST). In these landmark trials, CEA was compared to medical therapy, which for the most part was antiplatelet therapy with aspirin alone. Although ACST included antihypertensive and cholesterol-lowering therapy, the nature and the endpoints of this therapy were not specified.

Nevertheless, these important trials established the superiority of CEA compared to aspirin among low risk patients with carotid stenosis, since high risk patients were excluded (**Table 85-7**). Both NASCET and ECST confirmed a 65-67% reduction in the risk of ipsilateral stroke at 5 years after CEA for symptomatic patients with severe carotid stenosis. Each study used different definitions for stenosis severity, but it is widely accepted that symptomatic patients with carotid

### Table 85-7 • High Risk Criteria for Carotid Endarterectomy

**Anatomical criteria**

High lesion above C-2
Low lesion below clavicle
Radical neck dissection*
Neck radiation*
Contralateral carotid occlusion
Tracheostomy*
Contralateral cranial nerve palsy

**Clinical criteria**

Age >80 years
NYHA Class III-IV CHF
CCS Class III-IV angina
Severe CAD
LVEF <30%
Severe pulmonary disease
Severe renal dysfunction
Urgent heart surgery ≤30 days

*NYHA, New York Heart Association; CHF, congestive heart failure; CCS, Canadian Cardiovascular Society; CAD, coronary artery disease; LVEF, left ventricular ejection fraction*
*\* Often referred to as "hostile neck"*

stenosis >70% derive the most benefit from revascularization. In NASCET there was a gradient of stroke reduction at 5 years that was dependent on stenosis severity: CEA resulted in 65% reduction in stroke for patients with carotid stenosis >70%, 29% reduction for carotid stenosis 50-69%, and no reduction for carotid stenosis <50%.

One potentially important issue is the timing of CEA in symptomatic patients. Important considerations include the nature of symptoms, the duration between symptom onset and presentation, and the stenosis severity. In the past, standard recommendations were to delay CEA for 4-6 weeks after symptom onset to avoid the risk of intracranial hemorrhage. Unfortunately, this approach led to cerebral infarction while patient awaited revascularization. Contemporary approaches rely on early brain imaging to exclude intracranial hemorrhage at the time of symptom onset, followed by rapid risk stratification to identify patients at greatest risk for stroke. In general, the cumulative risk of stroke in symptomatic patients is 20% within 90 days, and is highest in patients presenting with motor deficits, neglect, or aphasia, and lowest in patients with pure sensory deficits or retinal syndromes. Urgent CEA within 2-14 days is recommended in patients with high risk symptoms, time interval <7 days between last symptom and presentation, and carotid stenosis >70%, after excluding intracranial hemorrhage by appropriate imaging studies.

In asymptomatic patients with carotid stenosis >70%, CEA resulted in a 46-54% reduction in the risk of ipsilateral stroke at 5 years compared to aspirin alone. In a meta-analysis of CEA in asymptomatic patients, the greatest risk reduction was observed in asymptomatic young men.

In contrasting the 5-year outcomes of CEA and medical therapy in low risk patients, several interesting observations emerge.

First, symptomatic patients have a two- to threefold higher risk of stroke than asymptomatic patients after CEA (10% versus 5%), and after medical therapy alone (25% versus 10%). Second, CEA results in ≥50% reduction in ipsilateral stroke compared to medical therapy alone for symptomatic (10% versus 25%) and asymptomatic patients (5% versus 10%). Third, the cumulative risk of stroke at 5 years after CEA is dependent on the perioperative risk of stroke within 30 days, plus the additive risk of stroke over the ensuing 5 years. About 60% of the risk of stroke is incurred in the first 30 days after CEA for symptomatic (6% of the 10%) and asymptomatic (3% of the 5%) patients. Finally, the risk of stroke after CEA is twofold higher in symptomatic than asymptomatic patients, including perioperative stroke within 30 days (6% versus 3%), and the subsequent risk of stroke over 5 years (1% per year versus 0.5% per year).

Although the merits of CEA and medical therapy have been studied in low risk patients, CEA was being performed in high risk patients without data from randomized trials to substantiate its safety and efficacy. Observational studies suggested that the perioperative morbidity and mortality after CEA was substantially higher in high risk patients than low risk patients, leading to interest in percutaneous techniques for carotid revascularization. Early studies of carotid angioplasty were hampered by inadequate equipment, technique, and experience, leading to unacceptably high risks of embolic stroke and need for "neurological rescue." In the last decade, there has been dramatic evolution of percutaneous carotid revascularization, resulting from the availability of embolic protection devices (EPDs), shift from neurologic rescue to neurologic protection, design and use of dedicated self-expanding stents for the carotid bifurcation, and improvements in operator experience and technique. Although initially designed and studied for high risk patients, carotid artery stenting (CAS) has been extensively studied in high and low risk patients in numerous nonrandomized and randomized trials.

The primary goal of CEA and CAS is stroke prevention and is accomplished by lumen enlargement and plaque passivation. From a technical standpoint, CAS is more dependent on the angiographic nuances of the aortic arch type and configuration, and the ability to achieve safe access to the carotid bifurcation. Most operators utilize a retrograde femoral artery approach, although brachial and radial artery approaches have been utilized as well. Access to the CCA can be achieved with a guiding catheter or interventional sheath, and equipment selection is largely operator-dependent. Patients should be pretreated with aspirin and clopidogrel, and anticoagulation during the procedure is achieved with heparin or bivalirudin.

EPDs have been incorporated into the standard of care for CAS, although their value has not been evaluated in randomized trials without EPD. However, it is unlikely that such trials will be performed. In general, EPDs fall into two categories, including proximal and distal devices, and both have advantages and disadvantages. Proximal EPDs rely on transient occlusion of the ECA and CCA, resulting in stagnant or reversed flow in the ICA. These devices are appealing because they establish embolic protection before the carotid stenosis is crossed with a guidewire. After stent deployment, blood is aspirated from the carotid bifurcation to remove debris, followed by deflation of the balloons and completion angiography. In contrast to proximal EPDs, distal EPDs must first cross the target lesion before deployment in the distal ICA. Distal protection is achieved with a filter or occlusion balloon on the end of the EPD. After completion of the intervention, the filter is recaptured and removed. If a balloon occlusion device is used, the ICA is aspirated first to remove debris, and then the balloon is deflated, prior to completion angiography. There are no comparative studies of different EPDs, and all devices are able to capture and remove debris. Although unusual, stroke may occur despite EPD due to incomplete capture or retrieval of debris.

The choice of stents for CAS is operator-dependent. Stainless steel or nitinol self-expanding stents are always utilized for the cervical portion of the carotid artery because of superior conformability and resistance to deformation that might occur with balloon-expandable stents. Angioplasty is used to predilate the lesion and postdilate the stent. The goals of CAS and PCI are different, and moderate residual stenosis after CAS is acceptable. Pursuit of a perfect angiographic result after CAS can increase the risk of complications and should be avoided.

Worldwide experience of CAS includes observational studies before EPDs, voluntary registries, prospective multicenter registries, and randomized clinical trials. The early observational studies before EPDs and the voluntary registries are notable for inclusion of nearly 20,000 patients, but were limited because the technique of CAS and independent oversight were not standardized. Nevertheless, these registries reported technical success rates >95%, neurologic events in 3-6%, and restenosis rates <4% at 5 years. In contrast to the voluntary registries, the prospective multicenter registries utilized predefined inclusion and exclusion criteria, clearly defined protocols, independent neurological evaluation before and after CAS, and special oversight committees to ensure safety and compliance. These registries were performed in high risk patients as part of IDE trials to acquire food and administration (FDA) approval in the United States, conformité européenne (CE) approval in Europe, or as part of FDA postmarketing approval. For comparison, these studies utilized a historically weighted estimate of strokes or death of 14.5% at 30 days after CEA (high risk patients). In all, there are about 20 high risk registries, including more than 30,000 patients. In most studies, the primary endpoint was major adverse cardiovascular events (MACE) at 30 days (death, stroke, myocardial infarction), and secondary endpoints included procedural success and ipsilateral stroke at 1-3 years. Many studies have been published, and others continue to actively enroll patients. Data from these high risk registries indicate procedural success rates >95%, a decline in 30-day MACE from 8% in early studies to <4% in more contemporary studies, and ipsilateral stroke at 1 year in 1-4%. Contemporary CAS experience suggests that symptomatic status, end-stage renal disease, and need for CABG within 6 weeks are independent predictors of MACE and stroke at 30 days. Anatomic complexity, such as complex arch anatomy, vessel tortuosity, and lesion calcification, is more common in the very elderly and may explain the excess of complications in octogenarians.

Numerous randomized clinical trials have been completed or are in active phases of enrollment, comparing CEA and CAS in high and low risk patients. Like the early randomized trials of CEA and medical therapy, early trials of CEA and CAS were limited by poor technology, inexperience, and lack of EPDs. The Stenting and Angioplasty with Protection in Patients at High Risk for Endarterectomy (SAPPHIRE) study is the only randomized trial of CEA and CAS in high risk patients that utilized contemporary stent technology and EPD, but was terminated prematurely due to slow enrollment. There was a trend toward lower MACE at 30 days after CAS (4.8% versus 9.8%, p = 0.09), low composite MACE and ipsilateral stroke at 1 year after CAS (12.2% versus 20.1%, p = 0.05), and similar 3-year rates of ipsilateral stroke (7.1% versus 6.7%, p = NS) and target vessel revascularization (3.0% versus 7.1%, p = NS) for CAS and CEA. Compared to CAS, CEA was associated with more procedure-related myocardial infarction and cranial nerve palsy. There are several randomized trials of CEA and CAS is low risk patients, including symptomatic (Stent-Protected Angioplasty versus Carotid Endarterectomy (SPACE), Endarterectomy versus Stenting in Patients with Symptomatic Severe Carotid Stenosis (EVA-3S), International Carotid Stenting Study (ICSS)) and asymptomatic (Asymptomatic Carotid Stenosis Stenting versus Endarterectomy Trial (ACT-1), Asymptomatic Carotid Surgery Trial-2 (ACST-2)) patients; one study enrolled both symptomatic and asymptomatic patients (Carotid Revascularization Endarterectomy versus Stent Trial (CREST)). These trials are in various stages of completion: SPACE and EVA-3S were terminated prematurely due to slow enrollment, and the results of both studies have been published. EVA-3S reported less stroke and death at 30 days after CEA compared to CAS (3.9% versus 9.6%, p = 0.01), but was limited by operator inexperience with CAS, poor CAS enrollment, and inconsistent use of EPDs and dual antiplatelet therapy. In SPACE, the incidence of death and ipsilateral stroke was similar after CEA and CAS (6.3% versus 6.8%, p = NS), despite the fact that 73% of CAS patients did not receive EPDs. In ICSS, the 120-day interim analysis showed that CAS resulted in similar rates of disabling stroke or death compared with CEA (4.0% vs. 3.2%, p= 0.23). In CREST, the incidence of stroke, myocardial infarction, or death was similar in the CAS and CEA at 4 years (7.2% vs. 6.8%, p= 0.51). While periprocedural and postprocedural ipsilateral stroke was higher with CAS compared with CEA (4.1% vs. 2.3%, p= 0.01), the majority of strokes were nondisabling. The incidence of cranial nerve palsy was much higher in the CEA group compared with the CAS group (4.7% vs. 0.3%, p< 0.001) and resulted in permanent disability. Enrollment in ACT-1 and ACST-2 is ongoing.

## Risk Assessment

In patients with CAD, the goal of therapy is to reduce the risk of stroke. A complete assessment of risk requires an understanding of the natural history of medically treated patients and determinants of the risk of revascularization. There are a number of important gaps in our understanding of the natural history of carotid stenosis, particularly regarding the risk of stroke in unrevascularized high risk asymptomatic patients and the relative benefits of medical therapies other than aspirin. Although the landmark studies of CEA and aspirin provide useful insight into the natural history of asymptomatic low risk patients, there are no randomized trials of "optimal medical therapy" and carotid revascularization (CEA or CAS) in high risk patients. Some observational studies suggest that certain high risk asymptomatic patients with carotid stenosis >80% may have a stroke risk >6% per year, so data from low risk patients in ACST and ACAS may not apply to high risk patients. Although statins, ACE inhibitors, and thienopyridines have been advocated as important therapies for stroke prevention, none have been specifically studied in patients with carotid stenosis, so their benefit relative to aspirin and impact relative to revascularization is unknown.

In contrast, the nature, frequency, and determinants of the risk of revascularization have been studied in high and low risk patients. For CEA and CAS, the types and incidence of complications are remarkably similar (**Table 85-8**). There are similarities and differences in the anatomical and

| Table 85-8 • Potential Complications of Carotid Revascularization | | |
|---|---|---|
| | **CEA** | **CAS** |
| Cardiovascular | Hypertension (20%), Hypotension (5%), MI (1%) | VV/VDR (5-10%), MI (<1%) |
| Carotid artery | Dissection, thrombosis (1%), Restenosis (5-10%) | Dissection (<1%), Thrombosis (<1%), Restenosis (3-5 %), |
| Neurological | HPS (<1%), ICH (<1%), seizures (<1%), TIA (1-2%) stroke (2-6%), cranial nerve injury (4-5%) | HPS (<1%), ICH (<1%), TIA (1-2%), stroke (2-3%) |
| General | Wound infection (1%) | Access site injury (5%), contrast reactions (1%), RCN (1-2%) |
| Death | 1% | 1% |

*CEA, carotid endarterectomy; CAS, carotid artery stenting; VV, vasovagal; VDR, vasodepressor reaction; MI, myocardial infarction; HPS, hyperperfusion syndrome; ICH, intracerebral hemorrhage*

clinical determinants of periprocedural stroke. Symptomatic stenosis, chronic renal failure, and age >80 years are clinical factors that may increase the risk of stroke after either CEA or CAS, whereas severe cardiopulmonary disease is a more important risk after CEA than after CAS. Anatomic factors such as complex arch and brachiocephalic anatomy and the presence of thrombus have significant impact on procedural success and complications after CAS, whereas CEA restenosis, severe bilateral carotid disease, contralateral carotid occlusion, and "hostile neck" can increase the risk of CEA.

## Treatment Recommendations

Medical therapy is appropriate for all patients with carotid stenosis, regardless of symptomatic status, risk profile, or plans for revascularization. Such therapy should include antiplatelet therapy for primary or secondary prevention, plus appropriate medical therapy for risk factor modification. Societal guidelines have established treatment recommendations based on symptoms status, risk for CEA, and stenosis severity, and these guidelines are further influenced by other patient and clinical factors and by insurance reimbursement.

Patients with symptomatic carotid stenosis should be risk-stratified according to stenosis severity and the risk for MACE after CEA. Patients with stenosis <50% should be treated medically. Patients with stenosis >50% who are low risk for CEA should undergo CEA; CAS may be considered if a clinical trial is available. Patients with high risk features may be considered for CEA or CAS, depending on the high risk criteria. For patients with severe cardiopulmonary disease and anatomic factors that are unfavorable for CEA, CAS may be a safer revascularization strategy.

Patients with asymptomatic carotid stenoses should also be risk-stratified according to stenosis severity and the risk of MACE after CEA. Patients with stenosis <70% should be treated medically. Low risk patients with stenosis >70% should undergo CEA; CAS may be considered if a clinical trial is available. Patients with high risk features may be considered for CEA or CAS depending on the high risk criteria. However, reimbursement for high risk asymptomatic patients is only available if a clinical trial is available, and if stenosis >80%. Medical therapy may be reasonable in high risk asymptomatic patients who are poor candidates for revascularization and for those who are ineligible for a clinical trial of CAS.

## Suggested Readings

1. Rosamond W, Flegal K, Furie K, et al. Heart Disease and Stroke Statistics—2008 Update: A Report from the American Heart Association Statistics Committee and Stroke Statistics Subcommittee. *Circulation.* 2008;117:e25–e146.

2. Qureshi AI, Alexanderov AV, Tegeler CH, et al. Guidelines for Screening of Extracranial Carotid Artery Disease: A Statement for Healthcare Professionals from the Multidisciplinary Practice Guidelines Committee of the American Society of Neuroimaging; cosponsored by the Society of Vascular and Interventional Neurology. *J Neuroimag.* 2007;17:19–47.

3. Eagle KA, Guyton RA, et al. ACC/AHA 2004 Guideline Update for Coronary Artery Bypass Graft Surgery. A Report of the American College of Cardiology and American Heart Association Task Force on Practice Guidelines (Committee to Update the 1999 Guidelines for Coronary Artery Bypass Graft Surgery). *Circulation.* 2004;110:e340–437.

4. Bates ER, Babb JD, Casey DE, et al. ACCF/SCAI/SVMB/SIR/ASITN 2007 Clinical Expert Consensus Document on Carotid Stenting: A Report of the American College of Cardiology Foundation Task Force on Clinical Expert Consensus Documents (ACCF/SCAI/SVMB/SIR/ASITN Clinical Expert Consensus Document Committee on Carotid Stenting) *J Am Coll Cardiol.* 2007;49;126–170.

5. Gurm HS, Yadav JS, Fayad P, et al. Long-term results of carotid stenting versus endarterectomy in high risk patients. *NEJM.* 2008;358:1572–1579.

# 86

# Pathophysiology of Arterial Thrombosis

WILLIAM P. FAY

## PRACTICAL POINTS

- Numerous antithrombotic drugs are used to prevent and treat cardiovascular disease. Physicians must have a sound understanding of the molecular and cellular components of the hemostatic system to use antithrombotic drugs effectively and safely.

- The primary activator of the blood coagulation system is tissue factor, a cell-membrane-anchored protein that is abundant in the adventitia of normal blood vessels and the necrotic core of atherosclerotic plaques.

- The prothrombinase complex, composed of factor Xa, factor Va, calcium, and phospholipid, converts prothrombin to thrombin. Thrombin clots fibrinogen and activates blood platelets.

- Endogenous anticoagulants, including antithrombin, protein C, protein S, and tissue factor pathway inhibitor, prevent over-activity of the hemostatic system and thrombosis. Deficiency of these factors can lead to thrombosis.

- Factor V Leiden (FVL) is a gain-of-function mutation (arginine$^{506}$→glutamine) in factor V. FVL has normal procoagulant function, but is resistant to inactivation by activated protein C. Hence, FVL is prothrombotic.

- Heparin anticoagulates blood by binding and activating antithrombin, which inhibits thrombin and factor Xa.

- P2Y$_{12}$ is the platelet receptor for adenosine diphosphate (ADP).

- Fibrinogen cross-links activated platelets by binding to integrin $\alpha_{IIb}\beta_3$ (GPIIb/IIIa).

- Plasmin degrades fibrin clots. Antiplasmin inhibits plasmin activity. Plasminogen activator inhibitor-1 (PAI-1) inhibits plasmin formation by inhibiting plasminogen activators.

- Atherosclerotic plaque rupture is the most common trigger of acute myocardial infarction.

The practicing physician needs a sound appreciation of the biologic systems that control blood clotting in order that he or she may adequately understand thrombotic disorders and rationally treat patients with antithrombotic drugs. This chapter will provide a focused review of the normal function of the blood clotting system and how abnormal function of this system contributes to the pathogenesis of arterial thrombosis.

## BLOOD COAGULATION CASCADE

Plasma contains multiple clotting factors that activate each other in a highly coordinated, cascade-like fashion to produce thrombin, which converts fibrinogen to fibrin and activates platelets (**Figure 86-1**).

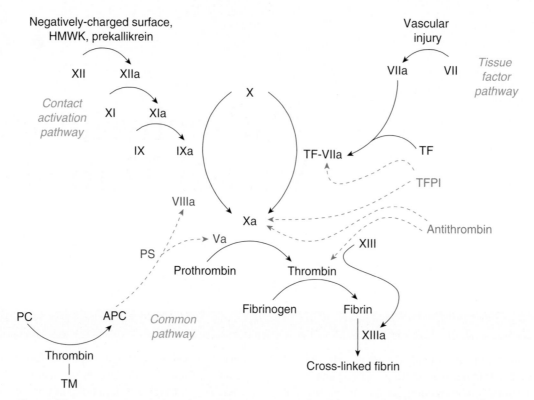

**Figure 86-1.** Diagram of key blood clotting proteins. The tissue factor and contact activation pathways converge at factor X, whose activation initiates the common pathway. Key cofactors for blood clotting (i.e., factors Va and VIIIa) and activated protein C (APC) activity (i.e., protein S (PS)) are shown in red. Inhibitors of blood clotting (e.g., tissue factor pathway inhibitor (TFPI) and antithrombin) are shown in blue. HMWK, high molecular weight kininogen; PC, protein C; TM, thrombomodulin.

The primary activator of the blood coagulation system is tissue factor (TF), a cell membrane-anchored protein that is abundant in the adventitia of normal blood vessels. In response to vascular injury, factor VIIa is exposed to and binds TF to produce a complex that activates factor X and factor IX. The TF pathway is also referred to as the extrinsic pathway, as under normal conditions active TF is not present in (i.e., is extrinsic to) the blood. The contact activation pathway (also referred to as the intrinsic clotting cascade), is activated by exposure of prekallikrein, high molecular-weight kininogen, factor XI, and factor XII to negatively charged surfaces, which eventually leads to formation of factor IXa, which, in complex with factor VIIIa, activates factor X. While TF plays an essential role in normal hemostasis, the contact activation pathway does not, as deficiency of some contact factors (e.g., factor XII) does not lead to abnormal bleeding. Nevertheless, the contact activation pathway plays an important amplification role in normal hemostasis and pathologic thrombosis. Factor Xa, in complex with factor Va, calcium, and phospholipid, converts prothrombin to thrombin. In addition to activating platelets and clotting fibrinogen, thrombin activates factor XIII, which crosslinks fibrin monomers. Thrombin also activates factor V and factor VIII, an example of "feedback amplification" of blood clotting.

While clotting factors circulate in plasma, blood clotting, whether adaptive (i.e., hemostasis) or pathologic (i.e., thrombosis) generally occurs on cell membrane surfaces. These surfaces provide the negatively charged phospholipid that is required for clotting factor complexes, such as the prothrombinase complex (composed of factors Xa and Va, phospholipid, and calcium ions) to assemble in the appropriate configuration necessary for efficient activation of substrates, such as prothrombin. Activated blood platelets, which form the initial hemostatic plug in response to tissue injury, are a major phospholipid-containing surface on which clotting factors assemble and activate. Other cell types, including activated endothelial cells, as well as cell fragments (i.e., microparticles) also are important biologic surfaces on which blood clotting occurs.

## ENDOGENOUS ANTICOAGULANT PATHWAYS

The blood clotting system requires intense regulation in order to respond rapidly to vascular injury yet remain quiescent under normal conditions. Anticoagulant pathways provide a critical braking effect on blood clotting, turning off thrombin production after hemostasis is achieved. Several anticoagulant

| Table 86-1 • Endogenous Anticoagulant Pathways | | |
|---|---|---|
| **Factor** | **Target(s)** | **Comments** |
| Antithrombin | Thrombin, factor Xa, and several other clotting factors | Protease inhibitor. Activity markedly accelerated by heparin |
| Thrombomodulin (TM) | Thrombin | Present on endothelial cells. Converts thrombin from procoagulant to anticoagulant |
| Protein C (PC) | Factors Va, VIIIa, and protease-activated receptors (PARs) | Activated to APC by thrombin-TM complex. De-activates clotting pathways and produces cytoprotective effect via PAR activation |
| Tissue factor pathway inhibitor (TFPI) | Xa and TF/VIIa/Xa complex | Inhibits TF (extrinsic) pathway |

proteins circulate in blood or reside on the surface of vascular endothelial cells (**Table 86-1, Figure 86-1**).

Antithrombin inhibits several activated clotting factors, with thrombin and factor Xa considered the most significant. The rate of inhibition of clotting proteases by antithrombin in markedly accelerated by heparin. Protein C is a vitamin K-dependent factor that circulates in plasma as an inactive zymogen. Binding of thrombin to thrombomodulin, an endothelial cell surface protein, alters the substrate preference of thrombin so that it activates protein C rather than converting fibrinogen to fibrin. Activated protein C (APC) cleaves and inactivates factor Va and factor VIIIa, thereby downregulating blood coagulation. APC also binds to endothelial cell protein C receptor (EPCR) and activates cell surface protease-activated receptors (PARs), such as PAR-1, which triggers intracellular signaling pathways and produces a cytoprotective effect. Protein S is a cofactor for the inactivation of factor Va and factor VIIIa by APC. Tissue factor pathway inhibitor (TFPI) is synthesized by vascular endothelial cells and circulates in plasma. TFPI inhibits blood clotting by inhibiting factor Xa and the TF-factor VIIa complex.

## BLOOD PLATELETS

Platelets form the initial hemostatic plug in response to vascular injury. They also play a central role in arterial thrombosis. Key activators of platelets include thrombin, which activates platelets by cleaving protease activated receptor-1 (PAR-1), a membrane-bound protein that is the main, but not exclusive, thrombin receptor on platelets and other vascular cells. Platelets also are activated by collagen, which is present in the subendothelial space and exposed by vascular injury. The main collagen receptors on platelets are glycoprotein VI (GPVI) and integrin $\alpha_2\beta_1$. Von Willebrand factor (VWF) circulates in plasma and binds to subendothelial collagen exposed by vascular injury. Platelets adhere to immobilized VWF, initially in reversible fashion via the platelet GPIb/GPV/GPIX surface receptor complex (GPIb/V/IX—*Note*: GPV and GPIX are distinct from plasma coagulation

factors V and IX), and, subsequently, in irreversible fashion via integrin $\alpha_{IIb}\beta_3$ (GPIIb/IIIa). VWF also mediates platelet-platelet interactions (i.e., aggregation) and growth of the platelet plug/thrombus. GPIIb/IIIa also binds fibrinogen, and this interaction plays a critical role in mediating platelet aggregation and thrombus growth. Under basal conditions, GPIIb/IIIa exists in an inactive conformation that does not bind fibrinogen. Upon platelet activation (e.g., by thrombin, collagen, or ADP), GPIIb/IIIa undergoes a conformational change that activates the receptor, enabling it to bind fibrinogen and VWF to trigger platelet aggregation. P2Y$_{12}$ is a G protein-coupled purinergic receptor that is activated by adenosine diphosphate (ADP). Thromboxane A2 (TXA2), produced from arachidonic acid by cyclooxygenase in response to platelet activation, activates platelets via a specific G protein-coupled receptor (thromboxane A2 receptor), thereby serving as a positive feedback amplification pathway to mobilize platelets after vascular injury. Key platelet agonists and receptors are summarized in **Figure 86-2**.

## LEUKOCYTES AND CELL-DERIVED MICROPARTICLES

Platelets are not the only cellular elements that control the hemostatic response to injury. Leukocytes, including monocytes, adhere to the injured blood vessel wall and are recruited to growing hemostatic plugs and thrombi. Microparticles, which are tiny membrane vesicles released from multiple cell types undergoing necrosis or apoptosis (including platelets, leukocytes, endothelial cells, and vascular smooth muscle cells), circulate in plasma and are recruited to growing thrombi. Intact leukocytes and microparticles express P-selectin glycoprotein ligand-1 (PSGL-1), which binds P-selectin on the surface of activated platelets, thereby leading to platelet-leukocyte and platelet-microparticle aggregates. Under some pathologic conditions, monocytes and microparticles express active TF. Recruitment of TF-bearing cells and microparticles to growing thrombi by P-selectin-PSGL-1 interactions may play an important role in supporting thrombus growth.

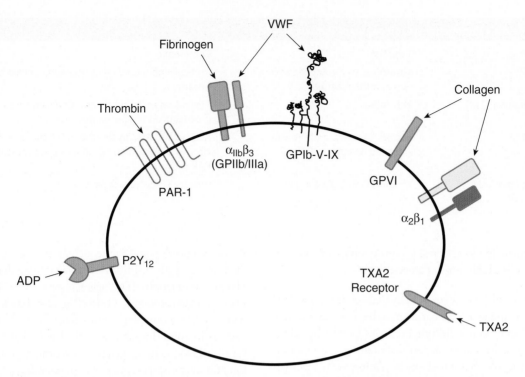

**Figure 86-2.** Key platelet receptors and agonists. ADP, adenosine diphosphate; PAR-1, protease activated receptor-1; GP, glycoprotein; VWF, von Willebrand factor; TXA2, thromboxane A2.

## ENDOTHELIUM

Under normal circumstances the vascular endothelium does not trigger platelet or clotting factor activation. However, in response to numerous pathologic conditions, including abnormal shear stress, dyslipidemia, oxidative stress, and cytokines, vascular endothelial cells become activated and express multiple prothrombotic and antifibrinolytic factors. For example, activated endothelial cells express: 1) P-selectin, which triggers leukocyte adhesion to the endothelium, and 2) plasminogen activator inhibitor-1 (PAI-1), an inhibitor of fibrinolysis.

## FIBRINOLYTIC SYSTEM

Fibrin formation and thrombosis depends not only on the balance of pro- and anticoagulant pathways, but also on the fibrinolytic pathway (**Figure 86-3**), which removes fibrin during vascular healing.

The central protein of the fibrinolytic system is plasminogen, which circulates in plasma and is activated by plasminogen activators (PAs). Urokinase (u-PA) and tissue-type PA (t-PA) are the two main endogenous PAs. Both are expressed in the vascular wall, though t-PA is the main plasma PA. t-PA is released by vascular endothelial cells. Activated plasminogen (i.e., plasmin) cleaves fibrin into soluble degradation products, thereby dissolving the fibrin clot. t-PA activates plasminogen rapidly when it is bound to fibrin, but slowly when it is free in plasma; hence, t-PA is a fibrin-specific PA. u-PA, which activates both free- and fibrin-bound plasminogen, is not fibrin-specific. Antiplasmin, which inhibits plasmin, and PAI-1, which inhibits t-PA and u-PA, are the main endogenous inhibitors of the fibrinolytic system. Fibrinolysis is also inhibited by thrombin-activated fibrinolysis inhibitor (TAFI), a plasma protein that is activated by thrombin. Activated TAFI (TAFIa) is a carboxypeptidase that removes lysine residues from the carboxy (C) termini of partially degraded fibrin fragments. Plasminogen binds avidly to C-terminal lysine residues within the partially degraded fibrin clot. Activation of bound plasminogen by t-PA stimulates continued fibrinolysis and eventually complete clot degradation. By removing C-terminal lysine residues from large fibrin fragments in the partially degraded clot, TAFI inhibits additional plasmin formation and fibrinolysis.

## VASCULAR TRIGGERS OF ARTERIAL THROMBOSIS

Atherosclerotic disease of the vascular wall is the most common determinant of arterial thrombosis in adults. Atherosclerotic plaque contains abundant amounts of TF within the necrotic core. Rupture of the atherosclerotic plaque, typically at sites with a thin-walled fibrous cap, exposes plasma to TF and initiates blood clotting (**Figure 86-4**).

Plaque hemorrhage can lead to the deposition of erythrocyte membranes within the plaque, which serve as a

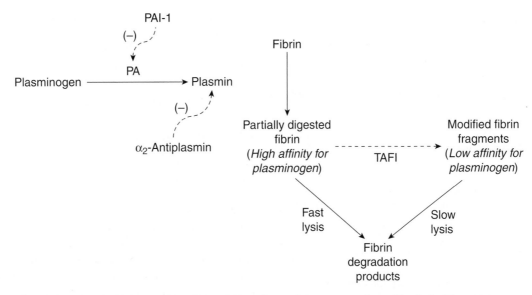

**Figure 86-3.** Fibrinolytic system. Actions of fibrinolysis inhibitors are indicated by dashed lines. PA, plasminogen activator; PAI-1, PA inhibitor-1; TAFI, thrombin-activated fibrinolysis inhibitor.

source of free cholesterol that leads to plaque growth, macrophage infiltration, plaque destabilization, rupture, and thrombosis. Plaque erosion, a distinct mechanism of arterial thrombosis, is characterized by loss of endothelial cell integrity and exposure of underlying vascular smooth muscle cells and extracellular matrix to flowing blood and blood clotting. Coronary vasospasm may play an important role in the pathogenesis of plaque erosion. Atherosclerotic plaque can calcify. Disruption of a calcified plate or nodule within an atherosclerotic plaque can also lead to contact of blood with thrombogenic surfaces within the plaque and thrombosis. Erosion of a calcified plate or nodule is more common in older men, and may occur more frequently in carotid arteries than in coronary arteries.

## ROLE OF ABNORMAL EXPRESSION OF HEMOSTATIC AND FIBRINOLYTIC FACTORS IN ARTERIAL THROMBOSIS

Arterial thrombosis in adults is generally a complication of atherosclerotic vascular wall disease. However, genetic or acquired alteration of expression of blood-borne factors may play an important role in arterial thrombosis, and often is considered in younger patients presenting with MI or stroke.

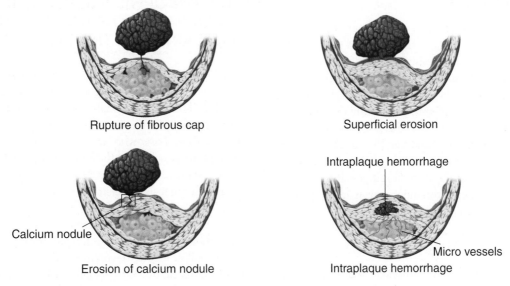

Rupture of fibrous cap

Superficial erosion

Calcium nodule

Erosion of calcium nodule

Intraplaque hemorrhage

Micro vessels

Intraplaque hemorrhage

**Figure 86-4.** Mechanisms of atherothrombosis. (Reproduced with permission from Libby, et al. *Circulation.* 2005;111.)

## Lupus Anticoagulant

Lupus anticoagulants are antibodies directed against complexes of plasma proteins and anionic phospholipids. Several prospective studies have demonstrated that antiphospholipid antibodies are associated with an increased risk of MI and stroke.

## Antithrombin Deficiency

Antithrombin deficiency is uncommon and is more often acquired (e.g., due to liver disease) than genetic in origin. There is no conclusive evidence that antithrombin deficiency is a risk factor for MI or stroke.

## Protein C/S

There are case and small series reports of ischemic stroke in young patients with protein C and protein S deficiency. However, larger studies have not convincingly demonstrated that protein C or S deficiency is a risk factor for arterial thrombosis, including MI or stroke.

## Prothrombin 20210A

A guanine to adenine (G→A) transition at nucleotide 20210 in the 3' untranslated region of the prothrombin gene results in prothrombin 20210A. Heterozygous carriers of prothrombin 20210A have 30% higher plasma prothrombin levels than do noncarriers, which may result from altered efficiency of mRNA processing and/or enhanced mRNA stability. Several case-control studies found an increased prevalence of the 20210A polymorphism in MI patients without atherosclerosis and/or other cardiovascular risk factors. Larger, prospective studies are currently not available.

## Factor V Leiden (FVL)

FVL results from a gain-of-function mutation (arginine[506]→ glutamine) in blood coagulation factor V. FVL has normal procoagulant function, but is resistant to inactivation by APC. Therefore, FVL enhances thrombin formation by reducing feedback inhibition of the blood clotting cascade. FVL is a key risk factor for venous thrombosis, particularly in Caucasians. One study suggested that FVL may increase MI risk in female smokers, and another study found that FVL plasma levels are increased in MI patients with angiographically normal coronary arteries. However, several studies suggested that FVL is not a risk factor for arterial thrombosis, even among patients who suffer vascular events at a young age.

## Homocysteine

Homocysteine is a modified amino acid that circulates in plasma. Homocysteine induces endothelial dysfunction and activates platelets. The strong majority of evidence supports a positive and independent association between plasma homocysteine level and risk of atherosclerosis and arterial thrombosis, including MI and stroke. However, B vitamin (i.e., folate, $B_{12}$, $B_6$) supplementation, despite its lowering effect on plasma homocysteine levels, has not been found to lower cardiovascular event rates.

## Lipoprotein(a) (Lp(a))

Lp(a) is composed of apoprotein(a), which is structurally related to plasminogen, and apo B100, an atherogenic lipoprotein. Most prospective studies suggest that elevated plasma levels of Lp(a) are associated with increased risk of MI. However, prospective studies examining the relationship between plasma Lp(a) and stroke/TIA have yielded variable results. It is unknown if lowering Lp(a) reduces risk. Estrogen, plasma apheresis, and niacin lower plasma Lp(a) levels. Statins generally have not been found to lower plasma Lp(a) levels.

## Fibrinolytic Factors

Elevated plasma levels of both t-PA and PAI-1 are associated with increased risk of myocardial infarction. While apparently paradoxical, the association of increased plasma t-PA levels with myocardial infarction may reflect a compensation of vascular endothelial cells (which secrete t-PA into plasma) to developing atherosclerotic plaque. Elevated plasma PAI-1 is strongly associated with insulin resistance. Hence, PAI-1 may represent an important mediator of the cardiovascular risk associated with diabetes mellitus. Elevated plasma TAFI levels have been associated with increased stroke risk. However, the role of TAFI in arterial thrombosis is not well-defined.

# THROMBOPHILIA SCREENING RECOMMENDATIONS FOR PATIENTS WITH ARTERIAL THROMBOSIS

The College of American Pathologists Consensus Conference XXXVI on Diagnostic Issues in Thrombophilia concluded that it is reasonable to measure antiphospholipid antibody and plasma homocysteine levels in patients with arterial thrombosis who are young and/or without documented atherosclerosis. Routine testing for FVL and prothrombin G20210A was not recommended in patients with arterial thrombosis associated with documented atherosclerosis, but can be considered in patients with unexplained arterial thrombosis without atherosclerosis or in young women who smoke. Routine testing for protein C, protein S, and antithrombin was not recommended for patients with arterial thrombotic disease associated with atherosclerosis, but can be considered in young patients with unexplained arterial thrombosis without atherosclerosis.

# 87

# Treatment of Arterial Thrombosis

RAJEEV GARG, SARAVANAN KUPPUSWAMY, RICHARD WEBEL, AND WILLIAM P. FAY

## ● PRACTICAL POINTS

- Aspirin, which inhibits platelet aggregation by inhibiting cyclo-oxygenase (COX), plays a key role in the prevention and treatment of acute myocardial infarction and other atheroembolic events.

- Thienopyridines, which inhibit platelet aggregation by inhibiting the $P2Y_{12}$ receptor, are often used in conjunction with aspirin to treat high-risk patients with coronary artery disease, and as sole therapy in aspirin-intolerant individuals.

- Unfractionated heparin (UFH), low-molecular-weight heparin (LMWH), and the synthetic pentasaccharide, fondaparinux, inhibit blood clotting by binding and activating antithrombin. UFH inhibits thrombin and factor Xa. LMWH preferentially inhibits factor Xa over thrombin. Fondaparinux exclusively inhibits factor Xa.

- Lepirudin, bivalirudin, argatroban, and dabigatran anticoagulate blood by directly inhibiting thrombin.

- Warfarin disrupts vitamin K metabolism by inhibiting vitamin K epoxide reductase (VKOR). Warfarin anticoagulates blood by inhibiting post-translational modification of vitamin K-dependent clotting factors.

- Fibrinolytic drugs convert plasminogen to plasmin, which degrades the fibrin clot.

- Percutaneous intervention (PCI) is preferred over fibrinolytic therapy in patients who can be transferred to the cardiac catheterization laboratory within 90 minutes of initial presentation. However, fibrinolytic therapy remains an excellent treatment option when cardiac catheterization cannot be performed in a timely fashion.

- Thrombolytic therapy is recommended for patients with acute ischemic stroke presenting within 3 hours of symptom onset. One study suggests that IV t-PA is also beneficial in patients presenting between 3 and 4.5 hours after symptom onset.

Thrombosis plays a critical role in the pathogenesis of numerous acute and chronic cardiovascular diseases. Consequently, antithrombotic drugs (see **Table 87-1** for a summary) are prescribed in a wide range of clinical settings, ranging from primary prevention of cardiovascular events to aggressive antithrombotic and fibrinolytic strategies in patients presenting with acute thrombosis. This chapter will review the use of antithrombotic and fibrinolytic drugs in coronary artery disease (CAD), ischemic stroke, and peripheral arterial disease (PAD).

## ANTIPLATELET DRUGS

Aspirin (ASA). Cyclooxygenase (COX) metabolizes arachidonic acid to thromboxane A2, a potent platelet agonist. Aspirin binds and irreversibly acetylates COX. Aspirin is a much more potent inhibitor of COX-1 than COX-2.

Thienopyridines. ADP activates platelets by binding to the $P2Y_{12}$ receptor. Thienopyridines, which include ticlopidine, clopidogrel, and prasugrel, inhibit platelet

| Table 87-1 • Classification of Antithrombotic Drugs |
| --- |
| 1. Antiplatelet drugs<br> • Aspirin (ASA)<br> • P2Y$_{12}$ inhibitors<br> • Glycoprotein IIb/IIIa inhibitors |
| 2. Anticoagulant drugs<br> • Heparins<br> • Vitamin K antagonists<br> • Direct thrombin inhibitors<br> • Other direct-acting clotting factor (e.g., Factor Xa, Factor IXa) inhibitors |
| 3. Fibrinolytic drugs |

aggregation by binding and irreversibly inhibiting the P2Y$_{12}$ receptor.

Dipyridamole. Dipyridamole inhibits adenosine reuptake and phosphodiesterase, thereby increasing platelet cAMP levels, which reduces intracellular calcium and inhibits platelet aggregation.

Glycoprotein $\alpha_{IIb}\beta_{IIIa}$ (IIb/IIIa) Inhibitors. These agents, which include tirofiban, eptifibatide, and abciximab, bind and inhibit the integrin receptor for fibrinogen, thereby blocking fibrinogen/fibrin-mediated platelet crosslinking and aggregation.

## Clinical Issues Relevant to Aspirin Therapy in CAD Patients

### Aspirin Resistance
Aspirin resistance is a laboratory phenomenon characterized by the lack of aspirin's efficacy in inhibiting platelet activation in vitro. *Aspirin treatment failure* is defined as the failure of aspirin to prevent clinical atherothrombotic events. Treatment failure does not imply aspirin resistance, as virtually no therapy is 100% effective in preventing vascular events. Aspirin resistance may have important clinical implications, and further research is necessary on this important topic. Currently available clinical guidelines do not advocate routine screening of patients for aspirin resistance when initiating aspirin therapy.

### NSAIDs, COX-2 Inhibitors, and Aspirin Use
Nonselective non-steroidal anti-inflammatory drugs (NSAIDs) such as ibuprofen and naproxen compete with aspirin for binding to COX-1, providing a mechanism by which the NSAID may blunt aspirin's antithrombotic effect. However, the clinical relevance of this interaction is not fully resolved. Selective COX-2 inhibitors do not block binding of aspirin to COX-1, but have the potential to promote thrombosis by inhibiting prostacyclin (PGI$_2$) production. In patients with or at risk of ischemic heart disease (IHD) who are taking aspirin, current recommendations are to limit nonselective NSAIDs and selective COX-2 inhibitors to those patients for whom no appropriate alternatives exist, and to use the lowest doses and shortest durations of NSAID and COX-2 inhibitors possible. Short-term use of NSAID appears safe, especially if aspirin is taken at least 2 hours before NSAID ingestion. NSAID and COX-2 inhibitors are contraindicated in acute MI.

### ASA and ACE Inhibitors
The overall evidence suggests that there is no deleterious interaction between ACE inhibitors and aspirin (at least when ASA is used in lower doses, such as 75 mg daily), and that ASA and ACE inhibitors can be used safely in patients at high risk for ischemic vascular events.

## ANTICOAGULANT DRUGS

## Heparin

Heparin is a polymeric, sulfated glycosaminoglycan that binds antithrombin and markedly accelerates its capacity to inhibit thrombin and Factor Xa. Heparin-antithrombin inhibits free thrombin, but not clot-bound thrombin. Unfractionated heparin (UFH) is derived from porcine intestine. Cleavage of UFH into smaller fragments yields low molecular weight heparin (LMWH), which preferentially (but not exclusively) inhibits factor Xa (via antithrombin) over thrombin. Fondaparinux is a synthetic pentasaccharide glycosaminoglycan that selectively inhibits factor Xa via antithrombin without inhibiting thrombin. Even when administered in weight-based doses, the anticoagulant effect of UFH can vary significantly among individuals due to variable binding to cells and plasma proteins, and, hence, undergo variable diversion of heparin from antithrombin. Therefore, UFH therapy is monitored with plasma or whole blood clotting time measurements, such as the activated partial thromboplastin time (APTT) and activated clotting time (ACT), so that the dose can be adjusted to achieve therapeutic anticoagulation. LMWH and fondaparinux have a more uniform anticoagulant effect due to less interaction with cells and plasma proteins. They also produce less of a prolonging effect on standard clotting times than UFH does. Therefore, LMWH and fondaparinux do not require monitoring of clotting times.

## Vitamin K Antagonists

Clotting factors II (prothrombin), VII, IX, and X, protein C and protein S, and some other factors are nonfunctional unless they undergo posttranslational modification (carboxylation of glutamic acid residues) by gamma-carboxylase, a liver enzyme that requires vitamin K in its reduced form as a cofactor. In the process of gamma-carboxylation of vitamin K-dependent factors, vitamin K is oxidized. Vitamin

K epoxide reductase (VKOR) is a microsomal liver enzyme that converts oxidized vitamin K back to a reduced form capable of cofactor function. Warfarin inhibits VKOR, which disrupts vitamin K recycling, and consequently inhibits gamma carboxylation of vitamin K-dependent factors. As warfarin does not inhibit circulating (i.e., already gamma-carboxylated) clotting factors, its anticoagulant effect is delayed for several days. Polymorphisms in VKOR and cytochrome P450 2C9 (CYP2C9, which metabolizes warfarin) account for much of the variability in warfarin dose requirements among individuals.

## Direct Thrombin Inhibitors

While structurally diverse, direct thrombin inhibitors share common features of direct inhibition of thrombin's active site and the capacity to inhibit both free and clot-bound thrombin. Lepirudin, a recombinant variant of hirudin (a natural compound isolated from leech saliva), selectively binds and irreversibly inhibits thrombin. Bivalirudin, a recombinant analog of hirudin, inhibits thrombin in a reversible manner. Argatroban is a small, nonprotein compound that inhibits thrombin's active site. Dabigatran, an orally available, reversible thrombin inhibitor, is under evaluation in clinical trials.

# FIBRINOLYTIC DRUGS

Fibrinolytic drugs dissolve fibrin indirectly by converting plasminogen to plasmin, a protease that degrades fibrin. Tissue-type plasminogen activator (t-PA) efficiently activates plasminogen that is bound to fibrin, but slowly activates plasminogen that is free in plasma. Hence, t-PA is a fibrin-specific agent that does not deplete plasma plasminogen levels. Urokinase activates both free (i.e. plasma pool) and fibrin-bound plasminogen. Streptokinase is a bacterial-derived PA that binds to plasminogen to form a complex that converts free plasminogen molecules to plasmin. Streptokinase is not fibrin-specific.

# ANTITHROMBOTIC THERAPY IN CORONARY ARTERY DISEASE

## Primary Prevention

Several antithrombotic agents have been studied in the context of primary prevention of myocardial infarction, most notably aspirin. The American College of Chest Physicians (ACCP) and American Heart Association (AHA) recommend aspirin for healthy men and women with a 10-year risk of a first MI or coronary death of ≥10%. The Thrombosis Prevention Trial evaluated low intensity

**Table 87-2 • Antithrombotic Therapy for Primary Prevention of Ischemic Heart Disease**

| Patient characteristics | Recommendations |
|---|---|
| Moderate or higher risk (>10% in next 10 years) for a hard CV event | Aspirin 75-100 mg daily |
| Particularly high risk of CV events in whom INR can be monitored without difficulty | VKA, target INR approx. 1.5, without aspirin |
| Aspirin allergy with moderate to high risk for CV event | Clopidogrel 75 mg daily |

*VKA, vitamin K antagonist; CV, cardiovascular*

oral anticoagulation with warfarin (target INR 1.5), low-dose aspirin, and combined therapy in the primary prevention of IHD. Aspirin reduced nonfatal ischemic heart disease. Warfarin reduced all IHD, mainly by an effect on fatal events. Combined warfarin and aspirin was more effective in reducing IHD than either agent alone was. The Charisma Trial found that addition of clopidogrel to ASA did not reduce the combined endpoint of myocardial infarction, stroke, or death from cardiovascular causes in individuals with multiple cardiovascular risk factors, arguing against combined ASA/clopidogrel therapy for primary prevention of IHD. 2008 ACCP Guidelines for antithrombotic therapy for primary prevention of IHD are summarized in **Table 87-2**.

## Secondary Prevention

Aspirin is recommended to reduce the risk of recurrent myocardial infarction, stroke, and vascular death in men and women with a history of stable or unstable angina, myocardial infarction, CABG, PCI, peripheral artery disease, stroke, transient ischemia attacks, or peripheral arterial disease. The CAPRIE Study compared the efficacy of aspirin versus clopidogrel in preventing vascular death, recurrent ischemic stroke, or myocardial infarction in patients with recent ischemic stroke, myocardial infarction, or symptomatic peripheral arterial disease. Study results supported the use of clopidogrel for secondary prevention of ischemic events, though aspirin is generally used for secondary prevention due to its low cost and small differences in efficacy compared to clopidogrel.

## Unstable Angina (UA)/Non-ST Segment Elevation Myocardial Infarction (NSTEMI)

Antiplatelet and anticoagulant drugs play critical roles in the management of patients with UA/NSTEMI. Just as there are multiple antiplatelet and anticoagulant agents, there are several antithrombotic treatment options for patients presenting with UA/NSTEMI. Key factors to consider in deciding which drugs to use include:

1. *Clinical risk assessment.* Clinical factors, including older age, persistent chest pain, angiographically documented coronary artery disease, hemodynamic instability, kidney disease, ventricular arrhythmia, elevated serum troponin, and marked ST-segment depression, predict high risk of adverse outcomes and advocate more aggressive antithrombotic therapy.
2. *Initially selected management strategy.* Based on assessment of clinical risk and other factors, patients with UA/NSTEMI are typically selected for either an *early invasive* or *early conservative* management strategy. For "early invasive" patients, the initial treatment plan is to proceed in timely fashion to coronary angiography and anatomy-based revascularization. For "early conservative" patients, the initial treatment plan is medical therapy-only, with plans to proceed to angiography only if recurrent ischemia is detected or if cardiac stress testing reveals high risk findings. Due to

other medical issues (e.g., recent surgery, acute renal failure), some patients are selected for a *delayed invasive* strategy. Initial antithrombotic management can differ significantly depending on which management strategy is selected.

3. *General medical status and bleeding risk.* Several factors, including age, gender, body weight, and hepatic and renal function, affect drug metabolism or risk of hemorrhagic side effects from antithrombotic therapy. Such factors, in addition to other clinical variables that affect bleeding risk (e.g., history of gastrointestinal bleeding, central nervous system pathology, history of recent surgery), must be considered in selection of, and dosing with, antithrombotic drugs.

Authoritative guidelines largely based on well-designed clinical trials are available to provide evidenced-based recommendations regarding patient management. **Table 87-3** summarizes key points of recently published guidelines.

## Table 87-3 • Antithrombotic Therapy in UA/NSTEMI

**Initial Early Conservative Management**

| Agent | Recommendation | Supporting trials |
|---|---|---|
| Aspirin | 162-325 mg p.o., then 81 mg daily | Antithrombotic Trialists' Collaboration, CAPRIE |
| Thienopyridine | Clopidogrel 300 mg p.o., then 75 mg daily | CURE, PCI-CURE, CREDO |
| GP IIb/IIIa inhibitors | Eptifibatide or tirofiban; abciximab not recommended | PURSUIT, PRISM, PRISM-PLUS, GUSTO IV |
| Heparin or heparin derivative | UFH, LMWH, or fondaparinux | ATACS, RISC, GUSTO-IIb, ESSENCE, INTERACT, TIMI IIb, A-Z, PENTUA, OASIS-5 |
| DTI | Consider if heparin contraindicated | None |
| Fibrinolytic drugs | Not indicated | TIMI III B, ISIS-2, Fibrinolytic Therapy Trialists' Collaboration |

**Initial Early Invasive Management**

| Agent | Recommendation | Supporting trials |
|---|---|---|
| Aspirin | Same as for early conservative management | |
| Thienopyridine | | |
| GP IIb/IIIa inhibitors | Use of a small-molecule i.v. GP IIb/IIIa inhibitor (eptifibatide or tirofiban) is preferred; abciximab not indicated unless coronary anatomy in known and PCI is planned within 24 h | PRISM -PLUS, PURSUIT, GUSTO-IV |
| Heparin or heparin derivative | UFH, LMWH, or fondaparinux | SYNERGY, ACUTE II, GUSTO-IVOASIS-5 |
| DTI | Bivalirudin can be used over UHF + GP IIb/IIIa inhibitor if clopidogrel is given >6 h prior to PCI and early angiography with PCI is performed | ACUITY |
| Fibrinolytic drugs | Same as for early conservative management | |

*Recommendations based on American College of Chest Physicians Evidence-Based Clinical Practice Guidelines (2008) on Antithrombotic Therapy for Non-ST-Segment Elevation Acute Coronary Syndromes and American College of Cardiology/American Heart Association 2007 Guidelines for the Management of Patients with Unstable Angina/Non-ST-Elevation Myocardial infarction. UFH, unfractionated heparin; DTI direct thrombin inhibitor.*

## Antiplatelet Therapy

Unless contraindicated, all patients with UA/NSTEMI should receive aspirin. Aspirin-allergic patients should receive a thienopyridine, such as clopidogrel. Patients with intermediate-high risk features and/or being managed with an early invasive strategy should receive either a thienopyridine or GP IIb/IIIa inhibitor in addition to aspirin prior to angiography. For many high risk patients, concomitant aspirin, thienopyridine, and GP IIb/IIIa treatment is appropriate. For UA/NSTEMI patients with intermediate-high risk clinical features in whom an initial conservative or delayed invasive strategy is selected, combined aspirin/thienopyridine therapy is reasonable. In high risk, conservatively managed patients, combined treatment with aspirin, thienopyridine, and a small-molecule GP IIb/IIIa inhibitor (i.e., eptifibatide or tirofiban) should be considered. Abciximab is not recommended in conservatively managed UA/NSTEMI patients based on the data from GUSTO-IV trial.

## Anticoagulant Drugs

Unless contraindicated, all patients with UA/NSTEMI should receive full antithrombotic doses of UFH, LMWH, fondaparinux, or bivalirudin. If UFH is given, an initial bolus of 60-70 U/kg (maximum bolus 5000 U), followed by an initial infusion rate of 12-15 U/kg/h (maximum initial infusion 1000 U/h) and subsequent dose titrations aimed at maintaining the APTT between 50 and 70 seconds is reasonable. Several studies support the use of LMWH as an alternative to UFH in UA/NSTEMI. Caution should be exercised when LMWH is used in patients with significant renal dysfunction. The Oasis-5 Trial demonstrated the effectiveness of fondaparinux in UA/NSTEMI. Due to an increased rate of catheter-associated thrombosis in patients whose anticoagulant therapy consisted solely of fondaparinux, it is recommended that additional UFH be administered to fondaparinux-treated patients that undergo cardiac catheterization. In patients managed with an initial conservative strategy, fondaparinux offers an advantage of a lower incidence of bleeding complications, supporting its use in UA/NSTEMI patients considered at high risk of bleeding. In patients with moderate-high clinical risk scheduled for very early coronary angiography, bivalirudin in combination with a thienopyridine may be selected as an initial antithrombotic strategy.

## Fibrinolytic Drugs

While thrombosis plays a key role in the pathogenesis of UA/NSTEMI, randomized clinical trials have demonstrated that plasminogen activators provide either no benefit or a higher incidence of adverse outcomes in ACS patients without ST-segment elevation on ECG. Therefore, there is no role for fibrinolytic drugs in this clinical setting.

## ST Elevation Myocardial Infarction (STEMI)

Aggressive antithrombotic therapy and early reperfusion of the infarct-related artery constitute the foundation of STEMI management. PCI is preferred over fibrinolytic therapy in patients who can be transferred to the cardiac catheterization laboratory within 90 minutes of initial presentation. However, fibrinolytic therapy remains an excellent treatment option when cardiac catheterization is not available or cannot be performed in a timely fashion. STEMI management is guided by abundant data from prospective clinical trials.

## Antiplatelet Therapy

Though measures to achieve early reperfusion dominate the treatment in STEMI, the role of antiplatelet agents should not be underestimated. Aspirin reduces mortality in patients with STEMI. Current recommendations are an initial dose of 162-325 mg, noncoated preparation, chewed and swallowed, followed by a maintenance dose of 81-162 mg daily. In patients who cannot tolerate aspirin, clopidogrel 75 mg can be substituted. In addition to aspirin, thienopyridine therapy initiated at the time of initial presentation improves outcomes as compared to aspirin therapy alone. Current recommendations are that patients with STEMI, whether undergoing PCI or receiving fibrinolytic therapy, receive a loading dose of clopidogrel (300 mg) followed by a maintenance dose of 75 mg daily (however, a loading dose of clopidogrel is not recommended in patients over 75 yrs of age who are treated with a fibrinolytic drug, due to increased risk of bleeding, based on data from CLARITY-TIMI-28 Trial). The optimal duration of thienopyridine therapy after hospital discharge of STEMI patients is less well-studied. A recommendation of long-term clopidogrel (i.e., up to 1 year) is based on extrapolation of data from NSTEMI studies. Combined therapy with a fibrinolytic drug and a GP IIb/IIIa inhibitor has been studied in STEMI, though increased bleeding risk and lack of sufficient decreases in adverse outcomes argued against such combined treatment. However, GP IIb/IIIa inhibitors are effective as an adjunct to PCI for STEMI. (**Table 87-4**).

## Anticoagulant Drugs

Inhibition of thrombin is important for maintaining patency of the infarct-related artery, whether achieved by PCI or fibrinolytic therapy. UFH administered i.v. (bolus of 60 U/kg, maximum 4000 U i.v.; initial infusion 12 U/kg/h, maximum of 1000 U/h) or LMWH should be administered to patients with STEMI, including those who are not treated with reperfusion therapy. Fondaparinux can be used as an alternative to heparin in STEMI patients being treated with a fibrinolytic drug or not receiving reperfusion therapy; however, fondaparinux is not recommended for STEMI patients undergoing primary PCI. Bivalirudin is not recommended in STEMI patients being treated with streptokinase, but can be considered in STEMI patients undergoing PCI

## Table 87-4 • Antithrombotic Therapy for STEMI

| Agent | Recommendation | Supporting Trials |
|---|---|---|
| Aspirin | 162-325 mg p.o., then 81 mg daily | GISSI, GUSTO |
| Thienopyridine | Clopidogrel 300 mg p.o. (if <75 years) or 75 mg (if >75 years), then 75 mg daily regardless of age, if bleeding risk acceptable | CLARITY-TIMI 28, COMMIT |
| GP IIb/IIIa inhibitors | For patients treated with PCI: recommended; for patients treated with fibrinolytic drug: not recommended | PCI trials: CADILLAC, RAPPORT, ISAR-2, ADMIRAL, ACE<br>Lytic trials: TAMI-8, IMPACT-AMI, PARADIGM, TIMI-14, GUSTO-V, ASSENT-3, ENTIRE-TIME-23 phase II |
| Heparin or heparin derivative | For patients undergoing PCI: UHF or LMWH recommended, but not fondaparinux; for patients receiving fibrinolytic drug, UFH, LMWH, or fondaparinux recommended | UFH: GISSI-2, ISIS-3, OSIRIS, GUSTO-I<br>LMWH: CREATE, ASSENT-3, ASSENT-3 PLUS, ExTRACT-TIMI-25<br>Fondaparinux: OASIS-6 |
| DTI | Bivalirudin not recommended with streptokinase; can be used in patients undergoing PCI | HERO-2, HORIZONS-AMI |
| Fibrinolytic drugs | See Table 87-5 | |

### Fibrinolytic Drugs

Fibrinolytic therapy continues to play a critical role in STEMI management, given its efficacy and the lack of timely access to cardiac catheterization laboratories in many areas. Numerous trials have compared the efficacy of the fibrinolytic drugs. **Table 87-5** summarizes the currently available agents. In general, fibrin-specific agents have shown superiority over non-fibrin-specific agents. Streptokinase is not frequently used in the United States. In patients meeting criteria for thrombolytic therapy, 2008 ACCP Guidelines recommend the following:

- In patients presenting within 6-12 hours of symptom onset and demonstrating persistent ST-segment elevation, treatment with SK, anistreplase, alteplase, reteplase, or tenecteplase is recommended over no fibrinolytic therapy. If it is an available option, prehospital administration of fibrinolytic therapy by appropriately trained and supervised personnel is recommended.
- In patients presenting within 6 hours symptom onset, alteplase or tenecteplase is recommended, and reteplase is suggested over streptokinase.
- A bolus agent such as tenecteplase is recommended because the ease of administration accelerates initiation of therapy, and because bolus therapy may decrease the risk of nonintracranial hemorrhage.

## Table 87-5 • Fibrinolytic Drugs

| Drug | Key Features | Dosing | Relevant Clinical Trials |
|---|---|---|---|
| Streptokinase | Streptococcal protein; antigenic; low cost; not FS | 1.5 million units over 60 min | GISSI-1, ISIS-2, GUSTO |
| Alteplase (tPA) | Recombinant form of human t-PA; FS; short HL | 15 mg bolus, then 0.75 mg/kg (max 50 mg) over 30 min, then 0.5 mg/kg (max 35 mg) over next 60 min | GUSTO I-III |
| Lanoteplase (nPA) | Deletion and point mutant of WT tPA; mutations produce long circulating HL (30-45 min) and greater fibrinolytic potency | | InTIME, InTIME-II |
| Reteplase (rPA) | Deletion mutant of WT tPA; less FS and longer HL than alteplase | 10 U over 2 min then repeat 10 U bolus at 30 min | RAPID I-II, GUSTO III, INJECT |
| Tenecteplase (TNK) | Multiple point mutant of WT tPA; longer plasma HL, more FS and resistant to inhibition by PAI-1 | Single weight-based bolus over 5-10 sec (<60 kg = 30 mg; 60-69 kg = 35 mg; 70-79 kg = 40 mg; 80-89 kg = 45 mg; >90 kg = 50 mg) | TIMI 10A,B, ASSENT-1,2,3 |

FS, fibrin-specific; WT, wild-type; HL, half-life; PAI-1, plasminogen activator inhibitor-1

## Table 87-6 • Contraindications to Fibrinolytic Therapy for STEMI

**Absolute**

Any prior intracerebral hemorrhage
Known structural cerebral vascular lesion
  (e.g., arteriovenous malformation)
Known malignant intracranial neoplasm
Ischemic stroke within 3 mo except acute ischemic
  stroke within 3 h
Suspected aortic dissection
Active bleeding or bleeding diathesis (excluding menses)
Significant closed-head or facial trauma within 3 mo

**Relative**

History of chronic, severe, poorly controlled HTN
Severe HTN (systolic BP >180 or diastolic BP >110 mm Hg)
Recent (<3 mo) ischemic stroke, dementia, or other major
  intracranial pathology
Traumatic or prolonged (>10 min) CPR or recent
  (<3 wk) major surgery
Recent (<2-4 wk) internal bleeding
Noncompressible vascular punctures
For SK/anistreplase: prior exposure (>5 days previous)
  or allergic reaction
Pregnancy
Active peptic ulcer
Current use of vitamin K antagonist and prolonged INR

*Modified from Acute ST Segment Elevation Myocardial Infarction: American
College of Chest Physicians Evidence-Based Clinical Practice Guidelines
(8th Edition). SK, streptonkinse; INR, international normalized ration;
HTN, hypertension; CPR, cardiopulmonary resuscitation*

**Table 87-6** lists contraindications to fibrinolytic therapy for STEMI.

## Elective Percutaneous Coronary Intervention (PCI)

PCI creates a milieu analogous to that which occurs spontaneously during acute coronary syndrome (ACS). By disrupting endothelial integrity, PCI exposes flowing blood to collagen and other procoagulant molecules that trigger thrombosis. Disruption of normal blood flow during balloon inflation and introduction of foreign bodies into the vasculature, including guide wires, catheters, and stents, also promote thrombosis during PCI. Hence, anticoagulant therapy plays a leading role in the management of patients undergoing PCI.

### Antiplatelet Therapy

Aspirin is routinely given prior to PCI, and following PCI it should be continued at a dose of 162-325 mg daily for at least 1, 3, and 6 months with bare-metal, sirolimus, and paclitaxel-eluting stents, respectively. Thereafter, aspirin 75-162 mg daily is recommended for secondary prevention of cardiovascular events, as well as for protection against late stent thrombosis. A thienopyridine, such as clopidogrel,

should be started before PCI. 2007 AHA/ACC Guidelines recommend an oral loading dose of clopidogrel of 600 mg. After PCI with a bare-metal stent, clopidogrel 75 mg daily is recommended for at least 1 month, and ideally for up to 12 months. After drug-eluting stent implantation, clopidogrel should be given for at least 12 months to patients who are not at high risk of bleeding complications. If clopidogrel is first given at the time of PCI, administration of a GP IIb/IIIa receptor antagonist can be beneficial to achieve more rapid platelet inhibition than that achieved with clopidogrel alone, and GP IIb/IIIa receptor antagonists can be considered in all PCI cases, regardless of timing of clopidogrel administration, particularly in patients with high risk coronary anatomy.

### Anticoagulant Therapy

UFH is recommended in addition to antiplatelet therapy for elective PCI. In low risk patients, bivalirudin can be considered as an alternative to combined therapy with UFH and a GP IIb/IIIa antagonist. Bivalirudin or argatroban are recommended in place of UFH in patients with heparin-induced thrombocytopenia.

## Coronary Artery Bypass Grafting (CABG)

Aspirin reduces vein graft occlusion within the first year after CABG and should be used indefinitely after CABG for prevention of myocardial infarction, death, and stroke. CABG can be performed safely in patients who take aspirin. For elective CABG, thienopyridine therapy is usually stopped at least 5 days before surgery to reduce bleeding risk. Initiation of aspirin should not be delayed after CABG, as the benefit on vein graft patency is lost if aspirin is initiated >48 hours after CABG. A thienopyridine should be used after CABG if aspirin is contraindicated. If CABG is performed in patients presenting with UA or acute MI, up to 9 months of combined aspirin and clopidogrel therapy is warranted, after which clopidogrel can be discontinued. Several months of combined aspirin and thienopyridine (e.g., clopidogrel) therapy is commonly used after CABG in patients without UA/MI, though data to support this strategy over aspirin alone are not available. Warfarin has not been shown to improve bypass graft patency over aspirin and may be associated with increased bleeding risk.

## ISCHEMIC STROKE

### Primary Prevention

Aspirin is not recommended by the AHA solely for primary prevention of stroke in men. Aspirin is recommended for primary prevention solely of stroke in women considered at higher risk. Aspirin is recommended for primary prevention of combined cardiovascular endpoints that include stroke in men and women considered at moderate or high risk of hard cardiovascular events, as defined by the Framingham criteria. Warfarin is effective for primary prevention of stroke in patients with nonvalvular atrial fibrillation and should be used in patient considered at moderate-high stroke risk, unless high risk of bleeding or other factors argue against its use. The ACTIVE W Trial showed that combined aspirin and clopidogrel treatment was inferior to warfarin for stroke prevention in patients with atrial fibrillation and at least one stroke risk factor (i.e., age ≥75 years, hypertension, prior stroke/transient ischemic attack, left ventricular ejection fraction <45%, peripheral arterial disease, or age 55-74 with coronary artery disease or diabetes mellitus). However, aspirin can be considered for primary stroke prevention in lower risk patients with nonvalvular atrial fibrillation (e.g., with CHADS2 score of 0-1) based on results of the SPAF III aspirin cohort study.

## Secondary Prevention

Patients who have sustained noncardioembolic stroke or TIA should receive an antiplatelet drug, with the combined preparation of aspirin 25 mg/extended-release dipyridamole 200 mg b.i.d. preferred over aspirin alone, and clopidogrel preferred over aspirin alone. Unless a coronary artery disease indication is present, long-term combined treatment with aspirin and clopidogrel is not recommended for secondary stroke prevention. A vitamin K antagonist such as warfarin is recommended for patients who have sustained a cardioembolic stroke—e.g., stroke secondary to atrial fibrillation. In patients with cryptogenic ischemic stroke and patent foramen ovale (PFO), antiplatelet therapy is recommended over warfarin or no therapy. If there is evidence of deep venous thrombosis (DVT) in patients with cryptogenic ischemic stroke and PFO, warfarin is recommended.

## Acute Ischemic Stroke

If initiated within 3 hours of symptom onset, i.v. t-PA is recommended. One study suggests that i.v. t-PA is also beneficial in patients presenting between 3 and 4.5 hours after symptom onset. For patients with angiographically demonstrated middle cerebral artery occlusion and without major early infarct signs on CT or MRI scan who can be treated within 6 hours of symptom onset, intraarterial tPA is recommended in centers with appropriate neurologic and interventional expertise.

# PERIPHERAL ARTERIAL DISEASE (PAD)

## Primary/Secondary Prevention

Primary prevention of PAD has not been studied as a sole endpoint. Aspirin and clopidogrel are each effective in reducing cardiovascular events in patients with PAD. The WAVE Study found that combined oral anticoagulant (target INR 2-3) and antiplatelet therapy (which was aspirin in >90% of patients), as compared to sole antiplatelet therapy: 1) was not more effective in preventing major cardiovascular complications, and 2) increased risk of life-threatening bleeding.

## Treatment of Acute Arterial Thromboembolism

2008 ACCP Guidelines recommend UFH in patients with acute arterial emboli or thrombosis, followed by long-term treatment with a vitamin K antagonist. In patients with short-term (<14 days) thrombotic or embolic disease, intraarterial thrombolytic therapy is recommended, provided the patient is at low risk of developing myonecrosis and ischemic nerve damage during the time required to achieve flow-restoring thrombolysis.

# 88

# Acute and Chronic Venous and Lymphatic Disorders

MARK NALLARATNAM AND ROBERT T. EBERHARDT

---

## ● PRACTICAL POINTS

- Deep vein thrombosis (DVT) presents an extraordinarily high risk for pulmonary embolism, as well as long-term complications such as post-phlebitic syndrome.

- Numerous clinical features encountered in hospitalized patients predispose to the development of DVT, thus warranting the use of various prophylactic measures based upon their specific risk.

- Venous duplex imaging remains the test of choice to exclude proximal DVT, but the D-dimer assay is being incorporated into many diagnostic algorithms.

- Treatment for DVT typically consists of antithrombotic therapy followed by anticoagulation for at least 3 months with a provoked proximal DVT and an evaluation for possible indefinite therapy with unprovoked DVT. In addition, the use of compression stocking for 2 years following a proximal DVT reduces the risk of post-phlebitic syndrome.

- Thrombophilia testing for inherited and acquired disorders may be considered for recurrent or unprovoked venous thromboembolism (VTE) or thrombosis in unusual territories.

- Chronic venous disease (CVD) is a common problem and may result in significant disability due to complications including edema, advanced skin changes, and ulcerations.

- Physical exam findings typically establish the diagnosis of CVD, but testing such as venous duplex imaging or air plethysmography may help to determine the pathophysiologic mechanism and guide management.

- Compression therapy remains the cornerstone in the treatment of CVD, whereas sclerotherapy and ablation are often used to treat superficial reflux disease with advanced manifestations.

- Lymphedema may be a primary disorder or secondary to other conditions such as infection or prior surgery.

- Techniques such as compression therapy, decongestive physiotherapy, and intermittent pneumatic compression are used to reduce edema; topical skin care also helps to reduce the risk of infection.

---

## VENOUS THROMBOEMBOLISM

Venous thromboembolism (VTE) represents a spectrum of diseases ranging from isolated calf vein thrombosis to fatal pulmonary embolism (PE). Deep venous thrombosis (DVT) most commonly involves the veins of the lower extremity but may arise within the venous system at numerous sites. An understanding of deep vein thrombosis affecting the lower extremity is the foundation for understanding this diverse disorder, venous thromboembolism.

### Epidemiology

The incidence of VTE has been reported to be 1 to 2 per 1000 in the generally population with nearly 500,000 cases in the United States annually. There is a strong age dependence with the incidence increasing exponentially with age (1000 per 100,000 for persons aged over 85 years). Approximately half of those with a DVT in the proximal lower extremity will experience a pulmonary embolism. In contrast, isolated calf vein thrombosis has a low risk for PE but 20% propagate to the proximal limb within 1 week. Overall, the 30-day mortality with thrombotic event is as high as 30%. After suffering an initial venous thromboembolic event, 30% of survivors will develop recurrent VTE within 10 years. Thus, therapy goals will include secondary risk reduction. In addition, the chronic sequelae of post-phlebitic syndrome with venous insufficiency is seen in about 30% of those following VTE.

## Pathophysiology

The prevailing view of the pathophysiology of VTE was described by Virchow in the late 1900s. Vichow's triad consists of the following:

- vascular injury
- stasis
- hypercoagulability.

Venous thromboembolic episodes may be classified as secondary if associated with one or more recognized risk factors, or idiopathic if unprovoked. Both inherited and acquired predisposing conditions have been described (see Thrombophilia section). Recognized clinical risk factors include advanced age (>60 years), prior VTE, surgery, trauma, malignancy, pregnancy, oral contraceptive pill, prolonged immobility, and systemic diseases such as congestive heart failure, nephritic syndrome, and inflammatory bowel disease.

- The highest surgical risk is with orthopedic and trauma surgery.
- The incidence of VTE with an active malignancy may be as high as 10% with an especially high rate for pancreatic, gastrointestinal, ovarian, and lung cancers.
- The use of oral contraception and hormone replacement therapy increases the risk (three- to fivefold and two- to threefold, respectively) in proportion to the estrogen dose.
- Pregnancy and puerperium is associated with an up to three- to sixfold increased risk.

## Clinical Presentation

The clinical presentation of VTE will depend upon the site of involvement and if a pulmonary embolism is present. Common symptoms and signs related to lower extremity DVT include the following:

- acute leg swelling
- leg pain and tenderness
- skin discoloration and temperature alteration
  - Most common is increased skin temperature and erythema

- Rarely *phlegmasia alba dolens*—or a cold and pale leg caused by obstructive ileofemoral thrombosis with compromised arterial perfusion
- Rarely *phlegmasia cerula dolens*—or marked swelling and cyanosis caused by obstructive ileofemoral thrombosis with severe venous congestion.

In general the physical exam findings of a DVT are nonspecific. Even the frequently described Homan's sign (or calf pain upon forced dorsiflexion of the foot) is neither sensitive nor specific.

Symptoms suggestive of PE include chest pain, shortness of breath, syncope, cough, and hemoptysis (see Chapter 18). Unique clinical presentations are seen with thromboses at other locations.

- Upper extremity venous thrombosis usually occurs as a complication of instrumentation or intravenous lines. Arm swelling is the key manifestation.
- Superior vena cava syndrome is most commonly seen with malignancy. This is characterized by marked swelling of the arms, neck, and face.

## Differential Diagnosis

There are a number of conditions that may mimic an acute lower extremity DVT. This includes the following:

- superficial phlebitis
- leg trauma (hematoma)
- arthritis of the knee or ankle
- ruptured Baker's cyst
- cellulitis
- myositis
- congestive cardiac failure
- low protein states such as cirrhosis, nephrotic syndrome, and protein-losing enteropathy
- peripheral arterial disease
- lymphedema.

## Diagnosis

There are significant limitations to establishing the diagnosis of a DVT based upon clinical findings alone. However, clinical signs and symptoms, established risk factors, and presence (or absence) of an alternative diagnoses may be used to establish the clinical probability even before any diagnostic testing. The Wells' criteria and its modifications are well-established models for predicting the pretest probability of DVT (see **Table 88-1**).

Venography was the gold standard modality for the diagnosis of DVT but has essentially been replaced by venous duplex imaging. Due to its invasive nature venography is now typically reserved for circumstances requiring endovascular therapies or to confirm a controversial diagnosis.

| Table 88-1 • Pretest Probability of Deep Vein Thrombosis | |
|---|---|
| **Clinical Features** | **Score** |
| Active cancer (treatment ongoing or within the previous 6 months or palliative) | 1 |
| Paralysis, paresis, or recent plaster immobilization of the lower extremities | 1 |
| Recently bedridden for more than 3 days or major surgery within 4 weeks | 1 |
| Localized tenderness along the distribution of the deep venous system | 1 |
| Entire leg swollen | 1 |
| Calf swelling by more than 3 cm when compared to the asymptomatic leg | 1 |
| Pitting edema (greater in the symptomatic leg) | 1 |
| Collateral superficial veins (nonvaricose) | 1 |
| Alternative diagnosis as likely or more likely than DVT | −2 |
| Previously documented DVT | 1 |
| **Probability** (add points from clinical features) | |
| DVT likely (moderate to high probability) | ≥2 |
| DVT unlikely (low probability) | ≤1 |

*Modified from Wells et al. N Engl J Med. 2003;349.*

Venous duplex has become the modality of choice for the diagnosis of DVT. The essential component of the exam is venous compressibility. This is supplemented by other elements such as venous flow, vein distention, and direct thrombus visualization. It has an excellent sensitivity and specificity (>95%) for the diagnosis of DVT in the proximal limb. The sensitivity is much lower, on the order of 70%, for a DVT in the distal limb (below the knee). Due to such limitations of calf vein imaging, it is often recommended that scans be repeated within 1 week to exclude the propagation of a calf vein thrombus into the proximal limb.

The D-dimer assay has become a popular test to assist in excluding the diagnosis of DVT. D-dimer is a degradation product of cross-linked fibrin which is elevated in the setting of active thrombus. However, elevated D-dimer levels may be seen in a number of other conditions, including infection, malignancy, trauma, bleeding, pregnancy and surgery. Thus, the assay has poor specificity but high sensitivity making it a useful test to exclude the diagnosis of a DVT (with a negative result). The assay seems to be most useful when a low clinical probability is present or if combined with venous duplex imaging (see **Figure 88-1**).

Other techniques have also been utilized. Impedance plethysmography had been used in the past with reasonable sensitivity and specificity (on the order of 80-85%) but now is rarely used. Magnetic resonance venography and computed tomographic venography are gaining experience but are more commonly used to assess venous outflow prior to intervention. In contrast, multidetector CT is being widely used in the diagnosis of PE with improving sensitivities (60-95%) and specificities (75-95%).

## Prevention

VTE is a major complication of hospitalization affecting up to 20% of general medical patients, with a significant

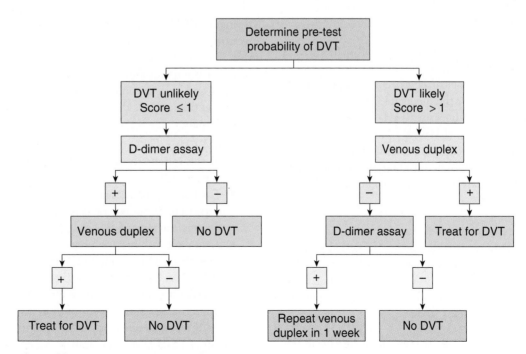

**Figure 88-1.** A suggested algorithm for suspected DVT.

| Table 88-2 • 2008 ACCP Guidelines for VTE Prophylaxis | | |
|---|---|---|
| **Risk Category** | **Clinical Feature** | **Prophylaxis Strategy** |
| Low | Medical – fully mobile Surgical – brief procedure with no risk factors | No specific prophylaxis Early ambulation |
| Moderate | Medical – bed bound Surgical – major general, urologic, and gynecologic | LMWH UFH-SQ Compression therapy for high bleeding risk |
| High | Medical – trauma Surgical – orthopedic | LMWH Fondaparinux Vitamin K antagonist (INR 2-3) |

*LMWH, low molecular weight heparin; UFH-SQ, subcutaneous unfractionated heparin*

impact upon health and health care delivery. Thus, there has been a focus on prevention with primary prophylaxis having been shown to reduce the rate of both VTE and PE. The American College of Chest Physicians (ACCP) Guidelines for VTE Prophylaxis were revised in 2008. DVT prophylaxis is currently divided into three groups (low, moderate, and high risk) for both medical and surgical issues (see **Table 88-2**).

The low risk category includes medical patients who are fully mobile and admitted for brief periods, and surgical patients who are mobile, undergoing brief procedures (<30 minutes) with no additional risk factors. No specific prophylaxis is recommended but early ambulation encouraged for the low risk group (Grade 1A).

The moderate risk category includes medically patients who are sick and confined to bedrest and surgical patients undergoing major general, urological, or gynecological procedures. Suggested prophylaxis for the moderate risk group includes low-dose unfractionated heparin (UFH) (Grade 1A), low molecular weight heparin (LMWH) (Grade 1A) or thromboembolic deterrent stockings or intermittent pneumatic compression devices in high bleeding risk (Grade 1A). Prophylaxis should start as soon as possible and continue until discharge.

The high risk category includes patients undergoing major orthopedic procedures or with trauma. Suggested prophylaxis for the high risk group includes LMWH (Grade 1A), fondaparinux (Grade 1A), or warfarin for an INR 2.0-3.0 (Grade1A-1B). Prophylaxis should begin early after postoperative and continue at least 10 days.

Aspirin and other antiplatelet therapy are ineffective in the primary or secondary prophylaxis of VTE.

## Treatment

Therapy for VTE should prevent clot propagation, embolization, and death while minimizing the risk of bleeding. Confirmed VTE requires the initiation of anticoagulation. The revised ACCP Guidelines for the Treatment of VTE in 2008 conclude that:

- Outpatient treatment of VTE is appropriate for patients without prior VTE, thrombophilic conditions, or substantial comorbidity.
- Inpatient treatment of VTE is suggested with prior VTE, comorbid medical conditions, or clinical instability.

### Heparins

Unfractionated heparin (UFH) binds to antithrombin III enhancing its affinity to inactivate thrombin (Factor IIa). Intravenous or monitored subcutaneous UFH has been shown to reduce morbidity, mortality, and recurrent thrombosis with greater efficacy upon achieving therapeutic levels within 24 hours. This is a prolonged activated partial thromboplastin time (aPTT) that corresponds to plasma heparin levels of 0.3 to 0.7 IU/mL anti-Xa activity. Careful use of weight-based nomograms allows therapeutic level to be achieved more rapidly but still carries a 5% risk of major bleed. An additional caution with heparin therapy is the risk of heparin-induced thrombocytopenia occurring in about 5% of those on heparin for 5-10 days. This requires the discontinuation of heparin and the use of alternative antithrombotic therapy.

LMWH binds to antithrombin III, yielding higher specificity for Factor Xa compared with thrombin. These agents have improved bioavailability, more predictable pharmacologic action, and do not require routine monitoring. LMWH is at least as effective as UFH in reducing recurrent thrombosis and mortality with lower bleeding risk. The major concerns with the use of LMWH are for those with renal dysfunction (as it is cleared through the kidneys and at a minimum its use requires dose adjustment), extremes of body weight (<50 kg and >100kg), and pregnancy.

- LMWH, UFH, or fondaparinux are recommended in the initial treatment of DVT for at least 5 days (Grade 1C).
- The use of LMWH is favored over UFH preferably for outpatient management (Grade 1C) or for inpatient treatment if necessary (Grade 1A).
- Treatment with heparin preparations should continue concurrent with a vitamin K antagonist until an INR of ≥2.0 for 24 hours (Grade 1A).
- LMWH appears to be more efficacious than warfarin in the initial treatment of those with cancer, thus being recommended for at least 3 months (Grade 1A). Either LMWH or a vitamin K antagonist should be continued as long as the cancer is active.

## Warfarin

Warfarin inhibits the vitamin K-dependent coagulation factors of the extrinsic clotting pathway. It is recommended that a heparin preparation be used during initiation of therapy with warfarin due to the theoretical risk of enhanced thrombosis with an early inhibition of the vitamin K-dependent antithrombotic factors (proteins C and S). The INR needs frequent monitoring with a target of 2.0 to 3.0. Duration of therapy has been a controversial issue, but in general unprovoked thrombosis should be treated for at least 6 months, while a provoked thrombosis with transient risk factors can be treated for 3 months. It has been shown prolonged treatment for idiopathic DVT with warfarin in the therapeutic range (INR of 2.0 to 3.0) for over 2 years was effective in reducing the recurrence rate of VTE by threefold but low intensity therapy (INR of 1.5 to 2.0) does not appear to be as beneficial.

- ACCP Guidelines suggest VTE caused by transient risk factors should be treated for at least 3 months (Grade 1A). Most other DVT should be evaluated all for potential indefinite therapy (Grade 1C) including first unprovoked DVT with low bleeding risk and most with a second unprovoked DVT (Grade 1A).
- Isolated calf vein thrombosis should be treated for 3 months rather than indefinite therapy (Grade 2B).
- A rare complication of warfarin therapy is skin necrosis seen with protein C deficiency.
- Warfarin should be avoided in pregnancy due to the risk for embryopathy and fetal bleeding.

## Compression Stockings

Post-phlebitic syndrome affects about 30% of those with a DVT. Manifestations of post-phlebitis syndrome include leg pain, swelling, and even ulceration. Compression stockings (with 30-40 mm Hg tension) have been shown to reduce the risk of post-phlebitic syndrome by 50% with 2 years of use. The use of compression stocking is recommended in the routine care of those with proximal DVT (within 1 month and continued for at least 2 years)(Grade 1A).

## Vena Cava Filters

The routine use of inferior vena cava (IVC) filters is discouraged. IVC filters are indicated with contraindications to anticoagulant therapy (Grade 1C), such as active bleeding, or failure of anticoagulant therapy. Complications of filter placement include dislodgement and thrombosis with a high risk of chronic limb sequelae. In theory, these issues may be reduced through the judicious use of removable or temporary filters, but the effect of this approach is not well established.

## Thrombolysis

Catheter-directed thrombolysis has been suggested for extensive proximal DVT to reduce symptoms and subsequent risk for post thrombotic syndrome (Grade 2B). The use of adjunctive devices as part of pharmacomechanical thrombolysis may be appropriate to shorten treatment time (Grade 2C). Even after effective thrombolysis, the same duration and intensity of anticoagulation is required.

## Treatment at Other Sites

Thromboses at other locations require site-specific workup and treatment.

- Upper extremity venous thrombosis requires removal of the intravenous lines.
- Spontaneous or effort-induced subclavian vein thrombosis requires anticoagulation using a regimen as suggested for lower extremity DVT, and consideration towards catheter-directed thrombolytic therapy with assessment for thoracic outlet compression (Grade 2C).
- Superficial thrombophlebitis is typically managed with the use of nonsteroidal antiinflammatory agents, warm compresses and leg elevation. However, extensive superficial venous thrombosis (for example, in close proximity to the saphenofemoral junction) may be treated with prophylactic or intermediate dose LMWH or intermediate dose UFH for 4 weeks (Grade 1B).

# THROMBOPHILIAS

Thrombophilias are inherited or acquired disorders that predispose to thrombosis. It is important to recognize that thrombosis does not develop in all those with a thrombophilia. Treatment of those with a thrombophilia occurs after the development of a VTE.

## Epidemiology

Acquired thrombophilias are the consequence of another medical condition or develop during an individual's lifetime (see **Table 88-3**). The most common acquired thrombophilia is antiphospholipid antibody syndrome. Antiphospholipid antibodies are seen in 5% of the general population and 10-50% of those with autoimmune conditions. The relative risk of thrombosis with antiphospholipid antibodies is 1.6 to 3.2.

| Table 88-3 • Acquired Thrombophilias |
|---|
| Antiphospholipid antibody |
| Neoplasm |
| Myeloproliferative disorder |
| Heparin-induced thrombocytopenia |
| Disseminated intravascular coagulation |
| Thrombotic thrombocytopenic purpura |
| Nephrotic syndrome |
| Paroxysmal nocturnal hemaglobinuria |
| Pregnancy |
| Use of estrogen hormone |

| Table 88-4 • Hereditary Thrombophilias |
| --- |
| Activated protein C resistance including Factor V Leiden mutation |
| Prothrombin gene mutation 20210A |
| Antithrombin deficiency |
| Protein C deficiency |
| Protein S deficiency |
| Hyperhomocysteinemia |

The most common inherited thrombophilias are Factor V Leiden and prothrombin gene mutation. Factor V Leiden mutation is seen in 4-8% of the general population and 20% of those with thrombosis. Similarly, prothrombin gene 20210A mutation is seen in about 2-3% of the general population and 4-8% of those with thrombosis. Other identified inherited disorders include protein C and S deficiencies, antithrombin deficiency, and dysfibrinogenemia (see **Table 88-4**). The cumulative lifetime incidence of thrombosis among carriers of familial disorders is about 10%.

## Pathophysiology

Inherited thrombophilias are generally disorders of the coagulation cascade with deficiency or dysfunction of an antithrombotic factor, or resistance of a prothrombotic factor to inactivation. Deficiency of antithrombotic factors includes protein C, protein S, and antithrombin deficiencies. Excessive activation of prothrombotic factors is seen with Factor V Leiden mutation, prothrombin gene mutation, and dysfibrinogenemia.

## Clinical Presentation

The most common clinical manifestation of thrombophilias is VTE both deep vein thrombosis and pulmonary embolism. These conditions should be suspected with unprovoked or recurrent VTE. Venous thrombosis in unusual territories such as cerebral, portal, mesenteric, or hepatic veins should also raise suspicion to a thrombophilia. Inherited thrombophilias may have a family history of VTE. These are also common among VTE occurring at a young age (<40 years old).

Arterial thrombosis (including stroke and myocardial infarction) are unusual complications of thrombophilias. Exceptions are the presence of an antiphospholipid syndrome, hyperhomocytinemia, heparin-induced thrombocytopenia, and certain myeloproliferative disorders. Acute limb ischemia due to arterial thrombosis has a differential that includes embolism and progressive arterial occlusive disorders such as the following:

- cardioembolism
- atherosclerosis
- fibromuscular dysplasia

- arterial dissection
- aneurysmal disease
- arterial entrapment
- ergots alkaloids.

Pregnancy-related complications may be seen with thrombophilias, particularly with antiphospholipid antibody syndrome. These include purpura fulminas neonatalis, recurrent fetal loss, still birth, pre-eclampsia, and, possibly, placental insufficiency and intrauterine growth retardation. Many of these conditions are included in the criteria to establish a diagnosis of antiphospholipid antibody syndrome. The fetal loss criteria are defined as 3 or more spontaneous abortions with no more than 1 live birth or unexplained second or third trimester fetal death.

## Diagnosis

Establishing a diagnosis of a thrombophilia begins with an understanding of the clinical indications that may prompt further testing. Established indication to evaluate for thrombophilias includes the following:

- unprovoked thrombosis
- recurrent thrombosis
- VTE at age <40 years old
- VTE with family history
- thrombosis in unusual vascular territories.

There is no single test for all thrombophilias, but there are several commonly measured assays. A thorough history and physical exam is of paramount importance for the physician to determine clinical risk factors and associated medical conditions. Routine laboratory investigations should include a complete blood count with differential, serum electrolytes, liver function, renal function, and coagulation tests including INR and PTT. Testing for the inherited thrombophilias includes the following:

- DNA-based testing for Factor V Leiden and prothrombin G20210A gene mutations
- activated protein C resistance assay
- functional assays for protein C, protein S, and antithrombin
- anticardiolipin antibody and lupus anticoagulant
- plasma homocysteine levels.

An important consideration is the timing of performing the testing for thrombophilias. Plasma coagulation factors should not be tested during the acute thrombotic phase as their levels can be transiently decreased. This is observed with protein C, protein S, and antithrombin. The use of anticoagulant medications may affect coagulation factors. In addition to the vitamin K-dependent procoagulation factors, warfarin reduces protein C and S levels. Heparin affects antithrombin levels and lupus anticoagulant testing.

In general, testing should be delayed for at least 6 weeks. Testing for protein C and S should be performed once warfarin therapy has completed.

## Treatment

### Primary Prevention

Primary prophylaxis is not recommended simply due to the presence of an inherited thrombophilia. The use of primary prophylaxis depends upon exposure to a thrombotic risk such as surgery, trauma, or immobilization. The prophylactic regimen in the presence of a thrombophilia is generally the same as without a thrombophilia. There are possible exceptions that warrant consideration:

- Antithrombin deficiency, combined thrombophilias, and homozygous mutations for Factor V Leiden or prothrombin gene should be treated throughout pregnancy and for 6-week postpartum with LMWH.
- Antithrombin deficiency may be treated with replacement of antithrombin prior to high risk situations such as surgery.
- Hyperhomocysteinemia should be treated with folic acid and supplemented with vitamin $B_6$ and $B_{12}$ until normalization of homocysteine levels.
- Avoidance of oral contraceptives and hormone replacement is controversial in the absence of a history of VTE.

### Acute Treatment

Treatment for VTE with a thrombophilia is generally the same as treatment without a thrombophilia. There are exceptions such as thrombosis with heparin-induced thrombocytopenia, disseminated intravascular coagulation and acute promyelocytic (M3) leukemia. Treatment of the underlying disorder is required for disseminated intravascular coagulation and acute leukemia. The treatment of thrombosis with heparin-induced thrombocytopenia has several unique features:

- Remove all heparin exposure.
- Don't use LMWH.
- Treatment requires a direct thrombin inhibitor such as argatroban or leupirudin, which may require renal dose adjustment. Fondaparinux has been used but is not FDA-approved for this indication.
- Warfarin should not be initiated until the platelet count exceeds 100,000.
- Overlap the direct thrombin inhibitor with warfarin for at least 5 days.

There are several issues with the treatment of thrombosis with antiphospholipid antibody syndrome. Use of either UFH or LMWH should be continued until 4 to 6 weeks postpartum, then may be converted to warfarin. The target INR is in the 2.0 to 3.0 range rather than a higher range, as once was the clinical practice.

### Secondary Prevention

Idiopathic or recurrent VTE should be considered for secondary prophylaxis with indefinite therapy. An identified inherited thrombophilia may modify the risk/benefit ratio to guide the duration of therapy (or need for secondary prevention). Most heterozygous mutations will be treated similar to those without an identified abnormality. In contrast, homozygous and mixed heterozygous mutations (or combined thrombophilias) favor the use of indefinite therapy.

# CHRONIC VENOUS DISEASE

Chronic venous disorders encompass a spectrum of venous abnormalities ranging from dilated cutaneous veins, such as spider veins and telangiectasias, to venous ulceration. The spectrum of disease consisting of varicose veins and more advance manifestations is referred to as chronic venous disease (CVD). The term chronic venous insufficiency (CVI) is most often used to indicate the most advanced forms of venous disease with skin changes or ulceration. CVI develops due to problems with valve incompetence or venous obstruction with resulting venous hypertension.

## Epidemiology

CVD is a common problem with varicose veins, affecting 5-35% of the United States adult population. There is a female predominance: women have an approximate two-fold increased risk over men. Risk factors associated with the development of CVD include age, female gender, family history of varicose veins, pregnancy, obesity, previous leg injury, and phlebitis. Other possible risk factors include occupational or environmental factors such as prolonged sitting, standing, or crossing legs.

The most serious complications venous ulcers, either active or healed, are seen in about 1% of the adult population. Almost 5 million people in the United States have CVI, of which 10% will develop venous ulcers. Risk factors associated with the first-time development of a venous ulcer include maternal family history and physical activity and history of deep vein thrombosis.

Complications of CVD have a significant impact on the health care system. The disability due to venous ulcers leads to loss of productive work hours as well as early retirement. Venous ulcer care has been estimated to cost up to 3 million dollars annually in the United States.

## Pathophysiology

The pathophysiology of CVI is best understood through appreciation of the normal venous anatomy and function. The venous system serves as a conduit to return blood to the heart even against gravity from the lower limbs. Blood is prevented from pooling in the lower limbs by a series of one-way valves within the superficial and deep veins, and the action of muscle pumps, forcing blood centrally. The superficial and deep veins are connected by a series of perforator veins, which also contain valves preventing blood from flowing from the deep to the superficial veins with muscular contraction. Proper functioning of these mechanisms will help to maintain a normal venous pressure around 15 to 30 mm Hg.

The principal superficial veins are the great saphenous vein, which runs from the ankle to join the common femoral vein at the saphenofemoral junction, and the small saphenous vein, which runs from ankle to join popliteal vein at the saphenopopliteal junction. The deep veins within the lower limb run beneath the facial layer. In the calf these include veins within the muscle architecture and paired axial veins running alongside the corresponding artery. These veins join to form a popliteal vein, which becomes the femoral vein (previously referred to as the "superficial" femoral vein) after passing through the adductor canal. The femoral vein is joined by the deep femoral vein in the upper thigh to form the common femoral and eventually iliac veins—providing the major venous outflow of the leg.

There are several possible mechanisms involved in CVI including the development of incompetent valves in the deep or superficial or perforator venous systems, or obstruction to venous outflow, or a combination. Chronic venous obstruction is increasingly recognized as an important cause of CVI (see **Table 88-5**). These processes ultimately lead to venous hypertension particularly during standing or prolonged sitting. Loss of the normal muscle pump function may exacerbate this problem. Chronic venous hypertension can lead to progressive varicose vein formation and various skin changes ranging from hyperpigmentation to lipodermatosclerosis to venous ulceration.

Varicose veins are classified as primary if only the superficial veins are affected. Those arising due to a coexisting problem, such as incompetence of perforator or deep veins, are termed secondary. Once varicose veins form,

---

**Table 88-5 • Causes of Venous Obstruction**

- Chronic deep vein thrombosis
- Malignancy
- Retroperitoneal fibrosis
- May–Thurner syndrome (or impaired venous outflow due to compression of the left iliac vein as crossed over by the right common iliac artery)
- Arterial aneurysms
- Pelvic masses
- Other rarer causes of venous obstruction include aplasia of the pelvic veins as seen in Klippel–Trénaunay syndrome.

---

progressive venous dilatation may cause dysfunction of the valves, thus perpetuating the cycle and causing more incompetence.

## Clinical Presentation

Chronic venous disorders most commonly present due to the appearance of telangiectasias, reticular veins, and/or varicose veins. The most common symptoms related to CVD are pain, swelling, and ulceration. The pain or discomfort of the leg is typically described as heaviness or aching that is aggravated by prolonged standing and relieved by elevation. Varicose veins may become sore due to venous distention. Varicosities are also prone to superficial thrombophlebitis. Edema begins in the perimalleolar region but extends up to leg with accumulation occurring in a dependent manner.

Chronic venous-related skin changes are a prelude to the development of venous ulcerations. This includes hyperpigmentaion due to hemosiderin deposition and lipodermatosclerosis with scarring and thickening of the skin due to fibrosis in the dermis and subcutaneous fatty tissue. In addition, atrophie blanche may be seen with atrophic skin surrounded by dilated capillaries. There is also an increased risk of other skin problems including eczematous dermatitis, cellulitis, and lymphangitis. Ultimately, cutaneous ulcers may develop typically in the perimalleolar region with delayed wound healing.

The routine venous exam should include an evaluation in both the supine and upright positions to induce maximal venous distention. Varicose veins are often in the distribution of the affected superficial veins with dilation of their branches. Edema is typically pitting, however protracted edema may become more resilient to palpation, thus referred to as brawny edema. The skin needs to be inspected for characteristic skin findings or ulcerations either active or healed. The Brodie–Trendelenberg test may help distinguish deep and superficial reflux. This bedside test uses a tourniquet or manual compression over the superficial veins followed by placement of the limb in the dependent position. The rapid appearance of varicose veins in the absence of compression but delayed appearance with compression implies superficial venous incompetence.

A consensus classification scheme, known as the CEAP classification, was developed for venous reporting standards to provide a basis for uniform reporting, diagnosis, and treatment of CVD (see **Table 88-6**). The basic elements of the CEAP classification include clinical class, etiology, anatomic and pathophysiologic classifications. Additional schemes have been developed to provide objective measures of disease severity, including the venous severity score (VSS). These seem most useful to assess longitudinal

### Table 88-6 • CEAP Classification of Venous Disease

| Class | Definition |
|-------|-----------|
| C | Clinical signs (grade 0-6), supplemented by (s) for symptomatic and (a) for asymptomatic |
| 0 | No visible or palpable signs of venous disease |
| 1 | Telangiectasias, reticular veins, malleolar flare |
| 2 | Varicose veins |
| 3 | Edema without skin changes |
| 4 | Skin changes ascribed to venous disease (pigmentation, lipodermatosclerosis) |
| 5 | Skin changes (as defined above) in conjunction with healed ulceration |
| 6 | Skin changes (as defined above) in conjunction with active ulceration |
| E | Etiologic classification (congenital, primary, secondary) |
| A | Anatomic distribution (superficial, deep, or perforator, alone or in combination) |
| P | Pathophysiologic dysfunction (reflux or obstruction, alone or in combination) |

changes in CVD with treatment or when comparing different modalities of treatment.

## Differential Diagnosis

The differential diagnosis for CVI includes conditions that may cause edema as well as those that may cause ulceration. This includes the following conditions:

- Congestive heart failure—especially right heart failure, which causes bilateral pitting edema.
- Systemic conditions such as nephrosis, cirrhosis and endocrinologic disorders.
- Medication side effect—may be seen with calcium channel blockers, nonsteroidal antiinflammotory agents, and certain oral hypoglycemics.
- Peripheral arterial disease—onset of critical limb ischemia results in rest pain and ulceration.
- Deep vein thrombosis and superficial thrombophlebitis—may cause pain and swelling but with a more acute onset.
- Lymphedema—typically with nonpitting edema (at least in the later stages) and without venous skin changes.
- Regional disorders such as ruptured Baker's cyst, soft tissue hematoma, gastrocnemius tear or cellulitis.

## Diagnosis

The diagnosis of CVD is made with history and physical exam, but noninvasive and rarely invasive testing may be required. The easiest and most cost-efficient method to confirm the diagnosis is venous duplex ultrasonography with reflux testing. Duplex is a very sensitive modality for the detection and exclusion of deep vein thrombosis, especially in the proximal limb. However, duplex reflux testing is also sensitive to detection of reflux in the venous systems. This technique most often uses rapid cuff inflation and deflation with patients in an upright (or semi-upright) position. Venous flow towards the head is augmented by cuff inflation then abnormal flow towards the feet may be seen following deflation, indicating venous reflux.

Several plethysmographic techniques may be used to assess for venous reflux including photoplethysmography and air plethysmography. Air plethysmography is particularly useful for assessing the contribution of each pathophysiologic mechanism, including reflux, obstruction, and muscle pump dysfunction. Photoplethysmography is most useful for establishing a diagnosis of reflux but provides limited additional information.

Invasive imaging such a contrast venography is rarely performed unless an intervention is planned. More commonly, computed tomography and magnetic resonance imaging are used to evaluate for central venous stenosis. In addition, intravascular ultrasound (IVUS) is rapidly gaining acceptance, being utilized to visualize periluminal vascular anatomy and guide interventions. Ambulatory venous pressure monitoring, the hemodynamic "gold standard" for the assessment of CVD, is rarely performed.

## Treatment (see Table 88-7)

### Medical Treatment

Medical treatment is generally aimed at minimizing the degree of edema and preventing complications. Behavioral measures may include elevation of the legs when at rest and weight loss programs. Skin care is important to prevent infection, with the use of emollients to keep the skin moisturized. Hyperkeratosis may respond to topical 20% urea cream. Ulcerations should be attended to by a wound care

### Table 88-7 • Treatment of Chronic Venous Disease

- Medical Treatment
  Behavioral measures
  Skin care
  Compressive garments
- Interventional Management
  Sclerotherapy
  Catheter venous ablation
  Venous stenting
- Surgical Therapies
  Venous ligation and stripping
  Subfascial endoscopic perforator ligation
  Venous bypass
  Valve reconstruction and transplant

specialist. There are a variety of topical dressings to control fluid drainage and local skin maceration, as well as biologic human skin substitutes to facilitate healing.

Compressive leg garments are the mainstay of treatment for nearly all stages of CVD. The most common garment is graded elastic compression stockings to provide external resistance to oppose the hydrostatic forces of venous hypertension. Pneumatic compression devices have been use to help reduce edema to allow for application of other garments or to promote healing of ulcers.

### Interventional Management

Chemical sclerotherapy may be used to obliterate venous abnormalities, such as cutaneous veins and varicose branches, by direct injection of a sclerosing agent into the vein. Ultrasound-guided foam sclerotherapy is being used more frequently even for the truncal superficial veins. Percutaneous venous ablation using radiofrequency or laser is being used to obliterate incompetent great or small saphenous veins. The procedure is effective in alleviating symptoms with a low complication risk for deep vein thrombosis and thermal injuries. Venous stenting, particularly of the iliac veins, has been used to restore venous outflow with venous obstruction, with good results in terms of patency and clinical improvement.

### Surgical Therapies

Surgical options should be considered for CVI refractory to medical and less invasive therapy, to complement compressive therapy. The surgical procedure will depend upon the underlying pathophysiolgic mechanism. The most common operative procedures are venous ligation and stripping, as well as vein avulsion to treat superficial incompetent and varicose veins. Subfascial endoscopic perforator surgery provides a means to ligate incompetent perforator veins from a site remote from an area with skin injury. Venous bypass may be considered for venous obstruction that is not amenable to an endovascular procedure. In rare circumstances, valve reconstruction and transplant have been performed in an attempt to restore valvular patency and function.

## LYMPHATIC DISORDERS

Lymphedema is the most commonly recognized disorder of the lymphatic system. It is a disorder characterized by limb swelling due to excessive accumulation of fluid in the extracellular space due either to inadequate drainage or overproduction of lymph. It may be classified into primary or secondary lymphedema based upon its etiology (see **Table 88-8**).

### Epidemiology

Primary lymphedema is an idiopathic condition resulting from inherited abnormalities in lymphatic structure and function. It has an incidence of 1 per 10,000 in people under the age of

| Table 88-8 • Causes of Lymphedema |
|---|
| **Primary** |
| Congenital |
| Familial |
| Syndrome-associated |
| Sporadic |
| Lymphedema praecox |
| Familial |
| Sporadic |
| Lymphedema tarda |
| **Secondary** |
| Infection |
| Post-surgical |
| Malignancy |
| Post-radiation |
| Post-traumatic |

20 years accounting for about 20% of affected persons. There is a strong female predominance with a female-to-male ratio of 4:1. Approximately 75% of primary lymphedema is due to lymphedema praecox, typically affecting females in their teenaged years to early twenties. Less than 10% of primary lymphedema presents after the age of 35 as lymphedema tarda.

Secondary lymphedema is an acquired disorder of the lymphatic system that is more common than primary lymphedema. It may result from damage to the lymphatic from processes such as malignancy, surgery, radiation, or infection. In fact, the most common worldwide cause of lymphedema is filariasis, caused by organisms including the parasite *Wuchereria bancrofti*.

### Pathophysiology

The pathophysiology of lymphedema may be divided into either low output failure with reduced lymphatic transport or high output failure with normal transport capacity overwhelmed by excessive lymph production. Insufficiency of the lymphatic vasculature may result from lymphatic dysplasia (as seen in primary lymphedema) or anatomic derangements with obstruction or obliteration of lymph channels (in secondary lymphedema).

Familial patterns of primary lymphedema have been described. Milroy's disease is a congenital disorder manifested in infancy. In this condition impaired lymphangiogenesis may be a consequence of a missense mutation in a gene-encoding vascular endothelial growth factor (VEGF)-3 receptor. Another disorder, called Meige's disease, is a familial form of lymphedema praecox. These disorders may be a result of agenesis, hypoplasia, hyperplasia, or obstruction of the lymphatic vessels.

Secondary lymphedema results from the loss, destruction, or obstruction of the normal lymphatic channels. In addition

| Stage | Clinical Features |
|-------|-------------------|
| 0 | Latent or subclinical |
| 1 | Early fluid accumulation<br>Subsides with limb elevation<br>Pitting may occur |
| 2 | Limb elevation rarely reduces swelling<br>Pitting is common until late stage |
| 3 | Encompasses elephantiasis<br>Pitting is absent<br>Trophic skin changes are common |

**Table 88-9 • International Society of Lymphology Classification**

to parasitic infection, recurrent bacterial infection may damage the lymphatic vessels causing lymphedema. Surgery with lymph node biopsy and excision is one of the most common secondary causes in North America. Other secondary causes include infiltration by malignant cells, radiation, trauma, and inflammatory diseases. Longstanding chronic venous insufficiency and even pregnancy may precipitate lymphedema.

## Clinical Presentation

Lymphedema results in swelling of the limb. It most commonly affects the lower limbs, although upper extremity disease may be seen particularly following surgery with lymph node dissection. During the early stages edema may subside with limb elevation but rarely in more advanced stages (see **Table 88-9**). Similarly, pitting may be present during the early stages but is not a feature of the later stages. The common description of lymphedema is as nonpitting edema. There may be extension of edema into the toes producing a classic 'square toe' sign. There may be induration with thickening of the skin creating an orange peel, or so-called "peau d'orange," appearance. An exam finding termed Stemmer sign (inability to pinch the skin at the base of the toe) is a specific but nonsensitive sign for lymphedema.

Lymphedema can be complicated by recurrent infection such as cellulitis and lymphangitis. Progressive trophic changes with fibrosis and induration of the skin may develop, leading to a cobblestone appearance called elephantiasis. It tends to cause severe swelling associated with immobility and can cause psychological strain. A rare complication is the development a highly lethal malignancy angiosarcoma.

## Differential Diagnosis

The differential diagnosis of lymphedema encompasses conditions that may produce chronic swelling of one or more limbs. This includes the following conditions:

- Chronic venous insufficiency and post-phlebitic syndrome

- Congestive heart failure—causing bilateral dependent pitting edema
- Myxedema—seen with both hypothyroidism and thyrotoxicosis (in pretibial region)
- Lipedema—caused by the excessive distribution of fat in the subcutaneous tissue
  - Onset is at puberty or pregnancy
  - Occurs more commonly in women
  - Unlike lymphedema, it spares the feet
  - Fat deposition is symmetric and the woody fibrotic skin changes are not seen
- Reflex sympathetic dystrophy and chronic limb dependency
- Factitious edema—caused by habitual application of a tourniquet.

## Diagnosis

The diagnosis is usually made based upon clinical history and physical examination. Testing is typically performed to exclude other conditions or to guide therapy. Perhaps the most important is an imaging study such as a CT or MRI to exclude secondary lymphedema due to malignant obstruction of the pelvic (or axillary) lymphatics. However, findings of lymphedema include thickened dermis and enlargement of the subcutaneous tissue with a characteristic honeycomb appearance. Ultrasonography may also be used to exclude other causes of limb swelling, such as acute or chronic venous disease. It may also be useful to visualize the extent of subcutaneous involvement with lymphedema.

Tests that may be performed to confirm the diagnosis of lymphedema include lymphangiography and lymphoscintigraphy. Lymphangiography involves the direct visualization of the lymphatic channels with injection of contrast, although is rarely performed as it requires a lymphatic cut-down. This is typically reserved for evaluation of candidates for lymphatic surgery. A more useful technique is lymphoscintigraphy, allowing for the visualization of the lymphatic system and assessment of lymphatic function. This is performed after an indirect injection of radiocontrast into the subcutaneous tissue of the hand or foot. Images are then obtained with a gamma camera after transport of contrast to lymph nodes creating a pattern of the lymphatic channels.

## Treatment (see Table 88-10)

Conservative measures are the mainstay of therapy for lymphedema, including interventions focused on edema reduction and preventive measures. Behavioral maneuvers such as elevation of the lower limbs is worthwhile but less effective than in venous edema. Compression therapy with wraps or stockings may be tried as tolerated. Lymphatic massage, particularly as part of a decongestive physiotherapy program,

| Table 88-10 • Treatment for Lymphedema |
| --- |
| **Edema reduction** |
| Compression wraps |
| Pneumatic compression device |
| Decongestive physiotherapy with lymphatic massage |
| Limb elevation |
| **Preventive measures** |
| Topical skin care |
| Antibiotics and antifungals |
| Exercise |
| Tumor surveillance |
| **Operative treatment** |
| Resection or "debulking" |
| Microsurgical reconstruction or shunting |

helps with lymphatic drainage and aids in discomfort relief. Intermittent pneumatic compression devices may help to force excess lymph fluid out from the subcutaneous tissues. There is limited or no role for diuretic therapy in the treatment of lymphedema.

The prevention of complications of unabated lymphedema is another focus in all patients. Skin hygiene is important with daily cleaning and use of emollients to prevent fissuring. Antibiotics should be used early if there are concerns for a bacterial skin infection. Similarly, fungal infections are common and require antifungal therapy. Exercise such as walking and swimming may be effective in reducing the swelling.

There is a limited role for operative methods tending to offer palliative rather than curative options. These are generally reserved for severe limb enlargement with deformity resulting in impairing function. The simplest operation is resection of the excessive skin and subcutaneous tissue known as a "debulking" procedure. This must be considered with caution as disruption of the superficial lymphatic channels may worsen the edema. Microsurgical techniques including reconstruction with a lymphatic collector or interposition vein and lympho-venous shunt have been tried with limited success.

## Suggested Readings

1. Consensus Document of the International Society of Lymphology. The diagnosis and treatment of peripheral lymphedema. *Lymphology.* 2003;36:84–91.

2. Eberhardt RT, Raffetto JD. Contemporary review in cardiovascular medicine. Chronic venous insufficiency. *Circulation.* 2005;111:2398–2409.

3. Kearon C, Kahn SR, Agnelli G, et al. Antithrombotic treatment of venous thromboembolic disease. American College of Chest Physicians Evidence Based Clinical Practice Guidelines (8th Edition). *Chest.* 2008;133:454S–545S.

4. Seligsohn U, Lubetsky A. Genetic susceptibility to venous thrombosis. *NEJM.* 2001;344:1222–1231.

# Special Topics

# 89

# Cardiac Tumors

FRANK SEGHATOL-ESLAMI

## ● PRACTICAL POINTS

- Cardiac tumors are rare lesions that may be intra-cavitary or intra-mural. Their clinical manifestations are protean and should be included in differential diagnosis. Echocardiography is used as screening test and allows a rapid diagnosis. Magnetic resonance imaging and CT scan play a role in delineating the nature and extent of cardiac tumors.

- Myxomas are the most frequent cardiac tumors; they usually are found in the left atrium, and rarely attached to the mitral valve.

- Papillary fibroelastomas are usually attached to the aortic or mitral valve and may cause stroke.

- The clinical context helps in differential diagnosis of cardiac tumors with thrombi and vegetations.

- Malignant neoplasms of the heart are also rare and one should think of metastasis to the heart from a remote site (melanoma, renal cell carcinoma) or by contiguity to the heart (lung, breast).

## INTRODUCTION

Primary and secondary cardiac tumors are rare cardiac lesions and include both benign and malignant neoplasia. It is important that the clinician be able to recognize cardiac tumors by different imaging modalities, but a definite diagnosis must await surgical excision. Nevertheless, their imaging features by either echocardiography or magnetic resonance imaging (MRI), their location in different cardiac chambers or in the myocardium, and other clinical features allow a presumptive presurgical diagnosis in most cases.

In this chapter, we describe the major imaging features of each of the cardiac tumors, with emphasis on echocardiographic-pathologic correlation. Newer technology, such as three-dimensional echocardiography and its role in delineating cardiac tumors, is described. We also give a differential diagnosis for other cardiac masses such as thrombi.

## CLINICAL PICTURE

Clinically, cardiac tumors come to attention because of a variety of symptoms: flow obstruction with signs and symptoms of heart failure, embolism, arrhythmias or constitutional symptoms. Echocardiography is the first imaging modality because it allows a rapid screening test and provides excellent anatomic and functional information. It can also be used for surveillance after resection. Recently, three-dimensional echocardiography has become a major imaging modality. However, some tumors may be differentiated better by contrast MRI or CT scan. For instance, because MRI has the highest soft tissue contrast, it can distinguish between hemangioma (high water content) and fibroma (low water content).

## CARDIAC TUMORS—CLASSIFICATION (TABLE 89-1 AND 89-2)

Cardiac tumors can be classified either by their prevalence according to patient age, or their location. For instance, myxomas are most often seen in the left atrium and sarcomas are seen in the right atrium. However, so the reader may be aware of the possibility that any cardiac tumor can also be encountered in an unusual location, we prefer to classify them by histologic type: benign, malignant, and metastatic type (**Table 89-1**).

*Primary cardiac tumors* are divided into benign and malignant lesions:

**Table 89-1 • Classification of Cardiac Tumors According to their Histological Nature**

| Benign | Malignant | Metastasis |
|---|---|---|
| Myxoma | Sarcoma | Lung |
| Papillary | • Angiosarcoma | Breast |
| Fibroelastoma | • Leiomyosarcoma | Melanoma |
| Rhabdomyoma | • Fibrosarcoma | Renal cell |
| Fibroma | • Rhabdomyosarcoma | Lymphoma |
| Lipoma | Lymphoma | |
| Hemangioma | Pericardial | |
| Teratoma | mesothelioma | |

- Benign tumors include: myxoma, papillary fibroelastoma, rhabdomyoma, fibroma, lipoma, hemangioma, and paraganglioma (An overview of several of these are given in **Table 89-2**).
- Malignant lesions are: sarcoma, lymphoma, and pericardial mesothelioma.

*Secondary cardiac tumors* are metastasized from a remote neoplasia that invades the heart either by local contiguity or by metastasis from a remote site.

# BENIGN CARDIAC TUMORS

## Cardiac Myxomas

- Cardiac myxoma is the most common primary tumor of the heart.
- About 75% of myxomas are found in the left atrium, 20% in the right atrium and rare cases in the ventricles or on cardiac valves.
- The majority of myxomas are attached to fossa ovalis by a pedunculated stalk; they may be sessile (**Figure 89-1**).
- On transthoracic echocardiography they manifest as spherical or polypoid mobile masses that may protrude into an atrioventricular valve (**Figure 89-2**).

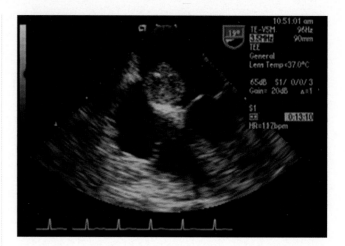

**Figure 89-1.** Left atrial myxoma. Note the heterogeneous nature of this spherical myxoma.

- A characteristic feature of myxoma is heterogeneity, which reflects hemorrhage, cyst formation and calcification.
- Polypoid myxomas are more likely to embolize (**Figure 89-3 A** and **B, 89-4**).
- Cardiac myxomas usually appear as sporadic lesions and, in about 10% of cases, as familial (as part of Carney complex with cutaneous lesions, Cushing syndrome, and Sertoli cell tumors).
- Because myxomas are potentially life-threatening lesions, urgent surgical excision is indicated. Surgical excision is considered safe, with excellent long-term results and low risk of recurrence.
- However, the risk of recurrence always exists and is more likely related to unsuspected multifocal myxoma rather than recurrence in situ. Nevertheless, postoperative serial follow-up with echocardiography is usually employed.

## Papillary Fibroelastoma

- Papillary fibroelastomas are the second most common primary benign cardiac tumor. They involve,

**Table 89-2 • Features of Major Benign Cardiac Tumors**

| Tumors | Location | Imaging Features | Clinical Presentation |
|---|---|---|---|
| Myxoma | 75% LA, 20% RA, 5% other | Spherical or polypoid mobile heterogeneous mass | Flow obstruction arrhythmias, constitutional symptoms |
| Fibroelastoma | Usually on cardiac valves | Pedunculated small mass with frond-like surface | TIA or stroke |
| Rhabdomyoma | Usually myocardium | Multiple well-circumscribed masses (hyperechoic) | Most often in children, 50% tuberous sclerosis |
| Fibroma | Usually myocardium | Single, round heterogeneous mass | Chamber obliteration, arrhythmias |

*LA, left atrium; RA, right atrium; TIA, transient ischemic stroke.*